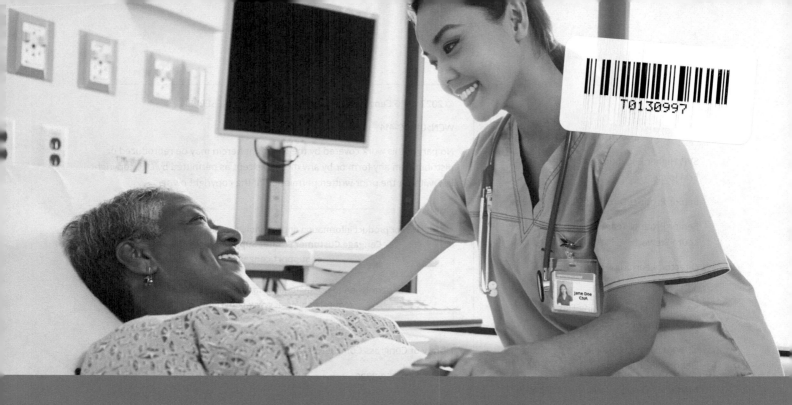

TWELFTH EDITION

NURSING ASSISTANT

A Nursing Process Approach

Barbara Acello, MS, RN

Independent nurse consultant
and educator

Barbara R. Hegner, MSN, RN

(Deceased)

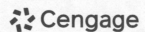

Australia • Brazil • Canada • Mexico • Singapore • United Kingdom • United States

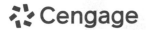

Nursing Assistant: A Nursing Process Approach, **12th Edition, Barbara Acello and Barbara R. Hegner**

SVP, Higher Education & Skills Product: Erin Joyner

Senior Product Director: Matthew Seeley

Senior Product Team Manager: Laura Stewart

Director, Learning Design: Rebecca von Gillern

Senior Manager, Learning Design: Leigh Hefferon

Senior Learning Designer: Deborah Bordeaux

Marketing Director: Michele McTighe

Marketing Manager: Courtney Cozzy

Director, Content Creation: Juliet Steiner

Senior Content Creation Manager: Patty Stephan

Senior Content Manager: Kenneth McGrath

Digital Delivery Lead: Allison Marion

Art Director: Felicia Bennett

Text Designer: Angela Sheehan

Cover Designer: Angela Sheehan

Cover images:
Monkey Business Images/ShutterStock.com
Rawpixel.com/ShutterStock.com
Monkey Business Images/ShutterStock.com
iStockPhoto.com/monkeybusinessimages

For product information and technology assistance, contact us at **Cengage Customer & Sales Support, 1-800-354-9706 or support.cengage.com.**

For permission to use material from this text or product, submit all requests online at **www.copyright.com.**

Library of Congress Control Number: 2020917872

ISBN: 978-0-357-37201-2

Cengage
5191 Natorp Boulevard
Mason, OH 45040
USA

Cengage is a leading provider of customized learning solutions. Our employees reside in nearly 40 different countries and serve digital learners in 165 countries around the world. Find your local representative at **www.cengage.com.**

To learn more about Cengage platforms and services, register or access your online learning solution, or purchase materials for your course, visit **www.cengage.com**.

Notice to the Reader

Printed Number: 7   Print Year: 2024
Printed in Mexico

Brief Contents

List of Procedures

ICON KEY: (O) = OBRA (P) = PPE

List of Tables

Contents

About the Authors

BARBARA ACELLO

Barbara Acello is currently an independent nurse consultant and educator in Denton, Texas. She is an active, contributing member of the Texas Nurses Association and the American College of Healthcare Administrators, where she was honored with the national Educator of the Year Award in 2007, the Journalism Award in 2009, and Chair's Award in 2018. Mrs. Acello's employment has evolved over her nursing career. Presently, she is involved with freelance consulting, lecturing, and writing. She has written and contributed to many textbooks, journal articles, instructor guides, computerized test banks, quick reference guides, and supplemental instructional materials for health care personnel. Geriatrics is her preferred area of clinical practice. She promotes the use of the nursing process and believes the nursing assistant is the most important caregiver in the health care facility. She is committed to improving working conditions and staffing, education, and professionalism for nursing assistants. She may be contacted at bacello@aol.com.

BARBARA HEGNER

Barbara Robinson Hegner, RN, MSN, was a graduate of a three-year diploma nursing program where direct and total care was the focus. She earned a BSN at Boston College and an MS in nursing from Boston University, with a minor in biologic sciences. She was Professor Emerita of Nursing and Life Sciences at Long Beach City College, Long Beach (CA).

Throughout her professional career, she had a deep interest in both hospital-based and long-term care nursing. It was Ms. Hegner's belief that ensuring the rights and well-being of all patients and residents requires the care of competent, caring nursing assistants under the supervision of professional nurses. The nursing assistants who provide this care should be thoroughly trained and consistently encouraged, evaluated, and given the opportunity for continued learning. Providing the tools to prepare these health care providers in the most effective and efficient way has been the goal of *Nursing Assistant: A Nursing Process Approach* through its many editions.

During the 1940s, nurses' duties involved tasks such as giving massages; preparing dressing packs, cotton balls, and applicator sticks; washing and sterilizing surgical gloves, dressings, syringes, and catheters for reuse; and sharpening the needles used on glass syringes. Physician supervision was required for taking blood pressure. World War II caused a shortage of nurses. Summer polio epidemics strained resources. Necessity is the mother of invention, so nursing responsibilities expanded. A new caregiver called the *nurse aide* was born. By the end of 1945, 212,000 women had become nurse aides. Hospitals began to make distinctions between skilled and nonskilled nursing care. How far we have come in 75 years!

Today's nursing assistants must possess critical thinking and technical skills. They have assumed more advanced responsibilities than ever before. Nursing assistants are important members of the nursing team, making valuable contributions to the nursing process. The nursing assistant of the twenty-first century must be prepared to use the nursing process to provide competent, patient-centered care in an advanced care setting. Selected advanced skills have been included in this revision to enhance nursing assistant knowledge and responsibilities. These skills are a routine part of the job description in many facilities.

Nursing Assistant: A Nursing Process Approach, 12th Edition is written for today's nursing assistants, providing information to support successful mastery of critical thinking and technical skills with a focus on providing excellent patient-centered care. Continuing its mission to emphasize the importance of treating those entrusted to care as total individuals who possess dignity, have value, and deserve respect, the ongoing goal of this text and supplement package is to provide tools that instructors can use to teach nursing assistants to meet high standards of personalized, patient-focused care. This will enable them to help patients achieve a desirable level of comfort, restoration, and wellness while protecting and respecting patients' rights as health care consumers.

ORGANIZATION

Long respected as a leading textbook for nursing assisting education, this 12th edition of *Nursing Assistant* is organized to bring the reader from the foundational concepts through detailed, step-by-step procedures for patient care. Section 1 is an introduction to nursing assisting, covering the role of the nursing assistant, rights and responsibilities in health care, and legal and ethical issues. Section 2 explores the foundational scientific concepts of medical terminology and body organization,

as well as the classification of disease. Communication skills and the critical skills of observation, reporting, and documentation are covered in Section 3, along with meeting basic needs and important coverage of developing cultural sensitivity. Section 4 thoroughly covers infection and infection control, which are critical to effective patient care. Section 5 presents detailed information on safety and mobility, including positioning, transfer skills, and ambulation. The important skills of measuring and recording vital signs, height, and weight are presented in Section 6. Admission, transfer, and discharge, as well as bedmaking, bathing, and general comfort measures, are covered in Section 7. Section 8 provides detailed but accessible information on nutrition and fluid balance. Section 9 covers a wide range of special care procedures that all nursing assistants will need to perform to provide quality patient care. Other health care settings, including the long-term care facility, home health care, and subacute care, are discussed in Section 10, which also contains a chapter on alternative, complementary, and integrative approaches. Section 11 provides comprehensive coverage of all body systems, common disorders, and related care procedures. The expanded role of the nursing assistant, including care of special populations, is presented in Section 12. Finally, Section 13 presents excellent resources for moving forward with professional practice, including employment opportunities and career growth.

FEATURES

The features of *Nursing Assistant: A Nursing Process Approach* have been carefully honed through its many editions to provide readers with the most important information in an easily digestible format.

- Chapter objectives help focus the reader on key learning outcomes.
- Key terms can be used to improve reading comprehension and to support study and exam prep.
- The "Guidelines" feature highlights important steps and considerations for specific care situations.
- Alerts highlight urgent information on infection control, safety, culture, difficult situations, Occupational Safety and Health Administration (OSHA), communication, age-appropriate care, and legal considerations.
- Clear, concise, step-by-step procedures are supported by full-color photographs and illustrations.
- Chapter Review and Nursing Assistant Challenge questions test and reinforce understanding.

New to This Edition

In addition to carefully updated content and numerous new, engaging, full-color photos, the following updated and enhanced content addresses the changing character of nursing assistant practice:

- Real on-the-job responsibilities
- Projecting a positive image
- Time management
- Managing and organizing assignments
- Handoff communication
- Career growth and advancement, and expanding the scope of nursing assistant practice
- Building relationships
- Professionalism
- Evidence-based practice
- Introduction to the Affordable Care Act (ACA)
- Social media
- Cell phones and other wireless handheld devices
- Electronic communication and documentation
- Differentiating between an electronic medical record (EMR), an electronic patient record (EPR), an electronic health record (EHR), and a personal health record (PHR)
- SBAR (situation, background, assessment, recommendation) communication
- Transitional care
- Biofilms
- Worsening problems with drug-resistant organisms
- Intergenerational care
- Understanding trends in health care due to an aging population
- Observation and reporting alerts
- Assistive transfer devices
- Basic sterile technique
- Dressings and bandages
- Preventing skin tears
- Negative pressure wound therapy systems and pulsatile lavage
- Intellectual disabilities and developmental disabilities
- Expanded home health care content
- Implantable cardioverter defibrillator
- Removal of an indwelling catheter

EXTENSIVE TEACHING AND LEARNING PACKAGE

Cengage Learning has provided a complete learning package to accompany *Nursing Assistant: A Nursing Process Approach*. Each supplement has been extensively revised to reflect the changes in the 12th edition of this textbook. Visit cengage.com to learn more.

Student Resources

The following resources were developed to help students learn and practice the information essential to becoming certified as a skilled nursing assistant:

MindTap for Nursing Assistant: A Nursing Process Approach, 12th Edition

MindTap is a fully online, interactive learning experience built upon authoritative Cengage content. By combining readings, multimedia, activities, and assessments into a single learning path, MindTap elevates learning by providing real-world application to better engage students and improve student outcomes. MindTap is device agnostic, meaning that it will work with any platform or learning management system and will be accessible anytime, anywhere: on desktops, laptops, tablets, mobile phones, and other Internet-enabled devices.

MindTap for Nursing Assistant: A Nursing Process Approach, 12th Edition includes:

- An interactive eBook with highlighting, note-taking, ReadSpeaker, and more.
- Flashcards for practicing key terms.
- Lecture slides in PowerPoint to review chapter material
- Computer-graded activities and exercises

Workbook to Accompany Nursing Assistant: A Nursing Process Approach, 12th Edition

The student workbook has been updated with new content and directly correlates to the textbook. This competency-based supplement includes challenging exercises and quizzes to help students understand essential content and master the definition of key terms. Certification style exam questions are provided to help students to prepare for taking a state certification exam.

Student Companion Website

Visit www.cengage.com for free online resources, including additional nursing procedures, and chapter support.

Instructor Resources

Instructor Companion Website to Accompany Nursing Assistant: A Nursing Process Approach, 12th Edition

The password-protected Instructor Resources Companion site allows you to spend less time planning and more time teaching. The Instructor Resources Companion site can be accessed by going to www.cengage.com/login to create a unique user log-in. Once your instructor account has been activated, you will have access to a comprehensive selection of digital support materials, including:

- The *Instructor's Manual to Accompany Nursing Assistant: A Nursing Process Approach, 12th Edition,* with instructor support and activities, answers to the chapter review questions, answers to the workbook questions, procedure evaluation forms, and more.
- PowerPoint® presentations for each chapter, high-lighting key concepts from each chapter.
- Cognero Testbank.

ACKNOWLEDGMENTS

Each new edition brings with it the pleasant task of acknowledging the contributions of a number of individuals who have believed in, supported, and contributed to this project.

First, my son Jon and grandson Chris have given greatly of themselves while I worked on this manuscript. I appreciate their assistance, love, and support.

Contributors

Virginia More, our beautiful 90-something patient/resident model understands the importance of realistic photos and graciously allowed us to photograph her during times of personal illness and injury. I sincerely appreciate her support, commitment to education, attention to detail, and generosity in allowing the intrusion into her personal life.

Robert More, of More and More, LLC, also generously allowed us to take numerous pre- and post-operative photographs for two surgical procedures, an acute care hospitalization, and home health care follow-ups.

My dear friend and frequent writing partner Laura More, LCSW of More and More, LLC, knows my strengths, weaknesses, likes, dislikes, and needs well. Although we did not collaborate on this book, I did not have to ask for help. She knows the process and jumped right in to take photos and locate resources, saving me time, improving the quality of your book, and helping ensure it contains the most current material available. I am fortunate to have such a generous, creative, and multitalented writing partner!

The following individuals provided valuable information, personal assistance, current technical photos, modeling support, suggestions, and resources for new content:

- Dwayne Carroll, Chief; Onega Group, Cherokee Nation of Texas
- Beverly Futrell, CNA
- Genevieve Gipson, RN, MEd, RNC; National Network of Career Nursing Assistants
- Laura More, LCSW; More and More, LLC
- Robert More; More and More, LLC
- V. Jean Morris, MS, FACHCA, LNHA, CALA; St. Mary Medical Center
- Steve Warren, Vice President; Skil-Care Corporation

A book of this size represents an enormous investment of time and talent by many dedicated individuals. I sincerely appreciate the support and assistance of Cengage Senior Content Manager Kenneth McGrath, whose vision, patience, and support was invaluable in manuscript construction and development; and Joseph Malcolm, Senior Project Manager, Lumina Datamatics whose consideration is sincerely appreciated. Many unnamed individuals handled the manuscript to bring it to fruition. I sincerely appreciate their care and attention to detail.

REVIEWERS

Reviewer A:
Linda Romano, BSN,RN
Health Science Educator/Nurse Aide Training
Program Coordinator
Newburgh Enlarged City School District

Reviewer B:
Carla Wright, MSNed, RN,
CNE Program Director College of Southern Nevada

Reviewer C:
Shelia Adams RN, MSN,
Dept. Chair, Program Coordinator,
Instructor Richmond Community College

Reviewer D:
Monica Tupper
Biological Science Teacher/HOSA Advisor
Lewis-Palmer High School

Reviewer E:
Joni Barry R.N. MEd.
CNA instructor Meridian Medical Arts Charter
High School

The 12th edition of *Nursing Assistant: A Nursing Process Approach* has been carefully designed and updated to make the study of nursing assistant tasks and responsibilities easier and more productive. For best results, you may want to become familiar with the features incorporated into this text and accompanying learning tools.

TABLE OF CONTENTS

For each chapter, the table of contents lists the chapter title, major topic headings, general guidelines for specific areas of care and topics of importance to the nursing assistant, and patient care procedures.

CHAPTER OPENING PAGE

Each chapter opening page contains objectives and vocabulary terms.

The **objectives** help you know what is expected of you as you read the text. Your success in mastering each objective is measured by the review questions at the end of each chapter.

The **vocabulary** list alerts you to new terms presented in the chapter. When each term is first used in the chapter, it is highlighted in boldface and color. Each term is defined at this point in the chapter. Read the definition of the term and note the context in which it is used so that you will feel comfortable in using the term. Note that the highlighted terms are also defined in the glossary at the back of the book.

TEXT ALERTS

The alerts provide important content on infection control, OSHA, communication, age-appropriate care, legal considerations, safety, difficult situations, critical thinking, and clinical information related to patient care. These alerts make the learner aware of best practices in patient care; include practical tips based on experience; and highlight critical infection control, safety, and other regulatory guidelines.

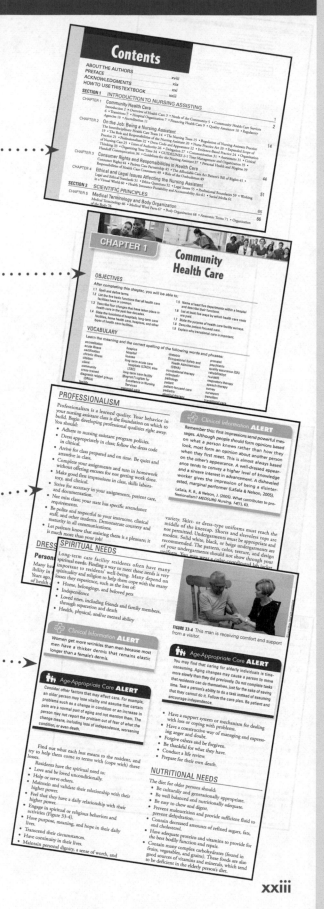

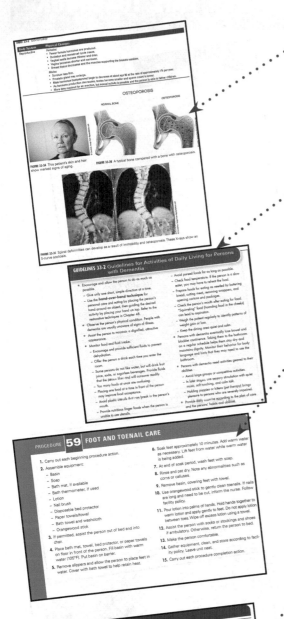

PHOTOGRAPHS AND ILLUSTRATIONS

Numerous color illustrations and photos help to clarify and reinforce the chapter content. Many figures are used in the procedures to help you visualize critical step-by-step information. Full-color anatomical drawings help you to locate body components and understand body organization.

GUIDELINES

"Guidelines for . . ." features highlight important points that you need to remember for specific situations or types of care. They are presented in an easy-to-use format that you can refer to repeatedly until you know the actions you must take when confronted with the situation.

PROCEDURES

The textbook sets out clinical procedures in a step-by-step format. Each procedure reminds you to perform both beginning and completion actions. Any relevant notes or cautions about performing the procedure are given. The steps take you carefully through the procedure, emphasizing at all times the need to work safely and to protect the patient's privacy. Each procedure is marked with icons to help you easily identify procedures that contain key OBRA (Omnibus Budget Reconciliation Act) and PPE (personal protective equipment) standards, as well as procedures for which a corresponding video is available in the MindTap.

CHAPTER REVIEWS AND TESTING MATERIAL

A variety of review questions at the end of each chapter test your understanding of the chapter content. This content has been expanded as a result of instructor requests. Each review contains a Nursing Assistant Challenge that presents a typical clinical situation and asks questions about your response to the situation. These questions help you master critical thinking skills and require you to integrate what you have learned to arrive at an appropriate solution or set of actions.

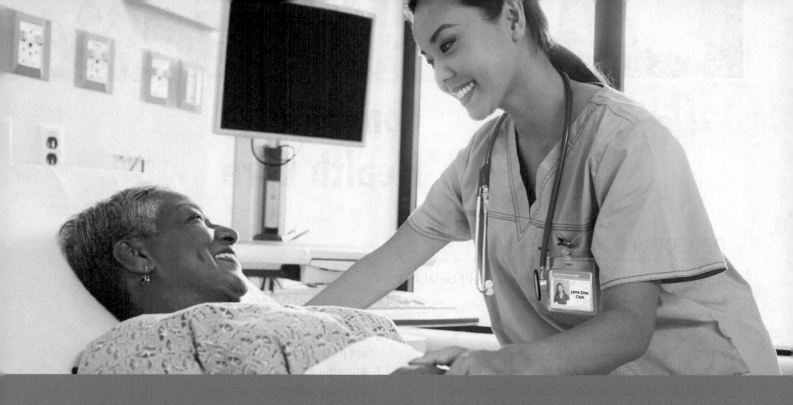

SECTION 1

Introduction to Nursing Assisting

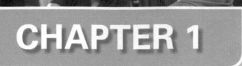

CHAPTER 1

Community Health Care

OBJECTIVES

After completing this chapter, you will be able to:

1.1 Spell and define terms.

1.2 List the five basic functions that all health care facilities have in common.

1.3 Describe four changes that have taken place in health care in the past few decades.

1.4 State the functions of hospitals, long-term care facilities, home health care, hospices, and other types of health care facilities.

1.5 Name at least five departments within a hospital and describe their functions.

1.6 List at least five ways by which health care costs are paid.

1.7 State the purpose of health care facility surveys.

1.8 Describe patient-focused care.

1.9 Explain why transitional care is important.

VOCABULARY

Learn the meaning and the correct spelling of the following words and phrases:

accreditation
acute illness
certification
chronic illness
citation
client
community
cross-trained
diagnosis related groups (DRGs)
facility
health care consumers
health maintenance organizations (HMOs)

hospice
hospital
license
long-term acute care hospitals (LTACH; also LTAC)
long-term care facility
Magnet Program for Excellence in Nursing Services
managed care
Medicaid
Medicare
multiskilled workers

obstetric
Occupational Safety and Health Administration (OSHA)
occupational therapy
orthopedic
pathology
patient
patient-focused care
pediatric
physical therapy
postanesthesia recovery (PAR)
postpartum

prenatal
psychiatric
quality assurance (QA)
rehabilitation
resident
respiratory therapy
speech therapy
survey
surveyors
transition
transitional care

INTRODUCTION

A nursing assistant is a paraprofessional health care worker with important responsibilities in providing comfort and care to people who are ill or injured. The nursing assistant is supervised by, takes directions from, and reports to licensed professional health care workers, such as physicians and nurses.

A **facility** is a place in which health care is given. A **hospital** is a complex organization that provides a full range of health care services. Some hospitals provide highly technical care. Others provide general care for patients with many different medical conditions. Some provide only specialized services, such as treatment for cancer or rehabilitation care. A **long-term care facility** provides care to persons whose conditions are stable but who need monitoring, nursing care, and treatments. Many of these residents are elderly, but facilities can accept persons of all ages who meet the legal admission criteria.

Functions of Health Care Facilities

All health care facilities have five basic functions:

1. Providing services for the ill and injured (Figure 1-1)
2. Reducing risk factors and preventing disease (Figure 1-2)
3. Promoting individual and community health
4. Educating health care workers (Figure 1-3)
5. Promoting research in medicine and nursing

OVERVIEW OF HEALTH CARE

Health care today emphasizes **patient-focused care**. This care focuses on the unique needs of each person. It includes several general areas of care:

- Keeping good communication
- Maintaining cost effectiveness and containing costs
- Making the patient a partner in their own care

- Respecting the patient's needs, values, beliefs, and decisions even if you disagree
- Meeting acceptable standards
- Promoting good health, a healthy lifestyle, physical care, and a clean, comfortable, and secure environment
- Supporting the patient's mental and emotional needs
- Coordinating care with others
- Limiting the number of people involved in patient care so workers are more familiar with the patient and the patient knows who their caregivers are
- Meeting the patient's needs efficiently
- Paying attention to the aspects of care that will help the person lead a fulfilling and satisfying life

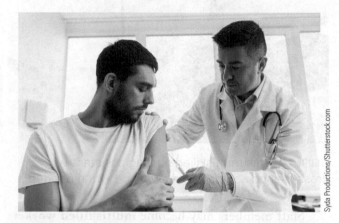

FIGURE 1-2 Vaccines are an important means of staying healthy. Unvaccinated health care workers can spread diseases to patients. You cannot get a disease from the vaccine.

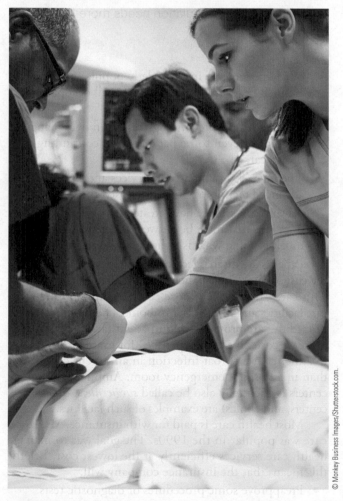

FIGURE 1-1 Health care facilities provide routine, emergency, and surgical services to many different types of patients.

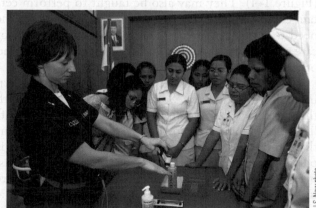

FIGURE 1-3 Health care changes regularly. Attending classes to learn new information helps you grow personally and professionally and enhances your knowledge and value as an employee.

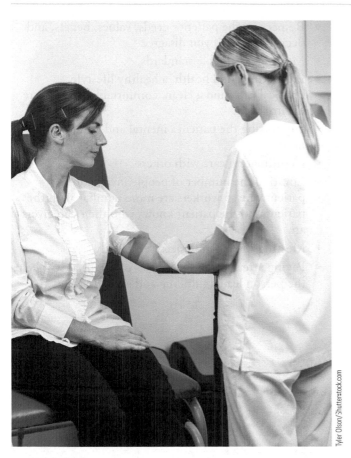

Tyler Olson/Shutterstock.com

FIGURE 1-4 This multiskilled nursing assistant was cross-trained so she can draw blood when needed.

Staff members may become **multiskilled workers** by cross-training to perform additional skills. Multiskilled workers can perform many functions, enabling them to do more than one kind of work. They usually learn skills from more than one discipline. For example, a multiskilled nursing assistant may be **cross-trained** to draw blood and/or obtain electrocardiograms (Figure 1-4). They may also be taught to perform certain clerical duties. This type of cross-training avoids the need to transfer the patient to another department for care and reduces the waiting time for necessary tests and other services.

Quality of life has become an important concern in health care delivery. Some decisions are made with the patient's future quality of life in mind. Quality-of-life policies focus on providing care in an environment that humanizes and individualizes each patient. Care is personalized to the person's needs. In some situations, preserving the quality of the patient's life is more important than increasing the length of life.

Many changes have occurred in health care within the past few decades. There are several reasons for this:

- People are living longer. People who are aging need more services. Demand for nursing assistants is high and is expected to continue growing rapidly because

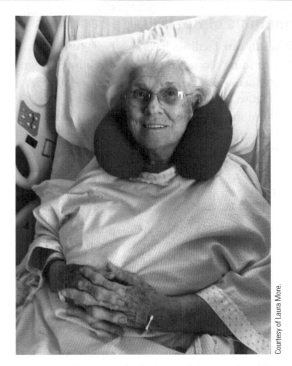

Courtesy of Laura More.

FIGURE 1-5 An aging population needs more health care services.

of a large increase in the elderly population. This is much faster than the average for all occupations (Figure 1-5).

- Use of advanced technology results in lives being saved. However, some patients need continuing health care.

- The increased demand for services and use of advanced technology have increased the cost of care.

- Advances in science have created many ethical (moral) questions that must be answered. Behaving ethically involves doing what is right in any given situation.

Patients are discharged earlier from hospitals to reduce the cost of care. These patients may still require health care. This care can be given more economically in long-term care facilities and in the person's home. Diagnostic tests and procedures are provided in outpatient facilities to further decrease costs. It is less expensive, for example, to receive treatment for a throat infection in an urgent care center than in a hospital emergency room. Ambulatory surgical centers (which may also be called *surgicenters*, urgent care centers, and clinics) are examples of such facilities.

Most health care is paid for with insurance. **Managed care** was popular in the 1990s. The goal was to manage health care services efficiently at the lowest cost. Briefly, this means that the insurance company will:

- Preapprove some procedures or diagnostic tests.

- Negotiate with some facilities and professionals to provide care and services at a lower cost to the company's members.

- Approve only a certain number of days of hospitalization for specific diagnoses. If the patient must stay longer, the hospital must get approval from the insurer or payment may be denied.
- Require that specific procedures be done on an outpatient basis rather than having the patient admitted to the hospital.

Although managed care is still alive and well, costs are increasing, and consumers have never been satisfied with the restrictive coverage. Today, managed care plans are offering more choices than they did in the past. Unfortunately, this has increased the out-of-pocket cost.

NEEDS OF THE COMMUNITY

People who live in a common area and share common health needs form a **community**. The community may provide services to keep the residents safe and healthy, such as waste disposal, safe drinking water, services to ensure that food in stores and restaurants is healthy, and some health services. Public health laws regulate these services and are enforced by government agencies.

Health care is needed throughout life. The care may be short term or long term and includes:

- Preventive care to maintain good health
- **Prenatal** care (care of the mother during pregnancy; Figure 1-6A)
- Well-baby checkups and immunizations (Figure 1-6B)
- Health education to teach individuals how to avoid disease and injury
- Physical examinations throughout life
- Emergency care for sudden illness or injury
- Surgery to repair an injured body part or remove a diseased organ
- Rehabilitation to help a person to regain abilities lost due to illness or injury (Figure 1-7)
- Long-term care for persons with chronic or incurable conditions
- **Hospice** care for persons who are dying and their families

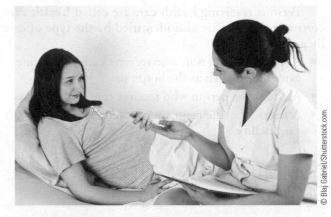

FIGURE 1-6A Prenatal care is essential for a healthy mother and infant.

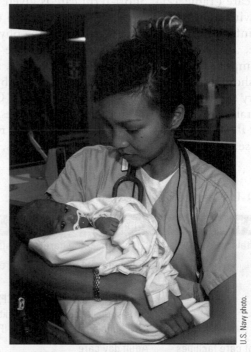

FIGURE 1-6B This infant will be scheduled for well-baby checkups and regular immunizations.

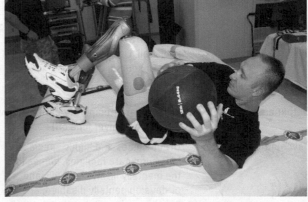

FIGURE 1-7 This amputee is performing abdominal training with a medicine ball during routine therapy.

Persons receiving health care are called **health care consumers**. They are also identified by the type of care they need:

- A **patient** is a person who receives care in an acute care facility, such as the hospital.
- A **client** is a person who receives care in their home.
- A **resident** is the recipient of care in a long-term care facility.

COMMUNITY HEALTH CARE SERVICES

There are two main types of health care facilities: those that provide short-term care and those that provide long-term care (Table 1-1). Short-term care is given to persons with routine or minor problems, such as a urinary tract infection. The care may be given in the physician's office, an outpatient clinic, or an urgent care center. Uncomplicated surgeries, such as hernia repair, require only short-term care and may be done in an ambulatory surgery center or outpatient surgery department. General hospitals provide short-term care for acute illnesses. An **acute illness** or injury comes on suddenly and requires intense, immediate treatment. Heart attacks, severe

TABLE 1-1 Types of Health Care Facilities

Short-Term Care	Long-Term Care
Hospitals	Long-term acute care hospitals
	Subacute and transitional care facilities
	Long-term care facilities (LTCF); these consist of skilled nursing facilities (SNF) and nursing facilities (NF)
Urgent care facilities	Adult day care
Surgicenters	Assisted living facilities (ALF) (A type of long-term care facility for people who can move about but who may need help with some activities of daily living. Most care is given by personal care assistants. Nursing staff is on call. Licensed nurses are not on duty 24 hours a day.)
	Rehabilitation centers
Outpatient clinics	Respite care (temporary care to allow a family caregiver time off)
Psychiatric hospitals	Group homes and highly specialized long-term care facilities, homes for the mentally ill, intellectually and/ or developmentally disabled, and psychiatric hospitals
Physicians' offices	Home care

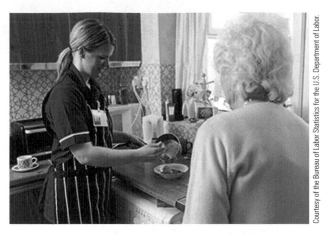

FIGURE 1-8 Home health care services are given in the client's home, eliminating the need for facility admission and reducing the cost of care.

burns, strokes, and uncontrolled diabetes are examples of acute conditions. The patient is expected to recover.

Long-term care is necessary for some persons who have chronic conditions. A **chronic illness** is one that is treatable but not curable and is expected to require lifelong care. This care may be given in a long-term care facility, adult day-care setting, respite care facility, assisted living facility, or the person's home (Figure 1-8). Alzheimer's disease, multiple sclerosis, Parkinson's disease, and diabetes are examples of chronic illnesses.

Hospitals

Most acute care hospitals accept and care for patients of all ages with a variety of medical and surgical problems. Some take care of patients with special conditions or care for specific age groups:

- **Pediatric** hospitals care only for children from birth to age 18.
- **Psychiatric** hospitals provide care for persons with mental illness.
- **Rehabilitation** hospitals provide rehabilitative and restorative services to patients following disease, illness, or injury. If complete restoration is not possible, the goal is to restore the patient to their highest possible level of function.
- **Long-term acute care hospitals (LTACHs; also LTAC)** are a rapidly growing segment of the health care market in the United States. The facility is licensed as a hospital but is designed for patients who are expected to stay 25 days or more. To be accepted in an LTACH, the patient must have a medically complex condition, need acute care services, and have a good chance of improvement. The level of care is higher than provided in long-term care facilities (nursing homes) or subacute care facilities.

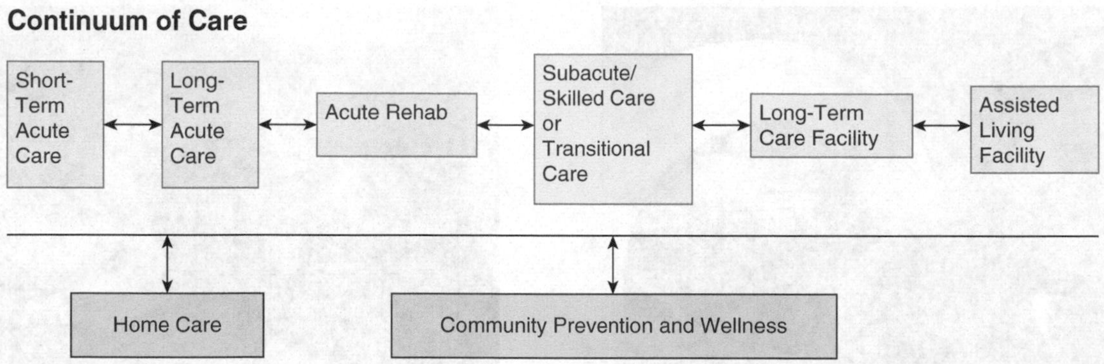

Continuum of Care

Short-Term Acute Care ↔ Long-Term Acute Care ↔ Acute Rehab ↔ Subacute/Skilled Care or Transitional Care ↔ Long-Term Care Facility ↔ Assisted Living Facility

Home Care

Community Prevention and Wellness

FIGURE 1-9 Patients move back and forth from one level of care to another as their needs change.

TRANSITIONS

A **transition** is the movement of a patient between various locations in which care is given as their needs change. This may involve moving to different levels of care within the same facility or moving to a completely different location (such as a long-term care facility or home; Figure 1-9). Transitional care includes:

- Educating the patient and family
- Coordinating health care services that will be needed after discharge
- Making phone calls and visits in the patient's new location
- Ensuring that the transition is safe and satisfying to the patient
- Providing important information to the patient's next care provider or setting to coordinate care and reduce the risk of errors

Each transition increases the risk of poor communication, lack of coordination, and the potential for errors across settings. Ensuring smooth transitions is part of patient-focused care. The safest transitions are carefully planned and patient centered.

HOSPITAL ORGANIZATION

Hospitals are designed to provide efficient delivery of service. Major departments in each facility meet the needs of patients with specific conditions (Figure 1-10). These units provide nursing care 24 hours a day, 7 days a week.

- Medical department: cares for patients with medical conditions such as pneumonia or heart disease.
- Surgical department: cares for patients before, during, and after surgery. The **postanesthesia recovery (PAR)** area is where patients are closely monitored after surgery. They remain in this area until they are stable enough to leave the surgical department.
- Pediatric department: cares for sick or injured children.

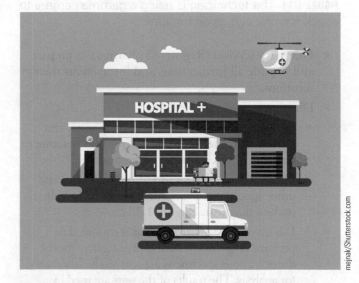

mejnak/Shutterstock.com

FIGURE 1-10 There are 6,210 hospitals in the United States. The largest hospital has 8,000 beds. The smallest hospital has 19 beds.

- **Obstetric** department: cares for newborns and their mothers. This department includes the labor and delivery unit, the **postpartum** unit (for mothers who have given birth), and the nursery for care of newborns.
- Emergency department: cares for victims of trauma, natural disasters (e.g., tornadoes and hurricanes), or medical emergencies.
- Critical care department: cares for seriously ill patients who require constant monitoring and care.

Larger hospitals have many specialized units to care for persons with problems such as cancer, cardiovascular disease, or kidney disease or for those requiring **orthopedic** (bones and muscles) surgery. Specialized health care workers provide services to the patients in these units. Specialized services include:

- Dietary services. A registered dietitian plans the meals for all patients and provides educational services to patients on special diets. The hospital's food service department prepares meals and delivers them to patients.

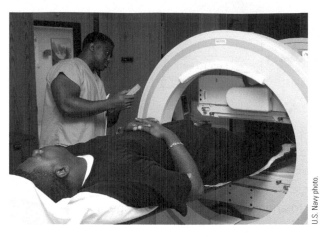

FIGURE 1-11 The technician is using a gamma camera to check for a hidden ankle fracture.

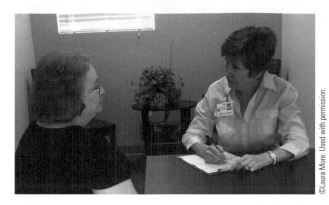

FIGURE 1-12 The social worker writes an assessment that will help the patient and the health care team make treatment plans.

- Pharmacy services. Registered pharmacists prepare and provide all medications and intravenous therapy solutions.
- Diagnostic services:
  - **Pathology** (study of disease). Diagnostic tests are done on specimens taken from body tissue to help the physician make a diagnosis.
  - Diagnostic imaging and radiology. X-rays and other specialized procedures are done to help make a diagnosis (Figure 1-11).
  - Laboratory. A department that is equipped to perform diagnostic tests and investigative procedures. Various specimens are sent to the laboratory for analysis. The results of the tests are used by physicians and others in the diagnosis and care of patients.
- Transitional care. The **transitional care** coordinator or department is responsible for ensuring continuity of care when a patient transitions from one location or facility to another.
- Rehabilitation services:
  - **Physical therapy.** Assists patients to regain mobility skills.
  - **Occupational therapy.** Helps patients to regain self-care skills.
  - **Speech therapy.** Helps patients to regain the ability to communicate and works with patients who have swallowing disorders.
  - **Respiratory therapy.** Provides care for patients who have disorders of the cardiopulmonary system, respiratory system, and sleep disorders that affect the patient's breathing.
- Social services. Staff members provide counseling for patients and their families, help needy families get financial assistance, plan for patient discharge, and arrange for patient transfers from one facility to another (Figure 1-12).

- Environmental services:
  - Housekeeping is responsible for the overall cleaning (Figure 1-13).
  - Maintenance cares for and repairs the building and equipment.
  - Laundry services provide and clean all linens.
- Business services. Responsible for patient billing, employee payroll, and other financial matters.
- Medical records. The department that transcribes and catalogs all patient records.
- Volunteers. Persons who provide services free of charge and perform tasks such as delivering mail

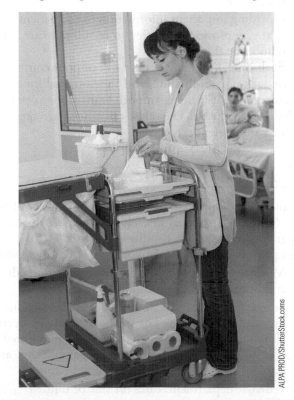

FIGURE 1-13 Housekeeping is responsible for the overall cleaning of the hospital.

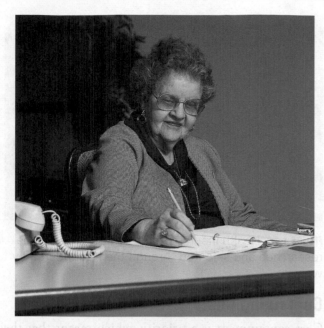

FIGURE 1-14 This independent older adult maintains her self-esteem and provides a valuable service by volunteering at the hospital.

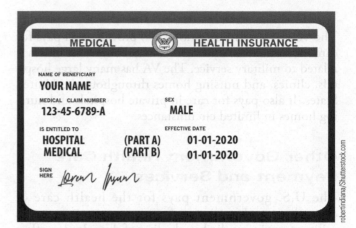

FIGURE 1-15 There are approximately 44 million people enrolled in the Medicare program. In 2018, the Medicare program cost $582 billion or about 14 percent of the total federal budget.

and flowers, running the gift shop, directing visitors, assisting in the surgery waiting area, and raising funds for the facility (Figure 1-14).
- Pastoral care helps meet patients' religious and spiritual needs and provides counseling.

FINANCING HEALTH CARE

Health care is paid for by:
- Insurance. Employers may offer a group insurance plan, or persons may buy individual insurance. Premiums are expensive, although an employer may pay all or a portion of the cost of a group insurance plan. **Health maintenance organizations (HMOs)** are one type of prepaid insurance. The HMO is a group of health care providers and hospitals. HMO members must see only certain doctors and go only to designated hospitals, except in emergencies.
- Out-of-pocket payments by the health care consumer who has no insurance or for expenses not covered by insurance.
- The federal government. The U.S. government pays for health care services for approximately 37 percent of the population of the United States.

Government Programs for Health Care Payments

Medicare

Medicare (Figure 1-15) is a federal government program that pays a portion of health care costs for persons aged 65 years and over and for younger persons who are permanently disabled and who qualify for the benefit.

A number of Medicare payment options are available. These vary depending on the person's eligibility, medical needs, and area of residence. Some procedures or treatments require prior approval and may have time limitations. Plans are available to pay for inpatient and outpatient services, home health care, physician services, therapy, diagnostic tests, some medical supplies and equipment, and prescription drugs.

Medicare payment to hospitals is based on **diagnosis related groups (DRGs)**. The actual cost of care is not considered. Rather, payment is based on studies that were done to determine the average length of stay required for various medical diagnoses, procedures, and treatments. Medicare set the payment rates based on these data. Although a hospital may charge variable rates for patient care, Medicare pays only the fixed amount that it has determined is fair for care based on the DRG.

Medicare does not pay for care of avoidable complications that began in the hospital, such as pressure injuries, surgical infections, catheter infection, and fractures that occur because of falls. If certain preventable events occur, the hospital must provide care for them free of charge.

Medicaid

Medicaid is a state and federal government program that pays health care costs for:
- Pregnant women
- Children and teenagers
- Individuals who are aged, blind, or disabled
- Those who fall into certain income categories

Veterans Administration

The Veterans Administration (VA) provides and pays for care for some military veterans whose injury or illness is related to military service. The VA has many large hospitals, clinics, and nursing homes throughout the United States. It also pays for care in private hospitals and nursing homes in limited circumstances.

Other Government Health Care Payment and Services

The U.S. government pays for the health care of dependents and survivors of persons who are in active military service or died in the line of duty. It also offers insurance plans to public-sector employees who work for the federal government.

A variety of other government agencies sponsor specialty health care services. For example, Title X funds reproductive health care. The State Children's Health Insurance Program (SCHIP) was established in 1997 to provide health insurance for children in low-income families. The Indian Health Service cares for certain Native Americans. The National Institutes of Health gives free treatment to patients who enroll in research trials and projects.

The Affordable Care Act

The Patient Protection and Affordable Care Act (PPACA) was signed into law on March 23, 2010. The Health Care Education and Reconciliation Act (HCERA) was signed on March 30, 2010. Together, the two acts make up the Affordable Care Act (ACA). The ACA is an important set of health care reforms that will help to ensure that people have access to health insurance.

The goals of the ACA are to:

- Reduce the number of uninsured Americans.
- Require employers to provide health care coverage.
- Require people to secure health care coverage.
- Expand Medicaid eligibility requirements.
- Require insurance companies to cover people with preexisting medical conditions.
- Prohibit insurers from dropping subscribers with expensive or chronic conditions.
- Require insurance companies to pay for preventive care (Figure 1-16).
- Require insurers to allow parents to keep their uninsured adult children under age 26 on their family coverage plan.

Some states have established state health care plans to provide affordable health care coverage to state residents. Although there are some exceptions, these states have certain coverage requirements.

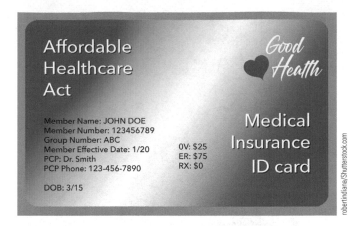

FIGURE 1-16 Health insurance through the ACA can be researched and selected through the HealthCare.gov website.

Containing Costs

Cost containment is a priority, which means that the maximum benefit of health care must be achieved for every dollar spent. Each worker must do everything possible to avoid waste and keep costs down.

QUALITY ASSURANCE

All health care facilities have a program called **quality assurance (QA)**. The QA committee conducts internal reviews to identify problems and then find and implement solutions. The committee meets to evaluate care and improve practices in the facility, such as restraint use, avoidance of pressure injuries, and infection control. Patient care should be continuously evaluated and adjusted to meet patient needs and comply with regulations. The QA program performs this important function.

The QA committee is very important to the operation of the facility, delivery of good patient care, and the facility's success in surveys. This self-improvement process prevents problems with regulatory agencies and improves the quality of care.

REGULATORY AGENCIES

Facilities must meet certain standards to operate. Many external agencies regulate health care facilities and set quality standards. Some regulatory agencies are branches of the state and federal government, but several are voluntary, private organizations.

The various agencies inspect the facility to ensure that it meets health and safety regulations and complies with accepted standards. A **survey** is a review and evaluation to ensure that facilities are maintaining acceptable standards of practice. Different types of facilities must meet different quality standards.

Each facility holds a state **license**, which permits it to conduct business. Most facilities also possess a **certification**. Certification is necessary to collect Medicare and Medicaid payments. Licensure and certification surveys are done by the state health department or human services agency. Occasionally, federal surveyors will inspect the facility. During a survey, a number of **surveyors** inspect conditions in the facility. Surveyors are representatives of the agency that reviews the facility.

ACCREDITATION

Accreditation is a voluntary process in which a professional organization recognizes a facility for demonstrating its ability to meet certain quality standards and criteria. Accreditation is an important means of measuring quality. Working to become accredited is part of QA. The health care organization identifies strengths and areas needing improvement and then determines the best ways to provide quality care.

The Centers for Medicare and Medicaid Services (CMS) has certain minimum health and safety standards that health care facilities must meet in order to participate in the Medicare and Medicaid programs and receive reimbursement. Although accreditation is voluntary, hospitals are not eligible to receive Medicare payment unless they are accredited. Medicare is an important source of revenue, and most hospitals could not survive financially without it.

Surveys

Surveys are done at varying intervals, depending on the purpose and type of the survey and the organization that is conducting the survey. Although there are many types of surveys, accreditation and licensure and certification surveys are the most common. Surveyors will arrive unannounced and will stay until they have finished. This may take a week or more, depending on the facility size, the type of the survey, and the findings. Accrediting organizations require facilities to periodically evaluate staff performance and maintain a record of these checks. They are also required to provide ongoing educational programs. This helps ensure that staff do their jobs correctly.

Surveyors review facility policies and procedures and determine whether staff are following them. They will ask questions and interview patients, families, and staff. They will monitor how staff:

- Give care.
- Practice handwashing and infection control.
- Treat patients, residents, families, and others.
- Maintain patient rights.
- Practice safety, dignity, and privacy.

Surveyors may:

- Ask you to demonstrate how to use patient care equipment.
- Ask you to demonstrate a procedure.
- Question you about how to respond in an emergency.
- Ask what the facility's code words are for emergencies such as fire, cardiac arrest, and others. (Some facilities print this information on the back of your identification badge.) If you don't know an answer to a question, be honest. Tell them you will find out and get back to them.

After the survey, a report is issued detailing the areas that require improvement. Accreditation is granted if the survey is acceptable. Surveyors will return to check the corrections if serious deficiencies are identified.

OSHA Surveys

The **Occupational Safety and Health Administration (OSHA)** also surveys health care facilities. OSHA is a government agency that protects the health and safety of employees. This organization does not evaluate patient care. OSHA inspectors review infection control, employee tuberculin testing, Material Safety Data Sheets, and other safety policies and practices. Surveyors will interview employees and tour all areas of the facility. The inspector will ask questions about health and safety practices. If the inspector identifies unsafe conditions, the agency may receive a citation or fine. A **citation** is a written notice that informs the facility of its violation of OSHA rules.

Magnet Hospitals

According to the American Hospital Association (AHA), 95 percent of all hospital care is given by nursing personnel. In recent years, the quality of nursing services has been closely studied and recognized for its effect on patient care. Facilities that adhere to the American Nurses Association (ANA) standards of practice have fewer negative outcomes than hospitals that are less supportive of the nursing staff. The **Magnet Program for Excellence in Nursing Services** is based on quality indicators and standards of nursing practice.

An award of Magnet status is a way of recognizing excellence. Research has shown that Magnet hospitals have higher percentages of satisfied staff, lower turnover, better clinical outcomes, and improved patient satisfaction.

Attaining the Magnet designation is not easy. The Magnet program recognizes quality patient care and nursing excellence. Hospitals that have achieved Magnet status are usually very progressive, desirable places to work. Nurses and others like to work in an environment that recognizes their professional status and contributions. Magnet status is reviewed every four years.

REVIEW

A. True/False

Mark the following true or false by circling T or F.

1. T F Nursing assistants work under the supervision of licensed professional health care workers.

2. T F Hospitals provide a full range of health care services.

3. T F Long-term care facilities provide care to persons who require monitoring, nursing care, and treatments.

4. T F The sole purpose of a health care facility is to care for the ill and injured.

5. T F Giving patient-focused care involves treating all patients as unique individuals.

6. T F Patients can remain in the hospital until they feel well enough to go home.

7. T F Persons receiving care in the hospital are called residents.

8. T F Well-planned transitions reduce the risk of errors.

9. T F Many procedures and treatments are done on an outpatient basis to reduce costs.

10. T F A chronic illness comes on suddenly and is usually curable.

B. Multiple Choice

Select the best answer for each of the following.

11. The general term for a person needing health care is:
    a. patient.
    b. Victim.
    c. consumer.
    d. provider.

12. Well-planned transitions:
    a. are special services given by multiskilled caregivers.
    b. involve stabilizing a patient when their needs change.
    c. involve transferring patients within the facility every few days.
    d. reduce the risk of errors and miscommunication.

13. Health care facilities:
    a. treat most patients on an outpatient basis rather than admitting them.

b. must obtain approval from the insurer before providing emergency care.

c. provide a variety of health care services to ill and injured persons.

d. allow patients to stay as long as they want if they cannot care for themselves.

14. Health care has changed because:
    a. there is less demand for services.
    b. people are living longer.
    c. the death rate is increasing.
    d. it is too expensive for most people.

15. Hospice care is provided to people who:
    a. are dying.
    b. have children.
    c. need surgery.
    d. are pregnant.

16. Managed care means that insurance companies:
    a. approve longer stays than private insurers.
    b. negotiate with providers to deliver service at a lower cost.
    c. require most surgery to be done on an outpatient basis.
    d. approve only patients with certain medical conditions.

17. The obstetrics department of the hospital cares for patients:
    a. with heart disease.
    b. who have mental illness.
    c. with conditions of the bones and muscles.
    d. before, during, and after childbirth.

18. Social services staff provide:
    a. nursing care 24 hours a day.
    b. diagnostic testing.
    c. counseling for patients.
    d. activities to relieve boredom.

19. Environmental services include:
    a. nursing.
    b. housekeeping.
    c. therapy.
    d. surgery.

20. One type of prepaid health care insurance is:
    a. Medicare.
    b. accreditation.

c. a health maintenance organization.

d. out-of-pocket payment.

21. Accreditation is:

a. required by the federal government.

b. a mandatory responsibility of the quality assurance committee.

c. a recognition for voluntarily meeting quality standards and criteria.

d. granted by the Centers for Medicare and Medicaid Services.

22. Medicare payment to hospitals is made based on:

a. diagnosis related groups.

b. services needed by the patient.

c. actual charges billed to the government.

d. the type of medical supplies used.

23. The purpose of quality assurance is to:

a. guarantee quality to the physicians.

b. identify and correct problems.

c. ensure that the facility receives payment.

d. pass the accreditation inspection.

C. Word Choice

Choose the correct word or phrase from the following list to complete each statement in questions 24–33.

ambulatory surgical center	pathology
	patient-focused care
hospitals	physical therapy
long-term care facility	prenatal
Medicare	residents
occupational therapy	

24. A _____ provides care to persons whose conditions are stable but require monitoring, nursing care, and treatments.

25. _____ are complex organizations that provide a full range of health care services.

26. _____ is given when the patient is considered a unique individual with specific needs.

27. _____ care is given to a mother during her pregnancy.

28. Persons living in a long-term care facility are usually called _____.

29. Uncomplicated surgeries may be performed in an _____.

30. _____ means the study of disease.

31. _____ helps patients regain self-care skills.

32. _____ helps patients regain mobility skills.

33. A federal program that pays health care costs for persons 65 years of age and older is called _____.

D. Nursing Assistant Challenge

Mrs. Hernandez is pregnant with her first child. She wants to do everything she can to make sure that she has a safe and uncomplicated pregnancy, labor, and delivery and that her baby is healthy. Consider how Mrs. Hernandez will move through the health care system to achieve this goal.

34. What is the first type of care that Mrs. Hernandez needs to help her meet the goal of an uncomplicated pregnancy?

35. In your community, where is this type of care provided?

36. What programs are offered to pregnant women in your community?

37. From which hospital departments do you think Mrs. Hernandez will receive services when she delivers her baby?

38. After the baby is born, what health care will the baby need?

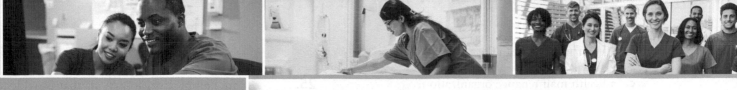

CHAPTER 2

On the Job: Being a Nursing Assistant

OBJECTIVES

After completing this chapter, you will be able to:

2.1 Spell and define terms.

2.2 Identify the members of the interdisciplinary health care team and the nursing team.

2.3 List the job responsibilities of the nursing assistant.

2.4 Explain how the Nurse Practice Act affects nursing assistant practice.

2.5 Discuss the importance of working within the established scope of nursing assistant practice.

2.6 List the federal requirements for nursing assistants working in long-term care facilities.

2.7 State the purpose of evidence-based practice.

2.8 Identify common nursing care delivery systems and briefly describe each.

2.9 Describe your facility's lines of authority.

2.10 Discuss the five rights of delegation.

2.11 Explain why good time management is a key to nursing assistant success.

2.12 Describe methods of organizing assignments to make the best use of your time.

2.13 State the purpose of shift report and handoff communication.

2.14 Explain why critical thinking is an essential skill for nursing assistants.

2.15 Describe the importance of good human relations.

2.16 List ways of building good relationships with patients, families, and staff.

2.17 Explain why projecting a professional image is important.

2.18 List the rules of personal hygiene and appropriate dress.

2.19 Explain why a healthy mental attitude is important.

2.20 Describe ways of relieving stress and preventing illness.

VOCABULARY

Learn the meaning and the correct spelling of the following words and phrases:

assessment	food handler	Nurse Aide Training and	partners in practice
assignment	handoff communication	Competency Evaluation	registered nurse (RN)
attitude	interdisciplinary health care	Program (NATCEP)	scope of practice
burnout	team	Nurse Practice Act (NPA)	shift report
career ladders	interpersonal	nursing assistant	
critical thinking	relationships	nursing team	
delegation	licensed practical nurse	Omnibus Budget	
empathy	(LPN)	Reconciliation Act	
evidence-based practice	licensed vocational nurse	(OBRA)	
(EBP)	(LVN)	organizational chart	

THE INTERDISCIPLINARY HEALTH CARE TEAM

The nursing assistant is an important member of the **interdisciplinary health care team** (Figure 2-1). Some facilities call this the *personal support team*. Others prefer the term *interprofessional team*. This team includes the patient, the physician, the nursing team, therapists, and other specialists trained to meet both general and specific patient needs (Figure 2-2). Members of the patient's family are also included, with the patient's permission. The physician (doctor) names the condition or illness (makes a diagnosis) and prescribes treatment. Healthcare professionals often specialize in one area of practice (Figure 2-3). Many specialties have subspecialties, or a narrow field of focus within a specialty. Table 2-1 lists common specialties, the name for the physician who practices each specialty, and a description of the care provided.

The **nursing team** provides skilled nursing care. The team consists of registered nurses, licensed practical (or vocational) nurses, and nursing assistants. Registered nurses plan and direct the nursing care of patients according to the physician's orders. All members of the team provide direct patient care.

Other specialists who may also be part of the team are listed in Table 2-2.

THE NURSING TEAM

The Registered Nurse

The **registered nurse (RN)** has completed a two-, three-, or four-year nursing program and passed a national licensure examination. They are identified by the initials RN. Registered nurses assess, plan for, evaluate, and coordinate the many aspects of patient care. They teach patients and their families about health practices, provide nursing care, and supervise performance of duties they delegate to others. Nurses may specialize in a certain area of nursing practice. Some of the many nursing specialties are:

- Administration
- Anesthesiology
- Cardiac care

- Dialysis
- Gerontology
- Gynecology
- Home care
- Independent practice (consultant, educator, nurse practitioner)
- Infection control
- Maternal and child health
- Oncology (cancer care)
- Public health
- Research
- Surgery
- Teaching
- Telemetry

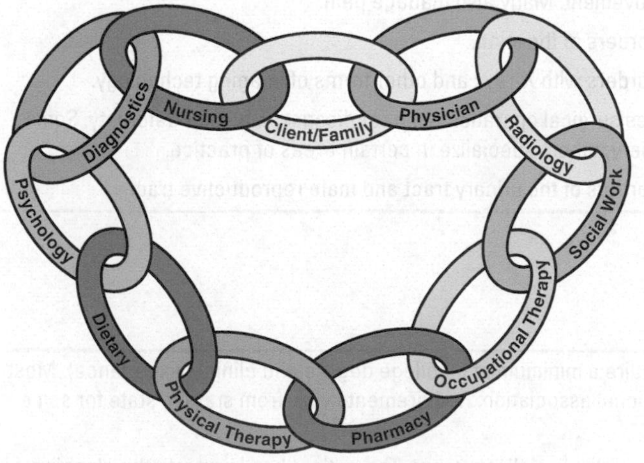

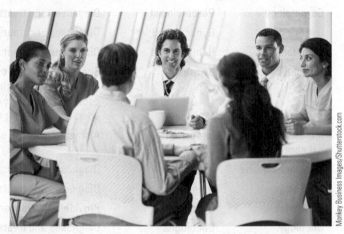

FIGURE 2-2 Each member of the health care team makes important contributions to the overall operation of the facility and the well-being of patients.

Monkey Business Images/Shutterstock.com

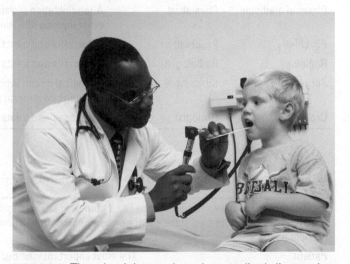

FIGURE 2-3 The physician makes the medical diagnosis and directs medical care. This physician specializes in pediatrics, which is the care of children.

FIGURE 2-1 The interdisciplinary team members are like the links in a chain; they work together in providing services to patients.

TABLE 2-1 Medical Specialties

Specialty	Physician	Type of Care
Allergy	Allergist	Diagnoses and treats patients who have an abnormal immune response to foreign agents, such as substances or drugs.
Anesthesia	Anesthesiologist	Provides anesthetics or drugs that cause unconsciousness prior to surgery. Specializes in airway management to ensure that patients receive enough oxygen during and after surgery.
Cardiovascular diseases	Cardiologist	Diagnoses and treats patients with disorders of the heart and blood vessels.
Dermatology	Dermatologist	Diagnoses and treats patients with disorders of the skin.
Endocrinology	Endocrinologist	Specializes in diabetes; diagnoses and treats other disorders of the endocrine system and glands that make hormones.
Family medicine	Family practitioner	Diagnoses and treats individuals and family of all ages, both sexes, each organ system, and every disease entity.
Gastroenterology	Gastroenterologist	Diagnoses and treats patients with disorders of the digestive system.
Gerontology	Gerontologist	Diagnoses and treats disorders of the aging person.
Gynecology	Gynecologist	Diagnoses and treats disorders related to the female reproductive tract.
Hematology	Hematologist	Diagnoses and treats patients with disorders of the blood and blood-forming organs.
Hospital care	Hospitalist	Specializes in care of persons who are in a hospital. The primary practice of these doctors is in the hospital rather than an office. The doctor admits patients through the emergency department and directs, manages, and reports on the hospital course of treatment to the patient's primary physician.
Intensive and critical care	Intensivist	A physician whose practice focuses on care of critically ill patients.
Internal medicine	Internist	Diagnoses and treats patients with disorders of the internal organs.
Neurology	Neurologist	Diagnoses and treats patients with disorders of the nervous system.
Obstetrics	Obstetrician	Provides care to women during pregnancy, childbirth, and immediately thereafter.
Oncology	Oncologist	Diagnoses and treats patients who have or may have cancer.
Ophthalmology	Ophthalmologist	Diagnoses and treats patients with disorders of the eyes.
Orthopedics	Orthopedist	Diagnoses and treats disorders of the bones, ligaments, tendons, and joints.
Pediatrics	Pediatrician	Diagnoses, treats, and prevents disorders in children.
Physical medicine	Physiatrist	A rehabilitation physician who diagnoses and treats nerve, muscle, and bone illnesses or other injuries affecting movement. Many also manage pain.
Psychiatry	Psychiatrist	Diagnoses and treats disorders of the mind.
Radiology	Radiologist	Diagnoses and treats disorders with X-rays and other forms of imaging technology.
Surgery	Surgeon	A medical doctor who uses surgical operations to treat disease, injury, or deformity. Some surgeons do general surgery; others specialize in certain areas of practice.
Urology	Urologist	Diagnoses and treats disorders of the urinary tract and male reproductive tract.

TABLE 2-2 Interdisciplinary Health Care Team Members

Each of these disciplines requires a specified course of study (many require a minimum of a college degree and clinical experience). Most require either licensing by a state agency or certification from a professional association. Requirements vary from state to state for some disciplines.	
Patient	The most important member of the interdisciplinary team. The patient has input into the planning and implementation of care. The family may participate in care planning if the patient gives permission or if the patient is unable to do so.
Physician (may be a medical doctor [MD] or Osteopathic Physician [DO])	Licensed by the state to diagnose and treat disease and to prescribe medications. Many specialty areas within medicine require additional education and certification.

(continues)

TABLE 2-2 *(continued)*

Specialty Services	
Clinical Nurse Specialist (CNS)	An advanced-practice registered nurse (RN) with a master's degree whose care focuses on a very specific patient population or type of care (e.g., medical, surgical, diabetic, cardiovascular, operating room, emergency room, critical care, pain management, geriatric, neonatal and others. The authority to write prescriptions varies from one state to the next.
Nurse Practitioner (NP)	An RN with advanced academic and clinical experience, which enables the NP to diagnose and manage common acute and chronic illnesses, either independently or as part of a health care team. All 50 states allow nurse practitioners to prescribe medication, but only 12 states and the District of Columbia allow nurse practitioners to prescribe medication independently without the oversight of a physician.
Physician Assistant (PA)	A health care professional licensed to practice medicine with physician supervision. PAs conduct physical exams, diagnose and treat illnesses, order and interpret tests, counsel on preventive health care, assist in surgery, and have limited authority to write prescriptions in all 50 states.
Registered Nurse (RN)	Licensed by the state to make assessments and plan, implement, and evaluate nursing care. Supervises other nursing staff and may coordinate the interdisciplinary health care team. Many specialty areas within nursing require additional education.
Licensed Practical Nurse (LPN) Licensed Vocational Nurse (LVN)	Licensed by the state to provide direct patient care under the supervision of an RN. Called *Licensed Vocational Nurse* (LVN) in Texas and California.
Nursing Assistant	Has completed a state-approved course, passed a competency examination, and is approved to provide direct patient care under the supervision of a licensed nurse.
Nutrition Assistant (Feeding Assistant)	After completing an approved class, may assist stable, long-term care facility residents with food and fluids, under the direction of a licensed nurse.
Medication Aide (MA)	A certified nursing assistant who has taken additional classes in medication administration and completed a state certification examination. Allowed to pass medications in nursing facilities and home health care in some states under the supervision of a licensed nurse.
Restorative Assistant (RNA)	A certified nursing assistant who has additional education in restorative nursing care. Helps patients attain and maintain their highest level of function and prevent physical deformities.

Specialty Services	
Chaplain—Pastoral Care	Provides services to meet the religious and spiritual needs of patients. Provides emotional support.
Dietitian	Licensed by the state to assess nutritional needs; plans menus and therapeutic diets and provides food services for patients.
Occupational Therapist (OT)	Licensed to provide rehabilitative services to evaluate and treat persons with physical injury or illness, psychosocial problems, or developmental disabilities. Occupational therapy assistants and aides work under the supervision of an occupational therapist. Most care is directed toward improving fine motor skills and activities of daily living.
Orthotist	Licensed by the state to design and fit braces and splints for the extremities.
Physical Therapist (PT)	Licensed by the state to provide rehabilitative services to evaluate and treat persons with physical injury or illness, psychosocial problems, or developmental disabilities. Physical therapy assistants and aides work under the supervision of a physical therapist. Most care is directed toward restoring gross motor skills, mobility, and ambulation.
Respiratory Therapist (also called Respiratory Care Practitioner or RCP)	Licensed to evaluate and treat diseases and problems associated with breathing and the respiratory tract. Cares for persons with sleep apnea.
Social Worker	Assesses need and provides services to meet the nonmedical, psychosocial needs of patients. Finds community resources. Responsible for discharge planning.
Speech Therapist (also called Speech-Language Pathologist or SLP)	Licensed by the state to provide services to individuals with speech and swallowing disorders caused by acute and chronic illness and trauma.

(continues)

TABLE 2-2 *(continued)*

Ancillary Clinical	
Pharmacist	Licensed by the state to fill prescriptions for medications as ordered by the physician. Acts as an information resource to nurses and physicians for updates on new medications and for maintaining safe drug therapy for patients.
Phlebotomist	Uses needles to puncture veins for the purpose of drawing blood.
Laboratory Technician	Laboratory worker who prepares specimens, operates automated analyzers, and performs manual tests.
Laboratory Technologist	Individual who performs complex laboratory tests and microscopically examines blood, tissue, and other body substances.
In addition to these members of the interdisciplinary health care team, other employees in the health care facility provide services that benefit patients.	
Administrator	Provides general administration and supervision.
Environmental Services	Maintain a clean and comfortable environment. Housekeeping keeps the facility clean. Maintenance cares for and repairs the building and equipment. Laundry services provide and clean all hospital linens.
Volunteers	Provide services free of charge and perform tasks such as delivering mail and flowers, running the gift shop, directing visitors, and raising funds for the facility.

The Licensed Practical/Vocational Nurse

The **licensed practical** or **licensed vocational nurse** has completed a one- to two-year educational program and has passed a national licensure examination. They are identified by the initials LPN or LVN. This nurse works under the supervision of the RN. The LPN is able to provide most of the care when the patient's nursing needs are not complex and also assists the RN in more complicated situations.

The Nursing Assistant

The **nursing assistant** helps with the care of patients under the supervision of either an RN or an LPN (Figure 2-4). Because the assistant's responsibilities and skills are not as great as those of the RN or LPN/LVN, the basic preparation is shorter. However, growth and learning will continue throughout your career. In the health care facility, the assistant is called by one of the following names:

- Patient care attendant (assistant) (PCA)
- Nurse aide (NA), nurse assistant (NA), nursing assistant (NA), state-tested nursing assistant (STNA), state registered nursing assistant (SRNA), certified nursing assistant (CNA), licensed nursing assistant (LNA), and others
- Clinical support associate
- Nurse extender
- Health care assistant
- Personal care assistant
- Patient care technician

- Unlicensed assistive personnel (UAP)
- _____ care technician (the first word of the title designates the unit on which the assistant works, such as critical care technician, surgical care technician, and so forth)

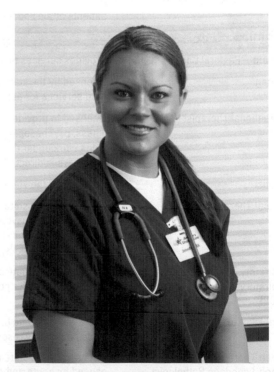

FIGURE 2-4 A registered professional nurse manages the nursing team and identifies nurses who will supervise nursing assistants and other team members.

REGULATION OF NURSING ASSISTANT PRACTICE

Federal and state legislatures write the laws that determine the scope of practice. Laws may also be called *statutes*. Legislators give state regulatory agencies the authority to make *rules*, which may also be called *regulations*. Rules are much more specific than laws because they determine how the law will be applied. Rules also set standards of conduct and can be updated and changed by state agencies whenever necessary.

Nursing assistants must know the scope of their duties and the laws governing their practice. Each state identifies the duties and responsibilities of the assistant and defines the education and level of competency required for safe practice.

In 1987, Congress passed a federal law that regulates the education and certification of nursing assistants. The law is called the **Omnibus Budget Reconciliation Act (OBRA)**. OBRA established the minimum requirements for nursing assistant programs. All persons working as nursing assistants in long-term care facilities must complete an approved educational course and competency evaluation. The education of nursing assistants is managed by each state, guided by federal regulations.

The National Council of State Boards of Nursing, Inc., developed the **Nurse Aide Training and Competency Evaluation Program (NATCEP)**. NATCEP meets the requirements of OBRA and serves as a guide for registering and awarding credentials to nursing assistants. NATCEP lists the skills to be achieved. Programs may exceed the state and federal minimum requirements.

The nursing assistant class must include a minimum of 75 hours of theory and practice. Some states require 80 to 175 program hours of written or oral and clinical skills in several areas. The mandatory content includes:

- Basic nursing skills, including infection control (Figure 2-5)
- Basic restorative services
- Mental health and social service needs
- Personal care skills

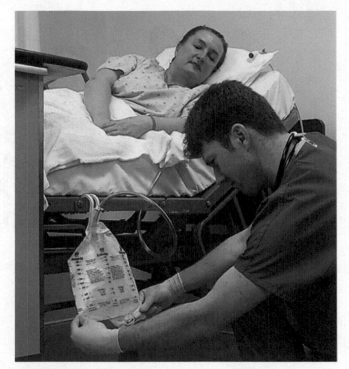

FIGURE 2-5 Responsibilities of the nursing assistant include direct patient care, making and reporting observations, and following infection prevention measures.

- Resident rights and good communication
- Safety and emergency care

Other rules that guide nursing assistant practice require:

- Successful completion of a competency evaluation program (skills test). Persons who have successfully completed the program have at least three opportunities to pass the state test
- Completion of a new program or retesting by nursing assistants who have not given nursing care for pay for a continuous 24-month period
- Continuing education (12 to 24 hours per year, depending on state rules)

Become familiar with the rules for nursing assistant practice in your state and facility and be sure you meet the requirements. In some states and facilities, you may be required to take special classes before being allowed to work on the nursing units. For example, your facility may require you to complete a cardiopulmonary resuscitation (CPR) class (Figure 2-6), or a certified **food handler** course. A food handler is an employee who works with unpackaged food, food equipment or utensils, or food contact surfaces. Some classes may be taken online.

You may be required to take additional classes to learn about care of persons with Alzheimer disease and abuse and neglect in people who are elderly or have disabilities.

⚖ Legal **ALERT**

OBRA nursing assistant requirements apply only to long-term care facilities, including skilled nursing units in hospitals. The federal requirements do not apply to acute care hospitals, although many states have voluntarily adopted the OBRA nursing assistant education requirements as the minimum entry standard for employment. Some states have established requirements for preparing nursing assistants for hospital and home health care practice.

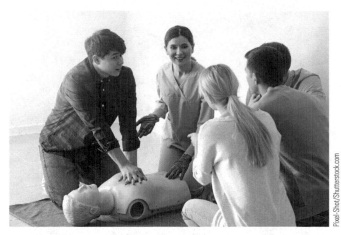

FIGURE 2-6 Learning cardiopulmonary resuscitation (CPR) is a job requirement when providing patient care.

THE ROLE AND RESPONSIBILITIES OF THE NURSING ASSISTANT

The nursing assistant provides physical care and emotional support to patients. You will make observations during care (Figure 2-7), report them to the nurse, and record them on the patient's chart (see Chapter 8). Nursing assistant responsibilities are based on the state **Nurse Practice Act (NPA)** and follow the job description and each person's plan of care. Each facility develops its own job descriptions. They will be similar, but not identical to, the job descriptions in other facilities.

An overview of nursing assistant responsibilities is provided in Table 2-3.

Nursing assistants are special people: they are interested in others, and they take pride in themselves and their work. They are willing to learn the skills necessary to care for those who are ill. Not everyone has these qualities.

Your interest and caring are valuable assets to the nursing team. You are the person the patient sees most often. You may observe and hear things that others will not. For example, the patient is far more likely to tell you of "minor complaints" that are not minor at all. Inform the nurse. Competent, caring nursing assistants make a valuable contribution to patient comfort and safety.

NURSE PRACTICE ACT

Nursing practice is regulated by a board of nursing, or other governing body, in each state. This agency establishes practice guidelines called a Nurse Practice Act (NPA) to describe the scope of nursing practice in that state. This may vary slightly from one state to the next. Facilities use the NPA as a guide when they develop job descriptions and determine which skills you can perform.

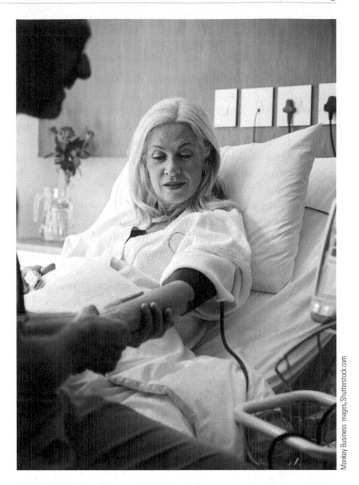

FIGURE 2-7 Nursing assistants measure vital signs and report abnormal values to the nurse in charge.

Scope of Practice

Scope of practice means the skills the nursing assistant is legally permitted to carry out according to state regulations and facility policies. If someone asks you to do something that is clearly outside of your scope of practice, such as giving medications, courteously explain that you have not learned to do the task. Report the incident to the nurse.

> ⚖ Legal **ALERT**
>
> Scope of practice is a very important legal concept. Your scope of practice is defined in the job description given to you by your employer. The policy and procedure manuals are an additional resource. Functioning within this scope of practice protects the nursing assistant and the facility. By state law, you may not be permitted to perform some of the advanced procedures discussed in this book. Consult with your instructor or supervisor to be sure you know your legal responsibilities. Do not perform or assist with any procedure unless your state's law permits you to do so.

TABLE 2-3 Typical Job Description for a Nursing Assistant

Nursing assistants commonly participate in the nursing process by carrying out the activities listed.

1. Assist with patient assessment and care planning.
   a. Check and record vital signs
   b. Measure height and weight
   c. Measure intake and output
   d. Collect specimens
   e. Test urine and feces
   f. Observe patient response to care
   g. Report and record observations of patients' conditions
2. Assist patients in meeting nutrition and elimination needs.
   a. Check food trays
   b. Pass food trays
   c. Feed patients
   d. Provide fresh drinking water and nourishments
   e. Assist with use of bedpans, urinals, and commodes
   f. Empty urine collection bags
   g. Assist with colostomy care
   h. Give enemas
   i. Observe feces and urine
   j. Monitor intake and output
3. Assist patients with mobility.
   a. Turn and position
   b. Provide range-of-motion exercises
   c. Transfer to wheelchair or stretcher
   d. Assist with ambulation
4. Assist patients with personal hygiene and grooming.
   a. Bathe patients
   b. Provide nail and hair care
   c. Give oral hygiene
   d. Provide denture care
   e. Shave patients
   f. Assist with dressing and undressing

5. Assist with patient comfort and anxiety relief.
   a. Protect patient privacy and maintain confidentiality
   b. Keep call signal within patient's reach
   c. Answer call signal promptly
   d. Provide orientation to the room or unit and to other patients and visitors
   e. Assist patients with communications
   f. Protect personal possessions
   g. Provide diversional activities
   h. Give backrubs
   i. Prepare hot and cold applications
6. Assist in promoting patient safety and environmental cleanliness.
   a. Use side rails and restraints appropriately
   b. Keep patient unit clean and clutter-free
   c. Make beds
   d. Clean and care for equipment
   e. Carry out isolation precautions
   f. Practice medical asepsis and infection control
   g. Practice standard precautions
   h. Observe oxygen precautions
   i. Assist in keeping recreational and nonpatient areas clean and free of hazards
   j. Participate in fire drills and patient evacuation procedures
7. Assist with unit management and efficiency.
   a. Admit, transfer, and discharge patients
   b. Transport patients
   c. Take specimens to lab
   d. Assist with special procedures
   e. Do errands as required
   f. Assist with cost-containment measures
   g. Answer the telephone
   h. Document care provided and assist with unit recordkeeping

EXPANDED SCOPE OF PRACTICE

In many states and facilities, experienced nursing assistants can expand their scope of practice by taking classes to gain information and learn new skills. This provides the opportunity for career advancement. Many facilities have special programs, such as **career ladders** or cross-training (see Chapter 1), or programs that provide an opportunity for upward mobility. You have chosen a career with unlimited opportunities for personal growth and satisfaction.

Avoid assuming that all nursing assistants are able and authorized to perform advanced procedures simply because those procedures are included in this textbook. Each facility has policies and supervisory practices that are consistent with state law and that ensure competency on the part of the caregiver and safety for the patient. Carry out procedures only after supervised practice and instructor or supervisor approval, in keeping with facility policy. Additional information supporting advanced procedures may be found in the chapters indicated.

 Clinical Information **ALERT**

Certified nursing assistants are responsible for preserving life, practicing and promoting good health, and treating all patients equally without discrimination (on the basis of religion, race, sexual orientation, gender, or age). Certified nursing assistants must carry out duties to the best of their abilities while treating each person with courtesy and respect. The nursing assistant must maintain the confidentiality of patients and families while on and off duty. Certified nursing assistants must avoid discussing their own personal business with patients. A well-groomed appearance and proper communication skills are essential. They must be loyal to their employers and patients. Professional nursing assistants regularly attend continuing education classes to learn new information and gain new skills.

PROFESSIONALISM

Professionalism is a learned quality. Your behavior in your nursing assistant class is the foundation on which to build. Begin developing professional qualities right away. You should:

- Adhere to nursing assistant program policies.
- Dress appropriately in class; follow the dress code in clinical.
- Arrive for class prepared and on time. Be quiet and attentive in class.
- Complete your assignments and turn in homework without offering excuses for not getting work done.
- Make good first impressions in class, skills laboratory, and clinical.
- Strive for accuracy in your assignments, patient care, and documentation.
- Not miss class; your state has specific attendance requirements.
- Be polite and respectful to your instructor, clinical staff, and other students. Demonstrate courtesy and maturity in all communications.
- Let patients know that assisting them is a pleasure; it is much more than your job!

DRESS CODE AND APPEARANCE

Personal Appearance

Many health care facilities allow employees great flexibility in selecting the type and style of their uniforms. Years ago, patients were able to identify the various types of health care workers by their uniforms, including nursing caps. Today, it can be very difficult to distinguish one type of worker from another.

Some states and many facilities require staff to wear a name badge or photo identification tag that lists the person's name and position or title so the patient knows who is taking care of them. As a safety measure for the workers, some facilities list only the first name and title on the name badge. A gait (transfer) belt (see Chapter 15) is a required part of the clinical uniform for nursing assistants in some facilities.

Uniform

Some facilities have a color code for employee uniforms (Figure 2-8). They may post a key to the colors in patient rooms, so all patients can see at a glance what service is caring for them. Wear a fresh uniform. Your uniform should fit loosely enough to prevent tearing. It must be color-coordinated, neat and clean in appearance, wrinkle free, and in good repair. Acceptable uniforms may be of the top-and-pants and/or skirt/dress

 Clinical Information ALERT

Remember this: first impressions send powerful messages. Although people should form opinions based on what a person knows rather than how they look, most form an opinion about another person when they first meet. This is almost always based on the other's appearance. A well-dressed appearance tends to convey a higher level of knowledge and a sincere interest in advancement. A disheveled worker gives the impression of being a disinterested, marginal performer (LaSala & Nelson, 2005).

LaSala, K. B., & Nelson, J. (2005). What contributes to professionalism? *MEDSURG Nursing, 14*(1), 63.

variety. Skirt- or dress-type uniforms must reach the middle of the kneecap. Shorts and sleeveless tops are not permitted. Undergarments must be appropriate and modest. Solid white, black, or beige undergarments are recommended. The pattern, color, texture, and design of your undergarments should not show through your uniform. You may wear a color-coordinated lab jacket or coat over your uniform. Most facilities permit you to wear a tank top or long-sleeved thermal shirt for warmth and/or modesty under your shirt. Your instructor or supervisor has full authority to send you home to change clothing if you are inappropriately dressed. (Time spent away from class while changing may be counted as hours absent.)

You must wear socks or stockings in the clinical area. For your safety, shoes worn in the clinical area must have closed toes. A comfortable, well-fitting white athletic shoe or nursing duty shoe with a slip-resistant sole works best. You will be on your feet much of the day, and your comfort is important. Your shoes and shoelaces must be clean.

Wear your uniform only while you are on duty. If your facility does not provide an area for changing, wear a cover-up (such as a lab coat) when traveling to and from work so you will not spread germs. When you get home, remove your uniform, fold it inside out, and put it into the laundry. This helps keep the dirtiest part of your uniform away from the other clothes in the laundry.

Maintain a professional appearance and project a positive image to patients and others (Figure 2-9). Well-groomed nursing assistants are likely to have the same pride and caring attitude about their work. Patients will feel more secure and confident, and other staff members will regard you as mature and reliable. As you develop good health and professional habits, you become a role model for your family, friends, and co-workers.

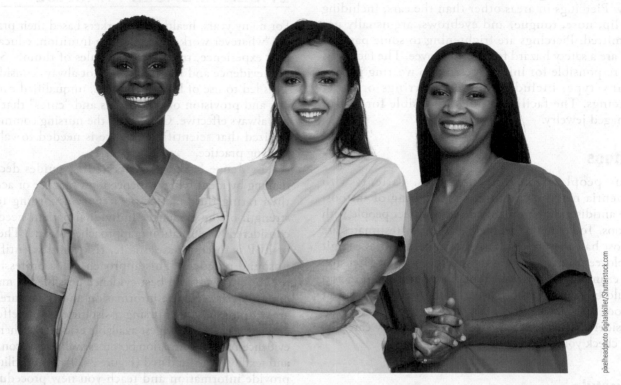

FIGURE 2-8 Some facilities have a color code for uniforms so that it is clear what function an employee serves. They may post a key to the colors in patient rooms.

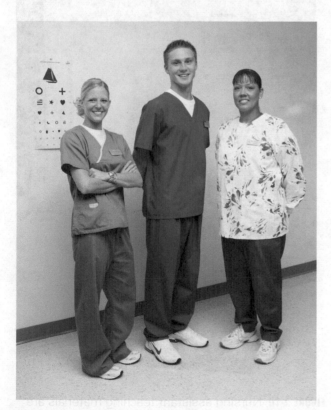

FIGURE 2-9 Well-groomed, professional-looking caregivers instill confidence in patients.

Head Covering

Most facilities permit employees to wear a head covering for religious purposes, but the permissibility of a head covering for religious purposes is decided by each facility and is beyond the scope of this book. Hats, scarves, and other ornamentation or hair covering may not be worn in the clinical area.

Sunglasses

Sunglasses may not be worn in the clinical area.

Jewelry, Earrings, and Body Piercings

Jewelry is a ready medium for bacterial growth. It may also injure a patient, especially if the person is confused, very old, very young, or has fragile skin. Small rings or wedding rings are limited to one ring or set per hand. Large settings, and those with sharp edges or stones, may not be worn. Bracelets and necklaces are not permitted unless they are the type used for medical identification. A watch with a second hand is part of your uniform. Avoid long, dangling earrings, hoops, and wires that can be easily caught in linen or pulled out by a patient. One set of small stud-type earrings may be worn in the lower earlobe only. Piercings in areas other than the ears, including the lip, nose, tongue, and eyebrows, are usually not permitted. Piercings are frightening to some patients and are a safety hazard for the employee. The facility is not responsible for injuries related to wearing jewelry of any type, including pierced earrings or other piercings. The facility is not responsible for lost or damaged jewelry.

Tattoos

Some people are fearful of tattoos. Patients with dementia may misinterpret the meaning of tattoos. The antidiscrimination laws do not protect people with tattoos. Today many people have tattoos (estimates are almost half the population) and some facilities permit employees to have them as long as they are not offensive. For example, tattoos with profanity, nudity, and racism would be considered offensive. Some facilities prohibit tattoos on the face and neck. Before getting a tattoo, consider the size, placement, and design very carefully and check your facility policy.

Hairstyle

A neat, natural hairstyle is part of a well-groomed appearance. Select a style that will not cover your face. Pull long hair back or wear it up. Extreme fashion statements such as shaving the head, Mohawk haircuts, or unusual or unnatural styles and neon hair colors are usually not permitted. Modest hair accessories (such as barrettes, combs, and hairbands) may be worn to keep hair out of the face. Accessories may be gold, silver, white, or any color that coordinates with the clothing.

Facial Hair

Each facility sets its own policy regarding facial hair of males. If permitted, facial hair must be neat and trimmed.

Makeup

Select shades that complement your natural skin coloring. Application must be light and well blended. Eye makeup, mascara, and lipstick must be subdued in color. Apply makeup carefully so it does not stain or bleed onto your uniform.

Fingernails

Fingernails must be clean and well-groomed and not exceed ¼ inch beyond the fingertip. Avoid acrylic and sculpted nails. Clear nail polish may be worn, and polish should be fresh without chips or cracks.

EVIDENCE-BASED PRACTICE

For many years, health care workers based their practice on "whatever worked," including intuition, education, past experience, tradition, and rules of thumb. Scientific evidence and research were not always considered. This led to use of home remedies, unqualified caregivers, and provision of treatments and "cures" that were not always effective. Over time, the nursing community realized that scientific evidence is needed to validate nursing practice.

Evidence-based practice (EBP) guides decision making by identifying evidence for a practice or activity, then rating the practice or activity according to the strength of the evidence. Individual patient needs are considered when planning approaches to care. The goal of EBP is to eliminate unsafe, risky, and scientifically unsound practices. This approach helps professionals use the strongest and best evidence possible for making clinical decisions. The information and procedures you are learning in your nursing assistant class are effective and based on the strongest available evidence. When new evidence-based information becomes available, lesson plans and textbooks are updated (Figure 2-10). Your facility will provide information and teach you new procedures if evidence results in changes in the way care is given.

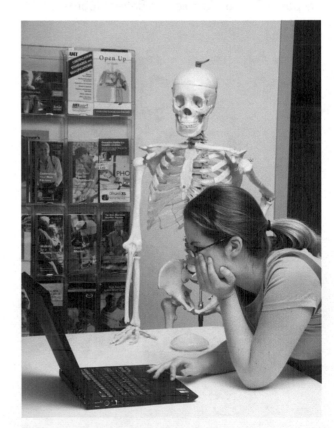

FIGURE 2-10 Nursing assistant teaching materials are updated with new evidence-based practices so students learn important, current information.

ORGANIZATION OF NURSING CARE

Each facility selects a method of providing nursing care to meet its patients' needs. The nursing assistant has a functional role in each method. No single delivery system is ideal. The facility determines job duties and the model of care based on the type of care provided, cost-effectiveness, and maximum patient benefit. The nursing care delivery system describes how care is organized in the facility. Remember that caring is the essence of nursing, regardless of the system of care being used.

Primary Nursing

In primary nursing, an RN is responsible for care of an assigned patient throughout the person's hospitalization. Licensed staff and assistants may help with the care under the RN's direction. The nurse plans and coordinates the nursing care, teaches, gives direct nursing care, carries out treatments, and plans for the patient's discharge. Patients appreciate primary nursing because it enables them to relate directly to one nurse. In the primary nursing situation, each RN is assigned to and responsible for six to eight patients.

Functional Nursing

Functional nursing is a task-oriented way to organize care. It was first introduced in the 1930s and is still being used today. In this method, the charge nurse is responsible for all patients. All other staff members are assigned specific tasks, such as giving medications, administering treatments, or providing personal care.

Patients may find this type of nursing confusing because many people are involved in their care. However, some facilities find that this method uses available, qualified personnel to their best advantage.

Team Nursing

Team nursing is one of the most common methods of delivering care. In this system, an RN team leader determines the nursing needs of all the patients assigned to the team for care. In some settings, the LPN or LVN is a team leader. They are supervised by an RN. Team members receive instructions and assignments from, and report back to, the team leader.

Patient-Focused care

Patient-focused care (see Chapter 1) is the practice of nursing that is individualized to the person's needs. Services that are traditionally provided by other departments are provided by nursing staff, reducing the number of people caring for the patient and reducing the cost.

Patients learn about their conditions and are empowered and involved in their care so they are able to guide decision making. Services are both clinically effective and cost effective.

Partners in Practice

In the **partners in practice** method of providing care, a registered nurse or primary nurse is paired with a nursing assistant or other team member. The team works together to meet the needs of their assigned patients. In many facilities, they work on the same schedule. The partners care for the same group of patients for the day, but may have a different group the following day.

Case Management

In the case management method, an RN (or social worker, in some facilities) is the designated case manager. They are responsible for assessing the patient and working with others to manage the care and for meeting the patient's health, wellness, and teaching needs from admission to discharge. The case manager helps identify services, providers, and facilities that the patient needs and ensures that resources are used in a timely and cost-effective manner. Care is given by nurses and nursing assistants. The case manager advocates for the patient and keeps the lines of communication open to achieve the best possible outcomes.

Progressive Patient Care

Facilities using progressive patient care move the patient from one unit to the next as the patient's health needs change. The staff on all units assist the patient to their highest level of function until partial or complete independence is restored. Each unit is set up and staffed to meet the needs of its patient population. For example, a patient is admitted to the intensive care unit for critical care and close monitoring. When the patient is stable, they are moved to an intermediate care unit. When they have adjusted and are medically stable, they move to a medical care unit. If they continue to need ongoing care, they may transfer to a long-term care unit (or facility) before finally being discharged home. Although this is an efficient system of care, moving from one unit to the next may be difficult and confusing for the patient.

Palliative Care

The concept of palliative care was introduced to provide comfort care and pain relief to persons who are dying. This type of care is given in some hospitals, long-term care facility units, hospices, and home health care. The goal of palliative care is to provide the best possible quality of life for patients and their families. It is not intended to be curative or to hasten death; rather, it is given to keep patients comfortable while nature takes its course. This system of care views dying as a normal part of life and helps all parties to accept and cope with death. A team of workers who specialize in different types of care are assigned to meet the patients' and families' needs. For example, the palliative care team may consist of nurses and nursing assistants and other persons who can provide services needed by the patient, such as a social worker, dietitian, chaplain, and physical therapist.

Teamwork

The various models of patient care are successful because they focus on cooperation and teamwork and provide many opportunities for personal growth. Learning to work with others as a member of a team is one of the most important skills to master during your nursing assistant career. You can be an effective member of the interdisciplinary team by:

- Recognizing the importance of all team members
- Appreciating each member's contribution to the team
- Learning as much as possible about patients and their families, to help you understand their feelings and concerns
- Attending care plan conferences and sharing your observations and ideas
- Attending in-service sessions to increase your knowledge
- Becoming cross-trained to increase your skills
- Cooperating with other team members to provide patient-focused care

Unit-Based Assignments

Many facilities use unit-based assignments. When this structure is used, nursing assistants care for all patients and assist all of the nurses on the unit rather than getting direction from just one. Assistants are responsible for carrying out certain activities each day, such as taking all patients' vital signs, monitoring patients' blood glucose values, checking routine pulse oximeter values (Figure 2-11), stocking cabinets so supplies that are routinely used are always available, checking the crash cart, making certain that the suction machine and other emergency equipment is clean and in working order, and collecting all the intake and output measurements at the end of the shift. They know these things must be done and are expected to organize their time and complete these tasks without being told or reminded to do so.

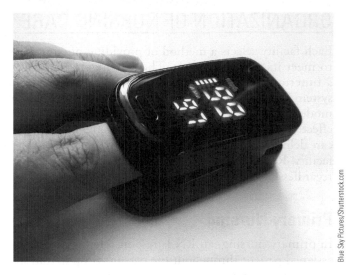

FIGURE 2-11 Nursing assistants routinely measure vital signs and record pulse oximeter values for stable patients.

Blue Sky Pictures/Shutterstock.com

LINES OF AUTHORITY

Nursing assistants receive their assignments from the nurse who supervises them. When they finish their assignments, they report to this same person. This represents the assistant's immediate line of authority and communication.

The assistant will work with a team whose leader is an LPN or an RN. In this case, the assistant's immediate superior is the team leader. The team leaders receive their instructions from the charge nurse. The charge nurse is responsible for the total care of a certain number of patients. Sometimes this includes all the patients on a wing, a unit, or a floor of the facility. Supervisors are responsible for several charge nurse units. They receive their authority and direction from the director of nursing or supervisor, depending on facility size. Health care facilities vary in the complexity of their staffing.

Organizational Chart

Each health care facility has a line of authority and communication. The **organizational chart** (Figure 2-12) is a guide for and spells out the line of authority. The chart illustrates how each department relates to other departments. Some of the larger departments, such as nursing, have their own charts that indicate the line of authority within the department. As a nursing assistant, you will need to use the lines of authority to communicate with staff in nursing and other departments.

The physician directs the patient's medical care. The RN carries out the physician's orders and plans the nursing care. The authority for nursing care

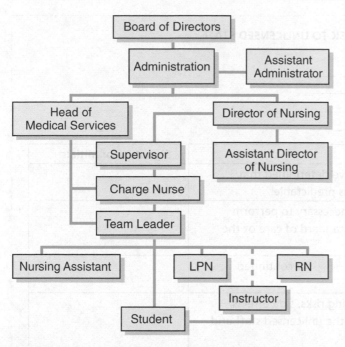

FIGURE 2-12 Typical model of nursing department lines of authority. The diagram may vary slightly from one facility to the next.

passes from the RN supervisor to the charge nurse, to the team leader, and then to the nursing assistant (Figure 2-13). The team leader may be an RN or LPN. Each facility has its own structure and titles for these positions. Assistants should learn the lines of authority in their health care facility, as shown in Figures 2-12 and 2-13. As a student, your immediate authority is your instructor or the person designated as your supervisor. When you accept the responsibility for an assignment, you must fully understand the assignment and be able to do it. If there is any doubt, discuss it with your supervising nurse, the team leader, or charge nurse.

DELEGATION

Delegation is the transfer of responsibility for the performance of a nursing activity from a nurse to someone who does not already have that authority. If a nurse delegates an activity to you, you are the only person with the authority to carry it out. You cannot ask someone else to do it. The nurse is responsible for the delegation decision and must be confident that you can complete the assignment correctly (Figure 2-14). However, they are not

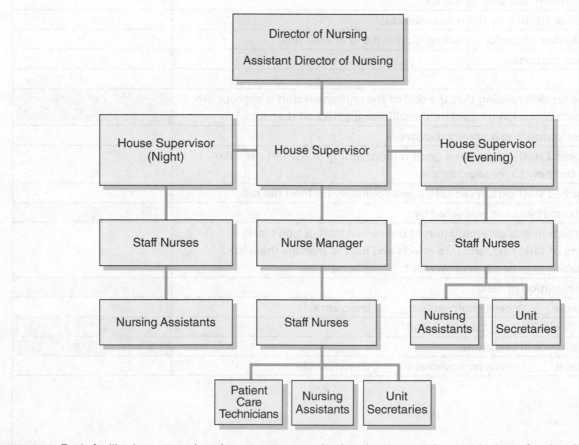

FIGURE 2-13 Each facility has a nursing department organizational structure that works best for that facility.

DELEGATION OF NURSING TASK TO UNLICENSED STAFF

Delegated task: _____

Patient: _____

Unlicensed staff: _____

Licensed Nurse: _____

Activity	Signature or Initials
After assessing the above named person's condition, I have determined that their condition is stable and the outcome of the activity is predictable.	
I have considered the complexity, the risks, and the skill necessary to perform this task and have determined that it is safe, within the standard of care of the unlicensed person, and acceptable to delegate.	
This patient's condition will be reassessed every _____ for continued appropriateness of delegating this task.	
The written instructions for the task noted above, including risks, side effects, and the appropriate response, have been reviewed with the unlicensed staff and are located at: _____.	
Methods of verifying competency for this procedure include (check methods used):	
— Review and discussion of the written material	
— Review of potential risks and side effects of the task	
— Demonstration of the task by the RN	
— Return demonstration by the unlicensed staff	
— Time for further discussion including question and answer time	
— Written test (optional)	
— Other:	
The rationale for determining that the skill of the unlicensed staff is appropriate for the patient's condition is based on the following (check all that apply):	
— The patient's condition is predictable/stable	
— The unlicensed staff person has a good understanding of the task, its risks/side effects, and how to manage them	
— The unlicensed staff person can safely and accurately perform the task	
Teaching outcome has been evaluated by:	
— Visual evaluation and determination of unlicensed staff person's level of understanding of task, risks, and side effects and how to manage them is: _____ acceptable _____ needs improvement _____ unacceptable	
Return demonstration of task:	
_____ acceptable _____ needs improvement _____ unacceptable	
Written test (if given): _____ pass _____ fail	
Overall competence in procedure:	
_____ acceptable _____ needs improvement _____ unacceptable	
Comments:	

FIGURE 2-14 Certain criteria must be met to ensure safe delegation.

(continues)

Delegation Approval—Supervision Statement

The unlicensed staff person has been instructed in the correct method of performing the above task and has successfully demonstrated understanding of the task, its risks/side effects, and management of both. It is my determination they can safely perform the task without direct supervision. I take responsibility for delegation of: _____ to_____.

I will provide supervision of the above unlicensed staff's performance of this task for as long as I am supervising the delegation of this activity. Re-evaluation and ongoing supervision will be performed and documented at least every 60 days unless otherwise noted.

Reason and rationale for supervision of unlicensed staff to exceed 60-day time frame:

_____

_____
                    (Delegating Nurse's Signature)

_____
                            (Date)

Unlicensed Staff Person's Statement

I understand that there are potential risks/side effects involved in the performance of this task and that I am prepared to effectively deal with the consequences of them.

I have been instructed that performing this task is specific to _____ and is not transferable to other patients or unlicensed staff.

_____
                (Signature of Unlicensed Staff)

_____
                            (Date)

FIGURE 2-14 *(continued)*

responsible for the flawless performance of a task. The person accepting the delegation is responsible for their own actions.

The NPA describes how nurses assign or delegate duties. Some states have passed laws that identify duties that are inside or outside the scope of nursing assistant practice. Your instructor will describe the requirements and restrictions in your state.

Five Rights of Delegation

The National Council of State Boards of Nursing has developed a guide called the five rights of delegation.

Nurses use this list to help them delegate correctly. Reading this list will help you learn if a delegation is appropriate. The rights are summarized in Table 2-4.

In some situations, patients need the assessment skills of a licensed nurse. Do not feel offended if the nurse provides the necessary care in a situation like this.

Delegated Activities

As you can see, delegating activities is a serious matter. When you accept the responsibility for a delegated task, you are responsible for your own actions. Discuss your feelings with the nurse if you think that the activity is

TABLE 2-4 Five Rights of Delegation

Delegation "Rights"	Meaning/Explanation	Activities
Right Task	A task that can legally be done by a nursing assistant who has been taught the proper way to do the procedure. A licensed nurse must have checked the assistant's competency and approved them to carry out the task on patients. The assistant must be allowed to perform the procedure according to state law and facility policy.	• The nurse believes that delegating the activity to a nursing assistant is legal and in keeping with facility policies. • The nurse may delegate data collection (such as weights and vital signs) and other parts of care but may not delegate the nursing process itself. • The task is appropriate for the patient. • The nursing assistant is permitted to perform the procedure in the facility. • The assistant has been taught to perform the procedure correctly. • A nurse has verified that the assistant can safely carry out the task without supervision. • If asked, the assistant can demonstrate the procedure.
Right Circumstances	The nursing assistant understands the purpose of the procedure, can perform it safely, and has the correct supplies or equipment to perform it properly.	• The nurse matches the complexity of the procedure with the nursing assistant's ability and the amount of supervision available. • The nurse believes that the nursing assistant can perform the task with the supervision, equipment, and supplies available. • The nursing assistant clearly knows the lines of authority and reporting.
Right Person	There are actually three rights associated with the "Right Person" rule: The *right person* delegates the right task to the *right nursing assistant*, to be performed on the *right patient*.	• The patient does not need frequent nursing assessments during the procedure. • The nurse believes the patient's response to the procedure is predictable. • The nurse believes that the nursing assistant will obtain the same or similar results as a nurse in carrying out the task.

Right Direction and Communication	The nurse gives the nursing assistant accurate and complete instructions, has clearly described the procedure, and has identified the limits (if any), and expected outcome(s). Always ask for instructions or clarification if you do not understand an assignment.	• The nurse must communicate the delegation decision in a culturally competent, individualized manner to the patient and nursing assistant. The level of detail and method of communication (oral and/or written) vary with the circumstances.
		• Communication should be clear, concise, correct, and complete.
		• Communication is a two-way process. The nursing assistant should have the opportunity to ask questions and/or to get clarification of expectations.
		• Situation-specific communication includes:
		  • Specific data to be collected and method and timelines for reporting
		  • Specific activities to be performed and patient-specific requirements, instructions, and limitations, if any
		  • The expected results of the activity
		  • The potential complications of the activity
		  • When and what information is to be reported
		  • The nurse's willingness and availability to guide and support the nursing assistant
		  • Verification that the assistant understands and accepts the delegation
		• The nursing assistant notifies the nurse if they are inexperienced or uncomfortable with the activity.
		• The nursing assistant asks for additional training or supervision, if needed.
		• The nursing assistant affirms understanding of expectations.
		• The nurse and nursing assistant agree on a method of communication and plan of action for emergency situations.
		• The nursing assistant's documentation is timely, objective, and complete.

(continues)

TABLE 2-4 *(continued)*

Right Supervision	The nurse delegating the activity answers the nursing assistant's questions and is available to manage changes in the patient's condition. The nursing assistant reports completion of the task and the patient's response to the nurse who delegated the activity.	The nurse: • Monitors performance • Obtains and provides feedback • Assists and/or intervenes if necessary • Ensures proper documentation • Evaluates the complete delegation process • Evaluates the patient • Evaluates the nursing assistant's performance of the activity The nurse answers the following questions: • Was the patient's desired and/or expected outcome achieved? • Was the outcome optimal, satisfactory, or unsatisfactory? • Was communication timely and effective? • What went well; what was challenging? • Were there any problems or concerns? If so, how were they addressed? • Is there a better way to meet the patient's need? • Was the delegation successful?

unsafe for the patient. Report your observations about the patient's condition, and be prepared to explain why you are uncomfortable with the task. Ask for help, if necessary.

You may refuse the delegation if:

- You believe that a procedure is not within your scope of practice.
- You have not been taught to do the task.
- You believe that the activity will harm the patient.

If you are unsure how to carry out a procedure, do not understand the instructions, or do not have the proper supplies, inform the nurse. Do not feel embarrassed. It is better to ask for help than to make an error and injure a patient. When your concerns have been addressed, you must perform the task. Do not refuse because you do not have time, or because the activity is unpleasant. Good communication is the key to successful delegation and patient safety. Be honest, tactful, and sensitive. If honest communication is ineffective, you can use the chain of command to address the problem with the next person in line. If you are assigned to a task, your supervisor depends on you to do it. Never ignore an assignment.

COMMUNICATION

Many names are used for the transfer of information from one worker to another in a health care facility. The titles for exchanging information include:

- Report
- Shift report
- Handoff
- Handoff report
- Handover
- Transfer of information
- Transfer of care

Information is provided about people you will be caring for. Impromptu reporting is also done for new admissions and patient changes in condition. A facility functions efficiently and care is best when information moves back and forth between caregivers and their managers frequently.

ASSESSMENT

A nursing **assessment** is a complete nursing evaluation of the patient, followed by an analysis and synthesis of the information. By law, the only member of the nursing team that can assess patients is the RN. This activity cannot be delegated. However, it is within the scope of nursing assistant practice to collect data for the assessment, such as blood glucose, intake and output, vital signs, height, and weight. Making observations and reporting them to the nurse is also a way of contributing to the assessment. The nurse uses all the data to identify the big picture and then makes a care plan that guides nursing care. The assignment will change as the patient's condition changes.

Your Workday: Managing an Assignment

Your workday will begin with communication, in the form of a **shift report**. Listen carefully to the report because it will help you plan your **assignment** (Figure 2-15). Oral reports are commonly used for routine reporting. Although facilities have different methods of reporting, as a rule the nurse who worked the previous shift will report

Patient Hernandez, Eric	Room 1264	Date June 11, 20___

DIAGNOSES, SPECIAL CARE, NOTES   CHF, COPD, IDDM, UTI

SAFETY   Fall Risk   Siderails Up   Bed Alarm   Chair Alarm   Low Bed
Wheelchair   Seatbelt   Front   Rear   Unable to Use Call Light

Comments:

TRANSFERS   Independent   Supervision   Limited   Extensive   Total Assists   One   Two
Manual Lift   Mechanical Lift   Hoyer Lift   Stand-up Lift   Pivot   Cane   Walker   Siderails

Comments:

AMBULATION/ LOCOMOTION   Independent   Supervision   Limited   Extensive   Total Assists   One   Two
Weight Bearing   Full   Partial   None   Ambulatory   Nonambulatory
Propels Own Wheelchair   Walker   Cane   Splint   Brace Prosthesis

Comments:

BED MOBILITY   Independent   Supervision   Limited   Extensive   Total Assists   One   Two
Turning Schedule   Siderails   Trapeze

Comments:

TOILETING   Independent   Supervision   Limited   Extensive   Total Assists   One   Two   Continent
Incontinent   Catheter Intake and Output   Bedside Commode   Urinal   Bedpan   Attends   Pads

Comments:

BATHING   Independent   Supervision   Limited   Extensive   Total Assists   One   Two
Tub   Shower Whirlpool   Bath Days_____   Shift_____

Comments:

DRESSING   Independent   Supervision   Limited   Extensive   Total Assists   One   Two
Laundry by   Facility   Family

Comments:

HYGIENE   Independent   Supervision   Limited   Extensive   Total Assists   One   Two
Dentures

Comments:

EATING   NPO Independent   Supervision   Limited   Extensive   Total Assists   One   Two
Diet   Regular   Chopped   Puree   Thickened Liquids   Assistive Devices

Comments:

FLUIDS   Push Fluids   Intake and Output
Fluid Restriction   Ice Chips   NPO

Comments:

RESTORATIVE   Range of Motion   Ambulation   Bed Mobility   Dressing   Hygiene   B&B

Comments:

SENSORY   Glasses   Hearing Aid   Right   Left

Comments:

COGNITIVE / BEHAVIOR   Short-Term Memory Problem   Impaired Decision Making
Confused   Occasionally Frequently   Always   Altered Sensory Perceptions

Comments:

FIGURE 2-15A The Nursing Assistant Care Sheet.

CNA ASSIGNMENT SHEET									Date	4-18-XX
Rm.	Patient	Bath	Pos. Sched.	ROM	V.S.	WT.	B+B	ADL Prog.	Transfer	Safety
101[A]	J. Damski	X	X	X			X	X	2+TB	X
101[B]	G. Jones		X	X	X	X			Mech Lift	
102[A]	C. Hernandez	X				X			Indep.	
102[B]	R. Lattini	X	X	X			X		2+TB	X
103	N. Goldberg	X			X	X	X		SBA	
104[A]	M. Welch		X	X					Mech Lift	
104[B]	L. Ordoni		X	X			X	X	1+TB	X
105	B. Brinzoski	X			X		X		Indep.	
106[A]	A. Feinstein	X				X		X	1+TB	
106[B]	D. Farmell		X	X	X		X	X	2+TB	
107	T. Green	X	X	X		X	X		2+TB	
108[A]	H. Johnson	X	X	X	X			X	2+TB	
108[B]	B. Miller		X	X		X			1+TB	X

FIGURE 2-15B The assignment sheet provides an overview of patient needs and activities.

to oncoming staff. In some facilities, the shift report is recorded. Your assignment tells you:

- Which patients you will care for
- The procedures you will need to do for these patients
- Changes in patients' conditions, if any
- Information about new patients
- Names of patients who were discharged or died
- Any incidents that occurred to patients
- New physicians' orders
- Special activities and events for patients that are scheduled during your shift

Each facility has a method for giving you the information needed to complete your assignment. It may be on the computer with your documentation files, or it may be printed on individual sheets of paper for each patient, or a single piece of paper listing the needs of all your patients.

Your supervising nurse will give you additional information, such as orders, care needs, appointments with other departments, and observations to make for specific patients. Chapter 8 gives additional information about reports.

In some facilities, Nursing Assistants may accompany patients to an appointment within or outside the facility. It's important to know your facility policy and procedure as well as your state's guidelines for scope of practice.

The CNA must know and understand the resident's physical and mental abilities before accompanying them to the appointment.

CRITICAL THINKING

A successful nursing assistant must apply critical thinking skills on the job. You will learn how to bathe and groom patients and make them comfortable, but your job involves much more than having excellent clinical skills. You can take direction from your facility procedure manual much of the time, but what will happen during the 1 percent of the time when the information is not in the manual or the information provided does not work? This is an especially important time when your critical thinking skills can be used to either cost a life or save a life.

Art and Science

Nursing is both an art and a science. Many of the things you do are a combination of both. As a nursing assistant, learning and applying **critical thinking** skills is an important responsibility that you will have as you work in a health care facility, provide excellent patient care, set priorities, and save lives. This involves using the nursing process and applying what you have learned in the classroom to real-life situations. First, you must identify the care wanted and/or needed by the patient. Then you must decide whether the care is appropriate and you are comfortable with the procedure. Next, you must analyze whether you are authorized to give this type of care. This includes evaluating the care needed, considering potential outcomes, conferencing with the nurse if necessary, and doing the procedure.

Applying the Nursing Process

What is different between the thinking of a nursing assistant and that of a TV reporter or office manager? It is primarily how you see the patient and the problems that you must deal with in your work. Thinking in this manner requires you to consider everything you have learned, including theories, concepts, and ideas that your instructors or other teachers have presented. The TV reporter wants a sensational story, and the office manager wants to make sure the chart is complete so the insurance company pays the bill. Of these, the nursing assistant is the only person who must use critical thinking to get the job done and ensure the patient benefits. Doing a quick mental content review is faster and easier if you have developed your skills to become very proficient in critical thinking. Nursing assistants who are proficient in critical thinking must be:

- Accurate
- Succinct
- Easy to understand
- Thorough and complete
- Consistent
- Analytical and logical
- Neutral
- Fair

Consider these attributes in all types of communication, including the spoken word; listening and interpreting a conversation; reading, writing, and role-play (acting); and demonstrating as needed for the patient. All these attributes must be true and accurate, regardless of who initiated the exchange. Protect and use these critical thinking skills and the nursing process. You will learn more about the nursing process in Chapter 8.

Focus on Outcomes

Focus on what you need to learn before, during, and after each lesson. Determine your personal ability to perform the skill. Identify the potential outcome and whether your action will accomplish the goal.

Your patient care experience may be limited at this point, but think about and apply critical thinking principles after each skills lab patient simulation, and each patient encounter in the clinical area. Think about opportunities to apply principles of critical thinking. For example, were you comfortably able to do everything the patient asked of you? Did you need to seek help with things you were not sure of? Ask someone else for feedback on your actions.

Completing an Assignment

Report the completion of your assignment and the patient's response to the nurse. You may be tempted to skip reporting if you will be documenting the activity. Reporting even simple tasks may be important.

ORGANIZING YOUR TIME

Successful time management is key to nursing assistant success. Time management skills cannot be mastered in the classroom. Your instructor will discuss ways of managing your time. Practice and use good organizational skills in the skills lab and clinical part of your class until good organization becomes automatic. Mastering good organization and time management skills helps you work more efficiently and reduces stress. Once mastered, organizational skills become a part of you, and you will not have to think about them. A bonus is that these skills are also very useful at home and in your personal life.

Time is something you borrow. Once used, it is gone forever. Each worker must manage their own time. However, good team players will help others who are behind. Each day begins with 86,400 seconds, 1,440 minutes, 24 hours. This equals 168 hours each week. If you work an 8-hour shift, you have:

- 28,800 seconds—480 minutes—in which to get your work done each day

If you work a 12-hour shift, you have:

- 43,200 seconds—600 minutes—in which to get your work done

Although your employer sets your working time, you must manage this time productively. Cutting corners, taking shortcuts, skipping breaks, and working longer hours are not good ways of managing time and may cause ethical and legal problems for you. At best, managing time in this manner is stressful. At worst, it is dangerous. You manage the time available. You must do this without working overtime. Never allow time to manage you. Practice *working smarter, not harder.*

Developing and Perfecting Time Management Skills

Lack of good organizational skills plagues health care workers at all levels. Avoid becoming so focused on "tasks" that you fail to see the big picture, which includes all of your work responsibilities, such as:

- Making patient observations as you circulate around the unit
- Checking patient needs and noticing if a patient's condition is changing, such as becoming sick or other issues
- Informing the nurse of patients' problems, complaints, and changes in condition

Making Rounds

If you do not manage your time, others will notice. The nurse may set a rigid schedule for you to ensure that your work gets done on time. This can be both difficult and stressful.

Making rounds is an important part of your time management strategy. Rounding saves you many trips up and down the hallway and provides a complete picture of patient needs. Checking on patients regularly will make them feel confident and secure. Setting priorities is a key to developing good time management skills. Avoid losing focus. Ensuring quality care and patient safety are high priorities.

GUIDELINES 2-1 Time Management and Organization

- Establish and develop a systematic daily routine for things.
  - Make rounds as soon as possible after report to identify patient needs and problems. Meet immediate needs during this round, such as assisting with toileting.
  - Develop your plan for each patient while making rounds.
- Practice good communication skills with patients and families while making rounds. Ask questions and obtain their input on your proposed plan.
  - Briefly visit with concerned family members. This may seem like a time waster, but it builds good relationships and may end up saving you time.
  - Families usually know the patient well. They may offer helpful and important information if you take time to listen.
  - Avoid becoming defensive if patients or family members complain (Figure 2-16). Report concerns, complaints, observations, and needs to the nurse. Listen to what patients have to say. Tell them what you will do about their concern, and give them a follow-up time if needed, such as, "I will come back to check on you in an hour." Thank them for sharing their concerns.
- Determine which patients need frequent monitoring.
  - *Monitoring* is simple oversight, such as looking in on or speaking with a patient, watching for new problems and changes in condition, and addressing known issues.
- Develop a personal plan for organizing your time by:
  - Planning and organizing your work. Be sure the plan is realistic.
  - Writing down your plan. Make a list every day. This step is important.

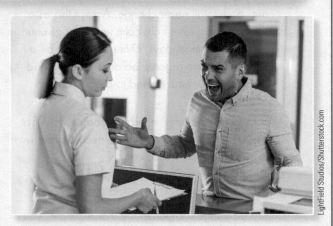

FIGURE 2-16 Monitor your body language and avoid becoming angry or defensive if a patient or family member complains.

  - Listing your main goals and deadlines for the day. Be sure they are realistic and achievable. This helps ensure that the most important priorities are done. Review each item on your list and ask yourself if it makes the best use of your time.
    - Complete your top priorities first.
    - Complete your next-level priorities as soon as your top priorities are done.
    - Breaks are important for reducing stress and preventing injury. Schedule your assigned break times into your plan. Avoid bringing work on your breaks. Do not spend your break time documenting at the computer.
- Be flexible. Expect the unexpected. Accept that you may have to change your plan if conditions and patient needs change.
- Accept that your priorities may change.
  - Identify "no options" activities that *must* be done during your shift, without exception.
  - Identify events that must be done by certain times, versus things you can do at any time.

(continues)

GUIDELINES 2-1 Time Management and Organization (continued)

- Ask yourself about the "what, where, when, why, who, and how" of your priorities; this will help you make a plan for completing them.
- Control the timing of events for which you are responsible.
- Emergencies, new admissions, and patient or family demands are imposed on you by others, and you cannot control them. This is part of health care, and it will never change. Accept this as a fact, and learn to remain calm when things change suddenly. On most days, changes will not be a burden if you do a good job of organizing and managing your time related to events you can control.
- Focus on the patients' *needs* instead of *tasks* that are to be done. Meeting patient needs is one way of giving patient-focused care.
- Avoid repetition. Do things right the first time so you don't have to redo them.
- Plan to do things simultaneously. For example, you must remain in the patient's room while they use the toilet and wash at the sink. Use the time productively! Provide privacy unless you must remain in the room with the patient. Make the bed or do another task instead of waiting impatiently.
- Set time limits when you have tasks to complete. Be realistic and reasonable.
  - Avoid becoming distracted. Focus on the task at hand.
  - Break activities down into small, manageable pieces, if possible.
- Evaluate your efficiency and time management skills regularly and work to improve them.

- Try to break your own record on time-consuming tasks. If a job takes 30 minutes today, try to get it done in 29 minutes tomorrow. Do this daily until you have streamlined the task as much as possible. One caveat, however: avoid cutting corners for the sake of saving time. The time you save is not worth the price you will pay for harming a patient or making a major error. If cutting corners is the only way you feel you can save time, try something else.
- Before beginning a task, organize what you will need.
  - Gather and organize your supplies in advance.
  - Bring everything you will need into the patient's room at once so you do not waste time and energy making trips up and down the hall to retrieve forgotten items.
- Communicate with peers, colleagues, and others throughout your shift. Good communication helps ensure success.
  - Be tactful and polite in all communications.
  - Treat others with dignity, respect, and integrity.
- Be assertive.
  - Help others when you can. Do not be afraid to ask for help when you need it. Other workers will be much more willing to help you if you are always available to help them when they need it. Negotiate a time that is convenient for both of you.
- Avoid wasting time; remain organized.
- Develop a plan of action if a patient's condition changes. Keep the nurse informed.
  - Take the blinders off! Continue to make important observations as you circulate around the unit. Help patients with immediate needs even if they are not part of your assignment.

HANDOFF COMMUNICATION

Handoff communication occurs when responsibility for a patient changes from one person to another. It is similar to your shift report, but the communication is about one patient. One worker communicates directly with the next person who will be caring for the patient (Figure 2-17). Transfer of care is a very vulnerable time for the patient and is one of the times when errors are most likely to occur. Handoffs are done at the desk in some facilities. In others, handoffs are part of walking rounds. Information in the handoff communication includes:

- The patient's situation and background
- Relevant observations and findings, especially changes and abnormalities
- Safety issues, high-risk conditions, and other concerns
- Recommendations and special orders or information for continuity of patient-focused care
- Scheduling issues
- Patient requests, wants, and needs

You will both give and receive handoff information. Be sure that your handoff communication is accurate, clear, and complete. Provide an opportunity to ask questions.

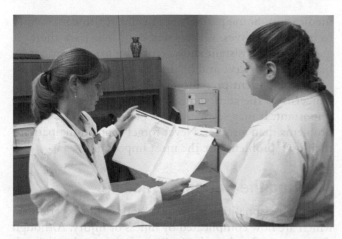

FIGURE 2-17 An accurate handoff is essential to patient well-being.

 Safety **ALERT**

Doing only tasks that you have been instructed to do in the way you were taught and avoiding shortcuts protects patients from injury. It also protects you from injury, legal exposure, and liability.

GUIDELINES FOR THE NURSING ASSISTANT

Only perform tasks that you have been taught to do. If you are unsure how to carry out a procedure, inform the nurse. Do not feel embarrassed. It is better to ask for help than to make an error and injure a patient.

Seeking Higher Authority

Sometimes your immediate supervisor may not act on a report you have made. This does not mean you are being ignored. The supervisor may have been busy and forgotten. They may not have taken your report seriously, but this is less likely. Make very sure of your facts and notify your supervisor again. Be tactful. This is a very sensitive issue. If you fail to get through and your information is very important, you can move up the chain of command. This situation should not occur often if there are good staff relations, but it can happen.

Personal Vocational Adjustments

You will have to make some personal adjustments to any new work situation. Obey facility rules and orders from supervisors even if you do not agree with them. Learn to accept and profit from constructive criticism. This shows

that you are willing to learn and grow. You show your maturity in many ways. You demonstrate:

- Dependability and accuracy by reporting for duty on time (Figure 2-18) and completing your assignments carefully
- Respect for your co-workers when you are ready and willing to help
- Understanding of human relationships by being empathetic, patient, and tactful with others

Interpersonal Relationships

Interpersonal relationships are interactions between people. You develop interpersonal relationships with everyone you know. Some relationships are deep and lasting, and some are only casual. But to some degree, you react to others and they react to you. Friendship is a good example of an interpersonal relationship that is satisfactory to two people.

Much of the satisfaction that a nursing assistant gets from work comes from the quality of the relationships that are developed with other staff members and patients. Good relationships with others begin with your own personality and attitudes. If you are polite, warm, accepting—and have a positive attitude—others will respond in the same way. If someone smiles at you, without thinking, your reaction is to smile back. Most human relationships are like this.

It is not necessary for you to like someone else personally in order to be pleasant and cooperative with them at work (Figure 2-19).

Attitude

Perhaps the single most important characteristic that you bring to your job is your **attitude**. Attitude is an outer reflection of your inner feelings. Body language is often a key to a person's attitude. Attitude develops throughout

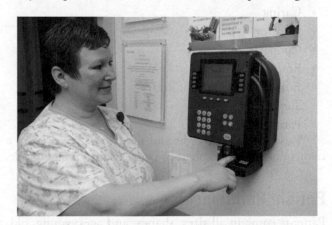

FIGURE 2-18 Reporting for work on time is a sign of responsibility and demonstrates dependability.

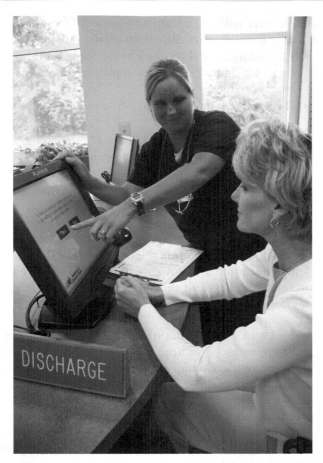

FIGURE 2-19 Smile, be pleasant, and cooperate with your co-workers. A positive attitude and spirit of cooperation are employee attributes that make the workplace pleasant.

your lifetime and is shaped by life experiences. Some people think having an "attitude" means being negative or opinionated, but all people show attitude through their behavior. Sometimes the attitude demonstrated is good and sometimes it is poor. Your attitude should reflect:

- Caring
- Courtesy
- Cooperation
- Emotional control
- **Empathy** (understanding)
- Tact
- Patience

Patients have the right and need to be cared for in a calm, unhurried atmosphere by people with a caring attitude.

Patient Relationships

Patients come in all sizes, shapes, and ages: young, old, and in between. Some have major, complicated illnesses. Others have problems that will improve with rest and

medication. Some patients are in the health care facility to begin their lives. Others will end their lives there. A good nursing assistant shows empathy for the patient by being eager to serve and by using a gentle touch.

Every patient presents a unique set of problems and concerns to the staff. These problems and concerns are important. It may seem as if one person has more serious problems than another. Never forget that, to the patient, their own problems are the most important.

Meeting the Patient's Needs

Patients' personalities are shaped by their life experiences, which are now complicated by illness or injury. Although they are confined to the facility, their social, spiritual, and physical needs must continue to be met. The restrictions imposed by illness may limit their ability to satisfy these needs through the normal channels. This is frustrating and can strain the patient's ability to establish and maintain good interpersonal relationships.

Some patients become irritable, complaining, and uncooperative because of:

- Fears about their diagnosis, disfigurement, disability, or death
- Pain
- Unrealistic perceptions of activities around them
- Uncertainties about the future
- Worries about family
- The loss or lack of social support systems
- Dependence on others
- Financial concerns
- Inability to tend to responsibilities due to illness and/or hospitalization

Offer emotional support, listen carefully, and report these concerns to the nurse.

Meeting the Family's Needs

Families and friends are extensions of the patient. They are usually very concerned when a loved one is in a health care facility, especially when that person is seriously ill or has a life-threatening illness. Sensitivity, awareness, patience, and tact are important at this time (Figure 2-20). This is a very stressful time, and they need to be reassured. Their anxiety may make them demanding and uncooperative.

Sometimes just quietly listening to a person or rephrasing your sentences can change an entire interaction. Try to be aware not only of the words used but also of the body language. As with words, clues such as the tone of a voice or a hand gesture reveal much about the inner feelings of other people. Always keep in mind that people are three-dimensional. They are physical, emotional, and social beings.

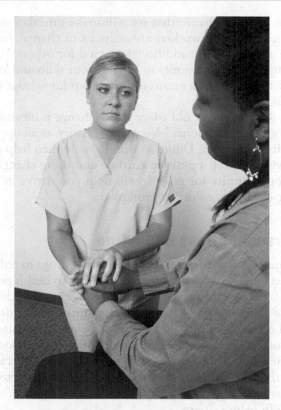

FIGURE 2-20 Concerned family members need a great deal of support and understanding.

Staff Relationships

All workers share a single goal: to help the patients. This single purpose unites the workers into a group that must work smoothly if your goal is to be accomplished. Keep your common goal in mind and recognize your co-workers as important members of the team. Good interpersonal relationships will make your working hours satisfying and productive. Good relationships can be formed if you:

- Remember that each person has a specific role to fulfill and jobs to carry out.
- Do not overstep your authority, criticize, or gossip about others.
- Listen to instructions carefully. Phrase questions about your assignment so it is clear that you are looking for clarification—not challenging authority.
- Promptly carry out orders and report if you feel you will be unable to finish your work.
- Offer help to others and accept help when you need it. Co-workers can often help one another when a task is particularly difficult or physically taxing (e.g., lifting a heavy patient or moving equipment). Simply being available when another member of the team gets behind in their work is a great help.

- Have a cheerful, positive attitude. This is as important for staff members' relationships as it is in establishing rapport (sympathetic understanding) with patients.
- Remember that your tone of voice and body language can change the message you are sending.
- Extend the same dignity and courtesy to every staff member that you would to patients.

PERSONAL HEALTH AND HYGIENE

You will be in close contact with others, so good personal grooming is essential. You should:

- Shower or bathe daily.
- Keep your hair clean and either short or tied back.
- Use an antiperspirant or deodorant. Antiperspirant prevents sweat and odor. Deodorant eliminates odor but does not prevent sweat.
- Keep your mouth and teeth clean.
- Avoid chewing gum on duty.
- Avoid odors caused by strong perfumes, aftershave lotions, and cigarettes that may be offensive to patients.

Reducing Stress

Your work as a nursing assistant is physically and emotionally demanding because you must give so much of yourself to those in your care. To stay healthy, prevent illness, relieve stress, and do your best, you should:

- Eat three well-balanced meals a day. Avoid crash diets and junk food.
- Avoid using alcohol, tobacco, and drugs.
- Avoid unhealthy habits such as smoking and chewing tobacco.
- Remain healthy and avoid alcohol and drugs. Each employer has a policy for drug testing. Keep your body healthy and clean.

🔓 Safety **ALERT**

Your hair is like a magnet for germs. Wash it regularly. Keeping long hair pulled back reduces the risk of injury from hair becoming entangled in equipment or being inadvertently pulled by a patient. This also reduces the risk that hairs will fall into patients' wounds or onto a sterile field when you are assisting with a procedure.

- Live in a clean environment.
- Get eight hours of sleep a night.
- Learn how to cope with stress and practice stress management.
- Find and practice satisfying leisure activities.
- Exercise regularly.
- See your doctor for regular checkups and other preventive health care and follow the doctor's advice.
- Make sure your immunizations (Chapter 12) are up to date.
- Practice testicular self-examination monthly if you are a man.
- Practice breast self-examination monthly and have mammograms as recommended by your physician if you are a woman.
- Use the safety practices you learned in class to avoid injury. You will find additional safety information in Chapters 14 and 30.

Burnout is total mental, emotional, and sometimes physical exhaustion. Burnout is common among those working in health care facilities. You can reduce the stress that leads to burnout by balancing your work with rest and recreation.

Some facilities offer employee assistance programs (EAP) to help employees reduce stress. Group discussions, exercise programs, and special counseling are available for general stress management and to meet special circumstances, such as personality conflicts or the death of a patient. Death is always a possibility, but the staff usually focus on improvement and recovery. The loss of a patient, especially a child, can be very stressful. Caring for an abused child can take a great toll on the staff as they try to work with the child and family.

Change

Change is a constant in health care. Many people resist change because the results are unknown. Venturing into the unknown can be both threatening and challenging. Change increases the risk of exposing our shortfalls and unmasking our weaknesses. We risk failure with each change. Avoiding and resisting change are much easier

than taking a chance that we will make mistakes or be criticized. When workers are resistant to change, negative attitudes cause additional turmoil for others. View change as an opportunity to expand your skills and learn new things and as a means of using your knowledge and skills.

Remember the old adage that "Change is inevitable, but growth is optional." View each change as an opportunity for growth. Doing so will do more than help you survive. Having a positive attitude and using change as an opportunity for growth will help you thrive in the ever-changing health care workplace.

Personal Stress Reduction

Some people use food, alcohol, or other drugs to reduce stress, but these substances can cause serious health problems. For example, some people use drugs or other chemicals to reduce stress. This is dangerous because drugs and other chemicals alter the body's chemistry, causing serious changes to thought, judgment, and behavior. In some cases, drug use becomes addictive and can cause death. You can learn healthful and effective personal stress-reducing techniques.

To reduce stress:

- Talk to your supervisor; a team conference may help.
- Try sitting for a few moments with your feet up.
- Shut your eyes and take some deep breaths.
- With your eyes shut, picture a special place you like and, in your mind, take yourself there.
- Take a warm, relaxing bath.
- Listen to some quiet music.
- Carry out a specific relaxation exercise.
- Make yourself a cup of herbal tea and drink it slowly.
- Exercise.
- Devote time to hobbies such as sewing, painting, woodworking, or playing a musical instrument.
- Go for a walk.
- Take advantage of available stress reduction programs.

REVIEW

A. True/False

Mark the following true or false by circling T or F.

1. T F The registered nurse plans and directs the nursing care of patients.

2. T F Interdisciplinary health care providers work as a team.

3. T F The LPN has completed a four-year college-based nursing program.

4. T F The nursing assistant gives physical care and emotional support to patients under the direction of the licensed nurse.

5. T F The nursing assistant is an important member of the nursing team.

6. T F Patients appreciate primary nursing because it allows them to relate directly to one specific registered nurse.

7. T F Team nursing is no longer used for providing patient care.

8. T F Nursing assistants are expected to work independently.

9. T F The State Nurse Practice Act affects nursing assistant practice.

10. T F Nursing assistants should project a positive image.

11. T F Caring about people is a valuable asset for a nursing assistant.

12. T F Being well groomed is not important for the nursing assistant.

13. T F All patients appreciate strong smells from after shave lotion and perfume.

14. T F Fingernails should be kept short and clean.

15. T F It is acceptable to wear your uniform to the grocery store after work.

16. T F How you look reflects the pride you feel in yourself.

17. T F Patient safety and comfort are main concerns for all caregivers.

18. T F Being a nursing assistant can be very stressful.

19. T F Smoking and eating are the best ways to reduce stress.

20. T F Evidence-based practice is used to guide decision making.

21. T F Professionalism is a learned quality.

22. T F Each member contributes to the patient care team.

23. T F Focus on tasks that must be done instead of patients' needs.

24. T F There is a high risk of incidents during transitions.

B. Multiple Choice

Select the best answer for each of the following.

25. Scope of practice refers to:
    a. things you are legally permitted to do.
    b. scheduling and staffing issues.
    c. activities of daily living.
    d. willingness to help others learn new tasks.

26. The nursing care approach that is task oriented is:
    a. primary nursing.
    b. functional nursing.
    c. team nursing.
    d. patient-focused care.

27. A nursing assistant who has a question regarding an assignment should ask the:
    a. physician.
    b. nurse.
    c. supervisor.
    d. administrator.

28. A patient tells you that they have difficulty making a fist because their hand feels weak. They did not mention this fact to the nurse. You must:
    a. advise them to tell the nurse.
    b. inform the nurse at the end of your shift.
    c. tell the nurse promptly.
    d. notify the physician.

29. Behavior in your nursing assistant class is the foundation on which to build:
    a. good grammar.
    b. pleasant manners.
    c. professional qualities.
    d. advanced skills.

30. The shift report is given by the:
    a. administrator.
    b. physician.
    c. nurse who worked the previous shift.
    d. director of nursing.

31. The purpose of the shift report is to:
  a. give information about all the patients on the nursing unit.
  b. discuss the social activities of the staff.
  c. tell the nursing assistants when they are scheduled for days off.
  d. rest before starting work.

32. Evidence-based practice:
  a. relies on tradition and rules of thumb.
  b. is used only when writing the care plan.
  c. ensures that everyone is treated the same.
  d. guides decision making based on evidence.

33. Palliative care:
  a. is very aggressive.
  b. hastens death.
  c. improves behavior.
  d. provides comfort.

34. The organizational chart:
  a. guides communication and identifies the line of authority.
  b. applies only to facility management.
  c. illustrates how evidence-based practice is used.
  d. is a tool used by the quality assurance department.

35. When a task has been delegated to a nursing assistant:
  a. they can perform the task if they have time.
  b. they can ask another assistant to perform the task.
  c. the nurse believes the complexity of the task is within their ability.
  d. the nurse believes they can perform the task without supervision.

36. The nursing assistant can refuse the delegation if:
  a. they do not want to do the task.
  b. they do not have time to do the task.
  c. the patient is confused and may be uncooperative.
  d. they do not know how to perform the task.

37. Your workday will begin and end with:
  a. making rounds.
  b. communication.
  c. an assessment.
  d. documentation.

38. An important part of time management is:
  a. documentation.
  b. making rounds.
  c. getting activities of daily living done early.
  d. meeting the patient's needs.

39. Empathy is:
  a. tact.
  b. patience.
  c. understanding.
  d. cooperation.

40. You must report to the nurse before you:
  a. prepare to take vital signs.
  b. complete each patient's care.
  c. begin your documentation.
  d. leave the unit for any reason.

41. Critical thinking has all of these attributes *except*:
  a. accurate.
  b. complete.
  c. inconsistent.
  d. understandable.

42. A fair critical thinking report is:
  a. judgmental.
  b. opinionated.
  c. incomplete.
  d. neutral.

43. You have been assigned to perform a procedure. Apply critical thinking to determine which of the following actions to take.
  a. Think about the procedure and consider whether it is appropriate.
  b. Ask another nursing assistant to do the procedure for you.
  c. Ask the nurse how to do the procedure because you have never done it.
  d. See if you can find the procedure in a procedure manual and print it.

C. Matching

Match the interdisciplinary team member and their function.

44. _____ Licensed to fill prescriptions for medications

45. _____ Qualified to test hearing

46. _____ Provides services to meet spiritual needs

47. _____   Licensed to fit and design braces and splints for extremities

48. _____   Licensed to provide rehabilitative services and to evaluate and treat persons with physical injury or illness, psychosocial problems, or developmental disabilities

  a. Orthotist

  b. Pharmacist

  c. Chaplain

  d. Occupational therapist

  e. Audiologist

D. Completion

Complete the following.

49. Why is it improper for nursing assistants to take orders directly from the physician? _____
_____

50. The benefits of a nursing assistant certification are:

  a. _____

  b. _____

  c. _____

  d. _____

E. Nursing Assistant Challenge

Read each clinical situation and answer the questions.

51. Enrique is given his assignment and has questions.

  a. He must check his assignment with
_____.

  b. One of his responsibilities is to bathe patients. Is this appropriate? _____

  c. One of his tasks is to give medications. Is this appropriate? _____

52. Felicia once worked as a part-time caregiver to an elderly woman but was never certified as a nursing assistant. What can you tell her about the requirements?

  a. Is a competency evaluation program required?
_____

  b. How many opportunities are there to meet requirements? _____

  c. How much continuing education is required once certification is granted? _____

53. Peggy reported for duty wearing bracelets, long earrings, and pale pink nail polish. Her uniform was clean and crisp, but the hem was hanging down on one side. Her shoes were dirty. State ways in which her appearance can be improved.
_____
_____

54. Who is the most important member of the interdisciplinary team? Explain why. Who acts as an extension of this person? How does this person affect patient care? What responsibilities do you have related to these individuals?
_____
_____

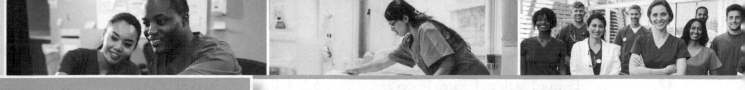

CHAPTER 3

Consumer Rights and Responsibilities in Health Care

OBJECTIVES

After completing this chapter, you will be able to:

3.1 Spell and define terms.

3.2 Explain the purpose of health care consumer rights.

3.3 Describe six items that are common to the Patient Care Partnership booklet, the Residents' Rights, and the Clients' Rights in Home Care documents.

3.4 List three specific rights from each of the three documents.

3.5 State the purpose of the Affordable Care Act and review the new Patient's Bill of Rights under that law.

3.6 Describe eight responsibilities of health care consumers.

3.7 List at least three responsibilities of the ombudsman.

VOCABULARY

Learn the meaning and the correct spelling of the following words and phrases:

advance directives	continuity of care	informed consent	Patient Care Partnership
Affordable Care Act (ACA)	grievance	ombudsman	Residents' Rights
Clients' Rights			

CONSUMER RIGHTS

All citizens in the United States have certain rights that are guaranteed by law (e.g., the right to vote). Health care consumers have rights to ensure that they will receive quality patient care. These rights are listed in a booklet called the **Patient Care Partnership**. There are different documents for patient rights, depending on where care is given. Facilities must have the rights booklet available in languages that are used in the community so that consumers can read and understand the document. The booklet is given to a close family member or other authorized person if the patient cannot read or understand the information. The person who is given the booklet must sign a paper acknowledging receipt of the rights document. Staff is expected to be familiar with and protect each person's rights.

A copy of the **Residents' Rights** is given to each person before they are admitted to a skilled care facility (Figure 3-1). The rights of residents in skilled care facilities were legislated by the federal government in the Omnibus Budget Reconciliation Act (OBRA) of 1987. Persons receiving care in their homes are given a copy of the **Clients' Rights**.

Each of these documents is similar and emphasizes the right of the patient, resident, or home care client to:

• Be treated with respect and dignity. This includes the rights to privacy and confidentiality.

• Have the benefit of open and honest communication with caregivers.

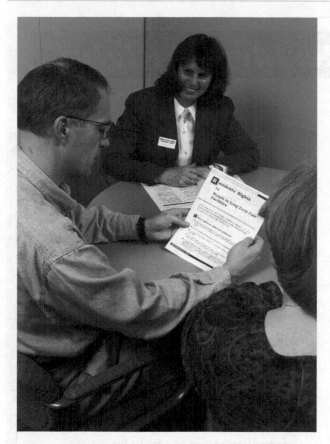

FIGURE 3-1 The Resident's Bill of Rights is presented to each resident (or the resident's legally responsible party) upon admission to a long-term care facility.

- Make health care decisions and participate in care planning. **Informed consent** means that the person gives permission for care after full disclosure of the purpose of the procedure, the benefits, and risks involved (Figure 3-2).
- Be advised of their rights about **advance directives** (documents that describe the consumer's wishes for treatment and end-of-life care if the person is unable to communicate or make health care decisions; see Chapter 32).
- Receive **continuity of care**. This core element of care means that health care is provided on a continuing basis from admission to discharge and beyond. A care plan is used to ensure that all caregivers understand their responsibilities to the patient.
- Be informed of resources for resolving conflicts or grievances. A **grievance** is a situation in which the consumer feels there are grounds for complaint.

Each rights document is reproduced in this chapter (Figures 3-3, 3-4, 3-5, and 3-6).

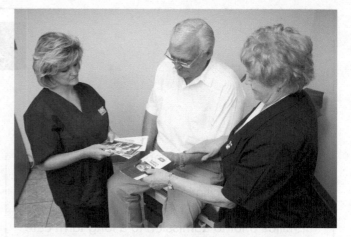

FIGURE 3-2 The nurse reviews information with a patient and spouse and provides an opportunity for asking questions. The nurse may also provide written instructions and information for later review.

PATIENT CARE PARTNERSHIP

"A Patient's Bill of Rights" was introduced by the American Hospital Association in 1972. After undergoing several revisions, it was renamed The Patient Care Partnership in 2003. The Patient Care Partnership booklet is given to patients at the time of hospital admission. Its contents summarize what the person should expect during the hospital stay. It also describes the patient's legal rights and responsibilities. It is available in many different languages.

Over time, many other bills of rights have been developed. Each focuses on a specific type of care. For example:

- EMS Patient's Bill of Rights
- Hospice Patient's Bill of Rights
- Indian Patient's Bill of Rights
- Mental Health Bill of Rights
- Pain Management Bill of Rights
- Pharmacy Bill of Rights
- Pregnant Patient's Bill of Rights
- Veterans Administration Code of Patient Concern

Some states have their own bills of rights for patients. Some insurance plans provide lists of rights for their subscribers. Become familiar with the rights guaranteed in your state and facility.

THE AFFORDABLE CARE ACT PATIENT'S BILL OF RIGHTS

The **Affordable Care Act (ACA)** (see Chapter 1) gives consumers control over their own health care. A new Patient's Bill of Rights developed under that law (Figure 3-6) provides the ability to make informed choices.

Residents' Rights

This is an abbreviated version of the Residents' Rights as set forth in the Omnibus Budget Reconciliation Act. This document must be given to all residents and/or their families prior to admission to a long-term care facility.

1. The resident has the right to free choice, including the right to:
   - choose an attending physician
   - full advance information about changes in care or treatment
   - participate in the assessment and care planning process
   - self-administer medications if the resident is able to safely do so
   - consent to participate in experimental research

2. The resident has the right to freedom from abuse and restraints, including freedom from:
   - physical, sexual, mental abuse
   - corporal punishment (the use of physical force) and involuntary seclusion (isolating a resident without a medical reason)
   - physical and chemical restraints

3. The resident has the right to privacy, including privacy for:
   - treatment and nursing care
   - receiving/sending mail
   - telephone calls
   - visitors

4. The resident has the right to confidentiality of personal and clinical records.

5. The resident has the right to accommodation of needs, including:
   - choices about life
   - receiving assistance in maintaining independence

6. The resident has the right to voice grievances.

7. The resident has the right to organize and participate in family and resident groups.

8. The resident has the right to participate in social, religious, and community activities, including the right to:
   - vote
   - keep religious items in the room
   - attend religious services

9. The resident has the right to examine survey results and correction plans.

10. The resident has the right to manage personal funds.

11. The resident has the right to information about eligibility for Medicare/Medicaid funds.

12. The resident has the right to file complaints about abuse, neglect, or misappropriation of property.

13. The resident has the right to information about advocacy groups.

14. The resident has the right to immediate and unlimited access to family or relatives.

15. The resident has the right to share a room with the spouse if they are both residents in the same facility.

16. The resident has the right to perform or not perform work for the facility if it is medically appropriate for the resident to work.

17. The resident has the right to remain in the facility except in certain circumstances.

18. The resident has the right to use personal possessions.

19. The resident has the right to notification of change in condition.

FIGURE 3-3 The Residents' Bill of Rights.

Clients' Rights in Home Care

The persons receiving home health care services or their families possess basic rights and responsibilities. As the client, you have:

The right to:

1. be treated with dignity, consideration, and respect
2. have your property treated with respect
3. receive a timely response from the agency to requests for service
4. be fully informed on admission of the care and treatment that will be provided, how much it will cost, and how payment will be handled
5. know in advance if you will be responsible for any payment
6. be informed in advance of any changes in your care
7. receive care from professionally trained personnel, and to know their names and responsibilities
8. participate in planning care
9. refuse treatment and be told the consequences of your action
10. expect confidentiality of all information
11. be informed of anticipated termination of service
12. be referred elsewhere if you are denied services solely based on your inability to pay
13. know how to make a complaint or recommend a change in agency policies and services

The responsibility to:

1. remain under a doctor's care while receiving services
2. provide the agency with a complete health history
3. provide the agency all requested insurance and financial information
4. sign the required consents and releases for insurance billing
5. participate in your care by asking questions, expressing concerns, and stating if you do not understand
6. provide a safe home environment in which care can be given
7. cooperate with your doctor, the staff, and other caregivers
8. accept responsibility for any refusal of treatment
9. abide by agency policies that restrict the duties our staff may perform
10. advise agency administration of any dissatisfaction or problems with your care

FIGURE 3-4 Home health care Clients' Bill of Rights.

Patients have the right to:

- Quality care
- Know who is caring for them
- Know if the caregivers are students
- Be informed of errors, significant events, and abuse or neglect
- Be notified of changes in care
- Be informed of their medical condition and given information about suitable treatment choices. Examples of this information include benefits and risks, whether the treatment is experimental or part of a research study, what to expect, and the financial impact of services and providers that are not covered by the insurer.
- Refuse treatment. However, they must be informed of the consequences of the refusal in a language and manner they understand.
- Consideration of their health care goals, values, and spiritual beliefs that are important to their well-being
- Make an advance directive and understand who will make medical decisions when the person cannot
- Privacy and confidentiality in care and documentation
- Information regarding how to manage care after hospital discharge
- Referral to community services and coordination of resources needed after discharge
- Billing and claims services through the hospital billing department
- More detailed notices and information when appropriate

Modified from Patient Care Partnership: Understanding Expectations, Rights and Responsibilities.

FIGURE 3-5 Summary of the American Hospital Association Patient Care Partnership: *Understanding Expectations, Rights and Responsibilities.*

The Affordable Care Act Patient's Bill of Rights provisions include:

- The ability to use the Health Insurance Marketplace to secure health care coverage.
- Requires insurance companies to cover people with preexisting medical problems. Insurers cannot charge extra for existing medical problems.
- Insurers cannot charge more because of gender. They are permitted to charge different prices based on age, tobacco use, family size, and geography.
- Provides information and assistance to help people understand their health care coverage.
- Holds insurance companies accountable for rate increases. Requires insurance companies to publicly justify any unreasonable rate hikes.
- Requires insurance companies to spend premium dollars primarily on health care—not administrative costs.
- Makes it illegal for health insurance companies to cancel your health care insurance if you get sick.
- Protects your choice of doctors by allowing subscribers to choose their primary care doctor from the plan's network.
- Allows young adults under age 26 to remain on their parents' health insurance plan.
- Requires insurers to provide free preventive care.
- Prohibits insurers from setting yearly and lifetime dollar limits on coverage of essential health care services.
- Prohibits insurers from cancelling coverage if a subscriber makes an honest mistake on an application.
- Guarantees the right to appeal denials.

FIGURE 3-6 The Affordable Care Act guarantees each patient certain rights related to health insurance.

RESPONSIBILITIES OF HEALTH CARE CONSUMERS

Consumers also have certain responsibilities that they must fulfill, including:

- Maintaining personal health care records so information is available when needed.
- Providing medical records when needed.
- Communicating openly and honestly with the physician and other caregivers. They must provide information regarding past hospitalizations and medications, for example.
- Informing the physician and other caregivers if they cannot follow the prescribed treatment plan.
- Learning how to manage their own health (Figure 3-7).
- Living a healthy lifestyle and avoiding unnecessary risks of illness or injury.
- Asking questions if they do not understand information, instructions, or explanations.
- Accepting responsibility for payment for health care and providing information for insurance claims.

The rights of health care consumers have both a legal and an ethical basis. Legal and ethical aspects of care are discussed in Chapter 4.

ROLE OF THE OMBUDSMAN

An **ombudsman** is a person who advocates for patients and residents of health care facilities. The ombudsman is a government employee or a volunteer and is not on staff at

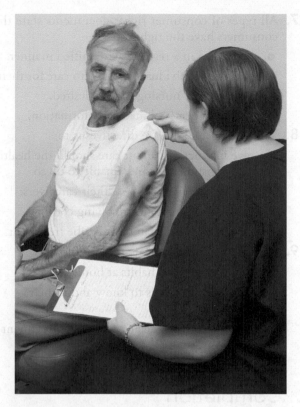

FIGURE 3-7 A teaching plan is developed by the nurse to help the patient manage personal health problems.

the facility. The ombudsman monitors facility conditions, assists with problems and complaints, and assists in finding quality care. Services are free of charge to the patients and residents. Facilities are required to post contact information for the ombudsman in a prominent location.

REVIEW

A. True/False

Mark the following true or false by circling T or F.

1. T F The rights of health care consumers are important only to patients in hospitals.
2. T F All U.S. citizens have certain rights that are guaranteed by law.
3. T F The Client's Bill of Rights is given to persons receiving home care.
4. T F The Patient's Bill of Rights has been in place since the 1970s.
5. T F Health care consumers in any setting have the right to prepare advance directives.

B. Multiple Choice

Select the best answer for each of the following.

6. The Residents' Rights document is given to persons before they are admitted to:
   a. home care.
   b. a skilled care facility.
   c. the hospital.
   d. hospice services.

7. All types of consumer rights documents state that consumers have the right to:

    a. be treated in a respectful, dignified manner.

    b. select the individuals assigned to care for them.

    c. private-duty nursing care, if desired.

    d. withhold personal medical information.

8. The purpose of advance directives is to:

    a. give instructions about care should the health care consumer become unable to do so.

    b. enable patients to choose their caregivers.

    c. provide a resource for resolving conflicts.

    d. permit the physician to prescribe treatment.

9. Health care consumers are responsible for:

    a. leaving their bad habits at home.

    b. learning all there is to know about their conditions.

    c. allowing the physician to make all treatment decisions.

    d. communicating openly and honestly.

C. Completion

Choose the correct word from the following list to complete each statement in questions 10–15.

advance directive	continuity of care
grievance	informed consent
privacy	respect

10. _____ means that the consumer gives permission for care or procedures after full disclosure.

11. A _____ exists when the consumer feels there are grounds for complaint.

12. A document that gives instructions about the consumer's wishes for treatment if the consumer is unable to communicate is called a(n) _____.

13. _____ is a core element of care, meaning that care is provided on a continuing basis.

14. By not opening and reading the consumer's mail, you are respecting the consumer's right to _____.

15. All health care consumers have the right to be treated with _____.

D. Check Your Knowledge

Identify benefits of the Affordable Care Act Patient's Bill of Rights by marking the following true or false by writing T or F on the line.

16. _____ Requires subscribers to see the primary care doctor assigned by the plan's network.

17. _____ Allows insurers to cancel coverage if a subscriber accidentally makes a mistake on an application.

18. _____ Allows parents to keep young adult children under age 26 covered under the parents' health plan.

19. _____ Prohibits insurers from placing lifetime limits on most benefits.

20. _____ Allows insurers to refuse coverage to adults with preexisting chronic conditions.

21. _____ Prohibits insurers from excluding children under age 19 with a health condition.

22. _____ Allows insurance companies to increase their rates at will.

23. _____ Requires insurance companies to spend premium dollars primarily on health care, not administrative costs.

E. Nursing Assistant Challenge

Mr. Delmonico was admitted to General Hospital for surgery to repair a fractured hip. After a few days in the hospital, he will be transferred to Memorial Nursing Center, a skilled care facility, for additional rehabilitation. After discharge from Memorial, it is expected that he will need home care for four to six weeks. Briefly explain how the different rights of each document will affect Mr. Delmonico's care.

24. Consider Mr. Delmonico's diagnosis and the services he will need for recovery. Which aspects of the Patient's Care Partnership booklet pertain to his hospital care?

25. Discuss the statements in the Residents' Rights document that pertain specifically to rehabilitation and independence.

26. For which items in the Clients' Rights document is the nursing assistant responsible?

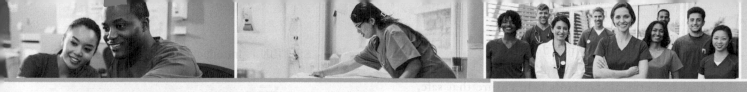

Ethical and Legal Issues Affecting the Nursing Assistant

CHAPTER 4

OBJECTIVES

After completing this chapter, you will be able to:

4.1 Spell and define terms.

4.2 Discuss ethical and legal situations in health care.

4.3 Describe the legal and ethical responsibilities of the nursing assistant.

4.4 Describe how to protect the patients' right to privacy.

4.5 Define abuse and give examples.

4.6 Define neglect and give examples.

4.7 Define sexual harassment and give examples.

4.8 Identify professional boundaries in relationships with patients and families.

4.9 Explain why working in a virtual world affects patient boundaries.

4.10 Give examples of boundary violations using the Internet and wireless media.

4.11 State the purpose of the HIPAA laws.

4.12 Explain why most facilities prohibit employees from posting work-related information on social networking sites.

VOCABULARY

Learn the meaning and the correct spelling of the following words and phrases:

abuse	Health Insurance Portability	need to know	relationship danger zone
aiding and abetting	and Accountability Act	neglect	sexual abuse
assault	(HIPAA)	negligence	sexual harassment
battery	informed consent	OBRA	slander
boundaries	invasion of privacy	physical abuse	social networking sites
coercion	involuntary seclusion	Platinum Rule	termination
confidential	legal standards	professional boundaries	theft
defamation	liable	protected health information	verbal abuse
ethical standards	libel	(PHI)	zone of helpfulness
euthanasia	malpractice	psychological abuse	
false imprisonment			

LEGAL AND ETHICAL STANDARDS

You must make decisions about your actions at work each day. Some of these involve being morally right or wrong. Others involve the legality of your behavior.

Two sets of rules help govern the moral and legal actions you will take:

• **Ethical standards** are guides to moral behavior. People who give health care agree to adhere to these standards. These rules must be followed in order to give safe, correct care.

• **Legal standards** are guides to lawful behavior. Workers who break the law may be prosecuted and found **liable** (held responsible) for injury or damage. This can result in the loss of nursing assistant certification, payment of fines, and/or imprisonment.

Legal and ethical standards help ensure that safe, quality care is given. Following them also protects the caregiver. Sometimes the rules that govern legal and moral actions cover the same issues.

ETHICS QUESTIONS

As a nursing assistant, you will take directions from the legal and ethical guidelines established by your facility. Ethical problems that health care providers must resolve include:

- When is life gone from a person on a life support system?

- When does life actually begin?

- Is assisting a patient before, during, or after an abortion right or wrong?

- Can a health care worker refuse to assist with a procedure for religious or moral reasons?

- Is **euthanasia** (assisted death) ever justified?

- Should food and water be withheld to speed death when the patient has expressed the desire to die?

- What should be done if an alert patient refuses to eat or drink for several days?

- Should a pregnant woman be removed from life support?

- Who makes decisions about removing life support systems when there is conflict between the facility ethics committee and a person's family?

- Can a person on dialysis stop at will, knowing that death will occur in a brief period of time?

- Can an alert person on a ventilator force the hospital to remove the ventilator, allowing them to die?

- How is the choice made when two or more people could benefit from an organ transplant but only one organ is available?

- Should marijuana be used for medicinal purposes?

- Should embryonic stem cells be used to cure serious and chronic diseases (Figure 4-1)?

- Should a person's DNA be tested for the presence of chronic illness or disease? If so, who should be permitted to see the results of the test?

- Should parents of a chronically ill child have another baby to use as a bone marrow donor for the child with chronic illness?

Most facilities have ethics committees (Figure 4-2) that advise the staff on ethical matters. Committee members include staff, clergy, interested community members, and advocates for the sick and elderly. The committee reviews the ethical problems and principles involved to help guide decision making. Sometimes the

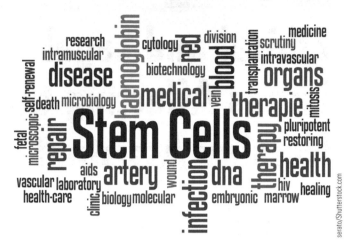

FIGURE 4-1 Stem cells have many uses in the treatment of infections and diseases.

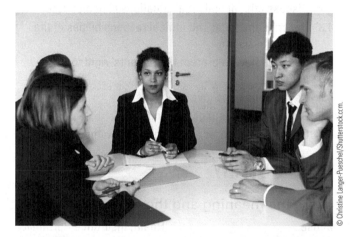

FIGURE 4-2 The ethics committee discusses complex patient situations and at times makes difficult decisions.

committee must handle difficult situations in which no single "right" decision is possible.

The ethics committee is responsible for resolving disputes in which one or both opposing parties may be unhappy with the decision. As you can see, these committees carry great responsibility, making their members' jobs difficult, sensitive, and very important to the operation of the facility. Respect for patients and their wishes is the primary concern. Part of this respect is shown by having patients actively involved in decisions about their care and future. As a nursing assistant, you will take direction from the legal and ethical guidelines established by your facility.

Respect for Life

One of the most basic rules of ethics is that *life is precious*.

The promotion of health and quality of life are primary caregiving goals. When death is certain, the major responsibility of medicine and all team members is to maintain quality of life and make the dying person comfortable.

Respect for the Individual

Respect for each patient as a unique individual is another ethical principle.

This uniqueness is demonstrated by differences in:

- Age
- Race
- Religion
- Gender
- Sexual preference
- Culture
- Attitudes
- Background
- Response to illness

If you respect each patient as a valuable person, you can learn to accept and work with each one in the best possible way.

You probably learned the Golden Rule—"Do unto others as you would have them do unto you"—when you were a child. An alternative to the Golden Rule is the **Platinum Rule**: "Treat others the way they want to be treated" (Figure 4-3). The Platinum Rule shifts the focus from treating everyone alike to providing individualized, patient-focused care. Find out what patients want and give it to them, as much as possible, in keeping with their plans of care.

Use both principles to guide your practice. There will be times when personal comfort and convenience could interfere with the care you give. By placing patients' interests ahead of your own, you are fulfilling the ethical and legal obligations of your practice, protecting patient safety, enhancing patient comfort and satisfaction with care, and reducing your personal risk of legal exposure. To provide proper care, you also have the ethical responsibility to maintain competence in your practice (Figure 4-4).

Patient Information

The ethical code asserts that *information about patients is privileged and must not be shared with others*. To observe this ethical rule:

1. Discuss patient information only in appropriate places.
   a. Avoid discussing a patient's condition while in the patient's room, even if the patient is unresponsive. The patient may be able to hear everything that is said, causing unnecessary worry.

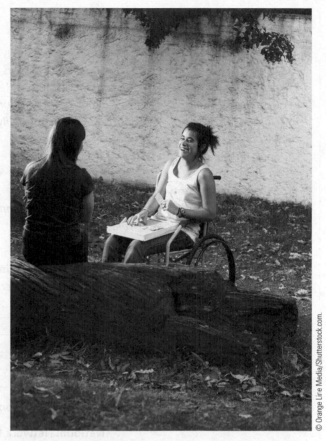

© Orange Lire Media/Shutterstock.com.

FIGURE 4-3 People with disabilities are often bullied. This young woman is treating her friend as an equal despite her disability.

   b. Never discuss patients during breaks, or in public areas of the facility.
2. Discuss information only with the proper people.
   a. You might be asked for information by other patients, family members, or members of the public, such as news reporters and others. Discuss patients only with persons who have a legal right to know (Figure 4-5).
   b. Even when it is appropriate to share information, provide information only about issues within your scope of practice, such as the patient's appetite or how well the patient slept.
   c. Never discuss patients with your family, friends, or others in the community.
   d. Discuss patients and their personal concerns only with your supervisor during conference or report, in a private area.
   e. Learn to evade inquiries tactfully by:
      • Stating that you do not know all the details of the treatment or the patient's condition.
      • Firmly, but politely, indicating that you do not have the authority to provide the answers and directing the inquirer to the proper person.

As a Career Nursing Assistant I Pledge to

1. Provide a high quality of care to the people in my care
2. Apply high moral and ethical values to daily tasks of care
3. Apply myself to the task at hand and attend to Residents' Rights and safety for the people in my care
4. Be an effective team member, support and encourage new NAs and my peers
5. Demonstrate good work habits and carry out daily tasks of care in a conscientious manner
6. Display a kind sense of humor
7. Seek out new information and training that will enable me to provide quality care to each individual person in my care
8. Help others to grow in positive ways
9. Take the initiative to serve on care-planning committees, safety committee, local, state and national nursing assistant organizations or related groups
10. Foster my own career growth

As a Career Nursing Assistant, I will work in the best interest of the people in my care, my peers, my supervisors, my employer, my professional organization, my career, and myself by upholding these commitments.

Signature _____

Facility_____

Address_____

City_____ State_____ Zip_____

Phone_____ email_____

~ A professional organization for nursing assistants since 1977 ~:

National Network Career Nursing Assistants
3577 Easton Road, Norton, Ohio 44203-5661
PH (330) 825 9342. FAX (330) 825 9378
Web - www.cna-network.org

National Network of Career Nursing Assistants. www.cna-network.org

FIGURE 4-4 The Career Nursing Assistant's Pledge upholds the highest ethical standards. It recognizes your commitment to your profession and the patients you care for. Follow the Career Nursing Assistant's pledge at all times.

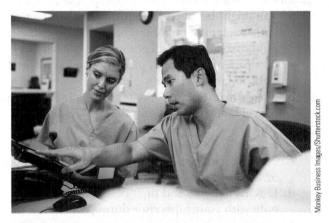

Monkey Business Images/Shutterstock.com

FIGURE 4-5 Patient information is disclosed only on a need-to-know basis.

3. Refer patient requests for personal medical information to the nurse or physician.
4. Never give information concerning the death of a patient to the patient's family. Respect patients'

personal religious beliefs (or absence of beliefs). You show your respect when you:

a. Inform the nurse if a patient requests a clergy visit.
b. Know and share correct information about the type of chaplain services available in your facility (Figure 4-6).
c. Know if a chapel is open for use by patients and families.
d. Respectfully treat patients' religious articles, such as a Bible, rosary, Koran, or holy pictures.
e. Avoid imposing your own religious beliefs on patients. Never argue with a patient whose beliefs differ from your own.
f. Assist patients to practice their religious beliefs and rituals, if requested. When a clergyperson visits, you should:
  • Be helpful and courteous.
  • Escort the clergyperson to the patient's bedside.
  • Draw the curtains or close the door for privacy.
  • Leave the room.

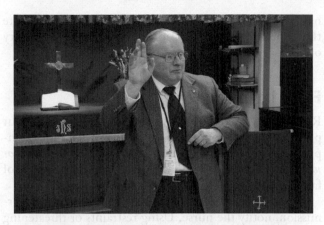

FIGURE 4-6 Respect patients' personal religious beliefs by providing correct information about the chaplain services and availability of a chapel in your facility.

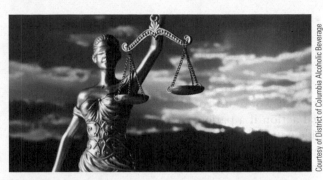

Courtesy of District of Columbia Alcoholic Beverage Control Board.

FIGURE 4-7 Lady Justice (Justicia) symbolizes that justice is fair and impartial, without favoritism or prejudice. The scales mean that both sides of a legal case must be carefully considered, similar to weighing them on a scale.

Tipping

If you follow the ethical code, the service you give will depend on need. It will *not* depend on the patient's race, creed, color, or ability to pay. There is no place for tipping within the health care system.

Patients are charged for the services they receive while in the health care facility. The salary you are paid is included in that charge. If a patient offers you money, firmly and courteously refuse.

LEGAL ISSUES

Laws are passed by governments and must be obeyed by citizens (Figure 4-7). Breaking the law may result in fines or imprisonment.

To avoid breaking the law, you should:

- Stay within your scope of practice (see Chapter 2). In this situation, the scope of practice is what a reasonable nursing assistant would do in a similar situation. Your job description, textbook, and facility policies and procedures are guides to the scope of nursing assistant practice. Your instructor is also an excellent source of information. You must comply with the law to remain out of trouble.

- Use good judgment. Policies and procedures are not the law. They are guiding principles that help staff work in a similar manner and approach situations consistently. However, they are never a substitute for using good judgment.

- Carry out procedures carefully and as you were taught.

- Keep your skills and knowledge up to date.

- Request guidance from the nurse before you take action in a questionable situation.

- Always keep the safety and well-being of the patient foremost in your mind, and act accordingly.

- Make sure you thoroughly understand directions for the care you are to give.

- Perform your job according to facility policies and **OBRA** guidelines.

- Attend inservices and obtain the required number of continuing education hours.

- Respect the patient's belongings (property).

Situations you must avoid are negligence, theft, defamation, false imprisonment, assault and battery, abuse, neglect, and invasion of privacy.

Negligence

Negligence is failure to exercise the degree of care that is reasonable in a particular situation. Negligence is also carelessness, which is often caused by rushing, taking shortcuts, or not focusing on the task at hand. It may be accidental or deliberate and result from either an action or an omission (failure to act). For example, not feeding a confused patient because they are a slow eater and you are short on time is negligence. However, forgetting to give a tray to a confused patient who feeds themselves is also negligent. Either way, the person is not given the expected level of care.

Reckless Behavior

Reckless behavior occurs when a worker knowingly and deliberately puts a patient at risk of injury. Workers who behave recklessly:

- Know the behavior is risky.
- Understand that the risk is great.
- Know that the behavior is not normal, and that other workers are not doing the same thing.
- Cannot justify placing the patient at risk, but does so anyway.

- Know that the supervisor, charge nurse, and peers would not approve of the behavior.
- Willfully ignore the risk(s) and act recklessly anyway.

Placing a patient at risk may result in disciplinary action at work and could result in criminal charges or legal action if a patient is injured. Let your conscience guide you and avoid risky behavior at all costs. Get help if you need it. A second worker is needed for safety in some situations.

Malpractice

Malpractice is improper, negligent, or unethical conduct that results in injury or loss to a patient. It often results from risky behavior. Staying within your scope of practice, following facility policies and procedures, and doing things in the way you were taught will help protect your patients from injury. Being discreet, respecting confidentiality, and avoiding gossip will help protect patients from hurt feelings and emotional harm. Be kind and polite. If a patient complains about something you have done, apologize and promptly correct the problem without becoming defensive.

You would be guilty of malpractice if you injured a patient by:

- Not performing your work as taught. For example, a patient is burned by an enema solution that you prepared that was too hot.
- Not carrying out your job in a conscientious manner. For example, the care plan states that Mr. Slotky transfers with the mechanical lift and two assistants. You fail to ask another worker to assist you with the transfer. The lift tips and the patient is injured.

Theft

Taking anything that does not belong to you is **theft**. The patient's and resident's rights documents refer to this action as the "misappropriation of property."

You are guilty of **aiding and abetting** if you see someone else committing a crime and do not report it.

People working in health care facilities must be honest and dependable. Despite careful screening, dishonest people are sometimes hired and things do disappear. These things range from washcloths, money, and patients' personal belongings to drugs and equipment.

Honesty and integrity are the hallmarks of the sincere and conscientious nursing assistant.

Defamation

Harming another person by making false statements is **defamation**. This is true whether you make the statement verbally (**slander**) or in writing (**libel**). For example, if you inaccurately tell a co-worker that a patient has AIDS, you have slandered that patient. If you write the same untrue information in a note, you are guilty of libel.

False Imprisonment

Restraining a person's movements or actions without proper authorization is **false imprisonment**. For example, patients have the right to leave the hospital *with or without* the physician's permission. You will be guilty of false imprisonment if you interfere.

If a patient plans to leave the facility without permission, notify the nurse. Using restraints or threatening to restrain the person is a form of false imprisonment. Restraints may be physical devices or chemical agents.

Sometimes it is necessary to support and restrain the movement of patients. Restraints cannot be used without a physician's order. The use of restraints is discussed further in Chapter 14.

Assault and Battery

Assault means intentionally attempting or threatening to touch another person's body without permission. **Battery** means actually touching a person without permission.

Care is always given with the patient's permission or **informed consent**. This means the patient knows and agrees to the plan before you begin. However, the patient may withdraw this consent at any time. For example, you are assigned to give a patient a warm foot soak. Despite your explanation of the reasons for the order, the patient refuses. You may not force the patient to comply. Doing so is battery. You commit assault if you threaten the patient by telling them that you will get others to hold them down if they refuse.

You can avoid legal pitfalls by:

- Informing the patient of what you plan to do
- Making sure the patient understands
- Giving the patient an opportunity to ask questions or refuse
- Reporting refusal of care to the nurse and documenting the facts
- Never forcing a patient to accept a treatment or procedure against their wishes

Coercion means forcing a person to do something against their wishes. Refusal of care creates a dilemma for the nursing assistant when the patient is mentally confused. When patients are confused, a family member or other responsible person consents to admission and treatment on the person's behalf. In this situation, we presume that the patient would agree to the care if they were mentally able to do so. The patient may refuse a procedure, such as a bath, but the legally responsible person has already consented to routine facility care, so you may bathe the patient. However, gaining the patient's cooperation and trust is always best. Return later and try again. Try to avoid forcing the person. Consult the nurse if you are in doubt about how to handle refusals of care.

Abuse

Abuse is any nonaccidental act or failure to act that causes (or could cause) harm or death to a patient. Abuse is always against the law and causes physical harm and/or mental anguish. Abuse can be verbal, sexual, physical, or mental. Involuntary seclusion is also a form of abuse.

Verbal abuse may be directed toward the patient or expressed about the patient. You are guilty of verbal abuse if you:

- Swear at a patient
- Raise your voice in anger at the patient
- Call the patient unpleasant, demeaning, or derogatory names
- Tease or embarrass the patient
- Use threatening or obscene gestures
- Make written threats or abusive statements
- Use inappropriate words to describe a person's race, religion, nationality, or lifestyle

Sexual abuse is inappropriate touching, forcing a person to perform sexual acts, or any behavior that is seductive, sexually demeaning, harassing, or reasonably interpreted as sexual by the patient. Examples of sexual abuse include:

- Tormenting or teasing a patient with sexual gestures or words
- Touching a patient in a sexual way
- Suggesting that a patient engage in sexual acts with you

Physical abuse is an intentional act that causes physical harm or pain to the patient. Examples include:

- Being rough with a patient (Figure 4-8)
- Hitting, slapping, pushing, kicking, or pinching the patient

Psychological abuse includes:

- Causing a patient to be afraid
- Threatening to withhold care or cause the patient harm
- Threatening to tell something to others that the patient does not want known
- Making fun of the patient (Figure 4-9). Calling the patient by names such as "pumpkin," "honey," "dear," and "grandma" is another way of belittling the patient
- Demeaning the patient by asking questions such as, "How did we sleep last night?" or "Have we moved our bowels yet?"
- Calling the attention of others to a patient's behavior

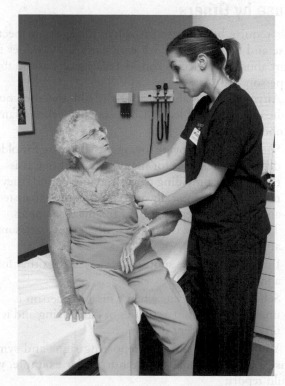

FIGURE 4-8 Being rough with a patient is one form of abuse.

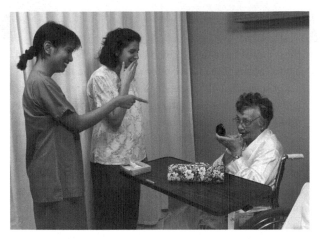

FIGURE 4-9 Making fun of a patient is psychological abuse.

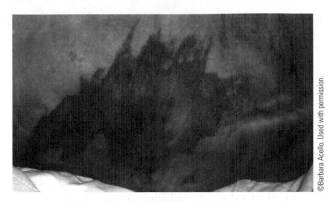

FIGURE 4-10 This patient's abuse occurred over a long period of time, but no one was aware of it because most of the bruises were hidden by clothing.

Involuntary seclusion is the separation of a patient from others against the person's will. Examples of involuntary seclusion are:

- Shutting the door to the patient's room when the patient wants the door open
- Leaving a patient without the signal cord or call bell

Separation is permitted when it is part of a care-plan approach to reduce agitation. The decision to use seclusion must be made by the nurse.

Abuse by Others

Laws require health care providers to report suspected abuse and neglect. A health care worker who does not report abuse or neglect is considered as guilty as the abusing person.

Anyone can be abused, but the old and the young are the most vulnerable. Usually, the caregiver or a family member is the abuser.

- Some families provide loving, capable care for older, dependent relatives for many years without assistance. After providing care for a long period, they may become physically and emotionally exhausted and may have depleted their financial resources. The risk of abuse is very high when these stressors are present.
- In some cases, one spouse has abused the other for a long time.
- Self-abuse may occur when a disabled person is unable to carry out activities of daily living and is unwilling to accept help.

You are responsible for reporting signs and symptoms of possible abuse to the nurse. For example, you should report:

- Statements by the patient suggesting that neglect or abuse may have occurred

- Unexplained bruises or injuries (Figure 4-10)
- Signs of neglect such as poor personal hygiene
- A change in personality

These are not conclusive signs of abuse, but they do require further nursing assessment.

When Your Patience Is Stressed

If you feel that your own tolerance level is being tested, you need to find ways of reducing your stress. Review the stress reduction techniques in Chapter 2. You might also:

- Try to identify the exact cause of your irritation.
- Talk with your supervisor about your feelings.
- Consider asking to be assigned to another patient.
- Try to reduce your overall stress and fatigue so that you are more positive and patient on the job.
- Request counseling through an employee assistance program.

Neglect

Neglect is the failure to provide necessary care to prevent discomfort, avoid physical harm, or prevent mental anguish. It is a failure to do something that you had a duty to do. The legal concept is related to negligence, but neglect usually involves deliberate withholding of care. The principles of neglect also apply to timeliness and failure to act in a timely manner. Simply put, neglect is not doing what you are supposed to do in the care of a patient. If you suspect that a patient is being neglected, inform the nurse. Examples of neglect include:

- Failing to turn the patient as often as needed, increasing the risk for pressure injuries
- Failing to carry out proper hygiene, such as not bathing a patient regularly (Figure 4-11)

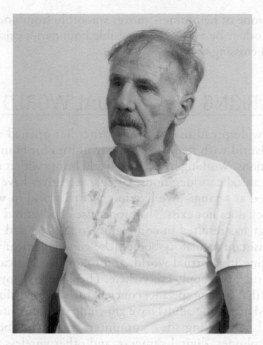

FIGURE 4-11 This patient's dirty shirt and bruise are signs of possible neglect.

- Failing to provide mealtime assistance to a dependent patient
- Failing to provide water to a patient who is on bed rest and has an order to encourage fluids

Invasion of Privacy

Personal information about patients must be kept **confidential**. Revealing personal information is an **invasion of privacy**, which is against the law. You can protect patients' privacy by:

- Protecting the patient from exposure of the body
- Knocking and pausing before entering a room
- Drawing curtains when providing care
- Leaving while visitors are with the patient
- Not listening as patients make telephone calls
- Abiding by the rules of confidentiality
- Not trying to force a patient to accept your personal beliefs or views
- Not discussing the patient's condition with others who are not authorized to know the information

Sexual Harassment

Sexual harassment is unwelcome sexual advances, requests for sexual favors, and other verbal or physical conduct of a sexual nature. The action may be physical, verbal, or nonverbal. The other party may be a patient or co-worker, of the same gender or another gender as the harasser.

Sexual harassment is illegal, but sometimes occurs despite the employer's best efforts to prevent it. Harassment of this nature has the potential to interfere with an employee's work performance and disrupt unit operation. It subjects employees to an intimidating, hostile, and offensive work environment. Facilities must respond promptly and appropriately when patients or employees make a claim of sexual harassment, whether the alleged harasser is another employee, an independent contractor, a patient, a visitor, a guest, or some other person. Your facility will have policies and procedures regarding actions to take and penalties if harassment occurs.

Examples of actions that may be considered sexual harassment include:

- Making comments about anatomy, such as the size or shape of the breasts, genitals, or areas of the body considered sexual
- Making suggestions of a sexual nature
- Staring at a person's body
- Unwanted touching, holding, grabbing, hugging, fondling, kissing, or pinching
- "Accidentally" colliding with or brushing up against another person
- Making lewd or sexually suggestive comments
- Using offensive gestures or motions
- Telling offensive, graphic jokes or using offensive language
- Making threats or comments, making fun of, or asking questions about a person's sexual orientation or personal sexual practices or behavior
- Displaying or circulating sexually suggestive material (written or pictorial, including cartoons)

If you believe you are being sexually harassed, or suspect that a patient is being sexually harassed, notify your supervisor promptly. Avoid conversations, gestures, and other behavior that may be offensive and perceived to be sexually harassing by patients and co-workers.

PROFESSIONAL BOUNDARIES

Boundaries are invisible lines that define healthy relationships and limit one's sphere of activity. Nursing assistants must stay within certain **professional boundaries** in the care of each patient. Boundaries are like driving down the street. Suddenly you find yourself in another town. You did not see a line when you left one town and entered another. Turning around is not possible. Being aware of boundaries is important with all patients, especially those who are emotionally stressed. Learn how to identify boundaries and avoid crossing them.

State law, licensing agencies, and the employer all establish boundaries. Respecting boundaries is an ethical responsibility and helps ensure that the contact is profes-sional and safe. Actively avoid crossing boundaries, even if you think you are meeting a patient's need. If in doubt, ask the nurse. If you feel that your relationship with a patient is too personal to discuss, you are probably cross-ing a boundary.

To avoid crossing boundaries, avoid thinking and acting as a family member or friend. Too much or too little contact can be unhealthy for both you and the patient. Use good judgment and determine the amount of contact that is right for each patient.

Ethical Behavior with Patients and Families

If any of the following occur, you are probably cross-ing professional boundaries and may be entering a **rela-tionship danger zone**. This occurs when you are close to crossing a boundary. The danger zone is an invisible area that threatens a relationship or causes ethical and legal problems. Examples of the relationship danger zone include:

- Keeping secrets with a patient and becoming defen-sive when someone questions your involvement in the patient's personal life
- Spending an inappropriate amount of time with the patient, including off-duty visits or trading assign-ments with others so you can be with the patient
- Reporting only partial information about the patient, because you fear disclosing unfavorable information

Consequences of Boundary Violations

There are many personal, legal, and professional conse-quences to boundary crossings.

Try to stay in the **zone of helpfulness** (Figure 4-12). This is a healthy relationship area where most patient contact should occur. Overinvolvement involves bound-ary crossing. Underinvolvement involves distancing yourself from the patient and may be viewed as neglect.

The zone of helpfulness moves smoothly from one area to another. Be aware that invisible boundaries exist and avoid crossing them.

WORKING IN A VIRTUAL WORLD

The widespread use of the Internet has opened a vir-tual world with many new opportunities for boundary violations. Working in a virtual world brings with it many new ethical considerations. Google executives have been quoted as saying: "We live in a virtual world in which privacy does not exist." Improper use of advanced tech-nology has resulted in complaints to nursing and nurs-ing assistant regulatory bodies. Use good judgment when working in a virtual world, and follow the ethical and legal rules that apply everywhere. There are so many vari-ables that writing specific, concrete rules is impossible.

Many young adults have grown up with the Internet, social networking sites, computers, tablets, webcams, smartphones, digital cameras, and other wireless com-munication devices. Because of this, some lead very trans-parent lives. They disclose things that people from older generations consider very private. They email and upload personal photos, with little thought to the appearance or consequences. For example, two Wisconsin nurses lost their jobs for posting a cell-phone photo of a sensitive x-ray on a social networking site. (They did not disclose the patient's identity.) During the investigation, the nurses stated, "We were just telling our friends about our shift at work." Nurses and nursing assistants have been prosecuted and jailed for taking cell-phone photos. Posting informa-tion and taking and/or posting photos without proper permission is always a boundary violation. (As a rule, both facility and patient permission is needed.) Patients expect health care workers to respect their dignity and act in their best interests. Making negative comments, shar-ing personal information, and taking and/or posting pho-tos of their bodies is not respectful or dignified.

You learn about patient confidentiality very early in your nursing assistant program because it is important and you are expected to apply the information for the

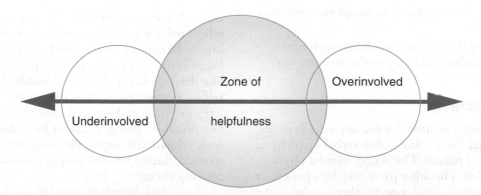

FIGURE 4-12 Most patient contact should occur in the zone of helpfulness.

rest of your career. Medical records and personal patient information are always privileged and confidential. All employees must protect patient information from access by unauthorized persons.

HEALTH INSURANCE PORTABILITY AND ACCOUNTABILITY ACT

In 1996, Congress passed the **Health Insurance Portability and Accountability Act (HIPAA)**. **Protected health information (PHI)** is the basis for the HIPAA rules. The purpose of HIPAA is to:

- Restrict use and disclosure of patient information
- Make facilities responsible for protecting PHI

Because HIPAA protects all identifiable health information, the rules apply to:

- Paper notes or records
- Photos, audio, and video recordings
- Verbal information
- Electronic communication such as email, tweets, and text messages
- Billing records
- Medical records

As you can see, HIPAA protects *all* communications regarding patients. Staff is given information only on the basis of their **need to know**. This means that information is revealed only if workers need it to carry out their duties. Staff cannot read charts out of curiosity. HIPAA guidelines extend to appointments within or outside a facility. If a CNA accompanies a patient to an appointment they must maintain HIPAA guidelines. Penalties for HIPAA violations range from $100 per person for a single violation, up to $25,000 per person per year for multiple violations. Criminal penalties may also apply. Refer to Chapter 8 for additional HIPAA information.

SOCIAL MEDIA

Most facilities have policies prohibiting employees from posting facility and patient information on any **social networking sites**, due to the risk of PHI disclosure. Social networking sites like Facebook and Twitter are Internet-based services that enable users to:

- Construct a public or private profile containing information they wish to share
- Make a list of other users with whom they share a connection
- View their personal list of connections and those made by their "friends" within the system

The nature of the information and connections varies from one site to the next. Many people are active on multiple social networking sites.

You might think that staff would know better than to post sensitive or personal information online, given their education and responsibilities concerning confidentiality rules and the rigid HIPAA regulations. However, many who use social networking sites believe that removing names is enough to avoid breaches of confidentiality and invasion of privacy. *This is not true.* Some employees bypass their employers' rules by bringing their own smartphones, tablets, and other wireless devices to work and using them without thinking about confidentiality. Persons who grew up with social media may not realize they are crossing electronic boundaries until it is too late.

Health care facilities expect employees to conduct themselves in an ethical manner that will reflect favorably on the facility, even if they are off duty. Facilities do not want people in the community to think that their employees:

- Lack empathy
- Are making fun of patients
- Are disrespecting patients
- Do not take patients' illnesses or misfortunes seriously

Facilities investigate reports of ethics and boundary violations to protect their reputation and image in the community. They must also prevent HIPAA violations. You may think you are anonymous and invisible when you are online, but you are not. Every computer and wireless device that connects to the Internet is identifiable through an Internet protocol (IP) number. Each time you go online, you leave footprints that can be traced. A number of health care workers have been disciplined for social media violations. Recent penalties include:

- Written warnings
- **Termination**, or loss of one's job
- Revocation of professional license or certification
- Formal charges of HIPAA violations
- Imprisonment

You are responsible for your actions and image. Avoid using personal electronic devices at work. You are being paid to work, not to use your phone to socialize, text, or conduct personal business. Follow your facility's policies. Never take photos of patients. Avoid posting information about patients or your employer online. Potentially damaging personal information or photos posted online (including on social networking sites) will find their way to a major search engine within 10 days. Because search engines also catalog images, any or all personal pictures they find will be archived in their database forever. You are a nursing assistant all the time, whether at home, work, or in the community. Protect your professional reputation. Although setting and maintaining boundaries may seem unnecessary, they are essential to successful nursing assistant practice.

REVIEW

A. Multiple Choice

Select the best answer for each of the following.

1. You overhear another assistant raise their voice when speaking to Mrs. Ryan. The assistant may be guilty of:
   a. negligence.
   b. theft.
   c. verbal abuse.
   d. invasion of privacy.

2. Mr. Deonne offers you two dollars as thanks for picking up a newspaper for him. Your response should be to:
   a. ignore the money and pretend not to see it.
   b. take the money—you earned it.
   c. report the matter to your supervisor.
   d. politely refuse because tipping is not allowed.

3. Mr. Chan's daughter is visiting and wants information about her father's condition. Your best response is to:
   a. give her the information.
   b. say you do not know.
   c. refer her to the nurse.
   d. write it down for her.

4. You observe another assistant slipping a patient's rosary into their pocket. Your best response is to:
   a. pretend you did not see it.
   b. inform the nurse.
   c. tell the patient.
   d. tell the patient's family.

5. Failure to exercise the degree of care considered reasonable in a given situation is:
   a. negligence.
   b. malpractice.
   c. neglect.
   d. coercion.

6. An assistant forgets that they are assigned to care for Mr. Olmsted, a patient with mental confusion. At the end of a 12-hour shift, the nurses do walking rounds during report. They discover that Mr. Olmsted has developed a pressure injury. This may be associated with not turning the patient due to:
   a. abuse.
   b. libel.
   c. involuntary seclusion.
   d. neglect.

7. Mrs. Rosario has very fragile skin that tears and bruises easily. The nurse instructed Tony, a nursing assistant, to handle the patient gently to prevent injury. Tony is in a hurry and bumps Mrs. Rosario's leg against the side rail, causing a large skin tear. This is an example of:
   a. slander.
   b. invasion of privacy.
   c. libel.
   d. negligence.

8. Mr. McNally tells you he is tired and does not want his bath right now. You should:
   a. tell him you will not have time to bathe him later.
   b. ask him when he would like you to return to assist him.
   c. advise him that the physician insists that he bathe.
   d. forget the bath for today.

9. Mr. Strong, a patient with mental confusion, has a visitor. After the visitor leaves, you discover a large bruise on the patient's arm that was not there previously. You should:
   a. call the physician.
   b. call the police.
   c. do nothing.
   d. notify the nurse.

10. A patient with cancer tells you that she no longer wants to live. She confides that she is collecting her medicine so she can take an overdose and die. You should:
    a. respect the patient's confidentiality and tell no one.
    b. notify the patient's husband when he visits.
    c. inform the nurse immediately.
    d. ask a more experienced assistant to reason with the patient.

11. Boundary crossings:
    a. are acceptable if you are meeting a patient's needs.
    b. do not apply to electronic communication.
    c. are not acceptable in any situation.
    d. do not apply to the relationship danger zone.

12. Posting a photo of a patient on a social networking site is acceptable if the:
    a. patient is not identified in the photo.
    b. patient's face is not in the photo.
    c. patient's family gives permission.
    d. patient and facility give permission.

13. An untrue verbal statement about another person is:
   a. battery.
   b. libel.
   c. defamation.
   d. slander.

14. An untrue comment that damages the reputation of another person is:
   a. assault.
   b. battery.
   c. defamation.
   d. libel.

15. Making a false written statement is:
   a. libel.
   b. defamation.
   c. slander.
   d. abetting.

16. Restraining a person's movements or actions without proper authorization is:
   a. aiding and abetting.
   b. false imprisonment.
   c. assault and battery.
   d. informed dissent.

17. Coercion is:
   a. consent.
   b. force.
   c. truth.
   d. entrapment.

18. A worker needs certain patient information to do their job. This involves the principle of:
   a. need to know.
   b. informed consent.
   c. open records.
   d. power of attorney.

19. Touching a person without permission is:
   a. consent.
   b. assault.
   c. battery.
   d. libel.

20. Most patient contact should occur within:
   a. the relationship danger zone.
   b. the zone of helpfulness.
   c. therapeutic boundaries.
   d. boundary excursion.

21. Making fun of a gay co-worker is an example of:
   a. mental abuse.
   b. verbal abuse.
   c. sexual assault.
   d. sexual harassment.

22. An example of invasion of privacy is:
   a. exposing areas of a patient's body unnecessarily.
   b. helping a patient read a letter.
   c. working in the patient's room when the family visits.
   d. assisting the patient when a priest gives communion.

B. True/False
Mark the following true or false by circling T or F.

23. T F   A patient may not refuse any treatment prescribed by the physician.
24. T F   You may learn much about a patient's personal life as you provide care.
25. T F   Lunchtime is the best time to discuss your patients with others.
26. T F   Accepting a tip is a form of abuse.
27. T F   You fail to follow an order to encourage fluids for Mr. Herrera. You are guilty of neglect.
28. T F   You forget to put side rails up when ordered, and a patient falls. You are guilty of negligence.
29. T F   Failure to report your observation of an illegal act makes you guilty of aiding and abetting the action.
30. T F   Leaving a portion of a patient's body unnecessarily exposed is an invasion of the patient's privacy.
31. T F   Use of restraints requires a physician's order.
32. T F   Ethics relates to moral rights and wrongs of behavior.
33. T F   Nursing assistants must respect professional boundaries.
34. T F   People give up their right to privacy when they are admitted to health care facilities.
35. T F   Boundaries are established by the employer, licensing agencies, and state law.
36. T F   Patients may cross professional boundaries.
37. T F   Every patient has the right to considerate, respectful care.

38. T F   Honesty and integrity are the hallmarks of a conscientious nursing assistant.

39. T F   Telling an off-color joke to a patient of the opposite gender may be considered malpractice.

40. T F   You may apply restraints to a patient who resists your caregiving.

41. T F   Patients may not be subjected to either verbal or physical abuse.

C. Nursing Assistant Challenge

In each of the following situations, describe the correct nursing assistant action.

42. Ms. Harvey is dying. Her physicians believe that she will live only a few days. What is your responsibility to this patient?

_____

_____

_____

43. Mrs. Wybok insists on saying her prayers every morning just as breakfast is ready.

_____

_____

_____

44. Mr. Bishop's daughter asks you what medicine the physician ordered for her father's heart condition.

_____

_____

_____

45. Boundaries can be electronic. List at least three devices that are potential sources of electronic boundary violations.

_____

_____

_____

46. Nursing assistants must protect their reputations at work only.

_____

_____

_____

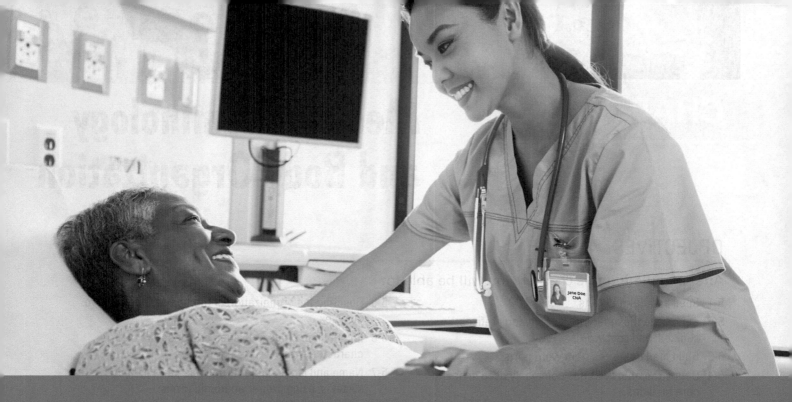

SECTION 2
Scientific Principles

CHAPTER 5
Medical Terminology and Body Organization

CHAPTER 6
Classification of Disease

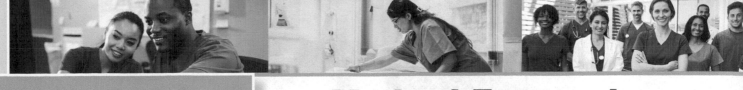

Medical Terminology and Body Organization

OBJECTIVES

After completing this chapter, you will be able to:

5-1 Spell and define terms.

5-2 Recognize the meanings of common prefixes, suffixes, and root words.

5-3 Build medical terms from word parts.

5-4 Define the abbreviations commonly used in health care facilities.

5-5 Describe the organization of the body, from simple to complex.

5-6 Identify four types of tissues and describe their characteristics.

5-7 Name and locate major organs as parts of body systems, using proper anatomic terms.

VOCABULARY

Learn the meaning and the correct spelling of the following words and phrases:

abbreviation	dorsal	muscle tissue	serous membrane
anatomic position	epithelial cell	nerve cell	skeletal (voluntary) muscle
anatomy	epithelial tissue	nervous tissue	smooth (involuntary,
anterior	health	organ	visceral) muscle
cardiac muscle	inferior	pericardium	suffix
cavity	lateral	peritoneum	superior
cell	medial	physiology	synovial membrane
combining form	membranes	pleura	system
connective tissue	meninges	posterior	tissue
connective tissue cell	mucous membrane	prefix	umbilicus
cutaneous membrane	mucus	proximal	ventral
disease	muscle cell	quadrant	word root
distal			

MEDICAL TERMINOLOGY

Medical science and health care have a special language called *medical terminology*. In this language, the terms are formed by building on common word parts (Figure 5-1). Terms are developed by combining:

- **Word root**—the foundation of a medical term. A word root usually, but not always, refers to the part of the body or condition that is being treated, studied, or named by the term.
- **Combining form**—a vowel may be added to the end of the word root to make it easier to form medical words. This combination of the word root and vowel is called a *combining form*.
- **Prefix**—word part added to the beginning of a word to change or add to its meaning.
- **Suffix**—word part added to the end of a word to change or add to its meaning.
- **Abbreviation**—shortened form of a word (often letters). You already know the abbreviation RN (for registered nurse). You will soon become familiar with additional abbreviations that are common to the world of medicine and health care.

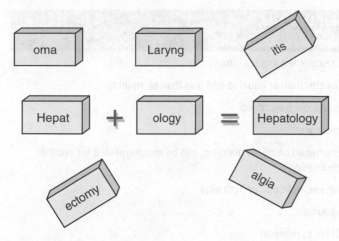

FIGURE 5-1 New words can be formed by combining different prefixes and suffixes.

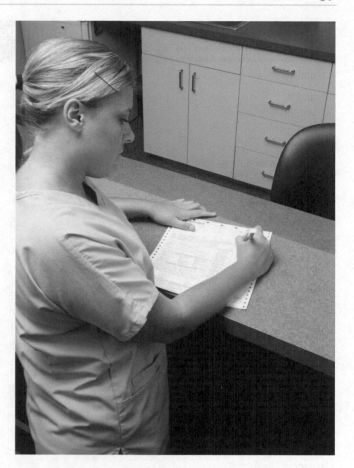

FIGURE 5-2B Handwriting must be clear and legible when paper documentation is used. Use only approved abbreviations.

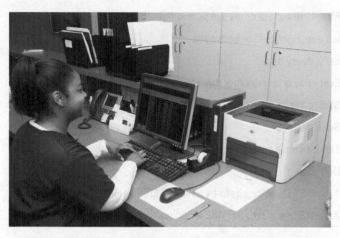

FIGURE 5-2A Most facilities use electronic patient records. Abbreviations are commonly used in documentation, assignment sheets, worksheets, and other formal and informal documentation. Use only approved abbreviations. Never invent your own.

Each health care facility also has special abbreviations that it uses (Figure 5-2A and 5-2B). Check the computer directory or procedure and policy manual of your facility to determine which abbreviations have been approved for use. A good medical dictionary is also a helpful tool.

Each facility will also have a list of abbreviations that should *not* be used (Figure 5-3). The facility adds abbreviations to the list every three months, so you must check it regularly. Abbreviations on the "do not use" list are

usually those that were formerly common and accepted, but they did not withstand the test of time. Over the years, the abbreviations on this list have been found to cause confusion and errors. The list is very important because it affects patient safety, but it is not uniform. Each facility makes its own list. The Joint Commission also publishes a list for their accredited facilities.

MEDICAL WORD PARTS

Word Roots

Familiarity with important word parts comes from study and repeated usage. You will gain experience with the word parts as you practice reporting and charting, and by communicating with your co-workers.

A single medical word root can sometimes be placed in different parts of a word and still have a specific meaning. For example, the root *cyte* means cell:

- *Cyt*ology—the study of cells
- Leuko*cyte*—a white blood cell
- Poly*cyt*osis—an illness in which there are too many red and white blood cells

---

⚖ Legal ALERT

Documentation is a means of communication. Abbreviations must be clear, and others must know their meanings, if the communication is to be effective and meaningful.

Example Do Not Use List	
Do Not Use This Abbreviation	**Meaning of Abbreviation**
> and <	Greater than and less than
≥ and ≤	Greater than or equal to and less than or equal to
ʒ, ℥	teaspoon, 5 mL, dram
Ug, μg, or μg	microgram
Any drug name abbreviations, such as HCl, AZT, DPT, HCTZ, MTX	Shortened name for the drug; can be misinterpreted for another medication
A.S., A.D., A.U.	left ear, right ear, or both ears
BT	bedtime
Cc, cc	Cubic centimeter
HS, hs	half strength, hour of sleep (bedtime)
IU	International Unit
MS, MS04, MgS04	Morphine sulfate or magnesium sulfate
O.S., O.D., O.U.	left eye, right eye, or both eyes
q1d	daily, every day
q.d, QD, QOD	Every day or every other day
ss	Sliding scale, one half
Subq, SC, or SQ	Subcutaneous
T.I.W. or t.i.w.	Three times a week
U, u, or u	Unit
Zero after decimal point (1.0mg)	1 mg. NEVER write a zero by itself AFTER a decimal point
Zero not placed in front of decimal (.5mg)	ALWAYS use a zero BEFORE a decimal point

FIGURE 5-3 Each facility has a "Do Not Use" abbreviation list that is appropriate for its documentation system.

No matter where the form *cyte* occurs in a medical word, it refers to cells. It may be a prefix, a suffix, or a word root. Word roots are often derived from Greek or Latin. For example, the word root *nephro* is derived from the word for kidney. This root may be used to form a variety of medical terms. For example:

- Nephroma—a tumor of the kidney
- Nephrectomy—surgical excision of the kidney
- Nephrolithiasis—presence of kidney stones

Give special attention to the exercises and activities in this chapter. Learning the new words and parts of words will make it easier for you to recognize meanings of medical terms.

Table 5-1 lists combining forms (word roots plus vowel).

Prefixes and Suffixes

Many medical words have common beginnings (prefixes) or common endings (suffixes). By learning some

of the more common prefixes (Table 5-2) and suffixes (Table 5-3), you can put together many new words.

Common Abbreviations

Table 5-4 lists abbreviations and their meanings. They have been grouped according to most common usage for easier learning. Other abbreviations are presented in the following chapters, within the context in which they are most often used.

BODY ORGANIZATION

All nursing care is directed toward helping patients reach optimum health and independence. **Health** is a state of well-being in which all parts of the body and mind are functioning properly. **Disease** is any change from the healthy state. Disease takes many forms. Medical science is the study of disease and its effects on the human body. These effects are easier to understand when you

TABLE 5-1 Combining Forms

Combining Form	Meaning	Example	Meaning
abdomin (o)	abdomen	abdominal	portion of body between the thorax and pelvis
aden (o)	gland	adenoma	a glandular tumor
angi (o)	vessel	angioedema	recurrent large areas of subcutaneous edema of sudden onset, commonly an allergic reaction to foods or drugs
arteri (o)	artery	arteriogram	X-ray of an artery after injection of contrast medium (dye)
arthr (o)	joint	arthritis	inflammation of a joint
bronch (i) (o)	bronchus (one of the larger passages conveying air to and from the lungs)	bronchiectasis	bronchi within the lungs become abnormally enlarged
cardi (o)	heart	cardialgia	pain in the region of the heart
cephal (o)	head	cephaloma	soft or encephaloid tumor
cerebr (o)	brain	cerebrovascular accident	another name for a stroke
chol (e)	bile	cholecystitis	inflammation of the gallbladder
col (o)	colon, large intestine	colectomy	excision of the colon
crani (o)	skull	craniotomy	opening of the skull
cyst (o)	bladder, cyst	cystitis	inflammation of the bladder
cyt (o)	cell	cytology	study of cells
dent (i) (o)	tooth	dentist	person licensed to practice dentistry
dermat (o)	skin	dermatitis	inflammation of the skin
encephal (o)	brain	encephaloma	herniation of brain substance
enter (o)	small intestine	enteritis	inflammation of the intestines
erythr (o)	red	erythroblastosis	presence of many red blood cells
fibr (o)	fiber	fibroadenoma	benign growth commonly occurring in breast tissue
gastr (o)	stomach	gastritis	inflammation of the lining of the stomach
geront (o)	elderly	gerontology	scientific study of process and problems related to aging
gloss (o)	tongue	glossodynia	burning or painful tongue
glyc (o)	sugar	glycosuria	urinary excretion of sugar
gynec (o)	female	gynecomastia	excessive development of male mammary glands
hem (o)	blood	hematuria	discharge of blood in urine
hepat (o)	liver	hepatitis	inflammation of the liver
hydr (o)	water	hydrocephalus	enlargement of the cranium caused by abnormal accumulation of fluid
hyster (o)	uterus	hysterectomy	surgical removal of the uterus
lapar (o)	abdomen, flank, loin	laparoscopy	examination of the contents of the abdomen through a scope passed through the abdominal wall
laryng (o)	larynx	laryngectomy	partial or total removal of the larynx by surgery
lith (o)	stone	lithiasis	formation of stones in any hollow structure of the body
mamm (o)	breast	mammography	imaging examination of the breasts
mast (o)	breast	mastitis	inflammation of the breast
men (o)	menstruation	menorrhagia	excessive menstrual flow
my (o)	muscle	myalgia	muscular pain
myel (o)	bone marrow, spinal cord	myelocele	protrusion of the spinal cord

(continues)

TABLE 5-1 *(continued)*

Combining Form	Meaning	Example	Meaning
nephr (o)	kidney	nephrolithiasis	presence of renal calculi (kidney stones)
neur (o)	nerve	neuropathy	any disease of the nervous system
ocul (o)	eye	oculodynia	pain in the eyeball
ophthalm (o)	eye	ophthalmoscope	instrument used to view the inside of the eye
oste (o)	bone	osteitis	inflammation of the bone
ot (o)	ear	otitis media	inflammation of the middle ear
ped (i) (o)	child	pedodontics	dental care of children
pharyng (o)	throat, pharynx	pharyngitis	inflammation of the pharynx
phleb (o)	vein	phlebitis	inflammation of a vein
pneum (o)	lung, air, gas	pneumonectomy	resection of lung tissue
proct (o)	rectum	proctoscopy	rectal exam with a proctoscope
psych (o)	mind	psychology	study of human behavior
pulm (o)	lung	pulmonary	pertaining to the lungs
py (o)	pus	pyogenic	producing pus
rect (o)	rectum	rectocele	hernial protrusion of part of the rectum into the vagina
rhin (o)	nose	rhinorrhea	discharge from nasal mucous membrane
splen (o)	spleen	splenomegaly	enlarged spleen
stern (o)	sternum	sternotomy	incision into or through the sternum
thorac (o)	chest	thoracotomy	opening of the chest
thromb (o)	clot	thrombocytopenia	abnormally small number of platelets in the circulating blood
tox (o)	poison	toxoplasmosis	disease produced by a parasite; can cause birth defects if acquired during pregnancy
trache (i) (o)	trachea	tracheotomy	incision of the trachea for exploration
ur (o)	urine, urinary tract, urination	urinalysis	analysis of the urine
urethr (o)	urethra	urethralgia	pain in the urethra
urin (o)	urine	urinometer	an instrument for determining the specific gravity of urine
uter (i) (o)	uterus	uterotonic	drugs that give tone to uterine muscle
ven (o)	vein	venostat	any instrument used to suppress venous bleeding

TABLE 5-2 Common Prefixes

Prefix	Meaning	Example	Meaning
a-	without	asepsis	without infection
brady-	slow	bradycardia	slow heart rate
dys-	pain or difficulty	dysuria	painful urination
hyper-	above, excessive	hypertension	high blood pressure
hypo-	low, deficient	hypotension	low blood pressure
pan-	all	pandemic	widespread epidemic
poly-	many	polyuria	excessive urine
post-	after	postoperative	after surgery
pre-	before	premenstrual	before the menses
retro-	behind, backward	retrograde	moving backward, degenerating
tachy-	fast	tachycardia	pulse rate above normal

TABLE 5-3 Common Suffixes

Suffix	Meaning	Example	Meaning
-algia	pain	arthralgia	pain in the joints
-ectomy	removal of	appendectomy	removal of the appendix
-emia	blood	anemia	lacking sufficient quality or quantity of blood
-gram	record	electrocardiogram	record produced by electrocardiography
-itis	inflammation	appendicitis	inflammation of the appendix
-logy	study of	hematology	study of blood
-oma	tumor	fibroma	a tumor containing fibrous tissue
-otomy	incision	tracheotomy	incision into the trachea
-plegia	paralysis	hemiplegia	paralysis of one side of the body
-pnea	breathing, respiration	apnea	temporary absence of respirations
-scope	examination instrument	otoscope	instrument for inspecting the ear
-scopy	examination with a scope-type instrument	proctoscopy	rectal exam using a proctoscope

have a clear picture in your mind of a normal and typically functioning body. The first step is to understand the organization of the body.

ANATOMIC TERMS

The **anatomy** (structure) and **physiology** (function) of the body are most easily understood and learned if they are studied in an orderly manner. Special terms are used to describe the relationship of one body part to another.

Whenever we describe the relationship of the body parts, we refer to the **anatomic position** (Figure 5-4), which is:

- Standing erect with feet together or slightly separated
- Facing the observer
- Arms at the sides with the palms forward

In our own minds, we should always position the body in this way before describing any body part or area. This gives everyone the same frame of reference.

Notice as you look at a patient's body or the pictures in this book or any other book about anatomy that you are seeing a mirror image of yourself. The patient's right side is opposite to your left, and your left is opposite to the right of the patient or the picture.

Descriptive Terms

Imaginary lines drawn through the body (Figure 5-5) provide us with other reference terms.

- A line drawn down the center of the body from head to foot (the *midline*) divides the body into

equal right and left sides. Note that the body has the same parts on either side. For example, there is an arm, a leg, an eye, and half of a nose on each side of the line.

- Parts close to this line are **medial** to the line.
- Parts farther away from the line are **lateral** to the line.

For example, in the anatomic position, the thumbs are more lateral to the line and the little fingers are more medial to the line.

Another line drawn parallel to the floor divides the body into upper and lower parts. This line can be drawn at any level on the body as long as it is parallel to the floor.

- Parts located above this line are **superior** to the line.
- Parts located below this line are **inferior** to the line.

For example, if the line is drawn between the knees and ankles, the knees are superior to the ankles, and the ankles are inferior to the knees.

A third line can be drawn to divide the body into front and back.

- Parts in front of this line are **anterior** or **ventral** to the line.
- Parts in back of this line are **posterior** or **dorsal** to the line.

Points of Attachment

The arms and legs are called the *extremities* of the body. The arms are attached to the body at the shoulders. The legs are attached to the body at the hips. Two terms are used to describe the relationship between the parts of the extremities and their points of attachment to the body:

TABLE 5-4 Common Abbreviations

Body Parts

ABCs	airway, breathing, circulation
abd	abdomen
ant	anterior
ax	axillary
bld	blood
BLE	both lower extremities
GI	gastrointestinal
GU	genitourinary
int	internal
lt	left
quad	quadrant
rt	right
sh	shoulder
vag	vagina, vaginal

Diagnosis

AFB	acid-fast bacillus
AIDS	acquired immune deficiency syndrome
AKA	above knee amputation
AMI	acute myocardial infarction
ASCVD	arteriosclerotic cardiovascular disease
ASHD	arteriosclerotic heart disease
BKA	below knee amputation
BPH	benign prostatic hypertrophy (hyperplasia)
CA	cancer
CAD	coronary artery disease
CBC	complete blood count
CHD	coronary heart disease
CHF	congestive heart failure
CHI	closed head injury
COPD	chronic obstructive pulmonary disease
CVA	cerebrovascular accident; stroke
DJD	degenerative joint disease
DVT	deep vein thrombosis
ESRD	end-stage renal disease
FUO	fever of unknown origin

Fx	fracture
GERD	gastroesophageal reflux disease

Disease

HBV	hepatitis B virus (infection)
HCV	hepatitis C virus (infection)
HIV	human immunodeficiency virus (infection)
HTN	hypertension
IDDM	insulin-dependent diabetes mellitus
IH	infectious hepatitis
KS	Kaposi's sarcoma
LBP	low back pain
MD	muscular dystrophy
MI	myocardial infarction (refers to the death of tissues due to loss of blood supply)
MRSA	methicillin-resistant *Staphylococcus aureus*
MS	multiple sclerosis
NB	newborn
NIDDM	non-insulin-dependent diabetes mellitus
NSU	nonspecific urethritis
OA	osteoarthritis
OBS	organic brain syndrome
PID	pelvic inflammatory disease
PUD	peptic ulcer disease
PVD	peripheral vascular disease
RF	renal failure
RO, R/O	rule out
SDAT	senile dementia of Alzheimer's type
STD	sexually transmitted disease
TBI	traumatic brain injury
TIA	transient ischemic attack
URI	upper respiratory infection
UTI	urinary tract infection

VRE	vancomycin-resistant *Enterococcus*

Patient Orders and Charting

ā	before
AAROM	active (actively) assistive (assisted) range of motion
abd.	abduction; abdomen
ACT	active, actively, activities
add.	adduction
ADL	activities of daily living
ad lib.	as desired
adm	admission; administer; administrator
ADT	admission, discharge, transfer
AEB	as evidenced by
AFO	ankle-foot orthosis
aka	also known as
AMA	against medical advice
amb	ambulate, ambulatory
AROM	active range of motion
ASAP	as soon as possible
assist	assistance
as tol	as tolerated
B, (B), Ⓑ	bilateral, both
BB	bed bath
bilat	bilateral
BLE	both lower extremities
B.M., bm	bowel movement
BP, B/P	blood pressure
BPM	beats per minute
B.R.	bedrest; bathroom
BRP	bathroom privileges
BS	blood sugar

(continues)

TABLE 5-4 *(continued)*

BSC	bedside commode	ext.	extension; extremity; external	max	maximum
BSE	breast self-examination	F	fair	meds	medications
BUE	both upper extremities	FB	foreign body	min	minimum
c̄	with	FE	Fleet's enema	mmHg	millimeters of mercury
cal	calorie	flex	flexion	mod	moderate
cath	catheterize, catheter	FM	flow meter	NA, N/A	nursing assistant; also means "not applicable"
CBB	complete bed bath	FU, f/u	follow-up		
CBR	complete bed rest	FUO	fever of unknown origin	N/C, no c/o	no complaints
ck or ✓	check	FWB	full weight bearing		
ck freq or ✓ freq	check frequently	FWW, fw/w	front wheeled walker	neg, ⊖	negative
				NG	nasogastric
cl liq	clear liquid	G	good	NKA	no known allergies
c/o	complains of	g/c, GC	geriatric chair	NN	nurses' notes
CP	care plan; chest pain	GT, g/t	gastrostomy tube	NPO	nothing by mouth
CPG	clinical practice guidelines	gt	gait	N/S, NSS	normal saline solution
CPM	continuous passive motion	H	hydrogen		
CPR	cardiopulmonary resuscitation	H_2O	water	N & V	nausea and vomiting
DAT	diet as tolerated	H_2O_2	hydrogen peroxide	NVD	nausea, vomiting, diarrhea
dehyd	dehydration	HOB	head of bed	NWB	no weight bearing
dep	dependent	HOH	hard of hearing	O_2	oxygen
Disch, d/c	discharge	HP	hot pack	occ	occasional
		ht	height	OOB	out of bed
D/C	discontinue	Hx	history	O, OS	oral; mouth
DNR	do not resuscitate	①, ind.	independent	P	poor, pulse
DOA	dead on arrival	I&O	intake and output	PB, PBB	partial bath, partial bed bath
doc	document, documentation	IM	intramuscular		
Dr	doctor	irrig	irrigation	per	by
drsg	dressing	isol	isolation	p.o.	by mouth
DSD	dry sterile dressing	IV	intravenous	postop	postoperative
Dx	diagnosis	JT	jejunostomy tube	preop	preoperative
E, en	enema	K^+	potassium	prep	prepare
EHR	electronic health record	Kcal	kilocalorie, calorie	PRN	whenever necessary
EMR	electronic medical record	L	left, liter		
EOL	end of life	lat	lateral		
EOLC	end-of-life care	LBP	low back pain		
et	and	lg, lge, L	large		
ETOH	ethanol (used to refer to alcoholic beverages)	liq	liquid		
		L/min, LPM	liters per minute		
Eval	evaluation				
ex	exercise, example	LOC	loss of consciousness		
exam	examination				

(continues)

TABLE 5-4 *(continued)*

prog	progress; prognosis
PROM	passive range of motion
PWB	partial weight bearing
Px	prognosis (prog)
q̄	each, every
q.s.	sufficient quantity
qt	quiet
R	rectal; respiration; right
re:	regarding
rehab	rehabilitation
resp	respiration
rot	rotated, rotation
rt (R)	right; routine
r/t	related to
RT	respiratory therapy
Rx	treatment; prescription
s̄	without
SBA	standby assistance
sm	small
SOB	short(ness) of breath
s/s, S & S	signs and symptoms
SSE	soapsuds enema
stat	at once; immediately
std prec	standard precautions
Sx	symptoms
T, temp	temperature
TIAN	toilet in advance of need
TKO	to keep open
TLC	tender loving care
TPN	total parenteral nutrition
TPR	temperature, pulse, respirations
trach	tracheostomy
TSE	testicular self-examination
TTWB	touch toe weight bearing
TWE	tap water enema
Tx	treatment
Ung or oint	ointment
vc	verbal cues

VS	vital signs
WB	weight bearing
WBAT	weight bearing as tolerated
w/c	wheelchair
wt	weight

Physical and History

CC	chief complaint
DOB	date of birth
EENT	eye, ear, nose, throat
ENT	ear, nose, throat
FH	family history
H & P	history and physical
LMP	last menstrual period
L & W	living and well
M & F	mother and father
MH	marital history
NB	newborn
PE	physical examination
PI	present illness
PMH	past medical history
R/O	rule out
SOB	short(ness) of breath
UCD	usual childhood diseases
UK	unknown
WDWN	well-developed, well-nourished
WFL	within functional limits
WNL	within normal limits
Y/O	years old
YOB	year of birth

Tests

ABG	arterial blood gas study
BS	blood sugar
C & S	culture and sensitivity
CBC	complete blood count
CXR	chest X-ray
FBS	fasting blood sugar
FSBS	fingerstick blood sugar
H & H, H/H	hemoglobin and hematocrit

spec	specimen
UA, U/A	urinalysis

Places or Departments

CS	central supply
DR, D/R	delivery room; dining room
ED/ER	emergency department/emergency room
ECG, EKG	electrocardiogram
EEG	electroencephalogram
EENT	eye, ear, nose, throat
GYN	gynecology
ICCU	intensive coronary care unit
IDT	interdisciplinary team
Lab	laboratory
LTC	long-term care
MRD	medical record department
OPD	outpatient department
OR	operating room
OT	occupational therapy
PAR	postanesthesia recovery
Peds, pedi	pediatrics
PT	physical therapy
RR	recovery room
RT	respiratory therapy
SNU, SNF	skilled nursing unit, skilled nursing facility
ST	speech therapy
XR, X/R	X-ray

Process Improvement

assess	assess, assessment
BNE	board of nurse examiners
BON	board of nursing

(continues)

TABLE 5-4 *(continued)*

CE	continuing education	AM	morning	oz, ℥	ounce	
CEU	continuing education unit	b.i.d.	twice a day	**Vital Signs**		
CQI	continuous quality improvement	d	day	TPR	temperature, pulse, respirations	
EBDM	evidence-based decision making	h, H	hour	VS, vitals	vital signs	
		noc, noct	night	**Weight/Height**		
EBR	evidence-based recommendations	OC, oc	on call	cm	centimeter	
		p̄	after	ft	feet	
eval	evaluate, evaluation	p̄.c̄.	after meals	ht	height	
HC	health care	PM	evening or afternoon	kg	kilogram	
HCI	health care improvement	q̄h, qh	every hour	lb or #	pounds	
HCQ	health care quality	q̄4h, q4h	every four hours	in or ″	inches	
ID	identify, identification	q.i.d.	four times a day	oz, ℥	ounce	
IDT	interdisciplinary team	t.i.d.	three times a day	wt	weight	
info	information	WA, W/A	while awake	**Temperature**		
IT	information technology	x, X	times	°	degree	
NAR	nurse aide registry, nursing assistant registry	x2, x3, …	two times, three times, …	Ax	axillary	
NP	nursing practice, nurse practitioner	**Roman Numerals**		C	Celsius	
		I	1	F	Fahrenheit	
NPA	nurse practice act	II	2	O	oral	
PI	performance improvement, process improvement	III	3	R	rectal	
		IV	4	**Symbols**		
PRO	professional improvement organization, process improvement organization	V	5	♂	male	
		VI	6	♀	female	
		VII	7	↑	up, increase	
QA	quality assessment, quality assurance	VIII	8	↓	down, decrease	
		IX	9	//	parallel	
QHC	quality health care	X	10	Δ	change to, change in	
QI	quality improvement, quality initiative	**Other Common Numbers**		Ø	zero, none, nothing	
QIO	quality improvement organization	1°	first; primary; first degree	*	important	
QM	quality management	2°	second; secondary to; second degree			
QR	quality review	3°	third; tertiary; third degree			
RCA	root cause analysis	1x, 2x,	one time, one person; two times, two people, …			
SIQ	sharing innovations in quality	**Measurements and Volume**				
SOC	standard(s) of care	amt.	amount			
SOP	standard(s) of practice	gtt	drop			
std, stds	standard, standards	mL	milliliter			
TQM	total quality management	L	liter			
Time Abbreviations						
ā.c̄.	before meals					

ORGANIZATION OF THE BODY

All parts of the body are interdependent. The basic unit of the body is the **cell**. Groups of similar cells are organized into **tissues**. Different tissues form **organs**. The organs are organized into **systems** that perform the body functions.

Cells

Each cell performs the same basic functions that the total body performs, but on a smaller scale (Figure 5-7). These functions are breathing (respiration), reproduction, intake and use of nutrients, and excretion (elimination of wastes).

The lungs take in oxygen and give off carbon dioxide (a waste product). All the cells in your body need the oxygen you inhale to function. The body gets energy from food by using oxygen. *Cellular respiration* occurs when the cells use oxygen to break down sugars. Carbon dioxide is produced and exhaled during this process that creates energy. Much of this energy is stored in chemical form for later use. In normal respirations, the blood picks up oxygen and releases carbon dioxide in the lungs. The opposite is true during cellular respiration: in this case the blood releases oxygen and picks up carbon dioxide. Your cells also reproduce, take in and use nutrients, and eliminate waste products.

Some cells perform different kinds of work necessary for the body as a whole to function. A few of the various specialized types of cells are:

- **Epithelial cells**, which are very close together, form protective coverings and sometimes produce body fluids.
- **Nerve cells**, which carry electrical messages to and from the different parts of the body, coordinating activities and making the person aware of changes in the environment.
- **Muscle cells**, which are special in their ability to shorten or lengthen, thus changing their shape and the position of parts to which they are attached. They also surround body openings, such as the mouth, to control the size of these openings.
- **Connective tissue cells**, which are present throughout the body in many different types. They support and connect body parts.

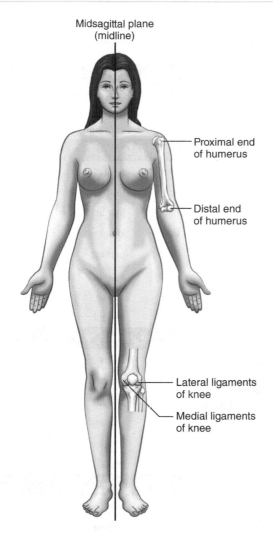

Midsagittal plane (midline)

Proximal end of humerus

Distal end of humerus

Lateral ligaments of knee

Medial ligaments of knee

FIGURE 5-4 All references to body parts are made in relationship to the anatomic position. The *midline* is the middle of the body. A *proximal* body part is located closest to the midline. A *distal* body part is located farthest away from the midline. *Medial* means closest to the midline, and *lateral* means on the side, away from the midline.

- **Proximal** means closest to the point of attachment
- **Distal** means farthest away from the point of attachment

The upper arm is proximal to the shoulder, which is the point of attachment for the arm. The fingers are distal to the point of attachment for the arm, which is in the shoulder.

Abdominal Regions

The abdomen is divided into four **quadrants**, with the **umbilicus** (navel) at the central point (Figure 5-6A). The abdomen can also be divided into nine regions (Figure 5-6B). Knowing these regions will be important as you report and document your observations.

Tissues

Groups of similar cells are organized into *tissues*. The basic tissue types are:

- Epithelial tissue
- Connective tissue
- Nervous tissue
- Muscle tissue

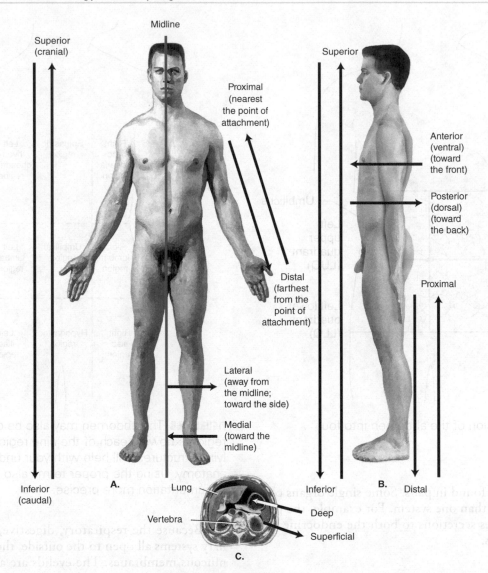

FIGURE 5-5 Imaginary lines are used to section the body to make it easier to locate parts. Directional terms relating to the anatomic position: (A) anatomic position; (B) lateral views of the body; (C) directional terms *deep* and *superficial.*

Epithelial tissue is specialized in its ability to absorb, secrete (produce) fluids, excrete (eliminate) waste products, and protect.

Nervous tissue forms the brain and spinal cord and the nerves throughout the body. This tissue is also found in the special sense organs such as the eyes, ears, and tastebuds. The activities of the rest of the body are directed and coordinated through the nervous tissues.

Three kinds of **muscle tissue** are found in the body:

- **Skeletal (voluntary) muscle** is attached to bones for movement (Figure 5-8A).
- **Cardiac muscle** forms the heart wall (Figure 5-8B).

- **Smooth (involuntary, visceral) muscle** forms the walls of body organs such as the stomach and intestines (Figure 5-8C).

Connective tissue forms blood, bone, and fibrous and elastic tissues to hold the skin on the body, attach muscles to bones, and support delicate cells throughout the body. Generally, connective tissues support and form connections for other tissue types.

Organs

Each organ is made up of more than one kind of tissue and performs special functions that contribute to the overall function of the body systems. Some organs, like

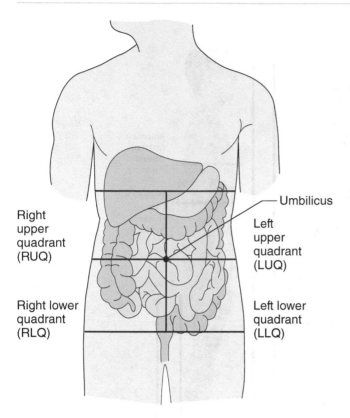

FIGURE 5-6A Division of the abdomen into four quadrants.

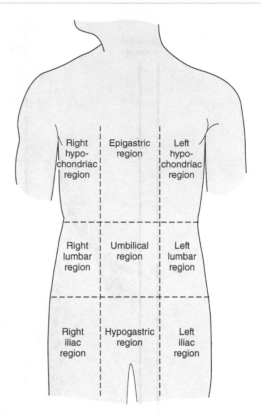

FIGURE 5-6B The abdomen may also be divided by region. Knowing each of the nine regions and underlying structures will help with your understanding of anatomy. Using the proper terms also makes your documentation more precise.

the kidneys, are found in pairs. Some single organs contribute to more than one system. For example, the pancreas contributes secretions to both the endocrine and digestive systems.

Systems

The body has 10 major body systems. Table 5-5 lists the organs that contribute to the function of each system. Notice that some organs are listed as being included in more than one system. For example, the ovaries contribute to the endocrine system by producing female hormones and to the reproductive system by producing the eggs.

Membranes

Membranes are sheets of epithelial tissues supported by connective tissues. Membranes:
- Cover the body.
- Line body cavities.
- Produce some body fluids.
  Important membranes include:
- **Mucous membranes**
  - Produce a fluid called **mucus**
  - Line body cavities that open to the outside

Because the respiratory, digestive, and genitourinary systems all open to the outside, they are lined with mucous membranes. The eyelids are also lined with a mucous membrane; another mucous membrane covers the eyeballs.

- **Synovial membranes**
  - Produce synovial fluid
  - Line joint cavities

The synovial fluid is a clear fluid resembling the white of an egg. It reduces the friction between the bones of active joints and the tendons.

- **Serous membranes**
  - Produce serous fluid
  - Cover the organs and line the closed cavities of the body

Serous fluid reduces friction as the organs work and move. Important serous membranes are the:

- **Pericardium**—surrounds the heart
- **Pleural**—surrounds the lungs and line the thoracic cavity
- **Meninges**—cover the brain and spinal cord, and line the dorsal cavity

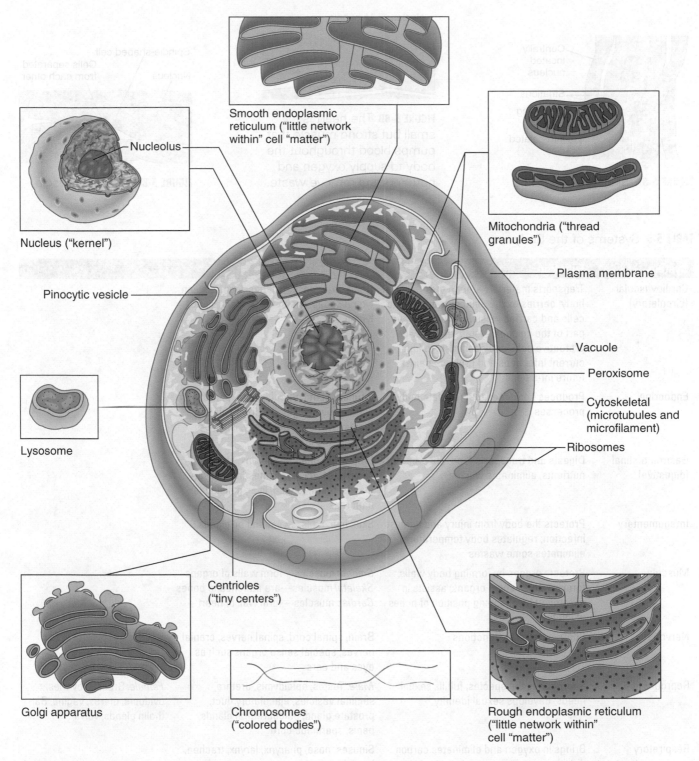

Nucleolus

Nucleus ("kernel")

Smooth endoplasmic reticulum ("little network within" cell "matter")

Mitochondria ("thread granules")

Plasma membrane

Pinocytic vesicle

Vacuole

Peroxisome

Cytoskeletal (microtubules and microfilament)

Lysosome

Ribosomes

Golgi apparatus

Centrioles ("tiny centers")

Chromosomes ("colored bodies")

Rough endoplasmic reticulum ("little network within" cell "matter")

FIGURE 5-7 This diagram shows the different parts of a cell. Each cell functions the same way that the body functions, but on a smaller scale.

- **Peritoneum**—covers the digestive organs and lines the abdominal cavity
- **Cutaneous** (skin)
  - Protects the body
  - Covers the entire body

- Helps to control body temperature
- Eliminates wastes through sweat glands
- Produces vitamin D when exposed to sunlight

Special epithelial cells in this membrane, called *glands*, secrete perspiration and oils.

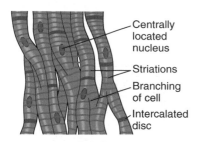

Centrally located nucleus

Striations

Branching of cell

Intercalated disc

FIGURE 5-8A Skeletal muscle.

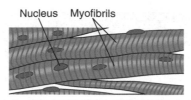

Nucleus   Myofibrils

FIGURE 5-8B The heart is a small but strong muscle that pumps blood throughout the body to supply oxygen and nutrients and remove waste.

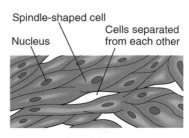

Spindle-shaped cell

Cells separated from each other

Nucleus

FIGURE 5-8C Smooth muscle.

TABLE 5-5 Systems of the Body

System	Function	Structures	
Cardiovascular (circulatory)	Transports materials around the body; carries oxygen and nutrients to the cells and carries waste products away; part of the immune system that provides protective cells and chemicals to fight current infections and protect against future infections	Heart, arteries, capillaries, veins, spleen, lymph nodes, lymphatic vessels, blood, lymph	
Endocrine	Produces hormones that regulate body processes	Pituitary gland, thyroid gland, parathyroid glands, thymus gland, adrenal glands, testes, ovaries, pineal body, islets of Langerhans in pancreas	
Gastrointestinal (digestive)	Digests and transports food; absorbs nutrients; eliminates wastes	Mouth, esophagus, pharynx, stomach, small intestine, large intestine, salivary glands, teeth, tongue, liver, gallbladder, pancreas	
Integumentary	Protects the body from injury and against infection; regulates body temperature; eliminates some wastes	Skin, hair, nails, sweat and oil glands	
Muscular	Protects organs by forming body walls; forms walls of some organs; assists in movement by changing position of bones at joints	*Smooth* muscles—form walls of organs *Skeletal* muscles—are attached to bones *Cardiac* muscles—form wall of heart	
Nervous	Coordinates body functions	Brain, spinal cord, spinal nerves, cranial nerves, special sense organs such as eyes and ears	
Reproductive	Reproduces the species; fulfills sexual needs; develops sexual identity	*Male:* Testes, epididymis, urethra, seminal vesicles, ejaculatory duct, prostate gland, bulbourethral glands, penis, spermatic cord	*Female:* Breasts, ovaries, oviducts, uterus, vagina, Bartholin glands, vulva
Respiratory	Brings in oxygen and eliminates carbon dioxide	Sinuses, nose, pharynx, larynx, trachea, bronchi, lungs	
Skeletal	Supports and protects body parts; produces blood cells: acts as lever in movement	Bones, joints	
Urinary	Manages fluids and electrolytes of body; eliminates liquid wastes	Kidneys, ureters, urinary bladder, urethra	

Cavities

The body seems like a solid structure, but **cavities** (spaces) within it contain the organs. Table 5-6 lists the two main cavities, the dorsal cavity and the ventral cavity.

Each of these cavities is lined by and divided into other cavities by serous membranes. These other cavities are also listed in the table, as are the organs contained in each. Figure 5-9 is a simple drawing of the location of these cavities.

TABLE 5-6 Body Cavities and the Organs Contained Within Each Cavity

	Cavity	Organs	
Dorsal Cavity			
	Cranial	Brain, pineal body, pituitary gland	
	Spinal	Nerves, spinal cord	
Ventral Cavity			
	Thoracic	Lungs, heart, great blood vessels, thymus gland	
	Abdominal (peritoneal)	Stomach, small intestine, most of large intestine, liver, gallbladder, pancreas, spleen	
	Pelvic	*Male:* Seminal vesicles, prostate gland, ejaculatory ducts, urinary bladder, urethra, rectum	*Female:* Uterus, oviducts, ovaries, urinary bladder, urethra, rectum
	Retroperitoneal space	Kidneys, adrenal glands, ureters	

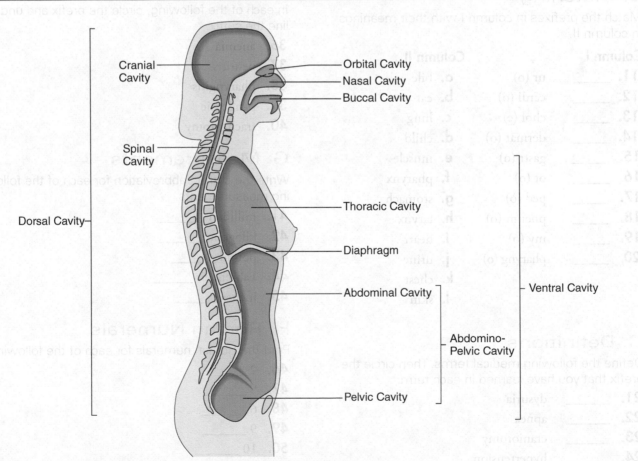

FIGURE 5-9 Lateral (side) view of the body cavities.

REVIEW

A. Matching

Match the definitions from Column II with the abbreviations in Column I.

Column I		Column II
1. _____	a̅.c̅.	**a.** three times a day
2. _____	b.i.d.	**b.** whenever necessary
3. _____	HCV	**c.** head of bed
4. _____	PRN	**d.** before meals
5. _____	NPO	**e.** hepatitis C virus
6. _____	stat	**f.** nothing by mouth
7. _____	HOB	**g.** after meals
8. _____	c̅	**h.** without
9. _____	ung.	**i.** twice a day
10. _____	s̅	**j.** at once
		k. ointment
		l. with

B. Matching

Match the prefixes in column I with their meanings in column II.

Column I		Column II
11. _____	ur (o)	**a.** bile
12. _____	cardi (o)	**b.** ear
13. _____	chol (e)	**c.** lung
14. _____	dermat (o)	**d.** child
15. _____	gastr (o)	**e.** muscle
16. _____	ot (o)	**f.** pharynx
17. _____	ped (o)	**g.** stomach
18. _____	pneum (o)	**h.** larynx
19. _____	my (o)	**i.** heart
20. _____	pharyng (o)	**j.** urine
		k. chest
		l. skin

C. Definitions

Define the following medical terms. Then circle the prefix that you have learned in each term.

21. _____ dysuria
22. _____ apnea
23. _____ craniotomy
24. _____ hypertension
25. _____ tachycardia

D. Definitions

Define the following medical terms. Then circle the suffix that you have learned in each term.

26. _____ neuralgia
27. _____ hemiplegia
28. _____ appendectomy
29. _____ hematology
30. _____ fibroma

E. Fill in the Blanks

Write the medical term for each item.

31. kidney stones _____
32. examination of the rectum using an instrument _____
33. incision into thorax _____
34. inflammation of the stomach _____
35. white blood cell _____

F. Identification

In each of the following, circle the prefix and underline the suffix.

36. anemia
37. neuritis
38. pharyngitis
39. pandemic
40. tracheotomy

G. Measurements

Write the correct abbreviation for each of the following measurements.

41. milliliter _____
42. kilogram _____
43. pound _____
44. Fahrenheit _____
45. inches _____

H. Roman Numerals

Print the Roman numerals for each of the following.

46. 2 _____
47. 5 _____
48. 6 _____
49. 9 _____
50. 10 _____

I. Multiple Choice

Select the best answer for each of the following.

51. When describing the relationship between the hand and the elbow, you should refer to the hand as being:

a. proximal.

b. posterior.

c. distal.

d. anterior.

52. The appendix is located in which quadrant of the abdomen?

a. URQ

b. RLQ

c. ULQ

d. LLQ

53. Which membrane covers the lungs?

a. Pleural

b. Pericardium

c. Peritoneum

d. Meninges

54. Which organs are located in the dorsal cavity?

a. Heart and liver

b. Kidney and spleen

c. Brain and spinal cord

d. Uterus and testes

55. Which organ pumps blood throughout the body?

a. Lungs

b. Heart

c. Liver

d. Adrenal glands

56. Which of the following is part of the skeletal system?

a. Ureters

b. Sternum

c. Gallbladder

d. Testes

57. The breasts are part of which system?

a. Muscular

b. Urinary

c. Cardiovascular

d. Reproductive

58. Membranes that line body cavities that open to the outside are called:

a. mucous membranes.

b. basilar membranes.

c. serous membranes.

d. fibrous membranes.

59. The eye and ear are part of which system?

a. Endocrine

b. Nervous

c. Cardiovascular

d. Digestive

60. The endocrine system:

a. eliminates liquid waste.

b. brings in oxygen.

c. transports blood.

d. produces hormones.

J. True/False

Mark the following true or false by circling T or F.

61. T F The urinary bladder and gallbladder are the same structure.

62. T F The pancreas functions in both the digestive and endocrine systems.

63. T F Muscular tissue enables the body to move.

64. T F Structures of different tissues acting together to carry out a specific function are called *organs*.

K. Nursing Assistant Challenge

Examine the sample care plan in Figure 5-10 and use your understanding of medical science and terminology to define each medical term and abbreviation used on the plan.

1.	**Patient Name**	Bruce Tratt	**Age** 47	**Rel** Prot		#876-3291-7	
2.	**Physician**	R. Morgan M.D.	**Dx** Splenomegaly—Diabetes Mellitus				
3.			**Orders**				
4.	**Preop orders**	3/18	on call for OR at 8 am 3/19				
5.	Stat CBC, ABG, FBS						
6.	UA						
7.	NG Tube at 6 am 3/19						
8.	Foley cath this pm.						
9.	Surg Prep.						
10.	NPO p̄ midnight						
11.	SSE at 9 pm.						
12.	Amb ad lib. this pm.						
13.							
14.	Anesthesiologist will call preop meds.						
15.							

FIGURE 5-10 Sample care plan.

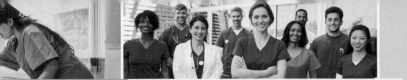

Classification of Disease

OBJECTIVES

After completing this chapter, you will be able to:

6.1 Spell and define terms.

6.2 Define disease and list some possible causes.

6.3 Distinguish between signs and symptoms.

6.4 List six major health problems.

6.5 Identify disease-related terms.

6.6 List ways in which a diagnosis is made.

6.7 Describe malignant and benign tumors.

VOCABULARY

Learn the meaning and the correct spelling of the following words and phrases:

acute disease
acute exacerbation
alternative
antibodies
autoimmune
benign
cachexia
carcinoma
chronic disease

complication
congenital
etiology
genetic
hypersensitivity
immune response
infection
inflammation
invasive

ischemia
malignant
medical diagnosis
metastasize
neoplasm
noninvasive
obstruction
predisposing factor
prognosis

protocol
risk factor
sarcoma
sign
symptom
therapy
trauma
tumor
vaccine

INTRODUCTION

The nurse uses and values your observations when making assessments and planning care as part of the nursing process. The information you provide will be more accurate if you understand the basic principles of disease.

DISEASE

The body is a complex chemical factory that depends on all of its parts to perform efficiently. It is subject to external and internal forces and stress that can interfere with normal function.

Disease is any change from a healthy state. The disease (illness) may be a change in structure or function, or it may be failure of a part of the body to develop properly. Each illness has:

- An **etiology**—cause of the illness or abnormality.
- A usual set of indications that the illness is in progress. These are called signs and symptoms.
- A usual *course*—the way in which the disease progresses.
- A **prognosis** or probable outcome of the process.

Predisposing factors to disease are general conditions, such as malnutrition, that may allow or contribute to the development of illness. Some diseases have related risk factors. **Risk factors** are conditions, behaviors, or circumstances that raise the possibility that a problem may develop or the patient's health will worsen. For example, smoking is a risk factor that increases the likelihood that a person will develop lung disease. Other risk factors and associated diseases include:

- Excess weight—high blood pressure, stroke, heart attack, diabetes (Figure 6-1)
- Poor nutrition—infection, skin breakdown
- Lack of exercise—osteoporosis
- High-fat, low-fiber diet—cancer of the colon
- Unprotected sex—hepatitis, AIDS, gonorrhea, syphilis (Figure 6-2)
- Family history—breast cancer, heart disease, diabetes mellitus
- Aging changes in the body

A young child who is malnourished and underweight is much more likely to develop an infection than one who is well nourished. The germs causing the infection are the actual cause of the illness, but the age and nutritional state of the child (risk factors) contribute to the development of the infectious process. Table 6-1 lists common causes of disease (both external and internal) and a number of risk factors for disease.

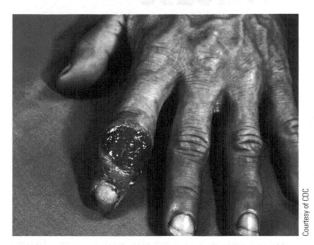

Courtesy of CDC

FIGURE 6-2 This patient has a painless chancre sore on the left index finger caused by syphilis. Although it is most common on the genital area, this is where the infection entered the body. A chancre will heal in three to six weeks but if not treated, the infection will progress to the secondary stage.

TABLE 6-1 Common Causes of Disease and Predisposing Factors

External Etiology	Internal Etiology	Predisposing Factors
Traumas	Metabolic disorders	Age
Radiation	Congenital abnormalities	Malnutrition
Microorganisms	Tumors	Heredity
Chemical agents		Previous illness

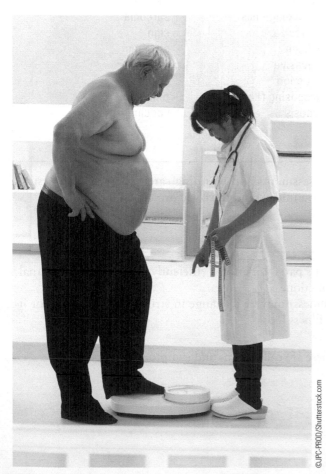

©JPC-PROD/Shutterstock.com

FIGURE 6-1 Many serious risk factors are associated with being overweight.

👪 Age-Appropriate Care **ALERT**

As a nursing assistant, you will be caring for patients of all ages. You must learn how to provide age-appropriate care to each age group. This means that you will meet the patient's age-related needs for communication, safety and security, and personal care and comfort. You will find that these measures vary slightly for each age group. Avoid treating adults as children, or children as adults. Meet each patient on their own level.

Signs and Symptoms

Signs of a disease can be identified by persons other than the patient. The color or condition of the skin is an example of a sign of disease (Figure 6-3). **Symptoms** are felt by the patient, who tells us about them. Pain is a symptom of many diseases.

The Course (Pattern) of Disease

The development and course of different illnesses vary greatly. **Acute disease** develops suddenly, progresses rapidly, and lasts for a predictable period, and then the person recovers (or dies). For example, the signs and symptoms of an infected finger may develop rapidly and last a relatively short period. Then, as the body controls the process, recovery is seen.

A person with a **chronic disease** will have periods when they experience signs and symptoms and periods when they seem to improve. During these times, evidence of the disease is less pronounced or disappears altogether. Rheumatoid arthritis (Figure 6-4A) and gout (Figure 6-4B) are examples of such diseases. At times the affected joints are red, hot to the touch, swollen, and painful. At other times, the signs and symptoms seem to go away. An **acute exacerbation** of a chronic disease is when the severity of signs and symptoms increases.

Complications

A **complication** makes the original condition more serious. For example, if a child who has measles also develops pneumonia (a serious lung infection), the pneumonia is a complication that makes it more difficult for the child to recover.

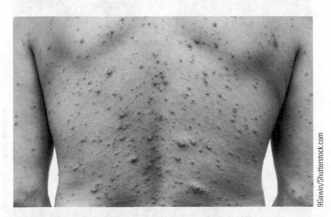

FIGURE 6-3 This patient has chickenpox. The blisters, which are itchy, will scab over in approximately a week. The condition is no longer contagious when all the lesions have scabbed over.

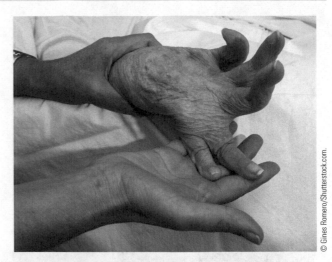

FIGURE 6-4A Rheumatoid arthritis is very painful and causes visible deformities.

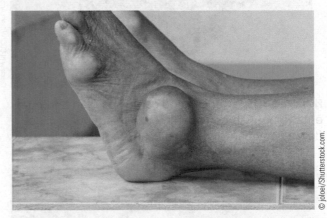

FIGURE 6-4B The first sign of gout is usually a bright red color on or near the big toe. Exacerbations and remissions are common with this painful condition.

MAJOR CONDITIONS

Some major conditions or illnesses that can affect the body's ability to function are:

- **Ischemia**—the lack of adequate blood supply to a body tissue, which prevents delivery of essential oxygen and nutrients (Figure 6-5). For example, a blood clot (thrombus) that has formed within a blood vessel wall can block the blood vessel.

Legal **ALERT**

Reporting and recording your observations are key nursing assistant responsibilities. Pay attention to details. Practice good communication skills. You will learn which observations must be reported immediately, and which can wait until the end of the shift. An alert, observant nursing assistant is invaluable in protecting patients' safety and well-being.

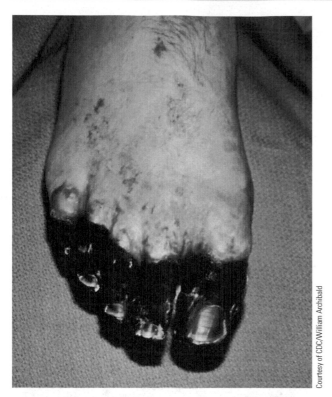

Courtesy of CDC/William Archibald

FIGURE 6-5 The arterial blood carries oxygen and nutrients to nourish body parts. Lack of adequate blood flow to any part of the body causes tissue death.

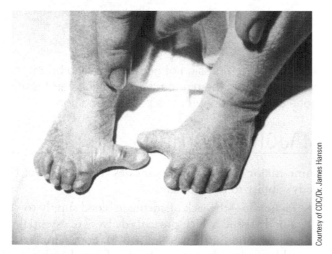

Courtesy of CDC/Dr. James Hanson

FIGURE 6-6 This infant was born with polydactyly which is an extra digit as shown on both feet. This condition can be helped with surgery.

- **Congenital** abnormalities—abnormalities that are present at birth (Figure 6-6). Some abnormalities occur while the baby is growing in the mother's uterus. Examples include:
  - Spina bifida—a birth defect in the spine and spinal vertebrae
  - Cleft lip—an imperfection in the formation of the upper lip

- **Genetic** abnormalities are due to defects in the information passed from the parents to the child. Examples include:
  - Sickle cell anemia—the red blood cells are improperly formed and take on a crescent shape.
  - Color blindness—the person is unable to distinguish between certain colors (Figure 6-7).
  - Hemophilia—the person lacks an important blood component needed for proper blood clotting.
- **Infection**—Infectious organisms or their products cause infection, including pneumonias, colds, measles, mumps, chickenpox, and abscesses. Inflammation is usually part of the infectious process.
- **Inflammation** is a localized protective reaction of tissue to irritation, injury, or infection (Figure 6-8).

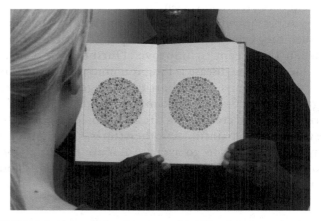

FIGURE 6-7 About 8% of men and 0.5% of women in the United States are color blind. This is the inability to see specific colors, the most common being red and green. Some people with color blindness cannot see the colors blue and yellow. A small number of people have a complete absence of seeing color. Testing for color blindness is done by reading numbers in a series of diagrams.

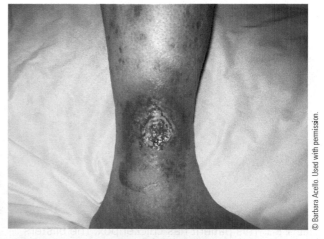

© Barbara Acello. Used with permission.

FIGURE 6-8 The red area surrounding this infected wound is hot to the touch and very painful. The redness is a good example of inflammation.

It is characterized by pain, redness, swelling, a feeling of heat on the skin, and loss of function. Inflammations that develop for reasons other than infection include:

- **Autoimmune** reactions—The body's protective mechanisms turn against the body and cause damage, resulting in conditions such as rheumatoid arthritis, systemic lupus erythematosus, and multiple sclerosis
- **Hypersensitivity** reactions—Allergic reactions such as hay fever, skin rashes, and asthma
- Irritations—May be caused by seeds in the intestinal tract, stones in the gallbladder or kidney, or the skin's exposure to chemicals

- Metabolic imbalances—Disturbances in the normal chemical processes in the body that cause conditions such as malnutrition, dehydration, edema, and diabetes mellitus.

- **Obstruction**—Tubes throughout the body carry a variety of materials that must flow continuously. Obstructions block the tubes and impede the flow. Examples of obstructions include blood clots in blood vessels, stones in the bile ducts or the kidneys, and blockages that occur when tubes become twisted, as in an intestinal obstruction.

- **Trauma**—Tissue damage resulting from an injury or blow to the body, such as an auto accident. Exposure to unusual pressure or extremes of temperature also causes trauma.

- Neoplasm—The word **neoplasm** means new growth. It is another term for **tumor**. Neoplasms are an important kind of disease that is usually progressive and uncontrolled. Neoplasms are discussed throughout this book, and you will find an overview of cancer in Chapter 47.

DIAGNOSIS

The **medical diagnosis** (the process of identifying and naming the disease) is made by the physician. To do this, the physician examines the patient; obtains a history of previous illnesses and injuries; reviews the results of the nursing observations, evaluations, and assessments; and carries out various laboratory and diagnostic tests. The physician matches the information to possible diseases, then makes the medical diagnosis.

Diagnostic Studies

Laboratory tests (Figure 6-9) and diagnostic studies give the physician valuable information for identifying the disease and planning treatment. The nursing staff prepares the patient for the tests and cares for the patient after testing is completed. The nursing assistant helps give this care and may be assigned to collect certain specimens.

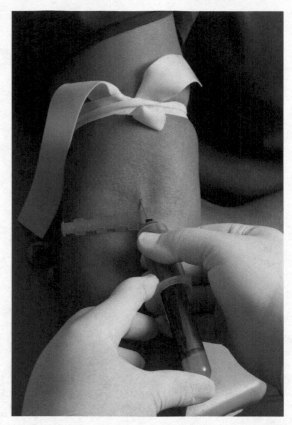

FIGURE 6-9 Performing laboratory tests on a blood sample is one method used to diagnose an illness.

Protocols are procedural standards and standards of care for the preparation and care of the patient for each test or study. For satisfactory results, follow protocols carefully. Improper preparation can result in:

- Inability to perform the test
- Inaccurate test results
- Inaccurate diagnosis
- Erroneous treatment
- Delayed diagnosis
- Increased costs
- Increased patient anxiety, pain, or discomfort
- Slower recovery

Noninvasive Tests

Some tests and studies are **noninvasive**. They do not break the skin or damage body tissues. For example, X-rays do not break the skin, but they do provide information about the inside of the body. Other common noninvasive tests include:

- Ultrasound—sound waves are bounced against the body to measure variations in tissue density (Figure 6-10). For example, a Doppler ultrasound probe measures the blood flow in blood vessels. Sonograms of a pregnant woman's uterus give information about the growing fetus.

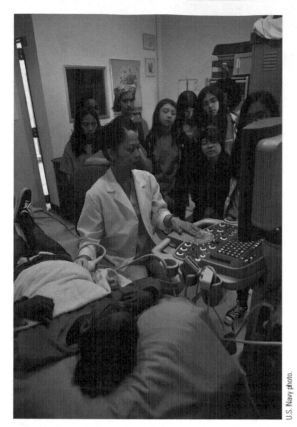

FIGURE 6-10 Ultrasound is used to identify harmful conditions inside the body. A technician at the U.S. Naval Hospital demonstrates how ultrasound equipment is used to a group of middle school students.

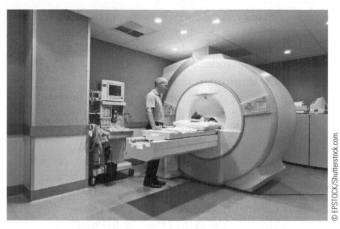

FIGURE 6-11 The *Magnetic resonance imaging (MRI)* uses a magnetic field to make pictures of the inside of the body.

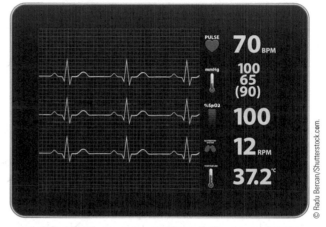

FIGURE 6-12 An electrocardiogram records electrical activity of the heart.

- Thermography—measures the temperature in body tissues. For example, thermograms of the breast indicate increased temperature in tumorous tissue.
- X-ray and fluoroscopy—use short-wavelength radiation to examine internal tissues. X-ray techniques are very advanced. Computerized axial tomography (CT scan or CAT scan) is an accurate procedure that provides a three-dimensional view of the internal structures of the body. A computer records and prints out information and images.

   Fluoroscopy is used to study and evaluate moving body organs such as the kidneys, heart, and lungs in many different types of exams and procedures. It also makes it possible to visualize the muscles, joints, and bones. A continuous X-ray beam passes through the parts being examined to a monitor so that motion can be seen in detail.
- Magnetic resonance imaging (MRI)—is an imaging technique that provides excellent pictures (images) of internal structures by use of radio waves (Figure 6-11). The body is placed in a strong magnetic field, which causes certain chemicals (ions) in body tissues to change position. The ions return to their original positions when the radio waves are turned off. The energy given off is recorded as the frequency returns to normal. The patient is unaware of this, does not feel the activity, and is not harmed.
- Recording of the electrical activity occurring in different body organs—is done on paper or on a screen for viewing. Such examinations include:
  - Electrocardiography (EKG or ECG)—records electrical activity of the cardiac cycle (Figure 6-12). This is further described in Chapter 40 of this book.
  - Electroencephalography (EEG)—records electrical activity of the brain.
  - Electromyography (EMG)—records electrical activity of muscles.

Invasive Tests

Some tests and studies require entry into the body and thus are known as **invasive** tests. Examples include taking tissue samples, introducing dye (contrast media), and probing deeply into body cavities.

A *sternal puncture* is a procedure in which a needle is used to draw a sample of blood-producing cells from the sternum. Iodine dyes, barium compounds, or air may be introduced into the body to produce contrast when making recordings and pictures.

Most invasive techniques are carried out in special areas, such as procedure rooms and laboratories that are designed for this purpose. Laboratories also examine patient specimens.

Other Techniques

Body tissues, secretions, excretions, and fluids are examined using chemical and microscopic studies. Invasive procedures are required to get some samples. Other sampling requires noninvasive procedures. The most common samples are:

- Blood
- Urine
- Sputum from the lungs
- Cultures from infected tissues
- Gastric secretions
- Feces (Figure 6-13)

Follow the instructions for collecting and storing any specimens you collect. As a rule, take specimens to the laboratory immediately. Specimens that remain on the unit usually need refrigeration. Make certain that the patient's name and other identifying information are on the collection container and laboratory requisition slip. You will find additional information in subsequent chapters of your book.

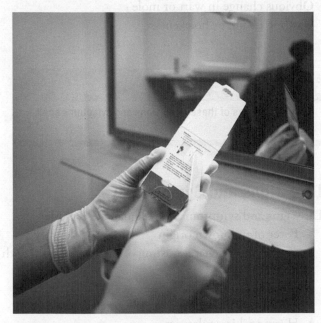

FIGURE 6-13 Testing stool specimens provides useful information about the gastrointestinal tract. This nursing assistant is testing the stool for blood that cannot be seen with the eyes.

THERAPY

Once the medical diagnosis is confirmed, the physician can predict the course of the disease and a probable prognosis (likely outcome). Then the physician decides on the best type of **therapy** (treatment).

There are four basic types of therapy. They may be used alone or in different combinations.

- Surgery—may remove unhealthy tissue, replace unhealthy parts, or repair injured, malformed, or defective areas. Prostatectomies remove unhealthy prostate glands. Coronary bypasses replace blocked arteries with other arteries.
- Chemotherapy—uses drugs and chemicals to improve body functions and control pain (Figure 6-14). For example, the patient with a fever is given a drug, such as acetaminophen (Tylenol), to reduce the temperature.
- Radiation—uses controlled radio waves or X-rays to destroy tumor cells.
- Supportive (palliative) care—is designed to keep the person healthy or support the patient's body in its attempt to return to health. For example, positioning a person upright makes it easier for them to breathe during an asthma attack. Pain control, rest, proper nutrition, fluid intake, and good hygiene all aid the body's own attempts to control the effects of illness.

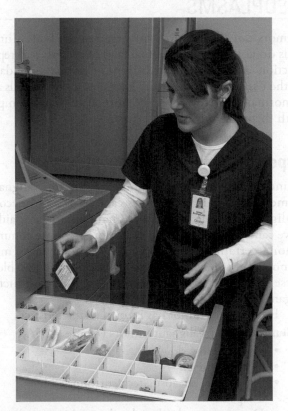

FIGURE 6-14 The nursing assistant reports the patient's problem to the nurse, who will use the nursing process to further assess the patient and provide medication, if indicated.

ALTERNATIVES TO MAINSTREAM HEALTH CARE

When most people in Western society think of medical care, they think of medical, surgical, pharmaceutical, and technological treatment of patients. In the United States, these are the accepted, traditional approaches to patient care and healing of illness; they constitute mainstream health care. Throughout history, people have used other means of healing the sick. Egyptian society used very advanced medical practices. Native American tribes had medicine men. These practices were considered mainstream before twentieth-century advances in medicine.

Today, some people prefer natural and spiritual treatments for illness. Others are afraid of the technology, drugs, and surgical procedures of today. Because of this, many people use **alternative** health care practices and products to prevent and treat illness. Alternatives are options to regular health care. Alternative therapies are used to treat every imaginable symptom and condition. Some people use alternatives to prevent illness. Others use alternative practices in addition to medical treatment. For safety, an alternative program should be supervised by a physician. Refer to Chapter 37 for additional information on alternative and complementary therapies.

NEOPLASMS

Tumors can affect almost any organ of the body. Tumor cells do not follow the normal laws of growth and reproduction, and may not stay within the normal boundaries of the tissue they come from. Excess numbers of cells and abnormal cells crowd out the normal cells and compete with them for nutrients.

Types of Tumors

Tumors can be benign (nonmalignant) or malignant. Some types of benign tumors can change and become malignant. People with a malignant tumor are said to have cancer. Different types of tumors are more common among certain groups of people. Children have more tumors of the nervous system, urinary system, and blood vessels. Adults have more tumors of the reproductive organs, lungs, and colon.

Each type of tumor has its own characteristics.

Benign or nonmalignant tumors (Figure 6-15A):
- Usually grow slowly.
- Do not spread.
- Are usually encapsulated (surrounded by a capsule).
- Do not cause death unless located in a vital area such as the brain.

- Are usually named by stating the part of the body involved and adding the suffix *-oma*. For example, *osteoma* names a benign bone tumor.

Malignant tumors or cancerous growths (Figure 6-15B):
- Grow relatively rapidly.
- Spread to other body parts (**metastasize**).
- If untreated, cause death.
- May be named sarcoma or carcinoma or have special names like leukemia or Hodgkin's disease or lymphoma.
- **Carcinomas** (Figure 6-15C) are spread primarily by way of the lymph nodes. They occur more commonly in people older than 40 years of age.
- **Sarcomas** (Figure 6-15D) are spread primarily by way of the bloodstream. They occur more commonly in people younger than 40 years of age.

Early Detection

Early detection of cancer may result in a cure. The sooner the cancer is found, the higher the rate of cure. Pain is usually a late symptom.

Early Signs and Symptoms

Early signs and symptoms of malignancies include:

Change in bowel or bladder habits
A sore that does not heal
Unusual bleeding or discharge
Thickening or lump in breast or elsewhere
Indigestion or difficulty in swallowing
Obvious change in wart or mole
Nagging cough or hoarseness

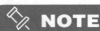

> **NOTE**
>
> The first letters of these early signs and symptoms spell **CAUTION**.

Late Signs and Symptoms

Late signs and symptoms of malignancies include:
- Fever of unknown origin
- **Cachexia** or general wasting of the body tissues with loss of weight
- Anemia
- Pain due to pressure, obstruction, and ischemia
- Hormonal irregularities
- Inflammations of the skin

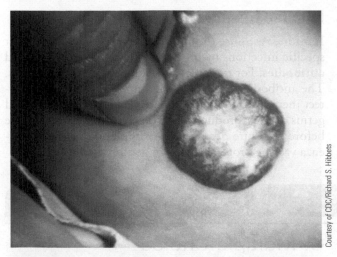

FIGURE 6-15A This is a strawberry hemangioma, a benign tumor that originates from cells that line blood vessels.

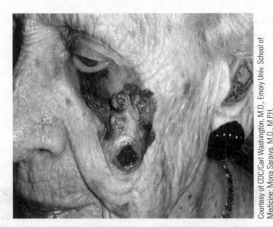

FIGURE 6-15B This irregularly shaped ulceration was diagnosed as malignant melanoma, a dangerous skin cancer that is usually the result of too much sun exposure.

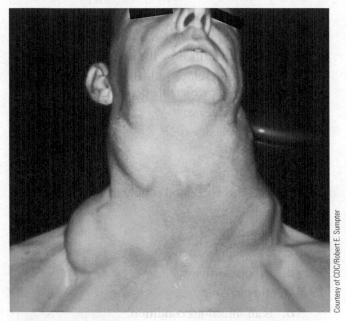

FIGURE 6-15C This patient has enlarged lymph nodes caused by Hodgkin's lymphoma or Hodgkin's disease which is a cancer of the immune system.

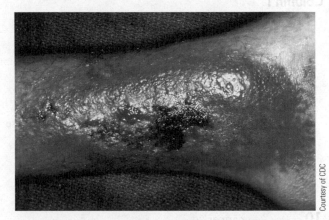

FIGURE 6-15D A Kaposi's sarcoma lesion is often mistaken for a venous leg ulcer.

- White blood cells, which surround and destroy foreign matter that enters the body
- Inflammation
- The immune response

BODY DEFENSES

The body has a natural line of defense against disease. Defenses include:

- Unbroken skin and mucous membranes, which act as mechanical barriers
- Mucus, which traps foreign particles, and cilia (small hairlike structures), which propel them out of the body
- The acidity of certain body secretions such as perspiration, saliva, and stomach juices, which slow the growth of microorganisms

Inflammation

The process of inflammation (which causes boils and abscesses) is an important part of the body's natural defenses. When anything foreign enters the body, small blood vessels (capillaries) in the area get bigger (dilate), bringing more blood to the infected part. The blood contains white blood cells and other protective substances. Fluid (serum) and white blood cells pass through the capillary walls into the area, gradually building a wall around the foreign object. The white blood cells try to destroy the invader, increasing pressure and forcing the material to the surface of the body. The inflammatory process takes place whenever injury occurs. The signs and symptoms of acute inflammation are:

- Redness
- Swelling
- Heat
- Loss of function
- Pressure
- Pain

Immune Response

Immune response (immunity) protects the body against specific infections by producing special chemicals called **antibodies**. For example, a person contracts the measles. The antibodies formed by the immune system will protect them from catching measles again. **Vaccines** (altered germs or their products) may be given to prevent disease before exposure occurs. For example, taking the influenza vaccine protects you from getting the flu.

REVIEW

A. Matching

Match the terms in Column II with the definitions in Column I.

Column I

1. _____ probable outcome
2. _____ color of the skin
3. _____ cause of disease
4. _____ noncancerous tumor
5. _____ pain as reported by the patient
6. _____ illness with sudden onset and short course
7. _____ injury
8. _____ inflammation
9. _____ condition transmitted from one generation to another
10. _____ cancer

Column II

- **a.** acute
- **b.** benign
- **c.** a natural body defense
- **d.** etiology
- **e.** genetic
- **f.** malignancy
- **g.** prognosis
- **h.** sign
- **i.** symptom
- **j.** trauma

B. Fill-In

For each of the items in questions 11–15, mark which is a sign and which is a symptom.

11. _____ dry, flushed skin
12. _____ nausea
13. _____ dizziness
14. _____ rapid pulse
15. _____ elevated temperature

C. Multiple Choice

Select the best answer for each of the following.

16. Signs of illness:
    - **a.** cannot be identified by nursing personnel.
    - **b.** are the patient's personal business.
    - **c.** are not important to a nursing assistant.
    - **d.** can be identified by the nursing assistant.

17. Disease that develops suddenly, progresses rapidly, and lasts for a predictable period is:
    - **a.** chronic disease.
    - **b.** neoplastic disease.
    - **c.** acute disease.
    - **d.** genetic disease.

18. Lack of adequate blood supply to a body part is:
    - **a.** ischemia.
    - **b.** infectious.
    - **c.** congenital.
    - **d.** hypersensitivity.

19. An obstruction:
    - **a.** is an infectious condition.
    - **b.** blocks flow of fluid in the body.
    - **c.** causes hypersensitivity.
    - **d.** is an autoimmune response.

20. Inflammation is:
    - **a.** a genetic condition.
    - **b.** nothing to worry about.
    - **c.** a localized protective response.
    - **d.** always the result of an infection.

21. Disturbances in the normal chemical processes in the body are:
    - **a.** genetic conditions.
    - **b.** hypersensitivity reactions.
    - **c.** traumatic responses.
    - **d.** metabolic imbalances.

22. A noninvasive test:

  a. may cut or burn the skin.

  b. penetrates internal structures.

  c. does not break the skin.

  d. withdraws fluid with a needle.

23. A protective mechanism that helps the body prevent infection is:

  a. immunity.

  b. trauma.

  c. radiation.

  d. ultrasound.

24. A malignancy:

  a. does not spread or grow.

  b. grows and spreads rapidly.

  c. is filled with pus.

  d. is not cancerous.

25. An autoimmune reaction occurs when:

  a. the body is fighting an infection.

  b. a noninvasive test is done.

  c. the person is diagnosed with cancer.

  d. the body turns against itself.

D. True/False

Mark the following true or false by circling T or F.

26. T F   The medical diagnosis is made by the supervising nurse.

27. T F   Nursing assistants may be assigned to collect certain specimens.

28. T F   Protocols are drugs given in diagnostic testing.

29. T F   Proper patient preparation contributes to the success of diagnostic testing.

30. T F   Improper patient preparation may cause inaccurate test results.

31. T F   Ultrasound provides information about a growing fetus.

32. T F   Thermography uses radio waves to test the electrical current of tissues.

33. T F   An upper GI series is an X-ray of the gallbladder.

34. T F   Nursing assistants may be asked to deliver specimens.

35. T F   Nursing assistants may contribute to the diagnostic testing process by offering emotional support to the patient.

E. Completion

Write out the early signs of possible malignancies.

36. C _____

37. A _____

38. U _____

39. T _____

40. I _____

41. O _____

42. N _____

F. Nursing Assistant Challenge

Read each clinical situation and answer the questions.

43. Your patient is 82 years old, is poorly nourished, and has a diagnosis of pneumonia.

  a. Name two risk factors for pneumonia.

  _____

  b. Will these factors make recovery more or less difficult?

  _____

  c. How would you classify the illness (pneumonia)?

  _____

44. Your patient is six years old and has a broken leg. They also have a condition that they inherited from their parents. This condition makes their bones brittle so they break more easily.

  a. What word would you use to describe their inherited condition?

  _____

  b. What term would you use to classify their inability to make strong bones?

  _____

  c. Do you think this kind of injury might occur often in this patient?

  _____

45. Your patient is 45 years old, is 40 pounds overweight, and gets little exercise. Their diagnosis is high blood pressure. They are scheduled for an ECG.

  a. What factors might contribute to their diagnosis?

  _____

  b. For what conditions are they at risk?

  _____

  c. What information will the ECG provide?

  _____

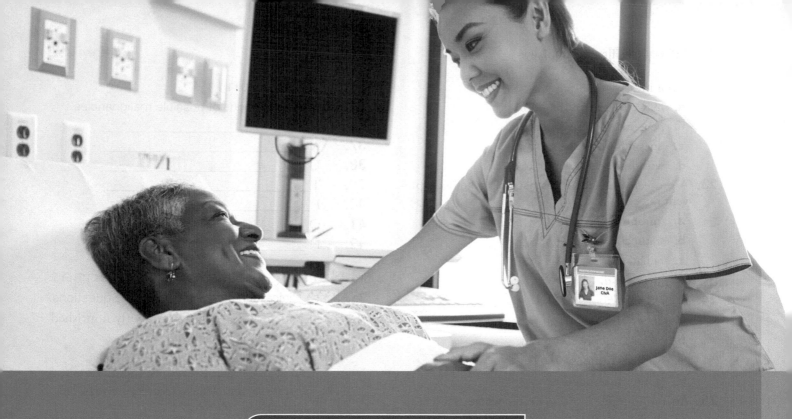

SECTION 3

Basic Human Needs and Communication

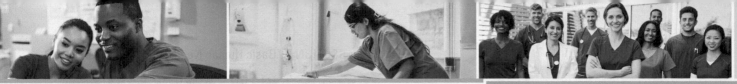

Communication Skills

OBJECTIVES

After completing this chapter, you will be able to:

7.1 Spell and define terms.

7.2 Explain types of verbal and nonverbal communication.

7.3 Demonstrate how to answer the telephone while on duty.

7.4 Describe four tools of communication for staff members.

7.5 Describe the guidelines for communicating with patients who have hearing loss.

7.6 Describe the guidelines for communicating with patients with impaired vision.

7.7 Describe the guidelines for communicating with patients with aphasia.

7.8 Describe the guidelines for communicating with patients with disorientation.

7.9 State the guidelines for working with interpreters.

VOCABULARY

Learn the meaning and the correct spelling of the following words and phrases:

aphasia	ethnic	message	sign language
body language	feedback	nonverbal communication	staff development
braille	interpreter	paraphrasing	symbols
communication	medical chart	receiver	verbal communication
disorientation	memo	sender	

INTRODUCTION

Communication is a two-way process in which we share information. We communicate orally, in writing, and through body language. Electronic communication is a relatively new means of sharing information. It may also be done orally or by using the written word. Nursing assistants communicate with their patients, with visitors, with their co-workers, and with their supervisors when they are working. As a nursing assistant, you will need to receive and send information about your:

- Observations and care of patients.
- Interactions with patients and visitors.
- Patients' feelings, problems, and complaints.

This information is received and sent through the process of communication.

Elements of Communication

Understanding the elements of communication will help you communicate effectively. Each message has four parts (Figure 7-1):

- **Sender**—the person who originates the communication
- **Message**—the information the sender wants to communicate
- **Receiver**—the person for whom the communication is intended
- **Feedback**—confirmation that the message was received as intended and understood

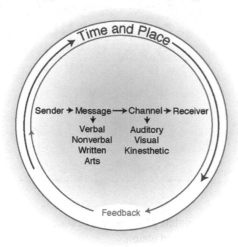

FIGURE 7-1 Nursing assistants communicate with patients in many different ways. However, all messages have a sender, a message, and a receiver. Giving feedback ensures that the message was received as intended

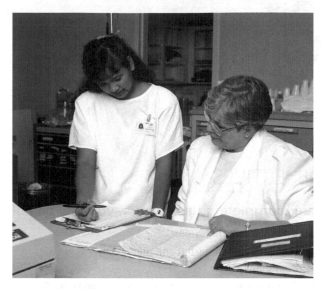

FIGURE 7-2 Verbal communication is the most common way of reporting observations to the nurse. In some cases, you may also provide written information, such as a piece of paper listing a patient's vital signs, intake and output measurements, height and weight, or amount of food consumed.

The *channel* is the medium through which the message is sent. Feedback may be verbal or nonverbal. An example of verbal feedback is asking a question or making a comment in response. An example of nonverbal feedback is a nod of the head, waving the hand, or some other movement indicating understanding.

COMMUNICATION IN HEALTH CARE

Communication between staff members must be effective if patients are to receive the safest and best care. Communication with patients and their visitors is also important. You and your patients must understand each other.

Verbal Communication

Words are used for **verbal communication**. They may be spoken or written. Written communication also depends on the use of **symbols**. Traffic signs are an example of symbols. You will use words to explain to a patient what you plan to do in carrying out a procedure and how the patient can help. You may also demonstrate nonverbally by using your hands or moving your body. The nurse will use words to explain your assignment. You will use words to report your observations (Figure 7-2), as well use words for written communication in your charting. You will use words to answer visitors' questions. Choose words carefully so that your message is clear. Avoid using slang. Whenever possible, avoid words that have the

same sound but a same or different spelling and a different meaning. These words are easily confused, such as:

* Pair (a couple, two) versus pear (a fruit).
* Fair (an event such as a state or county fair, or an activity like a health fair) versus fare (payment for something, such as bus fare or taxi fare).
* Lead (a metal object) versus led (guided).
* Accept (receive, take, obtain) versus except (excluding, omitting, leaving out).

Use words that the receiver is likely to be familiar with, particularly if this person's first language is not English. Speak slowly and clearly. Look at the receiver when speaking.

Paraphrasing

Paraphrasing is an effective method of showing that you understand what the speaker has said. When using paraphrasing, restate your understanding of what was said. Listening to the message and paraphrasing provide feedback and show that you are interested. Tone of voice, choice of words, and hand movements give clues to the real meaning of the message. Listen carefully to the message and watch the sender's facial expressions and body language.

Nonverbal Communication

Nonverbal communication is a message that is sent through the use of one's body, rather than through

Your message is:
7% words + 38% tone of voice
+ 55% body language
= Total Communication

FIGURE 7-3 Make eye contact during communication. Your body language should match the tone, pitch, and quality of your voice.

speech or writing. This kind of communication, called **body language**, can tell you a great deal. Nonverbal messages send even stronger signals than verbal messages.

When speaking with others, always remember the impact of nonverbal communication (Figure 7-3). Your words represent only 7 percent of your message. The remainder of the message is conveyed and interpreted through facial expressions, gestures, and overall body language. Your tone of voice represents 38 percent of the meaning. If the tone and pitch of your voice contradict the spoken words, the tone and pitch will overshadow the message. Be aware of the effect that the tone, pitch, and quality of your voice have on the way your message is interpreted. Gestures, facial expressions, and other body language represent 55 percent of your total communication.

Eye Contact

Eye contact makes the biggest impression and will be remembered best. You create a positive atmosphere by looking at the other person. In North America, eye contact is very important to communication. This is not true in all cultures. Be sensitive to cultural differences of patients and co-workers. Making eye contact can open communication channels and create a bond between two people. During conversation, eye contact communicates interest, concern, warmth, trust, feelings, and credibility. Eye contact can send many different messages.

Other Types of Nonverbal Communication

A patient who is in pain may protect the affected area. Tears may be a sign of depression. Some of the other ways your patients may "talk" to you through their body language include:

- Posture
- Hand and body movements
- Activity level
- Facial expressions
- Overall appearance
- Body position

OTHER METHODS OF COMMUNICATION

In Chapter 2 you learned that each health care facility has a line of authority for communication. In this chapter you will learn about other types of communication.

Answering the Telephone

Many telephone calls come into a health care facility. Families call to inquire about the condition of their loved ones. Physicians call to leave new medical orders. The laboratory may call to give test results. Nursing assistants are not allowed to take physicians' orders, to accept calls reporting results of diagnostic tests, or to give information to families. You must call the nurse to do this. If you answer the telephone:

- Smile! The caller will hear the difference if you "put a smile" in your voice (Figure 7-4).
- Identify the nursing unit: "third floor, north," for example.
- Identify yourself and your position: "Mary Smith, nursing assistant," for example.
- Ask the caller's name and ask the caller to wait while you locate the person requested or who can answer the caller's question.
- If the person requested by the caller is unavailable, take a message (Figure 7-5) and write down the following information:
  - Date and time of call
  - Caller's name and telephone number
  - Message left by caller
  - Whether the person is to return the call or whether the caller will telephone again later
  - Your signature

Some facilities have more complex telephone systems. You will be taught how to transfer calls or to

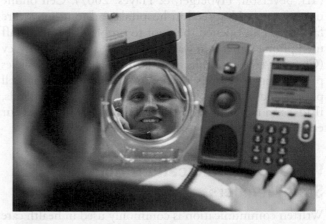

FIGURE 7-4 The caller will hear the smile in your voice!

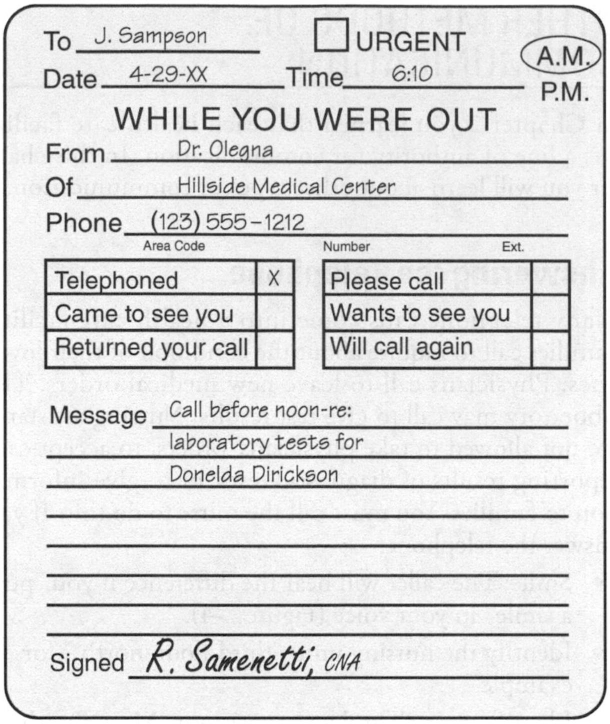

To J. Sampson   ☐ URGENT   A.M.
Date 4-29-XX   Time 6:10   P.M.

WHILE YOU WERE OUT

From Dr. Olegna
Of Hillside Medical Center
Phone (123) 555-1212
    Area Code   Number   Ext.

Telephoned	X	Please call	
Came to see you		Wants to see you	
Returned your call		Will call again	

Message Call before noon-re:
laboratory tests for
Donelda Dirickson

Signed *R. Samenetti, CNA*

FIGURE 7-5 Write an accurate and legible message and take it to the proper person. Do not leave it on a desk and assume it will be found.

voice-page. Most facilities do not allow employees to make or receive personal telephone calls while they are on duty, except in an emergency.

Cellular Telephones

In years past, cell phones were prohibited in health care facilities because they were believed to interfere with medical equipment. A 2007 Mayo Clinic study disproved this long-held theory and confirmed that normal cell phone use does not interfere with medical equipment (Tri, Severson, Hyberger, & Hayes, 2007). Cell phone use became widespread in hospitals and long-term care facilities. This opened the door to problems because staff used phone cameras in ways that violated patients' privacy (Chapter 4). As a result, most facilities developed policies prohibiting or severely restricting the use of personal cell phones and other wireless handheld devices, such as iPods, iPads, and tablets. Become familiar with and follow your employer's policies for wireless handheld devices.

Written Communications Among Staff Members

Written communication is commonly used in health care facilities. The ability to accurately read such communication is essential to providing patient care.

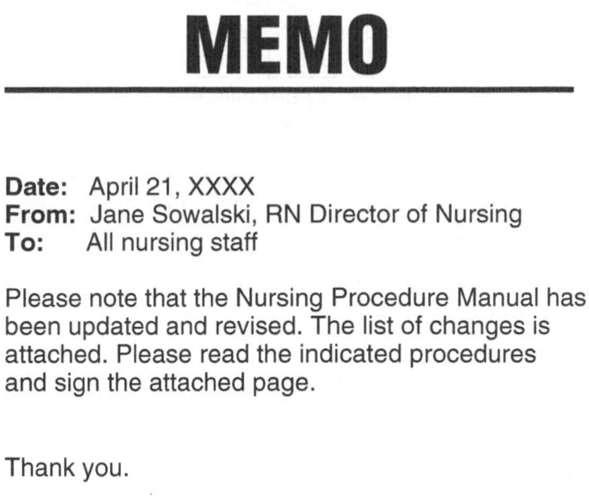

MEMO

Date: April 21, XXXX
From: Jane Sowalski, RN Director of Nursing
To: All nursing staff

Please note that the Nursing Procedure Manual has been updated and revised. The list of changes is attached. Please read the indicated procedures and sign the attached page.

Thank you.

FIGURE 7-6 Memos provide important information.

Memos

A **memo** (Figure 7-6) is a brief communication that informs or reminds employees of:

- Changes in policies or procedures
- Upcoming meetings or staff development programs
- Admission of new patients
- Promotions of staff members

Some facilities post memos immediately after your sign-on page in the computer. Others distribute memos in envelopes with paychecks. The latter method is much less popular because automatic deposit is being used by many facilities so that paychecks are deposited directly to your bank account.

Be sure you know where memos are posted so that you will be aware of the facility activities.

INTRANET MANUALS

The *intranet* is a private, password-protected internal communications network that uses World Wide Web software. Having everything online makes finding information quick and convenient. Become familiar with the procedures for accessing these materials.

Electronic documentation has become the norm in most facilities. This has affected the system for accessing facility manuals and other reference information. Although some paper manuals may be available, most facilities have added nursing manuals and nursing reference books to their intranet system, and they are available on every nursing computer.

Manuals

All facilities have reference manuals describing various policies and procedures (Figure 7-7). These may include:

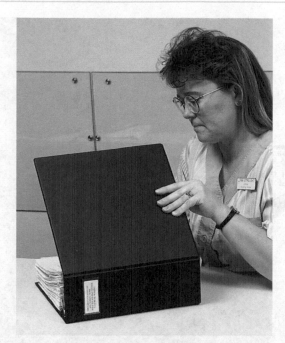

FIGURE 7-7 Manuals are an important source of information. Some facilities use printed manuals, some have electronic manuals, and many facilities have a combination of both. Become familiar with your facility's manuals and where to locate the information you need.

- Employee personnel handbook—describes all personnel policies and benefits.
- Safety and disaster manual—gives directions for actions to take in case of fire or other disasters.
- Procedure manual—gives directions on how procedures should be performed for patients.
- Nursing policy manual—describes rules and regulations pertaining to the care of patients. Sometimes this is combined with policies that affect nursing, so it is called a policy and procedure (P&P) manual.

⚖ **Legal ALERT**

Becoming familiar with the location and contents of facility policy and procedure manuals will help you do your job and practice within your scope of responsibility, within the limits of the law. Always follow the guidelines in these manuals. They may be slightly different from those of other facilities. Following your facility's policies and procedures will ensure that you give good patient care. The manuals will give you instructions for procedures and other facility requirements, and they will reduce your risk of legal exposure.

- Nursing procedure manual—describes steps of the various procedures so you can use them to learn procedures correctly and provide care according to your facility's requirements.
- Infection control manual—describes methods of preventing infection and procedures to follow for patients with known or suspected infection. Following these precautions protects many people, including caregivers, patient, patient's family and visitors, facility visitors, and other facility employees.
- Safety Data Sheet (SDS) manual—contains information on safe use and handling of chemicals and other substances used in the facility.

Your facility may have other types of manuals available, such as restorative care and quality assurance. You are not expected to memorize all the information in these manuals, but you should know where to find the manuals and be able to look up information when you need to.

Staff Development

Staff development is an educational process (Figure 7-8). Classes may be given to inform staff of:

- New rules and regulations
- New procedures, techniques, and information
- Recent research findings and evidence-based practices
- How to use new equipment
- New infection control information—that is, important information that has been released related to viruses, bacteria, and fungi in the past decade

The Patient Care Plan

The interdisciplinary health care team develops an individualized care plan for each patient. You will find more information on care plans in Chapter 8.

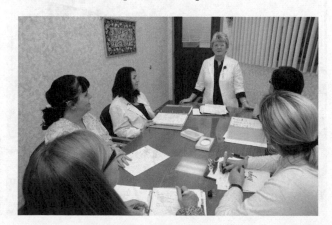

FIGURE 7-8 Attending regular staff development classes helps nursing assistants meet continuing education requirements and learn current information.

The Patient's Medical Chart

Each patient has a **medical chart** or record. The medical chart contains information about the patient, the care given, and the patient's response. It is usually organized by subject. Nursing assistants typically describe activities of daily living (ADL) care given, describing the patient's participation and response. They will also describe the person's dependence versus independence and response to care. Chapter 8 provides more information on the medical record and gives instructions for documenting (making notations) on the patient's chart.

Electronic Methods of Communication

Modern technology has increased opportunities for communication. You will see computers at the nurses' station and throughout the building.

Most facilities have one or more desktop computers at each nurses' station. Computers are used to document patient care, to maintain databases, to communicate with physicians' offices, to transmit payment information, to order supplies, and to maintain records of supplies and equipment.

Some facilities have computers mounted on the wall in every patient room (Figure 7-9A). Nursing staff can document before they leave the bedside. Other facilities use tablets or handheld computers. Some place computers on wheeled carts in the hallways (COW, computer on wheels) (Figure 7-9B). In some facilities, staff wears headsets with microphones. Speaking various commands into the microphone activates the documentation system, and the care given is entered in the patient's computerized medical record.

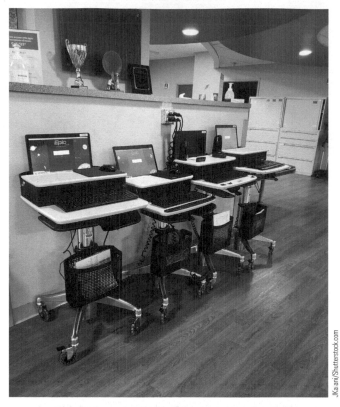

FIGURE 7-9B Computer systems on wheeled carts that can be transported to different locations to document patient care.

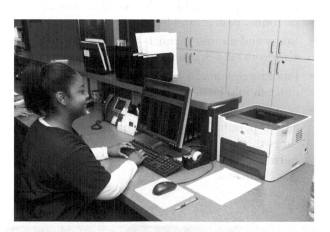

FIGURE 7-9C Most health care facilities depend on computers for data management, patient documentation, and communication.

If you are expected to use a computer, your facility will teach you to document using the medical records program it has selected (Figure 7-9 C).

Fax machines are also used in health care facilities (Figure 7-10). This type of technology uses telephone lines to send and receive information from physicians, laboratories, long-term care facilities, and others.

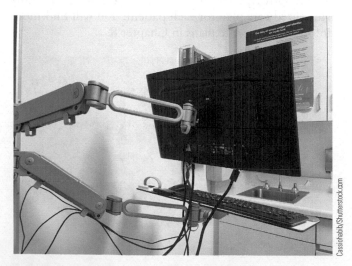

FIGURE 7-9A Computer monitor and keyboard attached to the wall to facilitate documentation in a patient's room.

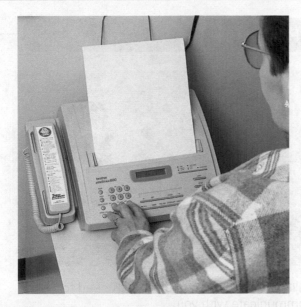

FIGURE 7-10 Fax machines are a convenient means of sending and receiving information. Protect patient privacy with fax transmissions. Do not leave papers on the fax machine. File or shred them when finished.

COMMUNICATING WITH PATIENTS

Your skill in communicating with patients will develop with experience. Remember that your choice of words may be less important to the meaning of the message than your tone of voice, facial expression, and the way you touch the patient. Your goal is to communicate a sense of honest caring to each person. Looking directly at patients as you speak and addressing them respectfully by name are also ways of showing that you care.

Active listening is an important part of communication. Listening actively is a great deal of work that requires more than just being physically present. When you listen actively, all of your attention is focused on the speaker. You maintain eye contact and do not interrupt while the other person is speaking. You ask questions that encourage the speaker to continue. You respond to specific questions your patient asks. Follow these guidelines to communicate effectively with patients.

Culture ALERT

Some cultures value periods of silence during conversation. Allow adequate time. Learn to overcome your personal discomfort with periods of silence.

Communicating with Patients Who Have Special Needs

Communication with patients may be impaired for many reasons. The patient may:

- Have a hearing loss
- Have a vision impairment
- Have aphasia
- Be confused or disoriented
- Be from a culture different from the nursing assistant's

Always check the care plan for special communication needs before attempting to communicate with a patient who has special needs. The care plan should list approaches for all staff to use. Lack of consistency in use of these approaches is confusing and frustrating to the patient.

Communicating with Patients Who Have Hearing Loss

1. Get the patient's attention first.
   - Make sure the patient sees you.
   - Touch the patient lightly to indicate that you wish to speak.
   - Recognize that individuals who are hard of hearing hear less well when they are tired or ill.
2. If the patient uses a hearing aid, be sure that they are wearing it and that the hearing aid is on.
3. If the patient has a "good" ear, stand or sit on that side.
4. Do not chew gum, eat, or cover your mouth while talking.
5. Keep the light behind the patient, so your face can be clearly seen.
6. Face the patient; many people with who are hard-of-hearing can read lips or otherwise interpret your facial expressions.
7. Reduce outside distractions. Speak in a quiet, calm manner.

Communication Highlight

Remember that one of the most important and powerful messages you send to patients is that you care about them. You do this in many ways, including your demeanor when you enter the room, your body language, your tone of voice, and your touch. Verbal communication with some patients will be very limited. Use nonverbal communication to send the message that you care to all patients.

GUIDELINES 7-1 for Communicating with Patients

- Be sure you have the patient's attention.
- Avoid chewing gum, eating, or covering your mouth with your hand when you speak.
- Use nonthreatening words and gestures that the patient is likely to understand.
- Speak clearly and courteously.
- Use a pleasant tone of voice.
- Make eye contact.
- Use appropriate body language.
- Be alert to the patient's need to communicate with you. Allow time for the person to talk and respond. Show interest and concern (Figure 7-11).
- Do not speak about the patient in front of the patient or other patients.
- Do not interrupt the patient.
- Reflect the patient's feelings and thoughts by rewording their statement into questions.
- Ask for clarification if you are unsure of what the patient is saying.
- Give the patient only factual information—not your personal feelings, opinions, or beliefs.
- Information concerning the patient's condition, medications, and treatments should be given by the physician or nurse.

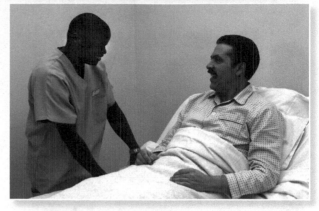

FIGURE 7-11 Recognize the patient's need to communicate with you.

- Do not argue with patients.
- Avoid using slang or cultural terms that are not familiar to the patient, and may be misinterpreted.
- Do not try to provide false reassurance, such as "Everything will be all right." The patient will not trust you when they learn you were not sincere.
- Wait long enough for a reply. Patients who are elderly, hard of hearing, or under the effects of certain medications may take longer to process a message and respond.

8. Start conversations with a key word or phrase so the patient has some clues as to what you are saying (context).
9. Avoid abrupt changes of subject, because your listener who is hard-of-hearing depends heavily on context to understand what you are saying. Also, do not interrupt your conversation with "small talk."
10. Keep your voice pitch low.
11. Speak slowly, distinctly, and naturally.
12. Form words carefully, use familiar words, and keep sentences short.
13. Pronounce words clearly. If a patient who is hard-of-hearing has difficulty with letters and numbers, use language such as "M as in Mary," "2 as in twins," "B as in boy." Say each number separately: "five six" instead of "fifty-six." Remember that *m, n; 2, 3, 56, 66;* and *b, c, d, e, t, v* are groups that sound alike.

14. Rephrase words as needed.
15. Avoid shouting, mouthing, or exaggerating words, or speaking very slowly. This only makes it harder for the patient to understand you.
16. Keep a notepad handy and write your words if the patient does not understand.
17. Use facial expressions, gestures, and body language to help express your meanings.
18. Some patients with who are deaf or hard-of-hearing use **sign language**.
    - Signing depends upon hand and finger movements and facial expressions.
    - This skill requires learning and practice (Figure 7-12).
    - There are different forms of sign language, just as there are different spoken languages.
    - There are some basic signs that may be helpful (Figure 7-13).

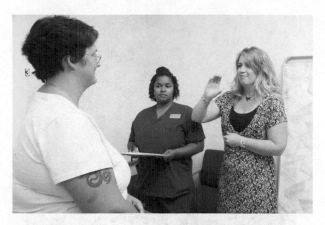

FIGURE 7-12 Learning sign language takes special education and practice.

19. Patients who have had hearing loss for several or more years may have speech that is difficult to understand.

20. Some people with hearing loss are embarrassed or reluctant to tell you when they do not understand you.

21. People who cannot hear may appear confused when they are not.

22. Never walk away, leaving a patient who has a hearing loss wondering what you said and thinking that you do not care. Avoid speaking from another room, when walking away, or with your back turned to the patient.

23. Always inform the patient before leaving the room, and be sure the patient has the call signal and other needed items.

Information and guidelines on caring for patients who use hearing aids are found in Chapter 43.

Communicating with Patients Who Have Visual Impairments

Patients who have visual impairments may have problems communicating because they are unable to see the sender or the sender's facial expressions and body language.

- When approaching a person who is visually impaired, address the person by name and then touch them lightly on the hand or arm to avoid startling them.

- Identify yourself and explain why you are there: "Hello, Mr. Smith. My name is Mary Jones and I would like to take your blood pressure."

- Be specific when giving directions: "I am putting your call light on the right side of your bed."

- When giving directions on how to find an area in the building, tell the patient how many doors they will pass and when to turn right or left.

- When you leave the patient, make sure you announce your departure. "I am leaving your room now. Can I get you anything else?"

- Offer to read mail to patients who are visually impaired.

- If the patient has a telephone, make sure they can use it. The patient can count the numbers or buttons on the number pad to make calls.

- Tactfully inform a person who has a visual impairment if clothing is soiled, mismatched, or in need of repair.

- Encourage the patient to listen to the radio or television to keep up with news and current events.

- If talking-book machines are available, make sure the patient is aware of this. Inform the nurse if the patient wishes to use one.

- Describe the environment and objects around the patient to establish a frame of reference. This helps avoid disorientation. Always ask the patient before changing the location of personal items or furniture.

- Some patients may read **braille**, a system that uses a series of raised dots to represent letters and words (Figure 7-14). The patient reads the letters and words by moving the fingertips over them.

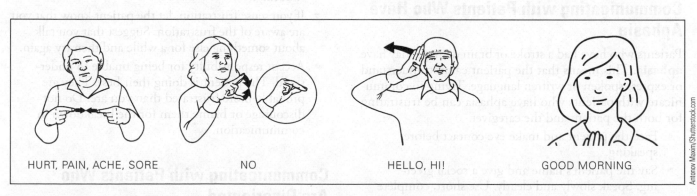

HURT, PAIN, ACHE, SORE   NO   HELLO, HI!   GOOD MORNING

Antonov Maxim/Shutterstock.com

FIGURE 7-13 These basic signs are essential to greetings, simple needs, and good manners. In addition to hand movement, facial expression is also important to sign language. Free videos are available online. Practice in front of a mirror until you master both hand signals and facial expressions. As a hearing person you will find it very useful and rewarding.

a	b	c	d	e	f	g
1	2	3	4	5	6	7

h	i	j	k	l	m	n
8	9	0				

o	p	q	r	s	t	u

v	w	x	y	z	Capital sign	Numeral sign

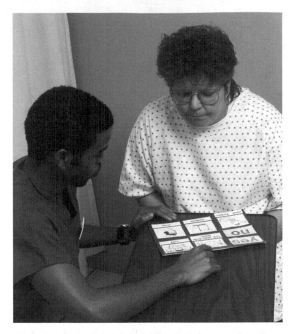

FIGURE 7-15 Patients with aphasia often use special communication boards and cards to make their needs known.

FIGURE 7-14 Many persons with visual impairment read by using braille.

Using the Telephone

The Telecommunications Act of 1996 requires phone companies to ensure that accessible telephones (including smartphones and cell phones) are available for people with hearing loss and visual impairments. Older phones with raised keys and braille phones are also available. If the patient inquires about phone availability, refer them to the social worker or notify the nurse.

Communicating with Patients Who Have Aphasia

Patients who have had a stroke or brain damage may have **aphasia**. This means that the patient cannot understand or express spoken or written language. Trying to communicate with patients who have aphasia can be frustrating for both the patient and the caregiver.

- Face the patient and make eye contact before speaking.
- Say the patient's name and give a social greeting. Speak slowly and clearly. Use short, complete sentences.
- Pause between sentences to allow the patient time to comprehend and interpret what you said.

- Check the patient's understanding. Ask a question based on information you just gave the patient.
- Use nonverbal cues to enhance spoken communication. Use gestures, facial expressions, or pictures.
- Ask questions that require only short responses or that can be answered nonverbally.
- Repeat what the patient just said to help them remain focused.
- Check the care plan to see if the speech therapist has made recommendations for nonverbal communication, such as communication boards or picture cards (Figure 7-15) or books.
- Speak to patients with aphasia even if they do not respond! Speak in a normal tone of voice; avoid shouting.
- If you sense frustration, let the patient know that you are aware of the frustration. Suggest that you talk about something else for a while and then try again.
- Accept responsibility for being unable to understand. The patient is doing their best. They are probably more frustrated than you are. Do not discourage or blame them for the breakdown in communication.

Communicating with Patients Who Are Disoriented

Some patients you care for may be disoriented. **Disorientation** means that the patient is confused about time, place (their physical location), or person who (they are). Disorientation can be caused by Alzheimer disease, stroke, or other disorders or injuries of the brain.

1. Begin the conversation by calling the patient by name and identifying yourself. Do not ask the patient if they remember you.
2. Talk to the patient at eye level and maintain eye contact.
3. Maintain a pleasant facial expression while you are talking and listening.
4. Place a hand on the patient's arm or hand, unless this causes agitation (Figure 7-16).
5. Make sure the patient can hear you. Avoid distractions of noise and activity.
6. Use a lower tone of voice.
7. Use short, common words and short, simple sentences.
8. Give the patient time to respond.
9. Ask only one simple question at a time. If you must repeat it, say it in exactly the same way.
10. Ask the patient to do only one task at a time.
11. Patients with dementia will eventually be unable to comprehend verbal communication.
    • Use pictures, and point, touch, or hand them things.
    • Demonstrate an action when you want them to complete a task.
12. The patient may use word substitutes. If these are consistent, try to find out what they mean. Use them yourself to see if the patient understands you better.

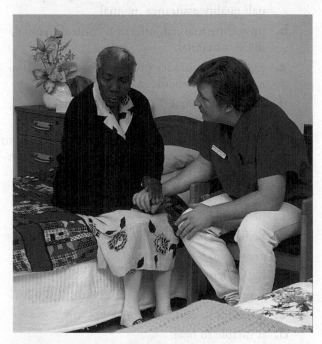

FIGURE 7-16 Gently touching a patient's hand or arm may be comforting.

13. Avoid abstract, common expressions. For example, "You can jump into bed now" may mean just that to the patient.
14. Repeat the patient's last words to help they stay on track.
15. Do not try to force the patient to understand. Avoid lengthy explanations and excessive verbal communication. This tends to agitate most people with dementia.
16. Use nonverbal praise freely and always respect the patient's feelings.

Communicating with Patients from a Different Culture

The persons you care for may come from other countries and have different customs, languages, and traditions. This is because they come from different cultures or have different **ethnic** backgrounds. Their interpretation of body language may be different from your own. For example, in some countries it is considered a sign of disrespect to maintain eye contact when speaking with another person. If you are assigned to someone from a different ethnic background, check the care plan for communication guidelines.

You will find additional information about culturally competent care in Chapter 11.

WORKING WITH INTERPRETERS

Gestures and body language are helpful when communicating, but they are not universal. For example, in the United States, we shake our head up and down to mean yes. We turn the head from side to side to signify no. In some countries gestures are just the opposite. Moving the head from side to side means yes, and shaking it up and down means no. Because of differences in culture and language, there may be times when you need the assistance of a communication professional.

Suggestions for Working with Interpreters

An **interpreter** is a communication professional who mediates between speakers of different languages. Interpretation is an activity that establishes oral or gestural communications between two or more persons who do not speak the same language. Some interpreters speak. Others use sign language to establish communication between a hearing person and a person with a hearing loss.

Facilities will use medical interpreters when they are available in the community. Try to avoid using patients' minor children or grandchildren as interpreters.

This may upset the child or family social order. The child's language skills and social experience may not be well developed in either language, causing inaccurate translation. Some medical subject matter may frighten children. Using a layperson as an interpreter may also cause problems. Persons who are unfamiliar with medical terms and procedures may not be able to interpret them correctly. A qualified interpreter is very familiar with the language, cultural values, beliefs, gestures, body language, and verbal and nonverbal expressions that are used in the languages they are interpreting. As you can see, this is a great responsibility. In health care, the terminology and technical information are complex. Health care interpreters receive special education to ensure that communication is accurate.

 Culture **ALERT**

Patients who are able to speak and read about their care in their native language usually feel more at ease and understand their care better.

The facility is required to furnish interpreters in certain situations, according to federal law. Some facilities use a telephone service for interpreting, so communication is not face to face. This service fills an important need because interpreters are "on call" personnel. The local interpreter may not be quickly available when services are needed.

REVIEW

A. Multiple Choice

Select the best answer for each of the following.

1. Paraphrasing involves:
   a. restating what the speaker said.
   b. keeping the body still when speaking.
   c. using accurate body language.
   d. giving patients the best and safest care.

2. Verbal communication includes:
   a. using gestures and smiling.
   b. interpreting facial expressions.
   c. speaking and using symbols.
   d. smiling and using gentle touch

3. For communication to be successful, all of the following elements must be present *except*:
   a. receiver.
   b. hearing.
   c. feedback.
   d. sender.

4. An example of nonverbal communication is:
   a. reading and using the patient's care plan.
   b. answering the telephone.
   c. listening to the shift report.
   d. conversing with patients.

5. A nursing assistant may give or take which information over the telephone?
   a. Report of a patient's condition
   b. Physician's orders

   c. Results of laboratory tests
   d. Name of person leaving a message

6. One purpose of a memo is to inform staff of:
   a. meetings or educational programs.
   b. patients' conditions.
   c. new physician's orders for specific patients.
   d. weather warnings.

7. Examples of manuals that are available for staff use include:
   a. computer manual, administrative policy manual, quality assurance manual.
   b. procedure manual, infection control manual, disaster manual.
   c. employee assistance program manual, personnel manual, benefits manual.
   d. isolation manual, X-ray manual, nuclear medicine manual.

8. A patient grimaces and holds their right arm close to their body when they move. You suspect they may:
   a. be right-handed.
   b. not want to get out of bed.
   c. be tired.
   d. be having pain.

9. A patient who is disoriented:
   a. has a mental illness.
   b. is unaware of place and time.
   c. is unable to communicate with you.
   d. is unable to hear.

10. Aphasia means that the patient:

   a. has a respiratory infection.

   b. has a hearing impairment.

   c. is disoriented.

   d. has problems with speech or understanding.

11. When working with patients who have hearing loss, you should:

   a. get the patient's attention before speaking.

   b. talk louder.

   c. avoid speaking if possible.

   d. speak very slowly.

12. When working with patients who have aphasia, it is best to:

   a. use only hand gestures to communicate.

   b. speak louder.

   c. face the patient and make eye contact.

   d. avoid communication if at all possible.

13. Persons with visual impairment should:

   a. stay in their rooms to avoid getting lost in the facility.

   b. be given directions for locating various areas in the building.

   c. have identification on their clothing so that everyone knows who they are.

   d. learn to use sign language.

14. When working with patients who are disoriented, you should:

   a. ask the patient if they remember you or know who you are.

   b. try to make the patient understand you.

   c. avoid distractions of noise and activity during communication.

   d. get as close as possible to the patient when talking or giving care.

15. Touching a patient can be a successful method of communication if you:

   a. are gentle and caring.

   b. ask the family's permission.

   c. are not offended by touch.

   d. always grasp the patient firmly.

B. Completion

Choose the correct word from the following list to complete each statement in questions 16–23.

aphasia	nonverbal
body language	communication
braille	paraphrasing
disorientation	verbal communication
memo	

16. Persons who cannot express themselves verbally or understand verbal communication have _____.

17. Loss of recognition of time, place, location, or person is called _____.

18. Restating your understanding of what was said is called _____.

19. A brief, written message that provides information is a _____.

20. _____ is an example of nonverbal communication.

21. _____ is a system of raised dots that persons who are blind use for reading.

22. Talking orally is _____.

23. _____ may be used for reading by persons with visual impairment.

24. A medical _____ is familiar with the patient's language and culture.

C. Nursing Assistant Challenge

Miss Johnson is one of your patients. She is visually impaired and in the hospital because she has a heart problem. Miss Johnson can feed herself and give herself a bath, brush her teeth, and comb her own hair if she has adequate assistance.

25. Using critical thinking and the information in this unit, describe how you can best get the ADLs done for this patient. Think about suggestions presented in this unit for communicating with persons who have visual impairment.

REFERENCE

Tri, J. L., Severson, R. P., Hyberger, L. K., & Hayes, D. L. (2007, March). Use of Cellular Telephones in the Hospital Environment. *Mayo Clinic Proceedings* *82*(3), 282–285. http://tinyurl.com/88k4ydo

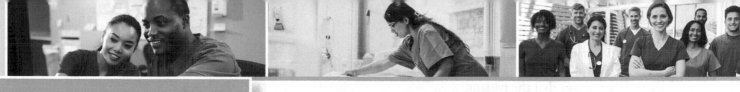

CHAPTER 8

Observation, Reporting, and Documentation

OBJECTIVES

After completing this Chapter, you will be able to:

8.1 Spell and define terms.

8.2 Define each component of the nursing process.

8.3 Explain the responsibilities of the nursing assistant for each component of the nursing process.

8.4 Describe two observations to make for each body system.

8.5 State the purpose of the care plan conference.

8.6 List three times when oral reports are given.

8.7 Describe the information given when reporting.

8.8 State the purpose of the patient's medical record.

8.9 Explain the rules for documentation.

8.10 State the purpose of the HIPAA laws.

8.11 Describe the difference between an electronic medical record (EMR), an electronic patient record (EPR), an electronic health record (EHR), and a personal health record (PHR).

8.12 List at least 10 guidelines for computerized documentation.

VOCABULARY

Learn the meaning and the correct spelling of the following words and phrases:

approach
assessment
care plan
care plan conference
charting
cloud
critical (clinical) pathways
cumulative
document
documentation
electronic health record (EHR)

electronic medical record (EMR)
electronic patient record (EPR)
evaluation
flow sheet
goal
Health Insurance Portability and Accountability Act (HIPAA)
implementation

intervention
nurse's notes
nursing diagnosis
nursing process
objective observation
observation
oral report
personal digital assistant (PDA)
personal health record (PHR)

planning
point-of-care testing (POCT)
SBAR (situation, background, assessment, recommendation) communication
subjective observation
tablet PC (TPC)

INTRODUCTION

Nursing assistants are responsible for collecting and communicating information about patients. You will communicate with patients and families and make observations while making rounds. Inform other team members by reporting and documenting. The **nursing process** is the mechanism used to carry out these actions.

NURSING PROCESS

Medicine and nursing are both necessary for positive patient outcomes (Figure 8-1). The physician collects information to diagnose and treat human illness. Nurses collect information, and then use it to diagnose and treat the *human response to illness*. Nursing diagnoses are very different from medical diagnoses.

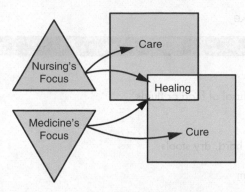

FIGURE 8-1 Medicine and nursing each have a separate focus, but both are essential for patients' well-being.

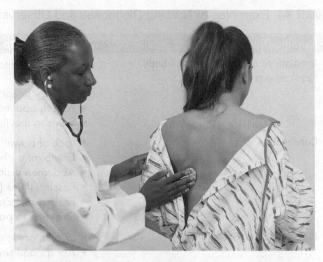

FIGURE 8-2 Part of the nursing assessment involves a physical examination. The nurse is auscultating (listening to) the patient's lungs.

The registered nurse is responsible for achieving positive outcomes by using the nursing process. They coordinate care and delegate responsibilities to other caregivers in an effort to achieve this goal. The nursing process consists of five steps:

1. Assessment—a nursing assistant cannot assess patients; however, your observations and results of care you report may be used by the nurse as part of the total assessment.
2. Problem identification and making a nursing diagnosis for each problem.
3. Planning care.
4. Implementation (giving the care that was planned).
5. Evaluation (evaluating the person's response to care to determine whether it was positive).

Assessment involves complete collection of data (information) about the patient. The registered nurse coordinates all assessments. The data are entered on a special form. Information is obtained from:

- Interviewing the patient
- The medical record
- The patient's family
- Physical examination (Figure 8-2)
- Collection of measurable data and information such as weight and vital signs (these data can be collected by other workers)
- Observations and information made by other members of the nursing team.

Proper use of the nursing process is essential in the delivery of effective health care. Nursing units run more efficiently if all staff understand and adhere to this model of care. If the nursing process breaks down, the risk of negative patient outcomes increases and the facility and its personnel are vulnerable to legal exposure. Understanding and fulfilling your role in the nursing process is an important responsibility.

The nursing assistant contributes to the assessment by collecting data and making and reporting observations. The nurse analyzes all the data, identifies the patient's problems, and formulates nursing diagnoses. A **nursing diagnosis** is the statement of a problem and the cause of the problem. For example, the nursing diagnosis may be impaired physical mobility (the problem) related to paralysis due to stroke (the cause of the problem). Nursing diagnoses may reflect:

- Actual clinical problems.
- At-risk problems.
- The person's vulnerability to certain new problems. The word *risk* is used to describe a problem in some diagnoses. The problem is not present, but nursing staff must take steps to prevent the condition from developing.
- Health promotion needs, such as things that will help improve the person's health. Nursing diagnoses associated with health promotion may have the phrase, "Expresses the desire to enhance."
- Wellness and teaching objectives.

The nursing diagnoses provide the foundation for nursing care. Table 8-1 gives a few examples of nursing diagnoses and what they mean. If you do not understand a nursing diagnosis, ask the RN.

After making the nursing diagnoses, **planning** (developing a care plan) is done. The purpose of planning is to:

- Identify possible solutions to the problems (nursing diagnoses).
- Develop **approaches** (what team members are going to do) that will help the patient solve the problems. Approaches may also be called **interventions**.
- Establish measurable **goals** (outcomes) for the patient so that caregivers will know whether the approaches are successful and whether the problems are being resolved.

TABLE 8-1 Examples of Nursing Diagnoses and Observations to Make

Nursing Diagnosis	Observations to Make
Imbalanced nutrition; less than body requirements	• Food/fluid intake • Weight loss • Inability to eat; dislike or refusal of food or fluids • Pain in abdomen or mouth • Sores in mouth
Constipation	• Lack of bowel movement or hard, dry stools • Complaints of feeling full • Abdomen distended and firm • Passing flatus (gas) • Feeling of rectal fullness • Straining to pass stool
Impaired urinary elimination	• Involuntary loss of urine associated with a strong sense of urinary urgency • Abrupt and strong desire to void • When the urge to void occurs, patient must go immediately and may be unable to suppress the urine • Once the bladder begins to empty, patient may be unable to stop or control the urine flow • Signs or symptoms of urinary infection, including incontinence, frequency, foul odor, pain, burning • Mucus, sediment, or blood in the urine • Voiding frequently in small amounts • Urine leakage after patient drinks small amounts of liquid or hears water running • Patient uses the bathroom many times each day; may get up at night to urinate • Retaining urine; unable to empty bladder completely
Decreased cardiac output	• Changes in blood pressure, irregular pulse, fatigue, difficulty breathing
Risk for aspiration	• Difficulty in swallowing, depressed cough and gag reflex, reduced level of consciousness
Impaired skin integrity	• Redness or destruction of skin
Impaired verbal communication	• Inability to speak or difficulty with speaking, difficulty breathing, disorientation
Ineffective coping	• Change in usual communication patterns • Inability to cope or meet basic needs • Change in behavior
Impaired adjustment	• Disbelief, anger, inability to solve problems • Actively complains of pain
Impaired comfort (This diagnosis is used to represent any uncomfortable situation in response to an unpleasant stimulus or order, such as being hungry and NPO)	• Reports or demonstrates discomfort • Guarding on movement • Facial expression and/or body language suggesting pain • Nausea and/or vomiting
Impaired physical mobility	• Reduced ability to move in bed, range of motion, balance, coordination, endurance
Activity intolerance	• Fatigue, weakness, shortness of breath • Irregular pulse
Disturbed sleep pattern	• Inability to sleep at night, or wakes frequently • Abnormal daytime sleepiness as a result of not sleeping at night • Changes in behavior or speech
Anxiety	• Shakiness, quivering voice, increased movements • Poor eye contact, helplessness

Planning may be done at a **care plan conference** (Figure 8-3A). This is a meeting of the members of the interdisciplinary team who care for the patient (Figure 8-3B). The patient and/or the family (if the patient consents) will be invited to attend the conference. The **care plan** contains a list of the nursing diagnoses, the approaches, and the patient's goals (Figure 8-4). You may be invited to attend the care conference. However, even if you are not present, the nurse will consider your observations and recommendations when developing a workable care plan. The nurse can update the care plan at any time if there is a significant change in condition. It is not necessary to wait for the next formal care plan meeting.

Implementation is the activation of the care plan. It means following your assignment and carrying out the approaches listed on the care plan in an effort to resolve the problems (nursing diagnoses) and to help the patient reach the goals (Figure 8-5). The approach states:

- Who is to carry out the approach
- When the approach is carried out
- How the approach is carried out

See Figure 8-4 for examples of approaches. Nursing assistants are responsible for knowing when and how the approach is to be carried out and for implementing each approach correctly.

Evaluation is the final step of the nursing process, but it is ongoing. The evaluation determines:

- Whether the patient is reaching the care plan goals, and if not, why not
- What should be done to assist the patient to reach the goals
- When goals are reached, whether they should be extended (e.g., if the patient reaches the goal of walking 200 feet, the distance may be increased to 250 feet)

The nursing assistant is responsible for reporting to the nurse when the:

- Approach cannot be carried out for any reason.
- Patient is having problems with the approach.

- Patient has met a goal.
- Patient refuses care listed in the approaches.
- Nursing assistant identifies a more effective approach (method of meeting a goal).

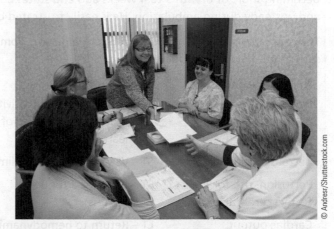

FIGURE 8-3A The care plan is developed during a care conference.

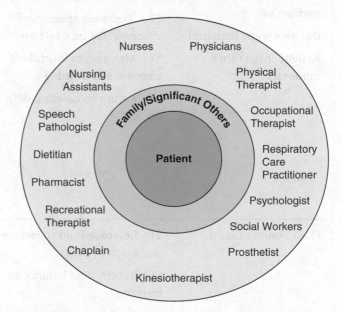

FIGURE 8-3B Members of the interdisciplinary team involved in the patient's care are invited to the care conference.

Patient information: Mr. Mario Herrera is an 81-year-old patient who was admitted to room 404 with a diagnosis of congestive heart failure (CHF). This condition causes the heart to be unable to pump enough nutrients and oxygen to meet the demands of the body. The patient is a retired teacher who has lived in his son's home for 15 years. He has had two heart attacks in the past. Mr. Herrera has gained 11 pounds in the past few weeks. He started becoming short of breath 3 to 4 weeks ago and states he feels "weak and tired all the time." He has become weak and unsteady during ambulation. He is easily frustrated because he becomes short of breath with activity.

The care plan is always individualized to the person. Some of the important nursing assistant orders for a patient such as Mr. Herrera may include:

Nursing Diagnosis	Goal	Nursing Assistant Approaches
Perfusion, ineffective peripheral tissue. Perfusion, risk for decreased cardiac tissue. Perfusion, risk for ineffective cerebral tissue. Cardiac output, decreased.	ST – Will participate in activities that reduce the workload of the heart. ST – VS within acceptable limits ST – Decrease fatigue & weakness LT – Return to hemodynamic stability	1. Vital signs q4h & PRN. 2. Observe for changes in mental status & LOC. 3. Monitor for changes in color. Monitor the color of the lips, gums, and nail beds. 4. Ensure he does not overexert himself during any activity.
Breathing pattern, ineffective. Gas exchange, impaired. Activity intolerance, moderate.	ST – Color WNL ST – Decrease episodes of dyspnea/SOB on exertion ST – Maintain as much independence as possible LT – Return to baseline with no SOB	1. Pulse oximeter: Notify nurse if SpO2 < 91% 2. Elevate HOB 3. O2 3 LPM via NC cont. 4. BRP with assist for BM or may use BSC 5. Encourage independent ADL; standby & assist if need 6. Report increase or decrease in activity intolerance 7. Amb with gait belt in room; use w/c for transport 8. Cool, comfortable, quiet environment 9. Encourage rest periods PRN 10. Monitor skin for red or open areas q shift & PRN d/t positional increase in pressure 11. 2 gm NA⁺ diet; assist PRN
Fluid Volume Excess.	ST - Decrease fluid to reduce workload of heart LT – Return fluid balance to baseline	1. Move as often as possible & position to relieve pressure 2. Fluids restricted to 1600 mL daily 3. Foley catheter 4. Strict I&O 5. Weigh daily at same time 6. Empty cath before weight 7. Notify nurse of weight gain/loss 8. Monitor skin turgor & mucous membranes 9. Monitor edema; notify nurse of increase or change 10. Elevate legs; check with nurse first if SOB 11. Oral care q2h & PRN

FIGURE 8-4 A computer-generated care plan. Some programs list approaches based on the nursing diagnoses, but the nurse entering the data can reject them or modify them to provide patient-centered care. The nurse may also add personal data to the plan based on the case presentation. Each facility has its own format. In some, all nursing care is listed together. Other facilities prefer to separate care given by nurses from care given by nursing assistants. They will print the pages and give staff copies during report. Keep your copies confidential and destroy them at the end of your shift.

Critical Thinking Activity

Nurses and nursing assistants must understand measurable goals. For example, Mrs. Milam has had hip surgery and must become strong enough to ambulate (walk) with a walker at home. The nursing assistant assignment sheet says:

Monday: Ambulate with wheeled walker twice daily.

The patient walked from the bed to the bathroom four times on your shift (6 a.m. to 6 p.m.) on Monday.

She has a small private room. You don't know how far she walked, but believe this is not important because she is getting good practice. She exceeded the number of times that were ordered.

The following day, the nursing assistant assignment sheet says:

Tuesday: Ambulate with wheeled walker and gait belt with one assist 50 feet in hallway twice a day.

Which of these nursing orders is most beneficial to the patient and easiest to follow?

You must document after completing your assignment. You must be sure that your documentation accurately reflects the care you gave. You must also document the patient's progress. There is tape along the floor of the unit. The distance is written on the tape.

Mrs. Milam walked 37 feet in the hallway at 10 a.m. You went for another walk at 2 p.m. and the patient walked 41.5 feet. You walked again at 6 p.m. and the patient walked 52 feet. You held the center back of the gait belt, and Mrs. Milam used the wheeled walker for each ambulation.

One of the best ways to write a measurable goal is to use numbers, pounds, distances, and so on that you can measure. For example, a goal that says "Patient's legs will get stronger" doesn't tell you much. However, you will know the legs are becoming stronger if the person meets or exceeds this goal: "Patient will walk 50 feet in the hallway twice a day."

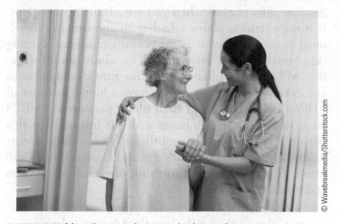

FIGURE 8-5 Nursing assistants help patients meet safety and mobility goals by assisting them with transfers and ambulation.

Critical (Clinical) Pathways

Many facilities use **critical (clinical) pathways** to direct care. The pathways are documents that detail the expected course of treatment and expected outcomes. New goals are set each day. The pathway lists actions and approaches to help the patient achieve the goals. Many of these interventions are the nursing assistant's responsibility. Review the care plan or critical pathway at the beginning of each shift to help plan your day.

MAKING OBSERVATIONS

An **observation** is information that is obtained by using one's senses: seeing, hearing, smelling, or feeling. Tasting is also a sensation but is not generally used for making health care observations. This information can help the care team determine:

- A change in physical condition, such as a blood sugar problem in a person with diabetes
- A new condition, such as a pressure injury (Figure 8-6)

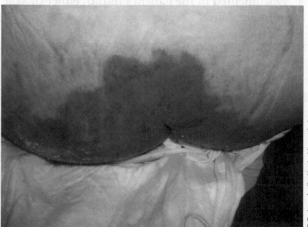

FIGURE 8-6 This is a pressure injury that developed from sitting in urine. The skin is also directly damaged from the urine.

- A change in mental condition, such as an alert patient who suddenly becomes confused
- A change in emotional condition, such as a patient crying and saying they do not want to continue living
- The effectiveness of a medication or treatment, such as a person whose pain level is the same as it was an hour ago, despite taking a pain pill

There are two types of observations: subjective and objective. An **objective observation** is one that is factual or measurable. For example, blood in the urine is factual. Blood pressure, temperature, pulse, and respirations are measurable. A **subjective observation** is a statement or complaint made by the patient. For example, "I have a headache," or "I feel sick to my stomach" are subjective observations.

You make observations by using:

- Your *eyes* to *see* observations:
  - Blood in the urine
  - Bruises or breaks in the skin (Figure 8-7)
  - The patient crying
  - A change in the way the patient walks
- Your *ears* to *hear* observations:
  - Wheezing when the patient breathes
  - Pulse or blood pressure (with a stethoscope)
  - Comments from the patient, such as "I am very tired today"
- Your *nose* to *smell* observations:
  - Body odor
  - Discharge from a wound or body cavity
  - Stool or urine when the patient is incontinent
- Your *hands and fingers* to *feel* observations:
  - A lump under the patient's skin (Figure 8-8)
  - Radial pulse
  - Warmth or coolness of the patient's skin

Remember that observations must be:

- Accurate and timely
- Reported to the nurse in a timely manner
- Documented in the patient's record, either by you or by the nurse

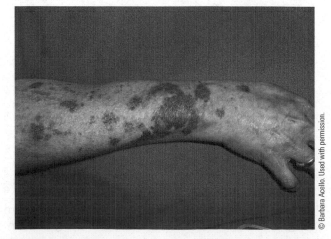

FIGURE 8-7 The purple-red spots are caused by bleeding under the skin.

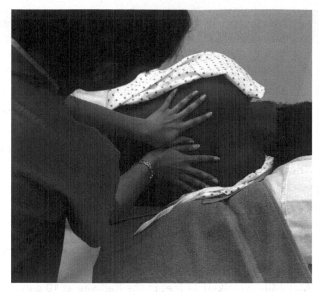

FIGURE 8-8 During a back rub, the skin can be observed for abnormalities that can be seen, such as bruised, red, or open areas. The skin can be felt for lumps, differences in temperature, or unusual areas under the skin.

Making Initial Observations

To make accurate observations, you must first know what is expected or normal for an individual. Collect baseline information when you are admitting a patient. It is important to know whether an abnormality developed at your facility or at the person's residence. Noting skin injuries is very important. The admission information will give you a basis for making future comparisons. For example, one patient may have a blood pressure of 110/68 on admission. If their blood pressure is 140/88 later, notify the nurse, because this is unusual for this person. Try to establish a routine way of making observations. Keep each patient's age and known illnesses in mind. It may be helpful to think of each body system and note the following:

- Integumentary system—skin, nails
  - Color: flushed, pale, jaundiced (yellow color), cyanotic (bluish, ashen, gray color); nails pale, pink, cyanotic (Figure 8-9)
  - Temperature: warm, hot, cool
  - Moisture: dry, moist, perspiring
  - Abnormalities: rashes, bruises, scars, pressure injuries, areas of redness (Figure 8-10)
- Musculoskeletal system—muscles, bones, joints
  - Posture: stooped, curled up in bed, straight
  - Mobility: ability to move in bed, to get out of bed, to stand, to walk, to maintain balance
  - Range of motion: ability to move all joints
- Circulatory system—heart, blood vessels, blood
  - Pulse: strength, regularity, rate
  - Skin: (see integumentary system)
  - Nails: (see integumentary system)
  - Blood pressure

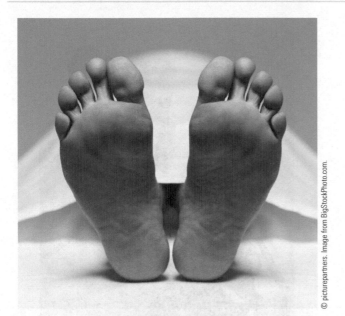

FIGURE 8-9 Cyanosis is an unusual blue or blue-gra-y color of the skin that indicates inadequate oxygen in the body.

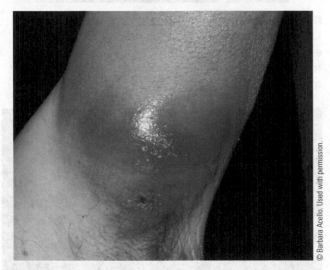

FIGURE 8-10 A raised, bright red area is a problem that should be reported to the nurse right away.

- Respiratory system—nose, throat, larynx, trachea, bronchi, lungs
  - Respirations (breathing): rate, regularity, depth, difficulty in breathing, shortness of breath upon exertion or while still, wheezing or crackling heard
  - Cough: frequency; dry, loose, productive; color and consistency of sputum (if any)
  - Hoarse
- Nervous system—brain, spinal cord, nerves
  - Mental status: orientation to time, place, person; ability to make verbal or nonverbal responses
  - Coordination: tremors, reaction time
- Senses—eyes, ears, nose, sense of touch; these are also part of the nervous system
  - Eyes: reddened, drainage, pupils equal in size

- Ears: drainage
- Nose: drainage, bleeding
- Sense of touch: ability to feel pressure and pain
- Urinary system—kidneys, ureters, bladder, urethra
  - Urination: frequency, amount, color, clarity, odor, presence of blood or sediment (Figure 8-11); ability to hold urine, incontinence
  - Pain on urination (dysuria)
- Digestive system—mouth, teeth, throat, esophagus, stomach, large and small intestines, gallbladder, liver, pancreas
  - Full or partial dentures
  - Dental caries (cavities)
  - Appetite: amount of fluids and food consumed (Figure 8-12); tolerance to foods; belching or burping
  - Eating: difficulty chewing or swallowing
  - Nausea and/or vomiting

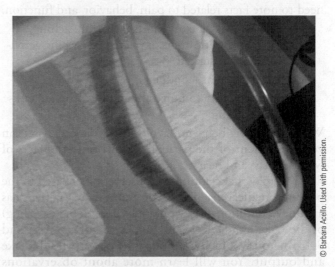

FIGURE 8-11 A large amount of sediment in the catheter drainage tube is a potentially serious problem.

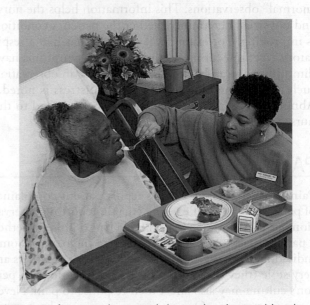

FIGURE 8-12 Accurately record the patient's meal intake.

- Bowel elimination: frequency, amount, consistency, color of stools; diarrhea, constipation, incontinence, flatus; difficulty in passing stool
- Endocrine system—glands
  - Signs and symptoms of diabetes (hypoglycemia, hyperglycemia)
- Reproductive system—male and female internal and external sex organs
  Female
  - Breasts: condition of nipples, presence of lumps, discolorations
  - Menstrual periods: frequency, amount, and character of bleeding; cramping
  - Vaginal drainage: amount, odor, and character
  Male
  - Testes: lumps
  - Penis: amount and character of drainage

In addition to the body systems observations, you also need to note facts related to pain, behavior, and function.

- Pain: location, type of pain (sharp, dull, aching), constant or intermittent or related to specific activities, time pain started
- Behavior: actions, conduct
- Function: ability to move about and complete tasks such as bathing

When reporting behavior, avoid using "labels" based on your judgment of the patient. Report only the facts of what you see and hear.

You may make additional observations related to the patient's medical diagnoses. For example, if a patient has a kidney condition, you would look for edema (swelling) of the face, hands, legs, and ankles (Figures 8-13A and 8-13B). You would also monitor the person's fluid intake and output. You will learn more about observations related to medical diagnoses as you study these conditions.

In some situations, you may be expected to report "normal" observations. This information helps the nurse and physician determine whether the patient's condition is improving. For example, if a patient has had a respiratory tract infection and the signs and symptoms have diminished, it can be important to report an observation such as "no coughing or respiratory distress is noted." Abnormal observations that should be reported to the nurse are listed in Table 8-2.

PAIN

Pain is never normal. Always report patient complaints of pain to the nurse. Be very factual in reporting observations of pain and behavior. Never try to judge whether a patient really has pain or how severe the pain is. Some individuals are very expressive about pain and others are very stoic (they try not to show their discomfort). A person's culture may also affect their response to pain. Never compare patients. One person may seem to have more

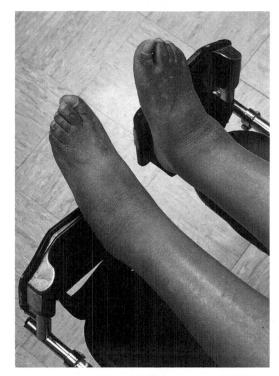

FIGURE 8-13A Patients with heart, circulatory, or kidney problems may develop edema of the lower extremities. The shoes were removed on this patient to demonstrate the edema. Remember that a patient must not get out of bed without proper footwear.

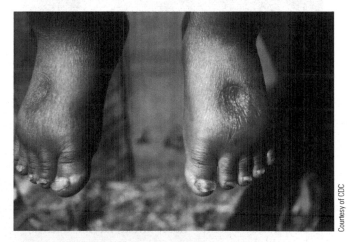

Courtesy of CDC

FIGURE 8-13B This picture demonstrates pitting edema.

pain than another person with the same diagnosis. It is not appropriate to think that they should both respond in the same way.

Determining whether pediatric patients or those who have cognitive impairments are in pain may be difficult because they may be unable to describe the nature of the problem. Pain is discussed in greater detail in Chapter 10.

REPORTING

Giving an **oral report** is one method used to relay information from one health care professional to another.

TABLE 8-2 Observation and Reporting Guidelines

General Signs and Symptoms of Illness That Should Be Reported to the Nurse		
Chest pain	Nausea or vomiting	Lethargy
Shortness of breath	Diarrhea	Unusual drainage from a wound or body cavity
Difficulty breathing	Cough	Changes in vital signs
Weakness or dizziness	Cyanosis or change in color	Profuse sweating
Headache	Change in mental status	
Pain	Excessive thirst	

System or Problem	Observation to Report	System or Problem	Observation to Report
Signs/symptoms of infection	Elevated temperature Sweating Chills Skin hot or cold to touch Skin flushed, red, gray, or blue Inflammation of skin as evidenced by redness, edema, heat, or pain Drainage from wounds or body cavities Any unusual body discharge, such as mucus or pus	Integumentary system	Rash Redness in the skin that does not go away within 30 minutes after pressure is relieved New, abnormally dark areas in patients with dark skin Pressure ulcers, blisters Irritation Bruises Skin discoloration Swelling Lumps
Evidence of pain (pain is not normal; all complaints of pain should be reported to the nurse)	Chest pain Pain that radiates Pain upon movement Pain during urination Pain when having a bowel movement Intensity of pain		Abnormal sweating Excessive heat or coolness to touch Open areas/skin breakdown Drainage Foul odor Complaints such as numbness, burning, tingling, or itching Signs of infection
Cardiovascular system	Abnormal pulse: below 60 or above 100 Blood pressure below 100/60 or above 140/90 Unable to palpate pulse or hear blood pressure Chest pain Chest pain that radiates to neck, jaw, or arm Shortness of breath Headache, dizziness, weakness, vomiting Cold, blue, or gray appearance Cold, blue, painful feet or hands Shortness of breath, dyspnea, or abnormal respirations Feeling faint or lightheaded		Unusual skin color, such as blue or gray color of the skin, lips, nail beds, roof of mouth, or mucous membranes Abrasions, skin tears, lacerations Skin growths Poor skin turgor/tenting of skin Sunken, dark appearance around eyes
		Gastrointestinal system	Sores or ulcers inside the mouth Difficulty chewing or swallowing food Unusual or abnormal appearance of bowel movement Blood, mucus, or other unusual substances in stool Unusual color of bowel movement Hard stool, difficulty passing stool Complaints of pain, constipation, diarrhea, bleeding Frequent belching Changes in appetite Excessive thirst Fruity smell to breath Complaints of indigestion or excessive gas Nausea, vomiting
Respiratory system	Respiratory rate below 12 or above 20 Irregular respirations Noisy, labored respirations Dyspnea Shortness of breath Gasping for breath Wheezing Coughing Retractions Cyanosis—blue color of lips, nail beds, or mucous membranes		

(continues)

TABLE 8-2 *(continued)*

System or Problem	Observation to Report	System or Problem	Observation to Report
Gastrointestinal system *(continued)*	Choking Abdominal pain Abdominal distention Coffee-ground appearance of emesis or stool	Nervous system	Change in level of consciousness, orientation, awareness, or alertness Feeling faint or light-headed Increasing mental confusion Progressive lethargy Loss of sensation Numbness, tingling Change in pupil size; unequal pupils Abnormal or involuntary motor function Loss of ability to move a body part Loss or lack of coordination
Genitourinary system	Urinary output too low Oral intake too low Fluid intake and output not reasonably balanced Abnormal appearance of urine: dark, concentrated, red, cloudy Unusual material in urine: blood, pus, particles, mucus, sediment (usually looks like sand) Complaints of difficulty urinating Complaints of pain, burning, urgency, frequency, pain in lower back Urinating frequently in small amounts Sudden-onset incontinence Edema, signs of fluid retention Sudden weight loss or gain Respiratory distress Change in mental status	Mental status	Change in level of consciousness, awareness, or alertness Changes in mood or behavior Change in ability to express self or communicate Mental confusion Excessive drowsiness Sleepiness for no apparent reason Sudden onset of mental confusion Threats of harm to self or others

The nursing assistant may participate in oral reports several times on a shift. Oral reports are given by the:

- Nurse going off duty to the staff coming on duty (Figure 8-14)
- Charge nurse to unit staff when explaining assignments, and as needed throughout the shift
- Nursing assistant to the nurse when leaving the nursing unit for any reason (including lunch and breaks)
- Nursing assistant to the nurse at the end of the shift
- Nursing assistant to the nurse if any unusual or new observations are made
- Nursing assistant to the nurse of outcomes from an appointment in which the nursing assistant accompanied the patient

Be specific when you report your observations. If you are relaying a subjective observation (something the patient has told you), repeat it exactly the way the patient told it to you. Here are some examples:

- Mr. Jones says it hurts every time he urinates.
- Mrs. Goldberg was wandering around the halls and said she did not know where she was.

To report objective observations, state your measurement or fact:

- Mrs. Dominick's blood pressure is 142/86.
- Mr. Hernandez ate 50 percent of his meal at lunch time.

When you report off duty at the end of your shift, report to the nurse:

- The condition of each of the patients you were assigned to

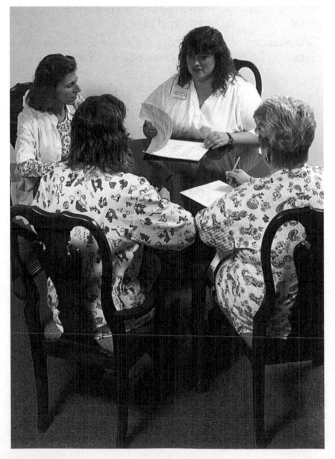

FIGURE 8-14 The nurse who worked the previous shift gives report to the oncoming shift.

- The care given to each patient
- Observations you made while giving care

SBAR Communication

Poor communication is a leading cause of important patient safety violations, including errors that result in serious injury and death. **SBAR communication** is a standard structure for concise, factual, effective, and meaningful reporting of patient information. SBAR stands for:

S—situation: what is happening at the present time that has triggered the SBAR communication?

B—background: what are the circumstances leading up to this situation? Put the situation in context.

A—assessment: what do I think the problem is?

R—recommendation: what should we do to correct the problem? How urgent is the situation, and when does action have to be taken?

Review the sample SBAR report in Table 8-3.

Practice reporting in SBAR format. Reporting is an essential part of the job. Preparing to give and receive report are critical activities. Although you may think you are simply transferring information, in most situations you are doing much more than this. You are transferring the responsibility for the patient to another individual, department, or shift. Practice your observation and reporting skills until you master them. This foundation will serve you well throughout your nursing career.

You will find additional information and guidelines for reporting in the online companion to this book.

TABLE 8-3 Sample SBAR Report

S	Javier is caring for Mr. Luna, who has a diagnosis of congestive heart failure. Mr. Luna has an order for daily weights. He weighs three pounds more than he did yesterday. When Javier walks Mr. Luna to the bathroom, he is markedly short of breath. The patient tells Javier that the shortness of breath started during the night but is a problem only when he is active. When Mr. Luna is finished in the bathroom, Javier seats him in the armchair and contacts the nurse on their cell phone to find out what to do.
B	When I walked Mr. Luna to the bathroom, he was short of breath. I was off yesterday. When I took care of him on Sunday, he was not short of breath. I weighed Mr. Luna. He weighs 3 pounds more than the weight recorded for Monday (yesterday). His fingers and ankles are swollen. When I press on the swollen ankles and remove my finger you can see the indentation. His color is good. His vitals are 98^2-78-22-158/94. His pulse oximeter reads 92.
A	He has a diagnosis of congestive heart failure. I think that is causing the problem because he has gained weight and become short of breath.
R	I would feel better if you will come and assess Mr. Luna.

DOCUMENTATION

You may be expected to record your observations on the patient's medical record (chart) (Figure 8-15). The medical record is a **document**. A document is a legal record. The process of recording the patient's care, response to treatment, and progress in the patient's chart is called **charting** or **documentation**. Nursing assistants may document on **flow sheets** (Figure 8-16A) in the chart or on a narrative record, such as the **nurse's notes** (Figure 8-16B) (sometimes called nurse's progress notes). Other documentation that may be recorded on a flow sheet is:

- Intake and output
- Food and supplement consumption (how much the person ate)
- Vital signs
- Elimination/bowel movement (BM) record
- Restorative nursing (see Chapter 48)

The charting must:

- Address the problems listed in the patient's care plan or critical pathway.
- Describe the approaches (interventions) listed in the care plan or critical pathway and note whether the interventions were effective.
- Indicate the progress the patient is making toward meeting the goals on the care plan or critical pathway.

Long-term care facilities periodically collect information for their assessment, called the Minimum Data Set (MDS). The MDS is the foundation for the care plan. Facility reimbursement is affected by the MDS, and quality of care scores is also measured based on MDS data. During the assessment period, you will document information about each person's ability to complete activities of daily living during a specific period of time. A numeric code is used to rate the person's self-performance

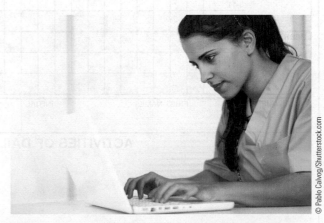

FIGURE 8-15 Observations are reported to the nurse and documented in the patient's medical record. This facility uses electronic documentation, and this nursing assistant is documenting on a laptop.

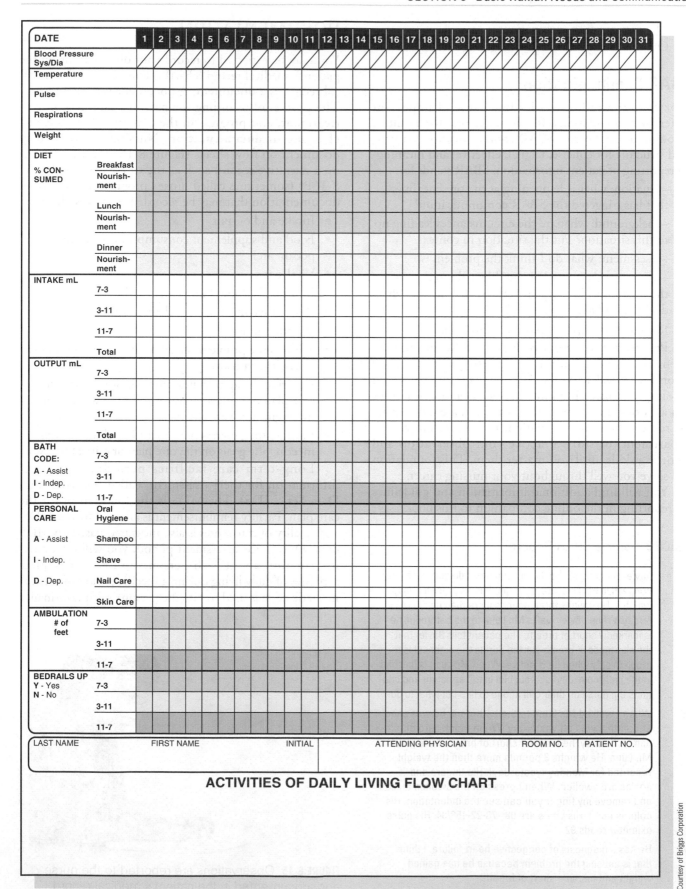

DATE		1	2	3	4	5	6	7	8	9	10	11	12	13	14	15	16	17	18	19	20	21	22	23	24	25	26	27	28	29	30	31
Blood Pressure Sys/Dia																																
Temperature																																
Pulse																																
Respirations																																
Weight																																
DIET % CON-SUMED	Breakfast																															
	Nourish-ment																															
	Lunch																															
	Nourish-ment																															
	Dinner																															
	Nourish-ment																															
INTAKE mL	7-3																															
	3-11																															
	11-7																															
	Total																															
OUTPUT mL	7-3																															
	3-11																															
	11-7																															
	Total																															
BATH CODE: A - Assist I - Indep. D - Dep.	7-3																															
	3-11																															
	11-7																															
PERSONAL CARE A - Assist I - Indep. D - Dep.	Oral Hygiene																															
	Shampoo																															
	Shave																															
	Nail Care																															
	Skin Care																															
AMBULATION # of feet	7-3																															
	3-11																															
	11-7																															
BEDRAILS UP Y - Yes N - No	7-3																															
	3-11																															
	11-7																															

LAST NAME	FIRST NAME	INITIAL	ATTENDING PHYSICIAN	ROOM NO.	PATIENT NO.

ACTIVITIES OF DAILY LIVING FLOW CHART

Courtesy of Briggs Corporation

FIGURE 8-16A Care provided and patient observations may be documented on a flow sheet. This flow sheet is for handwritten documentation, but a comparable form may be used for electronic documentation.

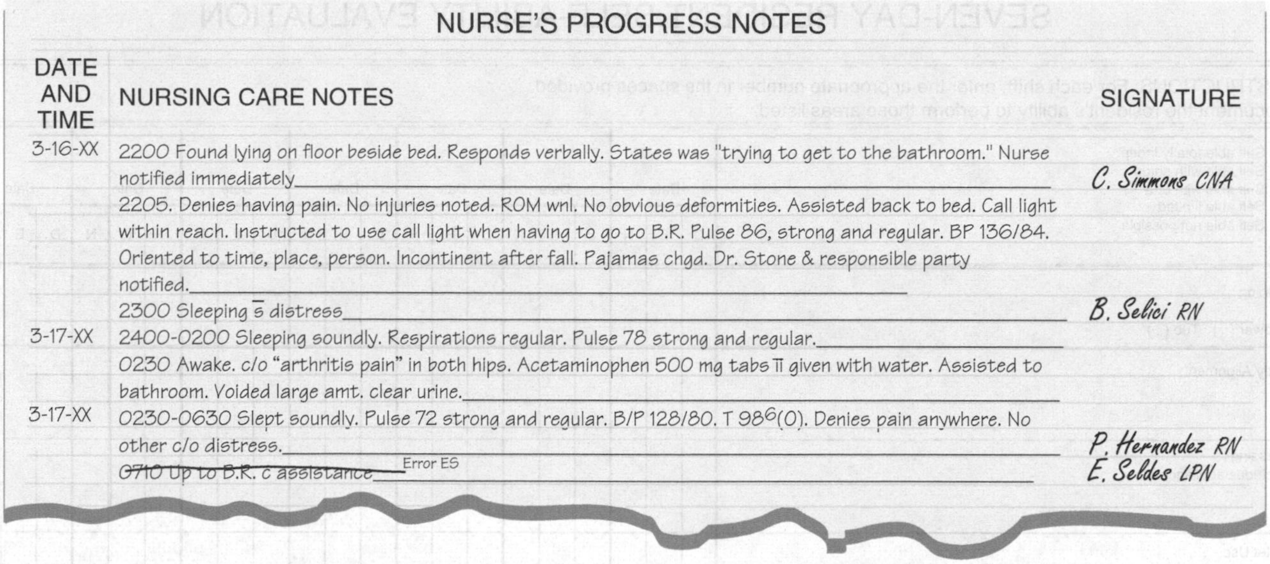

NURSE'S PROGRESS NOTES		
DATE AND TIME	NURSING CARE NOTES	SIGNATURE
3-16-XX	2200 Found lying on floor beside bed. Responds verbally. States was "trying to get to the bathroom." Nurse notified immediately_____	*C. Simmons CNA*
	2205. Denies having pain. No injuries noted. ROM wnl. No obvious deformities. Assisted back to bed. Call light within reach. Instructed to use call light when having to go to B.R. Pulse 86, strong and regular. BP 136/84. Oriented to time, place, person. Incontinent after fall. Pajamas chgd. Dr. Stone & responsible party notified._____	
	2300 Sleeping s̄ distress_____	*B. Selici RN*
3-17-XX	2400-0200 Sleeping soundly. Respirations regular. Pulse 78 strong and regular._____	
	0230 Awake. c/o "arthritis pain" in both hips. Acetaminophen 500 mg tabs II given with water. Assisted to bathroom. Voided large amt. clear urine._____	
3-17-XX	0230-0630 Slept soundly. Pulse 72 strong and regular. B/P 128/80. T 98⁶(0). Denies pain anywhere. No other c/o distress._____	*P. Hernandez RN*
	0710 Up to B.R. c̄ assistance_____Error ES_____	*E. Seldes LPN*

FIGURE 8-16B The nurse's notes are a narrative record of patient care and observations.

of the activity. Another code is assigned to the level of support provided. This information is important and must be very accurate. Most facilities use a form for collecting assessment information (Figure 8-16C).

> ## Communication Highlight
>
> You will learn when to report your observations about patients as you gain experience. In general, high-priority reporting items include abnormal vital signs, chest pain, difficulty breathing, change in color, change in mental status, bleeding, and pain. If you are in doubt about the urgency of reporting to the nurse, report your observation immediately. If the patient's condition changes after you have reported your observations, inform the nurse again.

Examples of items that should be routinely documented are listed in Table 8-4. Documentation must be accurate and timely.

Charting Guidelines

A patient's medical record (chart) is a legal document and may be used in court as evidence. Everything must be correct and legible. Use clear, simple, and accurate language. Entries must be printed or written neatly so that there can be no misunderstanding of the meaning. If you follow the established rules of charting, there will be no problem.

Each patient has an individual chart, so it is unnecessary to use the term *patient* or to use the patient's name. You should:

- Use phrases rather than full sentences.
- Avoid erasures and empty spaces on the record.
- Make all entries in black ink; no erasable ink or correction fluid is allowed.
- Use the correct medical terms and spell them correctly.
- Use only abbreviations that are approved for use by your facility.
- Chart only for yourself when the procedure or assignment has been completed. Never agree to document for someone else.
- Note the time when the entry is made.

Most health care facilities use international time (Table 8-5) to avoid confusion between a.m. and p.m. With international time, the 24 hours of each day are identified by the numbers 0100 (1:00 a.m.) through 2400 (12:00 a.m., midnight). The last two digits indicate the minutes of each hour (from 01 to 59). Thus, 0101 would be 1 minute after 1:00 a.m.; 1210 would be 10 minutes after 12 p.m. (noon); 1658 would be 4:58 p.m., and so on.

Many facilities use flow sheets for documenting routine patient care. Flow sheets save time and simplify documentation. To avoid problems, you should:

- Understand what you are supposed to be documenting. Read the flow sheet carefully.
- Never initial a procedure or observation that you did not do.
- Initial the right procedure, on the right day, on the right shift.
- Put your complete signature on each flow sheet (usually at the bottom of the page).
- Remember that flow sheets are legal records just like the other forms in the medical record.

SEVEN-DAY RESIDENT SELF-ABILITY EVALUATION

INSTRUCTIONS: For each shift, enter the appropriate number in the spaces provided.
Document the resident's ability to perform those areas listed.

1 = Self able totally Indep 2 = Self able with setup 3 = Self able with one 4 = Self able limited 5 = Self able not possible	Date			Date			Date			Date			Date			Date			Date		
	D	E	N	D	E	N	D	E	N	D	E	N	D	E	N	D	E	N	D	E	N
Bathing Shower ( ) Tub ( )																					
Body Alignment																					
Dressing (Includes appliances)																					
Toilet Use (Includes transfer, use of appliances)																					
Grooming (Nails, hair, face)																					
Ambulation (Includes use of wheelchair, walker, etc.)																					
Transfer Ability																					
Eating Tube feeding enter (T)																					
CNA Initials																					

CNA Signatures

_____   _____   _____

_____   _____   _____

_____   _____   _____

SUMMARY OF RESIDENT'S ABILITY TO SELF-PERFORM ADL ACTIVITIES - 7 DAYS:

_____   _____
              ChargeNurse   Date

Resident	Room/Bed	Physician

FIGURE 8-16C A separate form is used for collecting information on activities of daily living (ADLs) when a resident is admitted to a long-term care facility.

TABLE 8-4 Nursing Assistant Documentation

Information to Document	Details
Vital signs	Measure temperature, pulse, respiration, and blood pressure according to facility policy or as ordered. Report abnormalities to the nurse.
Height and weight	Measure height on admission. Measure and record weight as ordered.
Dressing	Putting on, fastening/unfastening, or removing clothing. Identify person's need for assistance, ranging from independent to totally dependent.
Feeding	Type and amount of assistance needed.
Meal and snack intake	Percentage of meal, snack, and supplement consumed.
Intake and output (I&O)	Offer fluids person likes each time you are in the room. Record only if ordered (listed on care plan). Document all fluid consumed during your shift. Record all liquid excreted via urine, emesis, etc.
Bathing	Type of bath given, amount of assistance needed.
Grooming	Assistance needed with grooming activities, such as combing and styling hair, applying makeup, shaving, nail care. Amount of assistance needed.
Oral care	Type of care given, such as brushing and flossing teeth, denture care, special oral hygiene, and so on. Amount of assistance needed.
Toileting	Assist with bedpans and urinals, toilet, commode; help to the bathroom; transfers; provide perineal or incontinent care; or changing brief for person who needs it.
Catheter care	Catheter care as needed: cleanse catheter and perineum, empty drainage bag, record I&O.
Bowel movement	Monitor for and document bowel elimination. Amount of assistance needed with incontinent care or bowel elimination.
Turning and positioning	Ensure that dependent persons are turned according to the plan of care (at least every two hours), to provide comfort and prevent skin breakdown. Ability of person to turn to sides, move from lying to sitting, reposition in bed.
Skin care	Apply lotion, follow care plan for pressure ulcer prevention, and protect from skin tears and other injuries.
Transfers	How the person transfers (bed, chair, wheelchair, standing), type and amount of assistance needed.
Ambulation	How the person ambulates, use of adjunctive devices, amount of assistance needed, location of ambulation (room, hall), distance ambulated.
Exercise, range of motion	Mobility, active (independent) movement or passive (dependent) exercise.
Routine check	Periodically check person to ensure that they are safe and all needs are met.
Linen change	Change bed linen according to facility policy and as often as needed.
Environment	Ensure environmental safety. Make beds and keep the person's rooms and belongings neat and organized.
Personal safety	Monitor persons with safety risks, including those with poor safety judgment and wanderers. Follow the plan of care.

- Chart after an event occurs or care is given. Be reasonable with the time you document. Make sure all your documentation is complete before you leave for the day. Documenting on another day is not acceptable.
- Never chart in advance.
- Notify the nurse if something is missing from a computerized flow sheet. The nurse will add missing information that is listed on the patient's care plan or critical pathway. For example, your facility routinely charts that patients are turned and repositioned every two hours. You routinely turn and reposition Ms. Avilla, according to her critical pathway. However, there is no place to document this important care on the flow sheet.

- If you forget to chart something or make an error, follow your facility's policy for making a late entry note or correcting the error.

Confidentiality and Privacy

Each patient has a right to expect that their medical information will be kept private. The medical record is private and confidential. Everyone is responsible for protecting patient information from access by unauthorized persons. Likewise, avoid the temptation to read charts out of curiosity. Medical records may be accessed only by those with a need to know the information.

TABLE 8-5 International Time

Standard Clock	Int'l. Time	Standard Clock	Int'l. Time
AM 12 midnight	2400	PM 12 noon	1200
1	0100	1	1300
2	0200	2	1400
3	0300	3	1500
4	0400	4	1600
5	0500	5	1700
6	0600	6	1800
7	0700	7	1900
8	0800	8	2000
9	0900	9	2100
10	1000	10	2200
11	1100	11	2300

In 1996, Congress passed the **Health Insurance Portability and Accountability Act (HIPAA)**. This law has many provisions. One portion applies to privacy, confidentiality, and medical records. The HIPAA rules:

- Increase patient control over personal medical records.
- Restrict the use and disclosure of patient information.
- Make the facility accountable for protecting patient data.
- Require the facility to implement and monitor its information release policies and procedures.

The HIPAA regulations protect all individually identifiable health information in any form, including paper, verbal, and electronic documentation; billing records; and clinical records. Because of this, patient information is provided to staff on a "need to know" basis. Information is disclosed only if staff needs it to carry out their duties. For example, the dietary department would need to know if a patient is on a diabetic diet. They would not need to know that the patient has an infected wound. The nursing assistant would need to know about both the diabetes and the infection. Facilities must monitor how and where they use patient information. Policies must protect patient charts, conversations and reports about patients and patient information, transmission of patient documents, and disclosure of other personal information.

The HIPAA rules ask providers to analyze how and where patient information is used and develop procedures for protecting confidential data. This includes the areas where patient charts are stored, the places where patient information is discussed, and how patients' personal health information (PHI) is distributed. The HIPAA policies and procedures for each facility are set by and specific to that facility.

 Communication ALERT

HIPAA requires facilities to protect all workstations, including desktops, laptops, and handheld devices. Seventy million smartphones are lost each year. About 7 percent of them are returned. One in 10 laptops is lost or stolen. In fact, a laptop is stolen every 53 minutes. Many of these contain work-related information and protected health information.

GUIDELINES 8-1 Guidelines for Charting

- Check for right patient, right chart, right form, right room, right time.
- Fill out new headings completely.
- Use a black or blue pen when documenting manually.
- Date and time each entry.
- Chart entries in the correct sequence.
- Make entries brief, objective, and accurate.
- Print or write clearly.
- Spell each word correctly.

- Leave no blank spaces or lines between entries.
- Do not use the term *patient*.
- Do not use ditto marks.
- Sign each entry with your first initial, last name, and job title.
- Make corrections by drawing one line through the entry; then print the word *error* on the line and your initials above.
- Late entries, which are made when you have honestly forgotten to document something, in a manner that does not appear to be self-serving.

ELECTRONIC RECORDKEEPING

The U.S. government has created an initiative to link medical information nationwide and make it easier for providers to collect, share, and report. Health care facilities and providers are required to convert their record-keeping from a manual paper-based system to a fully electronic computerized system.

The Electronic Health Record

Although you may hear the terms *electronic health record*, *electronic medical record*, and *electronic patient record* used interchangeably, there are differences in the definitions of each. An **electronic health record (EHR)** is a patient record in digital format. The EHR is not a complete medical record. It contains data that are part of a larger record collection, such as contact and insurance information, next of kin, a list of medications, and dates of hospitalizations. The information is **cumulative** or collected over a period of time. It is usually stored on an external server called a **cloud** that can be accessed online. Contributing organizations can use all or part of the information.

The Electronic Medical Record/The Electronic Patient Record

An **electronic medical record (EMR)** is the electronic version of one person's paper medical record. It is generated and maintained by one organization or provider. For example, a long-term care facility could create and maintain an organizational EMR. A small physician's office may also create an EMR. Information from the EMR contributes to the EHR. An organization can use EHR technology only if it has an EMR system that can communicate with other EMR systems. The term **electronic patient record (EPR)** is another term that is sometimes used to describe the electronic medical record.

A **personal health record (PHR)** is an EHR that the patient creates and controls. Most people store these digitally on a portable computer drive, on a handheld device, on a Web portal or gateway maintained by the employer or physician, or by leasing space on an online database. The PHR enables the patient to:

- Ensure that information about their medical condition and care is accurate.
- Keep important information in one location.
- Share medical information with their personal health care providers, caregivers, and family members.
- Quickly provide information needed for emergency treatment.
- Prevent duplication of procedures and tests.
- Maintain and update the PHR online as often as needed.

POINT-OF-CARE DATA CAPTURE

The most accurate documentation is done immediately after a change occurs or a procedure is done. Various devices have made it possible to obtain information, take action, and document at the bedside. **Point-of-care testing (POCT)** is testing done at the patient's location at the time care is required (Figure 8-17). The test result should enable a clinical decision to be made, resulting in action or treatment. Although there is no guarantee, the combination of the test result, the decision, and the action should lead to an improved health outcome. A blood glucose meter (see Chapter 42) is an example of a POCT device. Some POCT devices are for single use. Others are used repeatedly. Both types of glucose meters store the blood glucose values so that they can be uploaded to the computer and stored as part of the electronic health record.

Handheld Computers

Handheld computers were first introduced in 1995. Since then, they have become essential tools for many

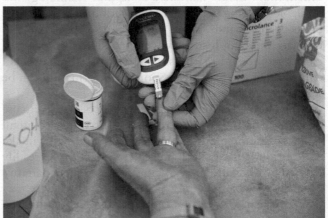

FIGURE 8-17 Point-of-care tests result in faster treatment and better outcomes.

Courtesy of CDC

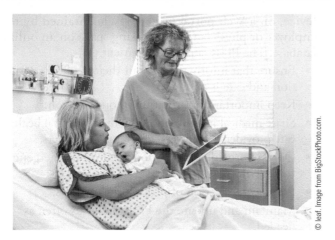

FIGURE 8-18 A tablet is a portable device used to document, teach, and obtain reference information. The screen is touched for some devices. For others, a stylus is used.

health care workers because they improve communication and make documentation easier.

Two major classes of portable computing devices that health care workers commonly use are **personal digital assistants (PDAs)** and **tablet PCs (TPCs)** (Figure 8-18). Many hospitals are using these small handheld computers as an integral part of their services. Some staff have purchased them for personal use. In addition to using the computer as a source of reference information, most are used for personal data, such as calendars and contact lists. Most PDAs also have a calculator function, camera, and various alarms and notifiers. Remember that if your device has a camera, you should not use it for taking photos at work (see Chapter 4).

Handheld computers use wireless Internet technology to transmit data. In many hospitals, handheld computers are used to transmit nursing notes and vital signs to the hospital's mainframe computer. These are also popular for home health agency recordkeeping and documentation. Before handheld computer technology was available, nursing personnel often scribbled notes on the backs of their hands, paper towels, and scraps of paper. If the data were not lost, they were transferred to patients' charts at the end of the shift. By using the handheld computer at the bedside, important information can be sent to the main computer immediately.

The keypad is tiny and a stylus may be needed to use it. Light pens and touch-screen data entry are also useful tools with some models. Data such as vital signs, intake and output values, and pain scale ratings can be readily entered by using the keypad. However, for longer narrative notes, the keypad may not be practical. The device may have a voice to text feature, and some handheld computers may be plugged into a larger keyboard, which is easier and faster to use. Some tablets use a heat-activated touch screen, so a fingertip must be used to record information.

In some facilities, each nurse and nursing assistant has a phone for patient communication. The primary caregivers' phone numbers are written on the whiteboard in each patient's room. The patient has a call light, but they may also call the caregiver on the telephone.

Handheld computers must be regularly charged and maintained so that they do not lose data. The term *hotsyncing* refers to linking the handheld computer to a full-size computer to update the information on both. Data are transferred by placing the PDA into a cradle, through which information is uploaded to the mainframe. This is essential for data preservation, especially if the handheld computer battery runs low. Many PDAs use rechargeable batteries, and placing the unit into the cradle also charges the battery.

Voice-Activated Systems

Personnel wear headsets when voice-activated systems are used (Figure 8-19). Such systems can be used for checking simple information (e.g., a diet order). They also provide access to more complex data, such as when you want to review the care plan. Patients are identified by room and bed number, not by name. Documentation is done by answering a series of yes/no questions. For example, the nursing assistant identifies the patient and the problem, such as a complaint of pain or need for repositioning. The computer asks a series of yes/no questions such as:

- The degree of assistance needed
- The number of persons assisting
- Props used
- Position

This information is immediately sent to the medical record. Most documentation is done in this manner, at the time of occurrence. This is the most accurate method of charting and saves a great deal of time at the end of the shift, when documentation is usually done. The drawback is that the nursing assistant must talk into the headset while giving care, making it difficult or impossible to communicate with the patient.

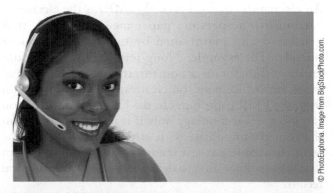

FIGURE 8-19 Voice-activated systems support accurate and timely documentation. The system may also be used to obtain information about a patient's care plan.

Computers and HIPAA Compliance

HIPAA affects all health care communication, especially *information technology* (IT). Because of this, hospital systems have layers of access to patient medical records. For example, you will be able to access the records for only those patients listed in your assignment. Information will be limited to that which is essential to patient care. The IT department can track who is accessing any patient's record and can readily identify misuse of the system. All of the electronic devices have online access. The facility will install a firewall to ensure that sensitive data are not being broadcast into cyberspace. Nevertheless, you must use good sense and take precautions to avoid letting viruses and malware onto your computer, cell phone, and other handheld electronic devices.

Having ready access to key nursing information is critical. Because of this, NANDA–I nursing diagnoses and classifications such as the Nursing Interventions Classification (NIC) and Nursing Outcomes Classification (NOC) are fully computerized, and data are available to nursing staff.

Legal ALERT

In health care, there is a saying: "If it's not charted, it wasn't done." The purpose of documentation is to communicate care given and the patient's response. Documentation is a true record of patient care and is the first line of defense in proving accountability for excellent care. Never chart care that you did not provide. For example, some assistants will chart that a patient was "turned every two hours" because they know that this is the care that is supposed to be given. Document only the facts. If you are unable to turn the patient according to your assignment, inform the nurse in advance, so they can arrange for help or adjust your assignment, if necessary. Do not be tempted to document care because it is supposed to be given. Document only what you have actually done. Always chart *after* giving care. If you forget to document, follow your facility's procedure for making a late entry. Specify the exact date and time the entry was recorded, as well as the exact date and time the event occurred. Clearly mark your documentation as a late entry.

GUIDELINES 8-2 Guidelines for Documentation in the Computerized Medical Record

- Do not be afraid of computerized charting. Make sure you enter the correct identification code for each patient.
- Do not give your identification code or password to others.
- Select a password that is not easily decoded, and do not give it to anyone. Do not write it down or leave it where it can be easily found, such as under the mouse pad, under the keyboard, or in an electronic file.
- Change your password promptly if you suspect it has been compromised.
  - Never let someone look over your shoulder when you are signing in or accessing patient data.
  - Turn or position the monitor so it is not visible to others.
- Document only in areas you are authorized to use.
- Remember that audit trails track the computer, user, date, time, and exactly which medical records are accessed, based on your user identification.
- The electronic record must note whether manual records are also being used, such as during a storm or electronic system failure. If this is the case, the records must cross-reference each other. Most

hospitals have policies about using paper documentation when the computer is down.
- Read and follow the directions on the screen.
- Do not print information unnecessarily. Print at the end of your shift or according to facility policy (Figure 8-20). Destroy printed copies that are not part of the permanent record. Placing them in the wastebasket is a violation of privacy laws. Records are commonly destroyed by shredding them in a paper shredder.

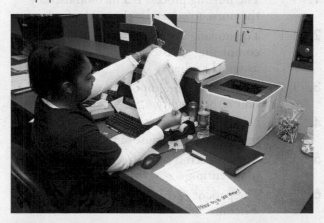

FIGURE 8-20 Print only essential information. The confidentiality laws protect all documents, even if they are incomplete.

(continues)

GUIDELINES 8-2 Guidelines for Documentation in the Computerized Medical Record (continued)

- Never delete information from the electronic medical record.

- The procedure for late entry and addendum documentation will be different than it is in a narrative system. Know and follow your facility's policies for this type of charting.

- Electronic documentation must be signed by the person giving care. Your facility will have a procedure for providing electronic signatures. These are valid as long as they are accessible only to the person identified by that signature.

- Protect patient data. Never send insecure identifiable patient information electronically.

- Always log off when you have finished using the computer.

- Wash your hands after using the computer. Many people use it, so the keyboard is a huge potential source of cross-contamination.

  - Some facilities cover the keyboard with a plastic cover. Users type through the plastic. Disinfect the cover with the recommended product after use.

  - Avoid products containing alcohol when cleaning the computer and accessories.

  - Some facilities use a handheld ultraviolet light to disinfect the keyboard (Figure 8-21).

- Stay current. Attend continuing education programs to learn how to maximize the use of computerized charting and information systems.

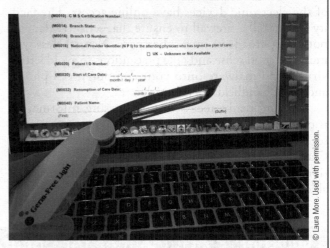

FIGURE 8-21 Ultraviolet light kills microbes in the environment, making it a useful tool for fighting infection.

REVIEW

A. True/False

Mark the following true or false by circling T or F.

1. T F   The nursing process is a method used by the nurse to supervise the work of others.

2. T F   The nursing assistant is responsible for completing an assessment on all patients assigned to them.

3. T F   Assessment is an important nursing assistant responsibility.

4. T F   A nursing diagnosis is a statement of a clinical problem and the cause of the problem.

5. T F   An approach is sometimes called an intervention.

6. T F   The patient's goal may be called an outcome.

7. T F   The care plan is developed at the care plan conference.

8. T F   Nursing assistants are not responsible for the implementation of the care plan.

9. T F   A patient's weight is an objective observation.

10. T F   The patient's chart is a legal document.

11. T F   Nursing diagnosis and medical diagnosis are the same thing.

12. T F   Implementation is the activation of the care plan.

13. T F   Evaluation is an ongoing step of the nursing process.

14. T F   In some situations, the nursing assistant may be expected to report "normal" observations.

15. T F   Pain is normal in some conditions.

B. Multiple Choice

Select the best answer for each of the following.

16. The purpose of the nursing process is to:
- **a.** make a medical diagnosis.
- **b.** achieve patient-focused care.
- **c.** make assignments.
- **d.** cure illness.

17. The nursing assistant contributes to the nurse's assessment of the patient by:
- **a.** listening to the heart and lungs.
- **b.** keeping the environment neat and tidy.
- **c.** establishing goals for the patient.
- **d.** reporting observations and vital signs.

18. The statement of a patient's problem and its cause is called:
- **a.** a medical diagnosis.
- **b.** an approach.
- **c.** an assessment.
- **d.** a nursing diagnosis.

19. The purpose of evaluation is to determine whether the:
- **a.** patient is reaching the goals on the care plan.
- **b.** laboratory tests are accurate.
- **c.** patient agrees with the critical pathway.
- **d.** family understands the patient's condition.

20. The purpose of making observations is to:
- **a.** make sure the nurse gets along with the patient.
- **b.** inform the doctor of how the patient's family is doing.
- **c.** note changes in condition or new problems developing.
- **d.** see if the medical diagnosis is accurate.

21. An example of an objective observation is that the patient:
- **a.** complains of abdominal pain.
- **b.** says they are feeling sad.
- **c.** has a pulse of 72 beats per minute (bpm).
- **d.** says they are not hungry.

22. When you offer to give Mrs. Jones a bath, she says, "Get out of here and don't come back." You report this to the nurse and say:
- **a.** "Mrs. Jones told me to leave her room and not come back."
- **b.** "Mrs. Jones is angry today."
- **c.** "Mrs. Jones is not cooperating with me."
- **d.** "Mrs. Jones does not want a bath today."

23. The form on which nurses enter daily information about the patient is called the:
- **a.** progress notes.
- **b.** nurse's notes.
- **c.** nurse's daily log.
- **d.** document.

24. Charting should always be:
- **a.** done in pencil.
- **b.** done after care is given.
- **c.** signed at least once each day.
- **d.** done before care is given.

25. In international time, midnight would be called:
- **a.** 12:00 a.m.
- **b.** 2400
- **c.** 1200
- **d.** 12:00 p.m.

26. The HIPAA rules:
- **a.** make it easier to share patient information with other health care workers.
- **b.** prohibit the sharing of patient information with unlicensed workers.
- **c.** empower the physician to specify information to disclose.
- **d.** restrict the use and disclosure of patient information.

27. The device that prevents patient information from being inadvertently transmitted over the Internet is the:
- **a.** firewall.
- **b.** PDA.
- **c.** hot-sync.
- **d.** radio frequency emitting device.

28. Audit trails:
- **a.** are used only if the computer is down.
- **b.** are done each day to identify and correct missing documentation.
- **c.** track the computer, user, date, time, and which records are accessed.
- **d.** are very difficult to establish and are seldom necessary.

29. Medical records and other patient data:
- **a.** may be accessed by nursing employees who are curious about the patient.
- **b.** should be accessed only by those with a need to know the information.
- **c.** should be accessed only by the physician and the RN.
- **d.** may be accessed by the patient's family members, if desired.

30. The evaluation step of the nursing process determines all of the following *except*:

    a. whether the patient is reaching the care plan goals.

    b. what should be done to assist the patient to reach the goals.

    c. identification of a patient's care plan problems and needs.

    d. whether goals should be modified or extended.

31. Critical (clinical) pathways:

    a. detail the course of treatment and expected outcomes.

    b. summarize the laboratory reports and diagnostic records.

    c. list the most important doctor's orders.

    d. describe the goals the patient has met.

32. An EHR is stored in:

    a. hard copy.

    b. digital format.

    c. a portable drive.

    d. several pieces.

33. A POCT device:

    a. requires a great deal of preparation.

    b. is used only by the physician.

    c. is used at the patient's location.

    d. guarantees a positive outcome.

34. When using SBAR reporting, you know that:

    a. the S is for reporting subjective information.

    b. B stands for background information.

    c. nursing assistants cannot assess.

    d. R stands for reporting and recording.

C. Nursing Assistant Challenge

Mr. Fensten is a 47-year-old patient on the medical floor. He has had a stroke. These events occur while you are taking care of him:

- He has trouble walking because of hemiplegia (paralysis) on the right side of his body. He had trouble picking up his right foot and stumbled. This caused him to lose his balance. He almost fell. The fall was prevented because he grabbed the sink and the nursing assistant maintained control with a gait belt.

- He refuses to eat his breakfast.

- He throws the washcloth across the room when you help him with his bath.

- His BP is 146/88.

- He smiles and hugs his wife when she comes to visit.

- You do range-of-motion exercises on all joints without any problem.

- You notice a persistent reddened area on his coccyx (tailbone). Nurse notified.

35. For each of these observations, write the documentation exactly as you would in the patient's medical record.

36. Think about these observations and consider how many examples of verbal and nonverbal communication are given.

37. Do any of these situations involve Mr. Fensten's rights as a patient? If so, describe them.

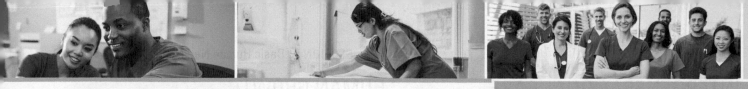

Meeting Basic Human Needs

CHAPTER 9

OBJECTIVES

After completing this chapter, you will be able to:

9.1 Spell and define terms.

9.2 Describe the stages of human growth and development.

9.3 Explain how the generation in which one is born affects the lives of its members.

9.4 List five physical needs of patients.

9.5 Define self-esteem.

9.6 Describe how the nursing assistant can meet the patient's emotional needs.

9.7 List nursing assistant actions to ensure that patients have the opportunity for intimacy.

9.8 Explain why cultural and spiritual beliefs influence patients' psychological responses.

9.9 Discuss methods of dealing with the fearful patient.

9.10 List guidelines to assist patients in meeting their spiritual needs.

VOCABULARY

Learn the meaning and the correct spelling of the following words and phrases:

adolescence	generation	neonate	sexuality
bisexuality	growth	personality	tasks
celibate	heterosexuality	preadolescence	tasks of personality
coitus	homosexuality	reflex	development
continuum	intimacy	self-esteem	toddler
development	masturbation	self-identity	transgender

INTRODUCTION

Each of us has things that we need to live successfully. These are called *needs* simply because we cannot get along without them. When a patient is admitted to the hospital, their needs come too. The difference is in the way those needs are expressed and fulfilled. Expression and fulfillment have to be different because of the hospital environment and the illness. Remember that the basic needs remain the same, regardless of how they are expressed or how they have to be met because of an individual's level of development or state of health.

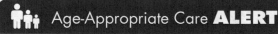 Age-Appropriate Care **ALERT**

Each patient is an individual with their own:

- Likes and dislikes
- Feelings, thoughts, and beliefs
- Limitations and abilities
- Life experiences

Avoid stereotyping patients based on their age or other characteristics, such as skin color, religion, or sexual preference. Provide patient-focused care by treating each patient as an individual. A key part of your job is the ability to recognize each patient's unique needs and abilities.

INTERGENERATIONAL CARE

You can learn much about your patients and co-workers by learning about the generation in which the person was raised. A **generation** is a group of individuals born within the same period of time. Each generation consists of individuals who have been influenced by the same social forces and occurrences, known as *markers*. One *generation* is the time that elapses between the birth of parents and the birth of their offspring (Figure 9-1).

The generation in which each person grows up helps define their characteristics, attitudes, beliefs, values, behaviors, expectations, habits, and motivators. As a group, these traits were shaped during the same time, by the same events and experiences. Events such as politics, wars, marketing, pop culture, and technology are defining measures of the group. Each group has music that its members consider their own. Although history molds generations, generations also mold history. Recognizing and addressing generational differences will help you understand your patients and meet their needs.

The "baby boomers" were the first U.S. generation to be given a label. This group was born into post–World War II (WWII) prosperity. The label was received well, so sociologists worked backward and labeled each previous generation based on its characteristics. Over time, generational labels became global.

HUMAN GROWTH AND DEVELOPMENT

Human beings change as they age, through the processes of growth and development. **Growth** refers to the changes that take place in the body over time. It is usually measured by height and weight, changes in texture and appearance of skin, and degree of system maturation. **Development** involves the changes that take place on a social, emotional, and psychological level. Developmental levels are shown in behavior and interpersonal skills.

People move from one level of development to the next (Table 9-1). At each level, they change in both the way they look and the way they think and act. Each level presents tasks that must be mastered before the person can move on to the next level.

The **tasks** to be mastered are those things that lead to healthy and satisfactory participation in society. The tasks are defined by the needs of the individual and the pressures of society.

Sometimes growth spurts occur and developmental skills must catch up. Both growth and development progress from simple to complex (Figure 9-2). Each depends on the other to achieve an orderly progression. For example, a child cannot be toilet trained until the nerve pathways have matured.

> ### 👪 Age-Appropriate Care **ALERT**
> Always introduce yourself by name (and title, when appropriate) to patients. Your communication must be appropriate for the patient's age and culture.

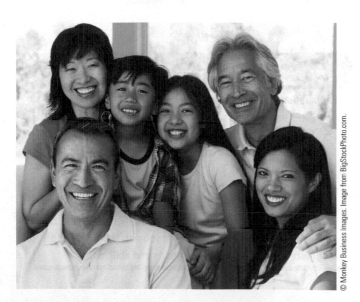

FIGURE 9-1 This family has members from three generations.

TABLE 9-1 Stages of Growth and Development

Neonate	Birth to 1 month
Infancy	1 month to 2 years
Toddler	2 to 3 years
Preschool	3 to 5 years
School age	5 to 12 years
Adolescence	12 to 20 years
Adulthood	20 to 49 years
Middle age	50 to 64 years
Later maturity	65 to 75 years
Old age	75 and beyond
Old old	Category used by some experts to describe those age 85 and older

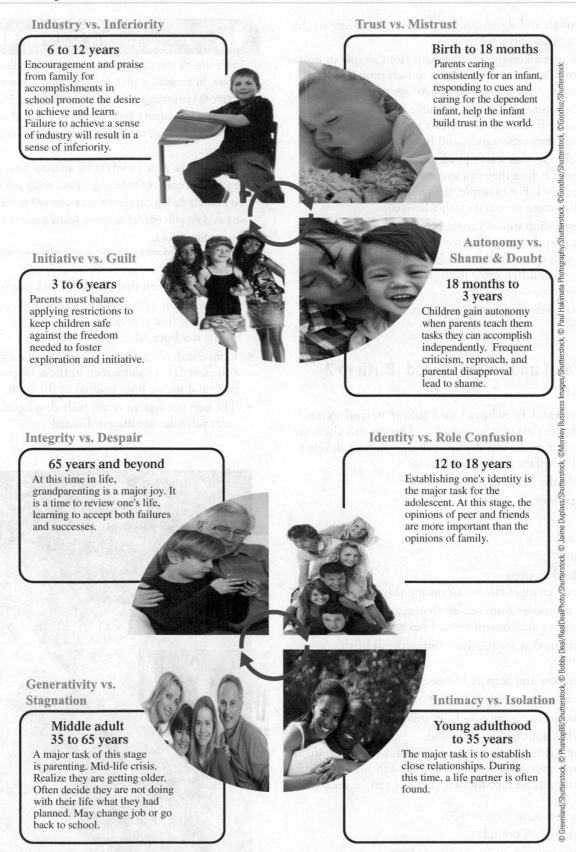

Industry vs. Inferiority

6 to 12 years
Encouragement and praise from family for accomplishments in school promote the desire to achieve and learn. Failure to achieve a sense of industry will result in a sense of inferiority.

Trust vs. Mistrust

Birth to 18 months
Parents caring consistently for an infant, responding to cues and caring for the dependent infant, help the infant build trust in the world.

Initiative vs. Guilt

3 to 6 years
Parents must balance applying restrictions to keep children safe against the freedom needed to foster exploration and initiative.

Autonomy vs. Shame & Doubt

18 months to 3 years
Children gain autonomy when parents teach them tasks they can accomplish independently. Frequent criticism, reproach, and parental disapproval lead to shame.

Integrity vs. Despair

65 years and beyond
At this time in life, grandparenting is a major joy. It is a time to review one's life, learning to accept both failures and successes.

Identity vs. Role Confusion

12 to 18 years
Establishing one's identity is the major task for the adolescent. At this stage, the opinions of peer and friends are more important than the opinions of family.

Generativity vs. Stagnation

Middle adult 35 to 65 years
A major task of this stage is parenting. Mid-life crisis. Realize they are getting older. Often decide they are not doing with their life what they had planned. May change job or go back to school.

Intimacy vs. Isolation

Young adulthood to 35 years
The major task is to establish close relationships. During this time, a life partner is often found.

FIGURE 9-2 Growth and development progress through different stages.

Growth and development progress according to the following basic principles:

- There is an ongoing movement from simple to more complex. For example, baby sounds progress to speech patterns and then fluent speech.
- Development and growth move from head to feet and from torso to limbs. The infant first raises the head, then sits, stands, and finally walks.
- Each stage has a set of tasks that the person must master before they can successfully move on to the next level. For example, the child learns to catch big balls before they can catch a baseball.
- Progression moves forward in an orderly manner, but the rate varies for each person. There are growth spurts in the preschool and teen years, but not all children grow to the same extent or at the same rate.
- Each person's growth progresses at an individual rate.

Neonatal and Infant Period (Birth to 2 Years)

The neonatal (newborn) and infant period extends through the first two years of life. During this time the child experiences rapid physical growth and development. The infant gradually learns to:

- Hold the head up
- Turn over
- Sit
- Crawl
- Stand
- Take first steps
  Other changes also occur during this period:
- Infant moves from self-awareness and parental or caregiver attachment toward ties with others.
- Systems that are relatively immature at birth stabilize.
- Alertness and activity increase.
- Teeth appear (erupt).
- Food intake progresses from milk to solid food.
- Verbal skills begin to develop.
  The primary caregiver of the infant is the central figure of emotional attachment. Growth and development progress so rapidly that changes can be seen each month.
  The **neonate** (Figure 9-3):
- Weighs 7–8 pounds
- Is approximately 19–21 inches long
- Has a head that seems disproportionately large compared to the body
- Has skin that is wrinkled, thin, and red

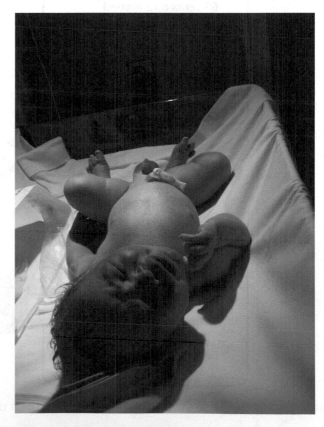

Age-Appropriate Care ALERT

There are no standard terms for describing the ages of babies. In general, a child is considered a newborn from birth to the beginning of the third month of age. The baby is considered an infant from 3 months to 1 year of age. However, many physical, social, and emotional factors affect the definition.

Communicate with an infant by smiling, being gentle, hugging, rocking, and touching. Speak softly and slowly or sing quietly during care. Introduce yourself to the parents and explain procedures to them. Allow parents to remain nearby during care.

- Has an abdomen that seems to stick out (protrude)
- Has dark blue eyes at birth that may change color during the first year of life
  In the newborn, the:
- Conversion of cartilage to bone (ossification) is not complete. This can be seen in the soft spots (fontanels) and suture lines (joints) of the skull
- The nervous system is not fully developed, so muscular activities are uncoordinated

FIGURE 9-3 A baby is considered a neonate (newborn) from birth to about 4 weeks of age.

- Vision is not clear, but hearing and taste are developed. Certain **reflexes** (automatic responses) are also developed. They are the:
  - Moro reflex—when the infant is startled, the arms extend outward with the thumbs flexed inward. The legs are extended and the head is thrust back. This response is also called the *startle reflex*. It usually disappears in 3 to 6 months.
  - Grasp reflex—touching the infant's palm causes the fingers to flex in a grasping motion. This reflex is strongest in premature infants and disappears several months after birth.
  - Rooting (sucking) reflex—stroking the cheek or side of the lips stimulates the infant to open the mouth and turn their head in the direction of the stroking. This is important in finding the nipple to suck the milk.
- Diet is milk or milk substitute.
- Routine is largely sleeping, eating, and eliminating.

The newborn is completely dependent on the caregiver. They must be handled carefully with the head well supported.

The 3-month-old infant:

- Has gained enough muscular coordination to hold their head up and raise their shoulders
- Has usually lost the Moro, rooting, and grasp reflexes
- Produces real tears
- Can follow objects with the eyes
- Can smile and coo

The 6-month-old infant:

- Can roll over
- Can sit for short periods of time
- Holds things with both hands and directs them toward their mouth
- Responds with verbal sounds when a caregiver speaks
- Is beginning to cut front teeth
- Eats finger foods and strained fruits and vegetables
- Recognizes family members
- Develops fear of strangers

The 9-month-old infant:

- Crawls and may begin to stand when supported
- Has more teeth erupt
- Can respond to their name
- Says one- and two-syllable words, such as *mama*
- Shows a preference for right- or left-hand control
- Eats junior baby foods

The 1-year-old infant:

- Understands simple commands such as "No"

- Begins to take steps—supported at first, then independently
- Eats table foods and can hold their own cup
- Weighs three times the birth weight

Toddler Period (2 to 3 Years)

The **toddler** period is a busy, active phase during which exploration and investigation are the main activities. The child also develops motor abilities (Figure 9-4). Vocabulary and comprehension increase.

During this period, the toddler:

- Learns to control elimination.
- Begins to become aware of right and wrong.
- Begins to become aware of themselves as a separate person and may respond negatively to attempts at socialization and discipline.
- Tolerates brief periods of separation from the caregiver, but the caregiver remains the source of security and comfort.

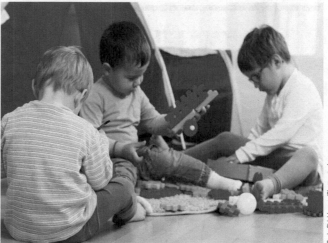

FIGURE 9-4 Toddlers play in the company of other children but do not interact with each other.

- May play in the company of other children but with no interaction. This age group is very possessive. *No* and *mine* are a major part of their vocabularies. At the end of this period, the toddler can:
- Walk and run.
- Display motor (manual) skills that include feeding themselves and riding toys.
- Put words together and speak more clearly. The average vocabulary of a 2-year-old is about 300 words.

Preschool Years (3 to 5 Years)

The 3- to 5-year-old (Figure 9-5) builds on the motor and verbal skills developed as a toddler. They are curious and ask many questions. During this period, the preschooler:

- Grows less reliant on the parent. Children in this age group begin to recognize their position as members of the family unit and their uniqueness from other members.
- Develops rivalries with siblings and forms greater attachments to alternate caregivers.

👪 Age-Appropriate Care ALERT

When caring for a preschooler, explain procedures to the child in simple language. Tell them what you will do each time, but do not expect them to remember. Demonstrate procedures on a doll or stuffed animal, whenever possible. Use simple words and short sentences. Smile often. Use familiar times, such as "before lunch" or "after dinner," rather than stating the time. Reward the child for positive behavior with attention and special treats, as allowed. Allow them to be as independent as possible.

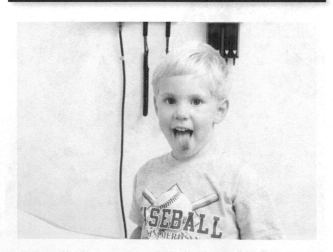

FIGURE 9-5 This preschool-age child cooperates during an examination by sticking out the tongue.

- Becomes more cooperative and gradually increases cooperative play. The child may seem eager to follow rules within limits.
- Develops a more active imagination.
- Becomes more sexually curious.

By the end of this period, children have become far more socialized than they were as toddlers. They are more cooperative. They enjoy interacting with family members and peers.

School-Age Children (5 to 12 Years)

The school-age child (Figure 9-6):

- Is able to communicate.
- Has developed small (fine) motor skills. With these skills, the child is able to master tasks such as writing.
- Develops an increased sense of self.
- Establishes peer relationships.
- Reinforces proper social behavior through games, simple tasks, and play.
- Begins to show concern for other living things (Figure 9-7).

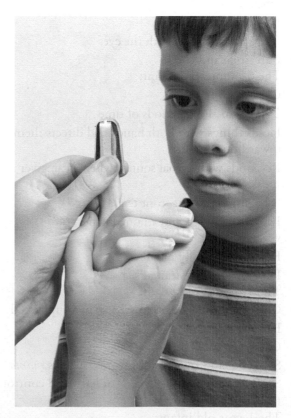

FIGURE 9-6 This school-age child closely observes as a splint is applied to an injured finger.

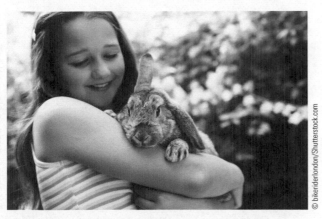

FIGURE 9-7 School-age children begin to show concern for other living things such as pets.

Preadolescence

Some experts recognize a transitional stage called **Preadolescence** that serves as an introduction to the teen years for 12- to 14-year-olds. Other experts do not recognize this stage. This is a period of great uncertainty. During this period:

- There is a growing awareness of and interest in the opposite sex.
- Hormonal changes stimulate the secondary sex characteristics. Many become sexually active.
- Feels on the verge of tremendous change (Figure 9-8).
- Mood swings and feelings of insecurity are common.
- Arms and legs seem out of proportion to the rest of the body.

Adolescence (12 to 20 Years)

Adolescence is marked by:

- The gradual development of sexual maturity.

Age-Appropriate Care **ALERT**

When caring for a school-age child, call the child by name. Explain procedures in simple terms, but use proper names for body parts. Encourage the child to ask questions. Allow the child to make decisions, as appropriate. Set limits on behavior, if necessary. Reason with the child, if necessary. Always speak during care. Allow the child to call or text friends on the phone, if desired. Be aware that the child may try to delay procedures. Stay with the child during painful procedures and provide comfort and reassurance. Distraction may be effective during procedures. Give the child as much control as possible.

Age-Appropriate Care **ALERT**

Preadolescent children are sensitive to the caregiver's body language; make sure yours is appropriate. Explain procedures in adult terms. Avoid talking down to the child, but simplify and clarify information as necessary. Spend time talking with the child. Maintain a nonthreatening demeanor. Avoid power struggles. Ensure that the child informs you of their whereabouts, if they leave the unit. Be as flexible as possible.

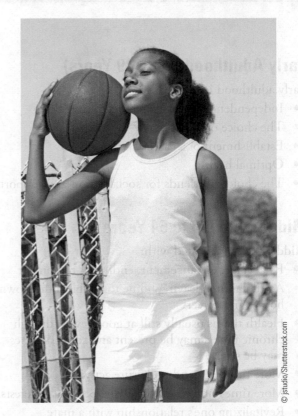

FIGURE 9-8 Preadolescent children begin to experience physical and emotional changes.

- A greater appreciation of the individual's own identity as a male or a female person.
- Conflicting desires for the freedom of independence and the security of dependence. Because of these conflicting desires, this can be a troublesome period.
- The establishment of personal coping systems and the ability to make independent judgments and decisions.
- Gradual success in mastering the developmental tasks of the age. The adolescent is able to make comparisons between the values they have been taught and reality.

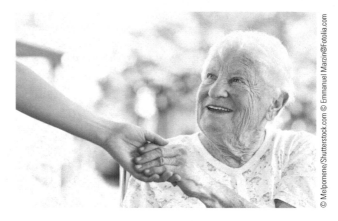

FIGURE 9-9 Older adults may become frail and need assistance from others.

Early Adulthood (20 to 49 Years)

Early adulthood is marked by:

- Independence and personal decision making
- The choice of a mate
- Establishment of a career and family life
- Optimal health
- The choice of friends for socialization and support

Middle Age (50 to 64 Years)

Middle age is associated with:

- Final career advancement, ending in retirement
- Adult children leaving home to establish their own homes and careers
- Health that is usually still at good levels, though chronic illness may be present and some declines may be seen
- More time to spend on leisure activities
- More time and money to pursue personal interests
- Revitalizing one's relationship with a mate
- Enjoying grandchildren
- For some middle-aged persons, being a member of the "sandwich" generation—caring for both their own parents and their children or grandchildren

Later Maturity (65 to 75 Years)

Later maturity is marked by:

- A gradual loss of vitality and stamina
- Physical declines related to the aging process, such as deterioration in vision and hearing
- Chronic conditions that develop and persist
- A period of gradual losses: loss of mate, friends, self-esteem, some independence
- Examination of one's lifetime

- More time to pursue personal interests
- Fewer responsibilities related to raising a family and holding a job
- Increased wisdom

Old Age (75 Years and Beyond)

Aging is a gradual process that begins at birth. Old age can be a period of development and enjoyment. Old age is frequently characterized by:

- Failing physical health and increased dependency (Figure 9-9)
- The acceptance of one's own mortality and need to deal with illness, disability, loneliness, and loss of friends and loved ones

Success in this period depends on the coping mechanisms that the person has developed over their lifetime. Having solid emotional and physical support is also important.

BASIC HUMAN NEEDS

Developmental skills and physical growth may vary during the life span. The basic human needs, however, are much the same for every individual.

Basic human needs are the things and activities required to live a successful, satisfactory life. All people have the same basic needs. Culture influences the expression of basic needs, as do native language, diet and food preferences, background, beliefs, values, spirituality, religion, hygiene, and health care practices. Avoid judging others for their beliefs. These cultural patterns are part of the uniqueness of each individual and must be considered when providing care.

Abraham Maslow and Erik Erikson are two leaders in the field of human behavior. They have helped us understand basic needs and how people go about satisfying them.

Age-Appropriate Care **ALERT**

When caring for elderly adults (age 65 and older), introduce yourself. Address the patient by title and last name unless they instruct you otherwise. Avoid use of demeaning terms, such as *honey* and *dear*. Speak slowly and clearly, making good eye contact. Be alert to vision and hearing problems, making adaptations as necessary, such as cleaning glasses or providing a pen and paper or white board for written communication. Avoid assuming that persons in this age group are confused, disoriented, or mentally impaired. Allow enough time for the person to respond to you. Be sensitive to the patient's need to communicate and allow time to talk. Be a good listener. Explain procedures honestly. Treat the patient with respect. Allow the patient to set their own routine, as much as possible. Adjust room temperature to the patient's preference. Maintain a quiet, well-lighted, safe environment. Inform the patient about policies, services, and routines. Avoid rapid changes in position. Allow the patient to dangle their legs at the bedside prior to transfer and ambulation.

Personality

Personality is the sum of ways we react to the events in our lives and satisfy our needs. It is gradually formed through experience and molded by cultural heritage.

Erikson suggested that our personalities are formed as we mature from infancy to old age. He believed that we pass through eight growing stages in search of **self-identity** (who we really are). Each stage has physical and mental tasks that must be accomplished before the person can move on to the next task. He called these the **tasks of personality development** (Table 9-2).

Maslow described human needs as physical, psychological, and sociological. He placed the needs on a **continuum** in which physical needs have to be satisfied first. According to Maslow's theory, realizing one's full potential is the goal of life. If something blocks the path to achieving this goal, the individual becomes frustrated. The psychological and sociological needs can be met only after the physical needs have been satisfied (Figure 9-10). The progression of needs is called a *hierarchy of needs*.

Physical Needs

The most basic human needs are physical needs. They include:

- Nutrition
- Rest
- Oxygen
- Shelter
- Elimination
- Activity
- Sexuality

Illness creates stress that makes meeting the needs a challenge. In fact, illness creates its own set of stresses (Table 9-3).

Meeting the Patient's Physical Needs

Meeting patients' physical needs is a key nursing assistant responsibility. These needs include oxygen, food, shelter, sleep, elimination, and physical activity.

Oxygen

The body cannot live without oxygen, which is found in the air. Most of us take breathing for granted until it becomes difficult. If a person is not getting enough oxygen, nothing else seems important. It may be necessary to give the patient extra oxygen by cannula, mask, or another device (see Chapter 39). Sometimes respirations can be eased by positioning and supporting the patient on pillows.

TABLE 9-2 Tasks of Personality Development According to the Stages Defined by Erikson

Physical Stage	Year of Occurrence	Tasks to Be Mastered
Oral-sensory	Birth to 2 years (infant)	To learn to trust (Trust)
Muscular-anal	2 to 3 years (toddler)	To recognize self as being independent from mother (Autonomy)
Locomotor	3 to 5 years (preschool years)	To recognize self as a family member (Initiative)
Latency	5 to 11 years (school-age years)	To demonstrate physical and mental skills/abilities (Industry)
Adolescence	12 to 20 years	To develop a sense of individuality as a sexual human being (Identity)
Young adulthood	20 to 35 years	To establish intimate personal relationships with a mate (Intimacy)
Adulthood	35 to 50 years	To live a satisfying and productive life
Maturity	50+ years	To review life's events and examine how they have influenced the development of a unique individual (Ego integrity)

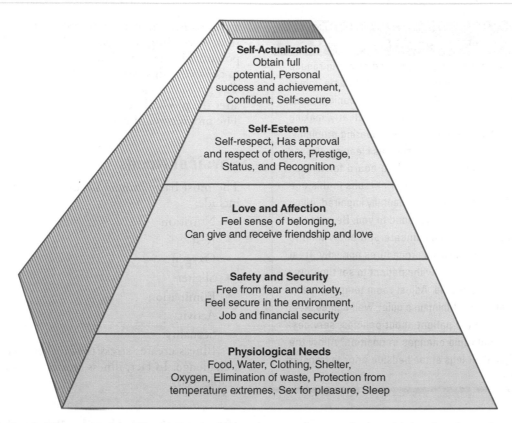

FIGURE 9-10 Maslow's hierarchy of needs. Lower-level needs must be met before higher-level needs can be addressed.

TABLE 9-3 Potential Stressors Caused by Illness

Threat	Potential Stressor
Physical threats	Fear of pain Fear of body changes Fear of changes in appearance Fear of death Procedures that cause actual pain
Mental threats	Self-image is threatened New situations are threatening Body-image changes are threatening Potential or actual life changes are threatening
Loss of control over environment and body	Feeling as if one has no say in important life changes Feeling as if one has no say in plan of care Loss of control affects self-esteem and increases anxiety Loss of control over body functions Lack of privacy in communication Loss of choice over foods
Unmet needs	Pain Hunger Thirst Uncomfortable position Inability to move unassisted Lack of privacy in bathing, dressing, toileting Inability to urinate Constipation Boredom; loss of preferred method of entertainment

Food

Patients may lose their appetite or sense of thirst due to:

- Inactivity
- Offensive odors
- Effects of some medications
- Pain
- Fear and anxiety
- Types of food served
- Illness
- Infection
- Aging changes (Chapter 33)

You will care for persons with a variety of nutritional problems, such as:

- Inability to feed self; need to be fed
- Need for special diets or foods
- Need for tube feeding
- Need for extra fluid replacement through a sterile tube inserted into a vein

Suggestions for improving nutritional intake:

- Assist patients to use the bathroom before meals
- Serve food at the proper temperature in pleasant surroundings.
- Close bathroom doors to eliminate unpleasant odors.
- Honor cultural preferences whenever possible.
- Assist with handwashing and positioning in bed or chair before (and after) meals, as permitted.
- Serve the food in a calm, pleasant manner.
- Encourage and assist patients to be as independent as possible, but be available to assist if needed.

Shelter

A safe and comfortable environment helps meet the need for shelter. For example:

- Ensure that the temperature is comfortable.
- Report the need for repairs to the proper person.
- Ensure floors are clean and obstacle free.
- Maintain a comfortable noise level (Chapter 10).

Sleep

See Chapter 10 for a discussion of the patient's sleep and rest needs.

Elimination

The body must be able to eliminate perspiration, urine, and feces. Promote elimination by:

- Bathing, which removes dirt and perspiration and keeps the skin healthy
- Encouraging the patient to drink six to eight glasses of fluids and, if possible, to eat foods high in fiber

- Helping patients who are unable to use the usual toilet facilities by providing them with bedpans, urinals, and bedside commodes

Physical Activity

Activity promotes improved functioning of all systems. Circulation and respiration are increased. Muscles, bones, and joints function more efficiently. The body as a whole responds in a positive way to activity. People, by nature, are active beings. Illness often limits activity, so the patient must stay in bed for a long time. Find ways of promoting activity for these individuals. Consider the patient's capability and treatment goals when planning activity.

Refer to Chapters 41 and 48 for additional information on the complications of inactivity and methods of reducing the risk of complications.

Security and Safety Needs

Once physical needs are provided for, safety and security become priorities. Security and safety for patients are provided by:

- Maintaining a safe environment (see Chapters 14 and 15)
- Taking measures that are necessary to prevent incidents and accidents
- Knowing how to respond to medical emergencies, such as patient falls
- Knowing how to respond to facility emergencies, such as fire
- Implementing the patient's care plan as indicated

Emotional Needs

The third and fourth levels of Maslow's hierarchy are related to emotional needs, including the need for love and belonging and the need for esteem. There is a need:

- To give love
- To feel love
- To be loved
- To be treated with respect and dignity
- To feel that self-esteem (our opinion of ourselves) is protected

All individuals—you, your co-workers, and your patients—have in their own minds an idea of how they appear and wish to appear to others. This idea is referred to as **self-esteem**. Protect self-esteem at all costs.

For example, a person might visualize and project to others the image of a very self-reliant person, capable of making important decisions and able to care for self and family. Suddenly that same person is scantily dressed in a hospital bed. A stranger is taking care of their most intimate physical functions. Even the times to eat and bathe are decided for them. This set of circumstances threatens even the most secure person's self-esteem.

A patient's response to this threat to self-esteem depends on two things. First, it depends on how often the patient has had these feelings of helplessness before, and how well they have dealt with them. Second, it depends on you and your ability to appreciate those feelings.

One patient may feel frustrated and angry. They may not even know that these feelings are based on fear. The patient may act out these feelings by complaining about the hospital, the staff, roommates, you, or the food. In fact, every aspect of the care may be cause for complaint. Be open and receptive to these actions, recognizing the underlying feelings.

Still another patient may react quite differently to the same emotional stress. That person may be quiet and withdrawn. They may be completely cooperative and uncomplaining. The behavior shown is a false front. It hides the patient's feelings of not being able to cope with the situation (Figure 9-11). Be aware of these feelings and the need for caring support.

Intimacy and Sexuality

Intimacy is a feeling of closeness with another human (Figure 9-12). It is a relationship marked by feelings of love and affection that are an integral part of the human response.

Sexuality is a lifelong characteristic that defines whether the person is male or female. This definition may be different for each person. All individuals are sexual, whether or not they have physical sexual relations. Sexuality has to do with the ability to develop relationships, to give of oneself to others, and to appreciate the giving by others. Intimacy is one aspect of sexuality.

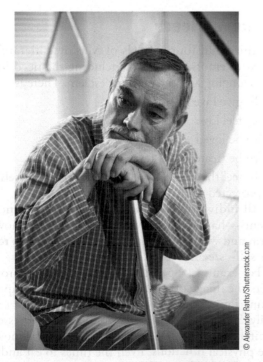

FIGURE 9-11 This patient appears vulnerable and alone.

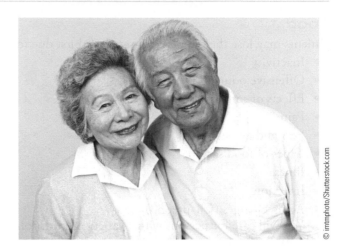

FIGURE 9-12 This couple appears to be happy.

Intimacy may be shared between friends or lovers. Also, a degree of intimacy is established when patient and caregiver learn to trust each other.

Sexual behavior is a personal choice, but intimacy is an important aspect of the human sexual experience. Moral standards, genetics, sexual orientation, and opportunity all affect intimate relationships and sexual identity.

Some patients will have same-sex partners. Others will select a partner of the opposite sex. One's choice of sexual partner and sexual preference is a very complex subject. Avoid judging the patient's choice of partner(s). This is especially important with members of the gay, lesbian, and transgender community. Most people worry about depending on strangers for intimate personal care. Many gay, lesbian, and transgender persons have been insulted, isolated, disrespected, and shunned when seeking health care services, and they fear that they will be mistreated or ignored again. They are human beings above all else, and as such deserve to be cared for with compassion and respect.

Commitment is an important part of each intimate relationship. Most couples make sexual intimacy part of their relationship, but some do not. For example, a loving couple may choose not to have sexual intercourse. Despite remaining **celibate** (no sexual intercourse), they still share an intimacy and commitment that is natural and fulfilling.

Our society tends to associate youth and beauty with sexuality. By these standards, persons who are old or have disabilities are not considered to be sexual beings. Old age, illness, and disability do not diminish human sexuality. The person within a human being does not change. Although the hair is gray, or the skin is wrinkled, the person inside still has needs for and feelings of love, affection, and intimacy. Help patients maintain their sexuality by:

- Assisting patients with hygiene, grooming, and an attractive appearance
- Conversing with patients on an adult level

It is important to recognize that not everyone has the same orientation, preference, opportunities, or moral standards. This does not mean that differences make one person wrong and another right. As a caregiver, you must be understanding of others who do not share your personal views.

Some terms related to human sexual expression are:

- **Heterosexuality**—sexual attraction between opposite sexes.
- **Homosexuality**—sexual attraction between persons of the same sex. Female partners are called lesbians. Male partners are often referred to as being gay.
- **Bisexuality**—sexual attraction to members of both sexes.
- **Transgender**—a person whose personal feelings about gender identity does not match the anatomical sex they were born with. These individuals feel as if they were born with a physical body of the wrong gender.
- **Masturbation**—self-stimulation for sexual pleasure.

You may hear the acronym LGBTQ used to describe the sexual orientation or gender identity of some persons. This means:

Lesbian

Gay

Bisexual

Transgender

Queer, Questioning

The terms *queer community*, *rainbow community*, or *LGBTQ +2 community* are also used. Please remember that this information does not affect the care you give. It is for your information and understanding only.

Love can be expressed in many different ways, including caressing, exchange of loving gestures, talking, hugging, and touching. **Coitus** (intercourse) is not always necessary for satisfaction.

Providing opportunities for patients to meet sexual and other intimate needs in a health care setting is not always easy. However, there are some actions that nursing assistants can do to help patients meet these needs:

- Respect patients' privacy. Always knock and wait before opening a closed door.
- Speak before opening curtains drawn around the bed.
- Do not judge behaviors and preferences that are different from your own.
- Do not discuss personal sexual information about a patient with others.
- Provide privacy if a patient is masturbating, and avoid passing judgment on this activity.
- Discourage patients who make sexual advances to you. State in a calm, matter-of-fact way that you are not interested and move on to other work. If a patient persists, report the matter to the nurse.

- Recognize that the need for intimacy is a basic human need that is expressed in many ways.

Human Touch

The need for human touch should not be overlooked. Pleasure and satisfaction are felt by a parent and child as they touch one another. Adults experience similar feelings.

Older adults tend to reserve touching for intimate friends and family members. They often feel sad, lonely, and deprived when circumstances change and opportunities for touching become fewer. These emotions are common in older adults who live alone or in long-term care facilities.

Be open to nonsexual touching. Avoid forcing attention on a patient. Help satisfy a patient's need for touch by:

- Giving a friendly hug and smile (Figure 9-13)
- Patting a person on the shoulder
- Holding or clasping hands
- Applying lotion to skin
- Giving a backrub

Nonsexual touching can mean much to the lives of those in your care. However, wearing gloves is sometimes necessary for safe and efficient care.

Each facility has policies and procedures for wearing gloves. Follow your employer's rules. In most facilities, nursing assistants are expected to use good judgment, applying gloves when necessary to reduce the risk of infection. Sometimes caregivers apply gloves upon entering the room, then wear these gloves until they are ready to leave. Although there are times when this is necessary, wearing gloves is not necessary or desirable for many patient care situations. In fact, wearing gloves may send a message that the patient is undesirable, untouchable, or highly infectious. Wearing gloves continuously has the potential for causing cross-contamination throughout the room. Make sure you are following standard precautions and guidelines for glove use. Avoid offending patients by the unnecessary use of gloves. Follow your employer's policies, but always remember the powerful need for human contact. Balance your infection control precautions (Chapter 13) with patients' emotional needs for love, belonging, and acceptance.

> ### ✚ Clinical Information **ALERT**
>
> The feeling of skin touching skin releases a hormone called *oxytocin*, causing a pleasurable sensation. Touch can send a variety of messages, depending on the nature and location of the touch. Of these, the most common messages we send are those of intimacy and love.

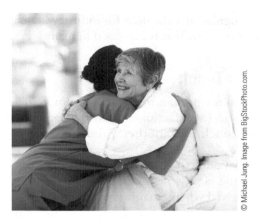

FIGURE 9-13 Hugging communicates caring and love.

Dealing with the Fearful Patient

The experienced nursing assistant does not take remarks from patients personally. The assistant realizes that the patient's complaints and refusal to cooperate may be a way of saying, "I need to be reassured and protected." Give the patient an opportunity to talk. Listen carefully to everything that is said (Figure 9-14). You may be able to convince the fearful patient to perform some personal care whenever possible. If help in feeding, shaving, elimination, or other such personal matters is needed, act in a very gentle, efficient manner and ensure the patient's privacy at all times.

To handle these situations successfully, the nursing assistant must:

- Recognize that this patient is a person with individual likes and dislikes.
- Give the quality of care that considers these likes and dislikes. Honoring the patient's preferences will enhance satisfaction. Meeting the patient's needs at this level is an excellent way of giving person-centered, individualized care.
- Help the patient find ways to fill the time while in the hospital. Boredom alone can lead to irritability. Some hospitals have volunteers who bring books and other activities directly to the bedside.

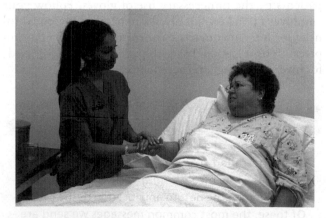

FIGURE 9-14 Tact and patience are necessary to break through a wall of fear and frustration.

Patient Privacy

Patients in the hospital give up a good bit of control over their lives. They put their lives and well-being into the hands of caregivers. In exchange, patients assume that certain of their rights will be assured. These rights include the right to privacy.

Patients must feel certain that their privacy will be protected. Even though you perform the most intimate procedures for them, you must do so in a way that neither exposes them unnecessarily nor embarrasses them. Privacy may be provided by means of:

- Curtains or screens placed around the bed
- Knocking and saying the patient's name before entering a room (Figure 9-15)
- Speaking to the patient before entering a screened area

Privacy must be provided for the patient whose body is exposed, such as during:

- Bathing
- Using the bedpan
- Receiving treatments
- Being visited by clergy

Be prompt at other times to recognize a patient's need for privacy and to provide it.

Patients must also be certain that you keep their personal information confidential. Treat them with the courtesy you would extend to a guest in your home. This adds to patients' sense of security. Understanding what patients are really trying to tell us is one of the most

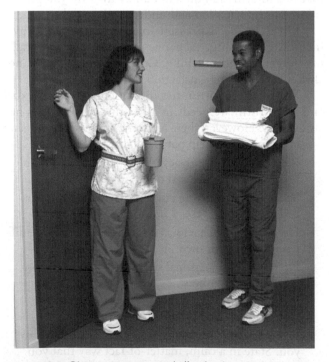

FIGURE 9-15 Show respect and dignity by always asking for permission to enter a patient's room.

difficult parts of giving care. When we are successful, it is probably the most rewarding. With this in mind, always remember to treat each patient as a unique individual.

Spiritual Needs

Spiritual beliefs are deeply held by some patients and disregarded by others. When beliefs are strongly held, they are apt to guide a patient's actions and responses in direct ways, such as praying, reading religious writings, and participating in ceremonies and celebrations. Some personal items may have special religious significance and must be treated with respect.

Patients' spiritual needs are often greater when they are fearful and ill (Figure 9-16). Be prepared to act on requests for clergy visits and spiritual support. Do not impose your beliefs on the patient.

You may be tempted to share your personal religious faith with others, especially when the patient directly asks your opinion. This is a challenging situation. Here are some guidelines to assist you:

- Remember that each person has a right to believe in any faith system or to deny the existence of any beliefs.
- Listen to the patient's thoughts and keep them confidential.
- Your role is to reflect the patient's ideas. Do not try to convince the patient of your ideas. For example, if the patient asks if you believe in God, reflect the patient's thinking with a statement such as "You have been thinking about God," or "Would you like to talk?"

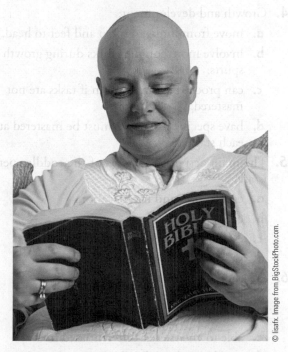

FIGURE 9-16 This patient appears to be peaceful and comforted by reading the Bible.

The patient may want to visit with a familiar clergy member, or may ask about the chaplain or clergy service available at the health care facility. Some health care facilities ask clergy from the community to make visits to patients who want such a visit but do not know a particular minister, priest, or rabbi. Larger facilities have chaplain educational residencies for people preparing for careers in the clergy. The residencies serve patients' spiritual needs while offering training for the chaplains.

Chapels are open in some facilities. Both visitors and ambulatory patients find comfort in visiting them. Religious services are sometimes broadcast to patients' rooms from these chapels.

Know what services are available to your patients. When asked, share this information, but do not recommend any particular service. Patients should be free to make their own choices. You should always be ready and willing to support their choices.

Social Needs

Some people have very poor self-esteem. Self-esteem affects all areas of a person's life. When primary physical, psychological, and spiritual needs have been met, the person is free to pursue the third level of social needs and activities that are unique to the individual. The goal of these activities is to make one feel good as a person, providing a sense of accomplishment and self-esteem. Sociological needs are met by successful positive interactions with others and opportunities for free personal expression.

One of the most basic needs of all people is the need to understand others and to be understood. We achieve this sense of understanding when we communicate successfully with others. We usually try to communicate verbally. Sometimes we also do this by the:

- Words we choose
- Way we say the words
- Tone of voice
- Facial expression
- Form of touch

Even the way we stand or reach out says a lot. We know it is not always easy to find the right words to express our thoughts and feelings. Thus, caregivers must be constantly aware of the patient's need to communicate effectively, too.

Volunteers and visitors, as well as television and reading, can provide entertainment and diversion. Learning about and supporting patients' interests helps prevent boredom and enhances self-esteem.

Appearing interested and unhurried when talking with patients makes it easier for patients to express their needs. It also makes it easier to find ways of meeting these needs.

REVIEW

A. True/False

Mark the following true or false by circling T or F.

1. T F   Growth and development go from the simple to the complex.

2. T F   Body development proceeds from the head toward the feet.

3. T F   All individuals move through the stages of growth.

4. T F   Growth and development progression are interdependent.

5. T F   Ossification of bones is not complete at birth.

6. T F   The Moro reflex occurs when the infant's palm is touched.

7. T F   The sucking reflex occurs when the infant is startled.

8. T F   A 3-month-old infant cries real tears.

9. T F   A 6-month-old infant can walk if well supported.

10. T F   First teeth begin to erupt about the sixth month of life.

11. T F   A 1-year-old infant has progressed to eating table foods.

12. T F   During the toddler period, children interact freely and play well with one another.

13. T F   Between the ages of 3 and 5 years, a child seems to have an endless list of questions.

14. T F   A school-age child is interested in and chooses members of the same sex as close friends.

15. T F   One of the developmental tasks of old age is to learn to deal successfully with loss.

16. T F   Basic human needs are the same at all ages, but different ways must be found to satisfy them.

17. T F   Erikson believed that one of the developmental tasks of infancy is learning to trust.

18. T F   Erikson states that the developmental task of the middle years is to integrate life's experiences.

19. T F   Patients who are fearful often show anger or frustration.

20. T F   Spiritual needs are part of basic human needs.

21. T F   Culture has no influence over how basic human needs are met.

22. T F   Each generation has music that they consider their own.

23. T F   The most basic human needs are psychosocial needs.

24. T F   Cultural patterns are part of the uniqueness of each individual.

25. T F   One generation is the time that elapses between the birth of the parents and the birth of their grandchildren.

26. T F   The tasks to be mastered are defined by the needs of the individual and the pressures of society.

27. T F   Culture does not affect the expression of basic needs.

28. T F   Treating each patient with approval and respect makes them feel valued.

B. Matching

Choose the correct chronologic age from Column II to match each lifetime period in Column I.

Column I		Column II
29. _____	old age	a. 65 years old
30. _____	adolescence	b. 16 years old
31. _____	later maturity	c. 7 years old
32. _____	school age	d. 35 years old
33. _____	adulthood	e. 80 years old

C. Multiple Choice

Select the best answer for each of the following.

34. Growth and development:
    a. move from limbs to torso and feet to head.
    b. involve more complex tasks during growth spurts.
    c. can proceed normally even if tasks are not mastered.
    d. have specific tasks that must be mastered at each stage.

35. The main activity/activities of the toddler period is/are:
    a. exploration and investigation.
    b. cooperative play.
    c. establishing peer relationships.
    d. showing concern for others.

36. Preschoolers are:
    a. less reliant on their mothers.
    b. able to join groups like Scouts.
    c. able to choose sex-differentiated friends.
    d. unable to tolerate brief separation from the mother.

37. The ways in which we react to the events in our lives are called:

   a. personality.

   b. self-identity.

   c. tasks of personality development.

   d. hierarchy of needs.

38. The members of a generation:

   a. are about the same age with the same interests.

   b. have been influenced by the same social markers.

   c. have the same problems, wants, and needs.

   d. are the same as those from other cultures.

39. The first U.S. generation to be given a label was:

   a. the GI generation.

   b. Generation X.

   c. the veteran generation.

   d. the baby boom.

40. Which of the following is true?

   a. Growth involves social, emotional, and psychological changes.

   b. Advances in behavior and interpersonal skills are examples of growth.

   c. Development describes social, emotional, and psychological changes.

   d. Height, weight, and system maturation are developmental levels.

41. Preadolescence spans ages:

   a. 5 to 12 years.

   b. 12 to 14 years.

   c. 14 to 20 years.

   d. 20 to 49 years.

42. The neonatal period:

   a. includes women of childbearing age.

   b. extends from birth through age two.

   c. involves teens and young adults.

   d. ends when a young couple marries.

43. Characteristics of later maturity include:

   a. new development of chronic disease.

   b. becoming a member of the "sandwich" generation.

   c. enjoying one's spouse, children, and grandchildren.

   d. acceptance of mortality and need to deal with disability.

44. According to Maslow:

   a. psychological needs must be satisfied first.

   b. physical needs are not as important as others.

   c. realizing one's full potential is the goal of life.

   d. the progression of needs is called egocentricity.

45. A person who is celibate:

   a. is attracted to members of the same sex.

   b. has elected not to have sexual intercourse.

   c. is physically unable to have intercourse.

   d. thinks they were born in the wrong body.

46. The sensation of skin touching skin:

   a. releases a hormone called oxytocin.

   b. can cause a painful sensation.

   c. stimulates release of blood glucose.

   d. stimulates production of testosterone.

47. Self-esteem:

   a. Is our opinion of ourselves.

   b. Describes how nice we look.

   c. Is how we feel about others.

   d. Applies to personal hygiene.

48. If you find a person masturbating

   a. tell the person to stop.

   b. provide privacy and leave.

   c. Inform the nurse.

   d. Cover them with a sheet.

D. Nursing Assistant Challenge

Mrs. Chen is a 35-year-old patient with a diagnosis of breast cancer. She recently had a radical mastectomy. She has lost most of her hair and has no appetite as a result of chemotherapy. Mrs. McClendon has lost weight and has occasional severe pain. She has a husband and three young children. Consider the needs that all people have and think about Mrs. McClendon as you answer the following questions.

49. Which physical needs may be difficult to meet? What can the nursing staff do to help Mrs. McClendon meet these needs?

50. Do you think her needs for safety and security will be met? What information do you have indicating that she has reason to feel fear and anxiety?

51. How might Mrs. McClendon's condition affect her relationship with her husband and children?

52. How do you think her sexuality may be affected?

53. Maslow states that human needs are on a hierarchy. Describe how this hierarchy may change throughout the day for Mrs. McClendon.

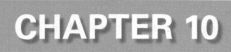

CHAPTER 10

Comfort, Pain, Rest, and Sleep

OBJECTIVES

After completing this chapter, you will be able to:

10.1 Spell and define terms.

10.2 Explain how noise affects patients and hospital staff.

10.3 Explain why nursing comfort measures are important to patients' well-being.

10.4 List six observations to make and report for patients having pain.

10.5 State the purpose of the pain rating scale.

10.6 Briefly describe how a pain scale is used.

10.7 Describe nursing assistant measures to increase comfort, relieve pain, and promote rest and sleep.

10.8 Name the phases of the sleep cycle.

10.9 Describe the importance of each phase of the sleep cycle.

VOCABULARY

Learn the meaning and the correct spelling of the following words and phrases:

analgesic
bruxism
comfort
enuresis
hypersomnia

insomnia
narcolepsy
nonrapid eye movement
   (NREM) sleep
pain

rapid eye movement (REM)
  sleep
rest
sleep
sleep apnea

sleep deprivation
somnambulism

COMFORT

All humans need comfort, rest, and sleep for physical and emotional health and wellness. **Comfort** is a state of physical and emotional well-being. The person who is feeling comfort is calm and relaxed and is not in pain or upset. Assisting patients with their comfort needs is a major nursing assistant responsibility. In fact, assisting patients with physical or emotional comfort needs is at the heart of nursing care.

Many factors affect patients' comfort. Environmental factors that interfere with comfort are unfamiliar environment, lack of privacy, noise, odor, temperature, lighting, and ventilation. Personal and uncontrollable factors that may increase or contribute to discomfort include age, activity, positioning, injury, illness, surgery, stress, and pain.

As a rule, patients are uncomfortable when their physical and emotional needs are not being met. Unmet needs cause tension and anxiety, and interfere with comfort and rest (Figure 10-1). Using basic nursing measures to meet patients' needs promotes comfort, reduces stress, and aids in relaxation, providing a sense of well-being.

NOISE CONTROL

Florence Nightingale is considered the founder of modern nursing (Figure 10-2). In *Notes on Nursing*, she wrote, "Unnecessary noise is the most cruel abuse of care which can be inflicted on either the sick or the well" (1859, pp. 26–27). Miss Nightingale would be aghast at the high-tech world of the twenty-first century. We have alarms on most medical equipment and electronic technology that did not exist in the nineteenth century that would cause her to question whether we are caring for patients or merely responding to alarms. Even without considering alarms, some medical equipment is very noisy.

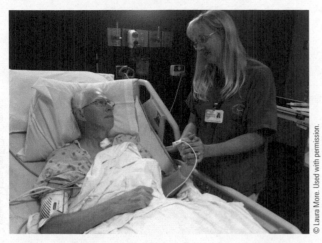

FIGURE 10-1 This patient appears to be content and relaxed, is in good body alignment, and has basic comfort needs addressed by the nursing assistant.

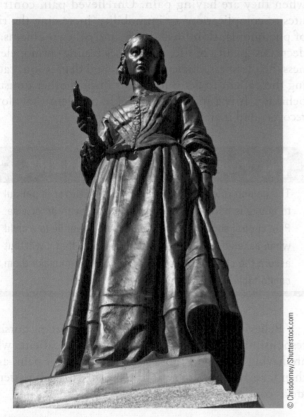

FIGURE 10-2 Florence Nightingale was called the "Lady with the Lamp." She insisted on nursing education and quality care.

Excessive noise delays healing, impairs immune function, and increases heart rate and blood pressure. Patients may feel very stressed or anxious and may not realize that noise is the cause of their distress. Patients who do not sleep well at night may be unhappy with care and be unable to stay awake during the day for therapy, diagnostic tests, physician evaluations, restorative nursing, meals, and activities. Some patients become confused and agitated when deprived of sleep. Confused patients may begin wandering to escape the noise.

The Occupational Safety and Health Administration (OSHA) has established noise standards stating that workers should not be exposed to 90 decibels of sound or higher for more than 8 hours. Decibel levels for common sounds include:

- 0 decibels—weakest sound heard by the normal human ear
- 30 decibels—whispered conversation
- 60 decibels—normal conversation
- 80 decibels—ringing telephone
- 90 decibels—hair dryer

Refer to Figure 10-3 for a list of examples of various noise levels. The Environmental Protection Agency (EPA) recommends that hospital noise levels not exceed 45 decibels during the day (see Figure 10-3).

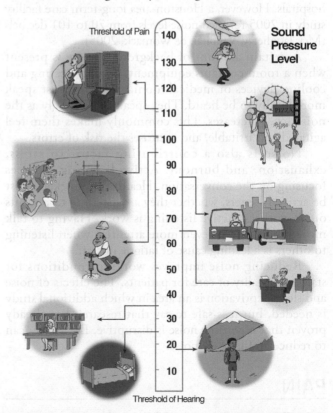

FIGURE 10-3 This chart identifies the intensity of sound created by various activities. Hospital noise at night can be equated with jackhammers and chainsaws and interrupts sleep. Actions to reduce noise include closing patient room doors and muffling sounds.

A study done by the staff of one hospital unit has direct implications for nursing assistant practice (Cmiel et al., 2004). In this study, nurse researchers were secretly admitted to the hospital as patients. Noise levels were measured with special instruments. The workers who were on duty did not know of the study or that noise was being measured. Study results were:

- Decibel levels as high as 113 were recorded at night.
- The noisiest time was at shift change, when more people were entering and leaving the unit.
- Two nurses who acted as patients noted that the noise from equipment alarms, phones, carts, X-ray machines, opening and closing doors, the paging and intercom systems, roommates, and nursing personnel interrupted their sleep.
- Noises that were tolerable during the day were more disruptive at night.

Some patients consider excess noise an invasion of privacy. This is a concern because the patient is powerless to control the disturbing noise. Noise inside the facility has been called an "invisible pollutant." It should never cause distress or anxiety, or interfere with patients' ability to hear.

A 1960 study at Johns Hopkins Hospital revealed that the average noise level was 57 decibels. A repeat study in 2005 found that the noise had increased to 72 decibels (Britt, 2005). In 1995, the World Health Organization (WHO) recommended keeping noise levels below 35 decibels in hospitals. However, a Houston-area long-term care facility study in 2005 revealed noise levels from 70 to 101 decibels (McClaugherty, Valibhai, & Womack, 2005).

A certain amount of background noise is present when a room contains equipment, such as heating and cooling devices or medical monitors. Staff must speak more loudly to be heard. They speak more loudly as the noise level increases. This commonly makes them feel agitated and irritable, and increases the risk of errors.

Noise is also a contributing factor to stress, exhaustion, and burnout. Active listening requires focusing on the conversation. Health care workers must be active listeners, whether they are listening to patients or co-workers. Active listening is work. Having to talk more loudly and be even more attentive when listening to others is a leading cause of fatigue in staff.

Reducing noise improves working conditions for staff and quality of care for patients. The effects of noise and sleep deprivation is an area in which additional study is needed, but it is safe to say that research has already proven that nighttime noise is disruptive. Do all you can to reduce and manage noise.

PAIN

Pain (Figure 10-4) is a state of discomfort that is unpleasant for the patient. It serves as a warning that something is wrong. It interferes with the patient's optimal level

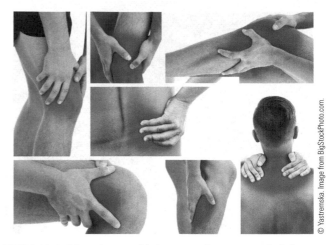

FIGURE 10-4 Muscles and joints can be very painful.

of function and self-care. Patients may limit movement when they are having pain. Unrelieved pain contributes to complications of immobility, increasing the risk of pneumonia, skin breakdown, and other problems. It decreases quality of life, and causes feelings of hopelessness, helplessness, anxiety, despair, and depression, causing the patient to act out, cry, or display other unusual behavior. It is a major preventable problem that slows recovery and increases health care costs.

Age-Appropriate Care ALERT

The golden rule for pain relief is that whatever is painful to adults is painful to children unless proven otherwise. Pain control should be evidence based. Never lie to a child when asked if a procedure will hurt. Admit that it will, but assure the child that you will do all you can to make them comfortable.

Relieving pain has always been an important nursing responsibility. Nursing staff must identify patients who are having pain, and those who are at risk for pain, and then take appropriate actions to ensure that all patients are as comfortable as possible.

Patients' Response to Pain

Each person responds to pain differently. Patients' reactions may be different from one moment to the next. Some individuals do not feel pain as acutely as others. Some try to ignore pain. Others may try to deny pain because they are afraid of what it means. Ignoring or denying pain increases the risk of injury because the normal warning that pain provides is overlooked or ignored.

Monitor for body language or other signs of pain in patients (Figure 10-5). Use nursing measures to make

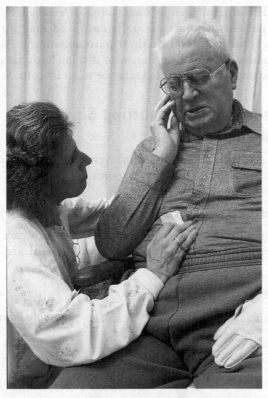

FIGURE 10-5 This patient's body language suggests the presence of severe pain.

the patient comfortable. Always report pain to the nurse. Your observations are a valuable contribution to the nursing assessment and patients' comfort.

Patients' responses to pain can be very individual. Some people are very emotional when they are in pain and some are stoic. Some think that showing pain is a sign of weakness.

Pain causes stress and anxiety, interfering with comfort, rest, and sleep. Rest and sleep are necessary for the body to repair itself and to restore strength and energy. Insomnia (inability to sleep), restlessness, and disturbed sleep may be caused by pain.

Identifying Patients in Pain and at Risk for Pain

Many factors affect patients' reactions to pain. Four types of pain are listed in Table 10-1. Monitor patients' body language for signs of pain.

Body language is often the first clue that a patient is having pain. Other signs and symptoms are:

- Pain on movement
- Change in facial expression
- Crying or moaning
- Rigid posture
- Guarded positioning; withdrawing when touched or repositioned

TABLE 10-1 Types of Pain

Type of Pain	Description
Acute pain	Occurs suddenly and without warning. Acute pain is usually the result of tissue damage, caused by conditions such as injury or surgery. Typically, acute pain decreases over time, as healing takes place.
Persistent pain (chronic pain)	Persistent pain lasts longer than six months. It may be intermittent or constant. Persistent pain may be caused by multiple medical conditions.
Phantom pain	Phantom pain occurs as a result of an amputation. For example, the patient has had a leg removed, but complains of pain in the toes of the missing leg. The pain is real, not imaginary.
Radiating pain	Radiating pain moves from the site of origin to other areas. For example, when a patient is having a heart attack, the pain may radiate from the chest and be felt in the jaw or arm.

- Restlessness
- Irregular or abnormal respirations
- Intermittent breath holding
- Dilated pupils
- Sweating
- Refusing to eat

Report your observations to the nurse and compare the new status with the patient's normal behavior. If the behavior changes back to normal after the nurse administers an **analgesic** (pain) medication, this confirms that the change in body language or behavior was caused by pain. Notify the nurse of this important observation. Signs and symptoms of pain to report to the nurse are listed in Table 10-2.

TABLE 10-2 Signs and Symptoms of Pain That Should Be Reported to the Nurse Immediately

Chest pain
Pain that radiates
Pain upon movement
Pain during urination
Pain when having a bowel movement
Splinting an area upon movement
Grimacing, or facial expressions suggesting pain
Body language suggesting pain
Unrelieved pain after pain medication has been given
Pain is **never** normal; **all** complaints of pain should be reported to the nurse promptly

Patients have the right to timely pain assessment and management. Avoid passing judgment about the presence or absence of pain if the patient is laughing, talking, or sleeping. Some patients may appear comfortable even while they are having severe pain. Vital signs may be normal.

Regularly ask patients if they are in pain. Some will not volunteer this information if not asked directly, so asking is the best way to find out. *The patient's self-report is the most accurate and reliable indicator of pain, and it should be respected and believed.* Never question the validity of a patient's complaints. Simply notify the nurse.

Make sure the patient can see and hear you when you ask about pain. Allow enough time for the patient to process your questions and respond. Be patient. Use language that is appropriate for the patient's age and mental status. Remember that patients may use different words for pain, such as *hurt, sore,* or *tender.* Children and patients who are mentally confused may surprise you. Some can describe their pain accurately. Always ask patients who are crying, who display body language suggesting pain, or whose behavior suggests pain.

Observing and Reporting Signs and Symptoms of Pain

Pain always requires further intervention. Always describe the pain in the patient's exact words.

Pain Assessment Scales

Many different pain scales are used in health care. The scales shown in Figures 10-6A and 10-6B are only

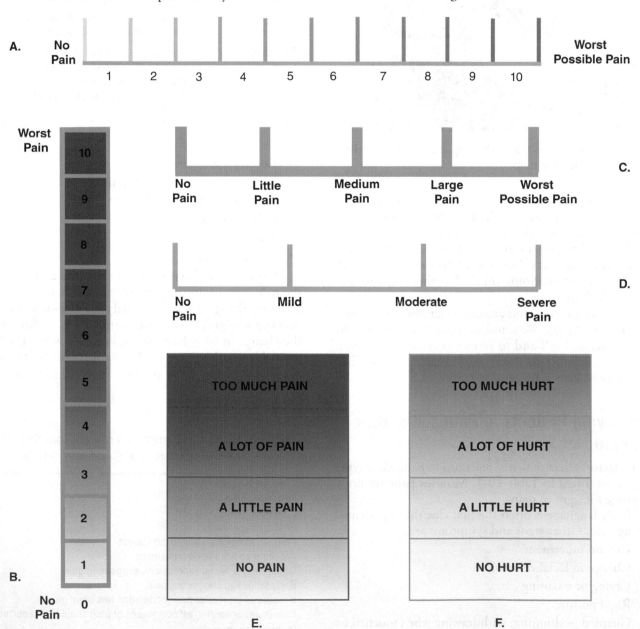

FIGURE 10-6 (A) Horizontal numeric pain scale; (B) vertical numeric pain scale; (C) verbal descriptor pain scale; (D) verbal pain scale; (E) verbal pain scale; (F) verbal pain scale.

examples. Your facility may use similar or different tools for evaluating pain. Pain scales use pictures, words, or numbers to help the patient describe pain intensity. Most scales range from no pain to very severe pain. Picture scales use a range from smiling faces to neutral faces to frowns and tears.

Although you will not directly assess patients' pain, you must understand the purpose of the scales used in your facility and how they are interpreted. Many facilities use a 0 to 10 scale, with 0 meaning no pain and 10 meaning intolerable pain. If the patient tells you that they are having pain at "level 5," for example, you must know what this means and inform the nurse. Likewise, if the patient complains of pain at "level 9" an hour after receiving pain medication, this suggests a potentially serious problem that must be reported immediately.

Managing Pain

Some patients may not complain of pain and may appear to be comfortable. Asking them if they are having pain is not offensive. Always ask instead of assuming. Likewise, if a patient has been medicated for pain, but continues to complain, inform the nurse. Do not assume that the pain has been relieved after a medication has been given. If the person continues to have pain, the nurse must assess the patient further.

Nursing Assistant Comfort Measures

Relieving discomfort helps reduce pain and anxiety. Nursing assistants can use many basic nursing measures to make a patient more comfortable. These include:

- Telling patients what you plan to do and how you will do it
- Providing privacy
- Assisting the patient to assume a comfortable position

- Repositioning the patient to relieve pain and muscle spasms
- Changing the angle of the bed to relieve tension on surgical sites or injured areas
- Avoiding sudden jerking motions when moving or positioning the patient
- Performing passive range-of-motion exercises to reduce stiffness and maintain mobility
- Using pillows to support the affected body part(s) (Figure 10-7)
- Providing extra pillows and blankets for comfort and support
- Straightening the bed and linens
- Giving a backrub (Figure 10-8)
- Washing the patient's face and hands
- Placing a cool, damp washcloth on the patient's forehead
- Providing oral hygiene
- Providing fresh water, food, or beverages as permitted (Figure 10-9)

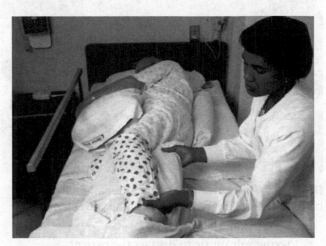

FIGURE 10-7 Place pillows to support the patient's body, maintain good alignment, and relieve pain.

Difficult Situations

Pain is very personal and subjective. One doctor tells a story of asking a patient to rate their pain using a 1-to-10 scale. The patient responded that the pain was a little more than level 2. When probed for information, the patient discussed their experiences in military service. They explained that their pain was a 2 when their finger was cut off with a dull knife. They described level 3 as the pain they felt when their leg was accidentally shot in a friendly fire incident, shattering the bones.

They said level 8 was like having dengue fever, an unusual disease that causes severe muscle and joint pain, feeling similar to bones breaking. They could not describe a level 10 pain. The point here is that everyone is different, and sometimes nurses must ask probing questions and consider many factors to rate the patient's pain intensity correctly. Even when a pain scale is used, avoid making judgments about the patient's pain. What is important is the patient's interpretation of the pain scale, which may differ from your own.

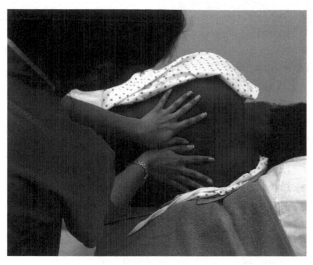

FIGURE 10-8 The relaxation of the muscles from a backrub reduces pain and enables the patient to rest comfortably.

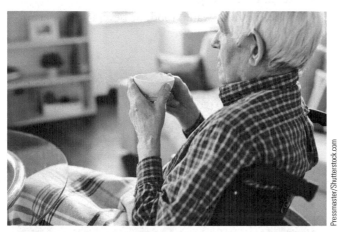

FIGURE 10-9 A patient may enjoy a decaffeinated beverage and light snack before going to sleep.

- Playing soft music to distract the patient
- Listening to the patient's concerns
- Providing emotional support
- Maintaining a comfortable environmental temperature

- Providing a quiet, dark environment
- Eliminating unpleasant sights, sounds, and odors from the environment
- Waiting at least 30 minutes after the nurse administers pain medication before moving the patient, performing procedures, or undertaking activities

Regularly incorporate these steps into your patient care. Follow the directions on the individual patient's care plan. The nurse may also direct you to apply warm or cold applications (see Chapter 27) to make the patient more comfortable.

REST

Rest is a state of mental and physical comfort, calmness, and relaxation. The patient's basic needs of hunger, thirst, elimination, and pain must be met before effective rest is possible. They should be dressed comfortably, and feel fresh and clean. The patient may sit or lie down, or may do things that are pleasant and relaxing (Figure 10-10). Some patients have rituals, such as reciting the rosary.

To promote rest, the environment should be calm and quiet. If basic care is tiring for the patient, allow

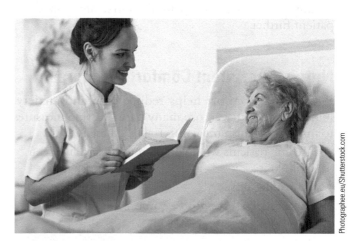

FIGURE 10-10 A family member reads to a patient who is resting in bed.

Difficult Situations

For many years, backrubs were almost a sacred part of routine nursing care. Over time, we have become much more dependent on technology. When we are busy or staffing is short, it seems as if there is no time for backrubs. Yet, calming the agitated patient who cannot sleep is time-consuming. The pregnant mother with a backache may use the call signal frequently. The patient with spasticity cannot get into a comfortable position. You may find that taking a few minutes to give a backrub will save you a great deal of time in caring for your patient. A good backrub is comforting and relaxing. Agitated patients often calm down. Uncomfortable patients become more comfortable and demand less attention. Do not omit this important part of nursing care—it pays dividends in patient comfort and satisfaction. Over time, it may even make your job easier.

them to stop and rest. Some patients feel refreshed after 15 minutes of rest. Others need more time. Some must rest frequently throughout the day. Plan your schedule and activities to allow for rest periods. Providing a backrub, nursing comfort measures, or other relaxation activities may assist the patient to rest. Follow the care plan and the nurse's instructions.

SLEEP

Sleep is a period of continuous or intermittent unconsciousness in which physical movements are decreased. Sleep is a basic need of all humans, as it allows the mind and body to rest so they can function properly.

Age-Appropriate Care ALERT

Children will often rest better if they have a personal comfort or security item with them, such as a special blanket, stuffed animal, doll, or toy. Treat this item with respect. Avoid making fun of the item, and do not tease the child for using it.

Sleep occurs in a cycle that lasts for several hours at a time. The body repairs itself during sleep. Because movement and activity are limited, the body's metabolic needs are reduced. The patient may become cold and need a blanket because they are not moving. Vital signs commonly decrease during sleep.

The need for sleep decreases as a person ages (Figure 10-11). Elderly patients require less sleep than younger or middle-aged adults (Figure 10-12). Infants and children require more sleep than adults. In fact, newborns may sleep as much as 20 hours a day. Sleep needs by age group are listed in Table 10-3. Weight loss may decrease the need for sleep, whereas weight gain often increases the need for sleep.

Sleep problems often result from a combination of several factors. Obvious problems that may interfere with the quality and quantity of sleep are:

- Pain, physical discomfort
- Hunger
- Thirst
- Need to eliminate
- Illness

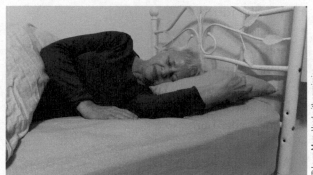

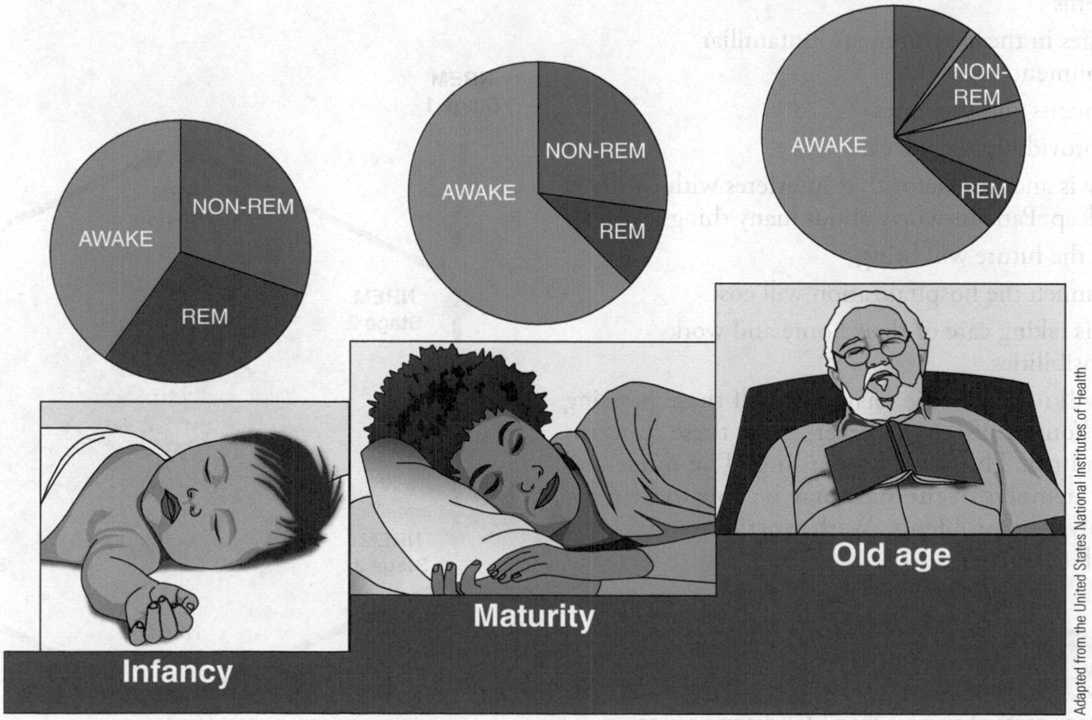

© Laura More. Used with permission.

FIGURE 10-12 Older adults require less sleep than *middle*-age and young adults.

AWAKE
NON-REM
REM
AWAKE
NON-REM
REM
AWAKE
NON-REM
REM
Infancy
Maturity
Old age
Adapted from the United States National Institutes of Health

FIGURE 10-11 Less sleep is required as we age.

TABLE 10-3 Sleep Needs Throughout the Life Cycle

Newborn infants sleep in 3- to 4-hour intervals for a total of 16 to 20 hours of sleep a day
Infants require 12 to 16 hours of sleep a day
Toddlers require 12 to 14 hours of sleep a day, usually broken into 10 to 12 hours of sleep at night, with one or more daytime naps
Preschool children require 10 to 12 hours a day
Elementary-school children require 10 to 12 hours a day
Adolescents require 8 to 10 hours a day
Young adults aged 18 to 40 require about 7 to 8 hours a day
Middle-aged adults aged 40 to 65 require about 7 hours a day
Elderly adults over the age of 65 require about 5 to 7 hours a day

- Sleep disorders
- Exercise
- Noise
- Temperature
- Ventilation
- Light intensity
- Some medications
- Caffeine intake
- Alcohol and/or drug use
- Some foods and beverages
- Lifestyle changes
- Anxiety, stress, anger, agitation, fear, emotional problems
- Changes in the environment, unfamiliar environment
- Treatments and therapies
- Staff providing routine care

Worry is another factor that interferes with comfort, rest, and sleep. Patients worry about many things, such as:

- What the future will bring
- How much the hospitalization will cost
- Who is taking care of their home and work responsibilities

You will not have the answers to all these pressing concerns. You can listen, however. Share these concerns with the nurse. This is not gossiping. The nurse and the other members of the staff may be able to help the patient solve the problems. With worries reduced, the patient will rest better.

Clinical Information **ALERT**

The average person has more than 1,460 dreams a year.

The Sleep Cycle

An internal biological clock tells each person when it is time to sleep and wake up. The sleep cycle (Figure 10-13) includes two types of sleep:

- **Nonrapid eye movement (NREM) sleep** is dreamless sleep. It has four phases, progressing from light to very deep. This part of the sleep cycle begins when the person first falls asleep. In the first two phases, the person is easily aroused. As they progress through the cycle, arousal becomes more difficult and sleep becomes deeper.
- **Rapid eye movement (REM) sleep** restores mental function. If you look closely, you will see the patient's eyes moving behind closed lids during this phase. Whenever possible, avoid awakening a patient who is in REM sleep. This is the part of the cycle in which dreams occur. Hospitalized patients often sleep for shorter periods than they do at home, causing them to feel less rested and more tired during the day.

The stages of the sleep cycle are further described in Table 10-4.

Sleep and the Older Adult

The need for sleep decreases with age. Older adults do not get as much REM sleep as those who are younger, despite the fact that the NREM stage takes longer to complete. Older persons often have trouble falling asleep. They awaken much more easily as well. It is not unusual for them to awaken several times during the night, then

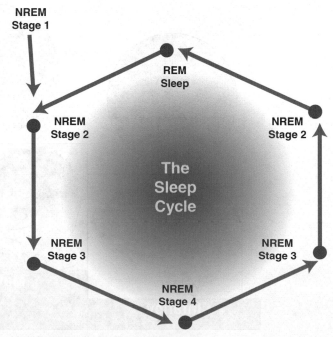

FIGURE 10-13 The sleep cycle.

TABLE 10-4 The Sleep Cycle

Stage 1: NREM Sleep

Lasts a brief time (a few minutes)

Lightest sleep; patient is easily awakened

Vital signs decrease progressively

Body metabolism gradually slows

Patient feels relaxed and drowsy

If aroused during this phase, patient may feel as if they had been daydreaming

Stage 2: NREM Sleep

Relaxation progresses, but patient remains easy to arouse

Progresses into sound sleep

Body functions and vital signs continue to decrease

Lasts 10 to 20 minutes

Stage 3: NREM Sleep

First stage of deep sleep

Patient is difficult to arouse

Little to no body movement

Muscles are completely relaxed

Vital signs continue to decrease

Lasts 15 to 30 minutes

Stage 4: NREM Sleep

Patient is very difficult to arouse

Deepest stage of sleep cycle

Body rest and restoration occur

Vital signs significantly reduced compared with waking values

Sleepwalking and enuresis (bedwetting)/incontinence may occur during this stage

Lasts about 15 to 30 minutes

REM Sleep

Rapid eye movements may be seen through closed eyelids

Begins about 50 to 90 minutes after first falling asleep

Full-color dreaming

Blood pressure, pulse, respirations vary

Limited or no voluntary movement

Patient is very difficult to arouse

Mental restoration occurs

Lasts about 20 minutes

wake up earlier in the morning than younger persons. Elderly patients who do not sleep well may become disoriented. This problem is preventable and correctable, and it may be mistaken for confusion!

 Critical Information **ALERT**

You may be surprised to find that patients who are ill have a higher fever in the evening and at night than they do during the day. Asthma, ulcers, and certain forms of arthritis worsen at night. Heart attacks and strokes may begin at night and become fully symptomatic in the morning. The study of how the time of day affects body functions is called *chronobiology*. This is a very new field. Science has much to learn about these body changes. Inform the nurse if you notice a change in a patient's condition during rest or sleep.

Sleep helps prevent fatigue, and is needed for healing of medical and surgical problems. Getting enough sleep and rest allows patients to function at their highest level. It also affects things such as longevity, weight maintenance, and good mental health. Moving through the stages of the sleep cycle uninterrupted is important. Some patients become irritable if they do not have enough sleep. Signs and symptoms of inadequate sleep are:

- Slow mental and physical responses
- Decreased attention span
- Forgetfulness or difficulty remembering things
- Reduced reasoning and judgment
- Puffy, red, swollen eyes
- Dark circles under eyes
- Disorientation
- Mood swings, moodiness
- Lethargy, sleepiness, fatigue
- Agitation, restlessness
- Clumsiness or lack of coordination
- Difficulty finding the right word
- Slurred speech
- Hallucinations in severe sleep deprivation

Sleep Disorders

Sleep has been studied extensively. Some facilities have units and clinics specializing in the diagnosis and treatment of sleep disorders. The most common sleep disorders are:

- **Insomnia**, a chronic deprivation of quality or quantity of sleep because sleep is ended or interrupted prematurely.
- **Hypersomnia**, a disorder characterized by sleeping very late in the morning and napping during the day. Causes can be physical or psychological.

- **Narcolepsy**, a condition in which patients have sudden, uncontrollable, unpredictable urges to fall asleep during the daytime hours. These individuals also get adequate sleep at night.
- **Sleep apnea**, a potentially serious condition in which air flow stops for 10 seconds or more. Untreated, this condition leads to severe medical problems.
- **Sleep deprivation**, which is prolonged sleep loss (inadequate quality or quantity of REM or NREM sleep).

High-Risk Conditions

Abnormal physiological problems cause several complications of the sleep cycle in some patients. These are:

- **Bruxism**—grinding of the teeth
- **Enuresis**—bedwetting
- **Somnambulism**—sleepwalking

Patients with these problems are at high risk of injury when they are asleep. To reduce the risk of incidents and injuries, special monitoring and safety measures will be listed on care plans of patients with these conditions.

Nursing Assistant Measures to Promote Comfort, Rest, and Sleep

Basic nursing comfort measures, such as those used to relieve pain, are also effective in helping patients to rest and sleep. Specific measures for each patient will be listed in the care plan. Measures that promote comfort, rest, and sleep include the following:

- Help the patient into loose-fitting, comfortable clothing or nightwear.
- Assist with toileting, cleanliness, oral care, and personal hygiene needs.

- Provide a warm bath or shower, if permitted.
- Avoid serving beverages containing caffeine after the evening meal.
- Provide a snack, if desired.
- Straighten the bed.
- Assist the patient into a comfortable position and provide pillows and props as needed for comfort.

 Critical Information **ALERT**

The gastrointestinal tract secretes more acid when the patient first goes to sleep. As a result, ulcer pain may worsen during this time, waking the patient up.

 Safety **ALERT**

Avoid warming blankets or other patient care supplies in a microwave; this can create hot spots and increase the risk of burns.

- Provide a comfortable environmental temperature and ventilation.
- Provide an extra blanket, if desired.
- Eliminate unpleasant odors.
- Eliminate noise.
- Adjust the lighting to a comfortable level, darkening the room as much as possible for sleep, and provide a nightlight if desired.
- Provide nursing comfort measures, such as a backrub or repositioning the patient into a more comfortable position.

Difficult Situations

Patients always rest better if they are comfortable. Many elderly patients are uncomfortable in a cool environment. Other problems, such as the open design of the hospital gown, lack of a blanket, incontinence, and some treatments, increase the feeling of coldness. The discomfort increases restlessness and muscle tension, aggravates pain, and decreases patient satisfaction with care. Most hospitals have commercial warmers that are used to warm IV solutions and bath blankets. Although these are usually in the perioperative department, they may be in other areas as well. Warmth promotes comfort, rest, and sleep, and reduces pain—especially in elderly persons. Because of this, nurse researchers studied the effects of applying warmed blankets to patients (ages 65 to 98) who were cold, anxious, or uncomfortable. They measured the level of comfort before and 1 hour after applying a warm blanket. They found that the patients were more comfortable after the warm blanket treatments (Robinson & Benton, 2002). Offering patients a warm blanket is a simple measure that can be implemented at any time. Helping to relieve pain and suffering is an important part of nursing assistant care. You will be rewarded with improved patient satisfaction, quality of care, and quality of life.

- Report pain to the nurse.
- If the patient is having pain, wait at least 30 minutes after pain medication is administered before performing procedures.
- If the patient is anxious, listen to what they says. Eliminate the cause of the anxiety, if possible.
- Avoid startling the patient.
- Handle the patient gently during care.
- Organize routine care to allow the patient uninterrupted sleep or rest.
- Avoid physical activity or activities that may upset the patient before bedtime.

- Assist with personal bedtime rituals, if any.
- Allow the patient to select their own bedtime.
- Allow the patient to read, watch television, or listen to the radio, if desired.
- Read to the patient from a favorite book.
- Assist with relaxation exercises and activities, as directed.
- If the patient receives a sleeping medication, make sure the patient is ready for sleep before the nurse administers the medication.
- Close the door to the patient's room.

REVIEW

A. True/False

Mark the following true or false by circling T or F.

1. T F Comfort is a state of self-actualization.
2. T F Lack of privacy can affect a patient's comfort.
3. T F Unrelieved pain can lead to complications of immobility.
4. T F Chronic pain never lasts longer than one month.
5. T F Acute pain results from tissue damage.
6. T F Phantom pain is imaginary pain.
7. T F Radiating pain always encircles the area in which the pain originates.
8. T F You can assume that the patient is not in pain if they do not complain.
9. T F Rest and sleep are necessary for the body to repair itself and restore strength and energy.
10. T F Pain always indicates that something is wrong.
11. T F Culture affects patients' responses to pain.
12. T F The patient's self-report of pain is the most accurate indicator of the existence and intensity of pain.

B. Matching

Choose the correct word or phrase from Column II to match each term in Column I.

Column I

13. insomnia
14. narcolepsy
15. rem sleep
16. sleep apnea

17. hypersomnia
18. bruxism
19. pain
20. enuresis

Column II

a. _____ sleeping all morning
b. _____ air flow stops for 10 seconds or more
c. _____ teeth grinding
d. _____ restores mental function
e. _____ bedwetting
f. _____ uncontrolled daytime sleeping
g. _____ chronic sleep deprivation
h. _____ state of discomfort

C. Completion

Complete the statements in questions 21 to 26 by writing the correct word from the following list.

comfort
hypersomnia
narcolepsy
REM
sleep apnea
somnambulism

21. Full-color dreaming occurs during the _____ phase of the sleep cycle.
22. _____ is a state of well-being.
23. A patient with _____ sleeps very late in the morning.
24. A patient with _____ may suddenly fall asleep at work during the day.
25. A patient with _____ stops breathing for 10 seconds or more.
26. The medical term for sleepwalking is _____.

D. Multiple Choice

Select the one best answer for each of the following.

27. The WHO recommends a noise level below _____ decibels in hospitals.

   a. 21

   b. 35

   c. 79

   d. 122

28. Speaking progressively more loudly to be heard over background noise causes staff to feel:

   a. energized, enthusiastic, and happy.

   b. determined to be heard.

   c. as if the communication is not important.

   d. frustrated, agitated, and irritable.

29. Loud noise:

   a. causes worker stress and fatigue.

   b. is to be expected in large facilities.

   c. can never be controlled in health care.

   d. is therapeutic for most patients.

30. Pain is:

   a. not the nursing assistant's responsibility.

   b. a sign of something wrong.

   c. an objective sign.

   d. a normal part of illness.

31. Pain:

   a. does not normally interfere with rest and sleep.

   b. is not stressful or worrisome.

   c. negatively affects well-being.

   d. can usually be ignored.

32. If a patient expresses their problems and worries, the nursing assistant should:

   a. stay out of the patient's business.

   b. not tell the nurse about the patient's concerns.

   c. allow them to talk about it and be a good listener.

   d. provide answers to the problems.

33. A state of mental calmness and relaxation is:

   a. comfort.

   b. sleep.

   c. leisure.

   d. rest.

34. A period of continuous or intermittent unconsciousness in which physical movements are decreased is:

   a. relaxation.

   b. comfort.

   c. sleep.

   d. diversion.

35. When a patient is sleeping,

   a. vital signs may be lower than usual.

   b. temperature increases.

   c. movement increases.

   d. the pulse decreases and respirations increase.

36. During the REM sleep cycle, the patient:

   a. dreams.

   b. awakens readily.

   c. progresses through four sleep phases.

   d. may feel hot to the touch.

E. Nursing Assistant Challenge

Mr. Huynh is grimacing and supporting his right side with his hands when you enter the room. He smiles and nods at you. Answer the following questions regarding this patient.

37. Can Mr. Huynh smile if he is having pain?

38. If Mr. Huynh's right side hurts, you may be able to position him for comfort and support by using

_____.

39. Should Mr. Huynh's body language be reported to the nurse?

40. Should you ask Mr. Huynh if he is having pain?

41. Use critical thinking and common sense to list six nursing assistant measures you can take to make Mr. Huynh more comfortable.

REFERENCES

Britt, R. R. (2005). Hospitals getting noisier, threatening patient safety. *Live Science*. Retrieved November 22, 2005, from https://www.livescience.com/3918-hospitals-noisier-threatening-patient-safety.html

Cmiel, C. A. et al. (2004). Noise control: A nursing team's approach to sleep promotion. *American Journal of Nursing, 104*(2), 40–48.

McClaugherty, L., Valibhai, F., & Womack, S. (2005). Physiological and psychological effects of noise on healthcare professionals and residents in long-term care facilities and enhancing quality of life. *Director, 13*(2).

Nightingale, F. (1859). *Notes on nursing.* London, UK: Harrison and Sons.

Robinson, S., & Benton, G. (2002). Warmed blankets: An intervention to promote comfort for elderly hospitalized patients. *Geriatric Nursing, 23,* 320–323.

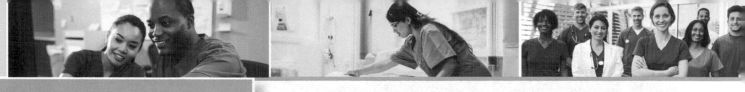

CHAPTER 11

Developing Cultural Sensitivity

OBJECTIVES

After completing this chapter, you will be able to:

11.1 Spell and define terms.

11.2 Name six major cultural groups in the United States.

11.3 Describe ways nursing assistants can develop sensitivity about cultures other than their own.

11.4 List ways the nursing assistant can help patients in practicing rituals appropriate to their cultures.

11.5 State ways the nursing assistant can demonstrate appreciation of and sensitivity to other cultures.

VOCABULARY

Learn the meaning and the correct spelling of the following words and phrases:

ablutions	ethnicity	race	standards
acupuncture	extended family	ritual	stereotype
belief	mores	sensitivity	talisman
culture	nuclear family	shaman	tradition
dialect	personal space	spirituality	

INTRODUCTION

America is a nation of immigrants whose ancestors came from other countries and indigenous people (Native (North) Americans), who have been here for 15,000 years or more. Each group brought its own cultural heritage that included language, beliefs, and customs. These people are your patients. Each one is a unique individual whose development is the result of their own culture, current lifestyle and community participation, and personal experiences. As a health care provider, you are expected to show sensitivity to the individuality and cultural heritage of each patient. You will work with health care providers from many different cultures as well (Figure 11-1). **Sensitivity** is the ability to be aware of and to appreciate the personal characteristics of others.

When members of different groups live and work in the same community, they sometimes form specific beliefs about the other groups. Rigid, unyielding beliefs that are based on generalizations are called **stereotypes**. Traits are stereotypes when applied to an entire group without consideration

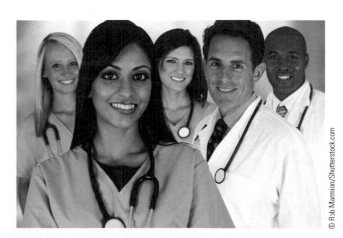

FIGURE 11-1 Health care workers come from many different cultures.

of the traditions and individual characteristics of the group.

Health care providers must avoid making assumptions about patients based on cultural stereotypes. Young immigrants and second- or third-generation

Culture **ALERT**

Treat each patient as an individual. Always consider culture. However, you must also:

- Avoid stereotyping.
- Consider other factors that may also affect care, such as age.
- Learn about the patient's unique views on health care.

Always consider the patient's cultural views on health. This is the patient's right, and considering culture shows your respect for the patient. Patients respond better to care when their culture is considered.

residents of the United States are often much closer to American culture than to their original culture.

RACE, ETHNICITY, AND CULTURE

The terms *race*, *ethnicity*, and *culture* are used to describe groups of people. **Race** is the classification of people according to shared physical characteristics such as skin color, bone structure, facial features, hair texture, and blood type.

Ethnicity

Ethnicity refers to special groups within a race as defined by national origin and/or culture. Members of an ethnic group share common:

- Heritage
- National origin
- Social customs
- Language

Six ethnic groups predominate in the United States (see Table 11-1).

Culture

Culture refers to the way a particular group views the world and the set of traditions that are practiced and passed from generation to generation. Culture enforces the **standards** (rules) established by the group based on their core values and beliefs. Cultural differences among ethnic groups may exist regarding:

- Family organization
- Personal space needs
- Communication
- Beliefs about health/illness and health care practices
- Beliefs regarding who is responsible for making health care decisions

TABLE 11-1 Major Ethnic Groups in America

Group	Some Countries and Areas of Origin
White/European American	England, Scotland, Ireland, Poland, Scandinavia, Italy, Russia
African American/Black	Africa, Haiti, Jamaica, Dominican Republic
Latinx	Spanish-speaking countries, such as Cuba, Puerto Rico, Mexico, Central and South America
Asian/Pacific	Pacific rim and Pacific islands; China, Japan, Philippines, Vietnam, Cambodia, Korea, Hawaii, Samoa
Native American	North America; one of more than 600 native tribes, such as Cherokee, Apache, Navajo, Blackfoot, Inuit (Alaskan)
Middle Eastern	Egypt, Iran, Yemen, Pakistan, India, Jordan, Saudi Arabia, Kuwait, Turkey, other Middle Eastern countries

- Religions
- Traditions, including weddings and other celebrations
- Death and dying

Cultural **mores** (customs) influence the way people interact. Ethnicity and culture contribute to an individual's sense of self-identity as they relate to the group and to other cultures. Cross-cultural nursing recognizes the individual within an ethnic and cultural group and provides nursing care that ensures cultural as well as individual acceptance and comfort.

Family Organization

Families form the basic social groups, but their structure varies from culture to culture. Family organization determines who will be the decision makers and who is responsible for providing health care. In some families, the father or oldest male is the authority figure. In others, both partners make decisions.

A **nuclear family** (Figure 11-3) consists of parents and their children living in the same household. An **extended family** (Figure 11-2) extends beyond the nuclear family and consists of parents and their children, uncles, aunts, cousins, and grandparents. Some families have only one parent. Some families have two same-sex parents. Many extended families live close to each other or in the same household.

Personal Space Needs

Personal space refers to the actual physical closeness that one person is comfortable with during social interaction with others. Personal space can be invaded by standing too close to another person, patterns of eye contact, and touching.

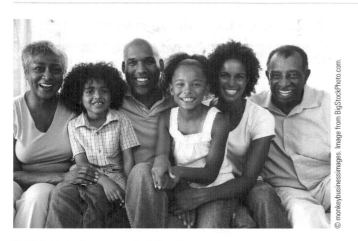

FIGURE 11-2 An extended family.

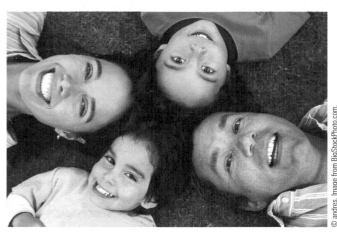

FIGURE 11-3 A nuclear family.

 Culture **ALERT**

Culture affects the type of care the patient expects to receive in the hospital. In some cultures, patients are comfortable doing self-care, if able. However, patients from other cultures may expect you to provide total care, even if they are physically able to do some things. They believe they should conserve their energy during illness. In some cultures, family members are expected to care for the patient. In other cultures, only caregivers of the same gender may care for the patient. The care plan should guide you in culturally sensitive care. Consult the nurse if necessary.

Personal Care

Touching a person is considered an invasion of personal space in some cultures.

Touching the body of another person may be even more restricted than the touching of hands in greeting. Mode of dress and body covering is very important to an individual's modesty. In some cultures, caregivers cannot care for members of the opposite sex.

Nursing assistants care for patients during very personal and private moments. Workers may not think about or be troubled by patients' bodies being exposed. However, many patients are very modest, and having the body exposed is quite traumatic. Cultural beliefs about keeping the body covered will affect the care you give. In some cultures, female patients must be fully covered, even when in bed. Traditional hospital gowns are not adequate. Some hospitals have long-sleeved gowns available that cover the patient from the neck to the ankles. However, these are not available at all facilities. Do whatever you can to keep patients covered and respect their modesty. The beliefs of some

patients from these religions and cultures require various garments:

- Amish—women must be covered from neck to ankles; a head covering is also worn.
- Mormons—adults of both genders who have attained religious status wear a short-legged, long-underwear-type garment at all times. Although the garment may be removed for hygiene, some patients believe it must be in contact with the body at all times because it is associated with God's protection.
- Muslims—males are covered from waist to knee. Women must be covered from neck to ankles; a head covering is also worn; some cover all but the eyes, whereas others show the full face (Figures 11-5A, 11-5B, 11-6A and 11-6B).
- Native (North) Americans—members of various Native (North) American tribes in the United States wear medicine bags around their necks. Avoid removing the bag, if possible.

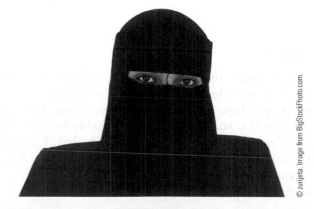

FIGURE 11-5A Traditional Muslim culture requires women to be completely veiled from head to toe. This woman is from a culture that requires the face to be covered.

© zurijeta. Image from BigStockPhoto.com.

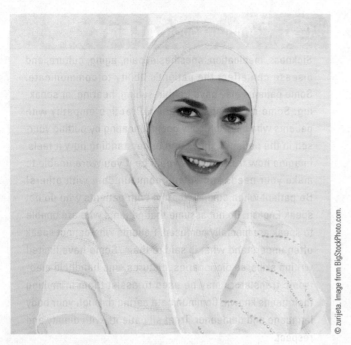

FIGURE 11-5B Young Muslim woman from a culture that does not require the face to be covered.

Courtesy of PatientStyle. Http://www.patientstyle.com/(510) 599-5273.

FIGURE 11-6A A modesty gown would be used by Muslim patients and others who must be covered from neck to ankles.

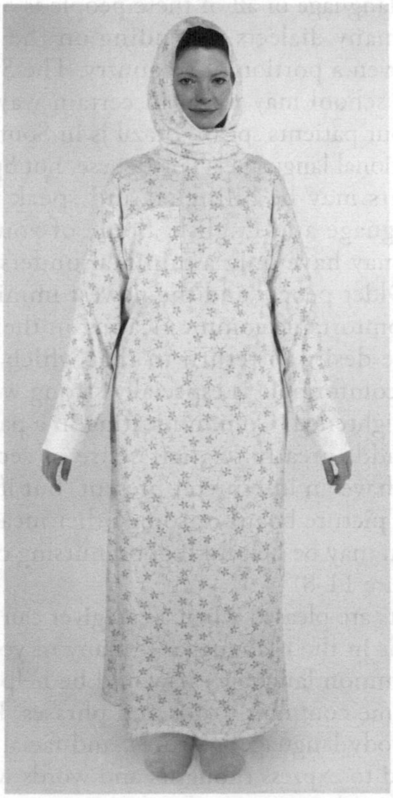

- Sikhs—adults of both sexes wear short pants called *kacchera* to symbolize modesty and morality. They may also wear bracelets called *kara* on the right wrist, symbolizing restraint from evil actions and unity with God and other Sikhs. Men wear turbans (Figure 11-7). Neither males nor females cut their hair or remove body hair.

Patients who are members of Islamic, Hindu, or Sikh religions have beliefs about ritualistic washing, water, and personal hygiene. Spiritual **ablutions** and washing are required at certain times of the day. *Ablution* is the practice of removing sins and diseases and cleansing negative energy from the body, mind, and spirit through the use of ritual washing. Physical cleanliness is associated with spiritual purity. Showering is preferable to a bath. The patient may refuse to eat until they have washed. Water for washing should be available to the patient whenever possible. Members of some cultures use the right hand for eating. The left hand only is used for personal hygiene after toileting.

As you care for patients from cultures other than your own, remember that the customs of the individual's culture greatly influence the acceptance of

Courtesy of PatientStyle. Http://www.patientstyle.com/(510) 599-5273.

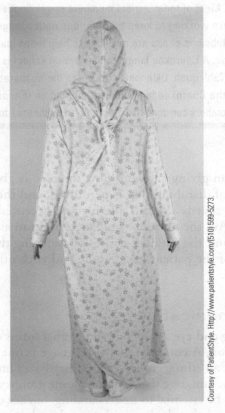

FIGURE 11-6B This example shows how a modesty gown would be tied in the back. The head covering can be removed.

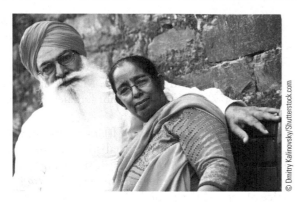

FIGURE 11-7 Sikhs who have been initiated must adhere to Five Ks: uncut hair (*kesh*), a bracelet (*kara*), a sword (*kirpan*), a cotton undergarment (*kacchera*), and a small wooden comb (*kangha*). Baptized males must wear a turban, whereas baptized females can choose to wear a scarf or turban.

 Communication ALERT

The Navajo language of American Indians was used to pass military messages during World War II because the enemy could not break the "code." The last living "code talker" died in 2014. Most of today's tribal members speak English, and tribes are working to keep their various native languages alive. Clubs and choirs are available to help teens learn the language. A Cherokee language immersion school is available in Tahlequah, Oklahoma. Thanks to the cooperation of Apple, the Cherokee language is included on iPhones, so tribal members can send text messages in their native tongue.

 Communication ALERT

Sickness, medication, anesthesia, pain, aging, culture, and disease can affect the patient's ability to communicate. Some patients may have trouble seeing, hearing, or speaking. Some do not speak English. Practice empathy with patients who have difficulty communicating by putting yourself in the patient's shoes and understanding how it feels. Imagine how frustrating it would be if you were unable to make your needs known and communicate with others! Be patient when communicating with patients who do not speak English. Do not assume that patients who are unable to speak are mentally confused. Patients who cannot speak often understand what is said to them. Some have limited writing skills, so dictionaries, pictures, and handheld electronic translators may be used to assist them in making their needs known. Communicate caring through your body language and demeanor. Treat all patients with dignity and respect.

the person giving care and how the care is given, the amount of disrobing that is permitted, and the degree of touch that is comfortable for and accepted by the patient. Ask the nurse for guidance. You can also learn much about the patient's desires by watching the interactions of the patient with family and with other staff members.

Communication

Touching and eye contact are nonverbal forms of communication. A common verbal language is one characteristic of an ethnic group. Silence may be an important part of the language. For example, some groups consider silence to be essential to understanding. Silence does not always mean that the listener has not heard or is inattentive to the speaker.

An ethnic group may share a common language, but local terminology and usage may vary (a **dialect**). For example, Hispanic Americans may have originated in

Puerto Rico, Mexico, Cuba, or Central or South America. The basic language of all of these people is Spanish, but there are many dialects depending on the country of origin or even a portion of a country. The Spanish you learned in school may differ in certain ways from the Spanish your patients speak. Brazil is in South America, but the national language is Portuguese, not Spanish.

Patients may be bilingual and speak both their native language and English. Some of your patients, however, may have only a minimal understanding of English. Older people and the newest immigrants will be most comfortable communicating in their own language. The desire to return to that which is familiar and most comfortable is especially strong when people are ill or frightened. Communicating in a patient's own language adds greatly to their sense of security. It is helpful to have an interpreter present, but if this is not possible, a picture board or some other means of communication may be helpful if good nursing care is to be given (Figure 11-8).

Patients are pleased when a caregiver can speak even a few words in their language. If many of your patients share a common language, it would be helpful for you to learn some common words and phrases. Remember, too, that body language, gestures, and facial expression can be used to express thoughts and words when verbal language is inadequate.

When communicating:

- Use a normal tone.
- Speak slowly.
- Use simple words.

Communication Flash Cards

NURSE	DOCTOR	BEDPAN
WATER	FOOD	PILL
BED	WHEELCHAIR	BOOK
PENCIL	PAPER	NEWSPAPER
BATHROBE	TV-RADIO	WATCH
HOT	COLD	FAMILY
OK / NO / YES	MONEY	PAIN

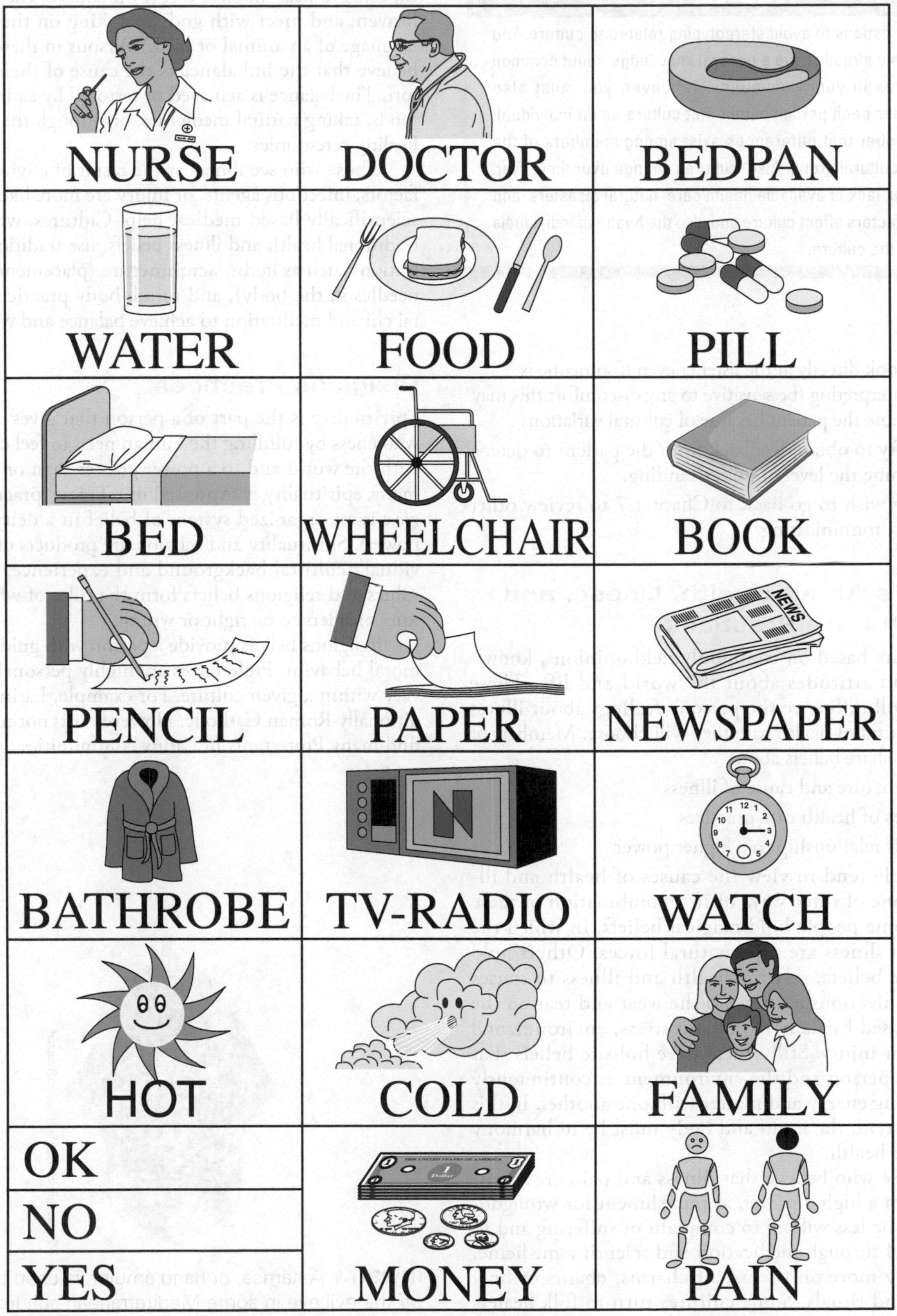

FIGURE 11-8 When using communication flash cards, the patient selects the card and points to the requested item. This tool improves accuracy and reduces frustration when communicating.

- Look directly at the listener even if someone is interpreting (be sensitive to any discomfort this may cause the patient because of cultural variations).
- Try to obtain feedback from the patient to determine the level of understanding.

You may wish to go back to Chapter 7 to review other ways of communicating.

Beliefs About Health, Illness, and Health Care Practices

Beliefs are based on commonly held opinions, knowledge, and attitudes about the world and life. These beliefs will influence the person's feelings about illness and the kind of health care they will choose. Members of a culture share beliefs about:

- The nature and cause of illness
- Types of health care practices
- Their relationship to a higher power

People tend to view the causes of health and illness in one of three ways or in a combination of these ways. Some people hold magical beliefs, in which the causes of illness are supernatural forces. Others hold scientific beliefs, relating health and illness to causes such as infectious agents and the wear and tear on the body caused by daily living and stress, environmental agents, or injury. Still others have holistic beliefs that view the person and the environment as continuously exchanging energy and matter with one another. In this belief system, the mind and body must be in harmony to ensure health.

Those who believe that illness and pain are a penance from a higher power, as punishment for wrongdoing, will be less willing to complain of suffering and to seek relief through medication and scientific medicine. They rely more on the use of charms, chants or holy words, and rituals. Some cultures turn to folk healers or shamans to help bring their bodies back into balance with nature. (A **shaman** is a traditional spiritual leader,

healer, or medicine man. In some societies, the shaman is expected to heal the sick, escort the souls of the dead into heaven, and meet with gods by taking on the shape or language of an animal or bird.) Persons in these cultures believe that the imbalance is the cause of their discomfort. The balance is achieved or restored by eating certain foods, taking natural medicines, or through the power of healing ceremonies.

Those who see illness as the result of environmental factors, infectious agents, or injury are more likely to seek scientifically based medical help. Cultures, which have traditional health and illness beliefs, use traditional medications such as herbs, **acupuncture** (placement of metal needles in the body), and mind–body practices such as tai chi and meditation to achieve balance and wellness.

Religious Practices

Spirituality is the part of a person that gives a sense of wholeness by fulfilling the human need to feel connected with the world and to a power greater than oneself. For many, spirituality is expressed in religious practice. *Religion* is an organized system of belief in a deity (higher power). Spirituality and religion are products of an individual's cultural background and experience. Spiritual values and religious beliefs form the rules of what a person considers to be right or wrong.

Religious beliefs provide a person with guidelines for moral behavior. Preferences are highly personal and can vary within a given culture. For example, Latinx are traditionally Roman Catholic. However, it is not unusual to find many Protestants in Latinx communities.

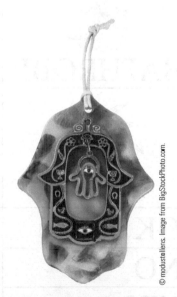

FIGURE 11-9 A hamsa, or hand amulet, is used to ward off the evil eye in some Mediterranean cultures. It has other special meanings to those who practice various religions throughout the world.

© modustollens. Image from BigStockPhoto.com.

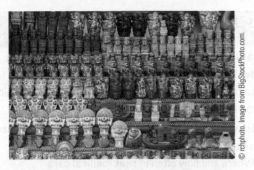

FIGURE 11-10 Traditional talismans for use in Aymara rituals at the Witches' Market in La Paz, Bolivia.

The major religions of the United States include:

- Protestantism (various denominations)
- Roman Catholicism
- Judaism
- Islam
- Hinduism

Religious items and **rituals** (solemn ceremonial acts that reinforce faith) are especially meaningful to practitioners. They must be treated with respect. For example, the crucifix, Bible, and religious medals are important to Roman Catholics. The prayer rug is significant to Muslims, who pray five times each day in the direction of their holy city, Mecca. Amulets and special charms are important to the religious beliefs of Native Americans and to some peoples in the Middle East. **Talismans** are engraved stones, rings, or other objects that are used to ward off evil (Figure 11-10). Copper or silver bracelets and religious medals are important and sacred to some cultures.

If a patient requests a visit from clergy, be sure the request is promptly relayed to the nurse. When the clergy visits, be sure to provide privacy. It is also important to provide privacy when the patient is engaged in a religious act such as praying. Refer to Table 11-2, which lists five religious faiths common in the United States and some

of their beliefs and religious items. Special religious rituals and practices related to dying, death, and care of the body after death are discussed in Chapter 32.

Foods are important in some religions. For example, members of the Orthodox Jewish faith may not be served milk and meat products at the same time. Roman Catholics restrict food intake on specific dates and some Baptists, Muslims, and others are not permitted to drink alcohol. Other food restrictions are discussed in Chapter 26.

An understanding of some of the major belief systems will help you be more sensitive to your patients' needs. You can support any patient's spirituality and religious practices by:

- Being a willing listener
- Respecting the patient's belief system
- Never trying to convert the patient to your belief system
- Respecting religious symbols
- Not interrupting during religious rituals
- Reading aloud the patient's favorite passages from religious books
- Providing privacy during prayers and meditation or when clergy visits

TRADITIONS

Traditions are customs and practices followed by members of a culture and passed from generation to generation. Often traditions are related to religious rituals and holiday celebrations. Foods are particularly traditional at holidays.

Numerous Native (North) American tribes exist in the United States today. Some live on reservations. Others live in communities. In fact, some tribal members may be your neighbors. Many work as nursing assistants. All are concerned with keeping their customs, traditions, and beliefs alive (Figure 11-11).

TABLE 11-2 Some Common Belief Systems (Religious)

Religion	Belief in a Deity	Value of Prayer	Belief in Hereafter	Special Practices, Symbols
Protestant	Yes	Important	Yes	Baptism, Holy Communion, cross, Bible
Roman Catholic	Yes	Important	Yes	Baptism, Holy Communion, Anointing of the Sick, Reconciliation, Bible, medals, pictures and statues of saints, rosaries, crucifix
Orthodox Judaism	Yes	Important	Yes	Torah, yarmulke (cap), tallith, menorah
Hinduism	Yes (many forms)	Important	Yes	No sacraments
Buddhism	Yes	Important	Yes	No sacraments
Islam (Muslim)	Yes	Important	Yes	Koran, prayer rug

Within the framework of each belief system, there are individual differences in the depth of belief and extent of practice.

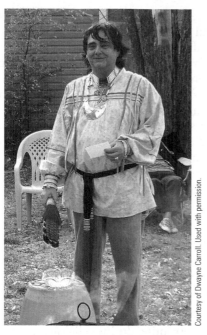

FIGURE 11-11 This Cherokee chief is conducting a ceremony to give a two-year-old child a tribal name.

Families carry out traditions from generation to generation. Holidays specific to cultures are celebrated each year.

 Culture **ALERT**

Learn about your own cultural beliefs and practices. Consider how your culture, the way you were raised, and family traditions affect you. For example, you may have opinions and beliefs about:

- How to be polite, how to greet someone in a polite manner, and use good manners in conversation with others
- Where and how often to seek medical care
- Punctuality (being on time)
- Preferred gender of caregiver
- Methods of expressing pain
- How children and elderly persons should be treated

Many traditions involve the coming to maturity of young people and are related to religious practice.

Honoring and practicing traditions gives people a sense of belonging, stability, and continuity. Traditions help to bind the people of a culture closer together.

Nursing assistants have a unique opportunity to learn about other cultures directly from their patients. There are ways to make this process easier for yourself and your patients (see Guidelines 11-1). Always remember that even though a person is part of an identifiable culture, they must always be recognized as an individual within the culture.

GUIDELINES 11-1 Developing Cultural Sensitivity

- Review your own belief systems.
- Consider how your own culture influences your behavior.
- Always view patients as individuals within a culture.
- Recognize that patients are a combination of heritage, culture, and community.
- Understand that culture influences how people behave and interact with others.
- Remember that personal space needs, eye contact, and ways of communicating are often culturally related.
- Recognize that some cultures have beliefs about health, wellness, and illness that are different from your own.
- Be willing to modify care according to the patient's cultural background and practices.
- Do not expect all members of a cultural group to behave in exactly the same manner.

- Remember that patients' health practices related to culture, values, and belief system are deeply ingrained and not easily changed.
- Avoid stereotyping people within a culture.
- Check with the nurse to learn special ways of communicating with patients of different cultural backgrounds.
- Treat religious articles with respect.
- Provide privacy when a spiritual advisor is visiting the patient or the patient is practicing a devotional act.
- Try to learn about the practices, beliefs, and cultural heritage of the people who are most likely to be your patients. A library and the Internet are good sources.
- Ask patients politely about practices that are unfamiliar.
- Attend staff development classes designed to promote cultural sensitivity.

REVIEW

A. Matching

Match each definition in Column II with the word in Column I.

Column I		Column II
1. _____	amulet	**a.** rules of conduct
2. _____	mores	**b.** charm against evil
3. _____	sensitivity	**c.** passed from generation to generation
4. _____	standard	**d.** awareness and appreciation of
5. _____	tradition	**e.** customs

B. Completion

Complete the following sentences by choosing the correct word.

6. Rigid, biased ideas about people are called _____. (stereotypes) (characteristics)

7. Classification by shared physical characteristics is based on _____. (ethnicity) (race)

8. The way a group views the world and the group's traditions are the foundation of a _____. (race) (culture)

9. Commonly held opinions, knowledge, and attitudes about life are called _____. (standards) (beliefs)

10. Solemn and ceremonial acts that reinforce faith are called _____. (rituals) (traditions)

C. Multiple Choice

Select the one best answer for each of the following.

11. The cultural language common to most Latinx is:
  a. English.
  b. French.
  c. Spanish.
  d. German.

12. You may expect that a person from the Middle Eastern culture was born in:
  a. Egypt.
  b. Russia.
  c. China.
  d. Poland.

13. The nursing assistant can show sensitivity and appreciation for the patient who does not speak your language by:
  a. Speaking in your language
  b. avoiding eye contact
  c. a comfortable degree of touch
  d. being silent and respectful

14. Sensitivity is the ability to be aware of a patient's:
  a. attractiveness
  b. individuality
  c. hair color
  d. intelligence

15. Second and third generation immigrants of the United States are usually close to:
  a. Their ancestral culture.
  b. The American culture.
  c. Their friends' culture.
  d. The culture of schoolmates'.

16. Cultural differences among ethnic groups may exist regarding all of the following except:
  a. Personal space
  b. Traditions
  c. Religion
  d. Appearance

17. Members of an ethnic group share:
  a. Hair and eye color
  b. hobbies
  c. Activities they enjoy
  d. Language

18. Women from cultures that must keep the body covered include all of the following except:
  a. Muslim
  b. Amish
  c. Sikh
  d. Mormon

19. Your patient speaks only a few words of English. When you speak to them, you should:
  a. raise your voice.
  b. speak slowly.
  c. use slang.
  d. look away.

D. Short Answer

20. You have a Catholic patient. Briefly explain how you can show sensitivity to their religious beliefs.

_____

_____

_____

21. Name your own culture. List two traditions that are common to your culture.

_____

_____

22. List two ways you can improve your cultural sensitivity to a new patient who has a culture different from your own.

_____

_____

E. Nursing Assistant Challenge

23. Mrs. Maraschino prays before breakfast every day. Her tray is the first one on the cart and she will not eat until she has said her prayers. You cannot hand out the other trays until she has finished with her prayers and you fear the food will be cold. What action will you take?

_____

_____

_____

24. Mrs. Maraschino finished her prayers and her food is cold. What action will you take?

_____

_____

_____

F. True/False

Mark the following true or false by circling T or F.

25. T   F   Financial hardship may prevent a patient from seeking treatment.

26. T   F   An extended family consists of parents and children living in the same household.

27. T   F   Personal space is the physical closeness a person has during social interaction.

28. T   F   Culture has no effect on the care a person receives in the health care facility.

29. T   F   Patterns of eye contact do not affect personal space.

30. T   F   Physical cleanliness may affect a person's feelings about illness.

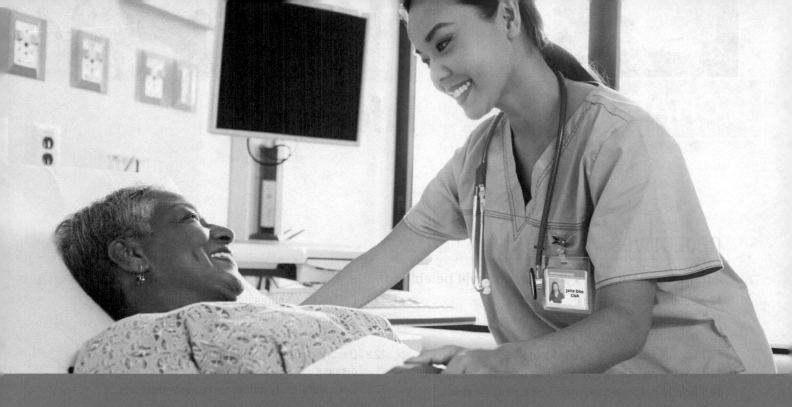

SECTION 4

Infection and Infection Control

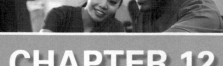
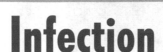

CHAPTER 12 Infection

OBJECTIVES

After completing this chapter, you will be able to:

12.1 Spell and define terms.

12.2 Describe the characteristics of the most common microbes.

12.3 List the links in the chain of infection.

12.4 List the ways in which infectious diseases are spread.

12.5 Briefly describe five serious infectious diseases.

12.6 Identify the causes of several important infectious diseases.

12.7 Explain how spores differ from other pathogens.

12.8 Explain how biofilms are different from other microbes.

12.9 Describe common treatments for infectious disease.

12.10 List natural body defenses against infections.

12.11 Explain why patients are at risk for infections.

VOCABULARY

Learn the meaning and the correct spelling of the following words and phrases:

acquired immunodeficiency syndrome (AIDS)
acute flaccid myelitis (AFM)
airborne transmission
allergy
antibiotic
antibiotic stewardship
antibody
antigen
bacillus, bacilli
bacteria, bacterium
bedbugs
biofilms
bioterrorism
carbapenem-resistant *Enterobacteriaceae* (CRE)
carrier
causative agent
Centers for Disease Control and Prevention (CDC)
chain of infection
coccus, cocci
colony
contact transmission
contagious
contaminated

2019 novel coronavirus (COVID-19)
culture and sensitivity
diplo-
droplet transmission
dysentery
Ebola
epidemic
Escherichia coli (*E. coli*) O157:H7
flora
fomite
fungi, fungus
hantavirus
head lice
hemoptysis
hepatitis
host
human immunodeficiency virus (HIV)
immune response
immunity
immunization
immunosuppression
incubation
infection
infectious

inflammation
jaundice
listeriosis
methicillin-resistant *Staphylococcus aureus* (MRSA)
microbe
microorganism
mite
mold
multidrug-resistant organisms (MDROss)
necrotizing fasciitis
nits
nonpathogen
organism
pandemic
parasite
pathogen
pediculosis
phagocyte
portal of entry
portal of exit
protozoa, protozoan
pseudomembranous colitis
reservoir
risk factor

rubeola (measles)
scabies
self-quarantine
sepsis
seropositive
social distancing
source
spirillum, spirilla
spores
staphylo-
strepto-
Streptococcus A
toxin
transmission
tubercle
tuberculosis disease
tuberculosis infection
vacciness
vancomycin-resistant enterococci (VRE)
vector
virus
World Health Organization (WHO)
yeast

INTRODUCTION

Humans are surrounded by a world of tiny **organisms** (living beings). We cannot see them without our eyes. They make their presence known by their effect, in much the same way we become aware of the wind. We cannot see the wind, but we feel its effects and see items blowing in the breeze.

These organisms can be seen only with a microscope. They are everywhere—in us, on us, and around us. They are:

- On our skin
- In our noses and mouths
- Within our bodies
- In and on the food we eat
- On what we touch or handle

Micro means small. Because these organisms (agents) are so tiny, they are called **microorganisms** or **microbes** (Figure 12-1). The organisms live in relationship to us and to each other.

Many of these microbes are useful to us. They are called **nonpathogens** because they do not cause disease. They help in the:

- Processing of cheese, beer, and yogurt
- Curing of leather
- Baking of bread

Other microbes are not useful. Microbes that cause disease in humans are called **pathogens** or pathogenic organisms. Pathogens grow best:

- At body temperature
- Where light is limited
- Where there is moisture
- Where there is a food supply
- Where oxygen needs can be met

Clinical Information **ALERT**

Ten percent of human dry weight is attributable to bacteria. About 100,000 bacteria per square centimeter live on the skin to help to protect the person from harmful pathogens. Hair traps dirt and other particles to keep them from entering the body. For example, the eyelashes and eyebrows shield the eyes from sun, dust, and perspiration. Nasal hairs protect the person from inhaling dust, pathogens, and other foreign bodies.

Infections occur when pathogens invade the body and cause disease.

MICROBES

Many different types of microbes are pathogenic to human beings. The major groups of microbes are classified as:

- Bacteria
- Fungi
- Viruses
- Protozoa

Bacteria

Bacteria (singular: **bacterium**) are simple one-celled microbes that cause infections in the skin, respiratory tract, urinary tract, and bloodstream. They are named according to their shapes and arrangement.

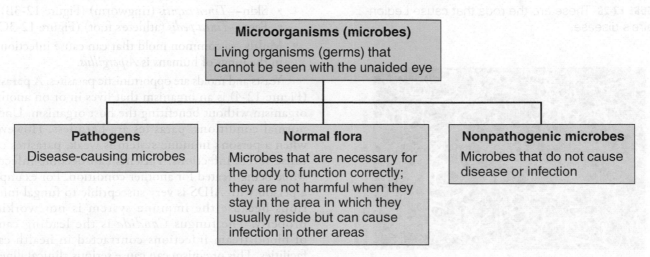

Microorganisms (microbes)
Living organisms (germs) that cannot be seen with the unaided eye

Pathogens
Disease-causing microbes

Normal flora
Microbes that are necessary for the body to function correctly; they are not harmful when they stay in the area in which they usually reside but can cause infection in other areas

Nonpathogenic microbes
Microbes that do not cause disease or infection

FIGURE 12-1 Various types of microbes.

Shape

In the following list, the first term is the singular form of the word. The word in parentheses is the plural form.

- **Coccus** (**cocci**)—round or spherical (Figure 12-2A)
- **Bacillus** (**bacilli**)—straight rod (Figure 12-2B)
- **Spirillum** (**spirilla**)—spiral, corkscrew, or slightly curved (Figure 12-2C)

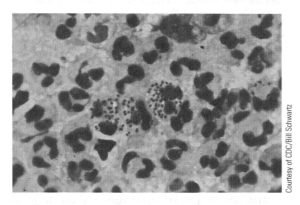

Courtesy of CDC/Bill Schwartz

FIGURE 12-2A These are the cocci that cause gonorrhea, a venereal disease.

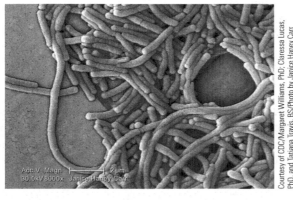

Courtesy of CDC/Margaret Williams, PhD; Claressa Lucas, PhD, and Tatiana Travis, BS/Photo by Janice Haney Carr

FIGURE 12-2B These are the rods that cause Legionnaire's disease.

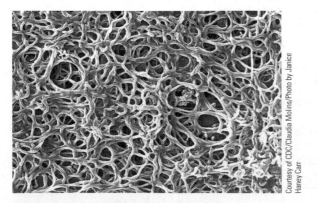

Courtesy of CDC/Claudia Molins/Photo by Janice Haney Carr

FIGURE 12-2C These spirochetes cause Lyme disease, a tick-borne illness.

Arrangement

Bacteria grow in groups called **colonies**. If we look at a small part of a colony under a microscope, we see that the bacteria typically are arranged in pairs, chains, or clusters.

- Single
- Pairs (**diplo-**)
- Chains (**strepto-**)
- Clusters (**staphylo-**)

The shape and arrangement of bacteria are important factors in identification. For example, round microorganisms grouped in chains are called streptococci. A very important member of this family is *Streptococcus hemolyticus*. It causes septic sore throat and rheumatic fever.

Round organisms grouped in a cluster are called staphylococci. An example of this family is *Staphylococcus aureus*. Staphylococci cause many infections, such as:

- Surgical wound infections
- Abscesses
- Boils
- Toxic shock syndrome

Round organisms in pairs are called diplococc *oeae*, a diplococcus, a diplococcus, causes gonorrhea (refer to Figure 12-2A).

Fungi

Two groups of **fungi** (singular: **fungus**) are most commonly associated with infection in humans:

- **Yeasts**—single-celled budding forms of a fungus. Yeast can infect areas of the body such as:
  - The mouth, vagina, underarms, and skin folds— *Candida albicans* (Figure 12-3A).
  - Skin—*Tinea capitis* (ringworm) (Figure 12-3B).
  - Feet—*Tinea pedis* (athlete's foot) (Figure 12-3C).
- **Molds**—a common mold that can cause infection in the lungs of humans is *Aspergillus*.

Yeasts and molds are opportunistic parasites. A **parasite** (Figure 12-4) is an organism that lives in or on another organism without benefiting the host organism. Under normal conditions, parasites are harmless. However, when a person's immune system is weak, parasites can cause severe infections. Patients can become infected while being treated for another condition. For example, a person with AIDS is very susceptible to fungal infections because the immune system is not working properly. The fungus *Candida* is the leading cause of bloodstream infections contracted in health care facilities. This organism can cause serious clinical illness, disability, and death. Many strains are drug resistant and very difficult to treat.

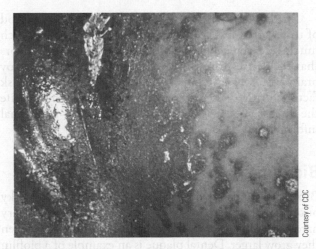

Courtesy of CDC

FIGURE 12-3A *Candida albicans* usually grows in warm, moist, dark skin folds. It can be quite painful.

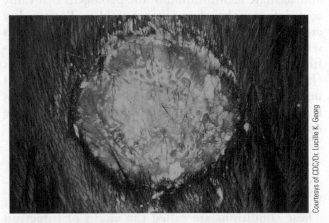

Courtesys of CDC/Dr. Lucille K. Georg

FIGURE 12-3B This condition is commonly called ringworm, but it is caused by a yeast, not a worm.

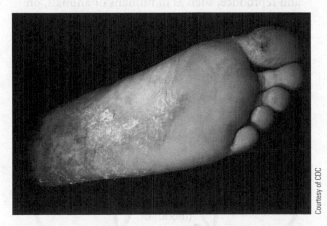

Courtesy of CDC

FIGURE 12-3C People who have poor hygiene, wear enclosed footwear such as tennis shoes, have prolonged wetting of the skin (e.g., from sweating during exercise), or have minor skin or nail injuries are more prone to experience tinea infections.

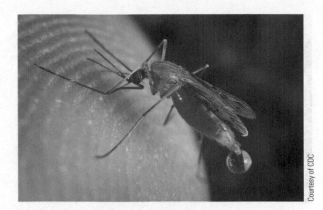

Courtesy of CDC

FIGURE 12-4 The mosquito is a parasite.

DRUG RESISTANCE

Drug resistance occurs when the same antibiotic is used repeatedly. The organisms defeat the drugs that are supposed to kill them. MDROs are microbes, typically bacteria, that are resistant to one or more classes of antimicrobial agents. **Multidrug-resistant organisms (MDROss)** develop when these organisms are all over the body, including on the skin, in secretions, in the nose, and other moist areas of the body. Antibiotics will not eliminate these organisms. Continuing to use them causes resistance to worsen. The world is in a state of multiple drug resistance, and experts have asked for everyone's cooperation to take control of the use of antibiotics. We must use antibiotics appropriately, or we will have none left that eliminate pathogens.

Antibiotic stewardship (also called antimicrobial stewardship) refers to a set of coordinated strategies being used worldwide. The goal is to improve the use of antibiotic medications to enhance patient outcomes, reduce drug resistance, and decrease unnecessary costs.

Viruses

A **virus** is a tiny microscopic pathogen that multiplies only within the cells of a living host (Figure 12-5). Viruses are classified by:

- Type of nucleic acid core (DNA or RNA)
- Host organism
- Clinical properties
- Type of disease
  Common viral infections include:
- Hepatitis
- Herpes
- Human immunodeficiency virus (HIV)
- Acquired immunodeficiency syndrome (AIDS)

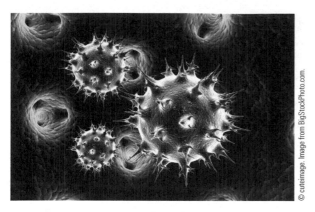

FIGURE 12-5 Viruses need body cells to survive. They are difficult to identify and are not treated with antibiotics. Some viral infections can be prevented through vaccinations.

- Chickenpox
- Influenza
- Common cold
- Measles
- Mumps

Protozoa

Protozoa (singular: **protozoan**) are one-celled organisms with a nucleus. They are classified by the way in which they move. For example, some move via whiplike tails, others via hairlike projections. They cause diseases such as:

- Malaria
- Toxoplasmosis
- African sleeping sickness
- Amebiasis

Some signs and symptoms of diseases caused by protozoa include:

- Diarrhea
- **Dysentery**—infection in the lower bowel
- Inflammation of the brain—encephalitis

Prions

Prion is a shorthand form of the term *proteinaceous infectious particle*. Mad cow disease (bovine spongiform encephalopathy, or BSE) is believed to be caused by prions. These recently identified pathogens may be ingested with infected food, such as meat. Wild game such as venison may present a higher risk. Other potential modes of transmission are blood transfusion and organ transplant.

Prions cause dementia and death in a brief period of time, often less than a year. This is an area in which much research remains to be done to identify factors that influence prion infectivity and how they destroy brain tissue. Researchers are also trying to identify risk factors for these conditions and determine when in life the disease appears. Refer to Chapter 33 for additional information.

Biofilms

Biofilms are colonies of bacteria that secrete a sticky outer coat that is hard to penetrate. Biofilms are very hard to identify. Some, but not all, become visible when they grow larger. Dental plaque is an example of a biofilm in humans. Some algae colonies on water and slime in drains are environmental biofilms. The pathogens in biofilms can break off, spreading to other areas. Complete and accurate identification of the pathogens that cause some infections has always been a problem. Because they are hard to detect, the presence and effects of biofilms seem to be underestimated. One study discovered biofilms in approximately 60 percent of chronic wounds (James et al., 2008). Of these, many of the microbes had never been identified through traditional methods. This is a new area of research, and much more work must be done in this area.

THE CHAIN OF INFECTION

Infections occur when certain conditions exist. These conditions are called the **chain of infection** (Figure 12-6A) and include a:

- Causative agent (pathogen) that causes the disease.
- Reservoir or source where the pathogen can live and reproduce, such as in humans or animals, on

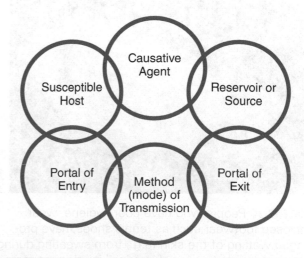

FIGURE 12-6A Chain of infection.

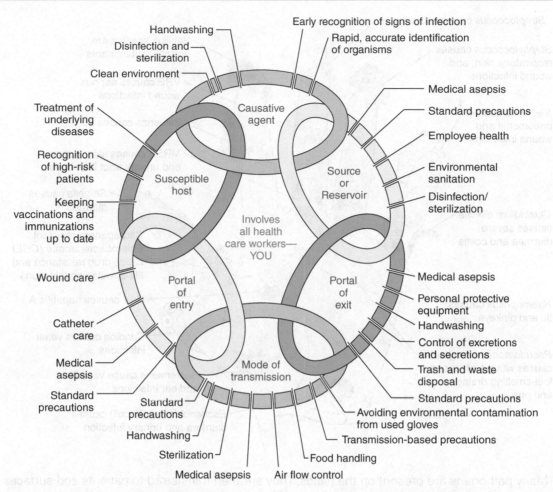

Handwashing
Disinfection and sterilization
Clean environment
Treatment of underlying diseases
Recognition of high-risk patients
Keeping vaccinations and immunizations up to date
Wound care
Catheter care
Medical asepsis
Standard precautions
Standard precautions
Handwashing
Sterilization
Medical asepsis

Early recognition of signs of infection
Rapid, accurate identification of organisms
Medical asepsis
Standard precautions
Employee health
Environmental sanitation
Disinfection/ sterilization
Medical asepsis
Personal protective equipment
Handwashing
Control of excretions and secretions
Trash and waste disposal
Standard precautions
Avoiding environmental contamination from used gloves
Transmission-based precautions
Food handling
Air flow control

Causative agent
Susceptible host
Involves all health care workers— YOU
Source or Reservoir
Portal of entry
Portal of exit
Mode of transmission

FIGURE 12-6B If one link in the chain is broken, infection cannot be transmitted to others. This diagram shows the chain of infection, with examples of various ways health care workers can break each link.

environmental surfaces, and **fomites**. These are objects that are **contaminated** with the pathogen, such as soiled linen.

- Portal of exit—a place that provides a way for the pathogen to leave the body, such as on the droplets in a sneeze.
- Method or mode of transmission—the manner in which the pathogen moves from one place or person to another.
- Portal of entry—the manner in which the pathogen enters another person or host.
- Susceptible host (also called **host**)—a person who is unable to resist the pathogen and will become ill from the entry of pathogens into the body.

Pathogens spread disease by leaving the body through a portal of exit and being transmitted to another person, where they invade a portal of entry. This cycle repeats over and over, with the potential for spreading disease to many people. The pathogens

enter the other person's body and can again cause disease. The purpose of infection control is to disrupt the chain of infection. Breaking one link in the chain (Figure 12-6B) is all that is needed to prevent the spread of disease.

Pathogens enter and leave the body through openings (portals of entry) such as:

- The eyes, ears, nose, or mouth
- Breaks in the skin or hand contact with the mouth or other mucous membranes (Figure 12-7)
- The penis, vagina, urinary meatus (bladder opening), or rectum

Infection Control **ALERT**

Breaking one link in the chain of infection will stop the infection from spreading.

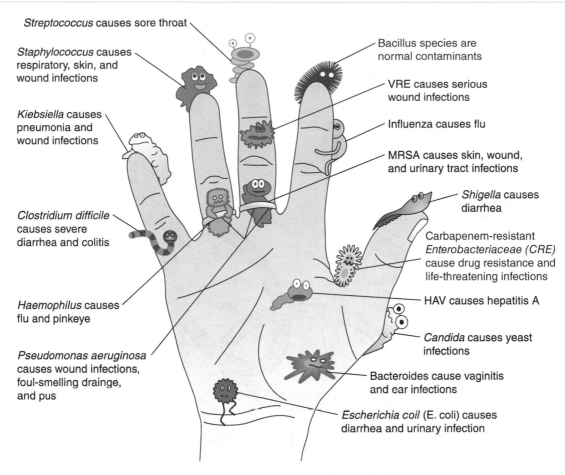

Streptococcus causes sore throat

Staphylococcus causes respiratory, skin, and wound infections

Klebsiella causes pneumonia and wound infections

Clostridium difficile causes severe diarrhea and colitis

Haemophilus causes flu and pinkeye

Pseudomonas aeruginosa causes wound infections, foul-smelling drainge, and pus

Bacillus species are normal contaminants

VRE causes serious wound infections

Influenza causes flu

MRSA causes skin, wound, and urinary tract infections

Shigella causes diarrhea

Carbapenem-resistant *Enterobacteriaceae (CRE)* cause drug resistance and life-threatening infections

HAV causes hepatitis A

Candida causes yeast infections

Bacteroides cause vaginitis and ear infections

Escherichia coil (E. coli) causes diarrhea and urinary infection

FIGURE 12-7 Many pathogens are present on the hands. They are then transferred to patients and surfaces through touch. They can also be introduced into the body by touching the eyes, nose, mouth, or other mucous membranes.

Causative Agent

The **causative agent** is the pathogen that causes the disease. The most common causative agents are:

- Bacteria
- Viruses
- Fungi
- Protozoa

Reservoir

The **reservoir** or **source** is where pathogens live. They may or may not multiply in the reservoir. The four most common reservoirs are:

- Humans—active cases and carriers
- Insects and animals (Figure 12-8)
- Environment
- Fomites—objects that become contaminated with material containing the pathogen. Fomites are anything that comes in direct contact with infectious matter, such as through contact with:
  - Bedpans and urinals
  - Doorknobs and faucet handles

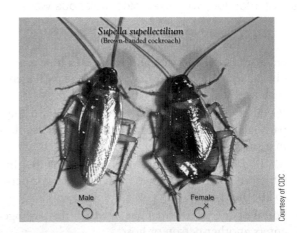

Supella supellectilium (Brown-banded cockroach)

Male   Female

FIGURE 12-8 Insects and other animals can transmit pathogens. Cockroaches live in sewers, bathrooms, kitchens, dining areas, and other areas where food is prepared and/or stored. They can contaminate food and spread many diseases. The roaches pictured here can produce up to 300,000 offspring in one year.

- Linens
- Instruments
- Containers with specimens for laboratory analysis

In the health care setting, reservoirs include the:
- Patient
- Health care worker
- Environment
- Equipment

Human Reservoirs

The two major human reservoirs are cases and carriers.

- Cases—people with acute illness and obvious signs and symptoms. An example is a person with chickenpox.
- **Carriers**—people who are infectious and can pass a disease to others. A person may not show signs of illness and may not know they are infected. The condition is not harmful to the carrier but may be harmful to others. Another type of carrier is one in whom the organisms are multiplying (incubating) before signs and symptoms develop. Some infections can be spread during this **incubation** period. Specific diseases can persist in humans for an indefinite period of time, such as salmonella, hepatitis B, hepatitis C, HIV, and typhoid.

Portals of Entry or Exit

Portals of Entry

Organisms enter the body through the following **portals of entry**:

- Breaks in the skin or mucous membranes. Many organisms that are part of the normal flora, such as staphylococci, enter through cracks and other breaks in the skin.
- Respiratory tract. Organisms that cause the common cold and many childhood communicable diseases (such as mumps and measles) may enter this way.
- Genitourinary tract. Organisms that cause syphilis, AIDS, gonorrhea, and other sexually transmitted infections enter this way.
- Gastrointestinal tract. Salmonellosis, typhoid fever, and hepatitis A are caused by organisms that enter the digestive tract.
- Circulatory system. Organisms that cause malaria, yellow fever, and meningitis can enter the blood directly through the bite of insects.
- Transplacental (mother to fetus). This is one means by which AIDS and hepatitis B are spread.

Portals of Exit

Infectious organisms leave the reservoir of the host through body secretions (**portals of exit**), including:

- Excretions of the respiratory tract (sputum, mucus) or genital tract (mucus, semen, or vaginal excretions)
- Draining wounds

- Urine
- Feces
- Blood and other body fluids
- Saliva
- Tears

In infected persons, these products must be considered **infectious** or capable of transmitting the disease agent.

Transmission of Disease

Transmission (spread) of infection may happen in one of three ways (Table 12-1):

- **Airborne transmission**—tiny particles remain suspended in the air or trapped in dust and move with air currents. The susceptible host breathes in pathogens carried in this manner.

TABLE 12-1 Ways in Which Microbes Are Spread from One Person to Others

Airborne Transmission
Pathogens carried by moisture or dust particles in air; can be carried long distances
Droplet Transmission
Droplet spread within approximately 3 feet (no personal contact) of infected person by: • Coughing • Sneezing • Spitting • Talking • Whistling • Laughing • Singing
Contact Transmission
Direct contact with infected person: • Touching • Sexual contact • Blood • Body fluids (drainage, urine, feces, sputum, saliva, vomitus)
Indirect contact with infected person through fomites: • Clothing • Dressings • Equipment used in care and treatment • Bed linens • Personal belongings • Specimen containers • Instruments used in treatment • Food • Water

Note that pathogens can also be carried by insects and animals (**vectors**) and passed to humans.

- **Droplet transmission**—droplets are moist particles produced by people coughing, sneezing, talking, laughing, or singing (Figure 12-9A). Pathogens are transmitted into the air with the droplets. Droplets usually stay within three feet of the source. However, the CDC may be changing this published distance to 6 feet in the future.

- **Contact transmission**—*direct contact* (Figure 12-9B) occurs via contact with a person who is the reservoir of pathogens. *Indirect contact* occurs via touching an item contaminated with pathogens, such as soiled linen.

Not all organisms are transmitted in the same way, and some organisms may be transmitted in more than one way.

Host

The person who harbors infectious organisms is the host. This person does not have enough resistance to the infectious agent. An infection develops in the host when infectious organisms:

- Penetrate the body
- Begin to multiply
- Cause damage to the host

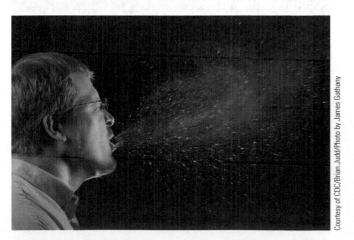

FIGURE 12-9A A sneeze expels a large cone-shaped spray of mucus approximately three to six feet from the mouth.

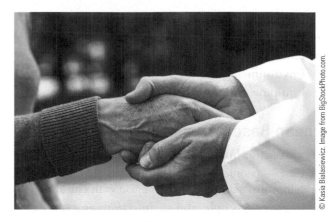

FIGURE 12-9B A handshake is one means of direct contact.

Rubeola

Rubeola (measles) was declared eliminated in the United States in the year 2000 because of the efficiency of the immunization program. Measles is one of the most contagious of all the infectious diseases. The number of cases has increased annually in the United States due to the of immunization. By early July 2019, there, were 1,100 cases in 28 states. This is the highest number since 2000. Some people have traveled abroad, contracted measles, then returned home with the disease. When they returned home, they were asymptomatic and naware of the problem. This is a serious condition that spreads rapidly via airborne transmission. The patients contract high fever (up to 105°F), pneumonia, and rash. The rash appears about 14 days after exposure. The person is considered contagious four days before the rash appears until four days after it develops. The rash begins at the head and spreads downward. There is no specific antiviral therapy for measles. Treatment is supportive.

Marissa gets the measles

Marissa has never been immunized. Although she doesn't know it, she is exposed to measles (rubeola), which is spread by a virus.

Mode of transmission

The measles virus resides in the mucus in the nose and throat of an infected person.

Portal of exit

The disease is usually passed when the infected person coughs or sneezes.

Portal of entry

When the infected person coughs or sneezes, the virus particles are expelled into the air on secretions (droplets from the nose or mouth), and the susceptible host (Marissa) inhales them.

Incubation period

Marissa does not get sick immediately. Because she has no signs or symptoms, she does not know she has been exposed. However, the measles virus is multiplying inside her body. The time from Marissa's exposure until signs and symptoms develop is called the *incubation period*. It appears that the rash first appears 14 days after exposure. Measles is highly contagious. There is some disagreement as to when measles becomes contagious. It seems to be most contagious and can be passed to others from four days before the rash becomes visible to four days after the rash appears. When the disease is transmitted to another person, the cycle begins again. One person can potentially infect many people.

Signs and symptoms of illness develop

Marissa woke up this morning feeling very ill. She has a high fever, hacking cough, and red and watery eyes, with swollen eyelids. These signs and symptoms first occur about 8 to 12 days from the date of exposure.

Mode of transmission and portal of exit

Measles is one of the most contagious of all infectious diseases. Marissa will spread the measles through the airborne method of transmission or by direct contact with infectious droplets. The virus is expelled during sneezing and coughing. If her close contacts have not been immunized, they will also probably contract the measles. Although Marissa knows she is feeling very ill, she still may not know she has the measles. Rash is a late symptom that will occur in about four days after the first symptoms develop. Touching the measles rash will not pass the infection. Marissa will be highly infectious from the time her first signs and symptoms occur until the rash develops, in about four more days. She will also be able to spread the infection for about four more days after the rash appears. Measles virus can remain infectious in the air for up to two hours after an infected person leaves the room.

Risk Factors

Marissa is young, healthy, well-nourished, and has normal fluid intake. She has no known underlying diseases. However, she has never been immunized to prevent measles. Measles is spread readily, so about 90 percent of those exposed will develop the disease unless they have been immunized. In this case, the lack of prior immunization is Marissa's only known risk factor.

Infection Control ALERT

In the United States, 1.7 million people develop sepsis each year. Approximately 270,000 Americans die from sepsis each year. One in k hospital patients that die have sepsis. Sepsis has many causes, so there is no single vaccine to prevent it. Get all recommended adult vaccines, practice good hygiene, and get immediate medical care if you have signs of infection that are not improving.

Risk Factors

Risk factors are conditions indicating that a problem may develop, causing the person's health to worsen. Some increase the likelihood that the person will develop an infection. Factors that increase the risk of infection are:

- Number and strength of the infectious organisms
- General health of the individual
- Age, sex, and heredity of the individual; adults over age 20 are believed to have the greatest risk of getting measles
- Condition of the person's immune system
  Emotional stress and fatigue also play a role in the progress of an infectious disease.

TYPES OF INFECTIONS

Infections can be:

- Localized (confined to one area)—such as boils, skin abscesses, or wound infections.
- Generalized—such as pneumonia (in one or both lungs).
- Systemic—widespread through the body or spread via the bloodstream (**sepsis**). Sepsis is the presence of pus-forming pathogens and other pathogens or their toxins in the blood. It is typically the most expensive condition treated in U.S. hospitals each year.

BODY FLORA

Different microbes live in and on our body surfaces. These microbes are the normal body **flora**. Flora are not the same in all body areas. For example, the organisms making up intestinal tract flora are different from those of the respiratory tract. Both are different from those in the urinary tract. Healthy individuals live in harmony with normal body flora. However, this balance may be disturbed by:

- Pathogenic organisms
- Normal flora becoming pathogenic organisms

- Drugs such as antibiotics that upset the normal balance of organisms within the body flora, allowing one group to flourish
- Flora from one area being transferred into a body area where they do not belong

When the organisms of one normal flora, such as those in the intestinal tract, remain within their normal environment, the related body areas function properly. However, when microbes from the intestines are transferred into the urinary tract, a serious infection may develop. Organisms that are nonpathogenic in their own environment may become pathogenic when they enter a different environment.

HOW PATHOGENS AFFECT THE BODY

The potential for infection depends on the risk factors listed previously. Two major factors are the susceptibility of the host and the amount of infectious agent that finds a portal of entry. Even then, an infection may not occur unless all elements of the chain of infection are present.

Microbes act in different ways to produce disease in the human body. Some pathogens:

- Attack and destroy the cells they invade; for example, invading the red blood cells eventually causes them to split
- Produce poisons called **toxins** that harm the body
- Cause sensitivity responses called **allergies**

BODY DEFENSES

The body has some natural defenses to protect it from infections. There are several natural external defenses. The most important of these is the skin. Intact skin acts as a mechanical barrier against the entry of pathogens. Other defenses include:

- Mucous membranes lining the respiratory, reproductive, gastrointestinal, and urinary tracts. The mucus is sticky and traps foreign materials before they can cause damage.
- Cilia (fine microscopic hairs) lining the respiratory tract, which propels mucus and trapped microbes out of the body.
- Coughing and sneezing, which remove foreign materials from the respiratory tract.
- Hydrochloric acid, a strong chemical that is produced in the stomach, which destroys many microbes.
- Tears, which provide a flushing action that protect the eyes by removing most microbes that enter the eyes.

The body also has a number of internal defenses against infectious agents, including:

- Fever.
- Special cells in the blood called **phagocytes** that destroy microbes. Phagocytes ingest foreign bodies, pathogens, bacteria, and dead or dying cells. In doing so, they fight infection and enhance immunity.
- **Inflammation**—a process that brings blood and phagocytes to the area of infection (Figure 12-10). A skin infection, for example, causes the affected skin area to become swollen, red, hot, and painful, signs that inflammation is occurring.
- Temperature—an elevated temperature is believed to increase the body's ability to fight infection.
- **Immune response**—the body develops protective proteins after having an infectious disease.

IMMUNITY

Immunity is the ability to fight off disease. A pathogen that enters the body is an **antigen**. The body responds to the presence of an antigen by forming **antibodies** to develop resistance to the disease caused by that particular antigen. For example, if a person has antigens in the bloodstream from measles (a virus), antibodies will prevent the occurrence of measles a second time.

> ⊕ Clinical Information **ALERT**
>
> One liter (about 1 quart) of human blood contains approximately six billion phagocytes.

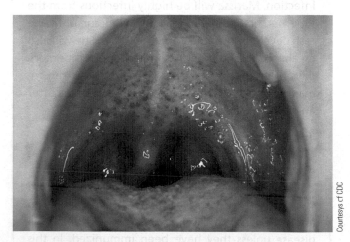

Courtesys cf CDC

FIGURE 12-10 Signs of inflammation include redness, swelling, pain, and loss of function. A sore throat is an example of a painful inflammation.

IMMUNIZATIONS

Immunizations are **vaccines** (medications) that protect against specific pathogens (Figure 12-11). Vaccines consist of artificial or weakened antigens that stimulate the formation of antibodies before the need arises. Vaccines are available to prevent most childhood diseases, such as measles, rubella (German measles), meningitis, mumps, polio, diphtheria, chickenpox, whooping cough, and tetanus. Pneumonia and influenza vaccines are given to both children and adults. Health care workers who have direct contact with patients are advised to get the hepatitis B vaccine. Federal legislation requires that employers provide this vaccine without charge to employees who are considered at risk.

Vaccination Overview

The Centers for Disease Control and Prevention (CDC) provides immunization guidelines. Booster doses of some vaccines are required throughout life. For example, tetanus is an acute, potentially fatal infectious condition caused by the release of a neurotoxin. Thus, tetanus is one of the mandatory childhood vaccines. Tetanus is one of the combined mandatory vaccines given in childhood. However, it is required throughout life. In adults, it may

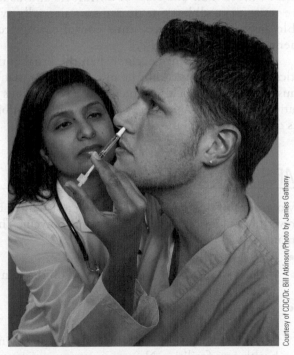

Courtesy of CDC/Dr. Bill Atkinson/Photo by James Gathany

FIGURE 12-11 The nurse uses a small syringe to deliver the flu vaccine mist into the nursing assistant's nostril. The nasal influenza vaccine should not be given to children younger than 2 years of age or adults 50 years and older.

be given as a tetanus toxoid shot or a diphtheria–tetanus (DT) shot. Many school districts check whether their students' vaccine history—including tetanus shots—is current; if not, children are not allowed to attend school. However, the risk of tetanus may not be considered for adults, and health care facilities seldom have a complete vaccination history for patients. Most adult patients do not know or do not remember the dates of their vaccinations, and many have not had vaccines or booster shots in years. This places the person with pressure injuries or other infected wounds at risk of yet another potentially serious problem. Adults with severe wounds and large pressure injuries may be given a tetanus vaccine to reduce the risk of yet another infection.

Resources

Keep your personal vaccinations current. You will find a copy of the most recent health care immunization guidelines and other information in the appendix of your book. Also refer to the resources at http://www.immunize.org/acip/.

IMMUNOSUPPRESSION

Immunosuppression occurs when the body's immune system is weak and cannot fend off pathogens that it should be able to fight successfully. A person who is immunosuppressed is at high risk of infection. Factors that increase the risk of this condition are:

- Very young or very old age
- Frailty
- Chemotherapy
- Infection with human immunodeficiency virus (HIV) or other disease that causes weakness of the immune system
- Injury to or removal of the spleen
- Radiation therapy

SERIOUS INFECTIONS IN HEALTH CARE FACILITIES

Serious infections are increasing in health care facilities as well as in the general public. Persons who are very old, very young, ill, frail, or have a weakened immune system are more likely to contract diseases. Signs and symptoms of infection to report to the nurse are listed in Table 12-2.

Bacterial Infections

Bacteria are often the cause of serious skin, respiratory, urinary, and gastrointestinal infections. If the physician

TABLE 12-2 Signs and Symptoms of Infection That Should Be Reported to the Nurse Immediately

System or Problem	Observation to Report
General Signs/ Symptoms of Infection	Elevated temperature Rapid pulse Rapid respirations Hypotension Fatigue New-onset mental confusion Sweating Chills Skin hot or cold to touch Skin flushed, red, gray, or blue Inflammation of skin as evidenced by redness, edema, heat, or pain Abnormal drainage from any part of the body Other abnormalities specific to the body system
Respiratory System Infection	Rapid respirations Irregular respirations Noisy, labored respirations Dyspnea Coughing Blue color of lips or nail beds, mucous membranes
Integumentary System Infection	Rash Redness Swelling Open areas/skin breakdown Drainage Foul odor
Gastrointestinal System Infection	Unusual or abnormal appearance or color of bowel movement Blood, mucus, or other unusual substances in stool Diarrhea Complaints of indigestion or excessive gas Nausea, vomiting Abdominal pain
Genitourinary System Infection	Urinary output too low Oral intake too low Abnormal appearance of urine: dark, concentrated, red, cloudy Unusual material in urine: blood, pus, particles Complaints of pain, burning, urgency, frequency, pain in lower back Edema Sudden weight loss or gain Respiratory distress Change in mental status
Mental Status Problems	Change in level of consciousness, awareness, or alertness Changes in mood or behavior Change in ability to express self or communicate Mental confusion

suspects a bacterial infection, a **culture and sensitivity** test may be ordered. The culture identifies the pathogen causing the infection. The sensitivity = identifies the **antibiotic** (antibacterial drug) that is most likely to eliminate the organism causing the infection.

Antibiotic Resistance

It is essential that patients take all prescribed antibiotics as ordered. Stopping the drug early may cause the pathogens to become resistant to the antibiotic. When this occurs, the antibiotics will no longer eliminate the infection. This is a serious problem. The antibiotics that are used to treat drug-resistant pathogens are usually quite expensive. They may cause serious side effects, such as hearing loss, liver failure, and kidney damage. It is possible that, in time, these infectious microbes may become resistant to the newer antibiotics as well. One thing is certain: we must do all we can to reduce the risk of drug resistance. Cleansing the hands and wearing protective apparel are some of the best methods of preventing drug resistance.

Antibiotics are some of the most commonly prescribed drugs in hospitals and nursing homes. Studies have shown that up to three-fourths of these prescriptions may be inappropriate, unnecessary, or even harmful to individuals who are frail and elderly. Resistant so more than one class of antibiotic and usually are resistant to all but one or two commercially available antimicrobial agents, thus complicating treatment of illnesses they cause.

Antibiotic resistance occurs when the usual antibiotics cannot eliminate (kill) the microorganism that has caused an infection. This is potentially a very serious situation because it is a point at which no known antibiotics can effectively kill the germ.

MRSA AND VRE

Two groups of organisms have become resistant to two powerful antibiotics, methicillin and vancomycin. These organisms are:

- **Methicillin-resistant** *Staphylococcus aureus* **(MRSA)**—which are normally found on the skin and mucous membranes.
- **Vancomycin-resistant enterococci (VRE)**— which are found in the gastrointestinal tract. They are a major cause of infections acquired in health care facilities. Newer strains are resistant to vancomycin.

Additional pathogens are developing resistance to methicillin and vancomycin, making it difficult to eliminate the infection.

Carbapenem-Resistant *Enterobacteriaceae* (CRE)

The community in early 2013 asking them to protect patients from a group of microbes called **carbapenem-resistant** *Enterobacteriaceae* (**CRE**). Carbapenem is an antibiotic that is given as a last resort to persons with very serious infections.

The CDC has tracked one form of CRE from a single health care facility to other facilities in at least 42 states. Under most circumstances, health care workers are concerned about problems caused by individual bacteria, such as MRSA and others noted in this chapter. CRE is an entire family, containing more than 70 bacteria. Most of these usually reside in the digestive tract and colon. They cause infection when they escape to other areas of the body.

CRE are usually spread on the hands of health care workers. Up to half of the patients who get bloodstream infections from this pathogen will die. In addition, one type of CRE bacteria can transfer drug resistance to other bacteria within the same family. This has the potential to cause many other life-threatening infections. CREs are most common in persons whose care requires ventilators (breathing machines), urinary catheters, intravenous (IV) catheters, and those who have been taking certain antibiotics for long periods of time.

Drug resistance of this type has made some infections impossible to cure. Prevention and early identification of the pathogens are the best approaches to patient care. To prevent the spread of CRE, the nursing assistant must:

- Begin by being alert to the presence of the organism in the facility. If it is identified in a laboratory test, take measures to stop it from spreading.
- Follow infection control recommendations for every patient.
- Use good handwashing and hand hygiene practices.
- Practice standard precautions and transmission-based precautions (Chapter 13). (In addition to standard precautions, persons with CRE require contact precautions.)

 Infection Control **ALERT**

Antibiotic-resistant bacteria develop as a result of repeated and/or improper use of antibiotics. Antibiotics will eliminate sensitive bacteria, but germs that are resistant will thrive. In some cases, an antibiotic eliminates helpful microbes that keep harmful microbes in check. Antibiotics are helpful for treating bacterial infections. They will not eliminate infections caused by viruses, such as colds, flu, and sore throats. Using antibiotics inappropriately in these and other situations promotes the spread of drug-resistant bacteria.

- Use good techniques when caring for persons who are incontinent; avoid environmental contamination.
- Report signs and symptoms of infection to the nurse.
- Attend classes to learn all you can about infection control.
- Follow instructions and use medical asepsis when caring for persons with tubes and other medical devices.
- Bathe patients in a soap called chlorhexidine, if ordered.

Other Bacterial Pathogens

Serious infections are also caused by the following types of bacteria:

- *Pseudomonas aeruginosa*—an organism und in water and on other environmental surfaces. It can infect any body tissue. It usually exploits a break in the host defenses to start an infection. It is rapidly becoming drug resistant.
- *Escherichia coli*—a bacterium commonly found in the intestinal tract, where it is normally harmless. Outside the intestinal tract, it often causes urinary tract infections or infections in pressure ulcers.
- *Klebsiella*—a bacterium that is a major cause of pneumonia, urinary tract infections, and wound infections. The bacteria are quickly becoming drug resistant. *Klebsiella* normally reside in the colon, where it takes part in normal bowel function. It usually infects patients with weakened immune systems.
- *Salmonella*—a group of bacteria that cause mild to life-threatening intestinal infections, including "food poisoning."
- *Listeria monocytogenes*—**listeriosis** is caused by ingesting these bacteria in contaminated food, especially uncooked meats and vegetables, hot dogs, cold cuts, soft cheeses, and unpasteurized (raw) milk.
- *Acinetobacter baumannii*—a bacterium that was contracted by many soldiers in Iraq and carried back on clothing and skin. It is a common cause of pneumonia, including 7 percent of hospital-acquired cases. Few drugs can treat it, and mortality rates can be 20 percent or more. Containing the spread of this infection has been very difficult.

Tuberculosis

Mycobacterium tuberculosis is the bacterium that causes tuberculosis (TB). Tuberculosis was a widespread disease with a high fatality rate before antibiotics were introduced. In the 1950s, the use of antibiotics markedly reduced the numbers of TB cases and deaths. The number of infections has increased since 1985 because some strains have become drug resistant. There has also been an increase in the number of people who are at risk for infection, including those who:

- Are HIV positive
- Are infected but fail to take their medication for the full treatment period
- Live in poverty and are malnourished
- Have immigrated to the United States from countries where tuberculosis is still common
- Have had inactive tuberculosis in their bodies become active

Tuberculosis Infection

Tuberculosis infection occurs when the bacterium that causes the disease enters the body. The body responds by containing the microbe in a barrier called a **tubercle** so it cannot spread. As long as the tubercle remains intact and no other tuberculosis bacteria enter the body, the infection is inactive. In this state the person is not **contagious** (able to pass the infection to others).

Tuberculosis Disease

Tuberculosis disease develops:

- If the person who is exposed to the bacterium has a weakened immune system and the tubercle does not form
- If an existing tubercle breaks down
- If more tuberculosis bacteria enter the body

When active tuberculosis occurs, the bacteria multiply, tissue damage increases, and the microbes may spread to other parts of the body. As the disease progresses, the person will show one or more of the following signs and symptoms:

- Fatigue
- Loss of appetite and weight
- Weakness
- Elevated temperature in the afternoon and evening
- Night sweats
- Spitting up blood (**hemoptysis**)
- Coughing

TB is spread only by the airborne method of transmission. A person with tuberculosis in the lungs can spread it to others through airborne pathogens in respiratory secretions. Most people know that tuberculosis affects the lungs. It also may affect any other part of the body, including the spine, the brain, or the kidneys. A person with tuberculosis is often very ill and may die without treatment. It was the leading cause of death in the United States at one time.

Diagnosis

The presence of the tuberculosis bacterium in the body can be shown by:

- A sputum culture—grows the organisms from a mucous specimen from the person's lungs. You will be collecting this specimen. Make sure the person coughs mucus up from deep in the lungs. Do not collect saliva from the mouth.
- Chest X-rays—show the extent of the disease process in the lungs.
- A positive skin test (Mantoux test)—shows the presence of antibodies to the tuberculosis organisms in the body (Figure 12-12).

Most health care workers must undergo a skin test for tuberculosis before employment. Many facilities use a two-step method of testing.

Treatment

A person with tuberculosis is treated with an antibiotic or combination of antibiotics. Because many TB organisms have become resistant to specific drugs, a combination

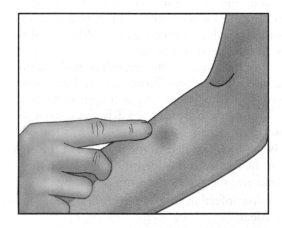

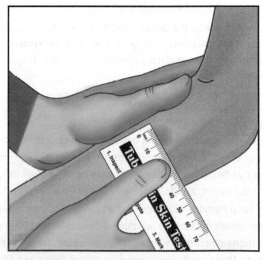

FIGURE 12-12 A positive Mantoux test shows redness and induration (swelling) 48 to 72 hours after the test.

of drugs must be used to control them. Once drug therapy starts, the patient usually becomes noncontagious (cannot spread the disease) within two to three weeks. However, the therapy must continue for six months to two years.

Streptococcus A

Streptococcus A (*Strep A*) is a bacterium that produces very powerful enzymes that destroy tissues and blood cells. At least 15 percent of people carry the bacteria in their respiratory secretions, but have no symptoms. They pass the infection to others by coughing or sneezin or by touching a susceptible person or environmental surface without washing their hands. *Strep A* (and some other organisms) cause a serious skin infection called **necrotizing fasciitis**. This condition is often called flesh-eating or man-eating strep. It occurs when bacteria enter the body through minor trauma or a tiny break in the skin. The toxin destroys muscle tissue. The injury worsens rapidly and can spread as much as an inch per hour, causing tissue death. Blood cannot reach or nourish the dead tissue. The wound turns black and gangrenous (Figure 12-13), requiring amputation. *Strep A* can be so serious that although the patient survives, they are scarred and has as many as all four extremities amputated. About 25 percent of cases result in death.

Escherichia coli O157:H7

You have learned that *Escherichia coli* (*E.coli*) can cause serious problems outside the intestinal tract. Another strain, *E. coli* O157:H7, has caused outbreaks resulting in serious illness and death. This form of the bacterium is found in the intestines of some cattle. It is spread in contaminated and undercooked meat. A small amount of these bacteria can contaminate a large amount of meat, particularly ground beef. The pathogen creates a situation in which blood flow to the brain, kidneys, and other organs is endangered. *E. coli* O157:H7 can be deadly, particularly to infants, children, elderly, persons with HIV, and others with weakened immune systems.

Pseudomembranous Colitis

A variety of bacteria live in the digestive tract of a healthy person. Most of these are harmless. Some are used for food digestion, but others are menaces with the potential for causing serious illness and major organ damage. The potentially harmful bacteria are usually outnumbered by good bacteria, so no harm comes to the person. **Pseudomembranous colitis** is a very serious condition in which a bacterium called *Clostridium difficile* (*C. difficile*) causes diarrhea. The shorthand term for this organism is *C. diff.*

Antibiotics have no way of knowing which microorganisms are helpful and which are harmful. Based on each one's specific characteristics, each antibiotic simply identifies microbes and kills as many as they can. Pseudomembranous colitis often develops in persons who have been on antibiotic therapy. The good bacteria die as a result of the antibiotic, and the bad bacteria grow out of control. Without the other friendly bacteria to keep *C. difficile* in check, it breeds rapidly, producing toxins that cause serious illness.

C. difficile is very common in health care facilities. It is picked up on the hands, bedpans, bedside commodes, toilets, sinks, countertops, bed rails, doorknobs, and other surfaces that have been contaminated by stool, even when the contamination is not visible. It most commonly enters the body through the mouth by contact with unwashed hands.

INFECTIOUS DIARRHEA

Spores are microscopic reproductive bodies and are responsible for the spread of some diseases. After leaving the body, they can survive in the environment in a dormant form for long periods of time, until conditions are ideal for reproduction. Once active, the spores will multiply and continue to spread infection. They are very difficult to eliminate. *C. difficile* is spread by spores. The condition of being dormant is similar to being in a deep sleep. When an organism is dormant, life functions are slowed. The spores are not growing or active, but they are able to return to a normal state of function in the future.

Norovirus (Norwalk virus) is a highly contagious pathogen that causes infectious diarrhea. You may have heard of these viruses on the news, as they have caused diarrhea outbreaks on many cruise ships, hospitals, and

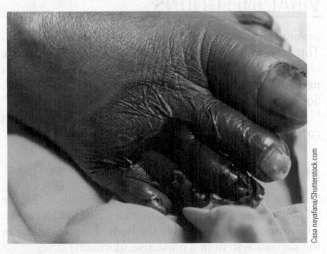

FIGURE 12-13 Gangrene occurs due to loss of blood supply to a body part. Amputation is the usual treatment.

Casa nayafana/Shutterstock.com

nursing homes. Very few particles are needed to transmit infection. The pathogen originates in the stool. Rotavirus is plentiful throughout environments in which many young children spend time (such as day care centers), especially during the winter months. Both viruses are highly resistant to disinfectants usually used for cleaning environmental surfaces. Norovirus and other organisms that form spores are highly resistant to alcohol-based hand cleaners. Rotavirus and norovirus remain active on the hands for at least 4 hours, on hard dry surfaces for up to 10 days, and on wet surfaces for weeks.

Patients with infectious diarrhea should be placed on contact precautions. When caring for patients with infectious diarrhea and other conditions known to be spread by spores, use good handwashing procedures. Friction and running water will remove spores and microbes from your hands.

ENVIRONMENTAL CLEANLINESS

When patients have infectious diarrhea or another condition spread by spores, special attention must be paid to hand hygiene and environmental cleanliness. These pathogens have the following features in common:

- *C. difficile* (Figure 12-14) and norovirus are usually plentiful in the environment (room or unit) of patients with infectious diarrhea.
- *C. difficile* and norovirus are spread by spores.
- Spores have been found on the hands of health care workers providing care to affected patients or touching items and surfaces in the patient's room.
- Spores are capable of surviving for days to months in the environment.
- *C. difficile* and norovirus are resistant to many chemical disinfectant products, including alcohol. They survive in a dormant state.

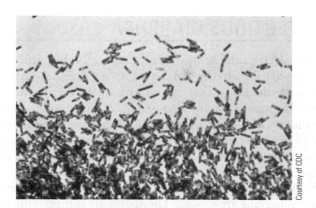

FIGURE 12-14 *C. difficile* is a spore-forming bacterium that causes pseudomembranous colitis and diarrhea. People become infected if they touch the mouth after touching contaminated items or surfaces. Health care workers can spread the bacteria to patients or contaminate surfaces through hand contact.

Courtesy of CDC

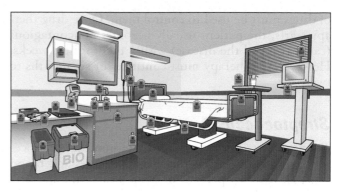

FIGURE 12-15 Points of environmental contamination. Studies have proven that infection can be passed through contact with common work surfaces.

- These organisms have caused outbreaks of infectious diarrhea in hospitals and long-term care facilities.
- They are transmitted through the digestive tract (usually entering through the mouth via the hands).
- Studies have shown that environmental surface contamination is a common source of infection (Figure 12-15).
- Good handwashing, with soap, water, and friction, is required to eliminate pathogens and spores from hands.
- Handwashing with soap, water, and friction loosens and removes spores from the hands, and running water washes them down the drain. This method is much more effective than alcohol hand sanitizer.
- Environmental cleaning is required, with friction and a disinfectant product known to kill the pathogen, such as those containing sodium hypochlorite (bleach).

VIRAL INFECTIONS

Several viral infections are discussed in this section. Topical products and drugs are available to treat the symptoms and make the person more comfortable, but no drugs have been developed to cure viral conditions . Some can be prevented through vaccinations.

Genital herpes (which is also a viral infection) is covered in Chapter 46.

Shingles

Shingles (herpes zoster) (Figure 12-16) occurs in people who were infected by the virus that causes chickenpox. The organisms did not leave the body. They remained in the nervous system in a nonactive (dormant) state.

Years later, when the person is in a weakened condition, the organisms may become active. Painful blister-like

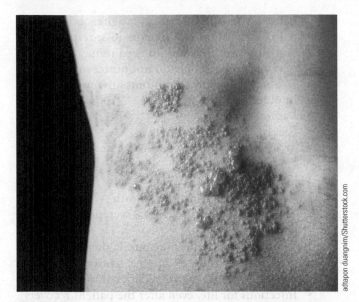

adtapon duangnim/Shutterstock.com

FIGURE 12-16 This rash is caused by shingles. The patient is infectious as long as the blisters are intact.

lesions containing infectious organisms develop on the skin along the nerve pathways on one side of the body. Health care providers who never had chickenpox, those who have not been immunized, and those who are pregnant should not enter the room of a patient with shingles. The person is placed in airborne precautions. When all the lesions have burst and crusted over, the patient is no longer infectious and will be removed from isolation.

Influenza

Influenza (the flu) is caused by a family of viruses. The infection can have serious consequences for elderly and/or frail people. Each year new types of viruses spread rapidly from person to person by way of respiratory secretions, causing many to become ill. Vaccines offer some protection against influenza viruses and are often given to residents in long-term care facilities. Hospitals and long-term care facilities both offer flu shots and pneumonia shots to their patients and employees each year.

 Infection Control ALERT

In 2014, West Africa experienced the largest outbreak of the **Ebola** hemorrhagic fever in history. The Ebola virus was first identified in the 1970s. It is very frightening because there is no cure, and 7 out of 10 people with the virus will die. Although experimental vaccines and treatments are under development, they are not ready for widespread use at this time. A person is contagious when signs and symptoms are present, even if they are mild. Proper use of protective equipment (Chapter 13) is key to protecting oneself.

In addition to making the person feel ill, the viruses may lower the patient's resistance to other infectious organisms. These other organisms can cause pneumonia and other life-threatening infections. You can help protect yourself and the patients in your care by:

- Getting the flu vaccine each year
- Staying healthy
- Not reporting for duty when you are ill
- Faithfully carrying out standard precautions
- Following the facility's policies regarding special precautions when a patient has a respiratory infection
- Encouraging the patients to drink fluids
- Reporting to the charge nurse when a visitor seems to be ill

Ebola Virus Disease (EVD)

Ebola virus disease (EVD) was formerly called Ebola hemorrhagic fever.

EVD causes severe bleeding, organ failure, and death. This condition has been a severe problem in Africa, but was never seen in the United States until 2014, when an emergency department patient was seen and diagnosed with sinusitis. He was sent home with antibiotics. ("Home" was his girlfriend's apartment. The patient was from Africa and was visiting his girlfriend and her five children.)

Two days later, the patient returned to the emergency department in an ambulance and was admitted to isolation observation. This time, he was correctly diagnosed with Ebola. Many people had already been exposed to the virus, which is spread through contact with blood and body fluids. The incubation period is believed to be 2 to 21 days, with the average being about 8 to 10 days. Contact may be direct (from human to human) or indirect. Animal bites and stings also spread this disease. The body can transmit disease after death.

Two nurses from the Texas hospital to which the patient sought treatment contracted Ebola. They were critically ill, but did survive. Both suffered tremendous personal losses because little was known about the mode of transmission at the time. Hazmat teams were sent to their apartments, where they took and destroyed all the nurses' property, including one nurse's engagement ring and the other nurse's wedding dress. Very little is known of their condition since the original illness, and they both live very private lives in unknown locations. At least one has experienced nightmares and severe headaches as a result of the Ebola.

Signs and symptoms of EVD include:

- Muscle pain
- Sore throat
- Headache
- Fever
- Vomiting

- Diarrhea, which may be severe
- Rash
- Signs of impaired kidney function
- Bleeding, including blood in the stool and oozing from the gums

As a result of this situation, the CDC has required facilities to use personal protective equipment (PPE) with a higher degree of protection. They have also changed the instructions for applying protective apparel to ensure that the caregivers' bodies are covered well. If the patient is known or suspected to have EVD, a supervisor must watch staff applying PPE to make sure the employee is covered and no skin is exposed.

Much remains to be learned about this condition. Health care facilities are doing a better job of screening when people are admitted, and there have been no active U.S. cases reported to the CDC since 2015. Health care workers must continue to be alert to the potential for this infection, which quickly can become an epidemic.

Hepatitis

Hepatitis is an inflammation of the liver caused by several viruses, including the:

- Hepatitis A virus
- Hepatitis B virus
- Hepatitis C virus
- Hepatitis D virus
- Hepatitis E virus
- Hepatitis G virus

Characteristics of these viruses include the following:

- Hepatitis A virus (HAV)
  - Most common.
  - Transmitted by feces, saliva, contaminated food, and sexual contact.
  - Signs and symptoms: **jaundice** (a yellow color of the skin and sclera; Figure 12-17), fever,

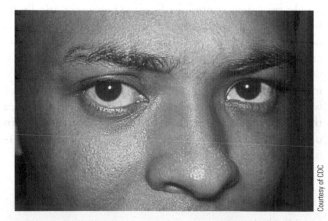

FIGURE 12.17 This patient has jaundice, which is seen by the yellowing of the eyes.

nausea, vomiting, diarrhea, fatigue, abdominal pain, dark urine, and appetite loss; respiratory symptoms, rashes, and joint pain may also develop; some people do not notice any signs of illness; as a rule, symptoms are more severe in older persons.
  - Vaccine available.
  - Rarely fatal.
  - Treated with bed rest and avoidance of alcoholic beverages.
- Hepatitis B virus (HBV)
  - Can cause liver cancer and death
  - Transmitted by blood, sexual secretions, feces, and saliva
  - Signs and symptoms may mimic the flu and include fever, aches and pains, nausea, fatigue, and urine that may turn a dark color
  - Infectious for life, even after the patient recovers from acute illness
  - Some patients have no symptoms at all but are still infectious
  - Vaccine available for protection
- Hepatitis C virus (HCV)
  - 50 percent of people infected develop chronic hepatitis
  - Transmitted mainly through blood, blood products, and body fluids
  - May be mistaken for the flu
  - Common signs and symptoms: extreme fatigue, depression, fever, mood changes, weakness, pain, loss of appetite
  - May cause liver cancer and liver failure
  - Disease may be present for years before patient becomes aware of it; during this time, it silently destroys the liver
  - Leading cause of need for liver transplants in the United States
  - Treated with alpha interferon; treatment not always successful

Other types of hepatitis—hepatitis D, hepatitis E, and hepatitis G—are less common. Infection with these organisms is not as serious as the other types.

Any infection of the liver is serious because the liver is a vital organ. Health care workers must take hepatitis very seriously because many individuals have no signs and symptoms of illness, yet are able to transmit the infection to others. You can best protect yourself by:

- Using standard precautions, including proper handling of sharps such as needles or razors (Chapter 13)
- Taking the vaccine, if available
- Practicing safe sex (using condoms)
- Not using illegal drugs

EMERGING INFECTIOUS DISEASE

You have probably been informally introduced to hundreds of new pathogens throughout your life and did not know it. Pathogens are microbes that can cause illness, but many variables affect whether persons exposed to them become sick. Some of these have probably made you and your contacts sick. Learning about new pathogens is an ever-changing subject.

The *coronavirus* has been with us for many years, but the strains have not been troublesome. In 2019, a new strain of this virus, the **2019 novel coronavirus (COVID-19)**, rapidly introduced itself to the world, causing serious illness, numerous deaths, and getting a great deal of attention. It has been identified on all continents but Antarctica. We quickly learned that people with this organism can be seriously ill or completely asymptomatic.

You must know the:

- *Incubation period*, which is believed to be within 14 days following exposure; most cases occur approximately 4 to 5 days after exposure.
- *Mode of transmission*, which is believed to be on respiratory droplets and direct or indirect contact on hands. Transmission is also prevented by **social distancing**. This means you should stay at least 6 feet away from other people. It also involves staying away from events with 10 or more people. You should also practice **self-quarantine**. This means you must stay at home unless you are leaving the house to seek a necessary service. Each community is specifying what services are considered necessary. Check with your city or county website or other official source of information.
- *Signs and symptoms of the illness*, which include fever, cough, shortness of breath, chest pain, new confusion, inability to arouse, and cyanotic lips or face.
- *PPE used to interrupt transmission*, which include an N95 mask and gloves.
- *Treatment*. Unfortunately, there is no known treatment or cure. Treatment is symptomatic until symptoms subside.

The **World Health Organization (WHO)** was appointed as the worldwide health authority by the United Nations. The **Centers for Disease Control and Prevention (CDC)** was appointed the health authority for the United States by the Department of Health and Human Services. Both organizations verified that in 2020 **pandemic** conditions related to the coronavirus were present, and alerted health care professionals about the potential for a worldwide epidemic. A disease is considered an **epidemic** when it spreads over a very large area and many people become sick at the same time. If the disease continues to spread, it becomes pandemic, affecting a larger geographical area and greater portion of the population.

Although your facility has an infection control nurse who will provide guidance, we are all responsible for infection prevention. Monitor compliance with infection prevention when you are making rounds. Basic methods of preventing infection include:

- Staying home from work when you are sick.
- Handwashing—this is the most important method of preventing the spread of infection.
  - Wash hands for at least 20 seconds before and after patient care and any time they are soiled or have had contact with a contaminated substance. If you are unable to wash your hands at the sink, use alcohol sanitizer for at least 20 seconds. Make sure hands are dry before touching anything. Alcohol will not kill spores or some microbes passed in the stool. Soap and water are the best method of cleansing your hands if spore contamination is a possibility or your hands have a substance on them.
- Apply the principles of standard precautions for actual or potential contact with blood, body fluids, mucous membranes, or nonintact skin. This includes both areas of the person's body and items in the environment. Remember that wearing gloves protects both you and the person you are caring for. Change them as often as necessary. Avoid touching clean environmental surfaces with soiled, contaminated gloves and vice versa. Staff have a tendency to apply gloves when they enter the room, provide patient care, then remove and discard the gloves prior to leaving. Unfortunately, this method may protect staff but it provides a great deal of cross-contamination in the environment and on the patient. Remember you are protecting yourself, the person receiving care, and others that enter and leave the room.
- Do not overdo it with the PPE. Use only what you need. If an organism is passed on the skin and the hands, there is no need to wear a mask. Wear gloves only. Wear a gown only if there is a risk of contamination of your uniform. Make sure PPE fits correctly. When caring for a person with both clean and soiled areas on the body, care for the cleanest sites first, and work toward the least clean areas. Remove gloves before leaving the room. Do not wear gloves in the hallway. Make sure that the protective apparel you are using fits correctly.

Acquired Immunodeficiency Syndrome (AIDS)

Acquired immunodeficiency syndrome (AIDS) is a viral disease transmitted through direct contact with the bodily secretions of an infected person. The virus that causes AIDS is the **human immunodeficiency virus (HIV)**.

The ways in which HIV is transmitted include:

- Blood to blood through:
  - Transfusion of infected blood. Note that federal regulations prohibit the use of untested and unregulated blood in the United States
  - Treatment of hemophilia with clotting factor from infected blood
  - Needle sharing among drug users
  - Prick from a contaminated needle or sharp
  - Unsterile instruments used for procedures such as ear piercing or tattooing
- Unprotected vaginal, oral, or anal intercourse when one partner is infected

HIV can be transmitted from infected mother to infant during:

- Pregnancy
- The birth process
- Breastfeeding

The AIDS Virus

The AIDS virus (HIV):

- Has many variants
- Does not live long outside the body
- Is affected by common chemicals such as bleach
- Depresses the immune system
- Makes the infected person more susceptible to infections
- Makes the infected person more likely to experience complications such as:
  - *Pneumocystis carinii* pneumonia (PCP)—a serious lung infection
  - Kaposi's sarcoma (Figures 12-18A and 12-18B)— a serious malignancy affecting many body organs
  - Brain involvement leading to dementia
  - Eye involvement leading to blindness
  - Tuberculosis
  - Other opportunistic infections

Incubation Period

Not everyone who comes in contact with the HIV virus becomes infected. For those who are infected, there is always a period of time between contact and the start of the signs and symptoms of infection. One-fourth to one-half of people exposed to HIV show evidence of disease within 5 to 10 years of antibody development (becoming seropositive).

- During this period, the virus is in infected cells but is not active. The body does not make antibodies to the virus.
- Most people become **seropositive**, or HIV positive (showing antibodies to HIV in the bloodstream), approximately three to six months after infection. They have developed HIV disease, which may progress to AIDS.

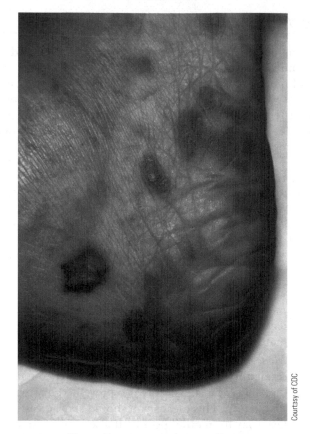

FIGURE 12-18A Kaposi's sarcoma is a malignant tumor caused by the human herpesvirus 8 (HHV8). It affects persons with weakened immune systems, such as those with HIV disease and AIDS.

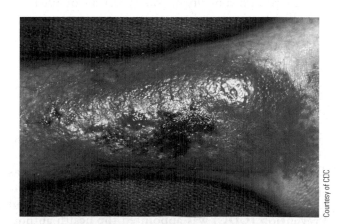

FIGURE 12-18B Kaposi's sarcoma may be hard to identify because it has so many different forms. This lesion looks much like a venous leg ulcer.

- The asymptomatic period (when no signs and symptoms are present) following infection may last months to years. AIDS does not always develop, but the person is an HIV carrier for life.

> ### Hepatitis B Infection
>
> Hepatitis B is much more contagious than HIV. Imagine that a quarter-teaspoon of hepatitis B virus is mixed into a 24,000-gallon swimming pool full of water. Someone draws a quarter-teaspoon of that water into a syringe and injects you with it. Despite the amount of dilution, everyone who receives such an injection will become HBV positive. By comparison, imagine that 10 people are in the room. Someone takes a quarter-teaspoon of HIV and mixes it into one quart of water. A quarter-teaspoon of that water is then injected into each person in the room. Statistically, only one person in the room will become HIV positive. Hepatitis B, then, is a much greater threat to health care workers than is HIV. Proper use of standard precautions (Chapter 13) will prevent the spread of HIV and hepatitis B, as well as many other diseases and infections. The threat of hepatitis B can be eliminated completely with proper vaccination.

Disease Progression

Progression of the disease process is determined by the effect of the viruses on special protective white blood cells known as CD4 cells (T cells). Over time, the number of these protective white blood cells drops. As a result, the immune system of the infected person becomes more suppressed (weaker) and less able to fight infection. When the number of CD4 cells drops to a critical level (below 200 cells/mm^3), the person is diagnosed with AIDS.

Treatment

At this time, there is no cure for AIDS. A combination of drugs currently in use reduces both the symptoms and viral activity. The virus becomes drug resistant quickly, so an ongoing supply of new drugs is needed.

Hantavirus

In May 1993, a cluster of unexplained deaths occurred among young Native Americans in the southwestern United States. An investigation revealed a virus that was previously unknown. This situation attracted a great deal of media attention. This strange disease is called **hantavirus**. It is spread by contact with rodents (rats and mice) or their excretions, including urine and stool. Once disturbed, viral particles in the excretions become airborne and are inhaled by the susceptible host. Signs and symptoms appear one to five weeks later and include high fever, chills, muscle aches, cough, nausea, vomiting, diarrhea, dizziness, and feeling very tired. As the disease progresses, the patient becomes very short of breath. When this occurs, the disease progresses rapidly, and the patient becomes seriously ill. Respiratory support may be necessary, and death may occur. Nonpulmonary cases were first identified in 2014.

Because rodents move about and are found everywhere, cases of hantavirus have been confirmed as far away as the state of New York in the United States.

Spread of this condition can be reduced by taking steps to prevent rodents from entering the home or eliminating them if they are present. Scientists have always thought that hantavirus is not transmitted from person to person. However, human-to-human spread has been reported in Argentina. There is much to learn about this virus, and scientists are studying the disease (Figure 12-19).

Acute Flaccid Myelitis (AFM)

Acute flaccid myelitis (AFM) is a serious condition affecting the nervous system and causing the person to become very weak. This condition first appeared in 2014, and instances been increasing gradually since that time. No one is quite sure of the cause, but it appears to be viral in origin. It is compared with polio, but the polio virus is shed in the stool. Stool specimens are negative in AFM. The problem is confined mostly to children, but has been seen in adults.

Sudden weakness and loss of reflexes and muscle tone are the most common symptoms. Some people have pain in the arms and legs, a drooping eyelid, slurred speech, and difficulty swallowing. At the present time, there is no specific treatment. This is another new condition that has quickly become problematic. Much more research is needed to determine the best method of management.

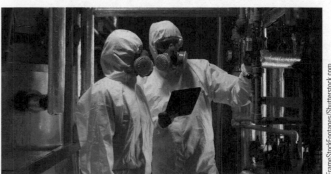

FIGURE 12-19 These scientists are wearing tight protective suits with a filtered, breathable air supply so they can study highly pathogenic viruses such as COVID-19

FrameStockFootages/Shutterstock.com

BIOTERRORISM

Bioterrorism is the use of biological agents, such as pathogenic organisms or agricultural pests, for terrorist purposes. Since October 2001, local, state, and federal public health authorities have been investigating cases of bioterrorism-related illness. Specifically, some individuals died from inhalation anthrax, a condition that was spread by a powdery substance containing anthrax spores sent through the mail. A number of other individuals developed the cutaneous (skin) version of this disease (Figure 12-20). Cutaneous anthrax is not fatal. Anthrax cannot be passed from one person to another. It is transmitted only through contact with spores. Fortunately, the number of workplaces and individuals contaminated was small, but it raised concerns regarding future terrorist attacks. Many individuals could be infected by a biological weapon before the exposure is detected and identified. Some of the diseases that can potentially be used as biological weapons have been considered eradicated for years, and today's health care professionals have never seen or treated them. Thus, bioterrorism is a significant threat.

Many health care facilities have developed disaster plans to address bioterrorism. The plans outline the steps necessary for responding to bioterrorism with the most common agents, including smallpox, botulism toxin, anthrax, and plague. The disaster plans include information for patients, employees, and visitors, and specify public health precautions and protocols to follow in the event of an emergency. Sadly, given the state of world affairs, health care facilities must be prepared for potential terrorist actions in the future.

PARASITES

You have already learned that yeast and mold are opportunistic parasites. Some insects are also parasites—they survive by feeding off another human or animal. Fleas and ticks are common examples of parasites.

Pediculosis

Pediculosis is another term for lice. Three common types of lice are seen in the United States:

- Head lice (*Pediculosis capitis*) (Figure 12-21)—found on the head, scalp, and behind the ears
- Pubic lice (*Pediculosis pubis*)—found in the pubic area; occasionally seen in underarm and eyebrow hair in humans
- Body lice (*Pediculosis corporis*)—found on the body and in clothing of infested people

Pediculosis can be seen with the eye. Body lice and pubic lice may look like many tiny scabs on the skin. They are spread by direct or indirect contact with an infected person. They can live for several days without food. Pediculosis can transmit disease. Inform the nurse immediately if you suspect that a patient is infected.

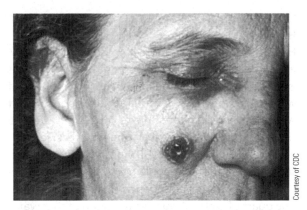

FIGURE 12-20 Cutaneous anthrax lesion on right cheek; lesion as seen on 11th day.

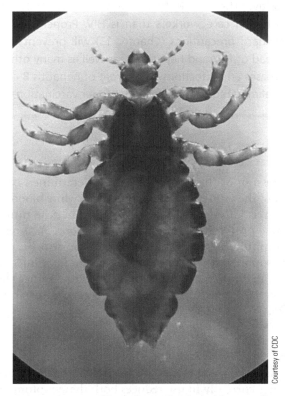

FIGURE 12-21 A magnified view of a head louse. Head lice are tiny, but can be seen with the unaided eye.

Head Lice

Head lice are parasites that spread primarily by direct contact with an infected person. They live very close to the scalp, where body heat is highest. They feed on blood from the scalp approximately five times per day. Lice live for about 40 days. During this time, females lay about 200 eggs (**nits**). The louse lays one egg per hair, using a strong adhesive to attach it close (about 3 mm) to the scalp (Figure 12-22). The egg will hatch in nine days. During this time the hair continues to grow, so eggs may be found 5 mm from the scalp. Hatched shells and infertile eggs may be found farther than this.

Head lice can also be spread by sharing personal belongings such as brushes, combs, ribbons, caps,

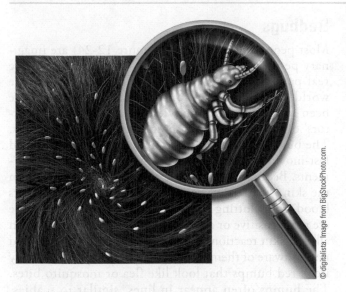

© digitalista. Image from BigStockPhoto.com.

FIGURE 12-22 The female louse lays her eggs close to the scalp. A sticky substance glues them in place, making them very difficult to remove.

clothing, and bedding with others. You cannot contract head lice from pets and animals. The lice do not hop, jump, or fly, but they can crawl very quickly.

When performing hair care, check patients for nits. Nits are tiny oval-shaped eggs that are yellow-white in color. They look like dandruff, but are firmly attached to the hair and are very difficult to remove. Dandruff brushes off readily. It may be difficult to differentiate nits from other conditions of the scalp. The nits hatch into live lice. Lice are tiny brown insects about the size of a sesame seed. They run away from light quickly. Notify the nurse for further assessment if you notice nits or other abnormalities.

Treatment for Head Lice

If nits or lice are suspected, you will wear a gown and gloves for contact with the patient until they have been treated. You must also wear gloves and a gown when handling the patient's clothing or linen. The physician will order a medicated shampoo to kill the parasites. Contact precautions will be used for 24 hours after the patient is treated.

Head lice have been with us for thousands of years. During this time many chemicals have been used to control them. The lice developed immunity to the chemicals, so the dosage was increased. This creates a health risk to children, elderly persons, and those with weakened immune systems.

As with other diseases, some head lice have become resistant to medicated shampoos. If the lice cannot be eliminated with a shampoo, the only way to remove them is by checking the head and eliminating them manually. This is a time-consuming task. Manual removal of lice and nits is done using a special comb, tweezers, or double-sided tape. Two people may need to check the head simultaneously, because the lice run very fast. Shining a flashlight on the

head may be helpful, as the lice will move away from the light source. A battery-operated comb may also be used on clean, dry, oil-free hair. This device will kill lice on contact, but will not eliminate nits. Before trying to manually remove the lice, comb the hair to remove tangles.

Bag the patient's clothing and tie the bags. Send the bags home with a family member, or follow the nurse's instructions. Send the linens and pillows to the laundry. You may be directed to check other patients for the presence of head lice.

Scabies

Scabies is a disease of the skin caused by a parasite called a **mite** (Figure 12-23A). A mite is a microscopic organism that cannot be seen with the naked eye. Scabies is highly contagious and is spread by direct and indirect contact. It causes a rash (Figure 12-23B) and severe itching of the skin. The rash may be seen between the fingers, inside the wrists, outside the elbows, and in the underarm, waist, and nipple areas. It is also sometimes seen in the genital area in men and around the knees and lower buttocks. One type of scabies causes scaling and crusts on the palms of the hands and soles of the feet. If you notice that a patient has a rash, notify the nurse immediately. As with head lice, you will be directed to wear a gown and gloves for further patient contact.

Treatment for Scabies

Special medicated creams and lotions are used to kill the mites. Some strains of scabies have become resistant to this treatment. If new lesions erupt after a patient has been properly treated, another product will be ordered. When treating for head lice or scabies, use the products exactly as directed. Products for treating lice and scabies are pesticides and repeated use can cause toxicity and other complications.

Clip the patient's nails before beginning. Work the medicated product into and around the fingernail area with a cotton swab. You may be directed to apply the lotion to the patient's entire body, not just the rash area. Avoid the eyelids or lips. Wear a gown and gloves when applying this treatment. The lotion remains on the patient's skin for 12 to 24 hours, then is washed off in the tub or shower. Reapply the lotion any time the patient's hands are washed. Another treatment may be required several days to several weeks later. The rash will disappear in about a month. The patient may experience itching even after the scabies is eliminated. You may be directed to check other patients for the appearance of a rash. Facility personnel may also be treated to prevent the spread of the mites.

The patient's room, clothing, and linens must also be cleaned. The room and furnishings should be vacuumed well to capture mites in the environment. Check the mattress and furniture for cracks, as the mites often crawl into foam padding. If items cannot be vacuumed,

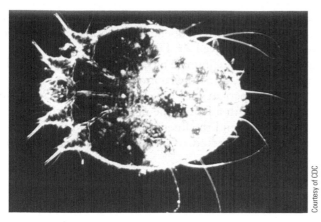

FIGURE 12-23A A microscopic view of the scabies mite, which cannot be seen with the unaided eye.

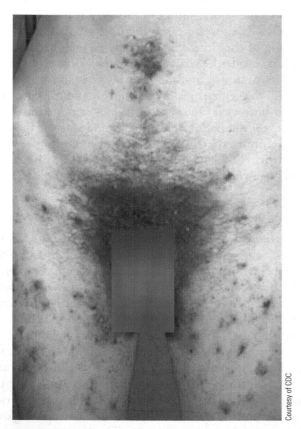

FIGURE 12-23B Scabies is commonly found at sites such as the wrist, elbow, armpit, between the fingers, nipple, penis, waist, belt line, and buttocks. Tiny blisters and scales may also be present. Scratching may cause skin sores that sometimes become infected.

they are contained in a sealed plastic bag for 14 days. The mites cannot live beyond this time without food. Some facilities expose the bags to extreme heat or cold to kill the mites more quickly. Contact precautions are used for 24 hours after the patient is treated. If the patient requires a second treatment, the cleaning procedure is repeated for clothing, linens, and furnishings.

Bedbugs

Most people think **bedbugs** (Figure 12-24) are imaginary pests from a nursery rhyme. In fact, bedbugs are real parasites that have been found throughout the world, with the exception of Antarctica. They have been found in hotels, movie theaters, hospitals, doctors' offices, and nursing homes in the United States. The bugs are usually seen at nigh and are stealthy and fast-moving. They can survive in hot and cold environments. Bedbugs bite, causing a painful rash-type area on the skin. Their saliva contains a chemical that prevents blood from clotting while they are eating. Some people are very sensitive or allergic to this substanc and have an allergic skin reaction. Others can live with bedbugs and not be aware of them. Some people develop welts or tiny itchy red bumps that look like flea or mosquito bites. The bumps often appear in lines, similar to scabies. Adult bedbugs can survive for up to a year without eating. Some are resistant to over-the-counter insecticides, and setting off pesticide bombs may cause them to scatter, even to other areas of the facility. Some exterminators have specially trained dogs to identify areas where bedbugs are hiding. They are quite sensitive to heat, so some exterminators successfully use this treatment instead of poisonous chemicals.

A bedbug is tiny, a little smaller than a sesame seed. They are flat, and clear or white in appearance before feeding. After eating a blood meal, they develop a

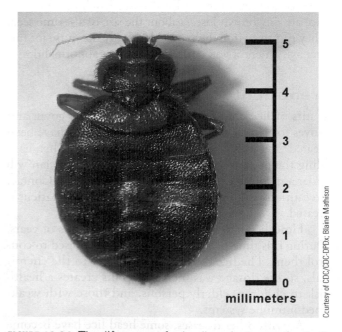

FIGURE 12-24 The life span of a bedbug is 4 months to 1 year. Bedbugs inject saliva into the host to temporarily numb the area and thin the blood. When the numbness wears off, the saliva acts as an irritant, causing severe itching and welts. The delay in the onset of itching gives the bedbug time to escape.

red-brown hue. They leave little excretions (droppings) on sheets and may give off a sickly sweet smell. Finding tiny bloodstains on linens from crushed bugs, or dark spots from the droppings, is a strong indication that bedbugs are present. They hide in the seams of clothing and furnishings, so the patient may have brought them from home and may not be aware of it.

Bedbugs can also live on bats, chickens, pigeons, other birds, laboratory animals, and some domestic pets. They run quickly and multiply quickly. They may hide in cracks and crevices in mattresses, on bed frames, behind headboards, inside nightstands, behind baseboards, and in window and door casings, pictures, and moldings. They have also been found hiding in furniture and clutter such as piles of books, papers, and boxes, and in items near sleeping areas. Shining a flashlight and aiming a hot hair dryer into crevices will help force the insects out.

If bedbugs are noted in a health care facility, a professional exterminator will be called to eliminate them. Everything in the room must be cleaned and washed. Items that cannot be washed should be sealed in plastic bags and exposed to very hot or freezing temperatures.

The eggs must also be found and eliminated, or more bugs will hatch. If you suspect that there are bedbugs in a patient's room, inform the nurse immediately.

OUTBREAK OF INFECTIOUS DISEASE IN A HEALTH CARE FACILITY

An outbreak of an infection in the facility can be serious. All patients, workers, volunteers, and visitors are at risk of exposure. Immediate steps must be taken to prevent the infection from spreading rapidly. Examples of common outbreaks include:

- Influenza
- Gastroenteritis, norovirus, diarrhea
- Hepatitis
- MRSA
- Scabies

Most of these are caused by viruses. Most facilities have an action plan for responding to an outbreak of infection. Nursing assistants will receive instructions from the nurse.

REVIEW

A. Matching

Match the terms in Column II with each definition in Column I.

Column I

1. _____ spiral-shaped bacterium
2. _____ organism that causes ringworm
3. _____ bacteria that grow in pairs
4. _____ organism that causes AIDS
5. _____ bacteria that grow as clusters
6. _____ colonies of bacteria and other microbes

Column II

a. staphylococci
b. protozoan
c. diplococci
d. streptococci
e. virus
f. fungus
g. spirillum
h. biofilms

B. Word Choice

Fill in the blanks for questions 7–11 with the correct word or phrase from the following list.

insects
method of transmission
portal of entry
portal of exit

reservoir
sexual contact
sneezing
susceptible host
water

7. Complete the chain of infection by naming the parts missing from the following figure.

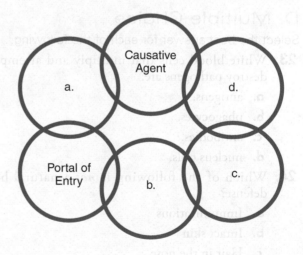

a. _____
b. _____
c. _____
d. _____

8. An example of transmission by direct contact is _____.

9. An example of transmission by indirect contact is _____.

10. A common vehicle for the transmission of microbes is _____.

11. Vectors, such as animals and _____, also transmit disease organisms.

C. True/False

Mark the following true or false by circling T or F.

12. T F   Normal body flora are the same in each part of the body.

13. T F   The fingernails are a common portal of exit for some infectious organisms.

14. T F   Biofilms are harmless substances.

15. T F   The general health of an individual is an important factor in determining if infectious disease will occur.

16. T F   Unbroken skin is a mechanical defense against infection.

17. T F   An abscess is an example of a generalized infection.

18. T F   Allergies are sensitivity reactions.

19. T F   The term *reservoir* may refer to a human body in which organisms live.

20. T F   Immunization causes the body to produce antibodies that protect the person against certain infectious diseases.

21. T F   MRSA infections are easy to control.

22. T F   Bandage scissors can act as fomites.

D. Multiple Choice

Select the best answer for each of the following.

23. White blood cells that multiply and attempt to destroy pathogens are:
    a. antigens.
    b. phagocytes.
    c. antibodies.
    d. nucleus cells.

24. Which of the following is *not* a natural body defense?
    a. Immunizations
    b. Intact skin
    c. Hair in the nose
    d. Tears

25. Biofilms:
    a. are helpful to the human body.
    b. are readily disinfected.
    c. contain many species of organisms.
    d. are not as strong as other organisms.

26. One patient's visitor is coughing and looks flushed. Your best action is to:
    a. ask the visitor to leave.
    b. put a mask on the visitor.
    c. put a mask on the patient.
    d. refer the matter to the nurse.

27. You woke up not feeling well this morning. You have an elevated temperature. Your best action is to:
    a. call in sick.
    b. go to work.
    c. stay home without notifying the facility.
    d. call a friend to go to work for you.

28. Infection with *Escherichia coli* O157:H7:
    a. is mildly uncomfortable.
    b. can cause renal failure and death.
    c. is caused by inhaling spores.
    d. is highly infectious to health care workers.

29. *Streptococcus A*:
    a. is spread only by the droplet method.
    b. is easily treated and eliminated with antibiotics.
    c. can cause gangrene, resulting in amputations.
    d. is a common cause of infectious diarrhea.

30. Spores:
    a. remain dormant until conditions are ideal for reproduction.
    b. can be eliminated by cleansing the environment with alcohol.
    c. are usually responsible for boils and skin abscesses.
    d. can be treated with antibiotics and increased fluids.

31. Head lice:
    a. can be treated and eliminated by antibiotics.
    b. can be passed from person to person on combs and brushes.
    c. are microscopic and cannot be seen with the eyes.
    d. require no special precautions beyond standard precautions.

32. Rotavirus and norovirus:
    a. die quickly after leaving the body.
    b. can be prevented by wearing a mask.
    c. are readily eliminated with alcohol-based hand cleaner.
    d. can remain on the hands for at least four hours.

33. Hantavirus is spread by:

   a. rodent excretions.

   b. indirect contact with fomites.

   c. direct contact with an infected person.

   d. inhalation of droplets from an infected patient.

34. Bioterrorism is:

   a. not a concern in the United States.

   b. the use of chemicals to cause illness.

   c. the use of biological agents for terrorist purposes.

   d. easily detected and treated.

35. Hepatitis B:

   a. is spread by oral–fecal transmission.

   b. can be readily cured with antibiotics.

   c. causes visible signs of serious illness.

   d. can be prevented by vaccination.

E. Nursing Assistant Challenge

36. Your patient, Mrs. Wallace, has a cold.

   a. What organism is responsible?

   _____

   b. Could Mrs. Wallace be immunized against this condition?

   _____

   c. How is the condition most likely transmitted?

   _____

37. Mr. Reynolds has a staphylococcal infection in his finger.

   a. What class of organisms are staphylococci?

   _____

   b. What shape are these organisms?

   _____

   c. How might Mr. Reynolds have acquired this infection?

   _____

38. Mrs. Steinbaum has a nonhealing wound. The nurse informs you that they suspect biofilms are keeping the wound from healing.

   a. Describe biofilms.

   _____

   _____

   b. Why are biofilms different than other types of pathogens?

   _____

   _____

   _____

39. Which of the following is true about biofilms?

   a. Biofilms are not very hard to identify.

   b. They are always visible when they grow.

   c. They usually remain in one area of the body.

   d. Biofilms are present only on the human body and food products.

   e. Biofilms have a sticky outer shell that helps protect them.

40. Which of the following is caused by a bacterium?

   a. Pediculosis

   b. HIV

   c. Scabies

   d. *Clostridium difficile*

REFERENCE

James, G. A., Swogger, E., Wolcott, R., et al. (2008). Biofilms in chronic wounds. *Wound Repair & Regeneration, 16*(1), 37–44.

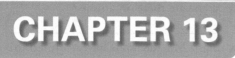

CHAPTER 13

Infection Control

OBJECTIVES

After completing this chapter, you will be able to:

13.1 Spell and define terms.

13.2 Explain the principles of medical asepsis.

13.3 State the purpose of standard precautions.

13.4 List the types of personal protective equipment.

13.5 State the purpose of each type of personal protective equipment.

13.6 Describe nursing assistant actions related to standard precautions.

13.7 Describe airborne, droplet, and contact precautions.

13.8 Demonstrate the following procedures:
- Procedure 1: Handwashing
- Procedure 2: Putting on a Mask
- Procedure 3: Putting on a Gown
- Procedure 4: Putting on Gloves

- Procedure 5: Removing Contaminated Gloves
- Procedure 6: Removing Contaminated Gloves, Eye Protection, Gown, and Mask
- Procedure 7: Serving a Meal in an Isolation Unit
- Procedure 8: Measuring Vital Signs in an Isolation Unit
- Procedure 9: Transferring Nondisposable Equipment Outside of the Isolation Unit
- Procedure 10: Specimen Collection from a Patient in an Isolation Unit (Expand Your Skills)
- Procedure 11: Caring for Linens in an Isolation Unit
- Procedure 12: Transporting a Patient to and from the Isolation Unit
- Procedure 13: Opening a Sterile Package

VOCABULARY

Learn the meaning and the correct spelling of the following words and phrases:

airborne infection isolation room (AIIR)
airborne precautions
airborne transmission
anteroom
asepsis
autoclave
biohazard
communicable disease
contact precautions
contact transmission
contagious disease
contaminated

dirty
disinfection
disposable
droplet precautions
droplet transmission
exposure incident
face shield
goggles
high-efficiency particulate air (HEPA) filter mask
isolation
isolation technique
isolation unit

medical asepsis
N95 respirator
National Institute of Occupational Safety and Health (NIOSH)
negative air pressure room
nosocomial infection
occupational exposure
personal protective equipment (PPE)
PFR95 respirator
other potentially infectious material (OPIM)

sharps
standard precautions
sterile
sterile field
sterilization
surgical mask
transmission-based precautions
ultraviolet germicidal irradiation (UVGI)
work practice controls

DISEASE PREVENTION

In the last chapter, you learned what infections are and some of their causes. In this chapter, you will be introduced to actions and procedures that can help prevent the transmission (spread) of infection to protect yourself, your co-workers, and those in your care.

GUIDELINES 13-1 Guidelines for Maintaining Medical Asepsis

To maintain medical asepsis, the nursing assistant should follow these guidelines:

- Wash hands thoroughly and at appropriate times. Protect the skin on the hands by using warm water, drying thoroughly, then applying lotion if needed.

- Treat breaks in the skin immediately by washing thoroughly, cleaning with an antiseptic, and covering. Report any breaks in the skin to your supervisor.

- Use gloves when required. Change gloves after handling excretions, body fluids, and contaminated items.

- Bathe or shower daily. Wear clean clothes each day. Keep your hair clean and away from your face and shoulders. Avoid artificial nails; keep fingernails short and clean. Do not wear rings, other than a plain wedding band.

- *Never* use one patient's personal items for another patient.

- Keep personal care items in the proper areas. The top drawer or shelf of the bedside stand is reserved for clean items, such as:

  - Toothbrush and toothpaste

  - Denture cup, if used

  - Comb and hairbrush

- Items such as a toothbrush, denture cup, wash basin, and emesis basin are considered clean. They should always be placed on a different shelf (or drawer) away from soiled items, such as a bedpan and a urinal.

- In the second drawer or on the shelf of the bedside stand, or in the bathroom, place clean items used for personal care:

  - Emesis basin

  - Wash basin

  - Soap and soap dish

- Store on the lower shelf:

  - Bedpan

  - Urinal for male patients

- Disinfect bathtubs and shower chairs after each use.

- Disinfect equipment that is used by more than one person, such as a stethoscope, before and after each use. Many facilities issue disposable supplies for each patient (Figures 13-1A and 13-1B), and then discard these items when the person is discharged. The patient may also elect to bring them home.

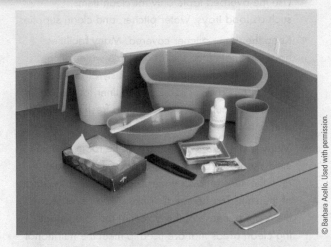

FIGURE 13-1A Most facilities issue disposable personal care items.

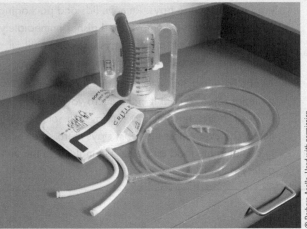

FIGURE 13-1B A disposable blood pressure cuff, oxygen cannula, and incentive spirometer. These items are sent home or discarded when the patient leaves.

- Note that the washbasin, bedpan, emesis basin, and other items used for ADLs are very inexpensive. Some facilities issue them so that patients use them once, then throw them away. Although it may seem wasteful, it is much less expensive than treating a nosocomial infection.

- Disinfect reusable personal care items such as bedpans, urinals, and commodes.

- If a clean item accidentally falls on the floor, replace it. Do not use it.

- Avoid spilling or splashing from bedpans and urinals. Cover when transporting.

- Avoid contaminating environmental surfaces by touching them while wearing used gloves.

(continues)

GUIDELINES 13-1 Guidelines for Maintaining Medical Asepsis (continued)

- Use the overbed table only for clean items, such as food trays, water pitcher, and clean supplies.

- Keep the water pitcher covered. Many facilities have eliminated the use of reusable water pitchers. Instead, they issue a covered styrofoam cup of ice water or a disposable plastic liner for the water pitcher. The cup is replaced with a fresh cup every shift and as needed when empty.

- Many facilities bring fresh ice to the room in a covered styrofoam cup. Some bring bottles of water to refill the cup. Leftover water is discarded at the end of the shift. The personal drinking cup never leaves the room because of the potential for contaminating clean areas that are used to meet the nutritional needs of everyone on the unit.

- Keep food and water supplies clean. Keep food covered when serving trays. Remove lids and packaging when serving trays. Remove used dishes immediately after use. Do not place used trays on a cart until all clean trays have been delivered to patients.

- At one time facilities would remove food from a patient's room, reheat it in the microwave, and return it. This practice has fallen out of favor in some facilities. Whatever enters the room stays there so as not to contaminate food and other clean items in the unit pantry and elsewhere.

- Do not allow patients to keep perishable food items such as puddings, eggs, milk, or mayonnaise from meal trays. Bacteria multiply rapidly in these foods when they are not refrigerated.

- Carry soiled equipment, supplies, and linens away from your uniform.

- Items that have touched the floor must be cleaned and/or disinfected before use. The floor is heavily contaminated. If you are in doubt about whether an item is clean, do not use it.

- Avoid raising dust, such as by shaking linens and other items. This scatters contaminated dust and lint. Gather or fold linens inward with the dirtiest area toward the center. Keep soiled linen hampers covered. Keep linens (even if soiled) off the floor.

- Keep clean and soiled items separated in hallways. For example, the soiled linen hamper and housekeeping cart must be separated from the clean linen cart and food cart by at least one room's width.

- Clean from least soiled areas toward those that are the most soiled.

- Keep work areas such as utility rooms clean. Return equipment to the proper storage area after use.

 Infection Control **ALERT**

Always work from the cleanest area to the least clean area. Avoid scrubbing back and forth. This way you will not move pathogens and soiled items into a clean area.

MEDICAL ASEPSIS

Asepsis is the absence of disease-producing microorganisms. Asepsis is achieved by using medical aseptic techniques and surgical aseptic techniques.

Medical asepsis may also be called *clean technique*. It reduces the numbers of microbes and interrupts transmission from one person, place, or object to another.

You will hear the terms *clean* and *dirty* applied to equipment and supplies used in the facility. For example, linen is *clean* when you remove it from the linen cart. After it is carried into the patient's room, it is considered *dirty*. If it is not used, the linen must still be washed before

being returned to the clean linen supply. This is because the linen has been exposed to the microbes in the patient's room. Keeping each patient's equipment and supplies separate from those used for other patients is an important part of medical asepsis. Articles that have contacted or have been exposed to potential pathogens are called **dirty** or **contaminated**. Articles that have been properly cleaned and disinfected are considered clean or uncontaminated.

Although we cannot eliminate all microorganisms from our bodies or the environment, we can reduce exposure by using medical aseptic technique:

- Handwashing or cleaning hands with an alcohol-based hand cleaner

- Using gloves when contact with blood, moist body fluids (except sweat), mucous membranes, or nonintact skin is likely

- Cleaning and/or disinfecting equipment

- Using disposable equipment whenever possible

- Storing items where they belong; not moving supplies or equipment from one room to the next

HANDWASHING

Handwashing is the single most important method of preventing the spread of infection. Handwashing is a short, vigorous rubbing together of all the surfaces of soap-lathered hands, followed by rinsing under warm running water. Warm water makes a good lather and is less damaging to the skin than hot water. Liquid soap is used because pathogens can grow in a wet soap dish and on the surface of bar soap.

Sinks in health care facilities vary in design. In most, you turn the water on by using faucets. The hands are soiled, so the faucets are a potential source of contamination to the next person who uses them. Because of this, holding a paper towel in your hand when turning the faucet on and off is a good idea. This way you will avoid picking up or depositing unwanted microorganisms. The water flow in some sinks is controlled by stepping on a foot pedal or pushing a knee lever to the right to turn the water on. Push the knee lever to the left to turn the water off.

Keep the fingertips pointed down when washing your hands. Avoid leaning against the sink or touching the inside of the sink with your hands.

The most important aspect of handwashing is the friction created by rubbing the hands together. This friction loosens and removes microbes from the hands, and water flushes them away and down the sink. Routine handwashing with soap, running water, and friction by all health care providers is the:

- Most significant control measure for the prevention of a **nosocomial infection** (infection acquired by a patient while being cared for in a health care facility). Nosocomial infections increase the cost of the stay and can be serious or life-threatening
- Single most important control measure to break the chain of infection

The recommended handwashing technique depends on the purpose of the handwashing. Hands can usually be washed effectively in a minimum of 20 seconds. More time will be needed, however, if hands are visibly soiled (refer to Procedure 1). Washing your hands for as long as possible is always best. You will continue to remove microbes the whole time. You are never microbe free.

Wash your hands (or use an alcohol-based hand cleaner):

- At the beginning of your shift
- After picking up any item from the floor
- Before handling food or beverages (Figure 13-2)
- After personal use of the bathroom
- After using a tissue
- After you cough or sneeze
- After handling a patient's belongings
- After touching any item or environmental surface that is soiled

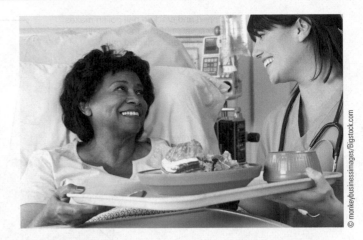

FIGURE 13-2 Wash your hands before serving meal trays and after stopping to assist a patient.

> Infection Control **ALERT**
>
> Using an alcohol-based hand cleaner is the *preferred method* of cleansing your hands if no visible soil is present. If hands are soiled, use soap and water.

- Before handling clean supplies
- Immediately before touching mucous membranes or nonintact skin; if you are already wearing gloves, change them
- Immediately after accidental contact with blood, moist body fluids, mucous membranes, or nonintact skin
- Before and after any contact with your mouth or mucous membranes, such as touching, eating, drinking, smoking, using lip balm, or manipulating contact lenses
- Before and after every patient contact
- Before applying and after removing gloves
- Whenever your hands are visibly soiled
- Anytime your gloves become torn
- At the end of your shift before going home

Most health care facilities do not permit caregivers to wear artificial fingernails of any type. Long nails (beyond the fingertips) are also not permitted. Long and artificial nails harbor bacteria and increase the risk of infection to both the patient and the worker. They are difficult to clean and may tear gloves. Rings with many stones and elaborate settings can also tear gloves. They hold harmful bacteria and are difficult to clean (Figure 13-3). Rings other than flat bands are better left at home when you are on duty.

> Infection Control **ALERT**
>
> Wear clear nail polish, if desired. Make sure it is freshly applied. Chipped polish allows microbes to hide.

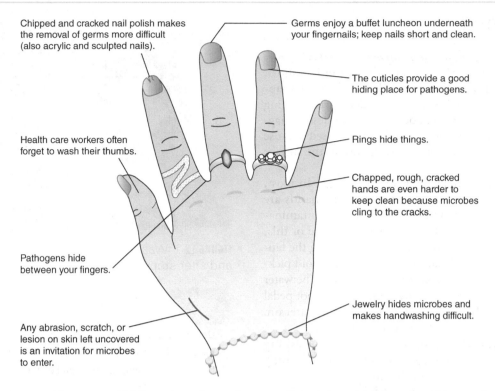

Chipped and cracked nail polish makes the removal of germs more difficult (also acrylic and sculpted nails).

Germs enjoy a buffet luncheon underneath your fingernails; keep nails short and clean.

The cuticles provide a good hiding place for pathogens.

Health care workers often forget to wash their thumbs.

Rings hide things.

Chapped, rough, cracked hands are even harder to keep clean because microbes cling to the cracks.

Pathogens hide between your fingers.

Jewelry hides microbes and makes handwashing difficult.

Any abrasion, scratch, or lesion on skin left uncovered is an invitation for microbes to enter.

FIGURE 13-3 Jewelry provides a good hiding place for pathogens. Practicing good handwashing and not wearing jewelry are the best methods of protecting both workers and patients.

  ### Infection Control **ALERT**

Recent studies show that hand disinfection using alcohol-based hand rubs (ABHRs) is more effective than soap-and-water handwashing *if* enough product is used to cover all hand surfaces and the rubbing is done for at least 20 to 30 seconds (until the hands are completely dry). Hand-rub products are also generally kinder to the skin.

Hand Lotion and Cream

Maintaining the integrity of the skin on your hands is very important to prevent injury and exposure to microbes. However, you must be careful when selecting and using hand care products. Lotions and creams from jars or squeeze bottles in which hands touch the dispenser opening become a source of contamination to everyone who uses them. Use a light, nonoily hand lotion. A personal-size bottle that you do not share is best. Avoid any product that comes in a jar. You may use bottles with pump dispensers and squeeze bottles, but avoid touching the dispensing spout.

PROCEDURE **HANDWASHING**

1. Check that there is an adequate supply of soap and paper towels. Be sure a waste container lined with a plastic bag is available near the sink.

2. Remove rings, if possible, or wash well underneath.

3. Remove watch, or push up over wrist.

4. Turn on the faucet. Use a paper towel to do so if this is your preference or facility policy.

5. Adjust water to a warm temperature. Once used, drop the paper towel in the waste container. Stand

back from the sink to avoid contact with your uniform. Wet your hands, keeping your fingertips pointed downward (Figure 13-4A).

6. Apply soap and lather over your hands and wrists, between fingers, and under rings. Use friction and interlace your fingers (Figure 13-4B). Work lather over every part of your hands and wrists. Clean your fingernails by rubbing them against the palm of the other hand to force soap under the nails (Figure 13-4C). Clean them with an orangewood stick or nail brush, if needed.

(continues)

PROCEDURE **1** CONTINUED

7. Rinse hands with your fingertips pointed down. Do not shake water from hands.

8. Dry hands thoroughly with a clean paper towel.

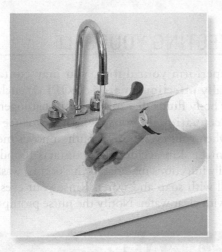

FIGURE 13-4A Wet your hands with your fingertips pointed down.

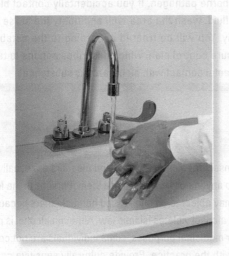

FIGURE 13-4B Interlace the fingers to clean between them.

9. Turn off the faucet with a clean, dry paper towel (Figure 13-4D); drop the towel in the waste container.

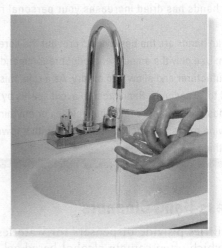

FIGURE 13-4C Clean under the nails by rubbing them against your palms.

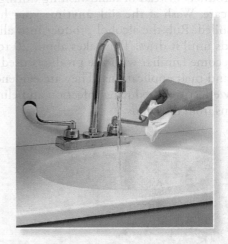

FIGURE 13-4D Turn the faucet off with a clean paper towel.

ICON KEY:
= OBRA

🔓 Safety **ALERT**

Alcohol-based hand sanitizer is very flammable. A small amount of alcohol will catch on fire when exposed to static electricity. Sliding a patient from a stretcher to a bed and sliding sheets on a plastic mattress can create enough static electricity to start a fire. Operating a light switch or other electrical appliance before the sanitizer on your hands has dried increases your personal risk of injury.

Clean hands are the best way to prevent the spread of infection. Use only the amount of product recommended by the manufacturer and allow it to air-dry. As a rule, this takes about 20 to 30 seconds. Remember to avoid sparks by making sure hands are dry before touching devices or anything metal. Do not wipe excess alcohol off your hands with a towel or your clothing.

Waterless Hand Cleaners

Many facilities provide dispensers for waterless hand cleaners, which often contain alcohol-based gel, lotion, or foam (Figure 13-5). Most also contain moisturizers that prevent drying of the skin. Follow facility policies for using the product. Most permit the use of alcohol-based products instead of handwashing during routine patient care. Wash at the sink anytime your hands are visibly soiled. Rub the alcohol product into all areas of the hands until it dries. This takes about 20 to 30 seconds. Become familiar with the products used by your facility and their applications. They are evidence-based and very effective in reducing infection and eliminating pathogens from the hands.

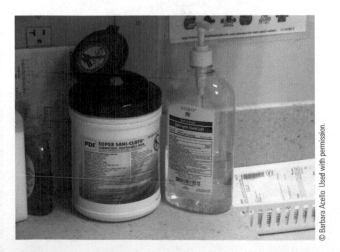

FIGURE 13-5 Alcohol-based hand sanitizer and disinfectant wipes may be placed in every room to be used for hand hygiene.

© Barbara Acello. Used with permission.

☣ Infection Control **ALERT**

Always wash your hands with soap and water if a patient has infectious diarrhea or another condition spread by spores. *Alcohol-based cleaners will not eliminate spores.* The mechanical action of soap, water, and friction used during handwashing will loosen and remove spores from your hands and wash them down the drain.

PROTECTING YOURSELF

As you perform your duties, you may contact **other potentially infectious material (OPIM)** such as blood or other body fluids that may contain pathogens. This is called **occupational exposure**. An **exposure incident** occurs when your eyes, nose, mouth, mucous membranes, or nonintact skin accidentally contacts blood or other potentially infectious material. If this occurs, wash exposed skin well with soap and water. Rinse your eyes, nose, or mouth with clear water. Notify the nurse promptly.

⚠ OSHA **ALERT**

Using proper medical asepsis and following standard precautions are the best ways to prevent infection with a bloodborne pathogen. If you accidentally contact blood or body fluid, wash the area well and notify the nurse immediately. You will be treated according to the established exposure control plan, which describes actions to take for accidental contact with biohazardous substances.

☣ Culture/Infection Control **ALERT**

Dispensers for alcohol-based hand cleaners are usually available to anyone who wants to use them. Persons of the Muslim faith may object to alcohol-based hand cleaners because the use of alcohol violates Islamic law. Although alcohol is permitted for medicinal purposes, some individuals are not comfortable with the practice. Provide culturally sensitive care and make sure that practicing Muslims have another, acceptable means of handwashing available to them. Triclosan was permitted at one time, but it is no longer recommended.

Standard Precautions

Standard precautions (Figure 13-6) are the infection control actions used for all people receiving care, regardless of their condition or diagnosis. All health care workers follow specific procedures, called **work practice controls**,

STANDARD PRECAUTIONS

Assume that every person is potentially infected or colonized with an organism that could be transmitted in the healthcare setting.

Hand Hygiene

Avoid unnecessary touching of surfaces in close proximity to the patient.

When hands are visibly dirty, contaminated with proteinaceous material, or visibly soiled with blood or body fluids, wash hands with soap and water.

If hands are not visibly soiled, or after removing visible material with soap and water, decontaminate hands with an alcohol-based hand rub. Alternatively, hands may be washed with an antimicrobial soap and water.

Perform hand hygiene:
    Before having direct contact with patients.
    After contact with blood, body fluids or excretions, mucous membranes, nonintact skin, or wound dressings.
    After contact with a patient's intact skin (e.g., when taking a pulse or blood pressure or lifting a patient).
    If hands will be moving from a contaminated-body site to a clean-body site during patient care.
    After contact with inanimate objects (including medical equipment) in the immediate vicinity of the patient.
    After removing gloves.

Personal protective equipment (PPE)

Wear PPE when the nature of the anticipated patient interaction indicates that contact with blood or body fluids may occur.

Before leaving the patient's room or cubicle, remove and discard PPE.

Gloves

Wear gloves when contact with blood or other potentially infectious materials, mucous membranes, nonintact skin, or potentially contaminated intact skin (e.g., of a patient incontinent of stool or urine) could occur.

Remove gloves after contact with a patient and/or the surrounding environment using proper technique to prevent hand contamination. Do not wear the same pair of gloves for the care of more than one patient.

Change gloves during patient care if the hands will move from a contaminated body-site (e.g., perineal area) to a clean body-site (e.g., face).

Gowns

Wear a gown to protect skin and prevent soiling or contamination of clothing during procedures and patient-care activities when contact with blood, body fluids, secretions, or excretions is anticipated.

Wear a gown for direct patient contact if the patient has uncontained secretions or excretions.

Remove gown and perform hand hygiene before leaving the patient's environment.

Mouth, nose, eye protection

Use PPE to protect the mucous membranes of the eyes, nose and mouth during procedures and patient-care activities that are likely to generate splashes or sprays of blood, body fluids, secretions and excretions.

During aerosol-generating procedures wear one of the following: a face shield that fully covers the front and sides of the face, a mask with attached shield, or a mask and goggles.

Respiratory Hygiene/Cough Etiquette

Educate healthcare personnel to contain respiratory secretions to prevent droplet and fomite transmission of respiratory pathogens, especially during seasonal outbreaks of viral respiratory tract infections.

Offer masks to coughing patients and other symptomatic persons (e.g., persons who accompany ill patients) upon entry into the facility.

Patient-care equipment and instruments/devices

Wear PPE (e.g., gloves, gown), according to the level of anticipated contamination, when handling patient-care equipment and instruments/devices that are visibly soiled or may have been in contact with blood or body fluids.

Care of the environment

Include multi-use electronic equipment in policies and procedures for preventing contamination and for cleaning and disinfection, especially those items that are used by patients, those used during delivery of patient care, and mobile devices that are moved in and out of patient rooms frequently (e.g., daily).

Textiles and laundry

Handle used textiles and fabrics with minimum agitation to avoid contamination of air, surfaces and persons.

FIGURE 13-6 Standard precautions.

to prevent the spread of infection. Standard precautions apply to situations in which care providers may contact:

- Blood, body fluids (except sweat), secretions, and excretions
- Mucous membranes
- Nonintact skin
  Some examples of secretions and excretions are:
- Respiratory mucus (phlegm)
- Sputum
- Cerebrospinal fluid
- Urine
- Feces
- Vaginal secretions
- Semen
- Vomitus

Standard precautions stress handwashing and the use of **personal protective equipment (PPE)**: gloves, gown, mask, and goggles or face shield.

TRANSMISSION-BASED PRECAUTIONS

Standard precautions do not eliminate the need for other isolation precautions. The goal is to interrupt the mode of transmission, which prevents the pathogen from spreading. A second set of precautions, called **transmission-based precautions**, is used with certain highly transmissible infections. *Standard precautions are always used in addition to transmission-based precautions.*

GUIDELINES 13-2 Guidelines for Personal Protective Equipment (PPE)

Keep in mind that PPE protects both workers and patients. You can transmit a pathogen to a patient just as easily as a patient can transmit a pathogen to you. You are responsible for knowing and applying standard precautions to protect yourself, patients, visitors, and others.

Type of PPE	Purpose
Gloves	Protect hands. Change gloves as often as necessary. Avoid environmental contamination with your used gloves. Wash hands before applying and after removing gloves.
Gown or apron	Covers skin and clothing. Must be resistant to fluid penetration. Protects worker from picking up pathogens. Protects patients from pathogens on workers' clothing.
Mask	Protects nose and mouth.
Respirator	Protects the respiratory tract/covers nose and mouth from tiny airborne pathogens.
Goggles	Protect eyes. Should fit snugly. If you wear glasses, remove them to wear goggles. If this is not possible, you may be able to use a face shield with wrap around sides. There are too many other variables to address in this book. See your doctor to discuss solutions.
Face shield	Protects face, eyes, nose, and mouth. Should cover forehead, extend below chin, and wrap around side of face. Wear a mask with the face shield. Many face shields fit comfortably over glasses, making removal of glasses unnecessary.
Cap (optional except in surgery)	Prevents hair from falling into sterile field. Protects head from splashes.
Shoe covers (optional)	Protect shoes from splashing and messes on floor.

GUIDELINES 13-3 Guidelines for Standard Precautions

1. Wash hands in the situations listed in the "Handwashing" section.

2. Wear gloves for any contact with blood, body fluids, mucous membranes, or nonintact skin, such as when:
   – Hands are cut, scratched, chapped, or have a rash.
   – Cleaning up body fluid spills.
   – Cleaning potentially contaminated equipment.

3. Wear gloves that fit properly. Gloves that are too large or small will not protect you.

4. Change gloves:
   – After contacting each patient.
   – Before touching noncontaminated articles or environmental surfaces.
   – Between tasks with the same patient if there is contact with open areas, mucous membranes, or infectious materials. If in doubt, apply fresh PPE.
   – Anytime your gloves become soiled for any reason.

5. Dispose gloves according to facility policy.

6. Wear a waterproof gown for procedures that are likely to produce splashes of blood or other body fluids.
   – Remove a soiled gown as soon as possible and dispose of it properly.
   – Make sure the gown covers your clothing and exposed skin.
   – Make sure the gown is tied or fastened properly.
   – Wash your hands.

7. Wear a mask and protective eyewear or face shield for procedures that are likely to produce splashes of blood or other moist body fluids. The surgical mask covers both the nose and the mouth. The mask is used once and discarded. Apply a new mask for each patient receiving care. If the mask becomes damp, change it. Masks lose their effectiveness when moist.

8. Goggles or a face shield help protect the mucous membranes of the eyes from splashes or sprays of blood and other body fluids. Wear a surgical mask with goggles or a face shield to protect the nose and mouth.

9. You should:
   – Know where to obtain PPE in your work area.
   – Be familiar with the principles of standard precautions and select the correct PPE for the task.
   – Remove the PPE before leaving the work area, whether the patient's room, an isolation unit, or the utility room.
   – Restock the supply closet. Make sure to replace items you have used. Never leave the stock of clean supplies empty.
   – Place used PPE in the proper container for laundering, decontamination, or disposal.

GUIDELINES 13-4 Guidelines for Environmental Procedures

1. Handle all patient care items so that infectious organisms will not be transferred to skin, mucous membranes, clothing, or the environment. Clean and decontaminate reusable equipment so it is ready to be used for another patient. Discard single-use items according to facility policy.

2. Follow facility procedures for routine care and cleaning of environmental surfaces, such as beds, bedside equipment, and other frequently touched surfaces.

3. Dispose **sharps**—needles, razors, and other sharp items—in a puncture-resistant, leakproof container near the point of use (Figure 13-7). The container should be labeled with the **biohazard** symbol (Figure 13-8) and color-coded red. Biohazardous waste disposal units contain items contaminated with blood or body fluids. Special precautions are taken to discard these waste containers.

4. Do not recap or handle used needles before disposal.

5. Mouthpieces or resuscitator bags should be available to eliminate the need for mouth-to-mouth resuscitation. Remember that you must be trained and qualified to use them.

(continues)

GUIDELINES 13-4 Guidelines for Environmental Procedures (continued)

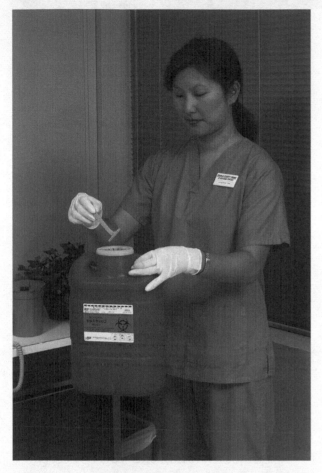

FIGURE 13-7 Carefully discard sharps in a safety container specifically designated for this use.

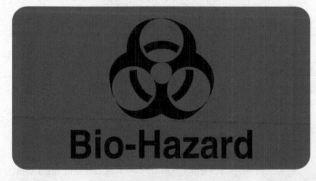

FIGURE 13-8 Containers for contaminated items are identified with the biohazard label. The symbol is black with a red or orange background.

6. Discard waste and soiled linen in plastic bags and handle the bags according to facility policy. Separate containers are used to discard regular waste and biohazardous waste. Containers for biohazardous

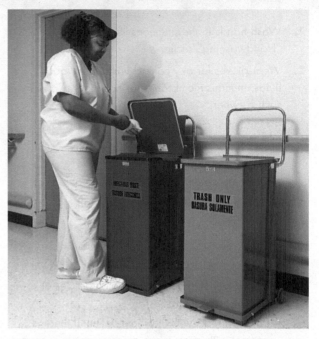

FIGURE 13-9 Discard all potentially infectious materials in the proper container. The container should be labeled if the contents contain biohazardous material. The lid must fit tightly with nothing overflowing or sticking out.

waste must be labeled with the biohazard symbol or be color-coded in red (Figure 13-9).

7. Wipe up blood spills immediately and disinfect the floor or other surface.
   - Use disposable gloves.
   - Do not touch your face or adjust PPE with used gloves.
   - For small spills, use bleach solution or facility-approved disinfectant.
   - For larger spills, use a commercial blood cleanup kit. Begin by sprinkling absorbent powder on the blood to absorb the spill. Use the scoop in the kit to pick up the solid substance. Discard the material and scoop in a biohazard bag (Figure 13-10).
   - Wipe with disinfectant and disposable cleaning cloths.
   - Discard gloves and cleaning cloths in a biohazardous waste container.

8. Dispose body fluids and contaminated articles according to facility policy.

(continues)

GUIDELINES 13-4 Guidelines for Environmental Procedures (continued)

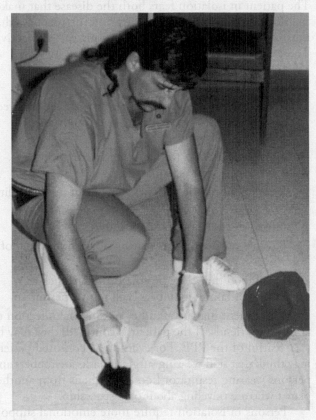

FIGURE 13-10 Clean blood spills immediately and then disinfect, using a 1:10 bleach solution (or 1:100, according to CDC guidelines and facility policy). Your facility may also have other disinfectants that are used for certain purposes. For larger spills, a blood spill kit can be used. The powder in the kit solidifies the blood so it can easily be scooped into a plastic biohazard bag.

9. Avoid eating, drinking, chewing gum, smoking, applying cosmetics or lip balm, or handling contact lenses in work areas where there may be exposure to infectious material.

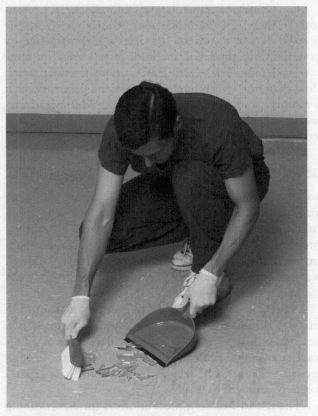

FIGURE 13-11 Wear gloves when cleaning up broken glass. Always use a broom and dustpan. Do not pick up the glass with the fingers. Discard the broken glass in a sharps container or other designated receptacle.

10. Store food and beverages in separate refrigerators and storage areas from laboratory specimens, chemicals and nonedible items, and other potentially contaminated items.

11. Use a brush and dustpan, tongs, or forceps to pick up broken glass (Figure 13-11). Discard according to facility policy.

 Infection Control **ALERT**

Items that have contacted blood or body fluids are biohazardous waste. Dispose these items in leakproof, tightly closed containers. Biohazardous waste is stored in special areas until it is removed for trash disposal and requires special handling during removal. This type of handling is very expensive, and storage space is often limited, so do not place nonbiohazardous materials, wrappers, or packages in the biohazard disposal containers.

Diseases may be transferred from one person to another either directly or indirectly. Such diseases are called **communicable** or **contagious diseases**. Some diseases are transmitted more easily than others. Specific precautions must be used to control their spread.

Communicable diseases may be spread:

• Through upper respiratory secretions by **airborne transmission** and **droplet transmission**

• By **contact transmission** (direct contact or indirect contact) with feces or other body secretions and excretions

- Through draining wounds or infective material such as blood on needles

Each mode of transmission requires special precautions to interrupt the movement of microbes from the infected person to others. If a disease is transmitted by more than one mode, all methods of transmission must be considered when selecting precautions for the patient. More than one type of precaution may be necessary, such as airborne and contact precautions for widespread herpes zoster (shingles). Table 13-1 lists transmission-based precautions and common diseases in each category.

Isolation

Isolation means being separated or set apart. The purpose of isolation is to separate the patient who has a communicable or contagious disease, to help prevent the spread of the infectious pathogens. The infectious organism need not be systemic. An organism that is localized to a wound, the bladder, or another area of the body can also be highly infectious.

A private room is used for persons in isolation precautions whenever possible. In some situations, two patients with the same disease may share a room. (This practice is called *cohorting*.) In rooms with more than one patient, the CDC recommends a three-foot separation between beds.

The use of isolation precautions is time-consuming and requires extra effort by all care providers, especially nursing assistants. The fear of infection also makes working with these precautions more stressful. Patients in isolation and their families and other visitors also feel stress.

Clinical Information **ALERT**

Who are you protecting? Breaking one link in the chain of infection prevents the infection from spreading. This is a great responsibility.

TABLE 13-1 Transmission-Based Precautions for Common Diseases

Transmission-Based Precautions Category	Disease or Condition
Airborne	Tuberculosis, measles
Airborne and contact	Chickenpox, widespread shingles
Droplet	German measles, mumps, influenza
Contact	Head or body lice, scabies, impetigo, infected pressure ulcer with heavy drainage

Psychological Aspects of Isolation

The patient in isolation fears both the disease that makes the isolation precautions necessary and the practices that must be followed for these precautions to be effective. These include:

- PPE worn by all who enter the isolation unit, including visitors
- Teaching visitors how to prevent the spread of infection, proper disposal of trash, and importance of good handwashing
- Special procedures for handling waste, specimens, food, linens, and personal effects of the patient
- Restrictions on the patient's movement in the facility
- Procedures to be followed when the patient is moved outside of the isolation unit
- Possible restrictions on visiting hours or number of visitors
- Likelihood that close personal contact, such as kissing of family members, will not be permitted

The patient may be afraid of passing the infection to family and friends. If the patient is confused, they may be very fearful of the PPE. For example, a confused patient may think that staff wearing surgical masks are robbers and persons wearing respirator hoods are aliens from another planet who are traveling about on a spaceship.

Persons in isolation require more emotional support and care. The extra time required to follow the isolation precautions could easily reduce the time available for providing emotional attention at a time when it is most needed. Be aware of your patients' needs and plan your work so you can spend the necessary time with each patient in isolation.

Transmission-Based Isolation Precautions

Standard precautions are used with all patients regardless of their condition. When patients are known to have or are suspected of having an infectious disease, *in addition to* standard precautions, isolation precautions are used to interrupt the mode of transmission. Guidelines from the Centers for Disease Control and Prevention (CDC) recommend three types of transmission-based precautions:

- Airborne precautions
- Droplet precautions
- Contact precautions

Airborne Precautions

Airborne precautions are used for diseases transmitted by tiny pathogens that are suspended on mucus or on tiny dust particles in the air. They can travel a long distance from the source by natural air currents and through ventilation systems. Tuberculosis is a disease that requires airborne precautions. Figure 13-12 shows the required precautions.

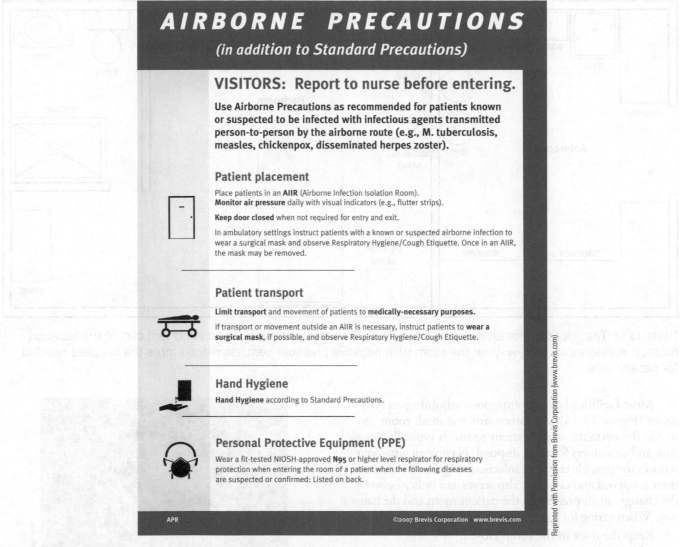

AIRBORNE PRECAUTIONS

(in addition to Standard Precautions)

VISITORS: Report to nurse before entering.

Use Airborne Precautions as recommended for patients known or suspected to be infected with infectious agents transmitted person-to-person by the airborne route (e.g., M. tuberculosis, measles, chickenpox, disseminated herpes zoster).

Patient placement

Place patients in an **AIIR** (Airborne Infection Isolation Room). **Monitor air pressure** daily with visual indicators (e.g., flutter strips).

Keep door closed when not required for entry and exit.

In ambulatory settings instruct patients with a known or suspected airborne infection to wear a surgical mask and observe Respiratory Hygiene/Cough Etiquette. Once in an AIIR, the mask may be removed.

Patient transport

Limit transport and movement of patients to **medically-necessary purposes.**

If transport or movement outside an AIIR is necessary, instruct patients to **wear a surgical mask**, if possible, and observe Respiratory Hygiene/Cough Etiquette.

Hand Hygiene

Hand Hygiene according to Standard Precautions.

Personal Protective Equipment (PPE)

Wear a fit-tested NIOSH-approved **N95** or higher level respirator for respiratory protection when entering the room of a patient when the following diseases are suspected or confirmed: Listed on back.

APR ©2007 Brevis Corporation www.brevis.com

Reprinted with Permission from Brevis Corporation (www.brevis.com)

FIGURE 13-12 Airborne precautions.

The patient must be in a private room with special air handling. Hospitals use many different methods of handling the air to reduce the risk that pathogens will escape into the ventilation system. A **negative air pressure room** is commonly used. Your facility may call this an **airborne infection isolation room (AIIR)** because of the type of air handling used. This means that air is drawn into the room and leaves the room through a special exhaust system to the outside. Air from the isolation room does not circulate directly into the facility.

Some isolation rooms have special **ultraviolet germicidal irradiation (UVGI)** lights in the room, in the air ducts, or suspended from the ceiling in the room and anteroom. In some facilities, these lights are in the hallway outside the room. UVGI uses ultraviolet-C light in the room air or air duct. It is not used for lighting the room. Rather, these lights are a secondary measure to kill or inactivate pathogens in the upper portion of the room or passing through the air duct. When the air is irradiated, droplets containing pathogens are inactivated so that they no longer pose a risk of infection. The lights are not on all the time, and their use is regularly monitored to ensure that the radiation is not a threat to the patient or health care workers.

Some facilities use portable ultraviolet lights to disinfect rooms after patients have been discharged (Figure 13-13). Some use handheld UVGI for disinfecting small surfaces such as computer tablets and keyboards.

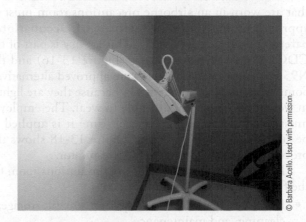

© Barbara Acello. Used with permission.

FIGURE 13-13 Portable UV light for cleaning the room.

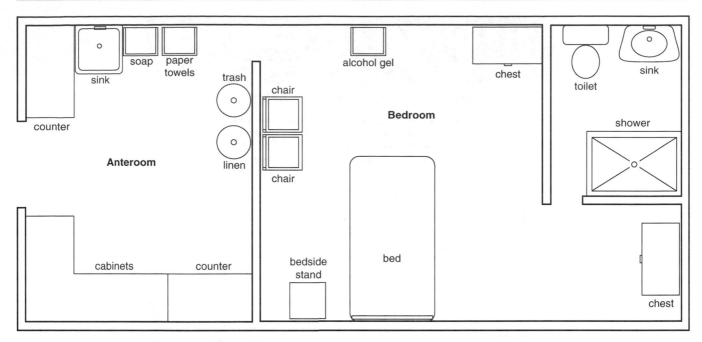

FIGURE 13-14 The floor plan for an isolation room. Note the anteroom, which is an important part of the isolation room. It serves as an entryway for the room with negative-pressure ventilation and stores the supplies needed for patient care.

Most facilities have an anteroom adjoining an AIIR room (Figure 13-14). An **anteroom** is a small room just inside the entrance to the patient room. It typically has a sink and containers for trash disposal. Having an anteroom reduces the possible escape of infectious organisms when the door is opened and closed. It also serves as a buffer between the changes in air pressure in the patient room and the hallway. When caring for a patient in airborne precautions:

- Keep the door to the room closed.
- Wear a **high-efficiency particulate air (HEPA) filter mask** or other specially filtered mask (Figure 13-15) for which you have been fitted by a professional.

The filter mask may be disposable or reusable. Men with facial hair cannot wear a filter face mask because the hair prevents an airtight seal. In this case, a special filter hood can be worn. The filter mask is the only mask that can be used in an airborne isolation room. Masks that are worn in an airborne precautions room must be approved by the **National Institute of Occupational Safety and Health (NIOSH)**. This agency is part of the CDC. The **PFR95 respirator** (Figure 13-16) and the **N95 respirator** (Figure 13-17) are approved alternatives. Some workers prefer these masks because they are lighter in weight and more comfortable to wear. The employee must self-test the respirator each time it is applied to be sure there are no air leaks. Figure 13-18 shows the procedure for self-testing the N95 respirator.

Before working in an airborne precautions room for the first time, employees must:

- Receive education about respirator use, fit, storage, cleaning, and maintenance.

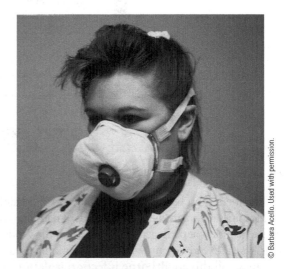

FIGURE 13-15 The HEPA respirator filter is individually fitted to the worker. The respirator is reusable. Store it according to facility policy.

- Have a medical examination to ensure that working in the mask will not harm the worker's personal health.
- Be fitted for the mask by a qualified professional.
  - The fit test involves performing several different activities while wearing a respirator, then demonstrating application and removal several times.
  - The respirator fits correctly if the user cannot detect the taste or smell of a test solution. Saccharin is usually used for this test.
  - After the professional fit test, workers must wear only the type and size mask approved by the fit tester.

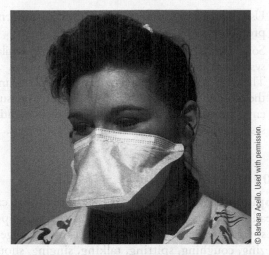

FIGURE 13-16 The PFR95 respirator filter is a NIOSH-approved respirator that is preferred by many health care workers because it is lightweight and comfortable.

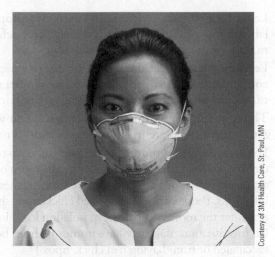

FIGURE 13-17 The N95 respirator is disposable. Some facilities store it for one shift, and then discard it. Be sure that both straps fit tightly and check the face for air leaks after applying.

Donning instructions (to be followed each time product is worn):

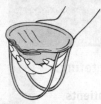

1 Cup the respirator in your hand with the nosepiece at fingertips, allowing the headbands to hang freely below hands.

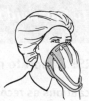

2 Position the respirator under your chin with the nosepiece up.

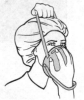

3 Pull the top strap over your head so it rests high on the back of head.

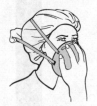

4 Pull the bottom strap over your head and position it around neck below ears.

5 Using two hands, mold the nosepiece to the shape of your nose by pushing inward while moving fingertips down both sides of the nosepiece. Pinching the nosepiece using one hand may result in less effective respirator performance.

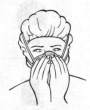

6 FACE FIT CHECK
The respirator seal should be checked before each use. To check fit, place both hands completely over the respirator and exhale. If air leaks around your nose, adjust the nosepiece as described in step 5. If air leaks at respirator edges, adjust the straps back along the sides of your head. Recheck.

NOTE: If you cannot achieve proper fit, do not enter the isolation or treatment area. See your supervisor.

Removal instructions:

1 Cup the respirator in your hand to maintain position on face. Pull bottom strap over head.

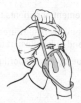

2 Still holding respirator in position, pull top strap over head.

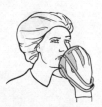

3 Remove respirator from face and discard or store according to your facility's policy.

FIGURE 13-18 Fit test the mask each time it is worn.

- Learn how to pack and store the mask in a properly labeled container that prevents damage and deformation of the face piece and exhalation valve.
- Learn how to protect the respirator from damage, contamination, dust, sunlight, extreme temperatures, excessive moisture, and damaging chemicals.

The following are points to remember when working with patients who are in airborne precautions rooms:

- People who are not immune to measles (rubeola) or chickenpox (varicella) should not enter the room of a patient known or suspected to have either of these infections. People who have not had chickenpox should not enter the room of a patient in isolation for shingles. (In this situation, staff may have immunity from being vaccinated or from having had chickenpox.)
- The patient should leave the room only when medically necessary. Apply a surgical mask to the patient's face before transport

- Use standard precautions in addition to airborne precautions.
- Some facilities do not have the special room ventilation systems required for airborne precautions rooms. These facilities use portable units that are placed in the room to filter the air, creating a negative pressure environment. They are slightly noisier than a ventilation system but are effective in eliminating pathogens.

Droplet Precautions

Droplet precautions are used for diseases that can be spread by means of large droplets in the air. A person can spread droplets containing infectious pathogens by sneezing, coughing, spitting, talking, singing, shouting, or laughing. Influenza is an example of a disease spread by droplets. Figure 13-19 shows the requirements for droplet precautions.

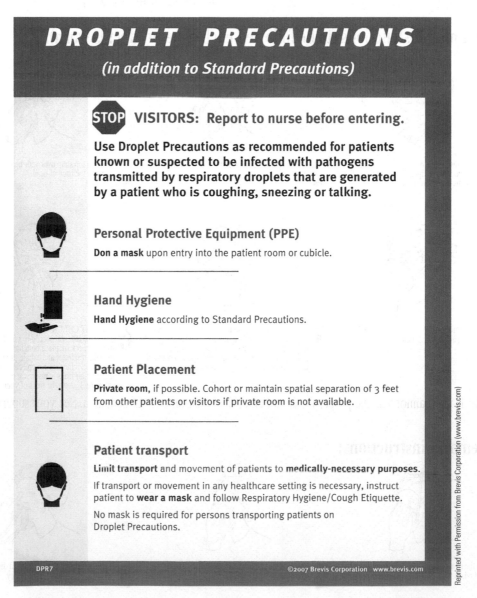

DROPLET PRECAUTIONS
(in addition to Standard Precautions)

STOP **VISITORS:** **Report to nurse before entering.**

Use Droplet Precautions as recommended for patients known or suspected to be infected with pathogens transmitted by respiratory droplets that are generated by a patient who is coughing, sneezing or talking.

Personal Protective Equipment (PPE)

Don a mask upon entry into the patient room or cubicle.

Hand Hygiene

Hand Hygiene according to Standard Precautions.

Patient Placement

Private room, if possible. Cohort or maintain spatial separation of 3 feet from other patients or visitors if private room is not available.

Patient transport

Limit transport and movement of patients to **medically-necessary purposes**.

If transport or movement in any healthcare setting is necessary, instruct patient to **wear a mask** and follow Respiratory Hygiene/Cough Etiquette.

No mask is required for persons transporting patients on Droplet Precautions.

DPR7   ©2007 Brevis Corporation   www.brevis.com

FIGURE 13-19 Droplet precautions.

When a patient's condition requires droplet precautions:

- Apply a mask when you enter the room.
- The patient should leave the room only when medically necessary. They should wear a mask when out of the room.
- Use standard precautions in addition to droplet precautions.

Contact Precautions

Contact precautions are used when an infectious pathogen is spread by direct or indirect contact. *Direct contact* occurs when the caregiver touches a contaminated area on the patient's skin or blood or body fluids containing the infectious pathogen. *Indirect contact* occurs when the caregiver touches items contaminated with the infectious material, such as the patient's environment, personal belongings, equipment or supplies, contaminated linens, and so on. Examples of infections requiring contact precautions are scabies, infected pressure injuries, and gastroenteritis. Figure 13-20 shows the requirements for contact precautions.

- The patient should be in a private room. If this is not possible, then patients with the same type of infection can be placed in the same room. The door can be open.
- Wear a gown and gloves for all patient contact and contact with potentially contaminated areas in the patient's environment. Apply PPE upon room entry and discard before exiting.
- Change gloves if you contact contaminated matter in the room. After care is completed, remove gloves and wash hands. Use a paper towel to open the door to leave the room and discard the towel in the trash container inside the room.

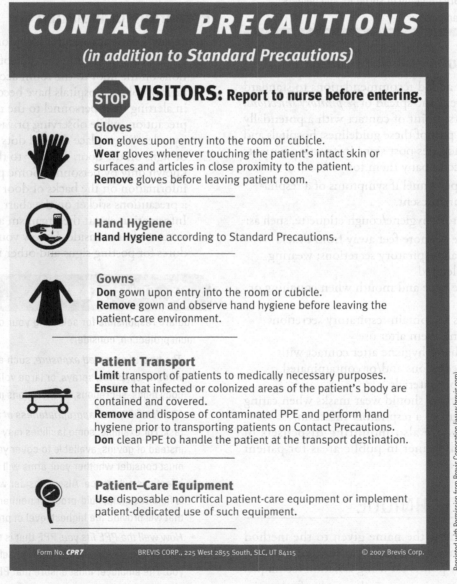

CONTACT PRECAUTIONS

(in addition to Standard Precautions)

STOP **VISITORS: Report to nurse before entering.**

Gloves
Don gloves upon entry into the room or cubicle.
Wear gloves whenever touching the patient's intact skin or surfaces and articles in close proximity to the patient.
Remove gloves before leaving patient room.

Hand Hygiene
Hand Hygiene according to Standard Precautions.

Gowns
Don gown upon entry into the room or cubicle.
Remove gown and observe hand hygiene before leaving the patient-care environment.

Patient Transport
Limit transport of patients to medically necessary purposes.
Ensure that infected or colonized areas of the patient's body are contained and covered.
Remove and dispose of contaminated PPE and perform hand hygiene prior to transporting patients on Contact Precautions.
Don clean PPE to handle the patient at the transport destination.

Patient–Care Equipment
Use disposable noncritical patient-care equipment or implement patient-dedicated use of such equipment.

Form No. *CPR7*   BREVIS CORP., 225 West 2855 South, SLC, UT 84115   © 2007 Brevis Corp.

FIGURE 13-20 Contact precautions.

- Transport the patient from the room only when medically necessary. Avoid contamination of environmental surfaces, other patients, and health care personnel. Cover or contain infected secretions. Remove your PPE before leaving the room.
- Use disposable equipment and supplies whenever possible. Noncritical, nondisposable equipment such as a stethoscope should be left in the isolation room. If equipment must be shared, clean and disinfect it between uses with different patients.
- Apply the principles of standard precautions in addition to contact precautions.

 OSHA ALERT

When wearing gloves:

- Avoid touching your face with contaminated gloves.
- Avoid unnecessary touching of surfaces and objects with contaminated gloves.

New Precautions and Screening

In 2003, the CDC added recommendations to standard precautions to prevent the spread of *respiratory infections*, beginning at the first point of contact with a potentially infected person. As part of these guidelines, hospitals and other health care facilities post signs instructing patients and persons who accompany them to:

- Notify facility personnel if symptoms of a respiratory infection are present.
- Practice respiratory hygiene/cough etiquette, such as:
  - Staying three or more feet away from others
  - Containing all respiratory secretions; wearing a mask, if tolerated
  - Covering the nose and mouth when coughing or sneezing
  - Using tissues to contain respiratory secretions and discarding them after use
  - Performing hand hygiene after contact with respiratory secretions and/or contaminated objects and/or materials

Health care workers should wear masks when caring for patients with signs of a respiratory infection.

Many facilities are also mounting dispensers of alcohol-based hand cleaner in public areas for patient and visitor use.

ISOLATION TECHNIQUE

Isolation technique is the name given to the method of caring for patients with easily transmitted diseases. Remember these key points for using isolation technique:

- Isolation technique interrupts the mode of transmission for disease.

- The nursing assistant must have a solid working knowledge of infection control to select the correct PPE and use proper isolation technique to prevent the spread of infection to self and others.
- All items that come into contact with the patient's excretions, secretions, blood, body fluids, mucous membranes, or nonintact skin are considered contaminated and should be discarded with the biohazardous waste.
- Apply the principles of standard precautions in addition to transmission-based precautions.

Isolation Unit

The **isolation unit** may be an area or a private room. A room with handwashing facilities and an adjoining room with bathing and toilet facilities is best. A private room is indicated.

Preparing for Isolation

To prepare a patient room for isolation, do the following:

1. Place a card indicating the type of isolation precautions on the door to the room according to your facility policy. Hospitals have become very creative in alerting their personnel to the need for special precautions while observing privacy and confidentiality rules. Some place colored dots on the door frame or signs on the door. The key to the color code is known only by personnel. Some place patient care information on the backs of door signs. Others place a precautions sticker on the chart cover or care plan. Information about the organism and special precautions are found inside. Follow your facility's procedures for posting signs and other information.

 OSHA ALERT

You are responsible for selecting your own PPE. For maximum protection, consider:

- *The type of expected exposure,* such as touch, or whether splashes, sprays, or large volumes of blood or body fluids, secretions, or excretions may be present.
- *The durability and appropriateness of the PPE* for the task. For example, some facilities may make aprons, instead of gowns, available to cover your clothing. You must consider whether your arms will be exposed to an infectious substance. Also, consider whether the fabric is fluid-resistant, fluid-proof, or neither. Select the item that will provide the highest level of protection.
- *How well the PPE fits you.* PPE that is too small or large will not provide optimal protection. Select items that fit you. The employer must ensure that PPE is available in sizes that will fit the workers.

2. Place an isolation cart outside the room, next to the door or in the location designated by your facility. Stock it with PPE as needed:
   - Gowns
   - Masks
   - Gloves
   - Goggles or face shields
   - Plastic bags marked for biohazardous waste
   - Plastic bags for soiled linen

3. Plastic trash bags. Line the wastepaper basket inside the room with a plastic bag labeled or color-coded for infectious waste.

4. Place a laundry hamper in the room and line it with a labeled or color-coded biohazard laundry bag.

5. Check the supply of paper towels and soap at the sink. Soap should be in a wall dispenser or foot-operated dispenser.

PERSONAL PROTECTIVE EQUIPMENT

PPE includes gloves, gown, mask, and goggles or face shield. The following sections describe the correct use of this equipment (see Procedures 2 through 6).

Cover Gown

A gown made of a moisture-resistant material is used when soiling or splashing with blood, body fluids, secretions, or excretions is likely (Figure 13-21). The gown prevents contamination of the uniform. Discard gowns in the patient's room after use. Never wear your PPE into the hallway.

> ⚠ OSHA **ALERT**
>
> PPE will protect you only if it fits properly, is free from defects, and is used regularly in the way you were taught. Never use equipment that is torn or defective. PPE is also worn during cleaning procedures when contact with blood, body fluids, secretions, or excretions is likely. PPE is discarded, laundered, or decontaminated after a single use. Be sure to replace what you have used so it is immediately available the next time it is needed.

> ⚠ OSHA **ALERT**
>
> Never wash your gloved hands. Handwashing damages the gloves, so they will not protect you. Remove gloves, wash your hands, and then put on a clean pair of gloves.

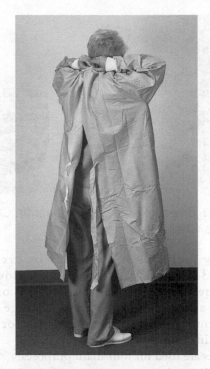

FIGURE 13-21 Apply a gown to protect the uniform if expecting contact with blood or body fluids.

Gloves

The use of gloves prevents the spread of disease. Gloves are worn for most health care procedures and are always worn when contact with blood, body fluids (except sweat), secretions, excretions, mucous membranes, or nonintact skin is expected. You should also wear gloves if you have cuts or open sores on your hands. Avoid touching your face or exposed skin when wearing gloves. Apply gloves prior to routine cleaning procedures. In this case, utility gloves may be worn (Figure 13-22). The use of gloves does not replace the need for handwashing. Always wash your hands before and after glove use. If you accidentally touch a potentially contaminated environmental surface after removing your gloves, wash your hands again.

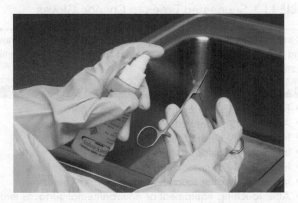

FIGURE 13-22 Wear utility gloves for routine cleaning duties.

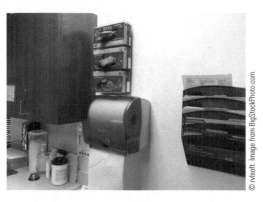

FIGURE 13-23 Select gloves with the best fit. Change the gloves when soiled.

Many facilities keep gloves in every room (Figure 13-23). However, do not wear gloves unless they are needed for standard precautions or wearing gloves is a facility requirement. Change gloves if they become soiled, become damaged, or are used for handling contaminated items.

Gloves are used for four main purposes:

- To avoid picking up a pathogen from a patient
- To avoid giving a patient a pathogen that is on your hands
- To avoid picking up a pathogen from a patient or the environment and carrying it to another patient on the hands
- To avoid picking up a pathogen on your gloves and depositing it anywhere that another person can pick it up on their hands or body and transfer it to the mouth, mucous membranes, or other surface where it can be transferred inside the body

To be effective, gloves must be intact and have no visible cuts, tears, or cracks. They must fit your hands well. Gloves come in different sizes. Select the size that most comfortably fits your hand. If the glove is too large or too small, a measure of protection is lost. Table 13-2 lists times when gloves should be changed. Remember to wash your hands every time you remove gloves. If you

TABLE 13-2 Suggested Times to Change Gloves

Remember to wash your hands before applying and after removing gloves. Never touch environmental surfaces with a contaminated (used) glove.

Change gloves:

- Before giving any patient care
- After giving patient care
- Immediately before touching mucous membranes
- Immediately before touching nonintact skin
- Immediately after touching secretions or excretions
- Immediately after touching blood or body fluids
- After touching equipment or environmental surfaces that are potentially contaminated
- Anytime your gloves are torn
- If your gloves become potentially visibly soiled

used alcohol sanitizer, make sure your hands are dry before reapplying gloves. Table 13-3 lists common nursing assistant tasks and the correct PPE to use for each job.

Gloves are for single patient use only. Wear them to care for one patient, and then discard. Avoid contaminating environmental surfaces with your gloves. Using the "one-glove technique" (Figure 13-24) reduces the risk of environmental contamination. Carry the contaminated item in a gloved hand. Remove the other glove. Use the ungloved hand to open doors, turn on faucets, and touch other environmental surfaces and supplies.

Health care facilities have many different policies regarding how and where gloves are discarded. Some facilities require the staff to discard gloves in sealed or covered containers instead of open wastebaskets (Figure 13-25). Tie the top of the trash bag and remove it when you leave the room. Place a fresh trash bag in the can. Know and follow your facility's policy.

Face Mask

Wear a **surgical mask** that covers the nose and mouth when exposure to droplet secretions may occur (Figure 13-26). For example, a mask would be worn when caring for a patient with influenza who is coughing and releasing droplets into the environment. It is also used whenever protective eyewear is worn. When a surgical mask is needed, it is:

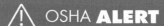

⚠ OSHA **ALERT**

Becoming familiar with the principles of standard precautions is one of the most important things you will learn. You need not fear contracting an infection if you apply precautions correctly. There are many variables in patient care situations, so there are no absolute guidelines for the use of PPE. Think about the situation and use good judgment. You are responsible for applying the principles of standard precautions and selecting the PPE according to the task to be done.

⚠ OSHA **ALERT**

Some health care facilities require staff to wear gloves for all contact with the patients or their bed linens, even if the contact is brief. If this is your facility's policy, wash your hands (or cleanse them with an alcohol-based product) and apply gloves immediately upon entering the room. Change gloves before and after exposure to blood, body fluid, secretions, excretions, mucous membranes, and nonintact skin. Remove gloves as soon as you have finished touching the patient or potentially contaminated items. Avoid touching clean items and environmental surfaces with used gloves.

TABLE 13-3 Personal Protective Equipment in Common Nursing Assistant Tasks

Nursing Assistant Task	Gloves	Gown	Goggles/Face Shield	Surgical Mask
Washing/rinsing utensils used for a bloody procedure in the soiled utility room	Yes	Yes, if splashing or uniform contamination is likely	Yes, if splashing is likely	Yes, if splashing is likely
Holding pressure on a bleeding wound	Yes	Yes	Yes	Yes
Wiping the shower chair with disinfectant	Yes	No	No	No
Emptying a catheter bag	Yes	No	No	No
Passing meal trays	No	No	No	No
Passing ice	No	No	No	No
Giving a backrub to a patient with a rash	Yes	No	No	No
Giving special mouth care to an unconscious patient	Yes	Yes, if facility policy	Yes, if facility policy	Yes, if facility policy
Assisting with a dental procedure	Yes	Yes	Yes	Yes
Changing the bed after an incontinent patient has an episode of diarrhea	Yes	Yes	No	No
Taking an oral temperature with a glass thermometer (gloves are not necessary with an electronic thermometer unless this is your facility policy)	Yes	No	No	No
Taking a rectal temperature	Yes	No	No	No
Taking an axillary temperature	No	No	No	No
Taking a blood pressure	No	No	No	No
Assisting an alert patient to brush teeth	Yes	No	No	No
Washing a patient's eyes	Yes	No	No	No
Giving perineal care	Yes	No	No	No
Washing the patient's chest and abdomen when the skin is not broken	No	No	No	No
Washing the patient's arms when skin tears are present	Yes	No	No	No
Brushing a patient's dentures	Yes	No	No	No
Assisting the nurse while they suction an unconscious patient who has a tracheostomy	Yes	Yes	Yes	Yes
Turning an incontinent patient who weighs 85 pounds	Yes, if linen is soiled	No, unless your uniform will have substantial contact with wet or soiled linen	No	No
Shaving a patient with a disposable razor	Yes, because this is a high-risk procedure	No	No	No
Shaving a patient with an electric razor	No	No	No	No
Cleaning the soiled utility room at the end of your shift	Yes	No	No	No

Note: Use this chart as a general guideline only. Add protective equipment if special circumstances exist. Know and follow your facility policies for using personal protective equipment.

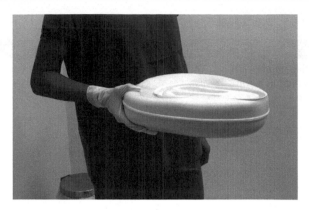

FIGURE 13-24 The one-glove technique is used to carry contaminated items. Use the ungloved hand for touching items in the room.

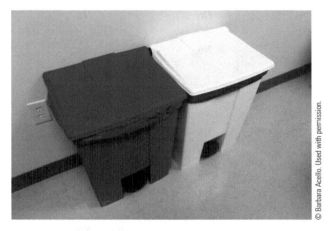

FIGURE 13-25 For safety, discard used gloves and contaminated supplies in covered containers.

- Used only once and discarded
- Changed if it becomes moist
- Handled only by the ties
- Never left hanging around the neck, because it can contaminate the uniform and the environment

> ⚠ OSHA **ALERT**
>
> A nursing assistant may wear a mask without eye protection. They may not wear eye protection without a mask.

Protective Eyewear

A full **face shield** (Figure 13-27A), or **goggles** (Figure 13-27B), are worn any time splashing of blood, body fluids, secretions, or excretions may occur. The eyewear does not protect the mucous membranes of the nose and mouth, so a mask is always worn along with eyewear. A good rule to follow is that a surgical mask may be worn without protective eyewear, but protective eyewear is never worn without a mask. Apply the mask first, followed by the protective eyewear. Some one-piece disposable masks have a protective eye shield attached to them (Figure 13-27C). Extra-large face shields are also available in some facilities. These may be worn without a mask only if the design is such that there is no risk of exposure from a splash or spray of fluid at the sides or bottom of the mask. Wearing a mask with all types of eye protection offers the highest level of defense. When removing the mask and eyewear, wash your hands, remove the eyewear, and then remove the mask.

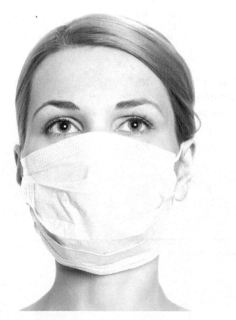

FIGURE 13-26 Wear a mask whenever it is needed to protect the nose and mouth from inhaling droplets or body fluids.

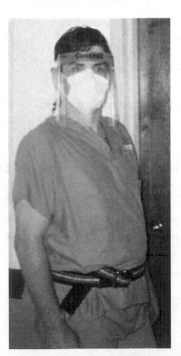

FIGURE 13-27A A surgical mask is always worn under a face shield.

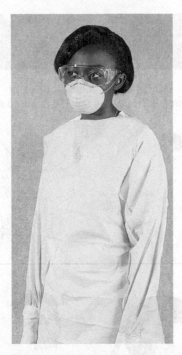

FIGURE 13-27B Always protect the nose and mouth with a mask when wearing goggles.

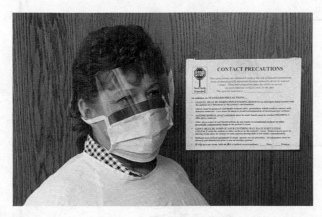

FIGURE 13-27C Some masks may have an attached face shield.

Sequence for Applying Personal Protective Equipment

1. Wash hands
2. Gown
3. Mask
4. Goggles or face shield
5. Gloves

Sequence for Removing Personal Protective Equipment

1. Gloves
2. Wash hands
3. Goggles or face shield
4. Gown
5. Mask
6. Wash hands

Figure 13-28 shows CDC recommendations for application and removal of PPE. Once applied, certain parts of the PPE are considered clean, and other areas contaminated. Clean areas are those that will be touched when you remove the apparel. Note that the CDC recommends removing PPE at the doorway to the patient room, or in the anteroom, if there is one. If a respirator is worn, remove it after leaving the patient's room and closing the door. Always wash your hands well or use alcohol-based hand cleaner immediately after removing PPE.

Equipment

Disposable (used once and discarded) patient care equipment is used by many facilities. It is ideal for patients on isolation precautions. Frequently used permanent equipment remains in the patient's unit. Most articles will not require special handling unless they are contaminated (or likely to be contaminated) with infective material.

SEQUENCE FOR PUTTING ON PERSONAL PROTECTIVE EQUIPMENT (PPE)

The type of PPE used will vary based on the level of precautions required, such as standard and contact, droplet, or airborne infection isolation precautions. The procedure for putting on and removing PPE should be tailored to the specific type of PPE.

1. GOWN

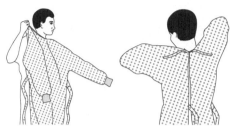

- Fully cover torso from neck to knees, arms to end of wrists, and wrap around the back.
- Fasten in back of neck and waist.

2. MASK OR RESPIRATOR

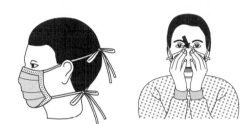

- Secure ties or elastic bands at middle of head and neck.
- Fit flexible band to nose bridge.
- Fit snug to face and below chin.
- Fit-check respirator.

3. GOGGLES OR FACE SHIELD

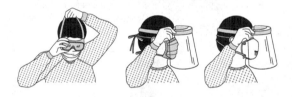

- Place over face and eyes and adjust to fit.

4. GLOVES

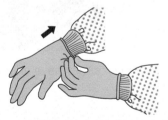

- Extend to cover wrist of isolation gown.

USE SAFE WORK PRACTICES TO PROTECT YOURSELF AND LIMIT THE SPREAD OF CONTAMINATION

- Keep hands away from face.
- Limit surfaces touched.
- Change gloves when torn or heavily contaminated.
- Perform hand hygiene.

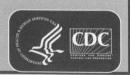

CS250672-E

FIGURE 13-28A Sequence for applying and removing personal protective equipment.

HOW TO SAFELY REMOVE PERSONAL PROTECTIVE EQUIPMENT (PPE) EXAMPLE 1

There are a variety of ways to safely remove PPE without contaminating your clothing, skin, or mucous membranes with potentially infectious materials. Here is one example. **Remove all PPE before exiting the patient room** except a respirator, if worn. Remove the respirator **after** leaving the patient room and closing the door. Remove PPE in the following sequence:

1. GLOVES

- Outside of gloves are contaminated!
- If your hands get contaminated during glove removal, immediately wash your hands or use an alcohol-based hand sanitizer.
- Using a gloved hand, grasp the palm area of the other gloved hand and peel off fitst glove.
- Hold removed glove in gloved hand.
- Slide fingers of ungloved hand under remaining glove at wrist and peel off second glove over first glove.
- Discard gloves in a waste container.

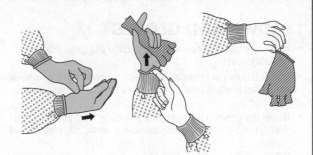

2. GOGGLES OR FACE SHIELD

- Outside of goggles or face shield are contaminated!
- If your hands get contaminated during goggle or face shield removal, immediately wash your hands or use an alcohol-based hand sanitizer.
- Remove goggles or face shield from the back by lifting head band or ear pieces.
- If the item is reusable, place in designated receptacle for reprocessing. Otherwise, discard in a waste container.

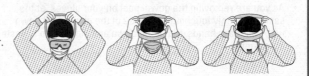

3. GOWN

- Gown front and sleeves are contaminated!
- If your hands get contaminated during gown removal, immediately wash your hands or use an alcohol-based hand sanitizer.
- Unfasten gown ties, taking care that sleeves don't contact your body when reaching for ties.
- Pull gown away from neck and shoulders, touching inside of gown only.
- Turn gown inside out.
- Fold or roll into a bundle and discard in a waste container.

4. MASK OR RESPIRATOR

- Front of mask/respirator is contaminated—DO NOT TOUCH!
- If your hands get contaminated during mask/respirator removal, immediately wash your hands or use an alcohol-based hand sanitizer.
- Grasp bottom ties or elastics of the mask/respirator, then the ones at the top, and remove without touching the front.
- Discard in a waste container.

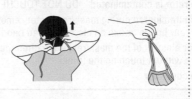

5. WASH HANDS OR USE AN ALCOHOL-BASED HAND SANITIZER IMMEDIATELY AFTER REMOVING ALL PPE

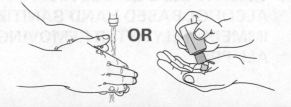

OR

PERFORM HAND HYGIENE BETWEEN STEPS IF HANDS BECOME CONTAMINATED AND IMMEDIATELY AFTER REMOVING ALL PPE

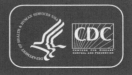

CS250672-E

FIGURE 13-28B *(continued)*

HOW TO SAFELY REMOVE PERSONAL PROTECTIVE EQUIPMENT (PPE) EXAMPLE 2

Here is another way to safely remove PPE without contaminating your clothing, skin, or mucous membranes with potentially infectious materials. **Remove all PPE before exiting the patient room** except a respirator, if worn. Remove the respirator **after** leaving the patient room and closing the door. Remove PPE in the following sequence:

1. GOWN AND GLOVES

- Gown front and sleeves and the outside of gloves are contaminated!
- If your hands get contaminated during gown or glove removal, immediately wash your hands or use an alcohol-based hand sanitizer.
- Grasp the gown in the front and pull away from your body so that the ties break, touching outside of gown only with gloved hands.
- While removing the gown, fold or roll the gown inside out into a bundle.
- As you are removing the gown, peel off your gloves at the same time, only touching the inside of the gloves and gown with your bare hands. Place the gown and gloves into a waste container.

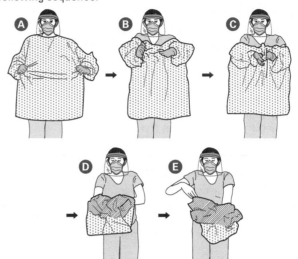

2. GOGGLES OR FACE SHIELD

- Outside of goggles or face shield are contaminated!
- If your hands get contaminated during goggle or face shield removal, immediately wash your hands or use an alcohol-based hand sanitizer.
- Remove goggles or face shield from the back by lifting head band and without touching the front of the goggles or face shield.
- If the item is reusable, place in designated receptacle for reprocessing. Otherwise, discard in a waste container.

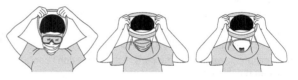

3. MASK OR RESPIRATOR

- Front of mask/respirator is contaminated—DO NOT TOUCH!
- If your hands get contaminated during mask/respirator removal, immediately wash your hands or use an alcohol-based hand sanitizer.
- Grasp bottom ties or elastics of the mask/respirator, then the ones at the top, and remove without touching the front.
- Discard in a waste container.

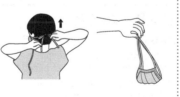

4. WASH HANDS OR USE AN ALCOHOL-BASED HAND SANITIZER IMMEDIATELY AFTER REMOVING ALL PPE

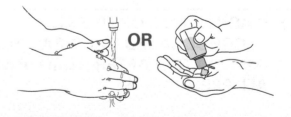

PERFORM HAND HYGIENE BETWEEN STEPS IF HANDS BECOME CONTAMINATED AND IMMEDIATELY AFTER REMOVING ALL PPE

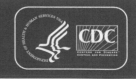

CS250672-E

FIGURE 13.28C (*continued*)

Containment of Contaminated Articles

Appropriately handle contaminated items to be taken out of the patient's room to avoid the spread of pathogens. Bag, label, and properly discard contaminated equipment. Place used articles in an impenetrable bag, such as plastic, before they are removed from the patient's room or unit. A single bag may be used if it is waterproof and sturdy enough to contain the article without contaminating the outside of the bag.

Soiled linen is a source of pathogens. Handle it with care. (Refer to Procedure 11.) Some facilities place contaminated linen in water-soluble bags that melt in the washer. If these bags touch wet linen before they are in the washer, they will begin to melt. Place them inside a regular plastic bag during transport to the laundry to prevent the bag from melting and the contents from contaminating surrounding items.

PROCEDURE 2 PUTTING ON A MASK

1. Assemble equipment:
   – Mask
2. Tie top strings of mask first, then bottom strings, or loop elastic over ears.
3. Adjust mask over nose and mouth by fitting the flexible bridge to the nose.

4. Adjust mask so it fits snugly around the face and chin.
5. Replace mask if it becomes moist during procedures.
6. Do not reuse a mask and do not let the mask hang around your neck.

PROCEDURE 3 PUTTING ON A GOWN

To be effective, a gown should have long sleeves, be long enough to cover the uniform, and be big enough to overlap in the back. Gowns should be waterproof.

1. Assemble equipment:
   – Clean gown
   – Paper towel
2. Remove wristwatch; place it on a paper towel.
3. Wash hands.
4. Put on the gown outside the patient's room. Put on gown by slipping your arms into the sleeves (Figure 13-29A).
5. Slip the fingers of both hands under the inside neckband and grasp the ties in back. Secure the neckband (Figure 13-29B).

6. Reach behind and overlap the edges of the gown. Secure the waist ties.
7. Take your watch into the isolation unit, leaving it on the paper towel.
   Remember, when using gowns:
   – A disposable gown is worn only once and then is discarded as infectious waste.
   – A reusable cloth gown is worn only once and then is handled as contaminated linen.
   – Carry out all procedures in the unit at one time.

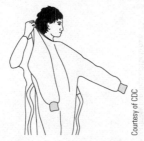

FIGURE 13-29A Select a gown that is the correct size. Unfold the gown, slip the arms in, and pull the gown up to the shoulders.

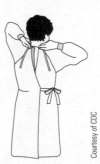

FIGURE 13-29B Slip the hands inside, under the neckband, and adjust to fit. Tie the neck ties. Then reach behind, overlapping the edges of the gown so that the uniform is completely covered, and tie the waist ties.

ICON KEY:

 = OBRA   = PPE

- Handle linen as little as possible.
- Fold the dirtiest side inward.
- Do not shake.
- Do not place soiled linen on the floor or tabletop.
- Bag linen before leaving the room.
- Keep soiled linen separate from general linen.
- Transport soiled, wet linen in a leakproof container or bag.

Transporting the Patient in Isolation

Sometimes a patient in isolation must be transported to another area of the facility for treatment or testing. Notify the receiving unit of your intention to transport the patient and describe the type of transmission-based precautions being used. If the patient is on airborne or droplet precautions, assist them to apply a surgical mask before leaving the isolation room. (Respirator filter and HEPA masks are not used on patients.) If the patient is on contact precautions, cover the infectious area of the skin before the patient leaves the room. You must wear PPE when picking up and returning the patient to the isolation room, but not during transport. (Refer to Procedure 12.)

You may remove your PPE after you have finished all tasks in the patient's room. Follow the instructions in Procedures 5 and 6. Table 13-4 summarizes some rules for nursing assistants in the practice of infection control.

PROCEDURE **4 PUTTING ON GLOVES**

1. Assemble equipment:
   - Disposable gloves in correct size
2. Wash your hands.
3. If a gown is required, put gloves on after applying the gown.
4. Pick up a glove by the cuff and place it on the other hand.
5. Repeat with a glove for the opposite hand (Figure 13-30).
6. Interlace fingers to adjust the gloves on your hands.
7. If wearing a gown, pull cuffs of gloves up over the gown sleeves.

8. Remember, when using gloves:
   - Wash hands before and after using gloves.
   - Remove gloves if they tear or become heavily soiled. Wash hands and put on a new pair.
   - Wear gloves whenever there is the possibility of contacting body fluids, blood, secretions, excretions, mucous membranes, or nonintact skin.
   - Change gloves between patients and wash hands.
   - Discard gloves immediately after removing them. Put them in a biohazardous waste container.
   - Avoid touching your face, exposed skin, or environmental surfaces with used gloves.

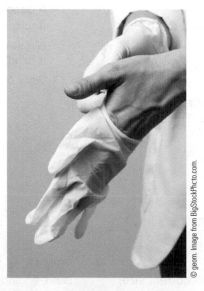

FIGURE 13-30 Put a glove on the opposite hand.

ICON KEY:

 = OBRA   = PPE

TABLE 13-4 Rules of Infection Control

Do
• Observe standard precautions and use barrier equipment (PPE) anytime contact with blood, body fluids, secretions, excretions, mucous membranes, or nonintact skin is likely. Contact may be with a patient or an environmental surface.
• Clean up dishes immediately after use.
• Damp-dust daily and be conscientious about cleaning while you carry out a task.
• Provide a bag for the disposal of used tissues.
• Turn the face to one side so that the assistant and the patient are not breathing directly on each other.
• Cover your nose and mouth when coughing or sneezing.
• Protect the skin on your hands by using warm water for washing, drying thoroughly, and applying lotion if needed.
• Treat breaks in the skin immediately by washing thoroughly, cleaning with an antiseptic, and covering. Report any breaks in the skin to the nurse.
• Disinfect equipment that is used by more than one staff member or patient, such as a stethoscope, before and after each use.
• Gather or fold used linen inward, with the dirtiest area toward the center.
• Clean reusable equipment immediately after use.
• Handle and dispose soiled material according to facility policy.
• Practice good personal hygiene.
• Wash your hands frequently.
• Keep clean and dirty items separate in patient rooms and storage areas.
• Bring only needed items into the patient's room.
• Keep soiled linen and trash covered in closed containers.
• Perform procedures in the manner in which you were taught.
• Empty wastebaskets frequently, if this is your responsibility.

Do Not
• Shake bed linens, because any microbes present could be released into the air.
• Allow dirty linen to touch your uniform.
• Eat or share food from a patient's tray.
• Borrow personal care items from another patient or employee, or use such items for another patient.
• Permit the contents of bedpans or urinals to splash when being emptied.
• Report for duty if you have an infectious disease.
• Permit linen to touch the floor, which is always considered dirty.
• Carry clean linen against your uniform or bring more linen than necessary into the patient's room.
• Store lab specimens in the refrigerator with food.

⚠ OSHA **ALERT**

To remove PPE safely, you must be able to identify what parts are clean and what are contaminated.

These areas are contaminated:

• The outside front and sleeves of the gown

• The outside front of the goggles, mask, respirator, and face shield

• The outside of the gloves

• Any area with visible blood, body fluids, or soiling

Touch only clean areas when removing PPE. These areas are clean:

• Inside the gloves

• The inside and back of the gown, including the ties

• The ties, elastic, or earpieces of the mask, goggles, and face shield

PROCEDURE **5** **REMOVING CONTAMINATED GLOVES**

1. Grasp the cuff of one glove on the outside with the fingers of the other hand (Figure 13-31A).

2. Pull the cuff of the glove down, drawing it over the glove (Figure 13-31B). Pull that glove off your hand.

   OR

   Grasp the palm of one gloved hand at the palm (Figure 13-32A). Pull the glove off (Figure 13-32B).

3. Hold the glove with the still-gloved hand.

4. Insert the fingers of the ungloved hand under the cuff of the glove on the other hand (Figure 13-32C).

5. Pull the glove off inside out, drawing it over the first glove.

6. Drop both gloves together into the biohazardous waste container (Figure 13-32D).

7. Wash your hands. Dry with a paper towel and discard the towel in the proper container. Use a dry towel to turn off the water faucet. Discard the towel.

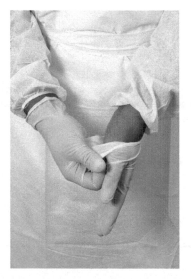

FIGURE 13-31A Grasp the outside cuff, and turn the glove inside out.

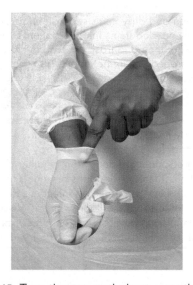

FIGURE 13-31B Turn the second glove over the first glove.

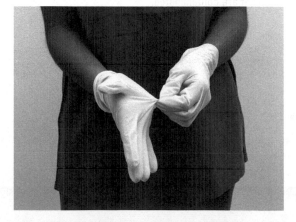

FIGURE 13-32A With the fingers of one glove, grasp the cuff or palm of the glove on the other hand.

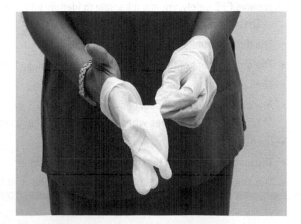

FIGURE 13-32B Pull the cuff of the glove down over the hand and fingers and remove it.

(continues)

PROCEDURE 5 CONTINUED 0

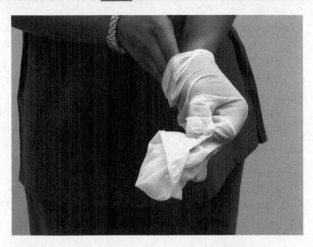

FIGURE 13-32C Hold the glove just removed in the gloved hand. Insert fingers of the ungloved hand inside the cuff of the other glove.

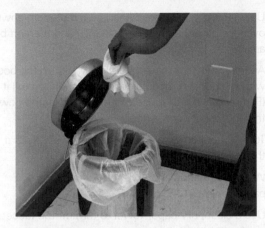

FIGURE 13-32D Pull the glove down over the hand and then pull both gloves off, holding the inside (clean side of glove). Discard the gloves in the proper container.

ICON KEY:
(0) = OBRA

PROCEDURE 6 REMOVING CONTAMINATED GLOVES, EYE (0) (P) PROTECTION, GOWN, AND MASK

1. Assemble equipment:
   – Biohazardous waste container for disposable items
   – Waste container for gown if it is not disposable
   – Paper towels

2. Undo waist ties of gown, if they are in the front. Follow Procedure 5 for removing contaminated gloves.

3. Grasp the earpieces or head strap of goggles or face shield and lift the eye protection outward, away from the face and up (Figure 13-33A). Discard or reprocess according to facility policy.

4. Undo waist ties of gown, if they are in the back (Figure 13-33B).

5. Undo the neck ties and loosen gown at shoulders.

6. Slip the fingers of your dominant hand inside the cuff of the other hand without touching the outside of the gown (Figure 13-33C).

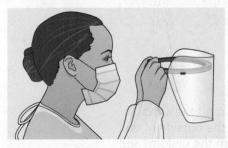

FIGURE 13-33A With ungloved hands, grasp the clean elastic strap or earpiece and lift the eye protection away from the face.

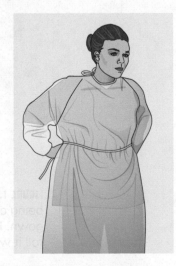

FIGURE 13-33B Untie the waist ties. *(continues)*

7. Using the gown-covered hand, pull the gown down over the other hand (Figure 13-33D) and then off both arms.

8. As the gown is removed, fold it away from the body with the contaminated side inward and then roll it up (Figure 13-33E). Dispose of the contaminated gown in the appropriate container.

9. Turn faucets on with a clean paper towel. Discard the towel.

10. Wash your hands and dry them with a clean paper towel.

11. Use a clean, dry paper towel to turn off the faucet.

12. If you brought a watch into the area (see Procedure 3), remove the watch from the paper towel. Hold the clean side of the paper towel and dispose of the towel in a wastepaper container.

13. Use a paper towel to grasp the door handle as you leave the patient's room. Discard the paper towel in an appropriate container before you leave the unit.

14. Remove mask:
    - Undo the bottom ties first and then the top ties.
    - Holding the top ties, dispose of mask in appropriate waste container.

15. Wash your hands.

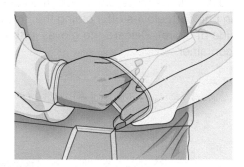

FIGURE 13-33C Slip the fingers of one hand inside the cuff of the other hand. Pull the gown down over the hand. Do not touch the outside of the gown with either hand.

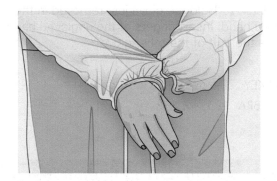

FIGURE 13-33D Using the gown-covered hand, pull the gown down over the other hand.

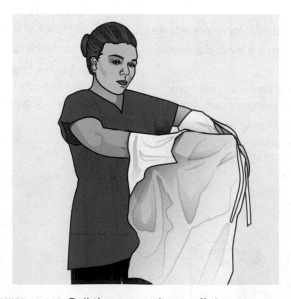

FIGURE 13-33E Pull the gown down off the arms, being careful to avoid touching the outside of the gown. Hold the gown away from the uniform and roll it with the contaminated side in.

ICON KEY:
O = OBRA **P** = PPE

Serving Meals to Persons in Isolation

At one time everyone in isolation was served meals using disposable dishes and utensils. Research and evidence-based practice have proven that using standard precautions, detergents, and hot water in the dishwasher is sufficient to eliminate microbes on dishes and utensils. Some facilities use disposables and isolation techniques for a variety of reasons. Because of this, we are including this procedure in the book, but its use is not mandatory. Your instructor will provide guidance. Follow your facility's policies and procedures.

PROCEDURE **7** **SERVING A MEAL IN AN ISOLATION UNIT**

1. Before entering the isolation unit:
   - Wash your hands.
   - Obtain the meal tray for the patient. Check the meal card on the tray and check that the correct menu was provided.
   - Ask for the assistance of another member of the team.
   - Place the tray on the isolation cart.
   - Put on PPE as required by the type of isolation precautions used.

2. Enter the isolation room and identify the patient.

3. Explain what you plan to do.

4. Provide privacy.

5. Allow the patient to help as much as possible.

6. Raise the bed to a comfortable working height.

7. Pick up the empty meal tray that remains in the room. Make sure the tray is clean.

8. Return to the door and open it. The team member assisting holds the meal tray while you carefully transfer items to the isolation tray.

9. Place the isolation meal tray on the overbed table. Prepare the patient for the meal.

10. Check the patient's identification band against the meal tray card.

11. Assist the patient with food preparation and feeding as needed.

12. When the patient finishes, note how much food and liquid have been eaten. Flush uneaten food (except bones) down the toilet.

13. Place all disposable items (bones, dishes, eating utensils, covers, plastic wrap, foil, napkins, cups, cartons) in the appropriate waste container.

14. Reusable dishes may be handled as follows:
    - Use a paper towel to open the door to the isolation unit.
    - Prop the door open with your foot. Transfer dishes to a tray held by another assistant outside the door.
    - The assistant outside the room covers the dishes and returns the tray to the food cart.

NOTE

The CDC does not require the use of disposable dishes for patients requiring transmission-based precautions. Either disposable or reusable dishes and utensils can be used for patients on isolation precautions. Personnel in the dish room routinely wear heavy-duty utility gloves when handling used (soiled) dishes. The combination of hot water and detergents used in hospital dishwashers is sufficient to decontaminate dishes, glasses, cups, and eating utensils.

15. Clean the isolation meal tray and store it in the isolation unit.

16. Carry out all ending procedure actions (see Chapter 15).

17. Remove PPE and discard in the appropriate container.

18. Wash your hands.

19. Use a paper towel to open the door to leave the isolation unit. Discard the towel before leaving the unit.

ICON KEY:
 = OBRA   = PPE

PROCEDURE **MEASURING VITAL SIGNS IN AN ISOLATION UNIT**

> ### ✍ NOTE
>
> Equipment to measure vital signs in isolation should be dedicated to the patient. (This means that the equipment will remain in the room with the patient.) It must be cleaned and disinfected before use with another patient.

1. Before entering the isolation unit:
   - Wash your hands.
   - Remove your wristwatch and place it on a clean paper towel.
   - Put on PPE as required by the type of transmission-based precautions used.
2. Pick up the paper towel with the watch. Enter the isolation unit.
3. With the watch still on the paper towel, place it where you can see it during the procedures.

4. Identify the patient and explain what you plan to do.
5. Provide privacy.
6. Allow the patient to help as much as possible.
7. Raise the bed to a comfortable working height.
8. Using the equipment dedicated to the patient, measure vital signs.
9. Note the readings so you do not forget them.
10. Clean and store the equipment.
11. Carry out all ending procedure actions (see Chapter 15).
12. Remove and discard PPE.
13. Wash your hands, dry them, and pick up your watch.
14. Handling only the clean side of the paper towel that the watch had been resting on, discard it in the appropriate container.
15. Pick up your notes. Use a clean paper towel to open the door and leave the isolation unit. Discard the paper towel before you leave the unit.

ICON KEY:

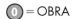 = OBRA   = PPE

PROCEDURE **TRANSFERRING NONDISPOSABLE EQUIPMENT OUTSIDE OF THE ISOLATION UNIT**

1. Nondisposable equipment used with a patient in transmission-based precautions may be dedicated to that patient. This means that the equipment remains in the isolation unit and is used only by that patient. Required cleaning is done in the room by the nursing assistant or housekeeping staff.
2. The equipment must be removed from the isolation unit and disinfected or sterilized before using with another patient.
3. Disinfect equipment after use before leaving the isolation unit.
4. Place the equipment in a plastic biohazard bag. In some facilities, a second person receives the items at the doorway. This person opens the large plastic bag and folds the top over into a cuff to cover their hands,

then stands outside the door and holds the bag open. The person inside the room places the disinfected item into the open bag. The second worker fastens the top of the bag to prevent possible contamination of the outside of the plastic bag.
5. Follow Procedures 5 and 6 for removing contaminated PPE.
6. Pick up the bag containing the equipment and leave the isolation unit.
7. Once outside the unit, follow facility policy for disinfecting or sterilizing the equipment.
8. Some equipment may be terminally (finally and completely) cleaned with disinfectant in the patient's unit when isolation is discontinued.

ICON KEY:

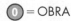 = OBRA   = PPE

EXPAND YOUR SKILLS

PROCEDURE **10** SPECIMEN COLLECTION FROM A PATIENT IN AN ISOLATION UNIT

1. Outside the isolation unit, assemble equipment:
   - Clean specimen container and cover
   - Paper towel
   - Biohazard bag for specimen container (Figure 13-34)
   - Two completed labels, one for the specimen container and one for the specimen bag

> **NOTE**
>
> The specimen bag may have a preprinted block on the bag that can be completed with the required information. In this case, a second label is not needed.

2. Place the equipment on the isolation cart while you put on PPE.

3. The biohazard bag for specimen transport remains outside the isolation unit.

4. Carry the specimen equipment into the isolation unit. Place the container and cover on a paper towel.

5. Identify the patient and explain what you plan to do.

6. Provide privacy.

7. Allow the patient to help as much as possible.

8. Raise the bed to comfortable working height.

9. Obtain the specimen. Place it into the container without touching the outside of the container.

10. Cover the container and apply a label.

11. Clean the equipment used to obtain the specimen.

12. Carry out all ending procedure actions (see Chapter 15).

13. Remove PPE as described in Procedures 5 and 6.

14. Wash your hands.

15. Use a paper towel to pick up the specimen container. Use another paper towel to open the door to leave the isolation unit.

16. Outside the unit, gather the paper towel in your hands so the edges do not hang loosely. Place the specimen container in the biohazard transport bag, being careful not to allow the paper towel to touch the outside of the transport bag.

17. Discard the paper towels in the appropriate container.

18. Follow facility policy for transporting the specimen.

19. Wash your hands.

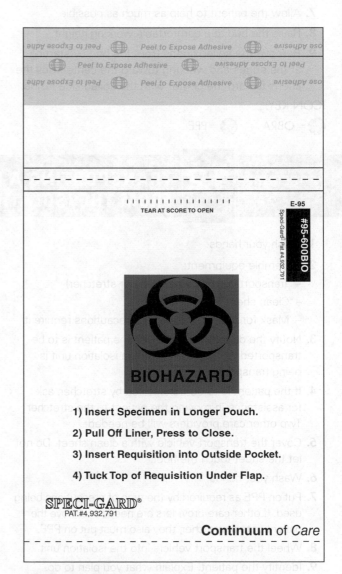

FIGURE 13-34 Transport specimens in the sealed, labeled transport bag.

PROCEDURE **11** CARING FOR LINENS IN AN ISOLATION UNIT

1. Assemble any linens required and place on a chair or stand outside the isolation unit.

2. Wash and dry your hands.

3. Outside the isolation unit, put on PPE as required by type of transmission-based precautions.

4. Once inside the isolation unit, place the clean linens on a chair.

5. Identify the patient and explain what you plan to do.

6. Provide privacy.

7. Allow the patient to help as much as possible.

8. Raise the bed to a comfortable working height.

9. Remove the soiled linens from the bed by starting at the edges and working toward the center. Roll the linens toward the center with the soiled side inside.

ICON KEY:

 = OBRA   **P** = PPE

10. Handle soiled linens as little as possible. Pick up the linens from the bed and hold them away from your uniform and gown (if used).

11. Place soiled linens in a meltaway laundry bag (a bag that dissolves in the wash water in the laundry), if used, or follow facility policy.

12. Place the meltaway bag in a laundry hamper lined with a biohazard plastic bag, or follow facility policy. The bag should be labeled biohazardous material for laundry.

13. Secure the bag and route soiled linen to the laundry.

14. If gloves are heavily contaminated from the soiled linens, remove gloves and dispose them in the appropriate container. Wash your hands, dry them, and put on a clean pair of gloves. Then remake the patient's bed with the clean linens.

15. Carry out all ending procedure actions (see Chapter 15).

PROCEDURE **12** TRANSPORTING A PATIENT TO AND FROM THE ISOLATION UNIT

1. Wash your hands.

2. Assemble equipment:
   - Transport vehicle (wheelchair or stretcher)
   - Clean sheet
   - Mask for patient, if isolation precautions require it

3. Notify the department to which the patient is to be transported that a patient from an isolation unit is being transported.

4. If the patient is to be transported by stretcher, ask for assistance in moving the patient to the stretcher. Two other care providers will be needed.

5. Cover the transport vehicle with a clean sheet. Do not let the sheet touch the floor.

6. Wash your hands.

7. Put on PPE as required by the type of precautions being used. If other care providers are needed to move the patient onto a stretcher, they also must put on PPE.

8. Wheel the transport vehicle into the isolation unit.

9. Identify the patient. Explain what you plan to do.

10. Provide privacy.

11. Allow the patient to help as much as possible.

12. If the patient is to be transported by wheelchair, the bed must be in the lowest horizontal position. For transport by stretcher, raise the bed to the same height as the stretcher.

13. Assist the patient into the wheelchair or onto the stretcher.

14. Put a mask on the patient, if required.

15. Wrap the patient in a sheet, if required for contact precautions. Make sure the sheet does not touch the floor.

16. Remove PPE and wash your hands. Open the door and take the patient out of the isolation unit (Figure 13-35).

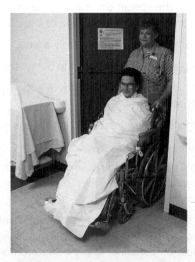

FIGURE 13-35 A patient on contact precautions is being transported out of the room. The receiving department is aware of the patient's precautions.

(continues)

17. To return a patient to an isolation unit, place the wheelchair or stretcher near the wall of the room as you put on PPE.

18. Enter the isolation unit, unwrap the patient from the sheet, and remove the patient's mask, if used.

19. Assist the patient from the wheelchair or stretcher (with the help of other caregivers) and return the patient to bed.

20. Carry out ending procedure actions (see Chapter 15).

ICON KEY:

O = OBRA   **P** = PPE

21. Place the sheet in the laundry hamper for contaminated linens and discard the patient's mask in the biohazardous trash container.

22. Remove PPE and wash your hands.

23. Remove the transport vehicle from the isolation unit. Follow facility procedure for cleaning and storing the vehicle used for the patient in isolation.

24. Report completion of procedure: transport of patient in isolation to another department and back to isolation unit.

DISINFECTION AND STERILIZATION

Disinfection is the process of eliminating harmful pathogens from equipment and instruments. A chemical called a *disinfectant* is used for this procedure. Do not use disinfectants on the human body. Disinfectants destroy bacteria, fungi, and viruses (but not spores) on surfaces. You may be required to disinfect personal care items such as washbasins, bedpans, and urinals. You may also use disinfectants to clean wheelchairs and other furniture items. Items are usually washed before they are disinfected. The procedure for disinfection depends on the chemicals used. Follow the directions of your facility for use of disinfectants. Wear gloves and a gown for completing these procedures. You may also need a face shield. Wear PPE that is appropriate to the procedure.

Sterilization removes all microorganisms from an item. This process can be completed in an **autoclave**, which uses steam and pressure to kill organisms (Figure 13-36). Gas sterilization is also used in some health care facilities. Sterilization procedures are used for nondisposable equipment that is exposed to potentially infectious materials. Facilities purchase many disposable sterile items. They are used once and discarded.

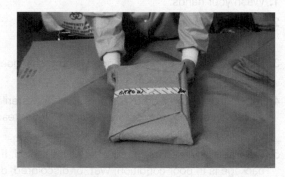

FIGURE 13-37 The stripes on the tape are not visible until they are exposed to heat and steam in the autoclave, indicating that the package has been sterilized.

Nondisposable items are washed and sterilized in the facility. Equipment to be sterilized is wrapped in special material. Tape on the packaging material changes color when the package is sterilized (Figure 13-37). Do not use the package if the tape has not changed color. Do not use a sterilized package that has been accidentally opened.

STERILE PROCEDURES

Surgical asepsis is the means by which the environment is kept free of all microbes, both pathogens and nonpathogens. In procedures where surgical asepsis is used, equipment and supplies must be **sterile**. In other words, items used in the procedure must go through a sterilization process.

In most facilities, you will not be expected to use sterile technique. If you are responsible for sterile procedures, you should first be given thorough education. Your responsibilities may include opening sterile packages. (See Procedure 13; also see Chapter 36.)

Sterile Field

The term **sterile field** refers to an area of sterile equipment and materials. When working with a sterile field and sterile equipment, keep the following points in mind:

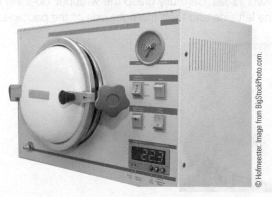

FIGURE 13-36 An autoclave uses heat, steam, and pressure to sterilize medical supplies and eliminate all microbes.

© Hofmeester. Image from BigStockPhoto.com.

- The sterile field may be a table covered with a sterilized sheet or a sterile towel placed on an overbed table. The table cover may be paper or cloth.
- Only the center of the table cover is actually used.
- Keep equipment two inches in from the edges all around, as an added precaution.
- Never reach for or pass anything that is unsterile over a sterile field. You might drop the unsterile article onto the field or touch the field. Instead, carry the unsterile object around the sterile field or hold it away from the sterile field.

- If there is even a suspicion that any nonsterile item has touched the sterile field, consider the field contaminated, and replace the entire setup.
- Coughing or sneezing while preparing a sterile field, or after the field has been set up, contaminates the field.
- Moisture means contamination. If a sterile item becomes wet, it is contaminated and must be replaced.

PROCEDURE 13 · OPENING A STERILE PACKAGE

1. Wash your hands.
2. Assemble equipment:
   - Sterile package
3. If the color code has not changed, or the seal does not look intact, do not use it.
4. Touch only the outside of the package. Only sterile surfaces contact other sterile surfaces. Never reach over a sterile field.
5. Commercially prepared products will be sealed. If the package is in poor condition, wet, or discolored, discard the item.
6. Place the package with the fold side up on a flat, clean surface.

7. Remove the tape.
8. Unfold the flap farthest away from you by grasping the outer surface only between your thumb and index finger (Figure 13-38A).
9. Open the right flap with your right hand using the same technique.
10. Open the left flap with your left hand using the same technique (Figure 13-38B).
11. Open the final flap (nearest you) (Figure 13-38C). Touch only the outside of the flap. Be careful not to stand too close. Do not touch the flap with your clothing or body as it is lifted free. Be sure the flaps are pulled open completely to prevent them from folding back over sterile items.

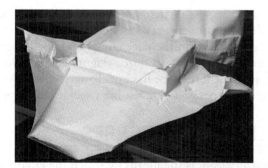

FIGURE 13-38A Touching only the corner, open the distal (top) flap away from your body.

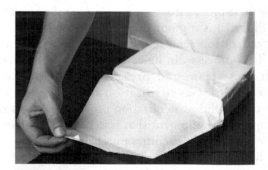

FIGURE 13-38B Carefully grasp the wrapper, opening first the left side and then the right side of the package.

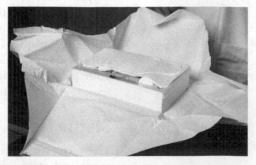

FIGURE 13-38C Open the proximal (closest) flap toward you. Avoid touching the flap or inside of the package with your hands or clothing.

ICON KEY:

0 = OBRA

REVIEW

A. True/False

Mark the following true or false by circling T or F.

1. T F When working in the droplet precautions room, always wear a NIOSH-approved respirator.

2. T F Surgical masks may be reused.

3. T F Wear gloves to care for one patient, then discard.

4. T F Food and drink may not be stored in the refrigerator with laboratory specimens.

5. T F Licensed nurses are solely responsible for carrying out isolation techniques for patients with transmission-based precautions.

6. T F Disposable patient care equipment is preferred when caring for a patient in isolation.

7. T F Droplet precautions do not require the use of a covering gown.

8. T F Wash your hands in cold water to prevent skin damage.

9. T F Always hold fingertips up when rinsing hands during handwashing.

10. T F Nonsterile items may touch the edges of the sterile field.

11. T F An alcohol rub is the preferred method of cleansing your hands if no visible soil is present.

12. T F Asepsis is the absence of all microbes.

13. T F A clean item is considered sterile.

14. T F Wearing a mask with all types of eye protection offers the highest level of protection.

15. T F Regular eyeglasses provide the same level of protection as goggles or a face shield.

16. T F Air from the airborne precautions room circulates directly into the facility.

17. T F After the professional fit test, workers must wear only the type and size mask approved by the fit tester.

18. T F Avoid contaminating environmental surfaces with your used gloves.

19. T F The exposure control plan describes actions to take for accidental contact with biohazardous substances.

20. T F Your mask fits correctly if you taste saccharin during the fit test procedure.

B. Completion

Complete the statements by writing the correct word(s).

21. The single most important health procedure a nursing assistant can carry out is _____.

22. Accidental contact with infectious or potentially infectious materials is known as a(n) _____.

23. Gloves, gowns, masks, goggles, and face masks are part of _____.

24. Small blood spills may be cleaned up by using. _____

25. Sharps and needles should be disposed of by placing them in the _____.

C. Complete the Chart

In addition to standard precautions, indicate the transmission-based precautions required by each disease or condition. Place an X in the correct column(s) to make your choice.

Disease/ Condition	Airborne	Droplet	Contact
26. Draining infected pressure ulcer			
27. Tuberculosis			
28. Mumps			
29. Infected surgical wound			
30. Influenza			

D. Multiple Choice

Select the best answer for each of the following.

31. Housing and caring for a person with an infection is known as:

a. segregation.

b. isolation.

c. sequestration.

d. separation.

32. After caring for a patient on contact isolation precautions, you should remove:

a. your gown first.

b. your gloves first.

c. your mask first.

d. PPE in any order.

33. The gloves stocked on your unit are size medium (M). You need size extra-large (XL). You know that having gloves that fit properly is important. You should:

   a. buy some XL gloves to use at work.

   b. not wear gloves when giving care.

   c. ask the facility to stock XL gloves.

   d. wear the size M gloves anyway.

34. The basic foundation of medical asepsis is:

   a. handwashing.

   b. isolation precautions.

   c. wearing a mask.

   d. wearing a gown.

35. If there is an exposure incident, you should:

   a. cleanse exposed skin with alcohol.

   b. report it at once to the supervisor.

   c. evacuate the area.

   d. tell other nursing assistants.

36. An AIIR isolation room:

   a. must have the air conditioner on at all times.

   b. has the window slightly open 12 hours each day.

   c. is connected to the facility's ventilation system.

   d. uses a negative pressure ventilation system.

37. Gloves are used for all of the following *except*:

   a. to avoid picking up a pathogen from a patient.

   b. to avoid giving a patient a pathogen that is on your hands.

   c. to avoid picking up a pathogen in one room and carrying it to another on the hands.

   d. to avoid the need for placing patients in isolation.

38. If a patient has signs of respiratory infection upon initial facility contact, they are:

   a. instructed to apply a surgical mask.

   b. asked to use respiratory hygiene and cough etiquette.

   c. promptly placed on airborne or droplet precautions.

   d. instructed to leave and return when symptom-free.

39. Isolation techniques:

   a. protect the portal of entry.

   b. prevent replication of the germ.

   c. interrupt the mode of transmission.

   d. improve the chain of infection.

40. Indirect contact occurs by:

   a. contact with a contaminated object.

   b. inhaling a pathogen in the air.

   c. touching a patient's skin.

   d. inhaling secretions from a sneeze.

E. Nursing Assistant Challenge

41. The doctor has just ordered contact precautions for Mrs. Minion. Your assignment is to set up the room. Write your answers in the blanks.

   a. What equipment should be assembled, and where is each item placed? _____

   b. What effect might being placed on isolation have on Mrs. Minion? _____

   c. What might you do to make her adjustment easier? _____

   d. How might her visitors feel? _____

42. You are reporting on duty. Some of your responsibilities will be handling food trays, making beds, straightening out your patients' overbed tables, and helping to change a patient who is wet with urine. During your shift, you will use a facial tissue and visit the restroom.

   List at least six times you will need to wash your hands.

   a. _____

   b. _____

   c. _____

   d. _____

   e. _____

   f. _____

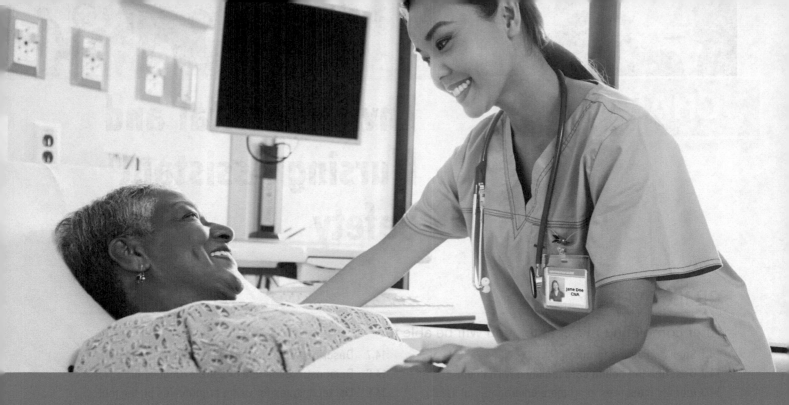

SECTION 5
Safety and Mobility

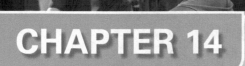

CHAPTER 14

Environmental and Nursing Assistant Safety

OBJECTIVES

After completing this chapter, you will be able to:

14.1 Spell and define terms.

14.2 Describe the health care facility environment.

14.3 Identify measures to promote environmental safety.

14.4 List situations when equipment must be repaired.

14.5 Describe the elements required for fire.

14.6 List five measures to prevent a fire.

14.7 Describe the procedure to follow if a fire occurs.

14.8 Demonstrate the use of a fire extinguisher.

14.9 List techniques for using ergonomics on the job.

14.10 Demonstrate appropriate body mechanics.

14.11 Describe the types of information contained in Safety Data Sheets (SDS).

VOCABULARY

Learn the meaning and the correct spelling of the following words and phrases:

concurrent cleaning	incident	private room	semiprivate room
environmental safety	incident report	RACE	side rails
ergonomics	PASS	Safety Data Sheet (SDS)	ward

INTRODUCTION

The hospital room is the patient's home while they are hospitalized (Figure 14-1). The room becomes the patient's world. Cheerful and pleasant surroundings give the patient a better sense of well-being. Attention to safety helps foster feelings of security in this unfamiliar environment. *Both* help speed recovery.

Many facilities provide an information board in each room that is updated daily. The nursing assistant helps keep the patient's unit safe and clean. All health care providers share the task of keeping the entire nursing unit safe and clean.

Environmental safety refers to the condition of an entire facility: patient rooms, hallways, and all departments. The environment includes:

- Temperature (heating and air-conditioning)
- Air circulation
- Light
- Cleanliness
- Noise control
- Walls, ceilings, and floors
- Plumbing
- Electricity
- Equipment and furniture

Prevention of injuries to patients, visitors, volunteers, and staff members is of primary concern.

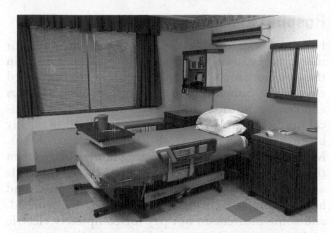

FIGURE 14-1 The patient's unit is home during the hospital stay.

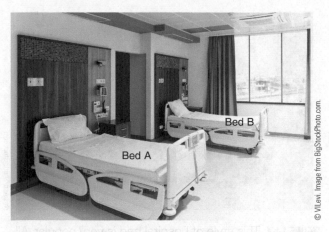

FIGURE 14-2 A semiprivate (two-bed) room.

 Infection Control **ALERT**

Some hospitals do not permit flowers in certain areas, such as the burn unit, intensive care unit, or rooms of patients with weakened immune systems. Flowers increase the risk for the spread of infection, especially *Pseudomonas* (see Chapter 12). Plants and flowers should be cared for by staff who are not involved in patient care or by the patient or a family member. If you must touch flowers or plants, wear gloves. Perform thorough hand hygiene with soap and water or an alcohol preparation when finished.

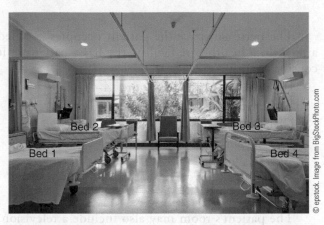

FIGURE 14-3 A four-bed ward. This type of room is not as common as it was in years past, but some hospitals and long-term care facilities still use them.

THE PATIENT ENVIRONMENT

Health care facilities have various types of rooms. A **private room** contains only one bed. **Semiprivate rooms** contain two beds (Figure 14-2). **Wards** are multiple-bed rooms, usually with three or four beds (Figure 14-3).

Hospitals have learned that having private rooms improves patient satisfaction. Other reasons that private rooms are desirable are:

- Improved confidentiality and privacy
- Reduced noise
- Reduced embarrassment
- More space
- Better accommodations for families who are spending a great deal of time at the hospital
- Improved opportunities for family to assist with care

Roommates can be a source of stress. Roommate problems often lead to transferring patients from one room or unit to another, which is costly and undesirable because new staff are often assigned who do not know patients.

Each room is numbered. The beds are marked by letters or numbers. For example, Room 871 in a large medical center may be a four-unit ward. The beds are labeled A, B, C, D (or 1, 2, 3, 4). The patient in the fourth bed is in Unit 871-D or Unit 871-4. The beds are usually numbered sequentially in a clockwise direction, beginning with the bed immediately to the left of the door. Using Room 871 as an example, this would be 871-A or 871-1. If two beds are on the right side of the room, the bed closest to the door is bed 1 or bed A. Refer to Figures 14-2 and 14-3. Four-bed units or wards were the norm for many years. Each nursing station had at least one. However, there is a much greater emphasis on privacy today than there was years ago. Hospitals have been remodeled and rebuilt and almost all of the four-bed (ward) rooms have been eliminated. Today's health care facilities have mainly one- and two-bed rooms. This is a positive change that has been well received and appreciated by patients. Older large military and veterans hospitals still depend on ward beds, but most others have phased them out.

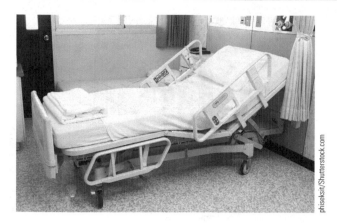

phisekit/Shutterstock.com

FIGURE 14-4 This style of hospital bed is very popular. All hospital beds are equipped with side rails. These are split rails that can be raised and lowered in any combination.

The personal space the patient occupies is called a *unit*. In a health care facility, the basic patient unit consists of a(n):

- Hospital bed with rails (Figure 14-4)
- Bedside table
- Chair
- Reading lamp
- Waste basket
- Overbed table
- Signal cord

The patient's room may also include a television, telephone, radio or clock. This equipment may be located in a single-, double-, or multiple-bed room.

The equipment from one unit should not be used by other patients. For home care, the same unit elements will be present, but they will be modified. For example, there may not be an adjustable hospital bed or an overbed table.

Hospital Beds

Hospital beds mostly have the same features, but there may be some differences. Hospital beds differ in the ways in which they operate. Most are controlled electrically. Some have special features such as scales and can be positioned in various ways to meet medical needs (Figure 14-5). A few are operated manually by turning cranks or gatch handles (Figure 14-6). Most facilities are phasing out manual beds when they purchase new equipment. However, manual beds are still in use in some long-term care facilities and home health care clients' homes. Medicare, Medicaid, and some insurers do not pay for completely electric high–low beds. Because of this, medical equipment rental companies continue to rent and sell manual beds, as well as beds that operate both manually and electronically. As a rule, the head and foot of these beds are operated electrically. The high–low feature of the bed (if there is one) is manually operated. To prevent injury, be sure to tuck the gatch handle(s) under the bed after you have finished caring for the patient.

Hospital beds:

- May be raised to a high horizontal position. In this position, there is less strain for those giving care. Return the bed to the lowest horizontal position when you leave the room.
- Are on wheels, to make it easy to move beds from one place to another. Always lock the wheels unless the bed is being moved.
- Break (or hinge) in the middle so that the head may be raised.
- Break (or hinge) behind the knees to increase physical comfort for patients who are confined to the bed.

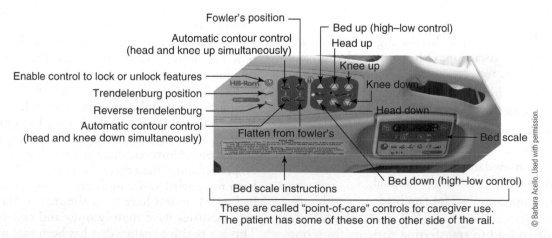

Fowler's position

Automatic contour control (head and knee up simultaneously)

Enable control to lock or unlock features

Trendelenburg position

Reverse trendelenburg

Automatic contour control (head and knee down simultaneously)

Flatten from fowler's

Bed up (high–low control)

Head up

Knee up

Knee down

Head down

Bed scale

Bed scale instructions

Bed down (high–low control)

These are called "point-of-care" controls for caregiver use. The patient has some of these on the other side of the rail.

© Barbara Acello. Used with permission.

FIGURE 14-5 This bed can be positioned in many different ways by using the electric controls. The bed has a built-in scale for bedfast patients.

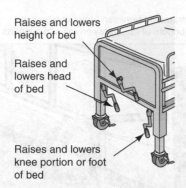

Raises and lowers height of bed

Raises and lowers head of bed

Raises and lowers knee portion or foot of bed

FIGURE 14-6 Gatch handles are used to change the position of nonelectric beds. Some stretchers also use handles similar to these.

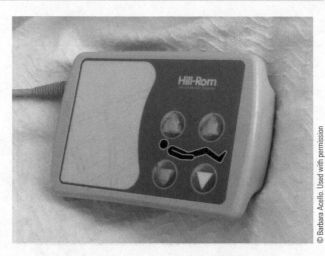

FIGURE 14-7 The bed control can be snapped into the side rail or removed and placed next to the patient.

⚠ OSHA **ALERT**

Elevating the bed to a proper working height is one of the most important measures to use for protecting your back. Always raise the side rails if you must step away from the bedside when the bed is in the high position. If a gatch handle is used to elevate the bed, use good body mechanics by squatting down when you turn the handle. For patient safety, make sure you lower the bed when you leave the room.

🔒 Safety **ALERT**

Always test the patient's ability to assist with moving procedures, unless contraindicated. The side rails are perfect tools for patients to use when moving in bed. When the patient uses the rail to assist in a move, your job is made easier and there is less strain on your back. Remember to lower the rail when you leave the room, according to facility policies or if indicated on the care plan.

Side rails are attached to the hospital bed. They protect the patient from falling. Side rails are restraints in some circumstances. (Refer to Chapter 15 for additional information.) Most health care facilities have policies, procedures, and guidelines describing their use. Potential benefits of side rails are that they:

• Provide support and a "handle" for the patient to use for turning and repositioning, and getting into and out of bed.

• Give the patient a feeling of security.

• Reduce the risk of the patient falling out of bed when they are being transported in the bed.

• Provide access to call light, bed, and television controls that are part of the bed rail design (Figure 14-7).

The potential risks of side rails include:

• Strangulation, suffocation, bodily injury, or death when the patient or part of the patient's body becomes entrapped between the bars of the side rails or between the side rails and the mattress (Figure 14-8)

• Serious injuries if the patient climbs over the rails and falls from this height

• Skin tears, bruises, cuts, and/or scrapes

• Agitation caused by a feeling of being trapped or caged in

• Feelings of isolation or restriction.

• Sadness because of loss of independence and having to call for help

• Actual loss of independence, such as the ability to get up to use the bathroom or to retrieve an item dropped on the floor

Several types of side rails are used on hospital beds (Figure 14-9). One type is a single rail that runs the length of the bed. Split rails are more common in acute care hospitals. Each side of the bed has two half-rails. One or both can be raised, depending on the patient's needs and plan of care. When side rails are used, they:

• Are positioned up or down, as noted on the plan of care

• Should be checked and attached securely

• Should be down only when the bed is in the lowest horizontal position

• Should never be used for the attachment of tubes or straps, such as restraints or catheters. Raising and lowering the side rails could put undue stress on such tubes and even pull them out

Zone 1 - Entrapment within rail

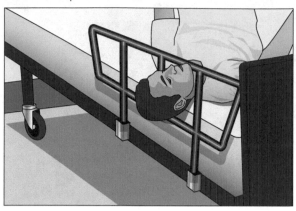

Zone 2 - Entrapment between top of compressed mattress to bottom of rail, between rail and supports

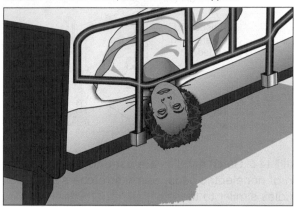

Zone 3 - Entrapment in horizontal space between rail and mattress

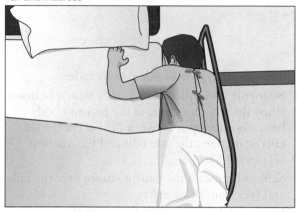

Zone 4 - Entrapment between top of compressed mattress and bottom of rail at end of rail

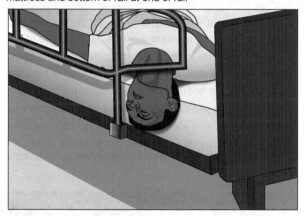

FIGURE 14-8 Patients can be seriously injured if they become trapped in the side rails. The risk is greater if an air mattress is being used to treat skin problems because it is compressed more easily.

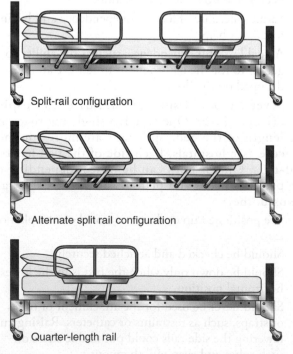

Split-rail configuration

Alternate split rail configuration

Quarter-length rail

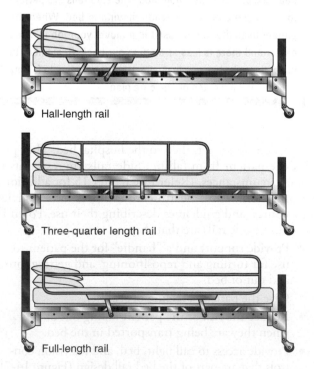

Hall-length rail

Three-quarter length rail

Full-length rail

FIGURE 14-9 Examples of the different types of side rails.

Temperature, Air Circulation, and Light

As you adjust and maintain the temperature, light, and ventilation, keep in mind the patient's condition, the patient's personal preferences, and the needs of any other patients in the room. The best temperature is about 71°F to 81°F, according to patient comfort and facility policy. Most patients are comfortable in the 71°F to 75°F range. Lower temperatures may cause chilling, and higher ones may cause discomfort.

Rooms in most hospitals and many long-term care facilities are air-conditioned. The thermostat may be set from a central location or set individually in each patient's room. Shield patients from drafts by using screens or curtains as necessary.

Lighting comes from several sources. There will be times when less light is desired. At other times, more light will be needed. Use as much light as needed to safely carry out your job and ensure patient safety.

Patients often find it difficult to sleep if lights are too bright. There should be only enough light at night to enable staff to work safely.

- Rooms are equipped with lights above each bed. These illuminate a single patient bed.
- There may also be a ceiling light.
- Flashlights may also be needed for some procedures, such as catheterization.
- The best lighting is indirect; glare causes fatigue.
- Be sure to return extra lights as soon as you are finished, because clutter in a room is hazardous.
- Night lights are often left on for very ill or elderly patients. If the room does not have a night light, turn on the bathroom light and crack the door slightly.

Cleanliness and Noise Reduction

You are responsible for the cleanliness, quiet, and order of the patient units to which you are assigned. Minimizing noise is very important (Chapter 10). To contribute to the comfort of the patient:

- Speak quietly.
- Report squeaky equipment wheels that should be oiled.
- Avoid banging equipment and trays against other surfaces.
- Keep the area neat as you work. Check its overall appearance before you leave.

 Infection Control **ALERT**

Make sure clean and soiled items are separated in patient rooms and storage areas. Keep the lids tightly closed on trash cans and linen hampers. Avoid putting biohazard-contaminated trash into open wastebaskets. Discard soiled items in a plastic bag or a covered trash can.

- Return equipment to its proper location after completing patient care.
- Do not turn the TV on or up while giving care to patients unless the patient asks you to do so.

You are responsible for keeping the patient supplied with fresh water, ice, disposable drinking cups, tissues, and straws. Make sure that all necessary pieces of equipment, such as the washbasin, emesis basin, bedpan, urinal, soap, and towels, are always available, clean, and in good condition (Figure 14-10). Store these items in the bedside table.

 Infection Control **ALERT**

When two or more patients share a room, make sure that all personal care items are labeled with each patient's name. Keep personal care items in the appropriate area. Store grooming supplies in a clean area. Avoid storing personal care equipment and supplies in community areas, such as bathrooms; storage in these areas increases the risk that personal care items will be used for the wrong patient(s).

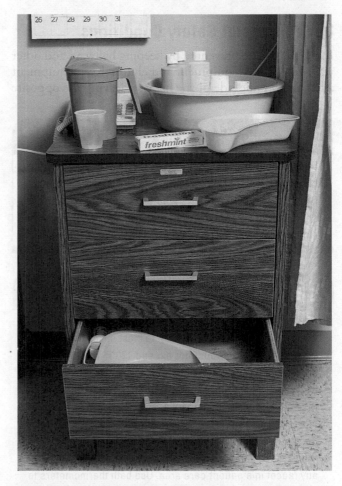

FIGURE 14-10 Make sure the items from the admission kit are readily available and stored correctly to reduce the risk of infection.

SAFETY MEASURES

Safety is the responsibility of everyone. A safe environment is essential for both patients and staff. Safety must be a part of everything you do. This concern extends to the safety of the unit and the entire environment. The number of accidents involving patients and staff can be greatly reduced if simple measures are followed.

An accident that occurs in a health care facility is referred to as an **incident**. An incident is any unexpected occurrence or event that interrupts normal procedures or causes a crisis. Incidents can harm a patient, employee, or any other person, but there are no injuries in some incidents. If you see an incident or are involved in one, notify the nurse. They will fill out an **incident report** (Figure 14-11) after obtaining information from the persons involved and witnesses. Prevention of incidents depends on employees:

- Knowing their jobs and following all safety policies and procedures
- Maintaining a safe environment
- Knowing the patients and implementing safety measures to decrease their risk of injury

Environmental Safety Conditions

Incidents can be prevented by keeping hallways and other walkways free of equipment and clutter. Keep equipment and carts on one side of the hallway, leaving the opposite

Age-Appropriate Care **ALERT**

Besides the safety practices specifically discussed in this chapter, keep sharp objects, chemicals, and plants away from children and patients who are experiencing mental confusion. If you are not sure about the safety of an item, check with the nurse.

Safety **ALERT**

Each state has laws governing the water temperature in patient care areas of the facility. In most cases, water temperature at sinks should not exceed 120°F. The regulators sometimes fail, sending excessively hot water into the facility. Water in bath and shower areas must be warm enough to comfortably bathe patients. Comfortable temperature for most people is 95°F to 105°F. Report water in bathing areas that does not warm up enough for comfortable bathing. Also report steaming water or water that feels excessively hot at any faucet in a patient care area. Use bath thermometers to check water temperatures before giving patient care, whenever possible.

side free so patients and visitors can use the handrail, if needed. Keeping equipment on the same side reduces the risk of falls and means that no one has to navigate through a maze of equipment to walk down the hallway. Report these potentially unsafe situations promptly:

- Burnt-out light bulbs and light switches or electric plugs that do not work
- Water leaks from faucets or pipes
- Handrails that are unclean or sticky to touch
- Faucets or water fountains that do not flow properly
- Loose or missing floor tiles
- Windows that do not close tightly or are cracked or broken
- Temperatures that are too hot or too cold and cannot be controlled within the room
- Water temperatures that are too hot
- Loose or missing ceiling tiles or leaks from the ceiling
- Toilets that do not flush properly

Equipment and Its Care

The daily or **concurrent cleaning** of equipment is an important part of your job. It contributes to the safety of your patients. The housekeeping department maintains environmental cleanliness. However, spills must be mopped up immediately to avoid falls. The nursing assistant is also responsible for keeping the patient's immediate area clean and safe.

In most health care facilities, equipment is tagged when it needs repair (Figure 14-12). That equipment is not to be used again until the tag is removed. Facility policy differs as to who is responsible for applying and removing these alert tags. Reporting broken or nonfunctioning equipment is the responsibility of everyone.

You can prevent accidents related to equipment by:

- Reporting needed repairs promptly. Possible hazards include:
  - Lost screws
  - Frayed straps
  - Loose wheels
  - Broken control knobs
  - Latches that do not hook
  - Side rails that do not fasten correctly
  - Faulty brakes on wheelchairs and stretchers
  - Frayed electrical cords, plugs, and sockets that are not working properly
- Reporting immediately if call lights (signal cords) are not working
- Disposing of used sharps in proper containers
- Never handling broken bits of glass with your hands
- Always knowing what you are handling and the proper method for its disposal
- Inspecting mechanical lifts (Figure 14-13) carefully before using

INCIDENT REPORT

Family Name	First Name	M.I.	Room No.	Hosp. No.

Address	City	State	Zip Code	Age	Sex M F

Date of Incident	Time a.m. p.m.	Place	Attending Physician

Status of person involved: Patient _____   Employee _____   Visitor _____   Other _____

Diagnosis: _____

_____

Describe condition before incident: Disoriented _____ Senile ____ Sedated ___ Normal ____ Other ____

_____

Was height of bed adjustable? Yes ___ No ___ Was bed up? Yes ___ No ___ Was bed down? Yes ___ No ___

Were bed rails ordered? Yes ___ No ___ Were they present? Yes ___ No ___ Were they up? Yes ___ No ___

Were they down? Yes ___ No ___ Other _____

Describe incident entirely, include part of body injured and treatment:

_____

_____

_____

_____

_____

_____

_____

_____

_____

_____

Vital Signs: Temp _____   Pulse _____   Resp _____   Blood Pressure _____

Indicate on diagram location of injury

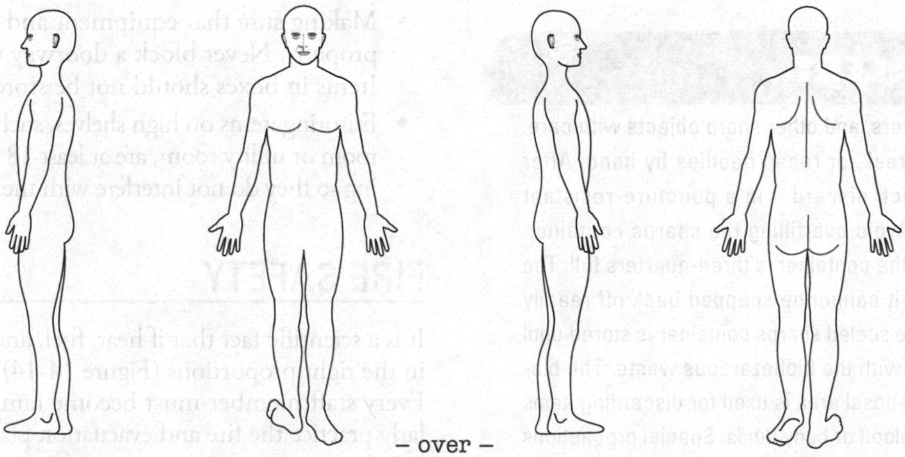

– over –

FIGURE 14-11 If an incident occurs, a special report is completed. This report is referred to as an incident report, an occurrence report, a variance report, or an accident report.

(continues)

Was physician called? Yes _____ No _____ Time_____ a.m.
                                                                                        p.m.

Who responded?_____ Time _____ a.m.
                                                                                               p.m.
                    Attending physician _____ On-call physician _____

Statement of physician _____

_____

_____

_____

_____

Was family called? Yes _____ No _____ Time _____ a.m. Who: _____
                                                                             p.m.

Give names, addresses, and phone numbers of any who witnessed incident _____

_____

_____

_____

A copy of this report will be sent to patient's physician.

Date of Report _____ Signed _____
                                                                  Signature and title of person preparing report

Nursing Office Review of Incident: Date _____ Signed _____

Comments: _____

_____

_____

_____

_____

_____

FIGURE 14-11 *(continued)*

- Making sure that equipment and supplies are stored properly. Never block a doorway with equipment. Items in boxes should not be stored on the floor

- Ensuring items on high shelves, such as in the linen room or utility room, are at least 18 inches from the ceiling so they do not interfere with the sprinkler system

FIRE SAFETY

It is a scientific fact that if heat, fuel, and oxygen are present in the right proportions (Figure 14-14), there will be a fire. Every staff member must become familiar with and regularly practice the fire and evacuation plans for the facility.

- Role-play the emergency procedures until you are completely secure. Remember that in any emergency, the welfare and safety of the patients are most important.

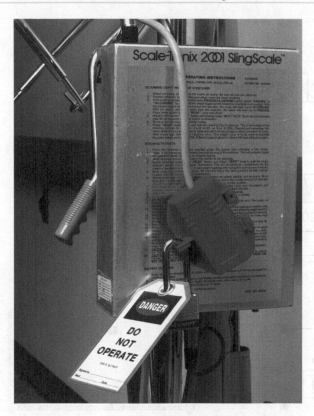

FIGURE 14-12 Unsafe electrical equipment is tagged and locked until it can be repaired.

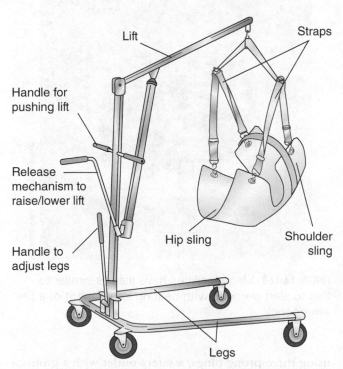

FIGURE 14-13 Carefully examine the mechanical lift before using it. If the lift is battery operated, also check the battery charge.

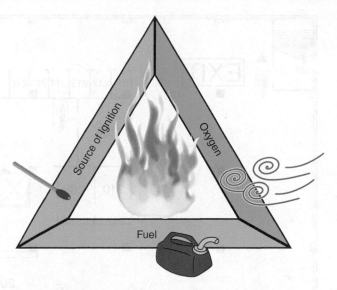

FIGURE 14-14 These three elements are needed to start a fire.

- Learn the location of escape routes and the location and operation of all fire control equipment (Figure 14-15), such as:
  - Fire alarms (Figures 14-16A and 14-16B)
  - Extinguishers
  - Sprinklers
  - Fire doors
  - Fire escapes
- Know and practice fire drill procedures conducted by your facility. Many patients could be injured during a fire because of confusion and their inability to help themselves.
- Keep alert to all possible fire hazards and report them immediately.

Fire Hazards

Improper use of electricity is a major cause of fire. The electrical equipment in a health care facility ranges from simple to complex. Improper use of electricity is a common cause of fire, so you must know how to use

---

🔓 Safety **ALERT**

In addition to knowing the location of fire extinguishers, become familiar with their ratings, which indicate the materials on which the extinguisher should be used:

Type A—wood, paper, household trash

Type B—grease, oil, liquids that will burn

Type C—electrical items

Type K—restaurant and large kitchen fires

Type ABC—any type of fire

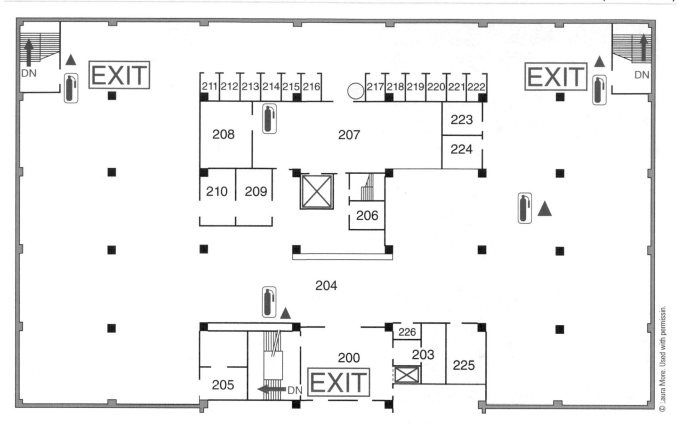

FIGURE 14-15 Become familiar with the facility evacuation plan.

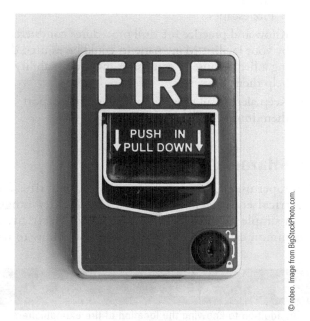

FIGURE 14-16A Learn the location of the fire alarms on the care area and how to use them.

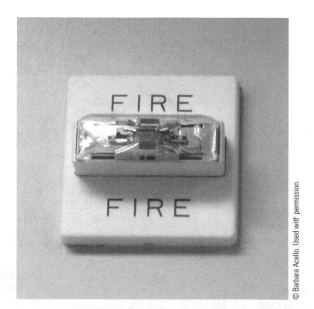

FIGURE 14-16B Many facilities have alarms similar to this to alert persons with hearing impairment of a fire emergency.

it safely. Medical equipment must be grounded so that stray currents are returned to the outlet, reducing the risk of electrical shock. An item that is grounded drains any unwanted electrical charge. Grounding is done by using three-prong plugs, a safety outlet with a ground-fault breaker, or a facility-approved power strip. In addition, check for frayed electrical wires, avoid lightweight extension cords, and do not overload electrical circuits.

Never use electrical equipment around water or any alcohol-based hand cleaner, make sure your hands are completely dry before handling electrical equipment, turning a light switch on or off, or creating static electricity.

Fire Prevention

Here are some other ways of preventing fires:

- Do not allow clutter to accumulate in doorways or traffic lanes.
- Empty wastepaper cans in proper receptacles.
- Report any possible hazards right away.
- Monitor for and report unauthorized smoking.
- Report smoke and/or burning smells.
- Keep all fire exits clear of equipment and debris.
- Know about and practice fire drill safety.
- Do not let visitors give smoking materials to patients.
- Follow all oxygen precautions.

Smoking

Most health care facilities do not permit smoking by anyone in any area. Some do not permit smoking anywhere on facility property. This applies to patients, visitors, and staff alike. Long-term care facilities that permit smoking usually store smoking materials at the nurse's station. In these facilities, residents must have direct supervision whenever they smoke. Some facilities will not accept new residents who smoke. Residents and staff must smoke outside at some facilities.

Oxygen Precautions

The use of oxygen presents a specific hazard. When oxygen is in use:

- Never permit smoking, lighted matches, or open flames in the area.
- Do not use flammable liquids such as oils, alcohol, nail polish, aftershave, lotions, perfume, or hair spray. Do not permit the patient to use alcohol-based hand cleaners.
- Do not use electrical equipment such as radios, hair dryers, electric razors, heating pads, or toys.
- Post signs indicating that oxygen is in use in designated areas, according to facility policy (Figure 14-17). Secondary "No Smoking" signs are not required in facilities that prohibit smoking and have signs at all major entrances stating that the facility does not allow smoking.

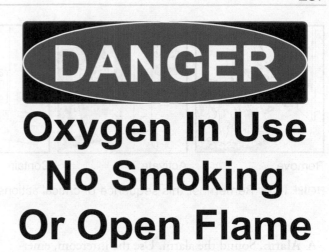

DANGER
Oxygen In Use
No Smoking
Or Open Flame

FIGURE 14-17 Each facility specifies where to post oxygen signs.

 Safety **ALERT**

Avoid stacking linens and supplies on upper shelves closer than 18 inches to the ceiling. If supplies are stacked too close to the ceiling, the sprinkler system will not be effective during a fire.

- Use cotton blankets and gowns for patients who use oxygen.
- Replace nonworking call signals with hand bells.
- Wear cotton uniforms and nonwool sweaters when providing care.
- Be certain there are no cigarettes, matches, or lighters in the room.
- Do not adjust the liter flow of oxygen. (Refer to Chapter 39 for additional information on oxygen therapy).

RACE System

In case of fire, remain calm. Move those in immediate danger to safety and sound the alarm. Follow the evacuation plan as you have practiced. Patients may be confused and frightened, so remaining calm and in control is important. In a fire emergency, remember **RACE** as defined here (Figure 14-18):

R Remove patients. Move patients to safety. Patients who can walk can be escorted. In some cases, they may be called upon to assist others to escape routes. Patients may have to be moved in their beds. If a person is unable to walk and the bed cannot be moved, bed sheets may be used as cradles to pull the patient to safety.

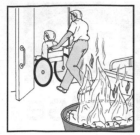
Remove

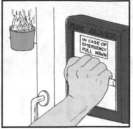
Activate

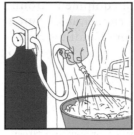
Contain

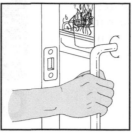
Extinguish or

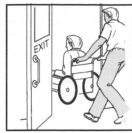
Evacuate

FIGURE 14-18 Remember this sequence of critical actions in case of fire.

A **Alarm.** Sound the alarm. Use the intercom, emergency signal bell, telephone, or fire alarm as directed by facility policy. Give the location and type of fire.

C **Contain fire.** Try to contain the fire to one area. Close windows and doors to prevent drafts, which will cause the fire to spread more rapidly. Before entering a closed door, touch the surface with the back of your hand (Figure 14-19). If the door is hot, do not open it.

E **Extinguish** the fire or *evacuate* the area.

Follow the fire emergency plan for your facility:

- Keep calm. Be prepared to follow directions when a person in authority takes charge.
- Shut off air-conditioning and other electrical equipment.
- Shut off oxygen.

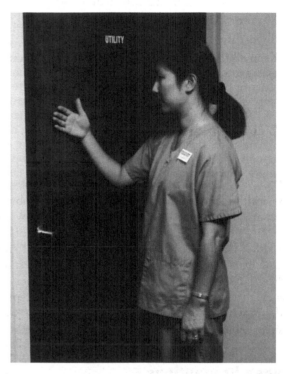

FIGURE 14-19 If a fire is suspected, touch the door with the back of the hand since it is more sensitive to heat than the palm. If the door feels hot, do not open it.

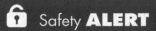 Safety **ALERT**

Oxygen is a prescription item, like a medication. It is safe as long as you follow facility policies and safety guidelines. Never change the fittings from one type of oxygen apparatus to another. Make sure you use the correct adaptor and plug for the unit. Always secure the oxygen cylinder in an upright position by chaining it to a carrier or placing it in a non-tip base. If it is accidentally knocked over, it has the potential to turn into a missile and cause great damage. If you have reason to believe that an oxygen tank or liquid oxygen canister is leaking, remove the patient from the room and close the door. Report the problem to the proper person immediately. Never attempt to carry or move an oxygen cylinder or canister that is leaking.

Safety **ALERT**

Bed linens can absorb oxygen. Avoid sparks when oxygen is in use. Static electricity can start a fire.

Safety **ALERT**

Health care facilities are built with safety features that aim to prevent fires from spreading. These features include doors that close automatically when the fire alarm sounds, an automatic sprinkler system, smoke detectors, and fire exits. Many materials used on the floors, doors, walls, and furnishings are fire-rated. This means that they will take longer to burn. Nevertheless, fire prevention is an important responsibility. Despite built-in safety features, health care facilities can catch fire. Many lives can be lost.

Safety ALERT

Removing patients from immediate danger is your first priority when a fire occurs. After sounding the alarm, contain the fire by closing doors and windows to slow the spread of fire. Move patients behind closed doors. The fire department may order evacuation if the fire is large and spreading rapidly.

- Do not use elevators.
- Close all doors into the hallway.
- Remove carts and equipment from the hallway. Get anything that may burn behind a door.

Use of a Fire Extinguisher

Carry a fire extinguisher upright. If you have been taught how to use a fire extinguisher, you may use it on small fires. Remember the letters **PASS**.

P—Pull the pin.
A—Aim the nozzle at the base of the fire.
S—Squeeze the handle.

Safety ALERT

Smoke from a fire is very dangerous. If you are in a smoke-filled area, stay as close to the floor as possible. If you can crawl to an exit, cover your mouth and stay on your knees. Because smoke rises, the area near the floor has the most oxygen. Touch the door with the *back* of your hand before entering a room. *If the door is hot to the touch, do not open it.* Stay in the room and place wet blankets or towels under the door to keep the smoke out. Opening the door could cause the fire to enter quickly and explosively.

Safety ALERT

For a widespread disaster, the facility disaster plan will also include managing the concurrent admission and treatment of multiple people from the community with injuries. The facility will have periodic disaster drills. The long-term care facility disaster plan will emphasize safe patient care during and after the disaster. It will also describe patient care in the event of the interruption of regular services, such as power failure and lack of water. In some communities, staff must be prepared to evacuate the facility. Learn your responsibilities in advance and remain calm if a disaster occurs. Follow the nurse's instructions.

S—Sweep back and forth along the base of the fire.
Do not attempt to fight a fire if:
- You are not sure which extinguisher to use.
- The fire is large and spreading and may block your exit.
- You do not know how to use a fire extinguisher.

OTHER EMERGENCIES

There may be other disasters for which you and your facility must be prepared. Tornadoes, hurricanes, floods, earthquakes, and bomb threats are examples of such disasters. In all emergency situations, get patients to safety, follow your facility's policy, and keep calm.

Interruption of Utilities and Services

Some emergencies may cause interruption of utility service. Your facility will have a backup generator to provide power to essential equipment. It may have battery-operated lights in strategic areas. The emergency generator is automatically activated in the event of a power outage. Some generators use natural gas. If this is the case, it will not operate if gas lines are damaged or disrupted. Earthquake-prone states such as California may use generators that are powered by other methods.

Respiratory support, such as oxygen concentrators and ventilators (Chapter 39), is a high priority. Locate the red outlets (Figure 14-20) to connect essential equipment to the power supply. Silver and white outlets will not have power when the facility is operating on generators. You should also know where emergency flashlights are stored. In the event of a power failure, obtain a flashlight and check on your patients.

Safety ALERT

If the facility has a weather – related power failure, stop what you are doing and check on all the patients. People with potential airway problems are your highest priority. Be sure that potentially life-saving equipment such as an oxygen concentrator are plugged into one of the red plugs that continues to supply electricity from the generator. If there are no red generator plugs available, obtain oxygen tanks. Persons using low air loss beds are the next priority. When power is lost, the beds lose air and the patient quickly sinks down to the frame. This is painful and potentially damaging to the skin. The bed must be inflated rapidly or the patient moved to a regular mattress. Patients using electrical medical equipment such as IV pumps, gastrostomy pumps, and other items are your next priority. Loss of electricity presents serious risk. Use good judgment and act quickly to prevent complications.

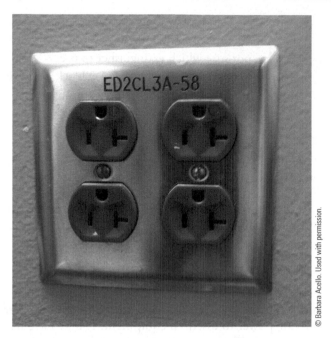

© Barbara Acello. Used with permission.

FIGURE 14-20 One type of emergency wall outlet that operates on the generator.

Areas that are usually equipped with emergency lighting are the:
- Front lobby
- Hallways
- Laundry room (lights only; will not operate appliances)
- Boiler room
- Stairways
  The facility generator does not:
- Provide heat or water.
- Provide power to laundry or kitchen.
- Operate the fire alarm system (this is on its own battery backup system).
- Operate the phone system.

Interruption of Water Service

The facility must also have at least a three-day supply of food and water. Disposable dishes may be used if water service is not available. The dietary department will distribute emergency meals and provide juice and other beverages that are on hand. At a minimum, the facility should have one gallon of water per day on hand for every patient and employee. Obviously, more is better if storage is available. Nonessential bathing and other water-consuming activities will be on hold until water service is restored. Waterless bathing products ("bag baths") will be used. Use alcohol-based hand cleaner unless hands have visible soil on them. Water in water heaters, storage tanks, and pools may be used for flushing commodes and bathing, if permitted by your facility disaster plan.

Tornadoes

Although rare in some parts of the country, a tornado can occur anywhere. A *tornado watch* means that conditions are favorable for a tornado to develop. During a tornado watch, someone is designated to monitor the weather in case the situation changes. Patients are not evacuated.

A *tornado warning* means that a tornado is actually in the area. Patients may be moved to a strong area in the center of the building. Tornadoes strike with little warning, so evacuation must be done very quickly. Move patients who cannot walk in wheelchairs or beds. Cover patients with blankets to protect them from flying debris. Close the room doors, fire doors, windows, and curtains. Do not go near windows during the storm.

NURSING ASSISTANT SAFETY

Ergonomics

The word **ergonomics** refers to adapting the environment and using techniques and equipment to prevent injury. If certain risk factors are present, it is more likely that an ergonomic (work-related) problem will occur. These risk factors include:
- Repeating the same motion or motion pattern every few seconds for more than two to four hours at a time
- Being in a fixed or awkward posture for more than two to four hours
- Using forceful hand exertions for more than two to four hours at a time
- Doing heavy lifting, unassisted, for more than one to two hours

Here are several ergonomic techniques you can use to reduce the risk of having an incident:
- Use correct body mechanics at all times, both at work and when you are off duty.
- Raise beds to a comfortable working height (remember to lower the bed when you finish your task).
- Use mechanical lifts when you need to transfer very heavy and/or dependent patients from a bed or chair.
- Use a back support belt if this is your preference. The use of back supports is controversial, but some nursing assistants find them helpful.
- Get another person to help when you need to transfer a patient who cannot bear their own weight fully.
- Use a cart to move heavy items.

🔒 Safety **ALERT**

Take fire and disaster drills seriously. In a real emergency, your actions will be automatic because you have practiced them during the drills.

Safety ALERT

The work performed by nursing assistants requires a great deal of lifting and moving of patients, objects, and equipment. You must use your body correctly to avoid injury.

⚠ **OSHA ALERT**

The back support belt works by keeping your spine in good alignment. You are less likely to be injured if your spine is straight and you are using good body mechanics. Using a back support belt does not make you stronger. Do not lift more than you would if you were not wearing the belt.

If you follow these eight commandments for lifting, you will reduce your risk of injury.
- Plan your lift and test the load (Figure 14-21A).
- Ask for help (Figure 14-21B).
- Get a firm footing (Figure 14-21C).
- Bend your knees (Figure 14-21D).
- Tighten your abdominal muscles (Figure 14-21E).
- Lift with your legs (Figure 14-21F).
- Keep the load close (Figure 14-21G).
- Keep your back upright (Figure 14-21H).

Warming up before working is another way to maintain a healthy body. Exercise before each work shift.

Check with your physician before beginning any exercise program.

Remember that you can avoid many problems if you also:
- Exercise every day.
- Eat a nourishing, well-balanced diet.
- Get adequate sleep.
- Avoid alcohol, cigarettes, drug use, and too much caffeine.
- Wear comfortable shoes with good support.

A.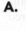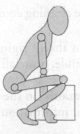

Plan your lift and test the load.
Before you lift, think about the item you are going to move and ask yourself:
"Can I lift this alone?" "Is it too awkward for one person?" "Is the path clear?" Also, test the load to see approximately how heavy it is before lifting.

B.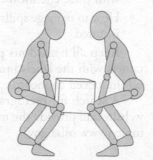

Ask for help.
If the load is too heavy or too awkward for you to lift, ask for assistance.

C.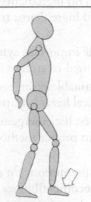

Get a firm footing.
Keep your feet apart for a stable base and point your toes out.

D.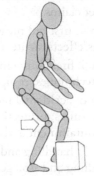

Bend your knees.
Don't bend at the waist. Keep the principles of leverage in mind at all times. Don't do more work than you have to.

E.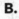

Tighten your stomach muscles.
Use intra-abdominal pressure to support your spine when you lift, offsetting the force of the load. Train your muscles to work together.

F.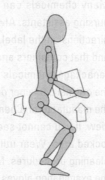

Lift with your legs.
Let your leg muscles do the work of lifting. Don't rely on your weaker back muscles.

G.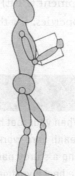

Keep the load close.
Don't hold the load away from your body. The closer it is to your spine, the less force it exerts on your back.

H.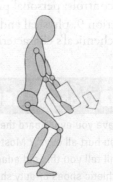

Keep your back upright.
Whether lifting or putting down the load, don't add the weight of your body to the load. Avoid twisting.

Reprinted with permission from Ergodyne

FIGURE 14-21A–H Eight rules for lifting and moving. (Reprinted with permission from Ergodyne Corporation, St. Paul, MN.)

Hazards in the Work Environment

All health care facilities have hazards in the work environment that can potentially cause injury to employees. Many of these items are chemicals that you may have in your own home (e.g., chlorine bleach). On a nursing unit, you might find cleaning supplies, disinfectants, and other products that are considered hazardous. Injuries can be prevented if you know what the hazards are and how to protect yourself and others. The Occupational Safety and Health Administration (OSHA) is a section of the federal government's Department of Labor. OSHA is responsible for employee safety. OSHA requires that all manufacturers of potentially harmful items supply **Safety Data Sheets (SDS)** with the products they sell. The SDS provide hazard communications that explain the following:

Section 1, identification: includes product identifier; manufacturer or distributor name, address, phone number; emergency phone number; recommended use; restrictions on use

Section 2, hazard(s) identification: includes all hazards regarding the chemical; required label elements

Section 3, composition/information on ingredients: includes information on chemical ingredients; trade secret claims

Section 4, first-aid measures: include important symptoms/effects, acute, delayed; required treatment

Section 5, firefighting measures: list suitable extinguishing techniques, equipment; chemical hazards from fire

Section 6, accidental release measures: list emergency procedures; protective equipment; proper methods of containment and cleanup

Section 7, handling and storage: list precautions for safe handling and storage, including incompatibilities

Section 8, exposure controls/personal protection: list(s) OSHA's permissible exposure limits (PELs); threshold limit values (TLVs); appropriate engineering controls; personal protective equipment (PPE)

Section 9, physical and chemical properties: list the chemical's characteristics

Section 10, stability and reactivity: list chemical stability and possibility of hazardous reactions

Section 11, toxicological information: includes routes of exposure; related symptoms, acute and chronic effects; numerical measures of toxicity

Section 12, ecological information

Section 13, disposal considerations

Section 14, transport information

Section 15, regulatory information

Section 16, other information: includes the date of preparation of the SDS or last revision

OSHA has also established other rules for a safe environment. Employers are required to inform employees of:

- The location of the SDS

- The hazards that exist in the work environment and where they are in the building

- The location of information related to the hazards

- How to read and understand chemical labels and hazard signs; all labels are required to have pictograms, a signal word, hazard and precautionary statements, the product identifier, and supplier identification

- What type of PPE should be worn while working with these chemicals, and where the PPE is stored

- How to manage spills and where cleaning equipment is stored

Keep all hazardous products in their original containers with the labels intact and legible. Store all chemicals in locked cupboards.

A search for pictograms and hazards on the OSHA website will provide the most current information on this topic (www.osha.gov).

 OSHA ALERT

Many chemicals can be hazardous to both patients and nursing assistants. Always use chemicals according to the directions on the label. Make sure they are properly diluted and that containers and surfaces are properly rinsed. Never repackage chemicals into unmarked containers. Use only the original container or special small containers provided by the manufacturer. Chemicals should always be stored within view. If you cannot see a chemical, it should be stored in a locked area. Wear utility gloves when using chemicals for cleaning procedures. Many chemicals will cause defects in the examination gloves used for patient care. This can irritate your hands, and the chemicals may be absorbed through your skin. Wear eye protection if there is a possibility of splashing or spraying chemicals during a cleaning procedure. Learn the locations of your facility's SDS, eyewash station(s), and body wash station(s).

🔒 Safety **ALERT**

Have you ever heard the expression "When your feet hurt, you hurt all over"? Most experienced health care workers will tell you this old adage is true. Buying a sturdy pair of athletic shoes or duty shoes is one of the best investments you will make in your uniform. Make sure that the shoe soles are appropriate for the floor surface in your facility. In most cases, this means having a nonslip sole. Having proper footwear will make you feel better and reduce your risk of falls and injuries.

REVIEW

A. Multiple Choice

Select the best answer for each of the following.

1. The patient's name is Phe Quan. She is in Room 116-B. From this information, you know that she is occupying a bed in a:
   a. private room.
   b. rehabilitation department.
   c. Special care unit.
   d. semiprivate room.

2. Side rails should be up and secure when:
   a. the bed is at the lowest horizontal height.
   b. the patient has a catheter.
   c. the bed is in the high position and you must step away.
   d. the patient does not have an order for restraints.

3. The best room temperature is approximately:
   a. 45°F.
   b. 65°F.
   c. 72°F.
   d. 88°F.

4. Which of the following represents a fire hazard?
   a. Frayed electrical wire
   b. Using three-prong plugs
   c. Supervised smoking
   d. Using UL-approved items

5. The elements needed to start a fire are:
   a. cigarettes, matches, and call signal.
   b. heat, fuel, and oxygen.
   c. electricity, oxygen, and matches.
   d. oxygen, linens, and electricity.

6. Which of the following contributes to unsafe conditions in a facility?
   a. Equipment in the halls
   b. Chemicals in locked cupboards
   c. Allowing patients to smoke with supervision
   d. Teaching patients how to use assistive devices

7. When oxygen is in use, you should not:
   a. use cotton blankets on the patient's bed.
   b. remove cigarettes from the room.
   c. adjust the liter flow.
   d. post a sign on the door.

8. Every staff member should know:
   a. how to open sealed windows in case of fire.
   b. the RACE procedure.
   c. the distance from the fire department to the facility.
   d. how to aim the extinguisher at the top of the flames.

9. The word that means adapting the environment to prevent body injury is:
   a. body mechanics.
   b. incident.
   c. ergonomics.
   d. RACE.

10. One principle of good body mechanics is to:
    a. bend from the waist when lifting.
    b. keep your feet close together when lifting.
    c. use the strong muscles of your legs for lifting.
    d. keep the load as far from your body as possible.

11. SDS are required to include information that:
    a. describes how to repackage the product.
    b. explains first aid measures to use if exposure occurs.
    c. describes how to use the product.
    d. lists other approved uses of the product.

12. Leonard Moltke is 77 years old. He becomes confused at night and believes people are in his room. The best approach to help this patient is:
    a. leaving the television on at night.
    b. turning the ceiling light on at night.
    c. leaving the bathroom light on.
    d. telling the patient he is alone.

13. An incident is:
    a. an unexpected occurrence.
    b. an accident that causes injury.
    c. an environmental emergency.
    d. a natural disaster.

14. Water temperature at sinks should not exceed:
    a. 80°F.
    b. 95°F.
    c. 120°F.
    d. 140°F.

15. Concurrent cleaning refers to:
    a. mopping the floor and washing the windows.
    b. keeping drawers and closets neat and clean.
    c. patient responsibilities for keeping their rooms neat.
    d. nursing assistant cleaning responsibilities.

16. A full sharps container should be discarded in the:
    a. biohazardous waste.
    b. housekeeping closet.
    c. utility room.
    d. outside dumpster.

17. Linen and supplies should be stored more than:
    a. 6 inches from the ceiling.
    b. 12 inches from the ceiling.
    c. 18 inches from the ceiling.
    d. 36 inches from the ceiling.

18. Several sparks shot from the wall when another nursing assistant unplugged the portable suction unit. The action you should take is to:
    a. put a lock and tag on it and report that it needs repair.
    b. clean the suction and return it to the patient's room.
    c. put it in an empty room so no one uses it.
    d. return the unit to the utility room.

19. When using a fire extinguisher on a small fire:
    a. aim the water source at the top of the fire and spray.
    b. sweep the hose from side to side at the base of the fire.
    c. push the pin in before beginning. Pull it out stop.
    d. point the hose at the flame and spray in a circular motion.

B. Completion

Choose the correct word from the following list to complete each statement in questions 20–28

body mechanics	mechanical lift
call light	OSHA
ergonomics	RACE
hips and knees	SDS
incident	

20. Using your body correctly while you are working is called _____.

21. Basic rules for lifting include bending from the _____, not from the waist.

22. An unexpected situation that can cause harm to an employee, a patient, or a visitor is called a(n) _____.

23. Adapting the environment and using techniques and equipment to prevent body injury is called _____.

24. You should use a _____ when you need to transfer very heavy or dependent patients.

25. All patients must have access to a _____ because it may be the only way they have to summon help.

26. All manufacturers must supply _____ with the hazardous products they sell.

27. The section of the federal government that oversees employee safety is called _____.

28. The acronym used to remember the sequence of critical actions in case of fire is _____.

C. True/False

Mark the following true or false by circling T or F.

29. T F The bed should be left in the lowest horizontal position when the patient is sleeping.

30. T F Side rails are restraints in certain circumstances.

31. T F There should always be enough light to enable staff to work safely.

32. T F Noise and clutter are very disturbing to most people.

33. T F Needed repairs should be reported immediately.

34. T F The signal cord is the patient's way of letting the staff know that they are in need.

35. T F It is all right to play while at work, as long as no one gets hurt.

36. T F You are responsible for knowing about and practicing fire drill procedures.

37. T F In case of a fire, follow your own plan of action.

38. T F It is wise to use an elevator during a fire emergency.

D. Nursing Assistant Challenge

Mary Hernandez is a new nursing assistant at Community Memorial Hospital. She has just completed her CNA course. Consider the information she needs to receive in orientation to help her be a safe and efficient worker.

39. What information does Mary need to learn about the facility to prevent fires and to follow correct procedures in the event of a fire?

    _____

    _____

40. Mary will need information about the equipment she will be working with. What items of equipment is she likely to be using on her job?

    _____

    _____

41. List two things Mary can do to prevent work-related injuries.

    _____

    _____

42. List two chemicals she is likely to be using.

    _____

    _____

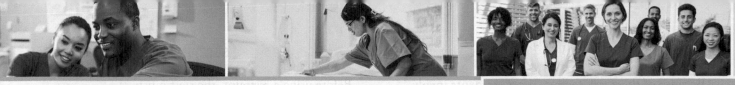

Patient Safety and Positioning

CHAPTER 15

OBJECTIVES

After completing this chapter, you will be able to:

15.1 Spell and define terms.

15.2 Identify patients who are at risk for having incidents.

15.3 List alternatives to the use of physical restraints.

15.4 Describe the guidelines for the use of restraints.

15.5 Demonstrate the correct application of restraints.

15.6 Describe two measures for preventing accidental poisoning, thermal injuries, skin injuries, and choking.

15.7 List the elements that are common to all procedures.

15.8 Describe correct body alignment for the patient.

15.9 List the purposes of repositioning patients.

15.10 State the purpose of assistive moving devices.

15.11 Demonstrate these positions using the correct supportive devices: supine, semisupine, prone, semiprone, lateral, Fowler's, and orthopneic.

15.12 Demonstrate the following procedures:

- Procedure 14: Turning the Patient Toward You
- Procedure 15: Turning the Patient Away from You
- Procedure 16: Moving a Patient to the Head of the Bed (Expand Your Skills)
- Procedure 17: Logrolling the Patient (Expand Your Skills)

VOCABULARY

Learn the meaning and the correct spelling of the following words and phrases:

90-90-90 position	enabler	postural support	slider
ambulate	Fowler's position	pressure injury	spasticity
aspiration	high Fowler's	procedure	splint
body alignment	laceration	prone	supine
caustic	lateral	seclusion	supportive device
chemical restraint	mobility	semi-Fowler's	transfer
coercion	orthopneic position	semiprone	trochanter roll
contracture	orthotic devices (orthoses)	semisupine	turning (moving) sheet
draw sheet	physical restraint	Sims' position	

PATIENT SAFETY

In Chapter 14, you learned how to maintain a safe environment and how to avoid personal injuries. The prevention of patient injuries is another very important part of your job as a nursing assistant. Patients in health care facilities are at risk for incidents because they may:

- Have impaired **mobility** (ability to move about) due to an injury, disease, or surgery
- Be receiving medications that affect mental status, balance, and coordination
- Be disoriented because of the change in environment or because of a medical disorder
- Have impaired hearing or impaired vision

Because of these risk factors, most incidents involving patients in any health care setting are falls. Falls may occur because the patient:

- Misjudges the distance from the bed to the floor
- Is in denial about their ability and does not call for help
- Feels weak or dizzy when trying to get up
- Changes position too rapidly and loses balance when trying to stand up
- Encounters hazards when walking
- Is walking in a poorly lit area

USE OF PHYSICAL RESTRAINTS

In the past, restraints were routinely used to prevent falls. However, many falls occur with side rails up and restraints intact. These injuries are often more severe than they would have been if the restraints had not been in use. Restraint-related accidents can result in serious injury and even death.

There are two types of restraints: chemical restraints and physical restraints. **Chemical restraints** are medications that affect the patient's mood and behavior. As a nursing assistant, you will be more concerned with the use of physical restraints.

A **physical restraint** is any manual method or physical or mechanical device, material, or equipment attached or adjacent to the patient's body that:

- The patient cannot easily remove
- Restricts the patient's movement
- Does not allow the patient normal access to their own body

OBRA (1987) states when and how chemical and physical restraints may be used in a long-term care facility. The Resident's Rights document states that "residents have the right to be free from physical and chemical restraints." According to this definition, many devices qualify as restraints if the resident does not have the physical or mental ability to remove the device readily.

Hospital patients have the right to be free from restraint or **seclusion**, in any form, imposed as a means of **coercion** (force), discipline, convenience, or retaliation by staff. *Seclusion* is separating a patient from others against their will. A patient who unexpectedly becomes violent or aggressive may be restrained as a last resort if the behavior places the patient, staff, or others in imminent danger. However, the restraint must be discontinued at the earliest possible time.

Before using a restraint, the staff must:

- Document why the restraint is needed.
- Document the unsuccessful approaches used to manage the behavior.
- Consult with the patient and/or responsible party when other options are not successful and obtain approval to apply a restraint (Figure 15-1).
- Obtain a physician's order for use of a restraint. Examples of physical restraints include:
- Wrist/arm (Figure 15-5) and ankle/leg restraints
- Vests (Figure 15-6)
- Hand mitts (Figure 15-7)
- Geriatric and cardiac chairs (Figure 15-8)
- Wheelchair safety belts, bars, and tables (Figure 15-9)
- Bed rails (if they meet the definition of a restraint)

Many devices and practices meet the definition of physical restraints if the patient does not have the physical or mental ability to remove the device. Examples of other practices that constitute restraint are:

- Tucking in, tying, or using Velcro to hold a sheet, fabric, or clothing tightly so that a patient's movement is restricted

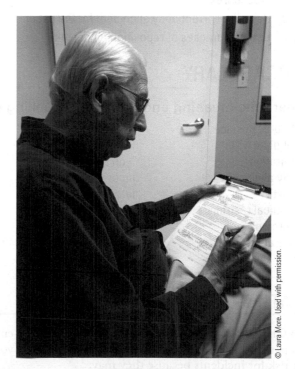

FIGURE 15-1 A responsible family member gives informed consent to apply restraints to the patient.

GUIDELINES 15-1 Guidelines *for* Preventing Patient Falls

- Always leave the bed in its lowest horizontal position when you have finished giving care.

- Keep brakes locked on bed wheels at all times, except when the bed is being moved.

- Check the care plan to see whether the side rails are to be raised.

- Check and adjust protruding objects such as bed wheels or gatch handles (Figure 15-2).

- Do not block or clutter open areas with supplies and equipment.

- Wipe up spills immediately.

- Encourage patients to use the handrails along corridor walls when walking (Figure 15-3).

- Monitor patients for signs of weakness, fatigue, dizziness, and loss of balance.

- Monitor patients for safe practice if they independently:

  - Propel their wheelchairs.

  - **Transfer** (get out of bed).

  - **Ambulate** (walk).

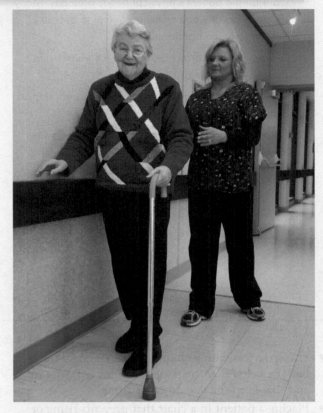

FIGURE 15-3 Encourage patients to hold rails on corridor walls when walking.

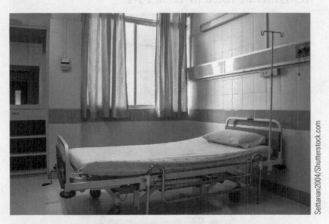

FIGURE 15-2 Medicare furnishes this home health care bed. An electric back and foot are provided. A manual handle is furnished for caregivers to raise and lower the bed.

Settanan2004/Shutterstock.com

- Provide adequate lighting.

- Eliminate noise and other distractions that may increase confusion and create anxiety.

- Avoid leaving patients alone in the tub or shower unless you are given specific permission to do so.

- Check patients' clothing for fit and safety. Loose shoes and laces, long robes, and slacks increase the risk of falling. Footwear should be appropriate for the floor surface. In general, this means using nonskid shoes on tile floor surfaces. For carpeted floors, consult the physical therapist if there is a question about appropriate footwear for the patient. Nonskid shoes may stick to the carpeting, causing falls. A leather or synthetic shoe sole may be more appropriate for a carpeted surface.

(continues)

GUIDELINES 15-1 Guidelines *for* Preventing Patient Falls (continued)

- Care for the patient's physical needs promptly. Many incidents occur when patients attempt to get out of bed to go to the bathroom.
- Always use the correct techniques for transferring and walking patients.
- Use a gait belt when assisting patients to transfer or ambulate (Figure 15-4).
- Follow the care plan when assisting patients with transfers and ambulation.

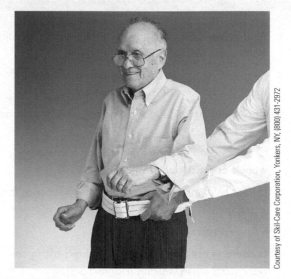

FIGURE 15-4 Use a gait belt to help provide balance and support.

- Using devices with a chair (such as trays, tables, bars, or belts) that the patient cannot remove easily and that keep the patient from rising
- Placing a patient in a chair that prevents rising or positioning a chair or bed close to a wall so the patient cannot get up

Restraints are medical devices. Avoid using them as a form of punishment, or for the convenience of the nursing staff. Take restraint use very seriously. Patients have been seriously injured and died as a result of restraint-related mishaps. Other potential complications of restraints are listed in Table 15-1.

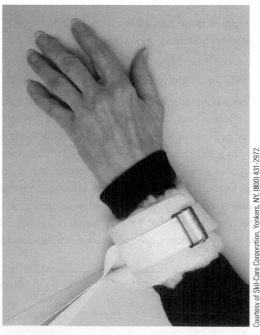

FIGURE 15-5 Wrist restraints may be used to prevent the patient from pulling on IVs and other tubes.

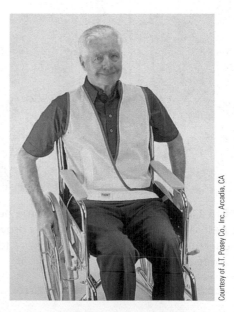

FIGURE 15-6 Vest restraints must be applied as pictured here, with the straps crossed over in front of the patient. Look closely at the strap placement, which is the key to keeping the hips down. The straps are threaded between the seat and the armrests, not through the armrests.

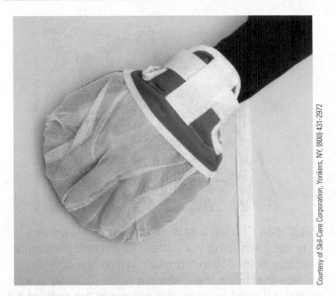

Courtesy of Skil-Care Corporation, Yonkers, NY, (800) 431-2972

FIGURE 15-7 Hand mitts may be applied to prevent the patient from scratching the skin or pulling on tubes.

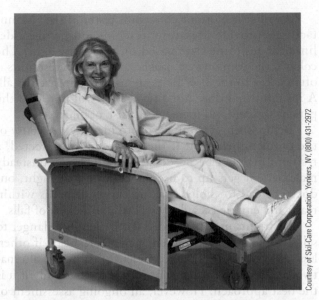

Courtesy of Skil-Care Corporation, Yonkers, NY, (800) 431-2972

FIGURE 15-8 A geriatric chair is a restraint if the patient does not have the ability to get out of the chair. In this case, no tray is being used and the seat is padded for comfort. The patient can stand at will and is not restrained.

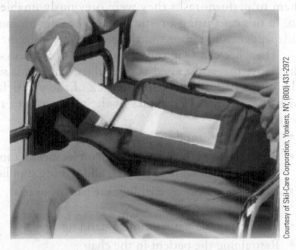

Courtesy of Skil-Care Corporation, Yonkers, NY, (800) 431-2972

FIGURE 15-9 Most wheelchair safety belts are designed to go over the patient's lap, not around the waist. If the patient has the ability to release the Velcro at will, the device is not a restraint.

🔓 Safety ALERT

The vest is a very secure restraint that crosses over in the front. Crossing the vest in the back can cause choking and other serious injury. It is used for patients at high risk of injury. Other similar restraints are pulled over the head. These are called by different names, such as *jacket* or *poncho*, but the principles of application are the same for all three devices. A vest restraint that fits properly, and is applied correctly, will safely and securely hold the patient.

TABLE 15-1 Complications of Restraints

Potential Physical Problems	Potential Psychosocial Problems
Decreased independence	Worsening of behavior
Pressure ulcers	problems
Weakness	Withdrawal, loss of social
Decreased range of motion	contact
Contractures (frozen,	Forgetfulness
deformed joints)	Fear
Loss of ability to walk	Anger
Edema (swelling) of ankles,	Shame
lower legs, feet, fingers	Agitation
Decreased appetite, weight	Mental confusion
loss	Combativeness
Dehydration	Restlessness
Urge to urinate frequently,	Sense of abandonment
dribbling	Frustration
Incontinence	Loss of self-esteem
Urinary tract infection	Depression
Constipation and fecal	Screaming, yelling,
impaction	calling out
Lethargy	
Pain	
Shortness of breath	
Pneumonia	
Bruising, redness, cuts,	
skin tears	
Falls	
Impaired circulation	
Blood clots	
Choking	
Death	

Another important concern is restraint size. Manufacturers provide literature, teaching aids, and guidelines for restraint size, based on patient weight. The color of the trim on vest, jacket, and poncho restraints is often a key to the size. Belts are usually one size fits all. A restraint that does not fit correctly will not hold the patient securely and increases the risk of injury.

Before using restraints, try to identify the cause of the problem behavior. If the cause can be corrected, a restraint may not be needed. For example, an unsteady male patient gets up to use the bathroom at night, but does not call for help. Making sure a urinal is within reach and emptied regularly will reduce the risk of falls.

Restraints may be needed if a patient is a danger to self or others or needs emergency medical care if other, less restrictive options are considered first. Many alternatives are available. A restraint should be used only if it is the best approach. However, an ongoing assessment of need is necessary, and personnel must work to reduce or eliminate the restraint.

 Safety ALERT

The wheelchair is an important piece of medical equipment in all health care facilities. Patients come in many shapes and sizes. Because of this, wheelchairs come in many sizes, and various accessories are available to meet medical needs. Attention to wheelchair size is important for comfort and safety. Restraints are sometimes used because the wheelchair does not fit the patient! Using a chair that fits properly often eliminates the need for restraints. You will find information about wheelchair size and safety in Chapter 17. Always consider the type and size of the wheelchair you are using when considering whether a restraint is needed.

If restraints are needed, the least restrictive restraint should be used for the least amount of time possible. The patient must be assessed after one hour by a nurse who is qualified to do this evaluation.

Using restraints requires careful application of the nursing process. A physician's order is needed. The care plan will describe the type of restraint to use, the time the restraint is to be applied, frequency of visual checks, and frequency of restraint release.

Enablers

Enablers are devices that help patients function at their highest possible level. For example, a patient in a wheelchair cannot sit up straight, so they are fed by staff. A supportive device that corrects their posture and allows them to feed themselves is an enabler. Enablers that maintain body position and alignment are commonly

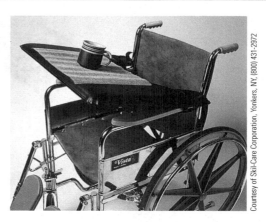

FIGURE 15-10 The lap tray is an enabler if it improves function, permitting the patient to eat independently. This tray is lined with a gripper, which is a nonslip surface that holds the dishes in place. The tray is a restraint if used to keep the patient in the chair and if it cannot be removed without assistance.

called **postural supports**. Used correctly, they give patients a higher degree of independence and enable them to perform tasks they were previously unable to do. In this case, using a restraint as an enabler promotes independence and improves the patient's self-esteem.

The wheelchair lap tray (Figure 15-10) is a restraint alternative that is also used as an enabler. The tray is simple to use: it is attached to the back of the wheelchair with Velcro straps. Examples of the many uses of this device are:

- Providing postural support
- Allowing patients to lean on it, and its surface can hold personal items or reading and writing supplies
- Moving food closer, enabling the patient to feed themselves
- Reminding the patient not to stand up
- Restraining the patient in the chair

If the tray promotes independence, it is an enabler. If it is used strictly to keep the patient in the chair, and the patient does not have the physical or mental ability to remove the tray, it is a restraint. If the patient can remove the tray, it is a restraint alternative.

SIDE RAILS AS RESTRAINTS

By definition, side rails are restraints. They can also be an enabler. Each facility sets criteria for side rail use. For example, some facilities consider the use of three half-rails an enabler, and four rails a restraint. (Refer to Figures 14-4, 14-8, and 14-9.) Many patients pull on rails to position and turn themselves in bed. Some feel more secure if the rails are up. Side rails must always be raised when patients are restrained in bed. In most facilities side rails may be raised only if requested by the patient or if an assessment reveals that the risk in use of side rails poses less danger than other interventions. The facility must continue to monitor for negative effects of side rail use and try to eliminate the rail use. In addition, patients must be monitored frequently for safety when side rails are used.

Side rails increase the risk of injury from both falls and entrapment. Up to 54 percent of all falls from bed occur over the elevated side rails. This is a common cause of hip fractures in confused elderly patients. When a patient climbs over the rails, they fall from a much greater height than they would from just the mattress. If the patient is wearing a restraint, they may be suspended in the air as the restraint tightens, resulting in suffocation. Leaving the restraint off and rails down may be a much safer alternative. Alarms are available that sound if the patient attempts to get up.

Entrapment

When side rails are used, it is important to check the space between the rail and the mattress. Hospital beds are permanent pieces of equipment that are used for years. Mattresses wear out and are replaced. There have been cases of injury and death in which patients became trapped between the mattress and side rails because the replacement mattress was not the same size as the original. Patients at high risk for entrapment include those with conditions such as confusion, restlessness, lack of muscle control, or a combination of these factors. Make sure that the gap between the mattress and the side rail is not large enough to cause injury. Figure 15-11 shows areas of potential entrapment.

Gaps between the mattress and bed frame or rails can also be caused by movement or compression of the mattress due to patient weight, movement, or bed position. This is a common problem with patients using low air loss mattresses (see Chapter 23) for pressure injury treatment. If you observe a gap that is wide enough to entrap a patient's head or body part, inform the nurse promptly. Another bed can be used or the mattress modified (Figure 15-12A) to prevent injury.

The nursing orders often specify the use of padded side rails for patients with seizure disorder, persons with some neurologic conditions, and those who are taking high doses of blood-thinning medication. In addition, patients who are at risk for climbing through the side rails may have orders for side rail padding. Bath blankets may be wrapped around the rails as a temporary measure, but these are easily pulled off and may worsen the patients' agitation because they cannot see through the bars. Using a commercial side rail pad (Figure 15-12B) is a good solution to the problem, if they are available in your facility. The pad is thicker than a bath blanket, and the patient can look through the space.

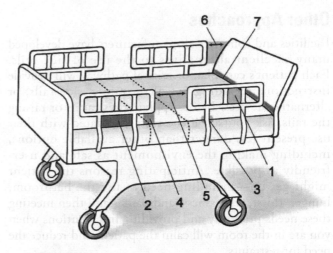

Courtesy of U.S. Food and Drug Administration

FIGURE 15-11 Seven zones of entrapment have been identified:

Zone 1: within the rail

Zone 2: between the top of the compressed mattress and the bottom of the rail, between the rail supports

Zone 3: between the rail and the mattress

Zone 4: between the top of the compressed mattress and the bottom of the rail, at the end of the rail

Zone 5: between the split bed rails

Zone 6: between the end of the rail and the side edge of the headboard or footboard

Zone 7: between the headboard or footboard and the mattress end

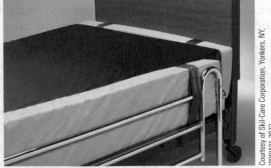

Courtesy of Skil-Care Corporation, Yonkers, NY, (800)431-2972

FIGURE 15-12A The mattress can be modified to fit the bed and decrease the risk of injury.

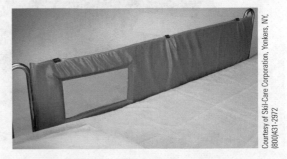

Courtesy of Skil-Care Corporation, Yonkers, NY, (800)431-2972

FIGURE 15-12B Padded side rails are a good safety feature for patients with seizure disorder, as well as those who might climb through the rail to get out of bed.

Other Approaches

Facilities and commercial manufacturers have developed many excellent alternatives to the use of side rails. Each patient's care plan or critical pathway will provide instructions regarding use of restraints, side rails, or alternative devices. Before applying restraints or raising the rails, ask yourself if the risks associated with their use present less danger than other available options, including making the environment as safe and user-friendly as possible. Anticipating reasons the patient might get up—including need to use the bathroom, hunger, thirst, restlessness, and pain—and then meeting these needs promptly and providing interventions when you are in the room will calm the patient and reduce the need for restraints.

Other possible alternatives to the use of side rails are:

- Keeping the bed in the lowest possible position with the wheels locked
- Using beds that can be raised and lowered close to the floor
- Placing mats on the floor next to the bed so that if a fall occurs, the patient will fall on a padded surface instead of the hard floor
- Using side rail bolster cushions
- Using pressure-sensitive bed and chair alarms that sound when a patient attempts to get up (Figure 15-13)

Some self-release belts sound an alarm immediately when the closure is released, to alert staff before the patient gets out of the chair or bed. Some pressure-sensitive mats can be placed on the floor next to the bed to sound an alarm if the patient's feet touch the surface.

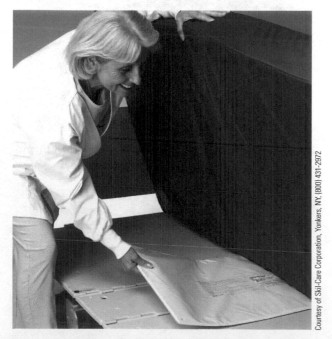

FIGURE 15-13 Many different pressure-sensitive pads are available. When the patient attempts to stand, an alarm sounds.

Each health care facility has policies addressing when side rails may be used. Know and follow your facility's policies.

Applying Restraints in Bed

When applying wrist, vest, poncho, jacket, or belt restraints to a patient in bed:

- Center the patient's hips in the middle of the bed. This is where the bed bends when the head is elevated.
- Make sure that when extended over the edge of the mattress, the straps are not at an angle. If the straps are angled even slightly, they will loosen if the patient moves up or down in bed.
- Wrap the strap around the frame deck (the movable part of the frame that supports the mattress) once or twice.
- Never wrap the strap around the lower frame, or the restraint will tighten and inhibit respiration when the head of the bed is elevated. Never tie the end of the strap to the outside of the frame where the patient can reach it.
- Loop the strap around itself again and tighten to form a slip knot.
- Always raise the side rails when the patient is restrained in bed. Never fasten the straps to the side rails or loop or wrap the straps around the side rails.

ALTERNATIVES TO RESTRAINTS

Alternatives to restraints should be tried before restraints are applied. Nursing assistants can take a number of actions to help reduce the need to use restraints:

- Care for patients' personal needs promptly.
- Take patients to the bathroom regularly.
- Provide adequate food and fluids to prevent hunger and thirst.
- Report signs and symptoms of pain or illness promptly.
- Follow all instructions for positioning and for assisting patients with exercise.
- Be sure that patients have their eyeglasses and hearing aids, if used.
- Answer call signals promptly.
- Check patients often to see if they need anything.
- Provide appropriate exercise and activities.
- Know which patients are at risk for falling. Monitor these patients regularly.
- Observe patients who walk and transfer independently. Sometimes falls occur because patients use incorrect and unsafe methods. Report these situations and learn how to teach patients the correct way.

Courtesy of Skil-Care Corporation, Yonkers, NY, (800) 431-2972

Safety ALERT

When applying restraints to a patient in a chair, make sure the patient's hips are all the way back on the seat. Most restraints are designed to keep the hips down. The straps are usually inserted between the seat frame and the armrest. A common mistake is threading the straps through the armrest. Patients in wheelchairs frequently try to stand or slide their hips toward the front of the seat while restrained, causing injury. Threading the straps through the armrest places the restraint straps around the abdomen and fails to keep the hips down. If the patient attempts to stand or slides forward, the chair may tip, or another injury may occur. Attention to the manufacturer's directions for strap placement in the wheelchair is very important for preventing injuries.

- Report any physical or mental change that could increase the risk of an incident, such as:
  - Disorientation (patient does not know time, place, or self)
  - Complaints of dizziness
  - Problems with balance and coordination
- Maintain a safe, quiet, calm environment.
- Provide comfortable chairs with arms. Use supportive devices as necessary.
- Apply a security device with an alarm to alert you if the patient stands. Devices are also available that set off an alarm when a wanderer tries to leave the unit or building.

Many commercial devices are available to use in place of restraints. Sometimes clothing or other items can be used as restraint alternatives. For example, a male patient who pulls at his urinary catheter can be fitted with boxer shorts. A patient with a feeding tube in the abdomen can be covered with a T-shirt or abdominal binder (see Chapter 29). A patient with an intravenous infusion in the arm can wear a long-sleeved shirt or a tube sock with the foot cut off. Covering the medical

device may be all that is necessary to keep the patient from pulling on it. Previously, wrist restraints would have been used to keep the patient from dislodging tubes. Giving the patient something to hold, such as a foam ball or gel pad (Figure 15-14), will occupy the hands and serve as a distraction.

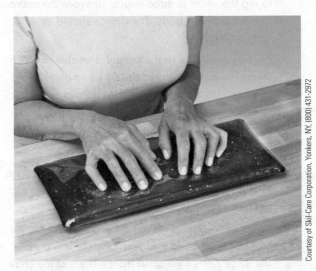

Courtesy of Skil-Care Corporation, Yonkers, NY, (800) 431-2972

FIGURE 15-14 A gel mat is a nice distraction that keeps the hands busy and maintains flexibility of the fingers.

Legal ALERT

The law is very clear regarding the use of restraints. It specifies that restraints must be applied according to manufacturers' directions. Each manufacturer determines the best way to apply its restraints. The directions for restraint application are sent to the government, which approves the instructions. There are many restraint manufacturers, so you must become familiar with the directions for applying the type of restraints used in your facility. You must also consider the size of the restraint. Restraints come in different sizes. Each manufacturer lists weight and size guidelines for its restraints. Some restraints have color-coded trim so you can tell the size at a glance. Using a restraint that does not fit correctly is dangerous.

GUIDELINES 15-2 Guidelines for the Use of Restraints

There are a few situations in which a patient may need a restraint, no matter how many alternatives are tried. When restraints are necessary, follow these guidelines:

- Be sure the nurse has instructed you on how to apply the device properly and has obtained a physician's order.

- Try the least restrictive device first.
- Use the right type and size of restraint. Apply it according to the manufacturer's directions.
- Check the device before use—do not use if it is frayed, is torn, has parts missing, or is soiled. Never apply a restraint next to bare skin. Make sure the breasts are not under the strap of the restraint.

(continues)

GUIDELINES 15-2 Guidelines for the Use of Restraints (continued)

- Always explain what you are doing, even if the patient does not seem to understand. After application, check the fit of the device. You should be able to slip the width of three fingers between the restraint and the patient's body. The device should never restrict breathing.

- Position the straps so the patient is unable to reach them. The restraint straps should be smooth. Avoid twisting. Pad the restraint if necessary to prevent irritation to the skin.

- Tie restraint straps with slip knots for quick release in an emergency.

- Make sure the patient has access to the signal light. Visually check every 15 minutes for the patient's comfort and safety. Make changes as needed.

- When the patient is restrained in a wheelchair, the brakes should be locked when the chair is parked. The large part of the small front wheels of the chair should face forward (Figure 15-15). This changes the center of gravity, making the chair more stable and less likely to tip.

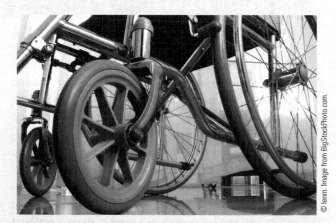

FIGURE 15-15 The large part of the small front wheels should face forward during transfers and whenever the chair is parked, to maintain the center of gravity and prevent tipping.

- Release the restraint at least every two hours (or more often) for at least 10 minutes to:
  - Check for irritation or poor circulation.
  - Change the patient's position.
  - Exercise—ambulate the patient or do passive range-of-motion exercises.
  - Take the patient to the bathroom.
  - Change incontinent patients and cleanse their skin.
  - Provide meals, fluid, or nourishment.
  - Attend to any other needs.
  - Document each of these actions.

- Maintain good body alignment whether the patient is in bed or a chair.

- When restraints are used in bed:
  - There must be full side rails on the bed, and they must be raised.
  - Position the patient in the middle of the mattress.
  - Always secure the restraint to the movable (upper) part of the bed frame so the restraint moves when the head of the bed is raised and lowered.

- Do not use medical restraints in moving vehicles or on toilets unless you are sure the device is intended for that use by the manufacturer. (This does not apply to safety restraints and seat belts that are part of the vehicle. Follow state laws.)

- Make sure the wheelchair is secured any time it is in a moving vehicle. As a rule, the frame of the wheelchair is fastened to the floor of the vehicle well near each wheel so the wheelchair cannot tip over. The person's upper body must also be secured so it does not lunge forward or shift to the side when the driver turns or applies the brakes. The shoulder harness for the vehicle will not hold the upper body of a person in a wheelchair securely. A separate device is needed for the wheelchair. This is also a safety device, not a restraint. It can be removed as soon as the person exits the vehicle.

Nursing Assistant Observations

The nursing assistant plays an important role in knowing the patient's needs and making recommendations for restraint alternatives. Making sure the patient is in touch with their environment reduces agitation and confusion. Other observations that will help eliminate the need for restraints are:

- Make sure the patient sees and hears well. If they wear eyeglasses, make sure they are clean. If they use a hearing aid, make sure it works. Check to make sure the ears are not plugged with wax. Behavior problems, balance problems, and other safety concerns may arise because the patient is out of touch with the environment. Correcting these problems may eliminate the need for a restraint.

- Be sure the person's needs are met, such as hunger, thirst, pain, or need to use the bathroom. Discovering the unmet need and meeting it may help you avoid using a restraint.
- Monitor the noise in the environment. Eliminating or reducing the noise may stop the problem behavior.
- Look for a pattern in the behavior, such as whether it occurs at a certain time of day, during a certain activity, or when a specific person is providing care.
- Boredom, loneliness, or looking for a misplaced item can cause unsafe behavior.
- If the patient tries to get out of bed or chair without help, they may benefit from an alarm. Be sure the call signal and other needed items are available.
- If you observe a condition that causes confusion or agitation, or discover an approach that is effective, inform the nurse.

PREVENTION OF OTHER INCIDENTS

Many situations can result in an incident that may harm the patient. Some incidents can be prevented when all staff members practice safety and are aware of appropriate preventive measures.

Accidental Poisoning

Common items, such as household chemicals, shaving lotion, plants, and cologne, are poisonous if ingested. Items such as denture tablets, some shampoos, and many cleaning products are **caustic**, or capable of burning living tissue, including skin, mucous membranes, and internal organs. Food kept in a bedside table may spoil and cause illness. Patients with poor vision and those who are disoriented may eat or drink any of these items. To prevent accidental poisonings:

- Keep all chemicals and cleaning solutions in locked cupboards.
- Do not store food in the same cabinet or refrigerator with chemicals or medications.
- Store patients' personal food items in the refrigerator in labeled, dated containers.
- Learn which personal care products are potentially harmful, such as denture cleaning tablets and some shampoos. Store these items in locked cupboards where high-risk patients cannot access them.
- Make sure products are clearly labeled.

Thermal Injuries

Thermal injuries are those caused by heat, cold, chemicals, or electricity; they result in burns (Figure 15-16). To prevent thermal injuries:

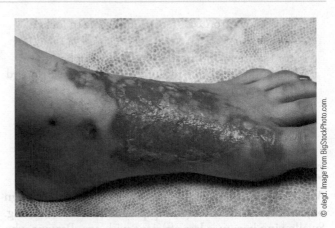

FIGURE 15-16 This burn was caused by dropping a hot container on the foot.

- Follow procedures accurately when administering warm or cold treatments.
- Check water temperatures before helping a patient into the bathtub or shower. Turn the hot water on last and turn it off first.
- Check food temperatures before feeding patients. Using a microwave oven to reheat food can be dangerous because of the uneven temperatures the oven produces.
- If smoking is permitted, store smoking materials in a safe place and supervise patients while they smoke.
- Monitor the temperature of heat treatments and other warm patient care supplies, such as bag bath, shampoo caps, and electrical appliances such as an aquathermia pad.

Skin Injuries

Skin injuries include **lacerations** (tears or breaks in the skin) and punctures (Figure 15-17). To prevent these injuries:

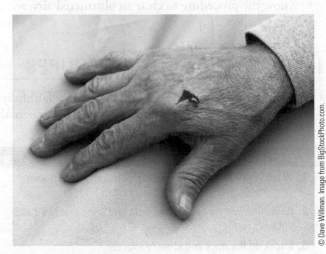

FIGURE 15-17 This patient has thin, fragile skin. The hand was lacerated by bumping it on the corner of a table.

- Store knives, scissors, razors, and tools in locked cupboards.
- Store syringes and needles in locked cupboards. These should not be recapped and must be disposed of in a sharps container immediately after use.
- Clean up broken glass immediately.
- Protect fragile skin with clothing, if possible.

Choking

Aspiration is the accidental entry of food or a foreign object into the trachea (windpipe). This causes choking. Swallowing becomes less efficient with age. Persons who are elderly, persons with impaired consciousness, persons who are disoriented and confused, and those with certain medical and neuromuscular conditions are at very high risk for aspiration and choking. To prevent aspiration and choking:

- Be aware of which patients have swallowing problems. Follow all instructions when helping with feeding:
  - Cut food into small pieces.
  - Feed slowly.
  - Offer fluids carefully between solid foods.
  - If the patient has had a stroke, place the food in the unaffected side of the mouth.
  - Use thickeners for liquids if ordered.
- Place patients upright in good body alignment before meals. Have them remain in this position for at least 30 to 60 minutes after eating.
- At the end of the meal, give oral care to patients who are known to keep food in their mouths. Food may remain in the mouth for several minutes after a meal and be accidentally aspirated if the patient coughs or goes to sleep.
- Refer to Chapter 26 for the care of patients with swallowing problems.
- Know the procedure to clear an obstructed airway. (See Chapter 26.)

INTRODUCTION TO PROCEDURES

Caring for patients safely means that you must faithfully and carefully carry out certain routines. The normal manner of carrying out a task is called a **procedure**. *Procedures* are the practices and processes used when following facility policies in patient care. The procedure lists your responsibilities when doing the task.

As you progress in your studies, you will learn the procedures for many nursing assistant tasks. You have already been introduced to the procedures for washing your hands and using PPE. The procedures that follow give you step-by-step directions for carrying out tasks that involve patients.

Certain things must be done before you begin patient care procedures. These actions are called *preprocedure* or *initial procedure actions*. At the end of each patient care procedure, you will carry out a standard series of *ending procedure (procedure completion) actions*.

COMMON STEPS IN ALL PROCEDURES

Certain steps are performed at the beginning and end of all nursing procedures. These are important and should not be omitted. Perform the steps in order, as appropriate to the patient and the procedure. This book calls these steps *initial procedure actions* and *ending procedure actions*.

Initial Procedure Actions

Perform these steps, in order, at the beginning of every procedure.

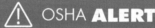

> ⚠ OSHA **ALERT**
>
> Some health care facilities require staff to wear gloves for all contacts with patients or their bed linens, even if contact is brief. If this is your facility's policy, apply gloves immediately upon entering the room and washing your hands (or cleansing with an alcohol-based product). Change gloves before and after exposure to blood, body fluid, secretions, excretions, mucous membranes, and nonintact skin. Remove gloves as soon as you have finished touching the patient or potentially contaminated items. Avoid touching clean items and environmental surfaces with used gloves.

Initial Procedure Action	Rationale
1. Wash your hands or use an alcohol-based hand cleaner.	Applies the principles of standard precautions. Prevents the spread of microbes and reduces the risk of cross-contamination.
2. Assemble supplies and equipment and bring them to the patient's room.	Improves efficiency, organizes your time, and ensures that you do not have to leave the room.
3. Knock on the door and identify yourself.	Respects the patient's right to privacy. Informs the patient who is giving care.

(continues)

Initial Procedure Action	Rationale
4. Identify the patient according to facility policy. Some facilities identify people via arm bands. Some ask the patient to recite their date of birth.	Ensures that you are caring for the correct patient.
5. Ask visitors to leave the room and advise where they may wait (as desired by the patient).	Respects the patient's right to privacy. Shows respect and courtesy to visitors.
6. Explain what you are going to do and what is expected of the patient. Answer questions. (Maintain a dialogue with the patient during the procedure, and repeat explanations and instructions as needed.)	Informs the patient of what is going to be done and what to expect. Provides information about the procedure and shows respect.
7. Provide privacy by closing the door, privacy curtain, and window curtain. (All three should be closed even if the patient is alone in the room during the procedure.)	Respects the patient's right to privacy. Protects modesty and dignity.
8. Wash your hands or use an alcohol-based hand cleaner.	Applies the principles of standard precautions. Prevents the spread of microbes and reduces the risk of cross-contamination.
9. Set up supplies and equipment at the bedside. (Use an over-bed table, if possible, or other clean area. Cover with a clean underpad, according to nursing judgment, to provide a clean work surface.) Open packages. Position items within convenient reach. Position a container for soiled items so that you do not have to cross over clean items to access it.	Prepares for the procedure and helps organize time. Ensures that equipment and supplies are conveniently positioned and readily available. Reduces the risk of cross-contamination.
10. Wash your hands or use an alcohol-based hand cleaner.	Applies the principles of standard precautions. Prevents the spread of microbes and reduces the risk of cross-contamination.
11. Position the patient for the procedure. Support with pillows and props as needed. Place a clean underpad under the area being treated, as needed. Make sure the patient is comfortable and able to maintain the position throughout the procedure.	Ensures that the patient is in the correct anatomic position for the procedure. Ensures that the patient is supported, is comfortable, and can maintain the position for the duration of the procedure.
12. Cover the patient with a bath blanket and drape for modesty. Fold the bath blanket back to expose only the area on which you will be working.	Respects the patient's modesty and dignity. Ensures that the patient is warm and comfortable. (This step is essential even if the door, window, and privacy curtains are closed.)
13. Raise the bed to a comfortable working height.	Prevents back strain and injury caused by bending at the waist.
14. Lock the wheels of the bed, stretcher, etc., if used during the procedure.	Prevents patient and caregiver falls and injuries.
15. Apply gloves if contact with blood, moist body fluids (except sweat), secretions, excretions, or nonintact skin is likely.	Applies the principles of standard precautions. Protects the assistant and patient from transfer of pathogens.
16. Apply a gown if your uniform will have substantial contact with linens or other articles contaminated with blood, moist body fluids (except sweat), secretions, or excretions.	Applies the principles of standard precautions. Protects your uniform and skin from contamination with bloodborne pathogens.
17. Apply a mask and eye protection if splashing of blood or moist body fluids is likely.	Applies the principles of standard precautions. Protects the assistant's skin, mucous membranes, and uniform from accidental splashing of bloodborne pathogens.
18. Lower the side rail on the side where you will be working.	Provides an obstacle-free area in which to work.

Ending Procedure Actions

Perform these steps, in order, upon completion of each procedure.

Ending Procedure Action	Rationale
1. Remove gloves.	Prevents contamination of the patient, the environment, and clean supplies from used gloves.
2. Reposition the patient to ensure that they are comfortable and in good body alignment.	All body systems function better when the body is correctly aligned. The patient is more comfortable when the body is in good alignment.

(continues)

Ending Procedure Action	Rationale
3. Replace the bed covers, then remove any drapes used. Place used drapes in a plastic bag to discard in trash or in soiled linen receptacle.	Provides warmth and security. Contains linen and drapes that have been contaminated during the procedure.
4. Elevate the side rails, if used, before leaving the bedside.	Prevents contamination of the side rail from gloves. Ensures patient safety. Prevents falls, accidents, and injuries.
5. Remove other personal protective equipment, if worn, and discard in a plastic bag or according to facility policy.	Prevents contamination of the patient, the environment, and clean supplies by used PPE.
6. Wash your hands or use an alcohol-based hand cleaner.	Applies the principles of standard precautions. Prevents the spread of microbes and reduces the risk of cross-contamination.
7. Return the bed to the lowest horizontal position.	Respects patient's right to a safe environment. Ensures patient safety. Prevents falls, accidents, and injuries.
8. Open the privacy and window curtains.	Privacy is no longer necessary unless preferred by the patient.
9. Position the call signal and needed personal items within reach.	Prevents accidents and injuries. Gives the patient a sense of security by ensuring that help is available. Provides for patient convenience. Eliminates the need to call out or reach for needed personal items (which could result in a fall).
10. Wash your hands or use an alcohol-based hand cleaner.	Applies the principles of standard precautions. Prevents the spread of microbes and reduces the risk of cross-contamination. (Although the hands were washed previously, they have contacted the patient and other items in the room. Washing them again before leaving prevents potential transfer of microbes to other patients, equipment, and surfaces outside the patient's unit.)
11. Remove procedural trash and contaminated linens when you leave the room. Discard in appropriate container or location.	Applies the principles of standard precautions. Prevents the spread of microbes and reduces the risk of cross-contamination.
12. Inform visitors that they may return to the room.	Shows respect, courtesy, and hospitality to visitors and patient.
13. Document the procedure, your observations, and the patient's response.	Provides a legal record of ongoing progress and care. Provides a record of what has been done and observations of the patient's condition. Serves as a vehicle for communication with other members of the interdisciplinary team.

So much handwashing may seem unnecessary, because of the short length of time that you are with the patient. Just remember that your hands can transmit germs. Patients already weakened by disease have a much lower resistance to germs. The risk of exposure to pathogens is much greater in health care facilities than it is in a home environment.

Because the initial procedure and ending procedure actions are the same for each patient care procedure, they are not restated in this book as individual steps with each procedure. Rather, a general reference is made to these steps at the beginning and end of each procedure. You must, however, learn and faithfully complete each of these steps for each patient care procedure you perform.

BODY MECHANICS FOR THE PATIENT

Body mechanics for the patient are very similar to those for the health care worker. Good posture for the patient means that moving in bed, getting out of bed, standing, and walking are done safely, with the body in good alignment.

Communication Highlight

Communicate with the patient throughout the procedure. Whenever possible, use age-appropriate terms and explanations. Talk to the patient even if they are young, are confused, may not understand, or cannot communicate verbally. Use gestures and body language to demonstrate, whenever possible. Make sure your terminology is also age-appropriate. For example, do not call an incontinent brief a *diaper*. Use the term *brief* instead. Continue to talk and smile throughout the procedure, regardless of the patient's age or level of understanding. This is important for the patient's well-being, and shows that you care. Remember that you also communicate with touch. Handle the patient gently to prevent injury and communicate caring.

Persons who are bedfast sometimes find it hard to stay in a desired position; they tend to slide toward the foot of the bed when the head of the bed is elevated (Figure 15-18). Patients who are dependent are not able

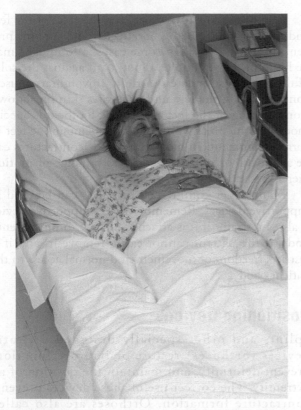

FIGURE 15-18 Patients frequently slide down in bed, causing poor body alignment and increasing the risk for injuries to the skin caused by friction and shearing.

to change their position. These patients need extra help to gain and maintain proper alignment. Remember to:

- Get help.
- Use turning or lifting sheets.
- Change the patient's position frequently, at least every two hours. Some people need more frequent positioning due to pain or musculoskeletal conditions. Reposition them if they ask and do not make them wait. Avoid creating friction (e.g., by dragging the patient's heels across the sheets). Elevate knees to reduce sliding.

Body Alignment and Positioning

Body alignment refers to a position in which the body can properly function. Patients who are weak, have impaired consciousness, are disoriented, have contractures and certain other medical conditions, or are in pain have problems keeping good alignment. Body alignment is maintained by moving, turning, and positioning the patient in a manner that:

- Helps the patient feel more comfortable
- Relieves strain
- Helps the body function more efficiently
- Prevents complications like contractures and pressure injuries

Complications of Incorrect Positioning

Complications can occur when body alignment is not maintained or when the patient's position is not changed often enough. The two most common complications are pressure injuries and contractures. **Pressure injuries** (bedsores) result when unrelieved pressure interferes with blood flow to an area. Pressure injuries are dangerous, painful, and expensive to treat. (These are discussed in Chapter 38.) **Contractures** occur when a joint is allowed to remain in the same position for too long (Figure 15-19). The muscles stiffen and shorten (atrophy), preventing the joint from moving fully. The joint becomes fixed in a bent position (position of flexion). Contractures are painful, are permanent, and interfere with mobility and independence with care.

Contractures can begin to develop within as few as four days of immobility and inactivity. After approximately 15 days, the patient loses the ability to move the joint freely. Contractures interfere with the patient's ability to move, complicate all nursing care, and interfere with proper positioning. They reduce blood flow to the joints, promoting the development of pressure injuries and making treatment of existing pressure injuries difficult. Voluntary movement of the joint becomes impossible as the contracture worsens. Contractures can be prevented, and some can be reversed, with proper care. (Additional preventive measures for contractures are discussed in Chapter 41.)

Supportive Devices

Supportive devices are used to maintain proper body alignment and position in bed or in a chair. Supportive devices include:

- Pillows and/or folded sheets, bath blankets, foam, wedges, or mattress pads to support the trunk and extremities

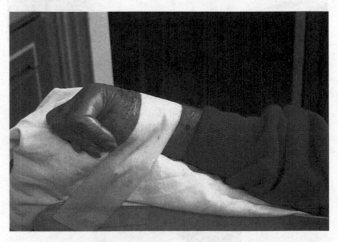

FIGURE 15-19 Contractures develop when joints are allowed to remain in the same position for too long. A contracture begins to develop within four days of immobility. Contractures are very difficult to reverse.

- Special boots or shoes that are worn in bed to keep the feet in alignment (Figure 15-20A)
- Bed cradles, which prevent pressure on the feet from the bed covers (Figure 15-20B)
- Footboards to maintain foot alignment (Figure 15-20C)

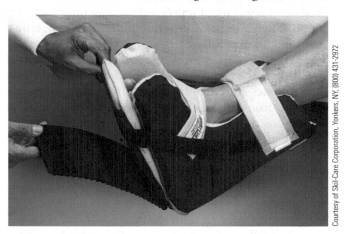

Courtesy of Skil-Care Corporation, Yonkers, NY, (800) 431-2972

FIGURE 15-20A Special boots will maintain the ankles and feet in good alignment. The boot prevents contractures of the feet and reduces friction and shearing of the skin upon movement.

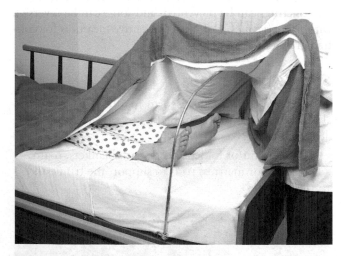

FIGURE 15-20B The weight of the bedding pushes the toes downward, increasing the risk for contractures. Patients with certain skin conditions also need to keep the bedding off the skin. Bed cradles elevate the bedding so it does not contact the patient's body.

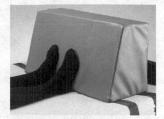

FIGURE 15-20C Supporting the feet maintains good alignment and prevents foot drop.

A folded pillow placed between the soles of the feet and the foot of the bed is an effective measure for preventing contractures. In some cases, a footboard may be harmful. For example, a footboard against the soles of the feet can stimulate **spasticity** (involuntary muscle contraction) in the legs and promotes skin breakdown from rubbing of the feet against the footboard. Special shoes are sometimes worn in bed to maintain the feet in correct alignment. In most cases, ankle contractures can be avoided by regularly doing passive range-of-motion exercises (see Chapter 41).

Many other commercial products can be used as supportive devices. Remember that a supportive device is also a restraint if it is attached or next to the patient's body, if the patient cannot easily remove it, and if it restricts freedom of movement and normal access to the patient's body.

Positioning Devices

Splints and other specially designed **orthotic devices (orthoses)** restore or improve function, prevent deformity, and maintain the position of an extremity. The correct use of these devices prevents contracture formation. Orthoses are also called **splints**. Figure 15-21A shows examples of orthoses for the upper extremities. The physician may also order splints or orthoses for the lower extremities. A common type is called the *ankle foot orthosis (AFO)*. The AFO provides support for an unstable ankle and helps reduce extensor spasticity (Figure 15-21B).

Patient Independence

You are responsible for ensuring that patients maintain independence whenever possible. The skills used in bed mobility form the foundation for many other activities. Observations to make and report about bed mobility are listed in Table 15-2.

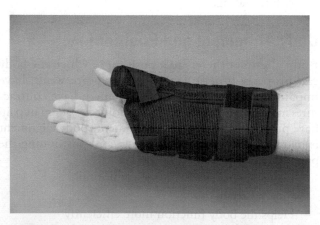

FIGURE 15-21A A wrist splint is used for treating many musculoskeletal conditions.

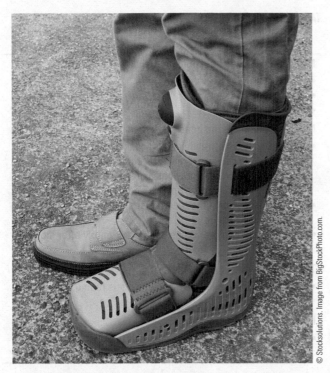

FIGURE 15-21B This AFO stabilizes an injury of the foot and ankle.

© Stocksolutions. Image from BigStockPhoto.com.

Basic Body Positions

There are four basic positions, with variations of each one. These are:

- **Prone** (on the abdomen), with a variation of **semiprone**
- **Supine** (on the back), with a variation of **semisupine**
- **Lateral** (on either side), with a variation of **Sims' position**
- **Fowler's position**, with variations of **high Fowler's**, **semi-Fowler's**, and **orthopneic position**

Changing a patient's position involves these steps:

TABLE 15-2 Observations to Make and Report About Movement, Bed Mobility, and Positioning

- Ability to position/reposition self
- Need for staff to reposition
- Special positioning aids
- Ability to move unassisted
- Presence of contractures
- Able/unable to move
- Movements shaky, jerking, tremors, muscle spasms, etc.
- Presence or absence of pain upon movement
- Deformity, edema
- Normal or abnormal range of motion
- Ability to sit, stand, move
- Paralysis in one or more extremities (hemiplegia, paraplegia, tetraplegia (quadriplegia), diplegia, etc.
- Need for side rails, trapeze, bed ladder, or other adjunct to enhance ability to move independently
- Need for pillows, props, or other device to maintain position
- Has contraindications/no contraindications for turning surfaces, such as pressure ulcer, stroke, operative site, etc.
- Cooperates/does not cooperate with positioning and maintaining position

1. Moving the patient into proper body alignment. You may have to move the patient up in bed or to one side of the bed. If the patient will be positioned on their left side, move them to the right side of the bed. If the patient will be positioned on their right side, move them to the left side of the bed. This ensures that they will not be too close to the edge of the bed after they are turned.

2. Turning the patient onto the back, onto the abdomen, or to the side.

3. Placing the patient's trunk and extremities in proper position and maintaining alignment with the use of supportive devices.

GUIDELINES 15-3 Guidelines for the Use of Splints

- The splint must be applied correctly. Follow the manufacturer's directions for each type of splint.
- Follow the care plan for the patient's wearing schedule.
- Keep the extremity that is under the splint clean and dry.

- If the splint becomes soiled, check with the nurse to see how it should be cleaned.
- Check the skin under the splint regularly for signs of redness, irritation, and skin breakdown.

MOVING AND LIFTING PATIENTS

Lifting, moving, and transporting patients is a major responsibility of the nursing assistant. Using proper body mechanics and following safety rules will protect both you and your patients from injury. *Always* find out whether help is needed to move a patient. If you are not sure you can move the patient alone, do not be afraid to ask for help. Always check the care plan to see if there are special instructions.

A **turning (moving) sheet** or **draw sheet** (folded large sheet or half-sheet) may be placed under a heavy or helpless patient to make moving easier. The sheet must extend from the shoulders to below the hips (about mid-thigh) to be effective. Tips for making moving procedures easier are listed in Table 15-3. Folding a flat sheet in half to create a draw sheet is not a good idea. Folding the sheet causes wrinkles, which increase pressure on the skin, creating pressure injuries and pain. Using a commercially made draw sheet is a much better idea.

Follow Procedures 14 to 17 when you are moving patients. As you practice these procedures, keep in mind the basic rules of good body mechanics that were described in Chapter 14.

 Safety **ALERT**

Avoid lifting as much as possible. Use assistive devices to move patients whenever you can. For example, using a turning sheet for moving a patient prevents injury to the skin and prevents pain that sometimes occurs when you pull on the patient's body. It also reduces the risk of back injury in nursing assistants. When moving a patient on a sheet, make sure you have enough help. Two or three assistants may be necessary. Usually, two assistants are needed to reposition the patient's torso. A third may also be needed to prevent friction and shearing on the feet if the patient is being pulled up in bed. One nursing assistant can usually move a patient by using a sling or a sheet. However, this creates friction on the patient's skin and often results in stage 1 pressure injuries.

ASSISTIVE MOVING DEVICES

Use devices to reduce the need for lifting and moving patients manually, whenever possible. Assistive devices

TABLE 15-3 Tips for Easier Movement of Bedfast Patients

Move the patient in segments to the side of the bed:
- Shoulders first
- Lower legs and feet next
- Hips and buttocks last

Move the patient to the head of the bed
- Tip the bed into the Trendelenburg position, with the head of the bed facing downward, and the feet elevated 20° to 30°, if permitted. This position provides a gravity assist, making moving easier and reducing strain on your body.
- Avoid this position if the patient uses oxygen or has respiratory problems.
- Return the bed to the supine position promptly after moving the patient

Turning the patient to one side
- Cross the far leg over the near leg so it is facing the direction of the turn

Moving a dependent patient
- Have the patient cross the arms over the chest and tuck the chin down

can be used for turning, positioning, and lateral transfers. Many of these have a slippery, low-friction surface. Because of this, the devices move easily. However, a dependent patient may slip off. Two or more nursing assistants are needed for safety.

A **slider** is a flat, slippery sheet (Figure 15-26A) or tube (Figure 15-26B), similar to a trash bag with the ends cut off. The tube is a two-surface device. They are made from low-friction fabrics that slide and glide over themselves during transfers. The inside is slippery, so it slides on itself. Other terms that may be used for the tubular device are *roller tube, roller sheet, sliding tube,* or *slide tube.*

The single-layer sliding sheet is also called a *slip sheet, slippery sheet, slide sheet, glide sheet,* and similar names. These reduce friction during lateral transfers and repositioning and reduce the amount of force needed during moving procedures. These sheets can be used in a flat (single) layer, by folding the fabric, or in conjunction with a second sliding device.

Sliders are available in various types, sizes, and lengths. Some are padded and some have handles. A one-way slider will prevent the patient from sliding back down if left in place. Some sliders move in both directions. Avoid leaving these under patients.

PROCEDURE 14 TURNING THE PATIENT TOWARD YOU

1. Carry out each initial procedure action.

2. Lower the side rail nearest to you. Cross the patient's far leg over the leg that is nearest to you.

3. Cross the far arm over the patient's chest. Bend the near arm at the elbow, bringing the hand toward the head of the bed.

4. Place your hand nearest the head of the bed on the patient's far shoulder. Place your other hand on the patient's hips on the far side. Brace your thighs against the side of the bed.

5. Roll the patient toward you (Figure 15-22A). Move slowly, gently, and smoothly. Help the patient bring the upper leg toward you and bend it comfortably.

6. Put up the side rail. Be sure it is secure.

7. Go to the opposite side of the bed.

8. Place your hands under the patient's shoulders and then the hips. Pull toward the center of the bed (Figure 15-22B). This helps the patient maintain the

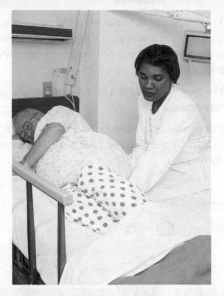

FIGURE 15-22B Move the patient to the center of the bed, keeping your back straight.

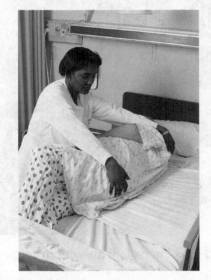

FIGURE 15-22A Place one hand on the patient's far shoulder and hip, and then turn the patient toward you.

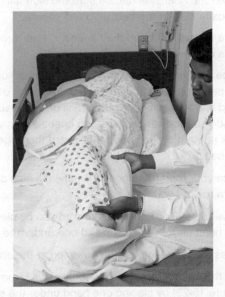

FIGURE 15-22C Place pillows to support the patient's body and maintain good alignment.

(continues)

PROCEDURE **14** CONTINUED

side-lying position. Make sure the patient is not lying directly on the lower arm. Tip the lower shoulder slightly, so pressure is not centered directly over the joint.

9. Make sure the patient's body is properly aligned and safely positioned.

10. A pillow may be placed behind the patient's back. Secure it by pushing the near side under the patient to form a roll.

11. If the patient is unable to move independently, support the extremities with pillows between the shoulders, hands and knees, and ankles to prevent friction and contractures (Figure 15-22C). If the patient has an indwelling catheter, make sure the tubing is not between the legs, to prevent undue stress on the catheter and to prevent pressure injuries.

12. Carry out each ending procedure action.

ICON KEY:

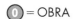 = OBRA   = PPE

PROCEDURE **15**   **TURNING THE PATIENT AWAY FROM YOU**

1. Carry out each initial procedure action.

2. Lower the near side rail. Be sure the side rail on the opposite side of the bed is up and secure.

3. Have the patient bend their knees, if able. Cross the arms on the chest.

4. Place your arm nearest the head of the bed under the patient's head and shoulders. Place the other hand and forearm under the small of their back. Bend your body at the hips and knees. Keep your back straight. Pull the patient toward the edge of the bed.

5. Place your forearms under the patient's hips and pull them toward you.

6. Move the ankles and knees toward you by placing one hand under the ankles and one under the knees.

7. Cross the near leg over the other leg at the ankles.

8. Roll the patient slowly and carefully away from you (Figure 15-23) by placing one hand under the shoulder and one hand under the hips.

9. Place your hands under the head and shoulders. Draw them back toward the center of the bed.

10. Move the hips to the center of the bed.

11. Place a pillow for support behind the back.

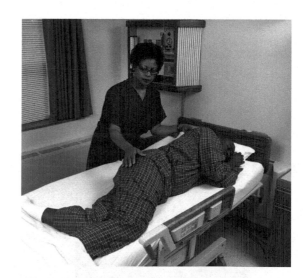

FIGURE 15-23 Roll the patient away from you.

12. Make sure that the patient's body is in good alignment. Support the upper leg with a pillow. Place the lower arm in a flexed position. Support the upper arm with a pillow.

13. Replace the side rail on near side of the bed. Return the bed to the lowest horizontal position.

14. Carry out each ending procedure action.

ICON KEY:

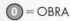 = OBRA

EXPAND YOUR SKILLS

PROCEDURE **16** MOVING A PATIENT TO THE HEAD OF THE BED

1. Carry out each initial procedure action.

2. Ask a co-worker to assist from the opposite side of the bed.

3. Lock the wheels of the bed. Raise the bed to a comfortable horizontal working height. Lower side rails.

4. Lower the head of the bed if the patient can tolerate this position. Remove the pillow. Place it at the head of the bed, horizontally on its edge, for safety.

5. Lift top bedding and expose the draw sheet. Loosen both sides of the draw sheet.

6. Roll the draw sheet edges close to each side of the patient's body (Figure 15-24).

7. Face the head of the bed. Grasp the draw sheet with the hand closest to the foot of the bed.

8. Position your feet 12 inches apart, with the foot that is farthest from the bed edge forward.

9. Place your free hand and arm under the patient's neck and shoulders, cradling the head from both sides.

10. Bend your hips slightly.

11. Together, on a count of three, raise the patient's hips and back with the draw sheet, while supporting the head and shoulders. Move the patient smoothly toward the head of the bed.

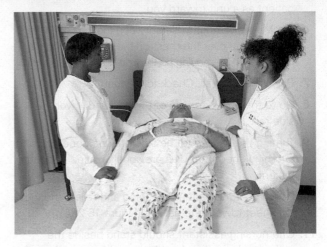

FIGURE 15-24 Using an overhand grasp, roll both edges of the turning (moving) sheet close to the patient's sides.

12. Replace the pillow under the patient's head.

13. Tighten and tuck in the draw sheet. Adjust the top bedding.

14. Carry out each ending procedure action.

ICON KEY:
 = OBRA

EXPAND YOUR SKILLS

PROCEDURE **17** LOGROLLING THE PATIENT

1. Carry out each initial procedure action.

2. Get help from another nursing assistant.

3. Raise the bed to waist-high horizontal position. Lock the wheels.

4. Lower the side rail on the side opposite to which the patient will be turned. Both assistants should be on the same side of the bed.

> **NOTE**
>
> This procedure is performed when the patient's spinal column must be kept straight, such as following spinal surgery or spinal cord or vertebral column injury. It is a good procedure to use with any dependent patient.

(continues)

PROCEDURE **17** **CONTINUED**

5. One assistant places hands under the patient's head and shoulders. The second person places their hands under the hips and legs. Then move the patient as a unit toward you.

6. Place a pillow lengthwise between the legs. Fold the patient's arm over the chest on the side to which the resident will be moving so they do not roll on top of it.

7. Raise the side rail. Check for security.

8. Go to the opposite side of the bed and lower the side rail.

9. Turning the patient to the side may be done by using a turning sheet that was previously placed under the patient.

10. Reach over the patient, grasping and rolling the turning sheet toward the patient (Figure 15-25A).

11. One nursing assistant should stand beside the patient to keep the shoulders and hips straight.

12. A second assistant should keep the thighs and lower legs straight.

13. If a turning sheet is not in position, the first assistant places their hands on the patient's far shoulder and hip.

14. The second assistant positions their hands on the patient's far thigh and lower leg.

15. At a specified signal, roll the patient toward both assistants in a single movement, keeping the spine, head, and legs straight. If a turning sheet is used, grasp the sheet and move the patient as a unit, onto their side (Figure 15-25B).

16. Place additional pillows behind the back to maintain the patient's position. A small pillow or folded bath blanket may be permitted under the patient's head and neck. Leave a pillow between the legs. Position small pillows or folded towels to support the arms.

17. Carry out each ending procedure action.

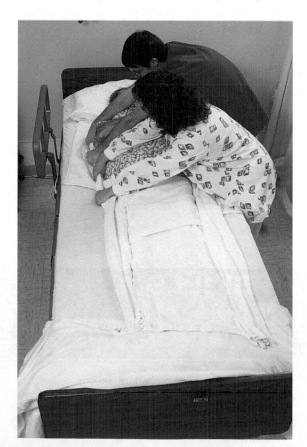

FIGURE 13.25A Roll the turning sheet against the patient.

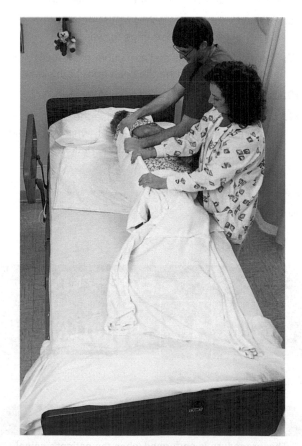

FIGURE 13.25B Pulling together, turn the patient to the side in one smooth motion.

ICON KEY:

 = OBRA

A maximum weight limit of 35 pounds is recommended for patient lifting tasks that are done under ideal conditions.[1] Your spine is one of the most important parts of your body, enabling you to maintain an upright position, move freely, stand, and walk. The vertebrae protect your spinal cord, a column of nerves connecting your brain with the rest of your body. Your organs would not function without it. Keeping your spine healthy is a vital concern for nursing assistants. Unfortunately, back injuries from improper lifting and moving are common in health care workers. Other contributing factors are rushing to get things done and not asking for help from others. Pay attention to your body and your position. Your back must last a lifetime.

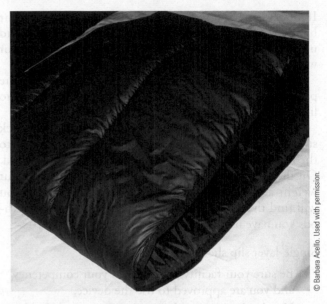

FIGURE 15-26B A tube rolls on itself to move the patient up and down or from one surface to another.

Guidelines for Moving Patients with a Slider or Tube

Use good judgment. Make the transfer only if you believe it is safe based on whether the patient can cooperate, follow instructions, and assist. Depending on the procedure, you may also have to consider the person's behavior, balance, space available, whether obstacles are in the way, and how many others will be assisting with the transfer.

When transferring from one surface to another, level the surfaces to be as close to the same height as possible. Moving uphill increases the difficulty of the task and risk of injury. Moving downhill is easier. Thus, if the height of the surfaces can be adjusted, adjust the surface you are transferring to so that it is an inch lower than the surface from which the transfer originates.

When sliding a person from one surface to another, bridge the gap with a sliding board or other firm device. Half of the fabric should be under the patient's body, on the surface of origin. Place the other half on the surface you are transferring to. Be sure the wheels are locked on both surfaces. Transfer toward the patient's good (stronger) side.

Know whether the device may be left in place or must be removed after the transfer. In most cases, you will remove the slide when you finish moving the patient. Follow the patient's care plan and your facility's policies. The low-friction surface results in minimal patient movement, even if the person is sitting in a chair. Avoid pulling the slider out toward the foot of the bed; doing so may cause the patient to slide down in bed.

If the device has webbing or handles, you may do best if you grasp the upper handle with an underhand grasp and the lower handle with an overhand grasp.

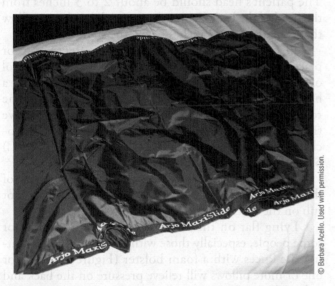

FIGURE 15-26A A slider is used to slide a patient in bed instead of lifting. It moves from side to side for turning, up and down for moving a patient up in bed, and for transferring a patient from a bed to a stretcher.

Never use a slider instead of a sling or lifting device. Sliders are not designed for lifting. However, they accomplish many of the same tasks by sliding instead of lifting. They move side to side for turning, and up and down for moving a person up in bed. Persons with good balance and arm strength can use sliders independently. Use short sliders for pivoting and repositioning, such as sitting (dangling) or moving the patient up in bed. Use long sliders for transferring supine patients from one surface to another, such as from bed to stretcher. Place the slider under the incontinent pad or draw sheet, if used.

[1]Waters, T. R. et al. (1994, January). *Applications manual for the revised NIOSH lifting equation* (DHHS (NIOSH) Publication No. 94-110). Cincinnati, OH: National Institute for Occupational Safety and Health. http://www.cdc.gov/niosh/pdfs/94-110.pdf; Waters, T. R. (2007, August). When is it safe to manually lift a patient? *American Journal of Nursing*, 107(8), 53–58; quiz 59.

If this seems awkward, switch the position of your hands. Try an overhand grasp for the upper hand and underhand grasp for the lower hand. The handles or webbing should be in the center of your palms.

Use a pulling and rocking motion to move the patient. You are not lifting! There is less of a tendency to lift if you are using a device with no handles.

Stand close to the patient or bed with your back straight, feet apart, knees bent, and the foot closest to the head facing the direction the patient is to be moved. On the count of three, slide the patient by shifting your weight and walking in the direction of the move. You will find that this takes much less effort than the methods you have used.

Single-layer slip sheet/slide sheet:

- Be sure your facility has checked your competency and you are approved to use the device.
- Use the device according to instructions and only for its intended purpose; never invent new uses.
- Select the correct size and type of slider for the task.
- Test the slider by rolling it on itself to learn if it slides in one or both directions, how well it slides, and whether there are signs of wear. This is especially important after laundering, as bleach and high temperatures can potentially damage the device. Do not use if it is worn or has bleach spots.
- Check the patient's skin for open or painful areas on the surface to be moved. If present, check with the nurse before moving the patient.
- Logroll the dependent person onto the device. A person with good balance can sit and lean to one side. You may also fan-fold the slider lengthwise, unfolding it from head to foot.
- Synchronize your movements with those of other workers.
- Use good body mechanics.
- Be sure the opposite rail is up when turning a patient in bed.

Using a tubular slide:

- Position the open ends of the tube facing the patient's head and feet when performing a sitting transfer from one surface to another.
- Position the open ends of the tube at the patient's sides when moving the patient to the head or foot of the bed.
- Center the tube under the patient's body (or at least from the shoulders to the hips) for bed mobility. A second tube may be needed to move the legs.
- Most tubular devices can be easily removed by pulling the bottom layer of fabric. Follow the manufacturer's instructions for the device you are using.

Sliders and tubes have special storage and washing instructions. Some are disposable and some are reusable. Follow the specific storage and infection control precautions recommended by the manufacturer.

Positioning the Patient

After you have turned and moved the patient into proper body alignment, you can place pillows and other supportive devices to maintain the position. Directions are given here for the basic four positions and their variations.

Supine Position

To place a patient in the supine position (Figure 15-27A), start with the bed flat and the patient lying on the back. The patient's head should be about 2 to 3 inches from the head of the bed. Center the patient's head on a pillow that extends about 2 inches below the shoulders.

Place a **trochanter roll** along the affected hip or place one along each hip if the patient has little control over the legs. A trochanter roll is devised by rolling a bath blanket into a shape about 12 inches long. The roll should be just long enough to reach from above the hip to above the knee (Figure 15-27B). The trochanter roll prevents external rotation (Figure 15-27C) of the hip.

Place pillows under the legs from above the back of the knee to the ankle so that the ankles and heels do not rub on the sheets.

Lying flat on the back is very uncomfortable for some people, especially those with low back pain. Elevating the knees with a foam bolster (Figure 15-27D) or one or more pillows will relieve pressure on the back and reduce discomfort.

Position a footboard or place a folded pillow to support the feet, if listed on the care plan. Position the ankles at 90° angles.

Extend the patient's arms and place small pillows that reach from the elbow to below the wrist. Align the hand with the wrist with the palm facing down.

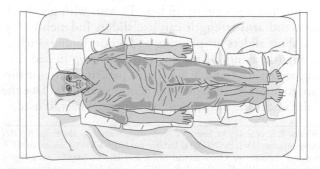

FIGURE 15-27A Supine position.

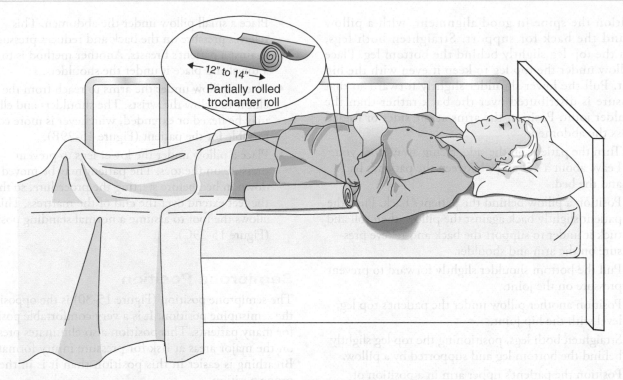

FIGURE 15-27B The trochanter roll should extend from the hip to just above the knee.

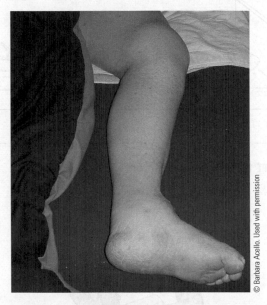

FIGURE 15-27C The side of this patient's leg is flat on the bed due to external rotation of the hip. A properly placed trochanter roll will turn the leg inward and hold it in place

Semisupine Position

The semisupine position (Figure 15-28) is also called the *tilt position*. It should not be confused with the lateral position. The patient is not lying directly on the side. When correctly used, the semisupine position relieves pressure from the hip, sacrum, coccyx, and buttocks. Before beginning, position the patient in the supine position and move them to the side of the bed that will be behind the back after you have finished.

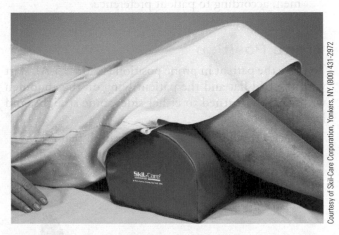

FIGURE 15-27D Supporting the knees relieves pressure and discomfort in the lower back.

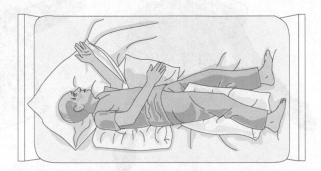

FIGURE 15-28 The semisupine position is a variation of supine that relieves pressure on the major pressure areas of the body.

Position the spine in good alignment, with a pillow behind the back for support. Straighten both legs, with the top leg slightly behind the bottom leg. Place a pillow under the top leg to keep it even with the hip joint. Pull the lower shoulder slightly forward so that pressure is distributed over the back rather than the shoulder joint. Position the arms at the sides or folded across the abdomen.

- Turn the patient on the side, facing away from you. Leave about a 45° angle between the patient's back and the bed.
- Position a pillow behind the patient's back. Push the patient slightly back against the pillow, then roll and tuck it under to support the back and relieve pressure on the arm and shoulder.
- Pull the bottom shoulder slightly forward to prevent pressure on the joint.
- Position another pillow under the patient's top leg, level with the hip joint.
- Straighten both legs, positioning the top leg slightly behind the bottom leg and supported by a pillow.
- Position the patient's upper arm in a position of comfort. The wrist may rest on a pillow or the abdomen, according to patient preference.

Prone Position

To place the patient in prone position (Figure 15-A), start with the bed flat and the patient lying on the abdomen with the head turned to either side, spine straight, and legs extended.

- Place a small pillow under the head so that it extends to the patient's shoulders and 5 to 6 inches beyond the face.

- Place a small pillow under the abdomen. This relieves pressure on the back and reduces pressure against a patient's breasts. Another method is to roll a towel and place it under the shoulders.
- Place a pillow under the arms to reach from the elbow to below the wrists. The shoulders and elbows may be flexed or extended, whichever is more comfortable for the patient (Figure 15-29B).
- Place a pillow under the lower legs to prevent pressure on the toes. The patient may be moved down in bed before starting the procedure, so that the feet extend over the end of the mattress. This allows the foot to assume a normal standing position (Figure 15-29C).

Semiprone Position

The semiprone position (Figure 15-30) is the opposite of the semisupine position. It is a very comfortable position for many patients. This position also eliminates pressure on the major areas at risk for pressure injury formation. Breathing is easier in this position than it is in the full prone position.

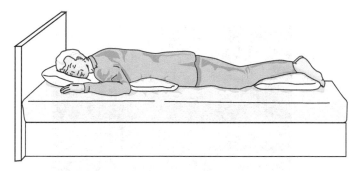

FIGURE 15-29A Prone position.

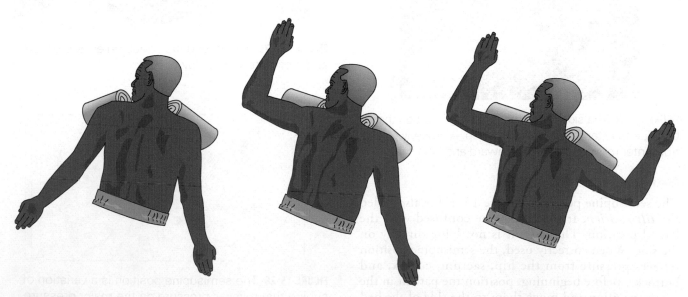

FIGURE 15-29B Position the arms for patient comfort.

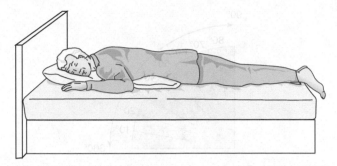

FIGURE 15-29C The patient may be moved down in bed so that the feet hang over the end of the mattress.

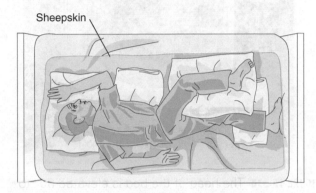

Sheepskin

FIGURE 15-30 The semiprone position is a variation of the prone position.

Begin the procedure by placing the patient prone. Lift the patient's chest and shoulder closest to you and place a pillow under them. Position the opposite arm behind the patient. Fold a second pillow in half and place it under the top leg. Keep the legs and spine straight. Turn the patient's head to either side and place it on a small pillow. Follow your facility's policy for use of the semiprone position. Like the prone position, some facilities require a doctor's order because lying on the abdomen may make breathing more difficult for some patients. Check the patient every 15 minutes to be sure they can tolerate the position.

- Turn the patient into the prone position as described earlier.
- Turn the patient's head to the side facing you, or according to patient preference.
- Gently lift the patient's near shoulder. Position a pillow under the chest and shoulder, with the patient's arm resting on the pillow. Position the other arm behind (but not underneath) the patient.
- Fold a second pillow in half and place it under the top leg.
- Straighten and extend both legs for comfort.
- Monitor the patient frequently for signs of respiratory distress.

 Safety **ALERT**

The semiprone and semisupine positions may be a source of confusion for some health care workers. These positions are not the same as the lateral positions. Patients in semiprone and semisupine positions are tilted at an angle so that pressure is not applied directly to the bony prominences, whereas the lateral position places pressure on many vital areas. The semiprone and semisupine positions are very comfortable and relieve pressure from all major pressure points on the patient's body.

Right Lateral Position

The right lateral position is shown in Figure 15-31. Reverse directions for the left lateral position.

- Start with the bed flat and the patient turned on the left side, with spine straight. Remember before turning to move the patient to the right side of the bed.
- Place a pillow under the head so it extends 5 to 6 inches beyond the patient's face and down to the shoulders.
- Position the right arm so the shoulder and elbow are flexed and the palm of the hand is facing up.
- Place the left arm so it is extended or only slightly flexed and rest it on the hip or bring it forward and place it on a pillow. Position the shoulder, elbow, and wrist at approximately the same height.
- Place a pillow between the legs, extending from above the knee to below the ankle. Position the hip, knee, and ankle at approximately the same height.
- A pillow may be placed behind the back to help maintain the position.

Sims' Position

Sims' position (Figure 15-32) is a variation of the lateral position with the person on the left side, left leg extended and right leg flexed. This position is often used for rectal examinations as well as treatments and enemas.

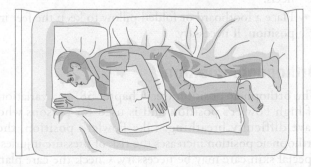

FIGURE 15-31 Right lateral position.

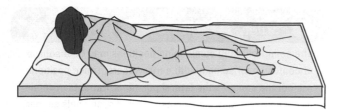

FIGURE 15-32 Sims' position.

- Place a pillow under the patient's head as for lateral position.
- Start with the bed flat and the patient moved and turned onto the left side.
- Extend the patient's left arm and position it behind the patient's back.
- Flex the right arm and bring it forward. Support the arm with a pillow.

Fowler's Position

This position, or a variation of it, is used for feeding patients in bed, for certain treatments and procedures, for the patient's comfort while visiting or watching television, and for those who have trouble breathing. This position increases pressure on the buttocks and increases the risk of skin breakdown and pressure injuries. Because of this, avoid leaving patients in Fowler's position for prolonged periods. Check the care plan for instructions.

- Start with the patient on the back, in the middle of the bed and in good alignment. Position the hips at the bend in the bed. Place the head of the bed at 15° to 30° for low Fowler's, 30° to 45° for semi-Fowler's (Figures 15-33A and 15-33B), 45° to 60° for Fowler's (Figure 15-33C), and 90° for high Fowler's (Figure 15-33D).
- Place one or two pillows behind the patient's head to extend 4 to 5 inches below the patient's shoulders.
- Flex the elbows and place a pillow under each arm to prevent pull on the shoulders.
- Place a pillow under each leg to extend from above the knee and to the ankle, to prevent pressure on heels.
- Place a footboard or folded pillow to keep the feet in position, if necessary.

Orthopneic Position

The orthopneic position (see Chapter 38) is a variation of high Fowler's position and is used for persons who have difficulty breathing. Like Fowler's position, the orthopneic position increases the risk of pressure injuries. Special skin care may be necessary. Check the care plan or ask the nurse for further instructions.

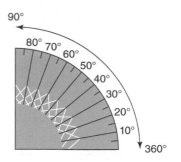

FIGURE 15-33A Degrees of elevation.

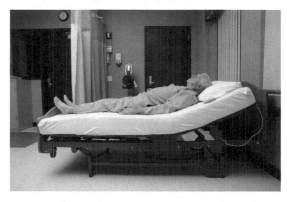

FIGURE 15-33B The head of the bed is elevated 30° to 45° in semi-Fowler's position.

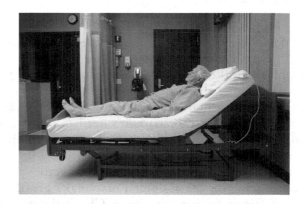

FIGURE 15-33C The head of the bed is elevated 45° to 60° in Fowler's position.

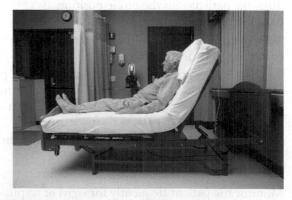

FIGURE 15-33D Orthopneic position.

- The position of the bed remains the same as for high Fowler's.
- Assist the patient to sit as upright as possible
- Have the patient lean slightly forward, supporting themselves with the forearms. Placing the overbed table in front of the patient and extending the arms over it provides a good means of support and helps ease respirations. This makes the thorax larger, enabling the patient to inhale more air.
- Place another pillow low behind the patient's back for support.

Sitting Position

Patients should be positioned in a comfortable, well-constructed chair so that the head and spine are erect (Figure 15-34A). The back and buttocks should be up against the chair back. Stabilizing the patient's feet on the floor or wheelchair footrests is the first step in good positioning. Solid foot support also prevents forward sliding in the wheelchair. For good posture and even weight distribution, the feet should be at a 90° angle to the lower legs. Each lower leg should be at a 90° angle to the corresponding thigh. The thighs should be at a 90° angle to the torso. This is called the **90-90-90 position** (Figure 15-34B).

- Pillows or postural supports may be needed to maintain the position.
- A small pillow may be folded and placed at the small of the back to add comfort and support.
- Do not permit the back of the patient's knees to rest against the chair.

> 🔓 Safety **ALERT**
>
> Patients can develop pressure injuries when sitting in a chair. If the person will be sitting for a long time, pad the chair seat. If the patient is able, remind them to push on the armrests and shift weight every 15 minutes. Ambulate, stand, or reposition the patient in the chair at least every two hours or more often to stimulate circulation and relieve pressure.

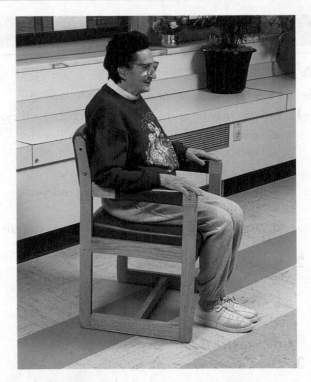

FIGURE 15-34A Orthopneic position.

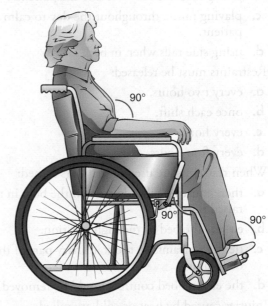

FIGURE 15-34B Use the 90-90-90 position when supporting a patient in a chair. The feet are at a 90° angle to the lower legs. Each lower leg is at a 90° angle to the corresponding thigh. The thighs are at a 90° angle to the torso.

REVIEW

A. Multiple Choice

Select the best answer for each of the following.

1. Patients may be at risk for incidents because they:
   a. ambulate independently in the hallway for exercise.
   b. use a wheelchair for long distances.
   c. keep one side rail up for turning independently when in bed.
   d. receive medications affecting balance, coordination, and mental status.

2. Falls can be prevented by:
   a. encouraging patients to remain in bed.
   b. using restraints when the patient is up.
   c. keeping the side rails up at all times.
   d. meeting the patient's needs promptly.

3. Alternatives to restraints include:
   a. taking patients to the bathroom regularly.
   b. giving medications to sedate the patient.
   c. playing music throughout the day to calm the patient.
   d. using side rails when in bed.

4. Restraints must be released:
   a. every two hours.
   b. once each shift.
   c. every hour.
   d. every four hours.

5. When restraints are used on patients in bed:
   a. there must be full side rails on the bed, in the raised position.
   b. elevate the bed to the high position.
   c. tie the restraints to the stationary part of the bed frame.
   d. the electric bed control should be removed.

6. Injuries caused by heat or cold are called:
   a. lacerations.
   b. bruises.
   c. thermal injuries.
   d. aspiration.

7. Choking may be prevented by:
   a. giving the patient only fluids.
   b. giving the patient finger foods.
   c. using thickeners for liquids.
   d. allowing only blended foods.

8. Initial procedure actions include:
   a. handwashing.
   b. raising side rails.
   c. placing the call signal within reach.
   d. opening the door.

9. Correct body alignment will:
   a. heal disease.
   b. prevent infection.
   c. help the body function efficiently.
   d. be harmful in some situations.

10. Examples of supportive devices include:
    a. belts.
    b. pillows.
    c. side rails.
    d. vests.

11. Supine position is:
    a. lying on the back.
    b. lying on the abdomen.
    c. lying on the side.
    d. sitting in the chair.

12. A position used for patients who have trouble breathing is:
    a. orthopneic.
    b. semiprone.
    c. lateral.
    d. supine.

13. Logrolling is a procedure performed for:
    a. persons who have had both legs amputated.
    b. ambulatory patients.
    c. all conscious patients.
    d. patients who have had spinal surgery.

14. A trochanter roll is used to:
    a. maintain the hip in alignment.
    b. maintain the feet in alignment.
    c. support the patient's back.
    d. prevent contractures of the hand.

15. Splints may be used to:
    a. maintain position of an extremity.
    b. provide support for a fractured femur.
    c. restrain the wrists.
    d. prevent pressure injuries.

16. The purpose of low-friction sliding devices is to:
   a. reduce the need for lifting and moving patients manually.
   b. enable patients to move in bed and transfer independently.
   c. eliminate the need for a sling or similar lifting device.
   d. increase the amount of resistance needed for moving patients.

17. After moving Mrs. Fedyn to the chair, you will:
   a. leave the two-way slider in place.
   b. leave the one-way slider in place.
   c. remove the one-way slider.
   d. fasten the slider to the chair.

18. When transferring from one surface to another:
   a. moving uphill works best.
   b. moving downhill is easiest.
   c. the surfaces must be the same height.
   d. do not adjust the height of the surfaces.

19. When sliding a person from one surface to another:
   a. transfer toward the patient's stronger side.
   b. use a nylon sling to bridge the gap.
   c. transfer toward the patient's weaker side.
   d. unlock the wheels on both surfaces.

20. Most tubular devices can be removed by:
   a. pulling the top layer of fabric.
   b. pulling the tube up on the weak side.
   c. pulling the bottom layer of fabric.
   d. carefully pulling from side to side.

21. Separating a patient from others against their will is:
   a. coercion.
   b. seclusion.
   c. ergonomics.
   d. aspiration.

22. When assisting a patient with a shower, the nursing assistant should:
   a. turn hot water on last and off first.
   b. turn cold water on last and off first.
   c. turn both faucets on at the same time.
   d. spray the person with hot water only.

23. The two most common complications of improper positioning are:
   a. pain and discomfort.
   b. pressure injuries and contractures.
   c. falls and immobility.
   d. weakness and limited movement.

24. Contractures:
   a. result from resting.
   b. are not painful.
   c. interfere with mobility.
   d. are easily reversed.

B. True/False

Mark the following true or false by circling T or F.

25. T F Restraints are attached to the side rails for security.

26. T F A slider is used to reduce the risk of injury when lifting.

27. T F A physician's order is not necessary before applying restraints.

28. T F Patients should be repositioned at least every two hours.

29. T F The left Sims' position is used for rectal treatments and enemas.

30. T F When turning a patient toward you, cross the patient's near leg over the leg that is farthest from you.

31. T F You must wash your hands before beginning and after completing every nursing assistant task.

32. T F Leave the bed in the highest horizontal position when patient care is complete.

33. T F Turning sheets make moving heavy patients an easier task.

34. T F You should always explain what you plan to do, even if the patient seems not to hear or understand.

35. T F Pressure injuries result from reduced blood flow to an area.

36. T F Atrophy improves joint mobility.

37. T F Pressure injuries are dangerous and expensive to treat.

38. T F There is a relationship between contractures and pressure injuries.

C. Matching

Complete the following by writing the letter of the matching term from Column II in the blanks in Column I.

Column I

39. _____ supine

40. _____ prone

41. _____ orthopneic

42. _____ trochanter roll

43. _____ splint

44. _____ contracture
45. _____ supportive devices
46. _____ physical restraints

Column II

    a. prevents external rotation of hip
    b. joint deformity caused by shortening of the muscles
    c. devices used to maintain patient's position
    d. device used to maintain position of an extremity
    e. position for patients with difficult breathing
    f. lying on the back
    g. lying on the abdomen
    h. devices that inhibit movement

D. Nursing Assistant Challenge

Sara Abrams is 76 years old, has Parkinson disease, and is a resident in a long-term care facility. She is ambulatory, with a shuffling walk, and has tremors of her hands related to the Parkinson's. She is disoriented and frequently walks into other patients' rooms.

47. Discuss safety issues related to Ms. Abrams's condition.

_____

_____

_____

48. Which of the Residents' Rights may be a special issue in this situation?

_____

_____

_____

49. What steps can you take to meet Ms. Abrams's physical needs? Will doing so lower her risk of falling?

_____

_____

_____

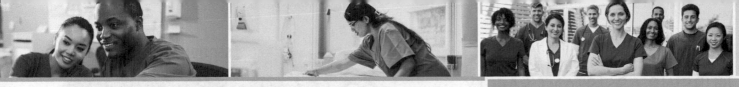

The Patient's Mobility: Transfer Skills

CHAPTER 16

OBJECTIVES

After completing this chapter, you will be able to:

16.1 Spell and define terms.

16.2 List at least seven factors to consider before lifting or moving a patient to determine whether additional equipment or assistance is necessary.

16.3 Demonstrate the principles of good body mechanics and ergonomics to moving and transferring patients.

16.4 List the guidelines for safe transfers.

16.5 Describe the difference between a standing transfer and a sitting transfer.

16.6 List the guidelines for using the manual handling sling.

16.7 List the guidelines for using the pivot disk.

16.8 Demonstrate correct application and use of a transfer belt.

16.9 Demonstrate the following procedures:
- Procedure 18: Applying a Transfer Belt

- Procedure 19: Transferring the Patient from Bed to Chair—One Assistant
- Procedure 20: Transferring the Patient from Bed to Chair—Two Assistants (Expand Your Skills)
- Procedure 21: Sliding-Board Transfer from Bed to Wheelchair (Expand Your Skills)
- Procedure 22: Transferring the Patient from Chair to Bed—One Assistant
- Procedure 23: Transferring the Patient from Chair to Bed—Two Assistants (Expand Your Skills)
- Procedure 24: Transferring the Patient from Bed to Stretcher (Expand Your Skills)
- Procedure 25: Transferring the Patient from Stretcher to Bed (Expand Your Skills)
- Procedure 26: Transferring the Patient with a Mechanical Lift (Expand Your Skills)
- Procedure 27: Transferring the Patient onto and off of the Toilet (Expand Your Skills)

VOCABULARY

Learn the meaning and the correct spelling of the following words and phrases:

contraindication	mechanical lift	partial weight-bearing	sliding board
full weight-bearing (FWB)	nonweight-bearing (NWB)	(PWB)	standing transfer
gait belt	paralysis	pivot	transfer belt
manual patient handling	paresis	sitting (lateral) transfer	weight-bearing (WB)

INTRODUCTION

As a nursing assistant, you will work with many patients who have impaired mobility. In Chapter 15, you learned how to move and position patients in bed. In this chapter, you will learn how to *transfer* patients (to move them from one place to another). Patients transfer:

- Out of bed into a chair and back to bed from the chair
- Out of bed onto a stretcher and back to bed from the stretcher
- Onto and off of a toilet or bedside commode
- Into and out of a car
- Into and out of a bathtub or shower

Refer to Procedures 19 through 27 later in this chapter.

NURSING ASSISTANT SAFETY

Nursing work is always one of the top 10 occupations for work-related musculoskeletal injuries. Having a previous history of back injury was identified as the biggest risk factor for either a new back injury or back pain. The rate of back injury in workers with a history of injury is about twice as high as the rate among workers with no history of back problems.

In 2005, the state of Texas passed the first state law requiring health care facilities to implement safe patient handling and movement programs. Since then, several other states have passed or are working on passing laws that protect health care workers against injury from patient lifting. The American Nurses Association (ANA) is working hard to get nationwide legislation passed.

Patient lifts and transfers are the tasks with the highest risk of injury. This is partly because workers often find themselves in awkward positions and must bend or reach while the back is flexed. High-risk patient handling tasks vary by clinical setting. Other factors that increase the risk of injury are:

- Patient weight
- Patient ability and willingness to cooperate and follow directions
- Transfer distance
- Confined workspace
- Lateral patient transfers
- Unpredictable patient behavior
- Stooping, bending, and reaching

To reduce the risk of worker injury, facilities have implemented various programs, such as lift teams. These are specially trained personnel who do all patient moving in the facility. Some facilities have "no-lift" policies. This does not mean that workers should never lift a patient, heavy box, or equipment. Instead, this term usually means that no manual lifting should be done. Facilities with no-lift or "zero-lift" policies depend on mechanical aids when moving patients. Some have a combination of mechanical, electrical, and ceiling-mounted lifts for moving patients vertically. Many require workers to use gait belts and mechanical aids for lifting and moving patients and heavy items. A no-lift policy is more of a pledge from management that equipment and/or personnel will be available to help with the task and reduce the risk of injury associated with manual patient handling.

Manual patient handling is moving a patient by hand or bodily force, including pushing, pulling, carrying, holding, or supporting the patient or a patient's body part. When moving a patient from one surface to another:

- Use an assistive device whenever possible.
- Know your limits.
- Get assistance from another worker whenever possible.

Safety ALERT

Remember that having the right equipment is only one part of an ergonomics program. Using good body mechanics, getting help when needed, reporting potential hazards, following facility policies and procedures, avoiding shortcuts, and using good judgment are all important to patient and nursing assistant safety.

The procedures in this chapter are an overview of the basic methods for moving and transferring patients. You must learn these before you can safely use a mechanical or friction-reducing device to assist with patient movement. Many new devices have been invented for lifting, moving, and repositioning patients to reduce the risk of worker injury. However, the types and availability of these devices vary widely from one facility to the next. You must adapt the procedures in this book to the policies, procedures, and equipment in your facility. Your facility will teach you how to match the equipment and type of transfer to the patient's size and needs. Still, the basic procedures you will use are the ones in this book.

In addition, practicing and using proper body mechanics is key to injury prevention. Before performing the procedures in this chapter, make sure you review and master the information on ergonomics, body mechanics, and safe patient handling in Chapter 14. Also, OSHA and ANA have ergonomic and patient handling information to reduce the risk of injury.

TYPES OF TRANSFERS

There are basically two types of transfers. With a **standing transfer**, the patient stands during the transfer with the help of one or two nursing assistants. With a **sitting (lateral) transfer**, the patient sits throughout the transfer, such as when a sliding board is used (see Procedure 21). A **sliding board** is a plastic or wooden board about two feet long that has a slippery surface. It is used for a sitting (lateral) transfer.

A mechanical lift may also be used for sitting patients, but this device is for *vertical* movement. The **mechanical lift** may be a manually operated hydraulic lift, an electrically (or battery) operated lift, or a ceiling-mounted lift. The mechanical lift is used to transfer dependent or heavy patients from one surface to another. Most facilities use battery-operated lifts. Medicaid and Medicare pay only for manual lifts for home care clients. Most lifts are used for patients who are seated or supine. Some are available for persons who are standing.

The nurse or the physical therapist determines which method is used to transfer a patient (Figure 16-1). Follow instructions carefully to avoid injury. The method selected depends on:

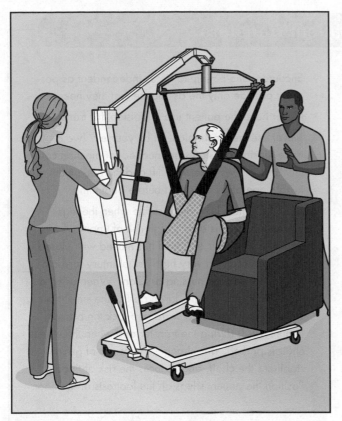

FIGURE 16-1 The physical therapist and nurse assess the patient to determine the best device to support patient safety and independence.

1. The patient's physical condition. This takes into consideration:
   - **Paralysis** (inability to move) of any extremity.
   - **Paresis**, which is weakness of an extremity.
   - Absence of an extremity due to amputation.
   - Recent hip surgery.
2. The patient's strength, endurance, and balance. These abilities may be affected by:
   - Respiratory (lung) disease.
   - Cardiac (heart) disease.
   - Neurological disease, such as multiple sclerosis or a stroke.
   - The ability to stand on one or both legs. This is called **weight-bearing (WB)**. For example, a patient may not be able to place full weight on a paralyzed leg. The physician may order the patient to be **nonweight-bearing (NWB)** or only **partial weight-bearing (PWB)** if the patient has had hip surgery. The ability to stand on both legs is called **full weight-bearing (FWB)**. For a standing transfer, the patient must be able to stand and have at least partial weight-bearing on one leg.
3. The presence of amputations, contractures, paralysis, or structural deformities (Figure 16-2).

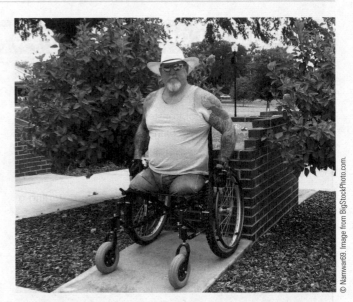

FIGURE 16-2 This person has bilateral above-the-knee amputations. Consider ways to safely transfer him from the wheelchair to a bed.

4. Whether the person needs to stand or sit during the transfer.
5. The patient's mental condition and ability to cooperate.
6. The patient's size. For example, transfer of a very tall or large person who cannot bear full weight would require two or more assistants or a mechanical lift.

Although the nurse or therapist selects the method of transfer, you will have to determine if you need another person or piece of equipment to assist you. When using the procedures in this chapter with the equipment available in your facility, key elements for you to consider at the time of the transfer are:

- The patient's ability to assist with the procedure.
- The patient's ability to bear weight.
- The patient's upper-extremity strength, if a sliding board or certain other transfers are used.
- The patient's ability to cooperate and follow directions.
- The patient's size (height and weight) compared with your size; in general, if the patient is larger than you are, you will need help from another assistant or a mechanical device. Even if the patient is smaller than you are, you may need help if the person is dependent or cannot cooperate.
- Special circumstances, such as presence of wounds, surgical sites, catheters, IVs, tubes, contractures, or other factors that restrict or interfere with mobility; always get help if there is danger of pulling on or displacing a tube or medical device during the transfer.
- Special physician orders or therapy recommendations for transfers and positioning, such as you would see for a patient who has had hip surgery.

GUIDELINES 16-1 Guidelines for Safe Patient Transfers

Moving dependent patients can result in injury to you or the patient unless all safety measures are followed.

- Know the method of transfer that has been ordered by the nurse or physical therapist.
- Know the patient's capabilities.
- Use correct body mechanics.
- Place the bed in the lowest position before starting a standing transfer. Make sure the wheels on the bed and the transfer vehicle (wheelchair, stretcher) are locked before the move. It is helpful to elevate the head of the bed for bed-to-chair transfers.
- *Never allow patients to place their hands on your body during a transfer.* This is a dangerous practice. A patient who is disoriented or frightened can cause you to lose your balance. If this happens, the patient can pull you down, possibly injuring both of you.
- *Never place your hands under a patient's arms or shoulders.* This practice can cause severe shoulder injury to the patient.
- Use a transfer belt for standing transfers unless contraindicated.
- Make sure the patient is wearing shoes with sturdy soles appropriate to the floor surface and that clothing is not too loose or dragging on the floor.
- Be aware of any tubes, orthoses, or other items that you must manage during the transfer.
- Transfer the patient toward the stronger side, if possible.
- Always explain what you are doing and how the patient can help.
- Test the patient's understanding and make sure they know what you expect them to do during the transfer.
- Allow the patient to see the surface to which they are being transferred. Encourage the patient to keep the head up.
- Stand close to the patient during the transfer.
- Brace the knee of a weak or paralyzed leg, using your own knee or leg. Support a paralyzed arm during the transfer to avoid dangling and pulling on the shoulder.

- Encourage the patient to be as independent as possible; provide only the assistance that they need.
- Never have the patient use a footstool for transfers.
- Never use the mechanical lift by yourself. Two or more nursing assistants are needed for mechanical lift transfers. Make sure the lift and the equipment are in safe operating condition before beginning.
- The mechanical lift is more stable when the legs are open. There is a very high risk of tipping if a patient is in the air or if the lift is moved with closed legs. This creates a very high risk of injury for both the patient and the nursing assistant. When using a wheelchair, position the large part of the small front caster wheels facing forward and lock the brakes (Figure 16-3) during the transfer and when the wheelchair is parked. This changes the center of gravity, stabilizes the chair, and reduces the risk of tipping. Position the patient's legs on the footrests or the floor.

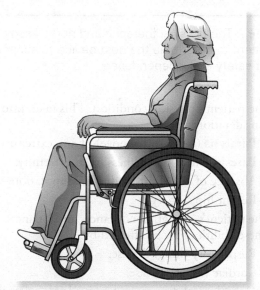

FIGURE 16-3 The large part of the small front wheels must face forward during a transfer and when the chair is parked. Lock the brakes. Changing the position of the front wheels makes the chair more stable. Fold the footrest up to prevent tripping during a transfer. Always lower the footrests after the transfer unless the patient uses the feet to move the chair. Avoid dragging the person's feet on the floor when moving the chair.

In some situations, you may be instructed to take the patient's pulse before they get out of bed and during the activity. If the patient has been inactive for a long time, the heart muscle may be deconditioned. Checking the pulse when the patient is active provides an evaluation of the heart's condition.

Patient Independence

Transfers and other mobility-related skills are listed on the care plan. Your contribution of information is important to the nursing process. Observations to make and report about the patient's ability to transfer are listed in Table 16-1.

TABLE 16-1 Observations to Make and Report About the Patient's Ability To Transfer

- Independent; no assistance required, but may use equipment such as side rails, trapeze, etc.
- Requires PRN assistance for transfers.
- One to transfer; continuously requires one person for physical or verbal assist on 60% or more of transfers. Specify when assistance is required and for what reason.
- Two to transfer; requires assistance of two or more during the entire activity on 60% or more of transfers. Specify when assistance is required and for what reason.
- Not transferred; may be transferred to a stretcher or chair once a week or less, excluding transfers to bath or toilet.
- Transfer belt used for transfers.
- Adjuncts such as slip sheet, transfer disk, sliding board, or the like used for transfers.
- Mechanical lift, standing lift, ceiling lift, or wall-mounted lift needed for transfers.
- Cooperates/does not cooperate with transfers.
- Willing and able to follow directions.
- Level of dependence or independence of the patient.
- Weight and need for special equipment or extra personnel to move the person safely.
- Physical conditions such as amputation or paralysis that affect stability.
- Person's ability to balance.
- Sensory deficits, such as loss of position sense, poor vision, or other problems (these are usually related to a condition of the nervous system).
- Consider weight limits of equipment, if used.
- Consider the push pull weight if a lift will be moved on carpeting.

TRANSFER BELTS

A **transfer belt** is a webbed belt. Most are 1.5 to 2 inches wide and about 54 to 60 inches long. Bariatric belts are 72 inches long (Figure 16-4). Some newer belts are padded and 4 to 6 inches wide. Some belts have handles. The transfer belt is an assistive and safety device used to transfer or ambulate patients who need help. (Refer to Procedure 18.) When it is used to assist with ambulation, it is called a **gait belt**.

Using a transfer belt avoids the need to grasp the patient around the ribcage or under the arms. Either of these methods can cause serious injury. The belt also allows you to have more control in directing the transfer. A transfer belt is not used to "lift" a patient. Another method should be used for transfers if the patient has no ability to bear weight.

Contraindications (situations in which something is not indicated, inappropriate, or potentially dangerous) for use of the transfer belt include:

- Abdominal, back, or rib injuries; fractures; or recent surgery
- Abdominal pacemakers
- Advanced heart or lung disease
- Abdominal aneurysms
- Pregnancy
- Colostomy

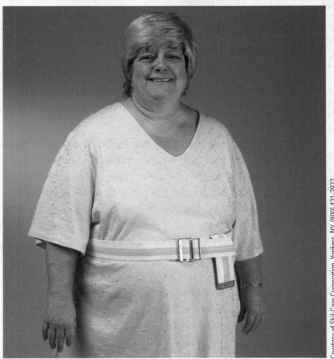

Courtesy of Skil-Care Corporation, Yonkers, NY, (800) 431-2972

FIGURE 16-4 The bariatric gait belt is 72 inches long. Two or more assistants are needed for transfers.

- Gastrostomy tube or jejunostomy feeding tube
- Recently implanted abdominal or spinal medication pumps (Figure 16-5)
- Other devices implanted into the spine, such as spinal catheters or spinal stimulators

Medication pumps may be implanted under the skin of the abdomen in some patients. If the surgical site is well healed, it is probably safe to use the transfer belt. However, always follow the care plan or check with the nurse or physical therapist before using a transfer belt to move a patient with any type of implantable device.

> ### ⚠ OSHA **ALERT**
>
> Each year more than 12.8 million Americans consult their doctors about back problems. In fact, as many as 8 out of 10 individuals will suffer back pain during their lifetime. A transfer belt is an inexpensive item that helps protect you from injury and makes transfers safer and more secure for patients. Make the transfer belt a permanent part of your uniform. Wear it when you are on duty so it is readily available when needed to move a patient.

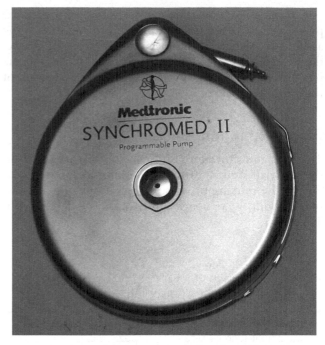

FIGURE 16-5 A medication pump is implanted under the abdominal skin. A tiny catheter is attached to the pump to deliver medication to the spinal canal.

PROCEDURE 18 APPLYING A TRANSFER BELT ⓞ

1. Carry out initial procedure actions.
2. Assemble equipment:
   - Transfer belt
3. Explain the procedure. Tell the patient that the belt is a safety device that will be removed as soon as the transfer is completed.
4. Apply the belt over the patient's clothing (Figure 16-6A). If the patient is undressed and being transferred from wheelchair to tub or shower chair, either leave the patient's shirt on, put the patient's robe on, or place a towel around the patient's waist and then apply the belt over the towel.
5. If the patient is going to transfer from bed to chair, the belt may be applied after the patient comes to a sitting position on the edge of the bed. The belt can be applied while the patient is lying down in bed if they have poor balance. You may need to readjust the belt after the patient sits up.
6. Keep the belt at the patient's waist level. Avoid placing it too high. Make sure the belt is right side out and is not twisted.

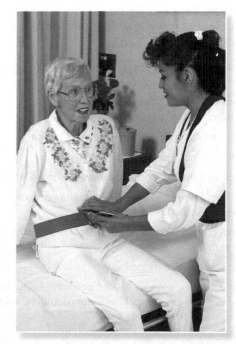

FIGURE 16-6A Always apply the transfer belt over clothing.

(continues)

PROCEDURE 18 CONTINUED

7. Buckle the belt in front by threading the belt end through the teeth side of the buckle first and then through both openings (Figure 16-6B). The buckle must be in front.

8. Check female patients to be sure the breasts are not under the belt.

9. The belt should be snug, so that it does not slide up, but not tight (Figure 16-6C). Check the fit of the belt by placing three fingers under it. There should be just enough space for your fingers to fit comfortably.

10. Before attempting to move the patient, be sure their feet are flat on the floor. If they are not, use the belt to assist the patient to the edge of the bed until their feet are resting firmly on the floor.

11. If you are transferring a patient into or out of a wheelchair, lock the brakes and keep the footrests out of the way during the transfer. After the patient is

seated, their legs should not dangle. The feet are supported on the floor or on the wheelchair footrests.

12. Teach the patient to assist by pushing off the bed or arms of the chair with their hands when you count to three.

13. Use an underhand grasp when holding the belt. For transfers, one hand should be on each side of the buckle in front.

14. Do not overuse the belt by pulling the patient up with force.

15. When the patient is standing, **pivot** (turn the entire body as one unit) to transfer.

16. The chair should be close enough so the patient can feel it with their hands after you pivot.

17. Remove the belt after the patient is safely moved.

18. Carry out ending procedure actions.

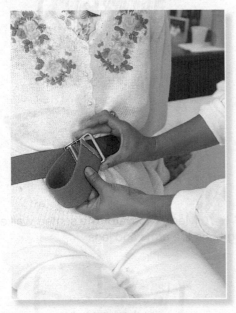

FIGURE 16-6B Thread the belt through the teeth side of the buckle first.

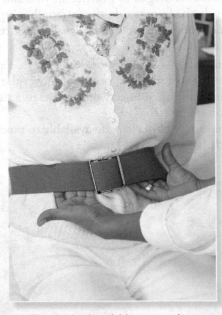

FIGURE 16-6C The belt should be snug but not tight.

ICON KEY:
 = OBRA

ASSISTIVE DEVICES

Avoid pulling on the patient's body during transfers, moving, and positioning. Use assistive devices such as sheets, a transfer belt, a sliding board, or the like to move patients. The goal is to keep patients moving and out of

wheelchairs. Hundreds of devices have been introduced in the past decade to make transfers and mobility easier and safer. Recapping all of them in a book is impossible, and the content would be meaningless to you unless your facility is using the equipment. If this is the case, they will teach staff how to use it. Common and useful devices are:

- Rollator—a frame with three or four large wheels, handlebars, and a seat that enables the patient to rest, if needed (Figure 16-7A).
- Merry Walker®—a black steel walker/chair combination that enables the patient to walk independently and then sit down to rest, if needed, or to prevent a fall. It gets patients walking after a period of immobility and reduces falls and pressure injury formation. This walker is available in 13 sizes (including bariatric sizes) to meet the individual needs of each patient (Figure 16-7B).
- Merry Motivator®—a height-adjustable, seated walker for patients who require two assistants to move from sit to stand. It decreases pressure injury risk because the patient's buttocks do not hang over the seat. The person strengthens the legs by moving them to walk and builds upper-body strength by pulling against the front cross arm to propel across the floor (Figure 16-7C).
- Merry Stand by Me®—a large black frame designed to retrain patients to get from sitting to standing in order to walk again. The wheelchair is placed inside the frame, with brakes locked, and the patient is encouraged to practice sit-to-stand activities inside the framework, thus strengthening the legs and working to get back to walking once again (Figure 16-7D).
- Standing lifter—a battery-operated lift that assists the patient to a standing position, moves the patient to a chair, and then lowers the patient to a sitting position (Figure 16-7E).

A large variety of devices are available to meet ambulation needs.

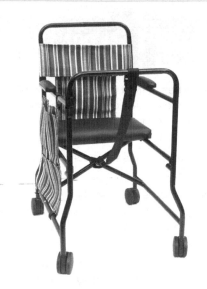

FIGURE 16-7B The Merry Walker enables patients to walk and sit to rest, if needed.

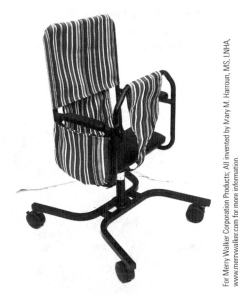

FIGURE 16-7C Merry Motivator is a seated walker that strengthens the arms and legs.

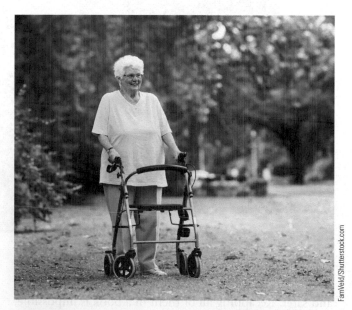

FIGURE 16-7A The Rollator provides balance and a surface for sitting.

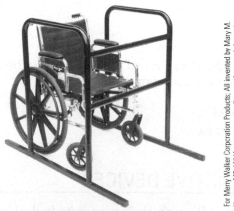

FIGURE 16-7D Merry Stand by Me enables patients to safely practice standing to strengthen the legs.

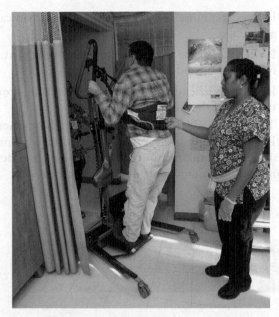

FIGURE 16-7E The standing lifter assists patients from a seated to a standing position. Standing helps maintain leg strength and mobility, and prevents osteoporosis.

Swivel Disks

Swivel disks (also called *turning disks, transfer disks,* and *pivot disks*) are round disks that turn, enabling you to pivot the patient. They can be used for both seated and standing transfers. The disk reduces the force needed for pivoting the patient. Disks are available in various sizes and may be flexible or solid. The flexible disks work well for sitting transfers. Rigid disks are used for standing transfers. Disks may be used with other devices, such as transfer boards and transfer belts. Wide transfer belts with handles work well for moving patients on a disk.

Swivel disks weigh about two to four pounds. The inner surfaces are made of low-friction materials. The outer surfaces consist of high-friction materials. The bottom remains stationary when the upper disk swivels. Some disks move by means of ball bearings. These move faster than other types of disks, and may be more difficult to control.

Swivel disks may be used for most pivot transfers. For standing transfers, use a disk only for patients who can stand and follow instructions. Persons who are unpredictable, are dependent, are combative, or cannot stand independently increase the risk of injury for both the nursing assistant and the patient. Heavy patients require excessive force during transfers. The maximum weight capacity of transfer disks is about 250 to 300 pounds. Learn the specifications for the device you are using.

When using a swivel disk, remember the following:

- Use the disk only in areas where you have enough space to use it safely.
- Do not use the disk if you must assume an awkward position.

- Maintain a wide base of support with your feet.
- The patient must be wearing shoes.
- Center the patient's feet on the disk.
- The patient's base of support is narrower on the disk. They are slightly less stable than if they were standing on the floor.
- Disks pose an increased trip hazard. Know where the disk is in relation to your feet and the patient's feet at all times. Remove and store the disk as soon as the transfer is complete. If the patient cannot be trusted to leave the disk alone, remove it from the room.
- Do not use the disk near water, as the surface may become slippery.
- Do not separate two-piece discs.

Manual Handling Slings

The manual handling sling is a small fabric or plastic sling (about 20 inches long and 8 inches wide) with handles on the long ends (Figure 16-8). This versatile moving aid is used for supporting patients during transfers and positioning. It has a number of patient handling applications. Some slings are used for moving amputated extremities. Some patients use them to assist with independent movement. The good news is that using a sling eliminates pulling and tugging on a patient's body and makes the task easier for the nursing assistant. The manual handling sling may be used to:

- Move patients up in bed
- Move the hips to one side of the bed in preparation for turning
- Move one or both of the patient's legs from the floor to the bed or position them within the bed
- Assist patients from the supine to sitting position in bed
- Assist with turning
- Assist a patient from the dangling position to standing position

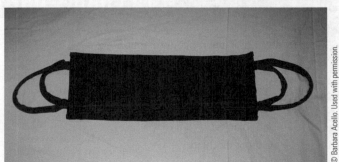

FIGURE 16-8 A sling may be used to guide a weight-bearing patient with transfers.

- Transfer a patient from bed to wheelchair
- Move a patient up in the wheelchair

The position of the sling is determined by:

- The nature of the procedure
- The patient's underlying medical problems
- The person's ability to assist and follow directions

The manual handling sling reduces your risk of injury. Other benefits of the sling for the nursing assistant are that:

- Your spine stays straighter.

- It gives you more control and a better mechanical advantage.
- It adds length for procedures in which your arms are used to guide and move a patient.
- It eliminates bending, twisting, and reaching around the back of the patient.

The patient side of some slings has a high-friction coating that prevents slipping. The two handgrips on the sides enable the nursing assistant to grip the device securely and maintain control of the procedure.

GUIDELINES 16-2 Guidelines for Moving Patients Using a Manual Handling Sling

- Follow the manufacturer's instructions for the device you are using.
- Do not use if the sling is torn or shows signs of wear.
- Be sure your facility has checked your competency and has approved you to use the manual handling sling.
- Use the sling only for its intended purpose; do not invent new uses.
- Use good body mechanics.
- Be sure the sling fits the patient. If it is too large or small, do not use it.
- The patient's skin should be dry; some plastic slings will slip on wet skin.
- Avoid powder on the patient's torso when using a plastic sling; powder becomes very slippery.

- Move the patient in segments and only in one direction. Avoid twisting.
- Avoid pulling on the patient's arms and legs during moving procedures.
- Synchronize the move with other workers. Move with the patient rather than away from the patient.
- Remove the sling when you finish moving the patient.
- The sling may be used with other mobility devices, such as transfer disks and sliding boards.
- Fabric slings have special storage and washing instructions. Plastic slings can be wiped clean and disinfected. Some are disposable and some are reusable. Follow the storage and infection control precautions recommended by the manufacturer.

PROCEDURE 19 TRANSFERRING THE PATIENT FROM BED TO CHAIR—ONE ASSISTANT

1. Carry out initial procedure actions.

2. Assemble equipment:
   - Transfer belt
   - Chair for patient
   - Bath blanket
   - Robe or clothing
   - Shoes and socks

3. Place the chair so the patient moves toward their stronger side. Set the chair parallel with the bed. Position the large part of the small front wheels facing forward. Lock the wheelchair and raise or remove the footrests (Figure 16-9A). Cover the chair with a bath blanket, unless the patient is fully clothed.

4. Lower the bed to the lowest horizontal position and lock the bed wheels.

(continues)

PROCEDURE **19** CONTINUED

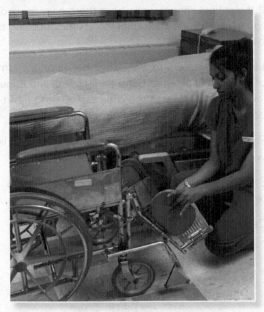

FIGURE 16-9A Lock the wheelchair and lift or remove the footrests before the patient transfers.

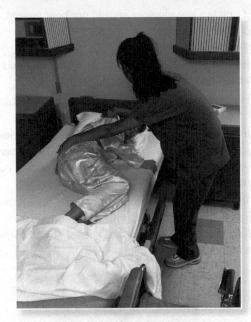

FIGURE 16-9B Instruct the patient to use the hands to push to a sitting position.

5. Stand against the side of the bed with the side rail down. Ask the patient to slide toward the side of the bed.

6. Have the patient roll over onto their side, flexing the knees and bending the right arm so it can be used for propping the upper body. Bend the elbow of the left arm so this hand can be used to push off from the bed (Figure 16-9B).

7. Instruct the patient to use the elbow to raise the upper body and to push with the hand so they come to an upright position.

8. Instruct the patient to let their legs slide off the bed at the same time.

9. If assistance is needed, place one arm under the shoulders (not the neck) and one arm over and around the knees (Figure 16-9C). Raise the patient's upper body at the same time as you move the legs off the bed.

10. Give the patient time to adjust to sitting up and then apply the transfer belt. Assist to put on shoes and socks. (If the patient has problems with balance, the shoes and socks can be put on while the patient is lying down in bed.)

11. If the patient has a weak or paralyzed arm, do not let it hang or dangle during the transfer. Put that hand in their pocket, or have them cradle that arm with their strong arm, or carefully tuck their weaker hand in the transfer belt or waist of the pants until they are again seated.

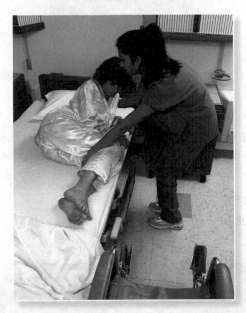

FIGURE 16-9C Place one arm under the patient's shoulders and one arm over and around the knees.

12. When the patient is ready to transfer:
   – Instruct them to move forward or closer to the edge of the mattress, to spread their knees, lean forward from the waist, and place their feet slightly back.

(continues)

- If one leg is weaker or should not bear weight, place this leg out in front with the strong leg slightly back.

- Remember to spread your feet apart and bend your knees and hips, keeping your back straight.

- Hold the belt with an underhand grasp, one hand on each side of the front of the belt.

- If the patient has a weaker leg, press your knee against their knee, or block the patient's foot with yours to prevent the weaker leg from sliding out from under them.

- Tell the patient on the count of three to use their hands (if able) to press into the mattress, to straighten their elbows and knees, and to come to a standing position (Figure 16-9D).

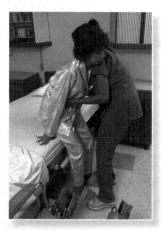

FIGURE 16-9D Instruct the patient to push on the bed and straighten the elbows and knees to come to a standing position.

ICON KEY:

 = OBRA

13. If the patient cannot walk, have them pivot around to the front of the chair until the chair is touching the backs of their legs.

14. Instruct the patient to place their hands on the arms of the chair (if able), to bend their knees, and to gently lower themselves into the chair as you ease them downward (Figure 16-9E). Replace the footrests.

15. Position the patient comfortably. Place the signal light within easy reach.

16. Straighten the bed and prepare it for the patient's return.

17. Carry out ending procedure actions.

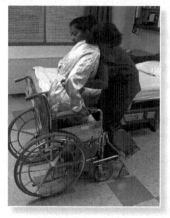

FIGURE 16-9E Pivot to the chair. Instruct the patient to hold the armrests and bend the knees when the back of the chair is felt on the legs. The patient can then safely lower the body into the chair.

EXPAND YOUR SKILLS

PROCEDURE **20** **TRANSFERRING THE PATIENT FROM BED TO CHAIR—TWO ASSISTANTS**

Two people may be needed to transfer patients who are weak, are disoriented, have limited weight-bearing ability, or are very large. Directions are given for transferring toward the patient's right side.

1. Follow steps 1 through 11 in Procedure 19.

2. The nursing assistants stand one on each side, facing the patient.

3. Each one places the hand closest to the patient through the belt, with an underhand grasp toward the front of the patient. The other hand of each assistant grasps the belt toward the back. Coordination of movement is necessary (Figure 16-10A).

(continues)

4. The nursing assistant closest to the chair (on the patient's right side) stands in a position to step or pivot around smoothly to allow the patient access to the chair. This person stands with the left leg further back than the right leg.

5. The other nursing assistant uses the left knee to brace the patient's weaker left leg. This assistant's left leg is further back than the right leg.

6. Instruct the patient to bend forward and place the palms of the hands on the edge of the mattress to push off.

7. The patient's knees should be spread apart, with both feet back and the stronger foot slightly in back of the weaker foot.

8. The nursing assistants bend their knees and give a broad base of support.

9. On the count of three, the patient stands. Allow them to stand for a moment and bear weight. Tell them to keep their head up. Both nursing assistants help the patient pivot by slowly and smoothly pivoting their feet, legs, and hips to their left.

10. To sit, have the patient bend forward slightly, bend the knees, and lower onto the chair. At the same time, have them reach for the arms of the chair with both hands (Figure 16-10B).

11. Complete the procedure as described for a one-assistant transfer (Procedure 19).

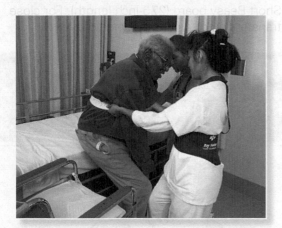

FIGURE 16-10A Coordination of movement is necessary.

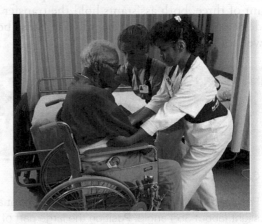

FIGURE 16-10B Instruct the patient to reach for the arms of the chair with both hands while being guided into a sitting position.

ICON KEY:
 = OBRA

A manual handling sling will not make you stronger. It is also contraindicated in patients who:
- Are totally dependent
- Cannot follow instructions
- Are combative

> 🔓 Safety **ALERT**
>
> Remember to lock the brakes before transferring a patient into or out of a wheelchair. Turn the small front wheels so the large part faces forward. Lock the brakes anytime the chair is parked. If you remove the wheelchair footrests during a transfer, remember to replace them. The patient's feet must be supported unless they use them to propel the chair.

SLIDING-BOARD TRANSFERS

A sliding-board transfer is used for patients who have good upper-body strength and sitting balance. This type of transfer is commonly used for patients with paraplegia, or weakness in both legs, such as those with postpolio syndrome or other neuromuscular diseases. The procedure involves doing a series of push-ups: The patient pushes with the hands and locks the elbows. To transfer, the patient must be able to lift the buttocks off the bed. After lifting the buttocks, they lower onto the sliding board, and then lifts and slides until the transfer is complete. Some patients perform this transfer independently, whereas others need help. If you will be assisting, use a transfer belt.

A wheelchair with removable armrests must be used for sliding-board transfers. The chair must also have removable or swing-away leg rests. The patient must have clothing on the lower half of the body. Bare skin will stick to the board, creating friction and shearing, and making the transfer very difficult or impossible. Blue jeans do not slide well on some boards. Cotton or synthetic slacks are best. If the patient has difficulty sliding on the board, draping a pillowcase across the board may be helpful. (Do not encase the board in the pillowcase as you would a pillow.) If a wooden board is used, it can be waxed to maintain a slippery surface.

The Beasy board is a transfer board with a movable round seat (Figure 16-11) that runs through a track in the center of the board. This type of board is helpful for more dependent patients. It may also be used for moving a patient up in bed.

Two assistants can move dependent patients by using a sliding board. However, this transfer works best when the patient can understand and cooperate with your instructions. For a two-person transfer, one assistant stands in front of and the other behind the patient. On the count of three, both assistants hold the transfer belt and slide the patient across the board. The Beasy board works well for this type of transfer.

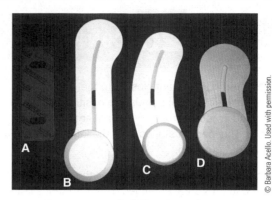

© Barbara Acello. Used with permission.

FIGURE 16-11 Four types of sliding boards:
A. Short wooden board. For close transfers, such as bed to wheelchair.
B. Long Beasy board (40-inch length). Used when there is a distance between the transfer surface and the patient. Works well for car transfers.
C. The curved Beasy board. Regular curved boards are also available. Works well for car transfers.
D. Short Beasy board (27.5-inch length). For close transfers, such as bed to wheelchair.

EXPAND YOUR SKILLS

PROCEDURE **21** | **SLIDING-BOARD TRANSFER FROM BED TO WHEELCHAIR**

1. Carry out initial procedure actions.

2. Position the wheelchair parallel to the bed, or at a slight (about 35°) angle. Position the large part of the small front wheels facing forward. Lock the brakes.

3. Remove the arm of the wheelchair closest to the bed. Remove the leg rests or fold them back.

4. Apply a transfer belt to the patient. Check the fit with two or three fingers.

5. Assist the patient to move close to the edge of the bed.

6. Tell the patient to lean away from the wheelchair. Place the sliding board well under the buttocks, with the beveled side of the board facing up. Avoid pinching the patient's skin between the board and the bed.

7. Place the opposite end of the board on the seat of the wheelchair.

8. Instruct the patient to push up with the hands, lock the elbows, and move across the board. Repeat until the patient is seated in the chair with one buttock on the board. You will assist by grasping the transfer belt

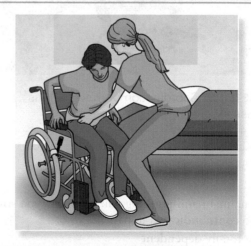

FIGURE 16-12A Grasp the transfer belt with an underhand grasp and assist the patient to slide to the wheelchair.

with an underhand grasp and sliding laterally when the patient pushes down on the bed (Figure 6-12A).

– The patient may pull or push on the opposite armrest of the wheelchair with one hand when they have moved close enough to reach it. This will make sliding easier or help achieve greater height

(continues)

PROCEDURE 21 CONTINUED   0

in the push-ups, depending on the method used. The patient may also push on the board. Caution the patient to avoid placing the fingers under the edges of the board.

9. Be prepared to assist by lifting the belt and/or patient's buttocks during the sitting push-up. If the patient is having trouble balancing, place your hands on the shoulders for support. Stop and allow the patient to balance before proceeding.

10. Support and move the patient's legs with your hands, if necessary.

11. Center the patient on the wheelchair seat (Figure 6-12B).

12. Instruct the patient to lean away from the bed when they are centered on the wheelchair seat. Remove the board.

13. Remove the transfer belt.

14. Replace the arm of the wheelchair. Position the patient's legs on the leg rests and foot plates, or as instructed.

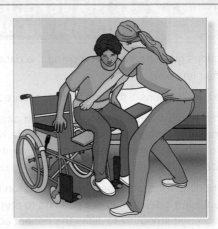

FIGURE 16-12B Center the patient in the wheelchair, and then remove the transfer belt.

15. Assist the patient with positioning for good body alignment.

16. Perform ending procedure actions.

17. Reverse the procedure to return the patient to bed.

PROCEDURE 22 TRANSFERRING THE PATIENT FROM CHAIR TO BED—ONE ASSISTANT   0

1. Carry out initial procedure actions.

2. Assemble equipment:
   – Transfer belt

3. Place the chair so the patient moves toward their stronger side. Set the chair parallel with the bed.

4. Move the bed to the lowest horizontal position and lock the wheels. Fanfold the top covers to the foot of the bed if necessary and raise the opposite side rail.

5. Lock the wheelchair and raise or remove the footrests. Position the large part of the small front caster wheels facing forward.

6. Have the patient place both feet flat on the floor.

7. Place the transfer belt around the patient's waist.

8. Instruct the patient to move forward in the chair, to bend forward, and to spread their knees apart. Both feet should be back, with the stronger foot slightly in back of the weaker foot. Both of the patient's hands should be on the arms of the chair.

9. Hold the transfer belt with an underhand grasp. Brace the patient's weaker leg with your knee or leg, as instructed in Procedure 18. Ask the patient to push off

the chair on the count of three and to stand up as you provide the necessary assistance.

10. Allow the patient to remain standing for a time to stabilize position. Keep your grasp on the transfer belt and continue to brace the weak leg if necessary.

11. To complete the transfer, instruct the patient to step or pivot around to stand in front of the bed, facing away from it. Tell the patient to sit when the edge of the mattress is touching the back of their legs. To sit, have the patient bend forward slightly, bend their knees, place the palms on the bed, and lower themselves onto the mattress.

12. When the patient is safely in bed, remove the transfer belt.

13. Remove the patient's slippers and robe. Assist the patient to lie down. Position the patient as necessary. Draw top bedding over the patient. Fold the bath blanket (if used) from the wheelchair and return it to the bedside stand. Make sure the signal light is within reach.

14. Move the wheelchair out of the way.

15. Carry out ending procedure actions.

ICON KEY:

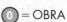 = OBRA

EXPAND YOUR SKILLS

PROCEDURE 23 **TRANSFERRING THE PATIENT FROM CHAIR TO BED—TWO ASSISTANTS**

The directions given here are for moving the patient toward their left side.

1. Follow instructions 1 through 8 in Procedure 21.

2. Each nursing assistant places the hand closest to the patient through the belt with an underhand grasp in front of the patient; both assistants grasp the back of the belt with an underhand grasp.

3. The nursing assistant closest to the bed (on the patient's left side) stands in a position to step or pivot around smoothly to allow the patient access to the bed. This person stands with the right leg further back than the left leg.

4. The other nursing assistant uses the left knee to brace the patient's weaker right leg. This person's right leg is further back than the left one (Figure 16-13A).

5. Ask the patient to push off the chair on the count of three and to stand up as you provide the necessary assistance.

6. Allow the patient to remain standing for a time to stabilize position. Keep your hands on the transfer belt and continue to brace the weak leg, if necessary.

7. To complete the transfer, instruct the patient to step or pivot around to stand in front of the bed, facing away from it. Tell the patient to sit when the edge of the mattress is touching the back of their legs. To sit, have the patient bend forward slightly, bend their knees, place their palms on the bed, and lower themselves onto the mattress (Figure 16-13B).

8. When the patient is safely in bed, remove the transfer belt.

9. Remove the patient's slippers and robe. Assist the patient to lie down and position as necessary. Raise the side rails if ordered. Draw top bedding over the patient. Fold the bath blanket (if used) from the wheelchair and return it to the bedside stand. Make sure the signal light is within reach.

10. Move the wheelchair out of the way.

11. Carry out ending procedure actions.

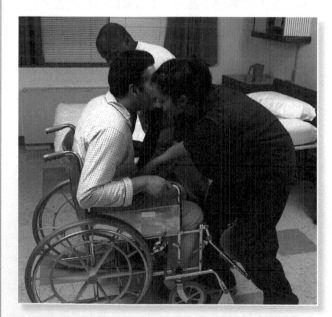

FIGURE 16-13A The nursing assistant uses the knee to support the patient's weaker right leg.

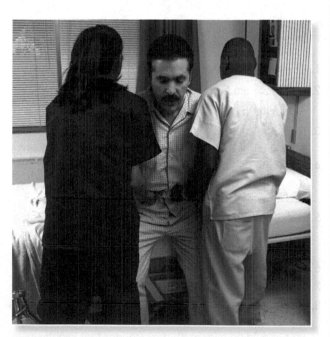

FIGURE 16-13B Instruct the patient to lean slightly forward, bend the knees, place their palms on the bed, and lower the body onto the mattress.

ICON KEY:
 = OBRA

EXPAND YOUR SKILLS

PROCEDURE **24** | **TRANSFERRING THE PATIENT FROM BED TO STRETCHER**

1. Carry out initial procedure actions.

2. Assemble equipment:
   - Stretcher
   - Bath blanket

3. You will need three to four people to transfer an unconscious or comatose patient from bed to stretcher.

4. Lock the wheels of the bed. Raise the bed to a horizontal position that it is *slightly higher than the surface of the stretcher.*

5. Lower the side rails.

6. Place a bath blanket over the patient and fanfold the top covers to the foot of the bed, out of the way.

7. Roll the turning sheet up against the patient on both sides. The sheet should be long enough to support the patient's head and shoulders during the move.

8. Position the stretcher close to the bed. Lock stretcher wheels.

9. Two or three people stand along the open side of the stretcher. The other person stands on the open side of the bed. This assistant may need to get on the bed, on their knees, to avoid overstretching their back.

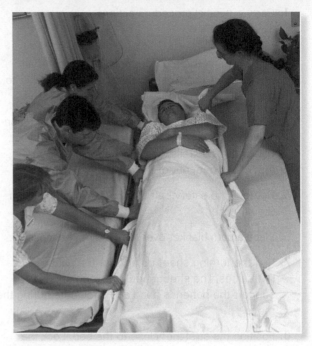

FIGURE 16-14 All persons slide the lifting sheet from bed to stretcher.

   - The middle assistant grasps the moving sheet by placing one hand by the patient's hips and the other hand by the patient's shoulders.
   - The assistant at the head of the bed grasps the turning sheet by the patient's shoulder and head.
   - On the count of three, all persons slide the moving sheet from bed to stretcher (Figure 16-14).

10. Center the patient on the stretcher in good body alignment. Secure the stretcher safety belt. Raise the side rails of the stretcher.

11. Transport the patient as directed.

12. Prepare the bed for the patient's return.

13. Carry out ending procedure actions.

Never leave a patient on a stretcher alone!

> ### ✎ NOTE
>
> Use an overhand grasp on the moving sheet to avoid wrist strain. Using a friction-reducing sheet, roller, lifting pad, or air-transfer device (Chapter 31) will make this task much easier and reduce the risk of personal injury.

   - The assistant at the end of the bed grasps the moving sheet by placing one hand by the patient's legs and the other hand by the patient's hips.

ICON KEY:
0 = OBRA

EXPAND YOUR SKILLS

PROCEDURE **25** | **TRANSFERRING THE PATIENT FROM STRETCHER TO BED**

1. Carry out initial procedure actions.

2. Assemble equipment:

3. You will need three or four people to transfer an unconscious or comatose patient from stretcher to bed.

4. Lock the wheels of the bed. Raise the bed to a horizontal position equal to the height of the stretcher. Lower the side rails. Fanfold the top covers to the foot of the bed, out of the way.

5. Remove the safety belt and lower the side rails on the stretcher.

6. Place a bath blanket over the patient, if necessary.

7. Roll the turning sheet up against the patient on both sides. The sheet should be long enough to support the patient's head and shoulders during the move.

8. Position the stretcher close to the bed. Lock the wheels and lower the side rails.

9. One person stands along the open side of the stretcher. The other two or three people stand on the open side of the bed. These assistants may need to get on the bed, on their knees, to avoid overstretching their backs.

✎ NOTE

Use an overhand grasp on the moving sheet to avoid wrist strain. Using a friction-reducing sheet, roller, lifting pad, or air-transfer device (see Chapter 31) will make this task much easier and reduce the risk of personal injury.

- The assistant at the end of the bed grasps the moving sheet by placing one hand by the patient's legs and the other hand by the patient's hips.

- The middle assistant grasps the moving sheet by placing one hand by the patient's hips and the other hand by the patient's shoulder.

- The assistant at the head of the bed grasps the turning sheet by the patient's shoulder and head.

- On the count of three, all persons slide the moving sheet from stretcher to bed (Figure 16-15).

10. Center the patient on the bed in good body alignment. Position the patient properly. Raise the side rails of the bed if ordered.

11. Carry out ending procedure actions.

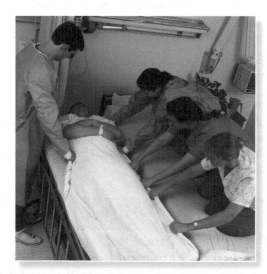

FIGURE 16-15 All persons slide the lifting sheet from stretcher to bed.

ICON KEY:
 = OBRA

⚠ OSHA **ALERT**

The mechanical lift is an important device for back safety. Using the mechanical lift for patients who are large or difficult to move is safer for both the patient and the nursing assistant. However, you should never use the lift alone. Make sure one or more other workers are available to assist you

STRETCHER TRANSFERS

This procedure is used to move a patient from their room to another room. Assure the patient that the procedure is safe.

NOTE

Procedure 23 is for moving an unconscious or semiconscious patient. For alert, fully awake patients, two people may be able to perform this procedure with one person against the stretcher and the other person on the opposite side of the bed. Instruct the patient on how to help you.

MOVING THE PATIENT WITH A MECHANICAL LIFT

A mechanical lift is used for moving heavy and dependent patients who have little or no ability to assist. Using a mechanical lift for transfers is safer for both the patient and the nursing assistant. Various types of slings are available so the patient can be moved in the sitting or supine position. Some mechanical lifts may be used to weigh bedfast patients.

Several types of mechanical lifts are available. Some are manually operated, and others are electric. The most common is the hydraulic lift. It is used when a patient is heavy, is unable to assist, is unbalanced, or has an amputation or other condition that makes transfer with a belt

 Safety **ALERT**

Some portable lifts are wheeled to the bedside. Some operate by using a ceiling-mounted hoist (Figure 16-16). The wall-mounted lift is similar to the ceiling lift and is used in rooms in which the ceiling will not support the weight of the hardware. Manual and electric hydraulic lifts are in widespread use. The principles of use are the same for all lifts, and showing instructions for every lift available on the market is impossible. The principles of patient safety and movement given here apply to other lifts with a sling seat. Follow your facility's policies and procedures for the lift you are using. Never use a lift until you have been instructed on how to use it and are approved to use it. Never use a mechanical lift alone. Be sure someone is available to assist before moving a patient.

 Safety **ALERT**

In addition to using the correct sling, make sure the resident falls within the weight guidelines for the seat. Facilities may have more than one brand of lift. Make sure the sling is compatible with the type (manufacturer's brand) of lift you are using. If you are caring for a bariatric patient, be sure to use bariatric equipment.

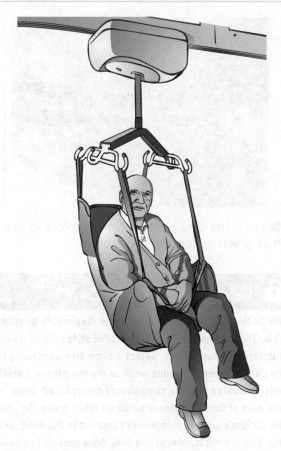

FIGURE 16-16 Some facilities permanently mount ceiling lifts in certain rooms. These rooms are reserved for patients who are dependent for transfers, such as those with paralysis.

difficult or impossible. Know and follow your facility's policy for use of the mechanical lift.

Check the care plan to ensure you have the right type of sling that is the correct size. Facilities usually have a variety of slings for various purposes. Some have a complete seat. Others have an opening in the seat for toileting. Others are U-shaped and can be applied and removed when the person is seated. These cross over the midline and wrap around the legs.

The sling will be fastened to the mechanical lift with chains or color-coded webbing (Figure 16-17). The color selected is determined by the most appropriate and comfortable position. For example, in the sling pictured, using the green loops at the top and purple loops at the bottom will position the person in the sitting position. Using the black loops at the top and bottom places the person in the supine position with the head supported. Check the strap length as soon as the person's body is above the surface of the bed. If the strap on one side is longer than the same strap on the opposite side, the sling is not centered correctly, which will make it difficult or impossible to position the person comfortably in the chair. Put the lift down and correct the problem before making the transfer.

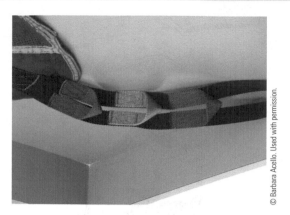

© Barbara Acello. Used with permission.

FIGURE 16-17 The care plan will list the colors to use, such as green on top, purple on bottom.

> ### 🔒 Safety **ALERT**
>
> Slings for the mechanical lift can be disposable or reusable. They are available in a variety of styles. Each meets a different patient need. Select a sling size according to the patient's weight. Visible wear on the sling (even a small hole) indicates that the sling should be replaced. Wear in one area of the sling places strain on other areas. Be sure the patient's body is completely centered in the sling, and that they are not leaning to one side. After tension has been applied to the straps, but before the person has been lifted, check to ensure that the straps are connected correctly and are secure. The sling must be washed before being used with another patient.

> ### 🔒 Safety **ALERT**
>
> Select a battery-operated lift whenever possible. This type of lift is easier to operate and causes much less wear and tear on your body compared with a manual pump–type lift.
>
> Check slings, chains, and straps for frayed areas or clasps that do not close properly. Check the hydraulic lift and the leg spreader to make sure they are both working. The leg spreader for a hydraulic lift must be opened wide when the patient is moved, or the lift will tip. Check the lift prior to each use by spreading the legs with the locking bar, then locking the handle into place. Next, hold pressure on the boom of the lift, while pressing your foot against the legs (Figure 16-18). If the legs close under this pressure, remove the lift from service until it can be inspected and repaired. Notify the nurse. A properly working locking mechanism should prevent the legs from closing under a load. Do not use the lift if there is oil on the floor or if equipment is defective. Report the need for repair and obtain safe equipment.

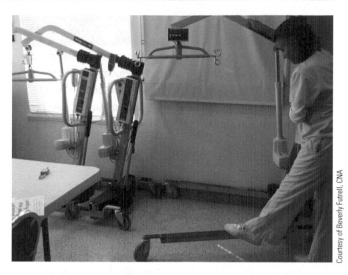

Courtesy of Beverly Futrell, CNA

FIGURE 16-18 Open the spreader bar. Position the far leg near a wall or stable piece of furniture. Hold your foot on the near leg while applying downward pressure to the boom. If the legs fold inward, the lift is not safe. Remove it from service until it is repaired.

Weight

If you will be using a mechanical lift with a scale feature, balance the scale to zero before obtaining the weight. Keep the person's body contained inside the sling. Make sure the feet and buttocks are not touching the bed.

TOILET TRANSFERS

The bladder empties much more efficiently if patients can use the toilet or commode rather than a urinal or bedpan. To use the toilet, the patient must possess transfer skills. Unless the patient has full weight-bearing on both legs and good balance, a wall rail is needed for support while transferring. (Refer to Procedure 27.) Towel racks are not safe for this purpose. Male patients may find it easier and safer to sit rather than stand while urinating.

TUB TRANSFERS

Showers with chairs, as well as tubs and whirlpools with hydraulic lifts, are available in many health care facilities. These are important safety devices. Follow directions when using them.

If the patient is at home, a tub chair, a rail on the wall beside the tub, and slip-proof mats in the tub are needed for safety. Add water to the tub after the patient has safely transferred, with cold water turned on first and off last. A handheld shower head attached to the faucet of the tub is safer and easier for self-bathing.

EXPAND YOUR SKILLS

PROCEDURE **26** **TRANSFERRING THE PATIENT WITH A MECHANICAL LIFT**

This procedure is used for heavy patients who have little or no weight-bearing ability.

 NOTE

The sling in this procedure is very popular and commonly used. It can be applied and removed when the patient is sitting. However, it is contraindicated in some medical conditions. Check the care plan before using it.

1. Carry out initial procedure actions.

2. Assemble equipment:
   - Mechanical lift
   - Sling
   - Chains—and bars, if needed—for the type of sling you are using
   - Chair or wheelchair

3. Place a wheelchair or other chair parallel to the foot of the bed, facing the head of the bed. Lock the wheelchair.

4. Elevate the bed to a comfortable working height. Lock the bed wheels. Lower the nearest side rail. Roll the patient toward you.

5. Position the sling beneath the patient's body behind shoulder, thighs, and buttocks. Be sure the sling is smooth (Figure 16-19A).

6. Roll the patient back onto the sling and position properly (Figure 16-19B). If the sling has inserts for metal bars, insert them now.

7. Position the lift frame over the bed with base legs in the maximum open position, and lock the lift legs (Figure 16-19C).

8. Attach suspension straps or chains to the sling (Figure 16-19D). Check fasteners for security. Lift the patient a few inches off the bed and check to be sure the sling is secure.

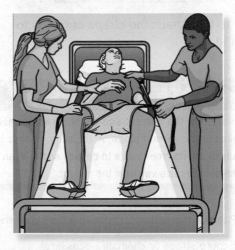

FIGURE 16-19B Roll the patient back onto the sling.

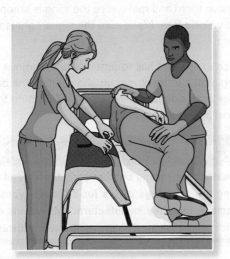

FIGURE 16-19A Position the sling under the patient.

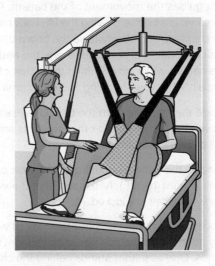

FIGURE 16-19C Position the lift frame over the bed.

(continued)

PROCEDURE **26** **CONTINUED**

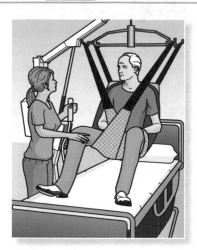

FIGURE 16-19D Attach the straps or chains to the sling.

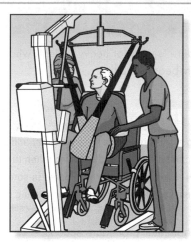

FIGURE 16-19E Position the lift frame over the chair and lower the patient into the seat.

15. Unhook the suspension straps or chains and remove the lift.

16. Position the footrests to support the patient's feet.

 NOTE

Be sure that the correct end of the strap or chain is hooked to the correct place on the sling. Always hook straps or chains from inside to outside so the open part of the hook faces away from the patient.

9. Position the patient's crossed arms inside the straps.

10. Secure straps or chains if necessary.

11. One assistant operates the lift and the other assistant guides the movement of the patient. Open the spreader bar before moving the lift. Lock the hydraulic mechanism, and slowly raise the boom of the lift until the patient is suspended over the bed. Talk to the patient while slowly lifting them free of the bed. Explain what you are doing and make small talk.

12. Guide the lift away from the bed. One assistant moves the lift, while the other supports and moves the patient's feet and legs.

13. Position the patient and lift over the chair or wheelchair (Figure 16-19E). Make sure that the wheels of the wheelchair are locked.

14. Slowly lower the patient into the chair or wheelchair. Pay attention to the position of the patient's feet and hands. One assistant stands behind the chair to pull and guide the patient's hips back into position at the back of the seat.

NOTE

Reverse these directions for moving a patient from chair to bed. When raising the patient from the chair, monitor the position of the S hooks (if used, depending on type of lift), to be sure they do not catch under the chair arms.

17. If the patient is in a chair, the sling can remain underneath the patient so it is in position for a transfer back to the bed. If the sling has metal bars, remove them and make sure the sling is smooth and wrinkle-free. Make sure the signal light is within reach.

18. Once the patient has returned to bed, remove the sling. Pull the top covers up and position the patient. Raise both side rails if necessary. Make sure the signal light is within reach.

NOTE

The method for raising and lowering the lift and for moving the base legs varies for different types of equipment. Read the manufacturer's directions and practice using equipment before using it with patients.

19. Carry out ending procedure actions.

ICON KEY:
0 = OBRA

CAR TRANSFERS

You may need to help a patient transfer into a car when they are discharged from your facility. If you are working in a patient's home, you may need to help the patient into and out of the car. A two-door car makes the transfer easier because the door is wider and gives more room for moving into and out of the car. With either a two-door or four-door car, the patient should always transfer onto the front seat. The front door is usually wider and opens wider.

 OSHA **ALERT**

OSHA restricts operating and assisting with lifting devices to those who are 18 years of age and older. Hospitals[1] and other institutions "primarily engaged in the care of the sick, the aged, or the mentally ill" are covered employers under Section 3(s)(1)(B) of the Fair Labor Standards Act (FLSA). Hazardous Order 7 of the FLSA prohibits minors under the age of 18 from operating or assisting in the operation of mechanical lifting devices. This rule has been amended slightly for health care facilities due to the high risk of back injuries. At the time of this writing, 16- and 17-year-old nursing assistants (who have completed the nursing assistant class) may assist workers over the age of 18 with use of a patient lifting device such as a mechanical lift, though they are still subject to a number of restrictions.

In some states, learning to use the mechanical lift is a mandatory part of the curriculum in the nursing assistant program. In these states, students under the age of 18 are required to use the lift and generally may use it to transport other students, but not patients. Check with your instructor for information regarding the rules for your state.

[1]29 C.F.R. pt. 570, subpart E. Effective on July 19, 2010. See http://www.dol.gov/whd/regs/compliance/whdfs52.pdf; http://www.youthrules.dol.gov/; http://www.dol.gov/whd/FieldBulletins/fab2011_3.htm.

 OSHA **ALERT**

Many health care facility bathrooms meet OSHA criteria for confined spaces. Confined spaces cause health care workers to work in awkward positions and use forceful movements because the spaces are small, crowded, or have obstructions. Lifting and moving in a confined space increases your risk of injury. If you are in a confined space, you may need to use a creative method of doing toilet transfers, such as using a ceiling-mounted lift or transferring the patient to a commode chair or shower chair outside the bathroom, then wheeling the chair in and positioning it over the toilet. Two or more workers will be necessary for this procedure.

 Safety **ALERT**

Many falls occur going to and from the bathroom, as well as in the bathroom. Assist patients with toileting regularly. Respond to call signals promptly. Do not leave the patient alone if you think doing so is unsafe.

 Safety **ALERT**

Patient transfers into and out of personal vehicles are considered high-risk tasks, especially if the patient is very weak, confused, or acutely ill. Another concern is having to transfer a patient with one-sided weakness or paralysis toward the weaker side. (For most transfers, the stronger side is the leading side.) Make sure you have enough help and supplies—such as a transfer belt, a friction-reducing sheet, or other special items—before transferring the patient.

EXPAND YOUR SKILLS

PROCEDURE **27** TRANSFERRING THE PATIENT ONTO AND OFF OF THE TOILET

1. Carry out initial procedure actions.

2. Assemble equipment:
   - Toilet tissue
   - Transfer belt
   - Disposable gloves
   - Commode if toilet is not available

3. Position the wheelchair at a right angle to the toilet or commode to face the wall rail. Position the large part of the wheelchair's front caster wheels facing forward, and lock the wheels. Raise or remove the footrests.

4. Place a transfer belt around the patient's waist. Use an underhand grasp with one hand toward

(continues)

the patient's back and the other hand toward the patient's front.

5. Tell the patient to lean forward slightly, to place the stronger foot slightly behind the other foot, to grasp the wall rail with both hands, and to bring themselves to a standing position by pushing off from the wheelchair (Figure 16-20A).

6. Have the patient pivot or step around until they feel the toilet or commode against the back of their legs.

7. Slide the pants and underwear down over the patient's knees. You may need to keep one hand on the transfer belt and use the other hand to manipulate the patient's clothing (Figure 16-20B).

8. Assist the patient to a sitting position on the toilet and allow them time to eliminate.

9. When the patient is finished, put on disposable gloves. Use toilet tissue to clean the patient if they are unable to do this themselves. If the patient is steady, remove and dispose of your gloves. Instruct the patient to stand and to reach for the wall rail. Then assist with pulling the patient's underwear and pants up.

10. If the sink is close enough, the patient can pivot or step to the sink to wash their hands before sitting down in the wheelchair. Otherwise, unlock the wheelchair, replace the footrests, and move the wheelchair to the sink so this step can be completed while the patient is seated.

11. Wash your hands.

12. Assist the patient to leave the bathroom. Make sure they are comfortable and have a signal light within reach.

13. Carry out ending procedure actions.

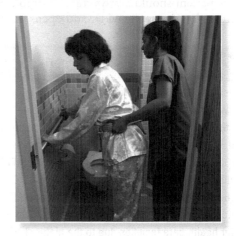

FIGURE 16-20A Tell the patient to grasp the wall rail with both hands.

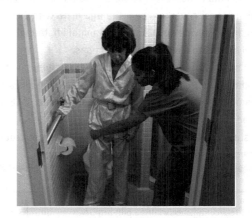

FIGURE 16-20B Keep one hand on the transfer belt and adjust the patient's clothing.

ICON KEY:
 = OBRA

REVIEW

A. Multiple Choice

Select the best answer for each of the following.

1. The method used for transferring a patient depends on:
   a. the availability of two nursing assistants.
   b. the patient's personal preference.
   c. the patient's size, strength, endurance, and balance.
   d. where the patient is going.

2. A transfer belt should never be used on patients who:
   a. take medications daily.
   b. have a colostomy.
   c. can stand on their feet.
   d. have an IV or catheter.

3. During a transfer, the patient should never:
   a. be allowed to help in the move.

b. place their hands on your body.

c. wear shoes.

d. be allowed to stand.

4. The Beasy board:

  a. is useful for independent patients.

  b. has a movable round seat in a track.

  c. should not be used by heavy patients.

  d. requires maximum staff assistance.

5. Using a manual mechanical lift requires that:

  a. two or more persons do the procedure.

  b. the patient be able to assist in the move.

  c. the patient be mentally alert.

  d. the patient weigh at least 300 pounds.

6. Which device is most useful for pivot transfers?

  a. Pivot disk

  b. Transfer board

  c. Slider

  d. Standing lifter

7. A manual handling sling is contraindicated in patients who:

  a. need minimum assistance.

  b. can follow instructions.

  c. are combative.

  d. do not need help moving.

8. The purpose of the colored loops on mechanical lift slings is:

  a. to match the sling to the correct lift.

  b. so you can color-code the sling for each patient.

  c. to position the person comfortably in the seat.

  d. so you can identify the sling for each patient.

9. When moving a patient in the hydraulic lift:

  a. open the leg spreader.

  b. lower the boom.

  c. close the leg spreader.

  d. wrap the person in a blanket.

10. Stan, age 17, and Melody, age 16, attend the nursing assistant class at XHN High School. Using the mechanical lift is part of the mandatory curriculum in their state. According to information in this chapter, they must have supervised practice and complete a skills checklist for each skill. During the lifting and moving content of their education, they will:

  a. skip all the mechanical lift content.

  b. use the lift for patients independently.

  c. use the lift for students in skills lab.

  d. learn the theory but skip skills practice.

11. When transferring a person into a car:

  a. use the rear passenger door because it works best.

  b. you must do a one-person standing pivot transfer.

  c. remember that the front passenger door is widest.

  d. a mechanical lift is the safest method of transfer.

12. A "no-lift" facility is a facility in which:

  a. workers should never move patients or heavy items.

  b. mechanical aids are available for moving patients.

  c. patients must be moved by hand or bodily force.

  d. no lifting equipment is available.

13. A vertical transfer could be done with a:

  a. Beasy board.

  b. mechanical lift.

  c. slider.

  d. sling.

14. A person who is FWB can:

  a. transfer independently.

  b. stand on one leg.

  c. walk in the hallway.

  d. stand on both legs.

15. When assisting with a bed-to-chair transfer, it is helpful to:

  a. have the patient place their hands around your neck.

  b. pull the patient up under the arms and shoulders.

  c. use a transfer belt unless contraindicated.

  d. elevate the bed to the highest horizontal position.

16. Positioning the large part of the small front wheelchair wheels facing forward during transfers:

  a. makes the chair less stable.

  b. is easier for the patient.

  c. is easier for the nursing assistant.

  d. reduces the risk of tipping.

17. A transfer belt is used to:

  a. lift the patient.

  b. supervise ambulation.

  c. control the transfer.

  d. pull the patient up.

18. To use a sliding board, the patient must have:
  a. paralysis of one or both legs.
  b. good upper-body strength.
  c. ability to direct the transfer.
  d. good lower-extremity strength.

19. When moving a patient in a mechanical lift, the:
  a. leg spreader must fold in when pressure is applied to the boom.
  b. boom must never be locked in the low position.
  c. brakes must be locked when the patient is in the air.
  d. leg spreader must be closed when the boom is elevated.

B. True/False

Mark the following true or false by circling T or F.

20. T F   Although mechanical lift slings differ in appearance; they are all very similar.

21. T F   During a transfer, the patient should place their hands on the nursing assistant's shoulders.

22. T F   A transfer belt should always be used for standing transfers unless contraindicated.

23. T F   Always transfer toward the patient's stronger side.

24. T F   During a transfer, the nursing assistant should place their hands around the patient's trunk.

25. T F   During a transfer, always explain to the patient how they can help.

26. T F   Towel bars are not safe to use as grab bars.

27. T F   Always inspect slings and straps for damage before using the mechanical lift.

28. T F   One person can safely transfer an unconscious patient from a stretcher to a bed if the correct type of moving device is used.

29. T F   Elevating the surface the patient is transferring from so it is slightly higher than the surface the patient is transferring to will make the transfer easier for all parties.

30. T F   Never transport an unconscious patient by stretcher.

31. T F   An unconscious patient should be secured with a safety belt during stretcher transport.

32. T F   A manual handling sling will make you stronger.

33. T F   A manual handling sling is contraindicated in patients who are totally dependent.

34. T F   The patient's feet must be supported in the wheelchair unless they use them to propel the chair.

35. T F   To use a hydraulic lifting device independently, workers must be 16 years of age or older.

C. Nursing Assistant Challenge

You are assigned to Mrs. McNeely, who is scheduled for surgery. She is alert and able to follow your directions. You know that when she returns from surgery, she will be semiconscious from the anesthesia and other medications. Consider the differences in procedures when she goes to surgery and when she returns to her room.

36. What instructions will you give Mrs. McNeely when she transfers from her bed to the surgical stretcher? _____

37. What will you need to do to transfer her back to bed after the surgery? _____

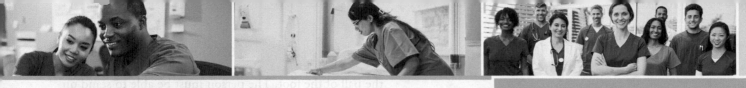

The Patient's Mobility: Ambulation

CHAPTER 17

OBJECTIVES

After completing this chapter, you will be able to:

17.1 Spell and define terms.

17.2 Describe the purpose of assistive devices used in ambulation.

17.3 List safety measures for using assistive ambulation devices.

17.4 Describe safety measures for using a wheelchair.

17.5 Describe nursing assistant actions for:
- Ambulating a patient using a gait belt.
- Propelling a patient in a wheelchair.

- Positioning a patient in a wheelchair.
- Transporting a patient on a stretcher.

17.6 Demonstrate the following procedures:
- Procedure 28: Assisting the Patient to Walk with a Cane and Three-Point Gait
- Procedure 29: Assisting the Patient to Walk with a Walker and Three-Point Gait
- Procedure 30: Assisting the Falling Patient (Expand Your Skills)

VOCABULARY

Learn the meaning and the correct spelling of the following words and phrases:

ambulate	gait	locomotion	prosthesis
assistive device	gait training	orthopedic	

AMBULATION

The term **ambulate** means to walk. Some patients may not be able to walk because of a disease or injury. Patients who cannot walk may be independent and goal-directed because they can self-propel their wheelchairs. Moving about in a wheelchair is called **locomotion**.

The term **gait** refers to the way in which a person walks. Many disorders can affect a person's gait, such as:
- stroke—one side of the body is paralyzed (hemiplegia) or weak (hemiparesis).
- Multiple sclerosis, postpolio syndrome—one or both legs are weakened and balance may be disturbed.
- Huntington disease—the patient has involuntary movements that disturb balance.
- Parkinson disease—the patient has stiffness, tremors, and slowness of movements, causing shuffling.
- Arthritis—the patient has pain and stiffness of joints.
- Amputation—the patient has a **prosthesis** (artificial limb) or the extremity is missing entirely. The patient may have difficulty balancing.
- **Orthopedic** issues—the patient has injuries or disorders of the musculoskeletal system and related structures.

Evaluation for Ambulation

Before initiating an ambulation program, the restorative nurse or physical therapist will evaluate the patient's:
- Tolerance to movement in bed
- Joint range of motion; ability to move freely (Figure 17-1)
- Ability to participate in active (as opposed to passive) exercise

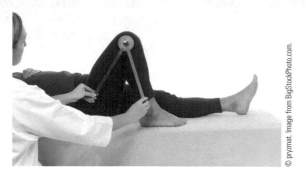

FIGURE 17-1 The physical therapist measures joint flexibility with an instrument called a goniometer.

- Ability to safely transfer with minimal assistance
- Ability to stand and bear weight
- Strength, endurance, and balance
- Mental state, to determine if the patient can follow directions
- Ability to walk alone (whether the assistance of a person or equipment is needed)

Normal Gait Pattern

There are two phases to a normal gait (walking). The leg is on the floor during the first phase and brought forward during the second phase. Walking begins with the ankle in *dorsiflexion* (toes pulled toward shin) and the heel striking the floor first (Figure 17-2), rolling onto

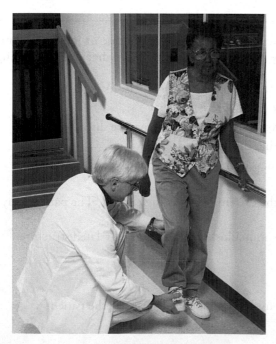

FIGURE 17-2 Walking begins with the ankle in dorsiflexion and the heel striking the floor first.

the ball of the foot. The person must be able to stand on this leg while bringing the other leg forward. Each arm swings slightly in the same direction as the opposite leg. To walk safely, the patient must have good strength and joint motion in the hips, buttocks, and knees. The physical therapist may work with the patient on exercises to promote movement and strength before the patient starts walking.

Gait Training

The physical therapist may work with the patient on **gait training** (teaching the patient to walk). The therapist will teach the patient how to:

- Walk correctly
- Walk on different surfaces, such as linoleum floors, carpet, grass, gravel, and so on
- Go up and down stairs
- Get in and out of a chair
- Use an assistive device if one is needed

The therapist also teaches the staff measures to assist the patient and special safety precautions to follow during nursing care, if needed.

Patient Independence

The patient's ability to ambulate safely and the amount of assistance needed are listed on the care plan. Observations to make and report about the patient's ability to ambulate and amount of assistance required are listed in Table 17-1.

TABLE 17-1 Observations to Make and Report About the Patient's Ability to Ambulate and Amount of Assistance Required

- Difficulty getting up and down
- Need for an assistive device, such as a cane or walker (does not have device and/or needs training)
- Safety awareness
- Gait steady, unsteady, shuffling, rigid, etc.
- Posture
- Environmental factors causing risk of falls
- Medical problems causing risk of falls, difficulty balancing
- Walks unassisted. Requires devices such as cane, crutch, or walker
- Requires assistance for uneven surfaces or difficult ambulation, such as stairs or ramps
- Uses wheelchair and may require physical assistance for difficult maneuvers such as elevators or ramps or longer distances (May be able to walk, but generally does not)

GUIDELINES 17-1 Guidelines for Safe Ambulation

- Encourage patients to use the handrail when walking.
- Always stand on the patient's affected (weak) side when walking.
- Always use a gait belt (transfer belt) if the patient needs assistance with ambulation. Grasp the center back of the belt with an underhand grip (Figure 17-3). Place your other hand on the patient's shoulder if balance is unsteady.
- Make sure the patient is wearing sturdy shoes appropriate to the floor surface. This is usually nonslip soles with laces tied. Clothing should not be too loose or drag on the floor.
- Check the floor for clutter or puddles that could cause a fall.
- If you are unsure of the patient's endurance or balance, ask another nursing assistant to follow behind

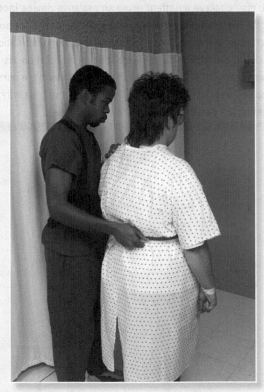

FIGURE 17-3 Hold the gait belt in back, using an underhand grip.

- you with a wheelchair. If the patient becomes weak, dizzy, or tired, they can sit in the wheelchair.
- Check the rubber handgrips and tips on the bottoms of canes, crutches, and walkers. Replace if the ridges are cracked, loose, or worn down. If the ridges are filled with debris, use alcohol and cotton swabs to clean them.
- Check screws, nuts, and bolts for tightness. Do not use any device that appears unsafe. Report the problem to the proper person.
- Practice good body mechanics for both yourself and the patient.
- Teach the patient to practice safety.
- Position your body so it moves with the patient's body. Match the person's stride and avoid interfering with the person's movement.
- Encourage the patient to stand upright and erect.
- Encourage the patient to take large, even steps while maintaining a wide base of support. The distance between the feet should be equal to the patient's shoulder width.
- Allow adequate time for ambulation. Avoid making the patient feel rushed.
- Allow the patient time to rest, if necessary.
- Provide only the amount of assistance needed.
- If the patient is not motivated, try goal setting. For example, place a chair ahead of them and ask them to walk to the chair.
- Stop ambulation immediately if the patient shows signs of illness, pain, extreme fatigue, shortness of breath, dizziness, sweating, or anxiety. Notify the nurse.
- Never leave the patient standing unattended. Assist the person to a chair when finished.
- Before leaving, quickly check the room for safety, such as items on the floor. Place the call signal and needed personal items within the patient's reach and remind the person to call for help, if needed.

ASSISTIVE DEVICES

An **assistive device** is often prescribed. These devices include:

- Crutches
- Canes
- Walkers

An assistive device helps compensate for walking problems. A walker or crutches may be ordered if the patient has only partial weight-bearing on one leg. Canes are usually ordered for persons who have problems with balance. There are several types of crutches, canes, and walkers (Figure 17-4). Each device is selected according to the needs of the patient and the cause and nature of the problem. The nurse or physical therapist will adjust the device to fit the patient. The gait is selected by the therapist and depends on the cause of the problem, the person's abilities, and the type of assistive device being used. Help the person use the device correctly during ambulation.

Use of Crutches

Standard crutches (Figure 17-5A) require good balance and two strong arms. They are seldom recommended for older adults. Metal forearm crutches are used by patients who have weakness of both legs, such as those with post-polio syndrome and other neurologic conditions. These crutches are also called *Lofstrand crutches* or *Canadian crutches*. The cuff of the crutch encloses the forearm so the person can release that hand without dropping the crutch (Figure 17-5B).

Forearm crutches with platforms permit weight-bearing on the forearms, providing stability. They are commonly used by persons with rheumatoid arthritis. During use, the elbows are at a constant 90° angle to the shoulder. The person may need help attaching the arm straps for the platforms. The nurse or therapist will teach you the gait for patients who use crutches.

Use of Canes

Several types of canes are available to meet patients' balance needs:

- Quad canes and tripod canes provide a wide base of support.
- Four-pronged pyramid canes have a broad base and are narrower at the top.

🔒 Safety ALERT

You may observe a patient using an assistive device incorrectly. For example, a patient may hold the walker for support when standing or carry the walker during ambulation. Assistive ambulation devices are used for ambulation. Using them for any other purpose may be unsafe. Inform the nurse, who will assess the patient and determine the best way of meeting the person's mobility and transfer needs.

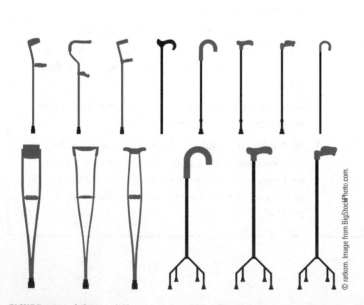

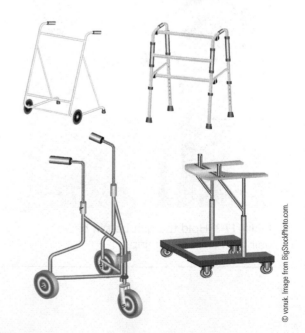

FIGURE 17-4 Many different mobility aids are available to meet patient needs.

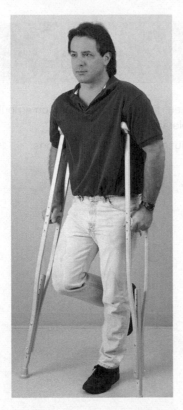

FIGURE 17-5A Standard crutches are used for injuries or amputation of one leg. They require good balance and upper-body strength and are usually not appropriate for elderly patients.

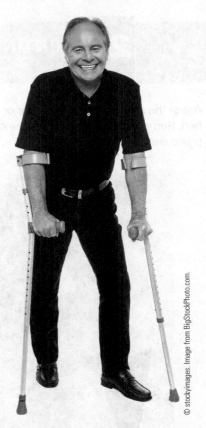

FIGURE 17-5B Forearm crutches are typically used for weakness in both legs.

PROCEDURE **28** ASSISTING THE PATIENT TO WALK WITH A CANE AND THREE-POINT GAIT

1. Carry out initial procedure actions.

2. Assemble equipment:
   – Cane as ordered
   – Gait belt

3. Make sure the patient has on sturdy shoes with non-slip soles. Check clothing to be sure it does not hang down over shoes.

4. Place the bed in the lowest horizontal position and lock the wheels. Assist the patient to sit on the edge of the bed. Place a gait belt on the patient and assist the person to a standing position. Stand on the affected or weaker side with your closest hand in the gait belt, using an underhand grip.

5. Instruct the person to hold the cane on their stronger side, with the tip about four inches to the side of

the stronger foot. Their weight should be distributed evenly between their feet and the cane (Figure 17-6).

6. Tell the person to shift their body weight to the strong leg and advance the cane about four inches so they are supporting their weight on the strong leg and the cane. Move the weak leg forward so it is even with the cane (Figure 17-7).

7. The patient then shifts their weight to the weak leg and the cane, moving the strong leg forward, ahead of the cane. Repeat this pattern while the person is walking.

8. Note the person's endurance, balance, and strength while walking. Stop immediately if the person has trouble and help them to the closest chair. Call the nurse.

(continues)

PROCEDURE 28 CONTINUED

9. Assist the patient to sit in the chair or to lie down in bed. Remove the gait belt. Store the cane in an appropriate area.

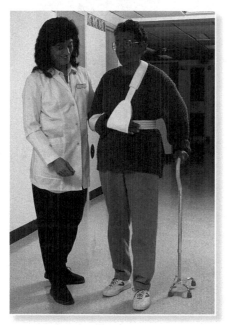

FIGURE 17-6 The patient holds the cane on the strong side of the body. The patient's weight should be evenly distributed between the feet and the cane before starting to walk.

ICON KEY:

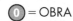 = OBRA

10. Document the distance the person ambulated and their tolerance of the procedure.

11. Carry out ending procedure actions.

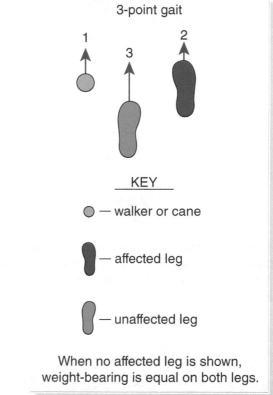

FIGURE 17-7 Three-point gait.

🔓 Safety **ALERT**

The procedures in this chapter assume that the facility has a tile or linoleum floor. You are instructed to apply nonslip footwear to the person. If the facility is carpeted, have the therapist or restorative nurse evaluate the person for appropriate footwear. A leather, synthetic, or plastic bottom may be more appropriate. Nonslip soles tend to stick to carpeting and may cause a weak or uncoordinated person to stumble. The therapist may slice tennis balls and cap some of the wheels if the person has a wheeled walker. These tend to move better on carpeting. As you can see, ambulation is an area where individual, assessment-based care is very important!

• Single-prong canes with T-handles or J-handles have straight handles and are easier to hold than half-circle handled canes.

For proper fit, the wrist must be even with the hip joint, with the elbow flexed 30°. Teach the person to hold the cane on the *strong* side of the body. The restorative nurse or therapist will develop a plan for safe ambulation.

Two-Point Gait with Cane

The steps for this procedure are as follows:

1. Follow steps 1 through 5 in Procedure 28.

2. Tell the person to move the cane and weaker leg forward at the same time, while their weight is on the stronger leg (Figure 17-8).

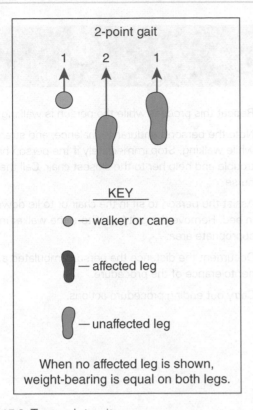

2-point gait

1   2   1

KEY

● — walker or cane

▮ — affected leg

▮ — unaffected leg

When no affected leg is shown,
weight-bearing is equal on both legs.

FIGURE 17-8 Two-point gait.

3. Instruct the person to shift their weight to the weak leg and cane, and move the stronger leg forward.

4. Repeat this pattern while the patient is walking. When using this gait, the person uses the left leg and right cane simultaneously, or right leg and left cane simultaneously, depending on which hand is holding the cane.

5. Follow steps 8 through 11 in Procedure 28.

Use of Walkers

Walkers also come in a variety of styles. Walkers are recommended for individuals who have general weakness of both legs, partial weight-bearing on one leg, or mild balance problems. The patient needs strength in both arms to pick up the walker. The walker must be wide enough to allow the person to walk into it. For proper fit, the elbow is flexed 30° when the hands are on the handgrip, and the top of the walker reaches the hip joint. Most walkers are adjustable. The nurse or physical therapist will make any necessary changes.

PROCEDURE 29 **ASSISTING THE PERSON TO WALK WITH A WALKER AND THREE-POINT GAIT**

1. Carry out beginning procedure actions.

2. Assemble equipment:
   – Walker as ordered
   – Gait belt

3. Make sure the person has on sturdy shoes with non-slip soles. Check clothing to be sure it does not hang down over shoes.

4. Place a gait belt on the person and assist them to a standing position. Place the walker in front of the person and have her grasp the walker with both hands. Stand on the person's affected side. Place your closest hand in the gait belt, using an underhand grip (Figure 17-9).

> ### ✎ NOTE
>
> The walker is not a transfer device and should not be used to help the patient stand up. The person grasps the walker after they are standing. To sit, the person releases their grip on the walker while still standing, and then places their hands on the arms of the chair or on the edge of the bed before sitting.

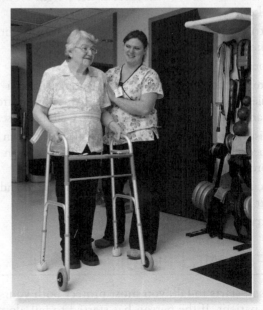

FIGURE 17-9 Stand on the patient's affected side as the patient grasps the walker with both hands. (Note the tennis balls on the rear legs of the walker.)

(continues)

PROCEDURE **29** CONTINUED

5. Instruct the person to stand with her weight evenly distributed between the walker and both legs, with the walker in front of her.

6. Have the person shift her weight to the strong leg as she lifts and moves the walker six to eight inches ahead. All four legs of the walker should strike the floor at the same time.

7. Advise the person to bring her weak foot forward into the walker. This may also be called a step-to or step-through pattern.

8. Now have her bring her strong foot forward even with the weak foot.

9. Repeat this process while the person is walking.

10. Note the person's endurance, balance, and strength while walking. Stop immediately if the person has trouble and help her to the closest chair. Call the nurse.

11. Assist the person to sit in the chair or to lie down in bed. Remove the gait belt. Store the walker in an appropriate area.

12. Document the distance the person ambulated and her tolerance of the procedure.

13. Carry out ending procedure actions.

ICON KEY:

0 = OBRA

Two-Point Gait with Walker

The steps for this procedure are as follows:

1. Complete steps 1 through 5 in Procedure 28.

2. Have the person shift their weight to the strong leg as they lift and move the walker and the weak leg six to eight inches ahead.

3. Now have them shift their weight to the weaker leg and the walker (with most of the weight on the walker).

4. Instruct them to move their strong leg six to eight inches ahead.

5. Repeat this process while the patient is walking.

6. Note the patient's endurance, balance, and strength while walking. Stop immediately if the person has trouble and help them to the closest chair. Call the nurse.

7. Assist the patient to sit in the chair or to lie down in bed. Remove the gait belt. Store the cane in an appropriate area.

8. Document the distance the person ambulated and their tolerance of the procedure.

9. Carry out ending procedure actions.

THE FALLING PERSON

If a person starts to fall, you must protect both yourself and the patient. If the person has started to fall, do not try to hold them upright. This will strain your back and may injure the patient. *If a person does fall, call the nurse to assess them for injuries before moving them.*

Fall prevention is a major concern in health care facilities. Patients with a previous history of falls are always at high risk. Other risk factors include advancing age, muscle weakness, gait and balance problems, urinary urgency, orthostatic hypotension (see Chapter 20), neurological and musculoskeletal disorders, some medications, mental confusion, dementia, lower extremity disability or foot problems, and visual impairment. Environmental risk factors include slippery surfaces, uneven floors, loose rugs, poor lighting, unstable furniture, food, water, or other liquids and objects on the floor.

Some elderly individuals have basic trust issues, particularly if the caregiver is young. They have their own way of doing things and believe they know best. The caregiver's way may be safest, but to gain cooperation, avoid telling the individual that they are wrong. Rather, try to incorporate the patient's method into a safer way of doing the task.

🔓 Safety **ALERT**

If you find a person on the floor, remain in the room and call for help. Leave the person on the floor. Deliver any emergency measures that you are qualified to provide. If the nurse suspects a fracture, they will instruct you on how to return the patient to bed. Rolling the patient onto a sheet or blanket will make the transfer less traumatic. After emergency treatment and positioning on the sheet, lift the patient back to bed with help.

EXPAND YOUR SKILLS

PROCEDURE 30 ASSISTING THE FALLING PATIENT

1. Keep your back straight, bend from the hips and knees, and maintain a broad base of support as you assist the falling person. Maintain your grasp on the transfer belt.

2. Ease the person to the floor, protecting their head.

3. As you ease the person to the floor, bend your knees and go down with the person (Figure 17-10).

4. Call for help.

5. Assist in returning the person to bed or chair.

6. Carry out ending procedure actions.

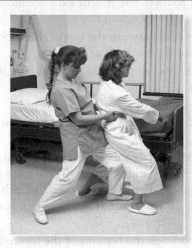

FIGURE 17-10 Ease the falling patient down your leg to the floor; bend your knees and go down with the patient.

ICON KEY:

= OBRA 　 = PPE

WHEELCHAIR MOBILITY

The wheelchair is an important piece of equipment in the health care facility. Many patients use wheelchairs for mobility. Some will progress to ambulation. Others will always use the wheelchair to move about. Whenever possible, the facility will restore the patient's ability to ambulate. Because patients spend so much time in wheelchairs, careful attention to fitting the chair to the patient is very important for comfort, pressure injury prevention, and restraint elimination. Sometimes wheelchairs are ordered or modified to meet special patient needs. For example, some patients with paralysis on one side of the body can propel the wheelchair independently by using their strong arm on the wheel and pushing the strong leg on the floor. The leg rest is removed on this side.

The wheelchair is a mobility device, not a transportation device. The goal is to keep patients ambulating independently. If a patient is weak and unsafe, restorative nursing should be notified. The restorative nurse and therapist will develop a plan of care to strengthen the person and restore their ability to walk.

Persons with medical conditions that require a wheelchair should move the chair independently. This is good exercise that promotes communication, independence, confidence, and self-esteem. Wheelchair mobility provides opportunities for patients to make choices and decisions. They can decide where they will go and what activities to attend. However, a facility emphasis on efficiency may create problems with wheelchair mobility. Pushing the chairs is faster for staff, but it deprives patients of much-needed exercise and independence. They lose the ability to make choices, which is very important. Some patients do not propel their wheelchairs because of physical problems, or because the chair does not fit correctly. However, adaptations may allow them to move independently. The therapy and restorative nursing departments will work with patients to fit their chairs correctly and teach patients to move the wheelchair independently. They may need to involve the wheelchair vendor if the patient has skeletal deformities or other special positioning needs. Assist and encourage patients to be as independent as possible in all activities of daily living.

Wheelchair Size and Fit

A wheelchair should fit the person who is using it. Correct fit and body alignment will prevent contractures and reduce the need for restraints, positioning aids, and body supports. A chair that fits correctly is also more comfortable and reduces the risk of skin breakdown. If the chair fits correctly, there will be:

- About four inches between the top of the back upholstery and the patient's axillae (armpits).
- Armrests that support the arms without pushing the shoulders up.
- Two to three inches of clearance between the front edge of the seat and the back of the patient's knee.
- Enough space between the patient's hip and the chair to slide your hand between the patient's hips on each side and the side of the wheelchair; the right amount of space avoids internal or external rotation of hips.
- Two inches between the bottom of the footrests and the floor.

- Ninety-degree angles between the feet and the legs, whether they are on the footrests or on the floor (when the footrests have been removed).

If the wheelchair does not fit the patient, check with the nurse or physical therapist to see how you can use pads or other devices to adapt the chair to the patient.

🔒 Safety **ALERT**

A wheelchair is not "one size fits all." Patients may have difficulty propelling a wheelchair that does not fit properly. A chair that does not fit correctly increases discomfort. Positioning problems are common. Patients may lean to the side, slide forward, or sit slumped in the chair. The risk of skin breakdown is increased. Positioning aids may be necessary. Sometimes unnecessary restraints are used to correct positioning problems. For many patients, a properly fit wheelchair eliminates the need for restraints! Inform the nurse if you suspect that the patient's problems are due to a wheelchair of the wrong size.

GUIDELINES 17-2 Guidelines for Wheelchair Safety

- Your first priority is ensuring that the wheelchair fits the patient. Use pillows, props, adaptive devices, or restraint alternatives if necessary to ensure that the patient maintains an upright position.

- Check the wheelchair to see that the brakes are working and the wheels are securely attached. If the patient needs footrests, make sure they are in place. Never transport a patient with the feet dangling or dragging.

- Replace the armrest of the wheelchair if it was removed during a transfer.

- Apply the brakes and lift the footrests out of the way when the patient is getting into or out of the wheelchair.

- When the chair is parked, position the large part of the front wheels facing forward to stabilize the chair and prevent tipping. Never park the wheelchair with the front wheels facing sideways.

- Position the patient in the 90-90-90 position, with the feet properly supported and the knees lower than the hips.

- Instruct the patient not to try to pick up an object from the floor. The restorative nurse or occupational

therapist may provide a reacher (also called a grabber) to safely enable the patient to retrieve dropped items or reach something on a high shelf (Figure 17-11). If the person has satisfactory trunk

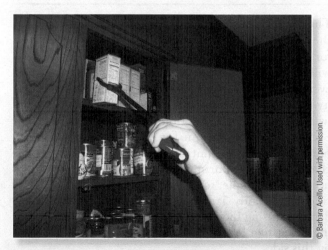

FIGURE 17-11 A reacher is an adaptive device that is like an extension of the arm, enabling the patient to reach things on high shelves or pick up items from the floor.

(continues)

GUIDELINES 17-2 Guidelines for Wheelchair Safety (continued)

stability and balance, they may be taught to pick up items with the hands, but instruct them to:

- – Avoid shifting weight in the direction of the reach.

- – Not move forward in the seat.

- – Not reach down between the knees.

- The safest method is to position the chair alongside an object that is to be reached for with casters in forward position, lock the chair, and reach only as far as the arm will extend.

- Check the patient's body alignment while in the wheelchair and reposition when necessary.

- Prevent bath blankets, lap robes, or clothing from getting caught in wheels.

- Be sure a paralyzed arm does not fall over the side of the wheelchair and become caught in the wheel.

- Guide the wheelchair from behind, grasping both handgrips.

- Approach corners slowly and look before you go around them.

- Take care when approaching swinging doors. Prop the door open to propel the chair through the door. If this is not possible, back through swinging doors.

- Always back over thresholds and into doorways and elevators (Figure 17-12).

- When leaving an elevator, push the stop button and ask others to step out. Turn the wheelchair around and back it out the door.

- Walk backward slowly when going down a ramp or incline. Periodically look over your shoulder, as you would when backing up in a car, to make sure that the path is clear.

- Always use the wheelchair entry button, if one is available on the door (Figure 17-13). The button will open

the door automatically and hold it open for about a minute to allow a wheelchair or stretcher to enter.

- When parking a wheelchair, avoid blocking a doorway. Apply the brakes.

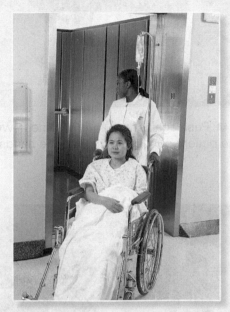

FIGURE 17-12 Always back over the threshold when entering doorways and elevators.

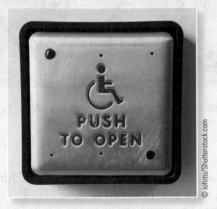

FIGURE 17-13 The automatic door opener allows passage through heavy doors safely and easily.

POSITIONING THE DEPENDENT PATIENT IN A WHEELCHAIR

The dependent person may slide down in the wheelchair, requiring assistance to regain body alignment. Several procedures can be used to correct the patient's position. Lock the drive wheels and position the caster wheels in the forward position before repositioning the patient.

- Stand in front of the patient; make sure that the feet are in alignment and the arms are on the armrests. Help the patient lean forward and push with the hands and legs as you push against the patient's knees (Figure 17-14A).

- For an alternate method, place a soft towel or small sheet under the patient's buttocks and use this as a pull sheet to move the patient up in the chair. This requires two people (Figure 17-14B).

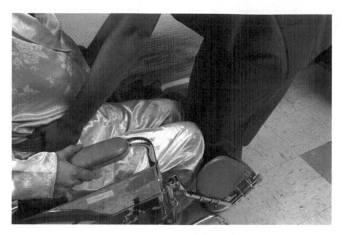

FIGURE 17-14A Push against the patient's knees with the legs as the patient pushes down with the hands and legs.

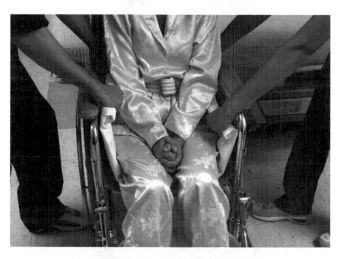

FIGURE 17-14B A draw sheet or lifting pad may be used to correct the patient's body alignment.

- Another method involves using a manual lifting device, such as a TLC pad (Figure 17-14C) or a lifting sling. The number of persons needed to lift is determined by patient size and the device you are using. Do not substitute a sheet for a manual lifting pad. The handles are necessary to coordinate the move and pull the patient safely. If the patient is uncooperative or heavy, two or more caregivers will be necessary. The TLC pad may also be used to turn a patient to the side or pull them up in bed. The pad is left in place when the patient is in a chair, wheelchair, or geriatric chair. Whether it stays in place when the patient is in bed is left to your discretion. The pad is soft and will not injure the skin, and some are quite absorbent in the event of incontinence. Those with a low-friction surface that tends to be slippery are best removed.

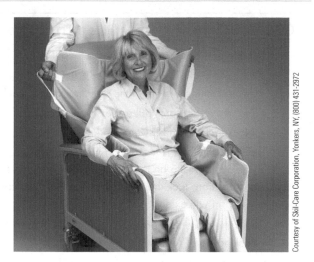

Courtesy of Skil-Care Corporation, Yonkers, NY, (800) 431-2972

FIGURE 17-14C One person can move a small or average-sized patient up in the geriatric chair by pulling the handles of the TLC pad. If unsure about the ability to move a patient, ask for help, since this will help prevent a back injury.

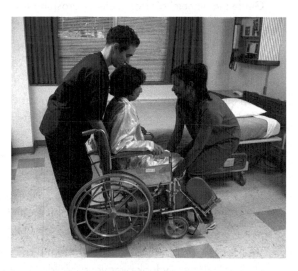

FIGURE 17-14D One assistant supports the lower extremities while the other uses the transfer belt to move the patient back in the chair. A sling may also be used (refer to Figure 16-8).

- This method also requires two people. Place the transfer belt around the patient's waist. One assistant stands behind the wheelchair and grasps the transfer belt with one hand on each side of the patient. The other assistant stands in front of the patient and places her hands and arms under the patient's knees. On the count of three, this assistant supports the lower extremities while the other moves the patient back in the chair (Figure 17-14D). This is not recommended for a heavy patient.
- Yet another method also requires two people. Stand behind the wheelchair and have another

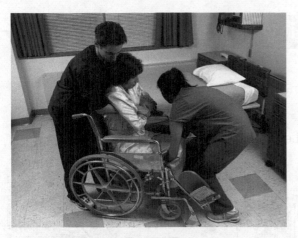

FIGURE 17-14E One assistant encircles the patient's legs with the hands and arms.

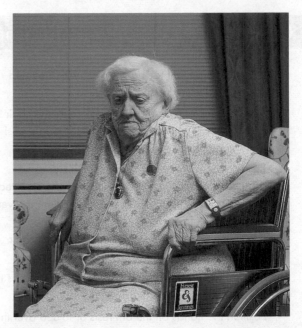

FIGURE 17-15 Wheelchair push-ups relieve pressure on the buttocks, preventing pressure injuries. If the patient cannot lift up enough to relieve the pressure every 15 minutes, the care plan will list instructions and times for staff to move the patient to eliminate pressure.

assistant in front. Both assistants work with knees and hips bent and backs straight. Lean forward with your head over the patient's shoulder. Instruct the patient to fold the arms, as if to hug herself. Place your arms around the patient's trunk. Grasp the patient's right wrist with your left hand and grasp the patient's left wrist with your right hand. The other assistant encircles the patient's knees with hands and arms. On the count of three, both assistants lift and move the patient up (Figure 17-14E).

If the patient can bear weight, it is easier and more beneficial to assist the patient to stand and then sit back down, getting the hips to the back of the chair. Wedge cushions placed in the wheelchair will prevent the patient from sliding forward.

WHEELCHAIR ACTIVITY

Pressure on the buttocks is dramatically increased when the patient is sitting. Teach the patient (and provide assistance if necessary) to periodically relieve the pressure by shifting weight every 15 minutes (Figure 17-15). *Be sure the wheelchair is locked, with the caster wheels in the forward position, before beginning any activities involving patient movement in the chair.*

Wheelchair Push-Ups

1. Teach the patient to place one hand on each armrest, keeping both elbows bent.
2. Have the patient lean forward slightly, pushing on the armrests and straightening the elbows while lifting the buttocks off the seat.
3. Instruct the patient to hold this position to the count of five if possible.

Leaning

If the patient cannot do push-ups, teach them to place the hands on the armrests or thighs and lean forward slightly and then to each side to relieve pressure on the buttocks. The caster wheels should be correctly positioned, with the brakes locked and the patient's feet on the floor, to prevent falling forward or chair tipping. Monitor patients who have balance problems.

Position the patient upright, without leaning to either side. Side leaning increases the risk for falls and other injuries, pain, discomfort, and deformities. Patients who lean to the side are often restrained to prevent injury. Avoid restraints whenever possible. Use pillows, pads, or other props to maintain alignment. Remember that good positioning begins with the feet. The feet must be well supported on the footrests, at a 90° angle to the lower legs. The lower legs must be at a 90° angle to the thighs. The patient's knees should not be higher than the hips. The thighs must be at a 90° angle to the torso. If the patient is positioned in this manner and continues to lean, an additional postural support is needed.

Leaning to one side or the other (lateral leaning) alters weight distribution, increasing pressure on the hips and buttocks. Many types of restraint alternatives may be used to keep the patient upright, avoid the use

GUIDELINES 17-3 Guidelines for Chair and Wheelchair Positioning

- Position the patient facing forward, with the head upright and erect (or supported).

- If the patient leans to the side, make sure the chair fits correctly. Support the person in an upright position using pillows, foam, or other props.

- Position the arms on the armrests if this does not push the shoulders up. If the shoulders are elevated, adding a seat cushion will boost the patient, preventing shoulder strain. Notify the nurse of this problem so the arms can be adjusted or another chair obtained.

- Support the arms on pillows, foam, or other props if the patient's shoulders are hanging.

- Position the hands on the armrests or folded over the patient's lap. Place a small pillow for support and comfort, if needed.

- The upper back of the wheelchair should be at the bottom of the shoulder blades.
  - If the chair back is too low, find another chair or ask the nurse about an extension.
  - If the chair back is too high, elevate the patient on a cushion.

- Place a folded bath blanket in the seat of the chair if the patient is wearing a hospital gown so the skin does not contact the vinyl. A bed protector may also be used to line the seat if the patient is wearing a hospital gown or is incontinent.

- Use a pressure-relieving pad in the seat if the patient plans to be up for a long time. The pressure-relieving cushion does more than make the patient comfortable. It has many hidden benefits:
  - The sling seat of the wheelchair tends to hammock (sag) in the center when a patient sits on it. The sagging causes rotation of the inner thighs, which increases pressure on the coccyx and buttocks, two common sites of pressure injuries.
  - Hammocking of the seat promotes sliding; the leveling pad at the bottom of many cushions corrects the sagging, distributing weight more evenly and reducing pressure.

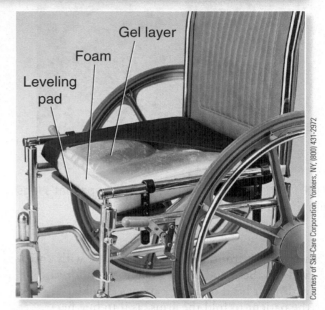

Courtesy of Skil-Care Corporation, Yonkers, NY, (800) 431-2972

FIGURE 17-16 A pressure-relieving gel and foam pad is comfortable, helps to prevent skin breakdown, and maintains skin integrity.

  - Although foam is comfortable and reduces pressure, it also traps heat, increasing the potential for skin damage. To counteract this, use a cushion with a gel layer on top, which cools the skin (Figure 17-16).
  - The gel also moves with the patient, which reduces the effects of friction and shearing.

- Position the hips at a 90° angle, at the back of the chair.
  - If the patient's hips slide forward, check the depth of the chair to make sure it fits. If the depth is correct, consult the nurse for postural supports or restraint alternatives. A gripper or wedge cushion may be placed on the seat to keep the patient from sliding.
  - Support the patient's weight with the legs and buttocks so that weight is equally distributed on both sides.
  - When positioning the male patient, make sure the scrotum is in front of the body, not underneath the patient.

(continues)

GUIDELINES 17-3 Guidelines for Chair and Wheelchair Positioning (continued)

- There should be at least three to four finger widths between the back of the knee and the seat of the chair.
- Support the feet on the floor or the footrests. If the patient's legs dangle:
  - Elevate the feet on a stool.
  - Use a commercial foot elevator (Figure 17-17).
  - Check with the nurse to see if the leg rests can be shortened to fit.
- When the wheelchair is parked, make sure the large part of the small front wheels faces forward. Lock the brakes.

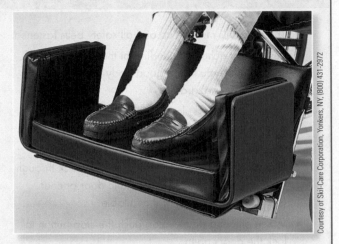

Courtesy of Skil-Care Corporation, Yonkers, NY, (800) 431-2972

FIGURE 17-17 The legs should never dangle. If the feet do not reach the foot plates, shorten the leg rests or apply a foot elevator to the chair.

of restraints, and maintain the patient's dignity and self-esteem. Devices such as lateral stabilizer bolsters are used on one or both arms to prevent patients with upper-torso weakness, paralysis, or deformities from leaning to the side and over the arm of the chair. The bolsters help maintain an upright position, use the arms to stabilize the torso, and provide armrest cushioning. Some bolsters are separate pieces, and others are fastened to the chair and fitted to the patient's skeletal deformities. They must fit under the patient's arm so they have functional range of motion.

Some patients require more support than pillows or foam bolsters can provide. Padded side wings (lateral supports, Figure 17-18) can be used on one or both sides of the body in a wheelchair or geriatric chair. A *side wing* is a semirigid device that provides additional support for patients with deformities and those who are difficult to maintain in an upright position. The side wings extend upward under the arms to provide stability to the torso. The padding prevents discomfort. The wings should extend to a few inches below the axilla on both sides. This maintains the patient in an erect, comfortable position and eliminates the need for straps, harnesses, and restraints, which are often used for patients who have positioning problems of the upper torso.

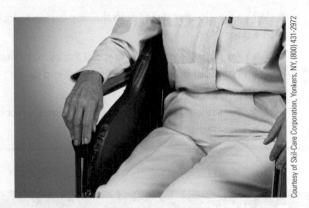

Courtesy of Skil-Care Corporation, Yonkers, NY, (800) 431-2972

FIGURE 17-18 Padded lateral supports (may also be called side wings) can be used on one or both sides of a wheelchair. This semirigid padded device provides support for patients with deformities and those who are unable to maintain an upright position.

TRANSPORTING A PATIENT BY STRETCHER

The guidelines for transporting a patient by stretcher are very similar to the guidelines for wheelchair safety. One major difference is that a person on a stretcher must *never* be left alone.

GUIDELINES 17-4 Guidelines for Stretcher Safety

- The side rails must be up and all safety belts fastened.
- Push the stretcher by standing at the patient's head. This enables you to use good body mechanics and see potential hazards.
- Approach corners slowly and look before you go around them.
- Prop swinging doors open to propel the stretcher through the door. If this is not possible, back through swinging doors. Use the automatic door opener (shown in Figure 17-13) if available.
- When entering an elevator, push the stop button to lock the doors open.
- Back the stretcher into the elevator by walking backward and pulling the head end of the stretcher (Figure 17-19).
- Stand by the patient's head while the elevator is in motion.
- When the elevator stops, push the stop button to lock the door open.
- Push the stretcher out so the feet exit the elevator first. If the threshold is uneven, go to the foot end of the stretcher and pull it out of the elevator.
- After the stretcher is safely out of the elevator, unlock the door mechanism.

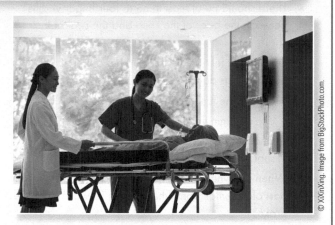

FIGURE 17-19 Lock the elevator doors into position as soon they open. Pull the head of the stretcher into the elevator first and then release the door lock. When exiting the elevator, lock the door open and push the stretcher out feet first. Then unlock the elevator doors.

- Walk backward slowly when transporting a stretcher down a ramp or incline. Guide the stretcher from the head end. Periodically look over your shoulder to make sure that the path is clear.
- Avoid blocking a doorway when parking a stretcher, for patient and facility safety.

REVIEW

A. Multiple Choice

Select the best answer for each of the following.

1. When ambulating a patient who has a weak right side, you should stand:
   a. in back of the patient.
   b. on the patient's right side.
   c. on the patient's left side.
   d. in front of the patient.

2. When ambulating a patient, you should hold the gait belt with:
   a. an overhand grasp in back of the patient.
   b. an underhand grasp in back of the patient.
   c. one hand on each side of the patient.
   d. one hand in front of the patient.

3. Before helping a patient to walk with a cane or walker, you should check the:
   a. distance between the patient's feet.
   b. screws and bolts for tightness.
   c. height of the wheelchair.
   d. length of each step.

4. Encourage the patient to hold the cane on/in their:
   a. stronger side.
   b. weaker side.
   c. dominant hand.
   d. nondominant hand.

5. When using a two-point gait with a cane, the patient will:
   a. place the strong foot forward, then the cane, then the weaker foot.
   b. place the weak foot and cane forward, then the strong foot.
   c. place the weaker foot and cane forward, then the stronger foot.
   d. place the strong foot forward, then the weak foot, then the cane.

6. If a patient starts to fall, you should:
   a. try to hold the patient upright.
   b. try to pull the patient to the bed.
   c. ease the patient to the floor.
   d. leave the room and run for help.

7. Mr. Herrera is ambulating with a walker. Encourage him to set it down so that:
   a. the front legs strike the floor first and then the back legs strike the floor.
   b. the back legs strike the floor first and then the front legs strike the floor.
   c. all four legs strike the floor at the same time.
   d. the walker slides across the floor with each step.

8. When transporting a patient in a wheelchair, always:
   a. stay to the right in corridors.
   b. guide the wheelchair from the front going down ramps.
   c. push the patient into an elevator frontward.
   d. position the patient's feet at a 45° angle.

9. Conditions that can affect a patient's gait include:
   a. diseases such as Parkinson disease.
   b. having a catheter.
   c. having hand surgery.
   d. transferring independently.

10. Assistive devices are usually selected by the:
   a. nursing assistant.
   b. physician.
   c. physical therapist.
   d. family.

11. You can expect your patient with a stroke to have:
   a. paralysis on one side of the body.
   b. a shuffling gait.
   c. phantom pain.
   d. paralysis of both arms.

12. You can expect your patient with Huntington disease to have:
   a. paralysis on one side of the body.
   b. involuntary movements and poor balance.
   c. phantom pains.
   d. a shuffling gait.

13. You can expect your patient with Parkinson disease to have:
   a. an endocrine system condition.
   b. a communicable disease.
   c. stiffness, tremors, and shuffling.
   d. paralysis of the lower body.

14. You can expect your patient with multiple sclerosis to have:
   a. weakness and balance problems.
   b. paralysis of the upper body.
   c. involuntary kicking of legs.
   d. a terminal prognosis.

15. You can expect your patient with arthritis to have:
   a. an endocrine system condition.
   b. pain and stiff joints.
   c. a history of injuries.
   d. an unstable gait.

16. You can expect your patient with a lower-extremity amputation to have:
   a. a nervous system condition.
   b. war injuries and mental problems.
   c. pain and stiff joints.
   d. a prosthesis.

17. You can expect your patient with an orthopedic disorder to have:
   a. a musculoskeletal system condition.
   b. paralysis on one side of the body.
   c. a genitourinary tract disorder.
   d. a congenital condition.

B. True/False

Mark the following true or false by circling T or F.

18. T F Always back in as you move a patient in a wheelchair into an elevator.

19. T F When transporting a patient in a wheelchair, always walk on the left of the corridor.

20. T F Wheelchair brakes should always be locked unless the patient is being moved.

21. T F A cane is held in the patient's weaker hand.

22. T F   The front two legs of the walker should strike the floor first, then the back two legs should strike the floor.

23. T F   When assisting a patient to ambulate, you need to use a gait belt only if the patient is using an assistive device.

24. T F   You should teach the patient how to do wheelchair push-ups or how to lean to relieve pressure on the buttocks.

25. T F   The patient should lean forward and reach down between the knees to pick an article up from the floor.

26. T F   A cane is used for patients who are unable to bear weight on one leg.

27. T F   The patient needs to be able to use both hands to manipulate a walker.

28. T F   The side rails and seatbelt are restraints that should not be used when transporting a patient on a stretcher.

C. Nursing Assistant Challenge

Mr. Santozi is 76 years old and has had right hip surgery. His physician does not want him to bear full weight on the affected leg. He uses a walker to assist his ambulation. He has been taught to use a three-point gait. When you help him out of bed, he reaches for the walker to help pull himself up from the bed. As you watch him walk down the hall, you note that he is setting the walker down by the front legs first and then the back legs. When he walks, he moves the walker and his strong leg ahead at the same time.

28. What errors is Mr. Santozi making, and how can you help him? _____
_____
_____

29. How will you position your body during Mr. Santozi's ambulation? _____
_____
_____

30. What gait will you use? _____
_____
_____

31. What will you do if Mr. Santozi loses his balance and starts to fall? _____
_____
_____

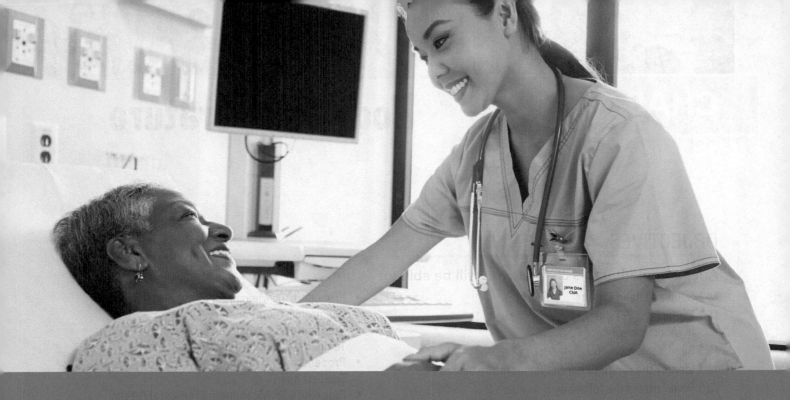

SECTION 6
Measuring and Recording Vital Signs, Height, and Weight

CHAPTER 18
Body Temperature

CHAPTER 19
Pulse and Respiration

CHAPTER 20
Blood Pressure

CHAPTER 21
Measuring Height and Weight

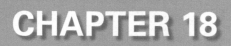

CHAPTER 18 — Body Temperature

OBJECTIVES

After completing this chapter, you will be able to:

18.1 Spell and define terms.

18.2 Explain the uses of three types of clinical thermometers.

18.3 Read a thermometer.

18.4 Identify the range of normal temperature values.

18.5 Demonstrate the following procedures:

- Procedure 31: Measuring an Oral Temperature (Electronic Thermometer)

- Procedure 32: Measuring a Rectal Temperature (Electronic Thermometer)
- Procedure 33: Measuring an Axillary Temperature (Electronic Thermometer)
- Procedure 34: Measuring a Tympanic Temperature
- Procedure 35: Measuring a Temporal Artery Temperature

VOCABULARY

Learn the meaning and the correct spelling of the following words and phrases:

body core
body shell
Celsius scale
clinical thermometer
digital thermometer

electronic thermometer
Fahrenheit scale
flagged
heat exhaustion
heat stroke

hypothermia
metabolism
Non-contact infrared
  thermometer (NCIT)
probe

temporal artery
  thermometer (TAT)
tympanic thermometer
vital (living) signs

INTRODUCTION

Measurement of body temperature is a common nursing assistant task. Body temperature is one of the **vital (living) signs**. The patient's other vital signs include pulse, respiration, and blood pressure.

Vital signs must be accurately measured because they tell us a great deal about the patient's condition. In most facilities, nursing assistants are permitted to inform the person of the results after taking vital signs. If the patient has further questions about the vital signs, advise that you will ask the nurse to discuss the results with them. Although they are usually determined as a combined procedure, each vital sign is discussed in a separate chapter of this text. Many facilities use electronic equipment that automatically registers four vital signs simultaneously.

TEMPERATURE VALUES

Temperature values may be expressed in either of two scales:

- **Fahrenheit scale**, which is indicated by an *F*. This is the scale that is generally used in the United States.
- **Celsius scale** (centigrade scale), which is indicated by a *C*. This is the scale that is used in Europe and other countries using the metric system.

A small ° (degree symbol) before either capital letter indicates degrees or levels of temperature.

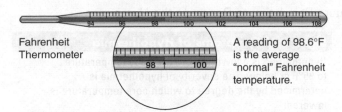

FIGURE 18-1 Fahrenheit thermometer.

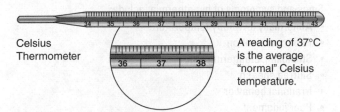

FIGURE 18-2 Celsius thermometer.

A formula can be used to convert temperature readings from Celsius to Fahrenheit and from Fahrenheit to Celsius. Figure 18-1 shows a reading from a Fahrenheit thermometer with a normal body temperature reading of 98.6 degrees Fahrenheit. Figure 18-2 shows a normal reading of 37 degrees Celsius. This type of thermometer is no longer used in patient care. The picture here is for example purposes only. Making a comparison scale with an electronic or **digital thermometer** is not possible.

DEFINITION OF BODY TEMPERATURE

Temperature is the measurement of body heat. It is the balance between heat produced and heat lost. Excessive body temperature stresses the vital body organs.

Body temperature is:

- Fairly constant. There is a daily variation of 1°F to 3°F. Body temperature is lowest in the morning. It is higher in the afternoon and evening.
- Lower the closer to the body surface it is measured. The temperature at the center of the body (**body core**) is much higher than the temperature at the surface of the body.
- Different in the same person when measured in different areas of the body. It is important to know the normal temperature for an individual because the normal may vary from person to person.
- Less stable in children.
- Affected by
  - Illness
  - External temperature/environment

- Medication
- Age
- Infection
- Time of day
- Exercise
- Emotions
- Pregnancy
- Menstrual cycle
- Crying
- Hydration

TEMPERATURE CONTROL

- Activities to control and regulate body temperature are managed by special cells in the brain.
- Heat is produced by chemical reactions (**metabolism**) and muscular contractions in the core of the body. For this reason, rectal temperature is highest.
- Heat is produced by cellular changes that occur when food is converted into energy. Muscle movement will also create heat. This explains why we feel hot during exercise. Involuntary shivering occurs to create additional heat when we are cold.
- Blood carries the heat to the skin (**body shell**). The heat is lost from the skin to the outside. Heat is also lost by sweating, breathing, and passing urine and feces.
- Heat loss is largely controlled by regulating the amount of blood reaching the skin and through perspiration.
- Average oral temperature range is 96.8°F (36°C) to 100.4°F (38°C). Average temperature is 98.6°F (37°C). Reportable values for adults are listed in Table 18-1.

Signs and symptoms of heat-related illness to report to the nurse are listed in Table 18-2.

TABLE 18-1 Reportable Temperature Values

Type	Report Values		
	Normal	*Below*	*Above*
Oral	98.6°F	97°F	100°F
Axillary	97.6°F	97°F	99°F
Rectal	99.6°F	98°F	101°F
Temporal artery	99.6°F	98°F	101°F
Tympanic	Tympanic values are set as oral or rectal equivalents. Use the reporting values for oral and rectal settings.		

TABLE 18-2 Signs and Symptoms of Problems with Temperature Regulation to Report to the Nurse

Signs and Symptoms of Heat Exhaustion

Heat exhaustion is caused by exposure to high temperature that causes the loss and imbalance of body fluids over time. It will progress to heat stroke and death if not treated promptly. Treatment is rest and fluids. Signs and symptoms are:

- Temperature normal or slightly below or above
- Headache
- Weakness
- Fatigue
- Dizziness
- Loss of appetite
- Nausea and vomiting
- Muscle cramps in the arms, legs, or abdomen
- Pale skin color
- Rapid pulse and respirations
- Orthostatic hypotension (Chapter 20)
- Skin cool and moist
- Excessive perspiration
- Confusion
- Clumsiness, incoordination

Signs and Symptoms of Heat Stroke

Heat stroke is a serious condition caused by inability to regulate temperature. It is caused by lengthy exposure to high heat. Early signs and symptoms of heat stroke are:

- Headache
- Dizziness
- Weakness
- Fatigue
- Skin hot and dry to touch

Unrecognized and untreated, the condition progressively worsens. Later symptoms are:

- Extremely high fever
- Shortness of breath
- Slow, thready pulse or strong, rapid pulse
- Blood pressure that is low or difficult to hear/palpate
- Absence of perspiration
- Bizarre behavior
- Combativeness
- Seizures
- Loss of consciousness
- Lethargy, stupor, or coma
- Heart abnormalities
- Death

Signs and Symptoms of Hypothermia

Hypothermia is a lowering of core body temperature to 95°F or below. The severity of hypothermia is determined by the degree to which core temperature is lowered:

Mild hypothermia, 93°F–95°F
Moderate hypothermia, 86°F–93°F
Severe hypothermia, less than 86°F

Signs and symptoms of hypothermia include:

- Abnormally low body temperature
- Poor coordination
- Stumbling, staggering gait
- Slurred speech
- Irrational behavior
- Poor judgment
- Amnesia
- Hallucinations
- Cyanosis
- Slight edema or puffiness of the skin
- Dilated pupils
- Decreased respiratory rate
- Weak or irregular pulse
- Stupor
- Tremors, intense shivering, and/or muscle rigidity (stops below 90°F)
- Fatigue
- Feeling of deep cold or numbness
- Disorientation
- Visual disturbances

Signs and Symptoms of Infection to Report to the Nurse

- Elevated temperature
- Rapid pulse and/or respirations
- Sweating
- Chills
- Skin hot or cold to touch
- Skin color abnormal-flushed, red, gray, or blue
- Inflammation of skin (redness, swelling, heat, pain)
- Drainage from any skin opening or body cavity
- Any other unusual body discharge, such as mucus or pus
- Other abnormalities specific to body system

MEASURING BODY TEMPERATURE

Temperature is usually measured in one of five body areas:

- Mouth (oral)—most common
- Ear (aural or tympanic membrane)—takes the least amount of time, but requires a precise technique for accuracy
- Rectal—believed to be the most accurate of commonly used sites (mouth, rectal, axillary);

rectal temperature registers 1°F (0.6°C) higher than oral

- Temporal artery (forehead)—a rapid, accurate method that has recently become popular
- Axillary or groin—least accurate; measures temperature under the arm or at the groin (this method is used only when the patient's condition or equipment available prevents the use of other methods); an axillary or groin temperature registers 1°F (0.6°C) lower than oral temperature

Facilities using the temporal artery method commonly use it for all patients except those who require special internal monitoring. If the temporal method is not used in the facility, a nurse will evaluate the patient's condition to determine which is the best site for measuring the temperature. The site used most often is the mouth. The mouth is not, however, always the best or safest site. In some situations, it is wiser to use another site. Notify the nurse if you believe something affects the site to use for taking the temperature.

CLINICAL THERMOMETERS

A patient's temperature is determined by using a **clinical thermometer**. There are several types of clinical thermometers.

The Glass Clinical Thermometer

The glass clinical thermometer is a slender glass tube containing liquid mercury. The mercury expands when exposed to heat and moves up or down the tube to measure temperature. This type of thermometer has been the gold standard for years. Now we know that mercury is dangerous to humans and the environment and should not be used. Other liquids have been used unsuccessfully. They are not as accurate as mercury for measuring the temperature. Glass also causes injury if it breaks. The U.S. government has various laws relating to the export, use, and disposal of mercury. Stores no longer sell glass thermometers, and health care facilities are not using them in clinical patient care.

Digital and Electronic Thermometers

The **electronic thermometer** (Figure 18-3) is most commonly used today. One unit can serve many patients because the nursing assistant simply changes the disposable sheath that fits over the probe.

- The electronic thermometer is battery operated. Batteries may be disposable or rechargeable. The temperature appears on the viewing screen in a few seconds.
- The portion called the **probe** measures the temperature.
- The probes are colored red for rectal use and blue for oral or axillary use.
- The probe is covered by a plastic sheath that is discarded after one use.

🔒 Safety **ALERT**

A disposable thermometer is made of rigid plastic. Remove the thermometer from the patient's mouth slowly. Pulling the thermometer out rapidly from between closed lips can cause tears of the lips and mucous membranes in the mouth.

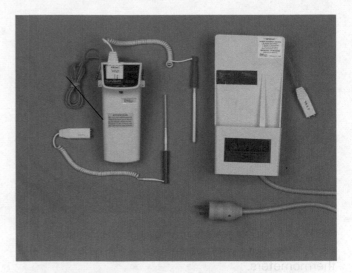

FIGURE 18-3 An electronic thermometer. The temperature is registered in large, easy-to-read numerals. The disposable protective sheath (probe cover) is placed over the probe tip. The probe is inserted in the patient's mouth in the usual manner. A plastic cord goes around the nursing assistant's neck when carrying the thermometer. The blue probe is used for oral, red for rectal. The thermometer is stored in its own charging unit.

Disposable Oral Thermometers

Plastic or paper thermometers (Figure 18-5) are used for oral temperatures in some facilities and clinics. Dots change color from brown to blue, according to the patient's temperature. Do not use this type of thermometer for rectal values. Discard this thermometer after one use.

Tympanic Thermometer

The **tympanic thermometer** is an instrument that measures the temperature from blood vessels in the tympanic membrane (ear drum) in the ear (Figure 18-6). The temperature reading obtained is close to the core body temperature. To obtain an accurate reading, place the probe solidly into the ear canal. The instrument has a built-in converter that provides the equivalent temperature in rectal or oral values (in both the Fahrenheit and Celsius systems). The type of temperature reading (mode) is selected by the user. Insert the disposable speculum into the ear canal, gently sealing the canal. Activate the instrument by pressing a button, and within a few seconds it registers the temperature of the blood flowing through the vessels in the eardrum.

When this thermometer was first introduced, it became instantly popular. However, many facilities stopped using it because user technique must be precise to obtain accurate values, and the margin of error is great.

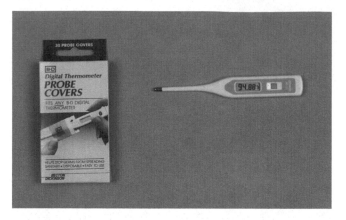

FIGURE 18-4 Probe covers may be used to reduce the risk of infection when using most stick-types of oral thermometers.

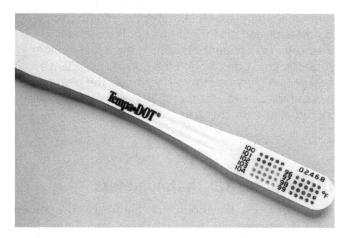

FIGURE 18-5 The chemical dot thermometer is used only for oral temperatures. It is used once, then discarded.

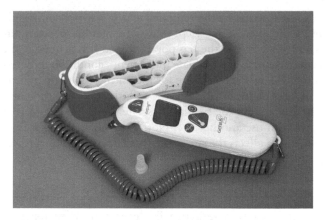

FIGURE 18-6 Handheld tympanic thermometer that measures the temperature deep within the ear. The window on the handset indicates the digital temperature reading. The thermometer can be set to provide an oral, rectal, Fahrenheit, or Celsius equivalent.

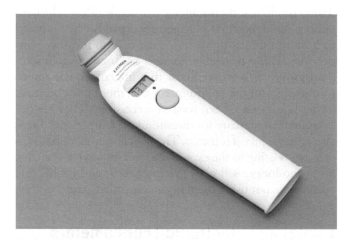

FIGURE 18-7 A temporal artery thermometer.

Temporal Artery Thermometer

The heart, lungs, and brain are vital organs. Blood flow to these organs is normally rich. During illness, blood flow to less essential areas slows to ensure that the vital organs are protected. The ideal location for measuring temperature is in the heart, but doing so is not possible. The temporal artery is a major artery in the head. This is the only major artery in the body that is close enough to the surface to measure an accurate internal temperature. In addition to being close to the heart, it has a high blood flow, making it well suited for measuring temperature. The **temporal artery thermometer (TAT)** (Figure 18-7) is battery operated. It measures temperature of the skin surface over the temporal artery. The TAT has become the most commonly used clinical thermometer. It is very accurate when used as directed and measurements are as close to the core temperature as those taken by a rectal thermometer.

The temporal artery thermometer has a wider range than other types of clinical thermometers and can measure temperatures from 60°F to 107.5°F. This is especially helpful for monitoring patients with below-normal

temperatures or cold exposure. Special error codes will appear on the screen to alert the user to values that are dangerously high or low.

When using the temporal artery thermometer, measure an area of the head that is not covered by a hat or blanket. Remove the hat or other covering so the entire head is exposed.

The temporal artery temperature is approximately 0.8°F higher than an oral temperature and is about the same as a rectal temperature. If the patient has a fever, the difference may be greater. This thermometer is more accurate than other types because it has less interference. Many factors interfere with the ability to obtain an accurate oral or rectal value during acute illness.

Other Types of Thermometers

A number of different thermometers are available. Many of these were designed with children in mind. For example, there is a pacifier thermometer and a thermometer tape that reads the skin temperature on the forehead. These thermometers are primarily for home use.

Using the Glass Thermometer

The glass thermometer is a long, cylindrical, calibrated tube that contains a column of heat-sensitive liquid.

- Starting with 94°F (34°C), each long line indicates a one-degree elevation in temperature.
- Every other degree is marked with a number.
- In between each long line are four shorter lines.
- Each shorter line equals two-tenths (²⁄₁₀ or 0.2) of 1 degree.

The liquid (the solid color line) in the bulb of the thermometer rises in the hollow center of the stem as heat is registered. To read the thermometer:

- Hold it at eye level.
- Find the solid column in the center.
- Look along the sharper edge between the numbers and lines.
- Read at the point at which the liquid ends.
- If it falls between two lines, read it to the closest line.

You will probably not use a glass thermometer in a clinical setting. You may encounter a home with glass thermometers if you work in home health.

Using a Thermometer Sheath

Cover reusable stick type thermometers with a sheath (Figure 18-8). An exception is the plastic chemical dot-type thermometer. These are used once and discarded.

NON-CONTACT INFRARED THERMOMETER (NCIT)

The **non-contact infrared thermometer (NCIT)** is an approved medical device (Figure 18-8A). Taking the temperature with a clinical thermometer requires close personal indirect or direct contact. This can be avoided by using the NCIT, which is faster and does not require close personal space for taking the temperature.

Sometimes it is necessary to quickly and efficiently screen people entering and leaving schools, airports, health-care facilities, and other businesses to identify people with potentially infectious conditions before they enter.

Guideline for using the NCIT

- Keep the unit clean and dry. Follow the manufacturer=s instructions for cleaning and using the device.
- Avoid drafts and direct sunlight. Place the NCIT in the facility screening area 10 to 30 minutes prior to use to allow it to adapt to the environment.
- Have the person entering remove any head covering.
- Hold the device 1½ to 6 inches perpendicular to the forehead.
- Take the temperature and document the reading. This documentation may be done on a clipboard instead of an individual medical record.

- The normal values are about the same as adult oral values. Your supervisor will provide instructions regarding reportable values.
- Ask the person to complete any screening documents required by the facility.

Documentation

In many facilities, temperatures are recorded on a worksheet on a clipboard, and then transferred to the individual patient charts. Always note which method was used when you document the temperature. Follow your facility's policy. For example, most facilities use "O" for documenting an oral temperature; "R" means a rectal temperature was taken; "A" or "AX" is used for an axillary temperature; and "T" is noted if a tympanic temperature was taken.

Changes in readings may be **flagged** (specially noted) by placing a circle around the reading or a star beside it. Report any changes from previous temperature readings directly to the nurse. Your accurate observations, reporting, and documentation contribute to the nurse's evaluation and assessment of the patient.

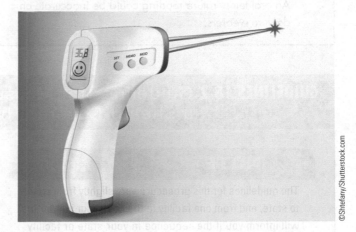

©Shtefany/Shutterstock.com

FIGURE 18-8A The non-contact infrared thermometer (NCIT) in an approved medical device that is faster and does not require close personal indirect or direct contact with the patient.

✚ Clinical Information **ALERT**

Each facility has policies and procedures about taking an oral temperature when the patient is using oxygen. In general, if the patient is using oxygen by mask, you should avoid taking an oral temperature. If the patient uses oxygen through a nasal cannula, the temperature reading may be slightly (approximately 0.3°F) lower because of the oxygen. Temporal artery and tympanic thermometers are ideal for these patients because the values are not altered by the use of oxygen. Consult the nurse if you are unsure of the method to use for taking the temperature of a patient who is using oxygen.

GUIDELINES 18-1 Guidelines for Using an Oral or Rectal Thermometer

Oral Thermometer

- Do not use if the patient is:
  - Uncooperative.
  - Restless.
  - Unconscious.
  - Chilled.
  - Confused or disoriented.
  - Coughing.
  - An infant or child under the age of six years.
  - A mouth breather/unable to breathe through the nose.
  - Recovering from oral surgery.
  - Irrational.
  - Very weak.
  - Receiving oxygen (except through nasal prongs).
  - On seizure precautions.
- An oral temperature reading could be inaccurate on denture wearers.

- If the person has been smoking, eating, or drinking, wait 15 minutes before taking the temperature.

Rectal Thermometer

- Do not use if the patient has:
  - Diarrhea.
  - Fecal impaction.
  - Combative behavior.
  - Rectal bleeding.
  - Hemorrhoids.
  - Had rectal surgery or rectal or colonic disease.
  - Recently had a heart attack.
  - Recently had prostate surgery.
  - A colostomy.
- Always hold a rectal thermometer in place the entire time.

GUIDELINES 18-2 Guidelines for Measuring Temperature Using a Sheath-Covered Thermometer

 NOTE

The guidelines for this procedure vary slightly from state to state, and from one facility to the next. Your instructor will inform you if the sequence in your state or facility differs from the procedure listed here. Know and follow the required sequence for your facility and state.

1. Carry out initial procedure actions.

2. Assemble equipment:
   - Gloves (standard precautions)
   - Clinical thermometer
   - Protective sheath (unopened package)
   - Pad and pencil

3. Have the patient rest in a comfortable position.

4. Ask the patient if they have had anything to eat or drink or has smoked within the past 15 minutes. If so, wait 15 minutes before taking an oral temperature.

5. Apply gloves.

6. Holding the thermometer in one hand, insert it into the marked end of a protective sheath wrapper.

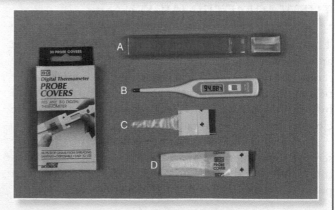

FIGURE 18-8B (A) Carrying case. (B) Digital thermometer. (C) Probe cover without backing. (D) Probe cover with backing.

7. Holding onto the sheath tab on the stem end of the thermometer, peel back the paper cover to expose the protective sheath.

8. Hold the paper wrapper in one hand. Twist the paper wrapper to break the seal with the tab and remove the paper wrapper, leaving the protective sheath on the thermometer.

(continues)

GUIDELINES 18-2 Guidelines for Measuring Temperature Using a Sheath-Covered Thermometer (continued)

9. Keeping the protective sheath over the thermometer, insert the bulb end of the thermometer under the patient's tongue, toward the side of the mouth.

10. Tell the patient to hold the thermometer gently, with lips closed, until the alarm sounds on the digital thermometer, indicating it has finished measuring the temperature.

11. Remove the thermometer and discard the used sheath. Read and record on notepad.

12. The thermometer can be stored in the patient's bedside stand for reuse with a new sheath. Disinfect the thermometer according to facility policy.

13. Remove your gloves.

14. Carry out ending procedure actions.

15. Report any unusual variations to the nurse at once.

PROCEDURE **31** MEASURING AN ORAL TEMPERATURE (ELECTRONIC THERMOMETER)

✎ NOTE

The guidelines for this procedure vary slightly from state to state, and from one facility to the next. Your instructor will inform you if the sequence in your state or facility differs from the procedure listed here. Know and follow the required sequence for your facility and state.

1. Carry out initial procedure actions.

2. Obtain an electronic thermometer, disposable probe covers, and gloves, if this is your facility policy. (Gloves are not necessary with an *oral temperature* using this type of thermometer. Know and follow your facility's policy.)

3. Ask the patient if they have had anything to eat or drink or has smoked within the past 15 minutes. If the answer is yes, wait 15 minutes before taking an oral temperature.

4. Cover the probe (blue) with a probe cover.

5. Insert the covered probe under the patient's tongue toward the side of the mouth (Figure 18-9A).

6. Hold the probe in position. Ask the patient to close the mouth and breathe through the nose.

7. When an audible signal indicates that the temperature has been determined, remove the probe from the patient's mouth.

8. Discard the probe cover in the appropriate container (Figure 18-9B). Remove and discard gloves.

9. Return the probe to its proper position.

10. Record the temperature on your pad.

11. Return the thermometer unit to the charger.

12. Carry out ending procedure actions.

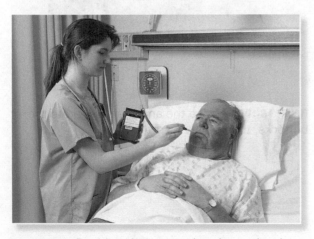

FIGURE 18-9A Position the covered probe under the tongue on one side of the patient's mouth.

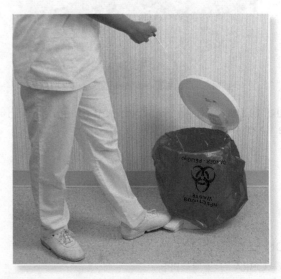

FIGURE 18-9B Discard the used probe cover according to facility policy.

ICON KEY:

 = OBRA

PROCEDURE **32** **MEASURING A RECTAL TEMPERATURE (ELECTRONIC THERMOMETER)**

 NOTE

The guidelines for this procedure vary slightly from state to state, and from one facility to the next. Your instructor will inform you if the sequence in your state or facility differs from the procedure listed here. Know and follow the required sequence for your facility and state.

1. Carry out initial procedure actions.

2. Assemble equipment:
   - Gloves
   - Electronic thermometer with rectal (red) probe
   - Probe cover
   - Lubricant

3. Lower the backrest of the bed. Ask the patient to turn on their side. Assist if necessary.

4. Put on gloves.

5. Cover the probe (red) with a probe cover.

6. Place a small amount of lubricant on the tip of the probe cover (Figure 18-10A).

7. Fold the top bedclothes back to expose the patient's anal area (Figure 18-10B).

8. Separate the buttocks with one hand. Insert the covered probe about 1 inch into the rectum, or as recommended by the thermometer manufacturer. With many thermometers, the rectal probe is inserted approximately ¼ inch. Hold in place. Replace the bedclothes for privacy as soon as the thermometer is inserted.

9. Read the temperature when registered on the digital display.

10. Remove the probe and discard the probe cover. Wipe lubricant from the patient. Discard tissue. Return the probe to its proper position.

11. Remove and discard gloves.

12. Record the temperature on your pad.

13. Return the thermometer unit to the charger.

14. Carry out ending procedure actions.

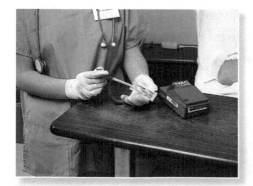

FIGURE 18-10A Apply a small amount of lubricant to the tip of the sheath.

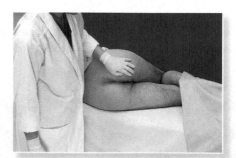

FIGURE 18-10B Expose the anal area, separate the buttocks, then gently insert the tip.

ICON KEY:
 = OBRA   = PPE

PROCEDURE **33** MEASURING AN AXILLARY TEMPERATURE (ELECTRONIC THERMOMETER)

NOTE

The guidelines for this procedure vary slightly from state to state, and from one facility to the next. Your instructor will inform you if the sequence in your state or facility differs from the procedure listed here. Know and follow the required sequence for your facility and state.

1. Carry out initial procedure actions.

NOTE

Use disposable gloves if there may be contact with open lesions, wet linens, or body fluids.

ICON KEY:

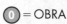

0 = OBRA

2. Equipment needed: same as for oral temperature measurement using an electronic thermometer (see Procedure 31).

3. Apply gloves if this is your facility's policy.

4. Cover the probe (blue) with a probe cover.

5. Wipe the axillary area dry and put the covered probe in place. Keep the patient's arm close to the body. Hold the probe in place until the temperature shows on the digital display and the audible signal indicates that it has been recorded.

6. Remove the thermometer probe. Discard the probe cover. Return the probe to its proper position.

7. Record the temperature on your pad.

8. Return the thermometer unit to the charger.

9. Carry out ending procedure actions.

GUIDELINES 18-3 Guidelines for Using a Tympanic (Ear) Thermometer

- Make sure the thermometer lens is clean and that there is no dirt or debris on the lens at the end of the probe tip (the lens is the shiny disc at the end of the probe tip through which the infrared energy must pass to be processed).

- Use each probe cover only once. Make sure the cover is tight, without ripples.

- Store the thermometer out of the path of any cold air flow. If the thermometer is in a cold area, allow it to warm up before use, or it may read low.

- Make sure the patient is not directly in the path of cold air or being fanned. This action cools the ears, which can cause a low temperature reading.

- If the patient is or has been lying on one ear, use the opposite ear.

- If the patient has a hearing aid, use the opposite ear or remove the aid and wait 15 minutes.

- The tympanic thermometer can be set to oral, core, or rectal mode. In most cases, oral is appropriate. The mode will be shown in the readout screen. If the

screen says "CAL," the thermometer is in the unadjusted mode, which is used only for calibration and other bench work.

- Insert the probe tip into the ear as far as possible, and then rotate the handle to the correct position in alignment with the jaw.

- Ear thermometers are similar to cameras. They provide the temperature of what you point them at. If the thermometer is not used correctly, you will get an inaccurate reading. Common causes of inaccurate tympanic temperatures are:
  - Pressing the scan button before the probe is fully inserted.
  - Using a probe cover more than once.
  - Using the thermometer without a probe cover.
  - Improper cleaning of the thermometer lens.
  - Not following manufacturer's instructions for placing the probe tip into the ear; following instructions for the thermometer you are using is important.
  - Using a thermometer with a broken or missing lens.

PROCEDURE **34** **MEASURING A TYMPANIC TEMPERATURE**

 NOTE

The guidelines for this procedure vary slightly from state to state, and from one facility to the next. Your instructor will inform you if the sequence in your state or facility differs from the procedure listed here. Know and follow the required sequence for your facility and state.

1. Carry out initial procedure actions.

2. Assemble equipment:
   - Disposable gloves if there may be contact with blood or body fluids, open lesions, or wet linens
   - Tympanic thermometer
   - Probe covers

3. Check the lens to make sure it is clean and intact (Figure 18-11A).

4. Select the appropriate mode on the thermometer.

5. Place a clean probe cover on the probe.

6. Put on disposable gloves if you may have contact with blood or body fluids, open lesions, or wet linens.

7. Position the patient so you have access to the ear you will be using.

8. Gently pull the ear pinna back and up (Figure 18-11B). This straightens the ear canal so the thermometer can be placed for an accurate reading.

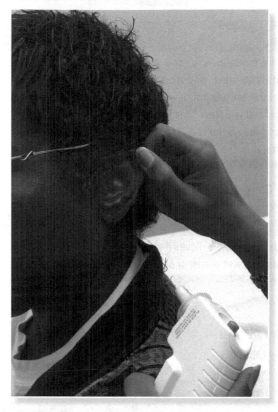

FIGURE 18-11B Gently pull the ear pinna back and up.

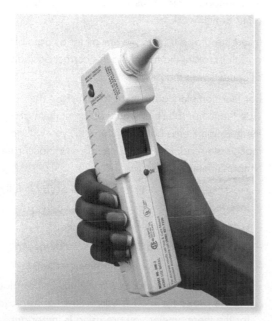

FIGURE 18-11A Check the lens of the tympanic thermometer to make sure it is clean and intact.

   - If the patient is a child under age three, pull the pinna down and back.
   - If the patient is a child over age three, pull the pinna up and back.

9. Place the probe in the patient's ear, aiming it toward the tympanic membrane. Insert the probe until it seals the ear canal (Figure 18-11C). Do not apply pressure.
   - Check the position of the probe. The tip should be inside the ear opposite the midpoint between the eyebrow and sideburn on the opposite side of the face.

10. Rotate the probe handle slightly until it is aligned with the jaw, as though the patient were speaking on the telephone.

11. Quickly press the activation button. Leave the thermometer in the ear for the time recommended by the manufacturer.

(continues)

PROCEDURE **34** **CONTINUED**

12. The display will blink when you have a reading. Remove the probe from the patient's ear and discard the cover. See Table 18-4 for normal ranges of tympanic temperatures by age group.

13. Record the temperature on your pad.

14. Return the thermometer unit to the charger.

15. Carry out ending procedure actions.

TABLE 18-3 Normal Ranges for Tympanic Temperatures

Years of Age	Fahrenheit	Celsius
0–2	97.5°F–100.4°F	36.4°F–38.0°C
3–10	97.0°F–100.0°F	36.1°F–37.8°C
11–65	96.6°F–99.7°F	35.9°F–37.6°C
>65	96.4°F–99.5°F	35.8°F–37.5°C

ICON KEY:

 = OBRA

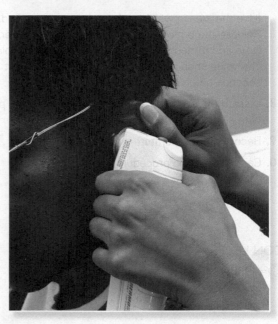

FIGURE 18-11C Place the covered probe in the patient's ear, aiming it toward the tympanic membrane. Insert the probe until it seals in the ear canal, and then rotate the handle until it is positioned like a telephone.

PROCEDURE **35** **MEASURING A TEMPORAL ARTERY TEMPERATURE**

 NOTE

The guidelines for this procedure vary slightly from state to state, and from one facility to the next. Your instructor will inform you if the sequence in your state or facility differs from the procedure listed here. Know and follow the required sequence for your facility and state.

1. Carry out initial procedure actions.

2. Assemble equipment:
   - Disposable gloves if there may be contact with blood or body fluids, open lesions, or wet linens (gloves are not necessary unless required by facility policy or potential exposure to body fluids)
   - Temporal artery thermometer
   - Probe covers
   - Alcohol sponges or disinfectant wipes

3. Check the lens to make sure it is clean and intact.

4. Apply a clean probe cover, or wipe the probe with alcohol or a disinfectant wipe.

5. Hold the thermometer as you would a pencil or pen. Gently press the probe (head) of the thermometer against the center of the forehead. Push the switch to the on position with your thumb. Keep this button depressed.

6. Slowly move the probe across the forehead to the hairline on one side of the head (Figure 18-12).

7. Push the hair back slightly with the opposite hand, if needed, and then lift the probe slightly. Quickly place the probe down just behind the ear lobe on the neck.

(continues)

PROCEDURE **35** CONTINUED

(Use the area in which perfume is usually applied.)
Release the button and remove the thermometer.
Note and remember the value on the digital display.
The value should remain on the display for about 30
seconds before disappearing.

8. Discard the disposable probe cover, or wipe the probe
   with an alcohol or disinfectant wipe.

9. Record the temperature on your pad.

10. Carry out ending procedure actions.

ICON KEY:

0 = OBRA

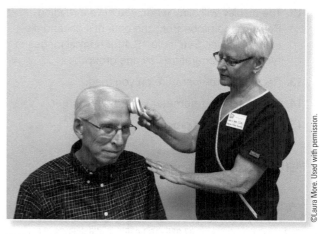

FIGURE 18-12 Hold the button down and move the
probe to the temple area. Push the hair back and
maintain good skin contact.

REVIEW

A. True/False

Mark the following true or false by circling T or F.

1. T F When charting an axillary temperature,
   always print *A* or *AX* after the reading.

2. T F Readings taken with a plastic thermometer
   may not be entirely accurate.

3. T F Temperature is the measurement of body
   heat.

4. T F The most common method of measuring
   the temperature of a cooperative adult is by
   mouth.

5. T F To measure a rectal temperature, the patient
   is best positioned on their back.

6. T F 96.8°F is an average oral temperature.

7. T F Only temperature variations of more than
   5°F should be reported to the nurse.

8. T F Clinical thermometers are always glass.

9. T F The probe of an electronic thermometer
   is covered with a red sheath for rectal
   use.

10. T F The axillary temperature of a patient will
    register approximately 1°F higher than their
    oral temperature.

11. T F The tympanic temperature reading is the
    most accurate.

12. T F Hold the temporal artery thermometer in
    place for three minutes.

13. T F Use a rectal thermometer for a 2-year-old
    child.

14. T F The temporal artery is deep within the
    body core.

15. T F Wait five minutes after the patient has
    taken hot liquids to measure an oral
    temperature.

16. T F Use hot water to wash used digital
    thermometers.

17. T F Always wipe the axillary area before placing
    a thermometer.

18. T F When using an electronic thermometer,
    you should not touch the tip of the probe
    sheath with your fingers.

19. T F All rectal thermometers should be lubricated before insertion.

20. T F The oral thermometer should remain in place until the unit signals that the temperature has been measured.

21. T F There may be times when a temperature has to be measured in the groin area.

22. T F Using a glass mercury thermometer is the most desirable method of taking an oral temperature.

23. T F The NCIT is the most accurate type of clinical thermometer.

24. T F Hold the NCIT firmly across the back of the head when taking a temperature.

25. T F Use the NCIT for all patient care.

26. T F Avoid using the electronic thermometer in children.

B. Completion

Complete the statements by choosing the correct words from the following list.

Fahrenheit   pulse
higher   temperature
less   tympanic

27. Vital signs include _____, _____, respiration, and blood pressure.

28. A normal temperature reading of 98.6° would be in the _____ scale.

29. A _____ thermometer is used to measure the temperature in the ear.

30. A temporal artery temperature might be expected to be slightly _____ than an oral temperature.

31. Temperature is _____ stable in children than in adults.

C. Nursing Assistant Challenge

32. Mrs. LeJune is having difficulty breathing and is very restless. The nurse asks you to measure her temperature. What type of thermometer would you choose if all were available?

a. Tympanic thermometer

b. Disposable plastic thermometer

c. Electronic oral thermometer

d. Temporal artery thermometer

33. Your patient tells you they do not feel good. They have no specific complaints. You check their vital signs, and their oral temperature is 94.8°F using a digital thermometer. What will you do next?

a. Ask the patient if they drank a cold beverage before you took their temperature.

b. Notify the nurse.

c. Recheck the temperature with the same thermometer.

d. Recheck the temperature with a different thermometer.

34. After finding a temperature of 94.5°F, your patient asks you if you found something wrong. How will you respond?

a. Yes, you found a broken thermometer.

b. You are just rechecking for accuracy.

c. Yes, you will notify the nurse right away.

d. No, there is nothing wrong with you.

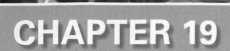

CHAPTER 19 — Pulse and Respiration

OBJECTIVES

After completing this chapter, you will be able to:

19.1 Spell and define terms.

19.2 Define pulse.

19.3 Explain the importance of monitoring a pulse rate.

19.4 Locate the pulse sites.

19.5 Identify the range of normal pulse rates.

19.6 Identify the range of normal respiratory rates.

19.7 Measure the pulse at different locations.

19.8 List the characteristics of the pulse.

19.9 List the characteristics of respiration.

19.10 List eight guidelines for using a stethoscope.

19.11 Demonstrate the following procedures:

- Procedure 36: Counting the Radial Pulse
- Procedure 37: Counting the Apical–Radial Pulse
- Procedure 38: Counting Respirations
- Procedure 39: Using a Pulse Oximeter

VOCABULARY

Learn the meaning and the correct spelling of the following words and phrases:

accelerated	expiration	rales	symmetry
apical pulse	inspiration	rate	tachycardia
apnea	pulse	respiration	tachypnea
bradycardia	pulse deficit	rhythm	thready pulse
Cheyne–Stokes respirations	pulse oximetry	stertorous	volume
cyanosis	radial pulse	stethoscope	wheezing
dyspnea			

INTRODUCTION

The patient's pulse and respiration rate are usually counted during the same procedure. Because breathing is partly under voluntary control, a person is able to stop or alter breathing temporarily for a short period. For example, when a patient realizes that their breathing is being watched and counted, they may alter their breathing pattern without meaning to do so. To avoid this, the respirations are counted immediately following the pulse count without telling the patient. Keep the patient's hand in the same position, with your fingers on the pulse point so it appears that you are still taking the pulse.

THE PULSE

The **pulse** is:

- The pressure of the blood felt against the wall of an artery as the heart alternately contracts (beats) and relaxes (rests)
- More easily felt in arteries that come fairly close to the skin and can be gently pressed against a bone
- The same in all arteries throughout the body
- An indication of how the cardiovascular system is meeting the body's needs

When taking a patient's pulse, check the rate, rhythm, and quality. The rhythm is the pattern that you feel, with pulsations and pauses between beats. If the pulse is normal, the length of the beat will be approximately equal to the length of the pause. The quality of the pulse is the volume you palpate. You can tell from touch whether it is weak, strong, or thready. A **thready pulse** is one that feels weak, like a piece of thread moving under your finger.

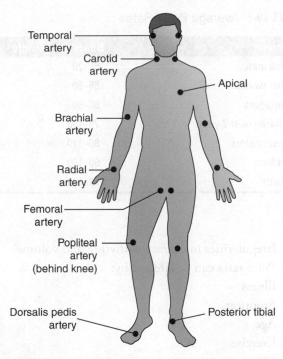

FIGURE 19-1 Common pulse sites of the body.

Radial Pulse

The **radial pulse** is the most commonly measured pulse. It is measured at the radial artery in the wrist. Figure 19-1 shows areas of the body where other large blood vessels come close enough to the surface to be used as sites for counting the pulse. Conscious patients can be checked at the radial artery (see Procedure 36). Unconscious patients should be checked at the carotid artery or apically (over the heart).

Pulse measurement includes determining the:

- Rate or speed:
  - **Bradycardia**—an unusually slow pulse (below 60 beats per minute)
  - **Tachycardia**—an unusually fast pulse (more than 100 beats per minute)

- Character:
  - **Rhythm** regularity
  - Volume or fullness

Report:

- Pulse rates over 100 beats per minute (bpm) (tachycardia)
- Pulse rates under 60 bpm (bradycardia)

PROCEDURE **36** **COUNTING THE RADIAL PULSE**

1. Carry out initial procedure actions.
2. Place the patient in a comfortable position. The palm of the hand should be facing down and the arm should rest on a flat surface.
3. Locate the pulse on the thumb side of the wrist with the tips of your first two or three fingers (Figure 19-2). Do not use your thumb—it contains a pulse that may be confused with the patient's pulse.
4. When the pulse is felt, exert slight pressure. Using the second hand of your watch, count for one minute. It is the practice in some hospitals to count for 30 seconds and multiply by two and to record the rate for one minute. A one-minute count is preferred and must be done if the pulse is irregular.

5. Remember the reading when counting respirations. Record the reading on your pad as soon as possible.
6. Carry out ending procedure actions.

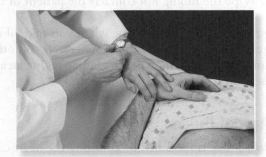

FIGURE 19-2 Locate the pulse on the thumb side of the wrist with the tips of the first two or three fingers.

ICON KEY:

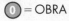 = OBRA

TABLE 19-1 Average Pulse Rates

Patient	Beats per Minute
Adult men	60–70
Adult women	65–80
Teenagers	60–90
Children over 7 years	75–100
Preschoolers	80–110
Toddlers	90–140
Infants	120–160

- Irregularities in character (rhythm and volume)
  Pulse rates can be affected by:
- Illness
- Emotions
- Age
- Exercise
- Elevated temperature
- Gender
- Position
- Physical training
- Lowered temperature
- Drugs
- Cigarette smoking
  Table 19-1 shows average pulse rates.

Using a Stethoscope

A **stethoscope** is a medical instrument used to listen to sounds inside the body. It intensifies sounds so they can be heard clearly. The parts of the stethoscope are pictured in Figure 19-3. Many health care workers use stethoscopes on many patients. This creates the potential for infection to be passed to both workers and patients. Before and after using the stethoscope, wipe the earpieces and diaphragm with an alcohol sponge or other disinfectant. Wipe the tubing if it contacts the patient or bed linens.

You will use the stethoscope when you take blood pressures. Your health care facility may teach you other procedures with the stethoscope, including taking an apical pulse.

The Apical Pulse

An **apical pulse** is measured by counting the heart contractions. Place the stethoscope over the apex (tip) of the heart. Listen for the heart sounds that indicate closing

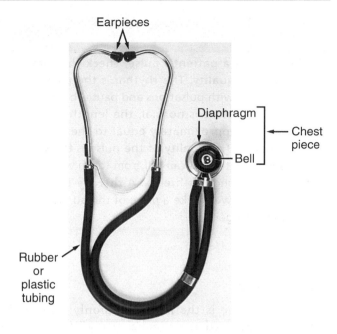

FIGURE 19-3 The stethoscope is used to listen to sounds inside the body.

of the valves as the heart pumps blood into the arteries. The sounds should occur at the same rate as the pulse that is felt as an expansion of the radial artery. The apex of the heart is found:

- On the left side of the front of the chest
- Between the fifth and sixth ribs
- Just below the left nipple
- In women, under the left breast

Listen carefully for two sounds: lub dub. The louder sound (lub) corresponds to the contraction of the ventricles pushing the blood forward through the arteries and the closing of the valves to prevent the backflow of blood. This is the sound to be counted. The softer sound (dub) corresponds to the relaxation of the ventricles as they fill with blood before the next contraction and the closing of the semilunar valves to prevent backflow from the arteries.

When documenting an apical pulse reading, write *AP* after the value.

Apical–Radial Pulse Rate

The apical–radial pulse rate is a comparison of the apical rate and the radial rate. Usually they are the same.

Sometimes the contraction of the heart is so weak that it fails to send enough blood to the arteries to expand them. When this happens, no pulse is felt. In this case, the number of loud sounds does not correspond with the number of pulses felt in the radial artery.

GUIDELINES 19-1 Guidelines for Using a Stethoscope

- Clean the earpieces and diaphragm of the stethoscope before using it.
- Clean the stethoscope tubing if it contacts the patient or bed linens.
- Check the earpieces of the stethoscope for wax, and remove it if present.
- Check the stethoscope tubing. Do not use if it has cracks or holes in it.
- The earpieces of the stethoscope should face forward.

- The diaphragm of the stethoscope should not come in contact with the patient's clothing, the blood pressure cuff, or any other device.
- Place the diaphragm of the stethoscope flat against the patient's skin and hold it in place. If the diaphragm is at an angle, you will not be able to hear the sounds.
  - Apply firm but gentle pressure when holding the diaphragm in place. If you press too hard, you may be unable to hear the sound.

The difference between the apical pulse (the loud sounds heard over the heart) and the radial pulse (the expansion felt over the radial pulse) is called a **pulse deficit**. Two people measure the heart rate and the radial pulse at the same time (see Procedure 37). The nurse measures the apical pulse, while the second person counts the radial pulse for one minute. The rates are then compared.

Apical pulse rates are checked:

- Whenever a pulse deficit exists or is suspected
- Before the nurse administers drugs that alter the heart rate or rhythm
- In children whose rapid rates might be difficult to count at the radial artery
- For one full minute

PROCEDURE 37 COUNTING THE APICAL–RADIAL PULSE

1. Carry out initial procedure actions.
2. Clean the stethoscope earpieces and bell or diaphragm with disinfectant.
3. Place the stethoscope earpieces in your ears with tips facing slightly forward for better fit.
4. Place the stethoscope diaphragm or bell over the apex of the patient's heart. If it is cold, warm the diaphragm with your hands before placing it on the patient's chest.
5. Listen carefully for the heartbeat.
6. Count the louder-sounding beats for one minute.
7. Check the radial pulse for one minute. The best way to obtain these numbers is to have the nurse count the apical pulse while you take the radial pulse (Figure 19-4).

8. Note results on a pad for comparison.

   Example: Apical pulse = 108

   Radial pulse = 82

   Pulse deficit = 26 (108 − 82 = 26)

9. Clean earpieces and bell of stethoscope with disinfectant.
10. Carry out ending procedure actions.

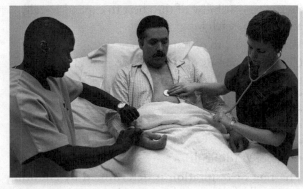

FIGURE 19-4 The nurse counts the apical pulse while the nurse assistant counts the radial pulse.

ICON KEY:

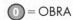 = OBRA   = PPE

- On any child 12 months of age or younger
- Whenever you are uncertain of the accuracy of the radial pulse or it is irregular

Pulse deficits are found in some forms of heart disease.

RESPIRATION

The main function of **respiration** is to supply the cells in the body with oxygen and to rid the body of excess carbon dioxide. When respirations are inefficient, there is less oxygen in the blood available for body needs. In addition, carbon dioxide is released less efficiently. The skin takes on a bluish or dusky color and the patient develops a condition known as **cyanosis**.

There are two parts to each respiration: one **inspiration** (inhalation) followed by one **expiration** (exhalation). Special terms describe different breathing patterns:

- Normal—regular, 12 to 20 breaths per minute
- **Tachypnea**—rapid, shallow breathing
- **Dyspnea**—difficult or labored breathing
- Shallow—breaths that only partially fill the lungs
- **Apnea**—periods of no respirations
- **Cheyne–Stokes respirations**—a period of dyspnea followed by periods of apnea
- **Stertorous**—snoring-like respirations
- **Rales** (crackles)—moist respirations; at times, fluid (mucus) will collect in the air passages; this causes a bubbling type of respiration; crackles are common in the dying patient
- **Wheezing**—difficult breathing accompanied by a whistling or sighing sound due to narrowing of bronchioles (as in asthma) or an increase of mucus in the bronchi

Respirations should be checked for:

- **Rate**—number of respirations per minute
- Rhythm—regularity
- **Symmetry**—ability of the chest to expand equally as air enters each lung
- **Volume**—depth of respiration
- Character—terms used to describe the character of respirations include:
  - Regular
  - Irregular
  - Shallow
  - Deep
  - Labored (difficult)

The rate of respiration is determined by counting the rise or fall of the chest for one minute, using a watch equipped with a second hand (see Procedure 38).

> ### Clinical Information **ALERT**
>
> When counting respirations, note whether the patient's breathing is normal (easy) or labored (dyspneic), shallow or deep, and quiet or noisy. Check the muscles of the neck and abdomen. If the patient is using these muscles for breathing, inform the nurse.

- The average rate for adults is 12 to 20 respirations per minute.
- If the rate is more than 25 per minute, it is said to be **accelerated**. Report accelerated respirations.
- If the rate is less than 12 per minute, it is too slow and should be reported.

Remember that respirations should be counted without the patient's knowledge. You might count respirations before or after counting the radial pulse. Continue pressing on the pulse area while counting.

The factors affecting respiratory rates include:

- Illness
- Emotions
- Elevated temperature
- Gender
- Age
- Exercise
- Position
- Drugs
- Cigarette smoking

Average respiratory rates are listed in Table 19-2.

Temperature, pulse, and respiration (TPR) rates and character are recorded in a note pad or on a clipboard and then transferred to the patient's chart. Abnormalities related to pulse and respirations to report to the nurse are listed in Table 19-3.

TABLE 19-2 Average Respiratory Rates

Age	Normal Respiratory Rate per Minute
Infant	30–60
Toddler	24–40
Preschool child	22–34
School-age child	18–30
Teenager	12–24
Adult	12–20

TABLE 19-3 Signs and Symptoms That Should Be Reported to the Nurse Immediately

Abnormal pulse: below 60 or above 100.
Pulse irregular, weak, or bounding.
Unable to palpate pulse.
Pain over center, left, or right chest.
Chest pain that radiates to shoulder, neck, jaw, or arm.
Headache, dizziness, weakness, paralysis, vomiting.
Cold, blue, or gray appearance.
Cold, blue, numb, painful feet or hands.
Blue color of lips or nail beds, mucous membranes.
Feeling faint or lightheaded, losing consciousness.
Also review the respiratory symptoms. These systems are closely related, and may be symptomatic at the same time.

Signs and Symptoms of Inadequate Breathing to Report Immediately

Movement in the chest is absent, minimal, or irregular.
Breathing movement appears to be in the abdomen, not the lungs.
Air movement cannot be detected by listening and feeling for breath sounds on your cheek and ear.
Respiratory rate is too slow (below 12) or rapid (more than 20), or there is a marked change in the rate.
Respirations are irregular, gasping, very deep or shallow, erratic, Cheyne-Stokes, or there is a marked change in the rhythm.
Dyspnea (difficult breathing).
Expelling respiratory secretions (note character, color, and amount).
Patient is unable to speak at all, or cannot speak in sentences because of shortness of breath.
Patient's skin, lips, tongue, ear lobes, mucous membranes, or nail beds are pale, blue, or gray.
Respirations are noisy, wheezing, whistling, crowing, or person has signs of respiratory distress.
Nasal flaring is present during inspiration.
The muscles below the ribs and/or above the clavicles retract inward during respiration.
Presence of cough; note whether productive (expelling secretions) or nonproductive (not coughing anything up).

PROCEDURE **38** COUNTING RESPIRATIONS

1. After you have counted the pulse rate, leave your fingers on the radial pulse and start counting the number of times the chest rises and falls during one minute (Figure 19-5). Count one inhalation and one exhalation as one respiration.

2. Note the depth and regularity of respirations.

3. Record the time, rate, depth, and regularity of respirations.

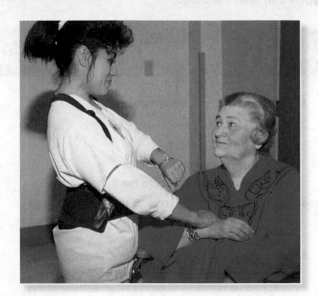

FIGURE 19-5 Keep the fingers on the radial pulse area while counting respirations.

ICON KEY:
 = OBRA

THE PULSE OXIMETER

Pulse oximetry (Figure 19-6) is a simple, painless test to determine how well the body is using oxygen. Hospital nursing assistants generally measure the pulse oximeter value when they check vital signs. We are including the information here, since it is part of the vital signs test. You will find expanded information on how well patients use oxygen in Chapter 39.

The pulse oximeter measures the level of saturation of the patient's hemoglobin with oxygen. *Hemoglobin* is the part of the blood that carries oxygen to the cells. The measurement may be continuous or intermittent. Having these data readily available enables the nurse to treat the patient quickly. Pulse oximetry will detect

critical changes in the patient's oxygen levels as soon as they occur. The outcome is better when early treatment is provided.

If supplemental oxygen is in use, document the liter flow before applying the continuous pulse oximeter. Attach the pulse oximeter to the patient's skin with a sensor. Several different types are available. They can be placed on the finger, toe, earlobe, foot, forehead, or bridge of the nose. The tip of the finger and the earlobe are most commonly used. In these areas, a clothespin-like sensor is attached to both sides of the body part. The finger and toe sensors work best with patients who have dark-colored skin. Poor circulation, cold extremities, and nail polish interfere with pulse oximeter values.

The pulse oximeter measures light as it passes through the tissue, and shows a numeric value for the

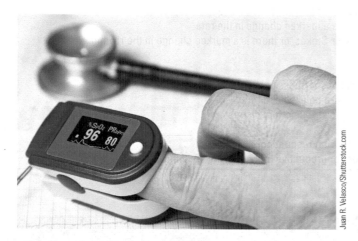

FIGURE 19-6 A pulse oximeter measures the amount of oxygen that is in the blood.

Juan R. Velasco/Shutterstock.com

 Safety ALERT

Always monitor the patient and not the equipment. For example, the continuous pulse oximeter alarm sounds and the oxygen saturation value reads 63 percent, suggesting that the patient is in severe distress. However, the patient is visiting with their family, smiling, and talking. Their color is good, and their nail beds and mucous membranes are pink. You are having an equipment problem, not a patient problem. If you cannot identify and correct the problem, ask the nurse or respiratory professional to help. Although your findings indicate an equipment problem, inform the nurse of the problem and your evaluation of the patient and situation.

PROCEDURE **39** **USING A PULSE OXIMETER** **O**

1. Carry out initial procedure actions.

2. Assemble equipment:
   – Pulse oximeter unit
   – Sensor appropriate to the site
   – Tape, if needed, to secure the sensor

3. Select and apply the sensor. If the sensor has position markings, align them opposite to each other to ensure an accurate reading.

4. Fasten the sensor securely, or the reading will not be accurate. Make sure the sensor is not wrapped so tightly with tape that it restricts blood flow.

5. Attach the sensor to the patient cable on the pulse oximeter.

6. Turn the unit on. If the audio is turned on, you will hear a beep with each pulse beat. Adjust the volume as desired. Some units also use light bars to indicate the strength of the pulse. Note the percentage of oxygen saturation. Inform the nurse and document according to facility policy.

7. Monitor the patient's pulse rate. Compare with the patient's actual pulse to make sure the unit is picking up each beat. Inform the nurse and document according to facility policy.

8. Monitor the patient's respirations and general appearance. Inform the nurse and document according to facility policy. If the patient's general condition changes at any time, notify the nurse.

9. Carry out ending procedure actions.

ICON KEY:
O = OBRA

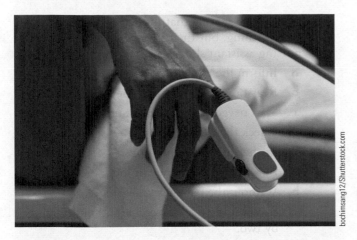

FIGURE 19-7 A pulse oximeter sensor applied to a finger.

TABLE 19-4 Pulse Oximeter Values

Pulse Oximeter Reading	Interpretation
95% to 100%	Normal
Below 90%	Suggests complications, impending hypoxemia
85%	Inadequate oxygen for body function; condition worsening, potential impending crisis
Below 70%	Life-threatening

amount of oxygen in the arterial blood (Figure 19-7). The percentage of oxygen saturation can be viewed on the digital display. Pulse oximeter values are listed in Table 19-4.

Never turn the pulse oximeter alarm off. (Refer to Procedure 39.)

Monitoring the Patient

Monitor the patient regularly when a pulse oximeter is being used. Reporting to the nurse is part of your ending procedure actions. In this case, make sure to report the patient's initial pulse oximeter reading and vital signs.

This is important information on which the nurse will act. They will further assess the patient and provide care for abnormal values. The nurse must know the initial values as a basis for comparison.

If the patient's vital signs or appearance change significantly from baseline values, notify the nurse promptly. Also inform the nurse immediately if the patient's pulse oximetry value declines markedly. Monitor the patient's supplemental oxygen, if used, each time you are in the room. Make sure it is set at the liter flow ordered by the physician. You are not expected to change the liter flow. If it varies from the ordered rate, notify the nurse.

Rotate the position of the tape finger sensor at least every four hours. Move the spring-clip sensor every two hours. Rotating the location of the sensor reduces the risk of skin breakdown and complications related to pressure.

REVIEW

A. True/False

Mark the following true or false by circling T or F.

1. T F   A pulse deficit results when there is a difference between the apical and radial pulses.

2. T F   The pulse is the pressure of blood against the arterial wall.

3. T F   Cheyne–Stokes respirations are deep and regular.

4. T F   Pulses differ when counted at different pulse sites.

5. T F   The pulse rate of an infant is 110 to 130 bpm.

6. T F   An apical pulse should be counted in children.

7. T F   The pulse site used most often is the carotid artery.

8. T F   The respiratory system rids the body of excess carbon dioxide.

9. T F   Mucus in the air passages causes crackles.

10. T F   A pulse is best counted using the thumb placed over the artery.

B. Matching

Choose the correct word from Column II to match the words and phrases in Column I.

Column I

11. _____   snoring types of respiration
12. _____   bluish discoloration to the skin
13. _____   regularity
14. _____   periods of no respiration
15. _____   difficult breathing
16. _____   rapid respirations
17. _____   increased or speeded up
18. _____   expiration
19. _____   speed
20. _____   slow pulse

Column II

a. accelerated

b. apnea

c. bradycardia

d. cyanosis

e. dyspnea

f. rate

g. rhythm

h. stertorous

i. tachypnea

j. inhalation

k. exhalation

C. Multiple Choice

21. If you find a crack in the stethoscope tubing, you should:

   a. Not use the stethoscope.

   b. Wrap the crack with tape.

   c. Not worry about it.

   d. Hold your hand over it.

22. When using a stethoscope:

   a. Apply very firm pressure to the diaphragm.

   b. Hold the diaphragm at a 45° angle.

   c. Straighten the clothing under the diaphragm.

   d. The earpieces should face forward.

23. A pulse oximeter value of 76%:

   a. Is normal in adult patients.

   b. Must be reported to the nurse immediately.

   c. Must be reported at the end of the shift.

   d. Suggests the patient is getting enough oxygen.

24. The pulse oximeter measures:

   a. The patient's red blood cells.

   b. The strength of the patient's pulse.

   c. The amount of oxygen in the blood.

   d. The patient's respiratory rate.

25. The patient reports that they cannot breathe. They are breathing, but their lips have a blue tinge. The nursing assistant should:

   a. Inform the nurse right away.

   b. Reassure the patient that they are fine.

   c. Start oxygen at 6 L per minute.

   d. Check their temperature.

26. Count the patient's respirations:

   a. By speaking each one out loud.

   b. Without the patient's knowledge.

   c. By counting for 15 seconds and multiplying by two.

   d. By counting for 30 seconds.

D. Nursing Assistant Challenge

27. Mrs. Morgan has a heart condition that makes her heart rate irregular and faster than normal. Her respirations are difficult or rapid, labored, and moist. She receives a medication that profoundly alters her heart action. Your orders are to assist in determining the pulse deficit. Complete the items below using the terms in the following list.

   apical   rales

   dyspnea   tachycardia

   radial   tachypnea

   a. The faster heart rate is described as _____.

   b. The difficult respirations can be charted as _____.

   c. Moist respirations are best described as _____.

   d. Rapid respirations are also called _____.

   e. Which pulse rate will you count? _____

   f. Which pulse rate will a second person count? _____

28. List two reasons a radial–apical pulse rate would be ordered.

   a. _____

   b. _____

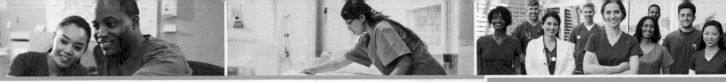

Blood Pressure

OBJECTIVES

After completing this chapter, you will be able to:

20.1 Spell and define terms.

20.2 Describe the factors that influence blood pressure.

20.3 Identify the range of normal blood pressure values.

20.4 Identify the causes of inaccurate blood pressure readings.

20.5 Describe how to select the proper size blood pressure cuff.

20.6 List precautions associated with use of the sphygmomanometer.

20.7 Demonstrate the following procedures:
- Procedure 40: Taking Blood Pressure
- Procedure 41: Taking Blood Pressure with an Electronic Blood Pressure Apparatus

VOCABULARY

Learn the meaning and the correct spelling of the following words and phrases:

aneroid gauge	depressant	hypertension	sphygmomanometer
antecubital area	diastole	hypotension	stimulant
auscultatory gap	diastolic pressure	orthostatic hypotension	systole
blood pressure	elasticity	prehypertension	systolic pressure
brachial artery	fasting	pulse pressure	

INTRODUCTION

Blood pressure is the measure of the force of the blood against the walls of the arteries. Blood pressure depends on the:
- Volume (amount of blood in the circulatory system).
- Force of the heartbeat.
- Condition of the arteries. Arteries that have lost their **elasticity** (stretch) give more resistance. The pressure is greater in these arteries.
- Distance from the heart. Blood pressure in the legs is lower than in the arms.
  Pressure varies with contraction (**systole**) and relaxation (**diastole**) of the ventricles of the heart.
- The systolic blood pressure reading indicates the period when the pressure within the arteries is the greatest, during contraction of the ventricles. The systolic blood pressure is the working pressure.
- The diastolic reading indicates the lowest point of pressure between ventricular contractions. The diastolic blood pressure is the resting pressure.

Blood pressure is elevated by:
- Sex of the patient (males slightly higher than females before menopause)
- Exercise
- Eating

Blood pressure is the fourth vital sign. Taking accurate blood pressures and reporting and documenting abnormal values saves health care dollars and improves patients' health. For example, high blood pressure causes 80 percent of all kidney failure, so the physician will treat the patient to control and reduce the hypertension. Controlling high blood pressure can delay the onset of renal failure by 4.5 years. The annual cost of treating renal failure is approximately $20 billion. Dialysis costs about $50,000 a year, so this control alone represents a potential savings of $225,000. Even more important, being in good health and not requiring dialysis maintains the patient's quality of life.

- Use of **stimulants** (substances that speed up body functions)
- Emotional stress, such as anger, fear, or sexual activity
- Disease conditions, such as arteriosclerosis (hardening of the arteries), elevated cholesterol, or diabetes mellitus
- Hereditary factors
- Pain
- Obesity
- Age
- Condition of blood vessels
- Some drugs

Blood pressure is lowered by:
- **Fasting** (not eating)
- Rest
- Use of **depressants** (drugs that slow down body functions)
- Weight loss
- Emotions such as grief
- Abnormal conditions such as hemorrhage (loss of blood) or shock

- Dehydration and fluid loss
- Some drugs such as antihypertensives (drugs that lower blood pressure in persons who have hypertension)
- Diuretics (drugs that lower the volume of body fluids)
Individual factors affecting blood pressure are:
- Age
- Sleep
- Weight
- Emotion
- Heredity
- Gender
- Viscosity of blood
- Condition of blood vessels
Average blood pressure values are listed in Table 20-1.

EQUIPMENT

The **sphygmomanometer** (pronounced sfig-moh-muh-nom-i-ter), which is a blood pressure measuring apparatus consists of:
- A cuff that fits around the patient's arm (different sizes are available). A rubber bladder is inside the cuff. A pressure control button is attached to the cuff. It is important to use the proper size cuff when measuring blood pressure. Cuffs that are too wide or too narrow will give inaccurate readings (Figure 20-1). To check the size of the cuff, compare the length of the rubber bladder inside the cuff with the patient's arm circumference. The bladder should be at least 80 percent of the circumference of the arm. If it is larger or smaller, obtain a different size cuff.
- Two tubes. One tube is connected to the pressure control bulb and to the bladder inside the cuff. The other tube is connected to the pressure gauge.
- A pressure gauge, which may be a column of liquid (Figure 20-2A) or a round **aneroid gauge** (Figure 20-2B) dial. Both are marked with numbers.
- Some nurses and home health agencies use wrist cuffs (Figure 20-2C).

TABLE 20-1 Average Blood Pressure Values

	Approximate Blood Pressure Value	
Age	Systolic	Diastolic
2–6 months	91	50 to 53
7–11 months	90	47 + age in months
1–5 years	90 + age in years	56
6–18 years	83 + (2 x age in years)	52 + age in years
Over age 18	120	80

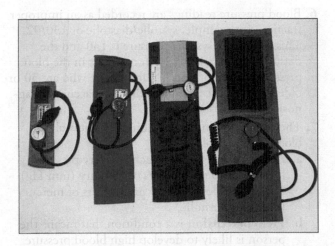

FIGURE 20-1 The cuff must fit properly to measure an accurate reading. A variety of cuff sizes are available.

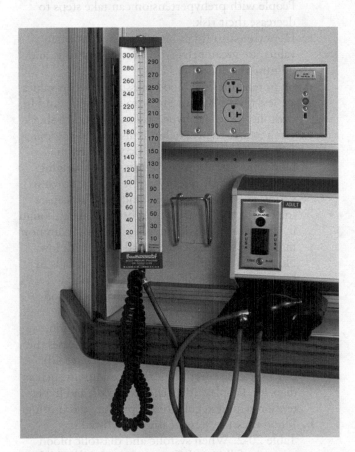

FIGURE 20-2A A mercury gravity sphygmomanometer that is still in use.

The stethoscope magnifies sounds. It consists of:

- A bell or diaphragm.
- Tubing that carries sounds to the listener.
- Earpieces that direct the sounds into the listener's ears. The earpieces and diaphragm must be cleaned with antiseptic before and after each use to prevent transmission of disease.

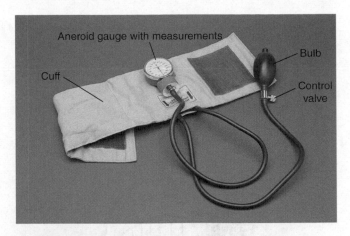

FIGURE 20-2B A dial (aneroid) sphygmomanometer.

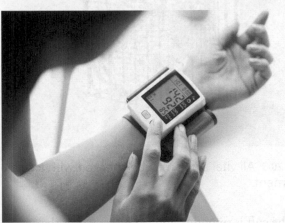

forma82/Shutterstock.com

FIGURE 20-2C Wrist cuffs have become quite common, especially in home health care.

Electronic sphygmomanometers with attached cuffs are used in some facilities. You do not have to use a stethoscope with these units, because they automatically register the readings on a digital display. Follow the manufacturer's directions for the type of unit you are using.

Some facilities use an instrument that measures pulse rate, temperature, blood pressure, and the pulse oximeter value (Figure 20-3).

MEASURING THE BLOOD PRESSURE

Blood pressure is usually measured in the upper arm over the brachial artery. Blood pressure readings taken anywhere else must be ordered by a doctor. The values are recorded in millimeters of mercury (mm Hg).

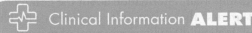
Clinical Information **ALERT**

Some facilities prefer measuring the blood pressure in the left arm, if possible, because it is closest to the heart.

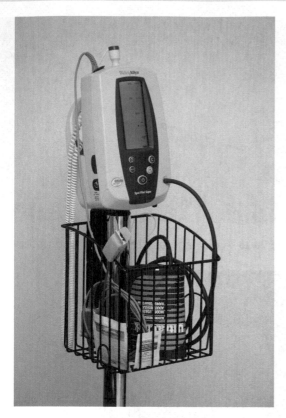

FIGURE 20-3 All vital signs may be checked with a single instrument.

1. The cuff is smoothly applied directly over the **brachial artery** (1 inch above the **antecubital area**).

2. The stethoscope diaphragm is placed over the brachial artery.

3. Pressure is then increased by inflating the rubber bladder in the cuff to stop the flow of blood through the artery.

4. The pressure is slowly released, and the sounds of heart valves closing can be heard. The sounds correspond to pressure changes in the blood vessel.

5. The blood pressure is measured:
   a. At its highest point as the **systolic pressure**. This will be the first regular sound you will hear. This is the sound of the bicuspid and tricuspid valves shutting.
   b. At its lowest point as the **diastolic pressure**. This will be the change or last sound you will hear. This is the sound of the semilunar valves shutting.
   c. The difference between systolic and diastolic pressure is called **pulse pressure**. The pulse pressure gives important information about the health of the arteries. The average pulse pressure in a healthy adult is about 40 millimeters (mm) of mercury (Hg) (range 30–50 mm Hg). However, factors related to both health and disease can alter the pulse pressure. An increase in blood volume or heart rate or a decrease in the ability of the arteries to expand may result in an increased pulse pressure.

6. Blood pressure readings are recorded as an improper fraction; for example, systolic/diastolic or 130/92. This means the systolic pressure is 130 and the diastolic pressure is 92. Both numbers in the blood pressure are important, but for people who are 50 or older, systolic pressure gives the most accurate diagnosis of high blood pressure.

7. There are some important things to know about blood pressure values:
   a. Average resting adult brachial artery pressure is less than 120 millimeters of mercury (mm Hg) systolic and less than 80 millimeters of mercury (mm Hg) diastolic.
   b. **Prehypertension** is a condition that means the person is likely to develop high blood pressure in the future. In this condition, blood pressure is between 120/80 mm Hg and 139/89 mm Hg. People with prehypertension can take steps to decrease their risk.
   c. **Hypertension** (high blood pressure) is when values are greater than 140 mm Hg systolic and 90 mm Hg diastolic.
   d. **Hypotension** (low blood pressure) is when values are less than 100 mm Hg systolic and 60 mm Hg diastolic. Excessive hypotension can lead to shock.
   e. **Orthostatic hypotension** is also called *postural hypotension*. This condition occurs when the blood pressure drops suddenly when changing position from sitting to standing, lying down to sitting, or stretching after standing. This causes the person to feel dizzy or light-headed. Although it can occur briefly in anyone, it is most common in persons who are elderly, and those with low blood pressure. It is a common cause of falls in long-term care facilities, especially at night.
   f. Record and report unusual or changed blood pressure readings (see Procedure 39).
   g. High blood pressure is a dangerous condition. There are no signs and symptoms. It increases the risk of several serious diseases (see Chapter 40). It can also cause complications of conditions such as diabetes. People with prehypertension and hypertension require regular blood pressure monitoring.
   h. Blood pressure classifications are listed in Table 20-2. When systolic and diastolic blood pressures fall into different categories, the higher category is used to classify blood pressure level. For example, 172/78 mm Hg would be stage 2 hypertension (high blood pressure).

Inaccurate Blood Pressure Readings

Causes of inaccurate blood pressure readings include:
- Using a wrong-size cuff
- Placing cuff over clothing
- Improperly wrapping the cuff
- Incorrectly positioning the arm

GUIDELINES 20-1 Guidelines for Preparing to Measure Blood Pressure

Before using the stethoscope:

1. Clean the earpieces with an alcohol wipe (Figure 20-4A) and clean the bell or diaphragm with a different alcohol wipe.

2. Point the earpieces forward when inserting them in your ears.

3. Use the diaphragm portion of the stethoscope.

4. Be sure the diaphragm portion is open so you will hear the beats.

Before using a sphygmomanometer:

1. If the silver substance in a mercury manometer moves up the column very slowly, it may have oxidized. Report this to the nurse and use another sphygmomanometer.

2. If using an aneroid manometer, make sure the needle is on zero before you inflate the cuff (Figure 20-4B). If it is not, report this to the nurse and use another sphygmomanometer.

3. Infection control is an issue with blood pressure cuffs. Facilities manage this problem in different ways:

   – Wiping the cuff with a disposable disinfectant wipe between patients.

   – Covering the cuff with a disposable paper cover that is discarded after one use.

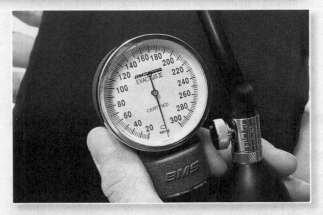

FIGURE 20-4B Make sure the needle is on zero before inflating the cuff on the aneroid sphygmomanometer.

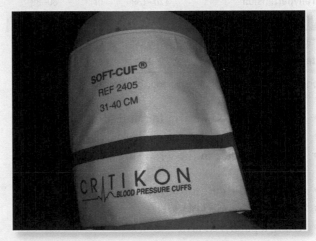

FIGURE 20-4C Many facilities issue a disposable blood pressure cuff to each patient. They are sent home with the patient or discarded upon discharge.

   – Issuing a disposable cuff to each patient (Figure 20-4C). Connect this cuff to the unit sphygmomanometer when vital signs are needed. Leave the cuff in the patient's room. Use it for the duration of the admission and discard on discharge.

Generally:

• Turn off radio and television when taking blood pressure. Ask the patient not to talk.

• Do not take blood pressure on an arm that:

   – Has an intravenous feeding or other device inserted.

   – Is being treated for burns, fractures, or other injuries.

   – Has a dialysis access device.

   – Is on the same side as the patient's recent mastectomy (breast removal) or other surgical procedure.

   – Has a pulse oximeter.

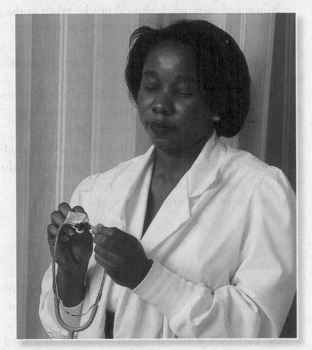

FIGURE 20-4A Clean the earpieces with an alcohol sponge before and after use.

Safety ALERT

Do not use a stethoscope that has cracks or holes in the tubing. Avoid contacting the patient's clothing with the bell or diaphragm of the stethoscope. Place the bell or diaphragm of the stethoscope flat against the patient's skin and hold it firmly, but gently, in place. You will not be able to hear the sounds if it is at an angle. If you press too hard, you will be unable to hear sounds.

Safety ALERT

Do not attempt to measure blood pressure using an arm that is the site of an intravenous infusion PICC (peripheral intravenous central catheter) line (see Chapter 36), is the site of a dialysis access device, is paralyzed, is injured, has edema present, is on the same side as a recent surgery, or has a pulse oximeter.

TABLE 20-2 Blood Pressure Classifications

Category	Blood Pressure Level (mm Hg)		
	Systolic		Diastolic
Hypotension	< 100	and	< 60
Normal	< 120	and	< 80
Prehypertension	120–139	or	80–89
High Blood Pressure			
Stage I hypertension	140–159	or	90–99
Stage II hypertension	≥ 160	or	≥ 100

Legend: < means less than; ≥ means greater than or equal to

- Not using the same arm for all readings
- Not having the gauge at eye level
- Placing the cuff in the wrong area, such as the forearm*
- Deflating the cuff too slowly
- Using a distended bladder
- Using a paralyzed arm
- Not supporting the arm
- Smoking
- Mistaking an **auscultatory gap** (sound fadeout for 10 to 15 mm Hg which then begins again) as the diastolic pressure

HOW TO READ THE GAUGE

The gauges on sphygmomanometers are marked with a series of lines. The large lines are at increments of 10 millimeters of mercury pressure. The shorter lines are at 2-mm intervals. For example, the first small line above 80 mm is 82 mm. The first small line below 80 mm is 78 mm (Figure 20-5).

---

*The effects of anatomical structures on adult forearm and upper arm noninvasive blood pressures. K. A. Schell, J. G. Richards, & W. B. Farquhar. (2007, February). *Blood Pressure Monitoring, 12*(1), 17–22.; K. A. Schell & J. K. Waterhouse. (2007). Comparison of forearm and upper arm: Automatic, noninvasive blood pressures in college students. K. A. Schell & J. K. Waterhouse. (2007). *Internet Journal of Advanced Nursing Practice, 9*(1).; J. Handler. (2009). The importance of accurate blood pressure measurement. J. Handler. (2009). *Permanente Journal, 13*(3), 51–54.

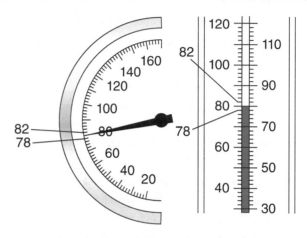

FIGURE 20-5 The aneroid gauge (left) and the mercury gauge (right). Take the reading at the closest line.

To properly read the mercury gauge:
- It should be at eye level.
- It should not be tilted.
- The reading should be taken at the top of the column of mercury. It should not be taken at the "hump" in the middle of the mercury when you hear the first sound.

To properly read the aneroid gauge, observe the gauge at eye level. Do not read it at an angle.

Following completion of the blood pressure measurement, you will record and report the following:
- If you were unable to hear the reading
- If blood pressure is higher than in a previous reading
- If blood pressure is lower than in a previous reading
- If the site where you took the reading was other than the brachial artery

Infection Control ALERT

Clean the manual or electronic blood pressure cuff and tubing with a facility-approved disinfectant after each patient. Alternatives are to use a disposable cuff that is issued to each patient and used throughout the hospital stay or to cover the cuff with a disposable sleeve.

PROCEDURE **40** **TAKING BLOOD PRESSURE**

Measuring the Blood Pressure: ONE-STEP METHOD

Blood pressure is usually measured in the upper arm over the brachial artery. Check with the nurse before taking blood pressure readings anywhere else. The values are recorded in millimeters of mercury (mm Hg). Here is the procedure for the one-step method of measuring brachial artery blood pressure:

1. Apply the cuff smoothly, directly over the brachial artery (1 inch above the antecubital area). This is the area on the inner surface of the arm, in front of the elbow.

2. Place the stethoscope diaphragm or bell over the brachial artery.

3. Begin inflating the bulb to increase pressure in the rubber bladder in the cuff to stop the flow of blood through the artery.

4. Slowly open the valve to release the pressure at a rate of 2 to 3 mm Hg per second. You will hear the sounds of heart valves closing. The sounds correspond to pressure changes in the blood.

Measuring the Blood Pressure: TWO-STEP METHOD

 NOTE

This is the "two-step" procedure that has been recommended by the American Heart Association (AHA) since 1993.* The AHA considers the two-step procedure the most reliable for normal blood pressure measurement. In some facilities and states, nursing assistants use the one-step procedure for measuring blood pressure.

1. Carry out initial procedure actions.

2. Assemble equipment:
   – Sphygmomanometer with appropriate size cuff
   – Stethoscope
   – Alcohol wipes

3. Remove the patient's arm from any sleeve or roll the sleeve 5 inches above the elbow; it should not be tight or binding.

4. Locate the brachial artery with your fingertips (Figure 20-6A).

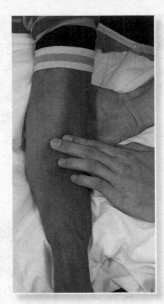

FIGURE 20-6A Locate the brachial artery with the fingertips.

5. Place the patient's arm palm upward, supported on bed or table, at heart level.

6. Wrap the cuff smoothly and snugly around the arm. Center the bladder over the brachial artery. The bottom of the cuff should be 1 inch above the antecubital space (inner elbow) (Figure 20-6B).

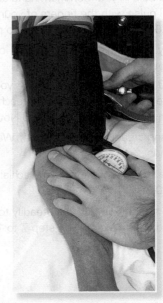

FIGURE 20-6B The bottom of the cuff should be at least 1 inch above the antecubital space (inner elbow).

*D. Perloff, C. Grim, J. Flack, E. D. Frohlich, M. Hill, M. McDonald, et al. (1993). Human blood pressure determination by sphygmomanometry. *Circulation, 88,* 2460–2470.

(continues)

PROCEDURE **40** CONTINUED   **0**

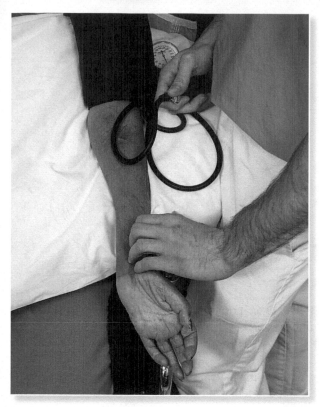

FIGURE 20-6C Hold the bulb in one hand and feel for the radial pulse with the fingers of the other hand.

7. Place the bulb in your dominant hand and feel for the radial pulse with the fingers of your other hand (Figure 20-6C). To find out how high to pump the cuff:
   – Rapidly inflate the cuff until you no longer feel the radial pulse.
   – Add 30 mm Hg to that reading. (If you no longer feel the pulse when the needle reaches 130, add 30 mm Hg, for a reading of 160.) Note that point.

8. Quickly and steadily deflate the cuff. Wait 15 to 30 seconds.

9. Place the stethoscope over the brachial artery (Figure 20-6D).

10. Reinflate the cuff quickly and steadily to the level you calculated (in the example in step 7, to 160).

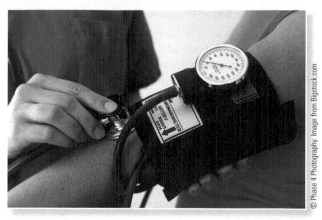

FIGURE 20-6D Hold the diaphragm of the stethoscope over the brachial artery.

11. Release the air at an even pace, about 2 to 3 mm Hg per second. Keep your eyes on the needle.

12. Listen for the onset of at least two consecutive beats. Note where the needle is on the sphygmomanometer when you first hear the sound. (Do not stop deflating the cuff.) This is your systolic reading.

13. Continue deflating the cuff. The last sound you hear is the diastolic reading. Continue to deflate and listen for 10 to 20 mm Hg more to make sure you have the correct diastolic reading.

14. Record the reading (blood pressure is always recorded in even numbers, with the systolic on top and the diastolic on the bottom; e.g., 128/82). Indicate the arm used and the position of the patient (sitting, lying down, or standing).

15. If you are not sure of the reading, or if instructed to obtain two measurements, wait 1 to 2 minutes before repeating the procedure. Average the two readings and document the average. If the first two readings differ by more than 5 mm Hg, the nurse may ask you to take a third measurement and average the three.

16. Clean the earpieces of the stethoscope with alcohol wipes. If the tubing has contacted the patient or linen, wipe the tubing as well.

17. Return equipment to the appropriate area.

18. Carry out ending procedure actions.

ICON KEY:
0 = OBRA

GUIDELINES 20-2 Guidelines for Electronic Blood Pressure Monitoring

Patient Selection

- This procedure can be done on patients of all ages and sizes. Be sure the cuff is the correct size for the patient.

- Take at least one blood pressure reading using the auscultation method before using an electronic blood pressure device. The auscultation value serves as a baseline with which to compare the values from the electronic device.

- The procedure is contraindicated in patients with:
  - Extreme hypertension or hypotension.
  - Very rapid heart rates.
  - Excessive body movement or tremors.
  - Irregular heart rhythms or atrial dysrhythmias.

  The care plan will note whether electronic blood pressure monitoring is contraindicated. If in doubt, check with the nurse.

- Do not place the cuff on an arm that:
  - Is paralyzed.
  - Is the site of an intravenous infusion (IV).
  - Has a pulse oximeter on it.
  - Has impaired circulation.
  - Is the site of a dialysis access device.
  - Is fractured.
  - Is burned.
  - Is on the same side as a recent mastectomy or other surgical procedure site.

Application of the Cuff

- Select the proper cuff size. The length of the bladder should be equal to 80 percent of the arm circumference.

- The upper arm is the preferred location for the monitoring cuff.

PROCEDURE **41** TAKING BLOOD PRESSURE WITH AN ELECTRONIC BLOOD PRESSURE APPARATUS

1. Carry out initial procedure actions.

2. Assemble equipment:
   - Electronic blood pressure device
   - Assortment of cuffs and tubes

3. Bring the electronic blood pressure unit to the bedside. Place it near the patient and plug it into a source of electricity.

4. Locate the on/off switch and turn the machine on.

5. Select the appropriate cuff for the machine and size for the patient's extremity.

6. Remove restrictive clothing.

7. Squeeze excess air out of the cuff.

8. Connect the cuff to the connector hose.

9. Wrap the cuff snugly around the patient's extremity, verifying that only one finger can fit between the cuff

and the patient's skin. Make sure the "artery" arrow on the cuff is correctly placed over the brachial artery.

10. Verify that the connector hose between the cuff and the machine is not kinked.

11. Set the frequency control to automatic or manual.

12. Press the start button.

13. If the cuff will take periodic, automatic measurements, set the designated frequency of blood pressure measurements.

14. Set upper and lower alarm limits for systolic, diastolic, and mean blood pressure readings.

15. Remove the cuff at least every 2 hours and rotate sites, if possible. Evaluate the skin for redness and irritation. Report abnormalities to the nurse.

16. Carry out ending procedure actions.

ICON KEY:

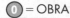 = OBRA

Pulse Oximeters

Some electronic vital sign monitors also measure the pulse oximeter value (Chapter 19). A spring clip slips over the patient's fingertip, and the unit displays the value. If the unit you are using also includes a pulse oximeter, apply the spring finger clip to the hand on the opposite side from the blood pressure cuff. (Applying it to an arm with an inflated blood pressure cuff will cause inaccurate values.) The spring finger clip may be applied to an arm with an IV, to one with a dialysis access device, or the side affected by a stroke or mastectomy without causing injury. The device will obtain a reading quickly, usually within a few seconds. If you obtain a value below 95, have the patient take a few deep breaths, and check the reading again. You may remove the spring clip as soon as the reading is obtained. Review the information in Chapter 19 on using the pulse oximeter so you are familiar with the reportable values.

REVIEW

A. True/False

Mark the following true or false by circling T or F.

1. T F   The volume of blood in the circulatory system affects the blood pressure.
2. T F   Exercise decreases blood pressure.
3. T F   To accurately measure manual blood pressure, you will need both a sphygmomanometer and a stethoscope.
4. T F   Blood pressures taken over arteries closer to the heart will be lower than those taken over arteries farther from the heart.
5. T F   A blood pressure below 100/60 suggests hypotension.
6. T F   The large lines on the blood pressure gauge are in increments of 20 millimeters of mercury pressure.
7. T F   Depressant drugs elevate the blood pressure.
8. T F   Using a blood pressure cuff of the wrong size will give an inaccurate reading.
9. T F   When measuring a blood pressure, always keep the gauge at eye level.
10. T F   Stethoscope earpieces should be cleaned both before and after use.
11. T F   The forearm is a good alternate location for taking blood pressure.
12. T F   Orthostatic hypotension is most common in middle-aged adults.

B. Matching

Choose the correct word from Column II to match each phrase in Column I.

Column I

13. _____   high blood pressure
14. _____   lowest blood pressure reading
15. _____   stretch
16. _____   artery most commonly used to determine blood pressure
17. _____   blood pressure apparatus

Column II

a. brachial
b. diastolic
c. stethoscope
d. femoral
e. sphygmomanometer
f. hypotension
g. hypertension
h. elasticity
i. systolic

C. Completion

Complete the statements by choosing the correct word.

18. The closing of the heart valves is heard as the _____ sound. (diastolic) (systolic)
19. High blood pressure is known as _____. (hypotension) (hypertension)
20. Blood pressure is lowered when weight is _____. (gained) (lost)
21. Blood pressure is raised with _____. (rest) (exercise)
22. The earpieces of the stethoscope should be pointed _____ as they are placed in the ears. (forward) (backward)
23. Postural _____ is a sudden decrease in blood pressure when changing position. (hypertension) (hypotension)

D. Nursing Assistant Challenge

You are assigned to take Mr. King's blood pressure at 12 noon. He is a very heavy man and has an IV inserted in his left arm. His blood pressure was 180/140 at 8 a.m. Answer the following questions.

24. What effect will his size have on your selection of cuff? _____
_____
25. On which arm will you apply the cuff? _____
26. Will you report your findings? _____
27. Why or why not?

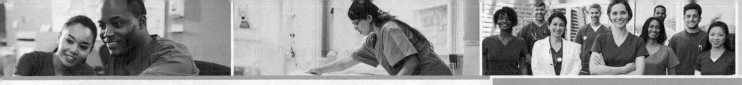

Measuring Height and Weight

OBJECTIVES

After completing this chapter, you will be able to:

21.1 Spell and define terms.

21.2 Understand why accurate weight measurements are important.

21.3 Describe the proper use of an overbed scale.

21.4 Demonstrate the following procedures:

- Procedure 42: Weighing and Measuring the Patient Using an Upright Scale (Expand Your Skills)

- Procedure 43: Weighing the Patient on a Chair Scale
- Procedure 44: Measuring Weight with an Electronic Wheelchair Scale
- Procedure 45: Measuring and Weighing the Patient in Bed

VOCABULARY

Learn the meaning and the correct spelling of the following words and phrases:

balance bar	increment	kilogram (kg)	pound (lb)
baseline			

WEIGHT AND HEIGHT MEASUREMENTS

Changes in weight are frequently used as an indicator of the patient's condition.

- **Baseline** (original) measurement of height and weight is obtained on admission. These measurements are usually noted on the Kardex.
- Patients who are taking drugs to increase their urine output (diuretics) often have an order for daily weights.
- Weight is an indicator of the patient's nutritional status.
- Weight and height values must be accurate. Document them promptly because many health care professionals depend on the accuracy of these measurements. The physician orders medications based on the patient's size.
- Height measurements may be recorded in feet (') and inches (") or in centimeters (cm).
- Weight measurements may be recorded in **pounds (lb)** or **kilograms (kg)**. The metric system may also be used for recording temperature.
- Use the upright scale for ambulatory patients who can stand unattended on the platform (Figure 21-1).

> **NOTE**
>
> Some facilities use the metric system, so you may be recording weight in kilograms and temperature in degrees centigrade. If your facility uses the metric system, the instruments will be calibrated for the metric system. You will not be required to convert the values to the metric system.

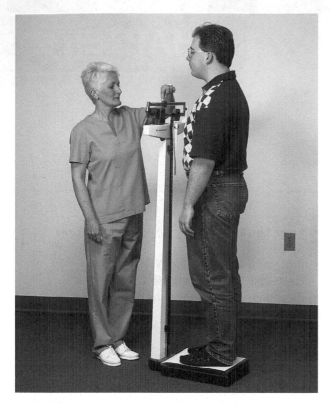

FIGURE 21-1 An upright scale is used only for patients who can stand on the platform unassisted.

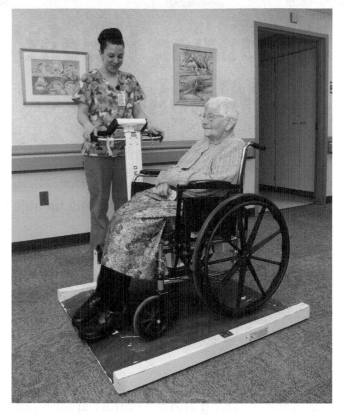

FIGURE 21-3 Electronic chair scales are used for patients who cannot stand on an upright scale.

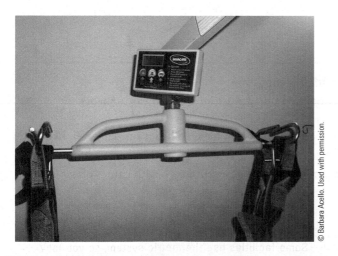

© Barbara Acello. Used with permission.

FIGURE 21-2 The scale on the mechanical lift is used for patients who cannot stand. The regular sling is used for most patients, but bed (supine) slings are available. Some of the slings that hang from colored loops may be used for both sitting and supine weights.

- A mechanical lift with scale can be used to weigh bedfast patients and those who cannot stand (Figure 21-2).
- Sling scales can be used to weigh patients whose condition does not permit the use of a mechanical lift/scale.

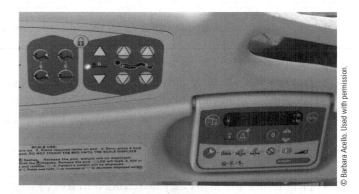

© Barbara Acello. Used with permission.

FIGURE 21-4 This hospital bed has a built-in scale.

- Electronic chair scales may be used to weigh patients in wheelchairs (Figure 21-3). Ramps and platforms are available for weighing persons in wheelchairs using an upright balancing scale.
- Some beds have built-in scales (Figure 21-4). Make sure that personal property and medical equipment are not in the bed when a bed scale is used. (See Procedures 42 to 45.)

GUIDELINES 21-1 Guidelines for Obtaining Accurate Weight and Height Measurements

To obtain an accurate weight measurement, you must:

- Always balance the scale before using it.
- Have the patient empty their bladder.
- Make sure the patient's incontinence brief is dry before obtaining the weight.
- Empty the catheter bag before weighing.
- Weigh the patient at the same time of day each time.

- Have the patient wear the same amount and type of clothing each time.
- Use the same method and the same scale each time, if possible.

If the patient has a cast, has recently had a cast removed, or has new-onset edema, consult the nurse about possible weight discrepancies.

Height is measured with a ruler attached to an upright scale or with a tape measure when the patient is in bed.

✚ Clinical Information **ALERT**

When weighing a patient who is in a wheelchair (see Figure 21-3), remove the lap tray and other wheelchair accessories before measuring the weight. If an accessory cannot be removed, weigh the empty wheelchair (with the accessory), and then subtract the combined weight from the total patient weight. Lap trays can add as much as 10 pounds to the total weight.

✚ Clinical Information **ALERT**

Some patients have orders for daily weights because of fluid balance problems. Weigh the patient at the same time, with the same amount and type of clothing, using the same scale, if possible. Empty the catheter bag before weighing the patient. A weight gain usually suggests fluid retention. A two-pound gain in a short time indicates that the patient is retaining an extra liter of fluid. Weight loss means that excess fluid has left the body.

You must learn to read the scale correctly. There are two bars on the upright scale (see Figure 21-1). The **balance bar** should hang free to start.

- The lower bar indicates weights in 50-pound **increments** (amounts).

- The upper bar indicates one-quarter-pound increments (Figure 21-5).
- The even-numbered pounds are marked with numbers.

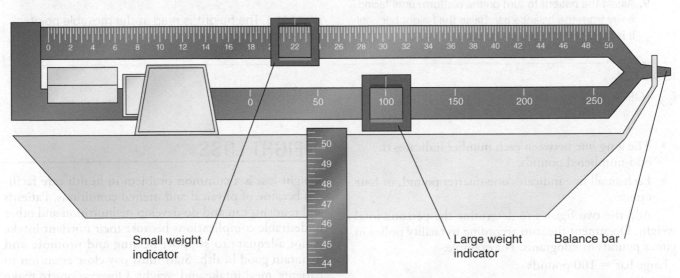

Small weight indicator

Large weight indicator

Balance bar

FIGURE 21-5 The upper bar indicates smaller pound weights. The weight shown on the lower bar is measured in 50-pound increments. This figure is added to the amount shown on the upper bar.

EXPAND YOUR SKILLS

PROCEDURE **42** WEIGHING AND MEASURING THE PATIENT USING AN UPRIGHT SCALE

1. Carry out initial procedure actions.

> ✎ **NOTE**
>
> Use disposable gloves if there may be contact with open lesions, wet linens, or body fluids.

2. Check notes or the chart for previous weight. Escort the patient to the scales.

3. Place a paper towel on the platform of the scale.

4. Be sure the weights are to the extreme left and the balance bar (bar with weight markings) is hanging free.

5. Assist the patient to remove shoes and step up onto the scale platform, facing the balance bar. The balance bar will rise to the top of the bar guide. Instruct the patient not to hold the bar or touch other parts of the scale.

6. Move the large weight to the right to the closest estimated patient weight.

7. Move the small weight to the right until the balance bar hangs freely halfway between the upper and lower bar guides.

8. Add the two figures and record the total as the patient's weight in pounds or kilograms, according to the type of scale used.

9. Assist the patient to turn on the platform until facing away from the balance bar. Raise the height bar until it is level with the top of the patient's head.

10. Take the reading at the movable point of the ruler (Figure 21-6).

11. Note the number of inches (or centimeters) indicated. Record this information in inches ("), feet (') and inches ("), or centimeters (cm), according to the type of scale and facility policy. The height shown in Figure 21-6 is 62 inches. This may be recorded as 62 inches or 5 feet 2 inches (62 ÷ 12 = 5 feet 2 inches). Record the value on your notepad.

12. Assist the patient off the platform. Help the patient to put on shoes, if necessary, and return to the room.

13. Carry out ending procedure actions.

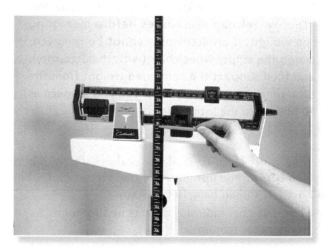

FIGURE 21-6 The height is read at the movable point of the ruler.

ICON KEY:

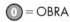 = OBRA

- The long line between each number indicates the odd-numbered pounds.
- Each small line indicates one-quarter pound, or four ounces.

Add the two figures to determine the person's total weight. Document the sum according to facility policy in either pounds or kilograms. For example:

Large bar = 100 pounds
Small bar = +22 pounds
Total = 122 pounds

WEIGHT LOSS

Weight loss is a common problem in health care facilities because of physical and mental conditions. Patients and residents can and do develop malnutrition and other undesirable complications because their nutrient intake is not adequate to support healing and promote and maintain good health. Staff must pay close attention to patients' meal intake and weight. Observations to make and report for persons with weight loss or reduced intake are listed in Table 21-1.

PROCEDURE 43 WEIGHING THE PATIENT ON A CHAIR SCALE

1. Carry out initial procedure actions.
2. Assemble equipment:
   – Chair scale

 NOTE

This procedure refers to a scale with a permanently mounted chair.

3. Take the patient in a wheelchair to the chair scale. Lock the brakes to the wheelchair. Be sure the chair scale is locked into place.

4. Apply a transfer belt to the patient and assist in a pivot transfer to the chair on the scale. Instruct the patient to sit down when the back of the legs touch the chair. Be sure the patient's feet are on the footrest of the chair once seated. Remove the transfer belt before obtaining the weight.

5. Walk behind the scale to obtain the reading.

6. Reapply the transfer belt. Transfer the patient back to the wheelchair.

7. Carry out ending procedure actions.

PROCEDURE 44 MEASURING WEIGHT WITH AN ELECTRONIC WHEELCHAIR SCALE

1. Carry out initial procedure actions.
2. Assemble equipment:
   – Wheelchair scale

 NOTE

This procedure refers to the scale pictured in Figure 21-3.

3. Determine and record the empty weight of a wheelchair by weighing it on the scale.

4. Take the wheelchair to the patient's room. Help the patient into the wheelchair and take the patient to the electronic wheelchair scale.

5. Open the metal ramp sides on the scale so that they rest on the floor. This allows wheelchair access to the scale.

6. Press the on button; the scale zeroes automatically.

7. Roll the wheelchair, with the patient in it, onto the platform of the scale (refer to Figure 21-3). Lock the wheelchair wheels.

8. The digital readout will show the weight.

9. Record the weight of the patient and wheelchair. Subtract the wheelchair weight to obtain the patient's weight.

10. Unlock the wheelchair wheels. Roll the wheelchair with the patient off the scale.

11. Fold the scale ramps back into place.

12. Carry out ending procedure actions.

PROCEDURE **45** **MEASURING AND WEIGHING THE PATIENT IN BED**

 NOTE

This procedure refers to the scale shown in Figure 21-2.

1. Carry out initial procedure actions.

2. Obtain assistance from a co-worker.

3. Assemble equipment:
   - Overbed (sling) scale
   - Sheet
   - Tape measure
   - Pencil

4. Check scale sling and straps for frayed areas or straps that do not close properly.

5. Lower the side rail on your side. Make sure the side rail is up on the other side.

6. Fan-fold the top linen to the foot of the bed.

7. Position the patient flat on the back with arms and legs straight and body in good alignment. Make sure the sheet under the patient is straight and wrinkle-free.

8. Make a small pencil mark at the top of the patient's head on the sheet.

9. Make a second pencil mark even with the heels.

10. Roll the patient on the side. Using the tape measure, measure the distance between the two pencil marks.

11. Note the patient's height in feet and inches on a pad.

12. Cover the canvas sling with a sheet. Balance the scale according to the manufacturer's directions. The scale should be balanced with the sheet, canvas sling, chains, or straps attached.

13. Remove the scale sling from the suspension straps and position half of the sheet-covered sling under the patient.
    - Turn the patient away from you.
    - Place the sling, folded lengthwise, under the patient.
    - Return the patient to the supine position and place the sling so that the patient rests securely within it.
    - Attach the sling to the suspension straps. Check to be sure attachments are secure.

14. Position the lift frame over the bed with base legs in maximum open position, and lock the frame.

15. Elevate the head of the bed and bring the patient to a sitting position.

16. Attach the suspension straps to the frame. Position the patient's arms inside the straps.

17. Slowly raise the sling so the patient's body is off the bed. Be reassuring.

18. Guide the lift away from the bed so that no part of the patient touches the bed.

19. Weigh the patient and remember or document the reading (weight).

20. Reposition the sling over the center of the bed.

21. Release the knob slowly, lowering the patient to the bed.

22. Remove the sling by reversing the process in step 13.

23. Assist the patient to a comfortable position.

24. Move the overbed scale out of the way.

25. Replace the top bed linen over the patient. Raise the side rail and lower the bed to the lowest horizontal height.

26. Carry out ending procedure actions.

TABLE 21-1 Observations to Make and Report for Persons with Unplanned, Undesirable Weight Loss or Reduced Intake

• Weight loss of > 5% in 1 month; > 7.5% in 3 months; > 10% in 6 months	• Symptoms suggesting depression
• Increase or decrease in food (caloric) intake	• Difficulty chewing
• Increase or decrease in body weight	• Difficulty swallowing
• Patients with diabetes who do not eat all their food, or who eat more than allowed on diet	• Poor position makes it difficult for patient to feed self (too far from table, food at shoulder height, no elbow support, etc.)
• Patients on restricted diets who do not adhere to their diet	• Needs help eating and drinking
• Refusal to accept meal, supplement, snack	• Dentures slip, do not fit, or lost
• Refusal to accept food substitute for meat or vegetable	• Wanders and paces during meal
• Meal intake of less than 50% (or 75%, according to facility policy)	• Becomes distracted and does not eat
	• Inability to see or difficulty seeing food
	• Drinks supplement during or immediately before meal, suppressing appetite

REVIEW

A. True/False

Mark the following true or false by circling T or F.

1. T F The lower bar on the scale indicates pounds in increments of 25.
2. T F Always check the overbed scale for needed repairs before use.
3. T F To obtain a proper reading, the scale balance bar must hang freely.
4. T F The scale used most often to weigh ambulatory patients in health care facilities is the upright scale.
5. T F A patient who cannot get out of bed cannot be measured.
6. T F When using an overbed scale, the patient's body must be free of the bed.
7. T F To measure a patient who is confined to bed, first help them assume the left Sims' position.
8. T F Patients and residents can and often do develop malnutrition during a stay in a health care facility.
9. T F Weight loss is a common problem in health care facilities because of physical and mental conditions.
10. T F Ill-fitting dentures have no effect on weight.
11. T F Disconnect the catheter bag before weighing the patient.
12. T F Many health care professionals depend on the accuracy of patient weight and height measurements.

B. Short Answer/Matching

Write the correct word from the following list on the blank to complete each statement.

    ambulatory
    away
    centimeters
    dependent
    inches
    independent
    kilograms
    pounds

13. Weights may be measured in _____ or _____.
14. Height measurements may be recorded in feet and _____ or in _____.
15. The upright scale is used to weigh _____ patients.
16. A scale that is calibrated for the metric system will express weights in _____.
17. When a patient is measured on a balance scale, they should face _____ from the scale.
18. The mechanical lift scale is used for weighing _____ patients.

C. Nursing Assistant Challenge

Mrs. Haughn is in bed recovering from a stroke. She is unable to walk or stand. She is receiving diuretics. Her doctor wants to order some new medication that is given according to the patient's size. You are assigned to weigh and measure the height of this patient. Answer each of the following by selecting the correct answer.

19. The best way to weigh this patient is with:
    a. an upright scale.
    b. an overbed scale.
    c. a wheelchair scale.
    d. a chair scale.

20. The best way to measure this patient is:
    a. with a height bar.
    b. with a tape measure.
    c. to ask the patient.
    d. to estimate the height.

21. One reason the physician might have asked for the patient's weight is because the patient:
    a. is receiving diuretics.
    b. has had a stroke.
    c. cannot stand.
    d. cannot walk.

22. The patient is 63 inches tall. This may be expressed as:
    a. 5 feet 6 inches.
    b. 5 feet 8 inches.
    c. 5 feet 3 inches.
    d. 6 feet 3 inches.

23. Some patients have orders for daily weights because they:
    a. eat too much.
    b. have fluid balance problems.
    c. need less medication.
    d. do not eat enough.

24. A two-pound gain in 24 hours suggests that the patient is:
    a. retaining an extra liter of fluid.
    b. retaining an extra gallon of fluid.
    c. not eating their meals.
    d. trying to lose weight.

25. Allen Nissen is 6'2" and weighs 140#. He usually eats about 70 percent of each meal. He enjoys sweets and always eats dessert. You know that he:
    a. is 62 inches tall.
    b. takes in 70 calories per meal.
    c. weighs 140 pounds.
    d. is 62 centimeters tall.

26. Mr. Nissen has a wound that is not healing. The nurse tells you they suspect this is because:
    a. his nutrient intake is not adequate to support healing.
    b. staff is not taking proper care of him.
    c. he is eating too much junk food.
    d. he has experienced many aging skin changes.

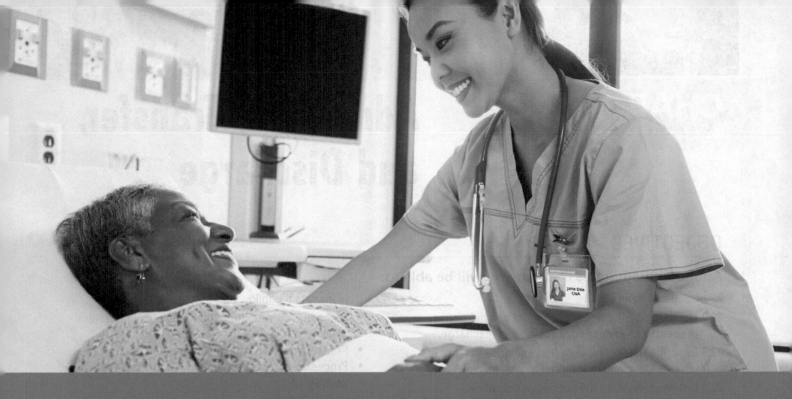

SECTION 7
Patient Care and Comfort Measures

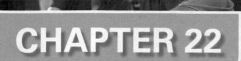

CHAPTER 22

Admission, Transfer, and Discharge

OBJECTIVES

After completing this chapter, you will be able to:

22.1 Spell and define terms.

22.2 List the ways the nursing assistant can help in the processes of admission, transfer, and discharge.

22.3 Describe family dynamics and emotions that occur when a loved one is admitted to the hospital.

22.4 List ways in which the nursing assistant can develop positive relationships with a patient's family members.

22.5 Demonstrate the following procedures:
- Procedure 46: Admitting the Patient (Expand Your Skills)
- Procedure 47: Transferring the Patient
- Procedure 48: Discharging the Patient (Expand Your Skills)

VOCABULARY

Learn the meaning and the correct spelling of the following words and phrases:

admission

baseline assessment

discharge

risk assessment

transfer

INTRODUCTION

The nurse is responsible for overseeing and carrying out procedures and physician's orders regarding all admissions, transfers, and discharges. You will usually help the nurse by carrying out the routine procedures associated with these activities.

An employee, such as a nursing assistant, volunteer, admitting clerk, or licensed nurse will escort them to the unit for admission. In many facilities, someone must always escort the patient from the unit during transfer or discharge as well.

You can do much to make these activities easier for the patient, family, and other staff members by:

- Having equipment and materials prepared for the activity.
- Being very observant during each activity.
- Documenting observations carefully and accurately. These make a valuable contribution to the nurse's initial **baseline assessment** of the patient's condition.
- Contributing to the nursing process by reporting information that the nurse will use in admission risk assessments, such as pressure ulcer risk and fall risk. A **risk assessment** is a careful evaluation of problems that have the potential to cause harm to a patient, such as falls or pressure ulcers. The nurse uses the assessment information for planning care.
- Reporting observations directly to the nurse.
- Giving attention to the details of each procedure.
- Being aware of the emotional stress these activities cause patients and their families.
- Being courteous to everyone.

ADMISSION

When a person enters a health care facility for treatment of an illness or injury, the **admission** process often causes concern or stress to the patient, family, and friends. You will be one of the first staff members the patient sees, so it is important that you be courteous, confident, and efficient (see Procedure 46).

Open the unit and prepare the bed as soon as you are notified of a new admission. If the patient will be admitted by ambulance or stretcher and put to bed, elevate the bed to the highest horizontal height, and open the bed. Move furnishings, if necessary, so the stretcher can be positioned next to the bed.

When a patient is ready for admission, ask the nurse if:

- The patient requires a stretcher or wheelchair to reach the unit
- Any special equipment, such as oxygen or a fracture bed, is needed
- There are any special instructions, such as withholding fluids or foods

Introduce yourself to the patient and observe them carefully. Listen for complaints as you escort and assist the patient to the room and to bed. Initial observations are very important. They become the basis of comparison for future observations.

The nurse will assess the patient on admission and begin a care plan. Your observations and your measurements of vital signs, height, and weight contribute to this assessment. You should also note and report your observations about:

- Rashes
- Bruises
- Pressure ulcers
- Other skin problems
- Vision problems
- Hearing problems
- Communication problems, including ability to make needs known and call for help
- Ability to ambulate and transfer safely
- Ability to use the bathroom safely

Inform the nurse and document your findings on the admission record, or according to facility policy.

Offer to assist in unpacking and storing the patient's belongings. Complete a personal belongings inventory (Figure 22-1), if used by your facility, and ask the patient or responsible party to sign it. Inform the nurse if no one is available to sign the form. Fill in all the forms for which you are responsible at the time of admission and make the patient and family as comfortable as possible.

If it is necessary to ask visitors to leave, do so in a kind and polite manner. They will be most anxious to remain and see the patient settled and comfortable, so:

- Show them where they may wait.
- Let them know about how long they will have to wait.
- Tell them where they can get refreshments.
- Answer questions they may have about visiting hours, and where to find a chapel, refreshments, and restrooms.
- After you have completed your part of the admission procedure, locate visitors and let them know they may return to the patient's room.

The nursing assistant is frequently the person who admits patients to the facility. This may be a difficult, stressful, frightening time for the patient. There is a common expression that "first impressions are usually lasting ones." The patient's perception of what is happening may be affected by illness, pain, and fear (Figure 22-2). Making a good first impression on the patient and family members is important. A negative first impression of the nursing assistant affects the patient's impression of all health care workers, and even the whole facility. Think about this and do your best to provide a positive, professional impression.

FAMILY DYNAMICS

The family is an extension of the patient. They must make many adjustments when the patient is admitted to the hospital. Admitting a loved one can be a very emotional time. Family members may feel relieved because the patient is getting help. They may also feel guilty for being unable to care for the loved one at home. Other common emotions that family members experience are:

- Fear—some family members will feel fearful and afraid to leave their relative in the facility.
- Anger—some families become angry about the admission. This is usually because they feel a loss of control. Occasionally they may take their anger out on the staff.
- Uncertainty—the family may feel uncertain about what will become of their loved one, causing them to feel afraid, worried, nervous, and tense.
- Sadness—the family may have difficulty coping with being separated from the patient.
- Guilt—the family may feel guilty for turning the care of the patient over to complete strangers. They may compensate by staying at the hospital most of the time to care for and protect the patient.
- Helplessness—family members may feel helpless because the patient's condition has worsened, and despite their best efforts, they cannot change the situation.
- Worry—family members worry about their loved one's well-being (Figure 22-3). They may have other worries and demands on their mind, such as how to pay the bills, or what to do with the patient's house or pets. They often feel overwhelmed with all the decisions and responsibilities.

Personal Belongings Inventory

Instructions: Nursing assistant completes upon admission. The Nursing assistant, patient, or responsible party sign. File in the medical record. Records and information concerning each person in care shall be maintained in such a manner as to preserve confidentiality.

PATIENT'S NAME	NAME OF PATIENT'S GUARDIAN	DATE OF ADMISSION
CONTACT LENSES	DENTURES	
EYEGLASSES	HEARING AID	
JEWELRY	WATCH	
MONEY/CHECKBOOK/CREDIT CARDS	OTHER	

		CLOTHING LIST	
NUMBER	ITEM		DESCRIPTION
	Bathrobe		
	Belt		
	Blouse		
	Brassiere		
	Coat		
	Dress		
	Gloves		
	Handkerchief		
	Hat		
	House coat		
	Laptop		
	Necktie		
	Nightgown		
	Pajamas		
	Pants		
	Shirts		
	Shoes		
	Skirts		
	Slippers		
	Slip		
	Smartphone		
	Socks		
	Stockings		
	Stylus		
	Suit		
	Suspenders		
	Sweater		
	Tablet		
	Undershirt		
	Underpants		
	Underwear–long		
	Vest		
	Other:		

		MISCELLANEOUS	
NUMBER	ITEM		DESCRIPTION
	Brush		
	Cane or crutches		
	Clock		
	Luggage		
	Radio		
	Television (model and serial number)		
	Walker		
	Wheelchair (model and serial number)		
	Other:		

Statement: I have read and agree that this is an accurate list of my belongings.

NURSING ASSISTANT'S SIGNATURE	DATE	PATIENT'S OR GUARDIAN'S SIGNATURE	DATE

FIGURE 22-1 Nursing assistants may be asked to complete a personal belongings inventory when a person is admitted to a hospital or long-term care facility.

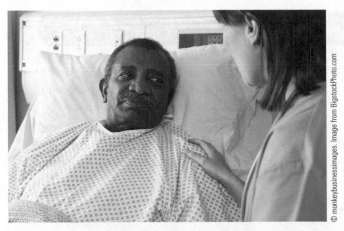

FIGURE 22-2 Treat patients and families with courtesy, respect, compassion, and understanding. Remember that admissions can be stressful for both the patient and family. First impressions are lasting ones, and you represent your facility to the patient.

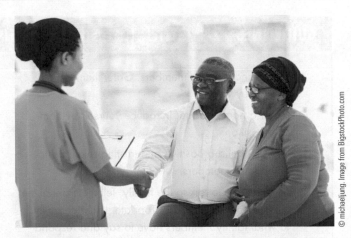

FIGURE 22-4 Make it a point to speak with family members when they visit. Treat each family member with warmth, courtesy, kindness, and respect.

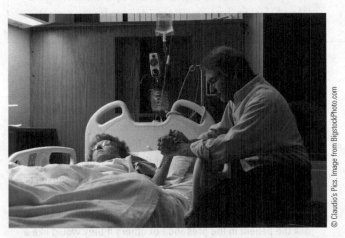

FIGURE 22-3 Family members worry about their loved one's well-being and may have many other problems related to the hospitalization.

Working to understand the emotions that families experience should give you an appreciation of why making a good first impression is so important. In addition, you must use good communication skills and show that you care. Greet each family member with warmth, courtesy, kindness, and respect. Introduce yourself and explain your responsibilities as a nursing assistant in the care of their loved one (Figure 22-4). Introduce the patient and family to roommates and other staff members. Make them feel welcome and show that you are sincerely interested in the patient. If appropriate, make comments such as, "I know this must be very difficult for you." Admission to a health care facility does not have to be a negative experience. A competent, caring, professional staff will calm family members' fears and turn a potentially negative experience into a positive one.

Communication **ALERT**

Security and Personal Identity

Many people bring their own pajamas and personal nightwear to the facility with them. If this is the case, allow them to wear it unless they are having surgery or a procedure in which they need a hospital gown. Wearing their own clothing makes them feel more secure and gives them a sense of identity. If tubes or the placement of medical devices interferes with using personal nightwear, help the person feel as comfortable and secure as possible. Make sure the body is covered and not exposed unnecessarily.

Culture **ALERT**

The patient's religion may affect important issues, including admission to the hospital. In some cultures, patients are cared for at home. Other issues that may be affected by culture are consent to treatment, routines, schedules of care, bathing and toileting routines, exposing the body for treatments and procedures, gender of caregivers, food preferences, room arrangements (because of certain religious practices), and birth and death practices. Look for clues to the patient's practices and

TRANSFER

It may be necessary to move the patient to another unit or facility. Preparations for the **transfer** will be handled by the nurse, but you may be asked to assist (see Procedure 47).

GUIDELINES 22-1 Guidelines for Family Dynamics

- Get to know family members. Greet them warmly when they visit.
- Wear a name badge. Introduce yourself by name and position.
- Work to build a positive and trusting relationship with family members.
- Be available to talk to the family. Tell them about the patient's activities, as appropriate. Listen carefully to what family members have to say and respond appropriately.
- Let the family know that you respect and support their role as their loved one's caregivers.
- Familiarize the family with facility routines and services.
- Refer questions of a medical or personal nature to the nurse.

- Listen to family members' suggestions, complaints, and comments. Inform the nurse of family concerns, or refer the family to the nurse, as appropriate.
- If the family has been caring for the patient at home, they often know what works best. Listen closely to their advice about patient care. Pass the information on to the nurse.
- Inform the nurse if a visit is stressful or tiring to a patient.
- Avoid judging the family and decisions they make. Stay out of family disagreements.
- Avoid gossiping with the family, and do not discuss facility business with family members.
- Allow the family to participate in the patient's care, if the patient does not object. However, avoid making the family feel as if they must provide care for the patient.

 Age-Appropriate Care **ALERT**

Pediatric patients may fear separation from the parents. Explain unit policies for visiting or rooming in. Orient the child and family to the playroom, bathroom, and other areas as appropriate. Speak directly to the child. Show the child how to use the signal to call for help. Ask them questions about normal routines. Allow the child to respond before questioning the parents. A primary goal on admission is to make the child and parents as comfortable as possible, relieving anxiety about separation.

 Safety **ALERT**

Never leave the room until the patient is safe, has the call signal within reach, and knows how to use it. If an ambulance service is delivering the patient, remain in the room until they have left the facility. Make certain that the patient has the call signal and everything else they need before leaving the room.

 Communication **ALERT**

Knowing when and how to ask a visitor to leave the room takes tact and diplomacy. Consult the nurse if you are unsure of how to handle a visitor situation. Try to schedule your care for when the patient is alone, if this is possible. If not, ask visitors to leave anytime the patient's body will be exposed or a procedure will be performed. If the patient requests that a visitor be allowed to stay, honor the request. However, do not ask the patient in the presence of others if they would like a visitor to stay. For a patient who is an infant or a young child, parents are generally permitted to remain in the room during procedures. Some adolescent and teenage children will be uncomfortable if parents remain in the room during personal care. Ask the parents to leave unless the child asks that they be allowed to stay. Make sure to ask the child their wishes privately. If parents are in the room, do not ask the child if they want the parents to stay.

The transfer may be the patient's own preference, or may be done because a change in the patient's condition requires a different type of care. The transfer may be temporary or permanent. If it is permanent, the patient is discharged from one unit or facility, and then admitted to another. The patient may or may not fully understand the reasons for the transfer. Be positive and supportive. Recognize that the patient may be feeling very anxious. It would be helpful to know what the patient has been told about the reasons for the transfer. You may learn this from the nurse and by carefully listening to what your patient says.

All details must be taken care of. Following facility policy ensures that there is no interruption of health care services. Some facilities have transportation services for transferring patients.

EXPAND YOUR SKILLS

PROCEDURE **46** **ADMITTING THE PATIENT**

1. Wash hands.

2. Assemble equipment:
   - Equipment for urine specimen collection
   - Equipment for taking temperature
   - Pad and pencil
   - Patient's chart or worksheet
   - Stethoscope
   - Admission kit:
     - Water pitcher
     - Glass
     - Liquid soap
     - Washcloth
     - Towel
     - Basin
     - Lotion
     - Mouthwash
   - Scale
   - Blood pressure cuff and manometer
   - Watch with second hand
   - Disposable gloves (if urine specimen is required)

3. Prepare the unit for the patient by:
   a. Making sure that all necessary equipment and furniture are properly placed and in good working order (Figure 22-5).
   b. Checking the unit for adequate lighting.
   c. Loosening the top sheet at the foot of the bed.
   d. Opening the bed.

4. Identify the patient by both asking the name and checking the identification bracelet.
   a. Introduce yourself.
   b. Take the patient and the patient's family to the unit.
   c. Do not appear to rush the patient.
   d. Be courteous and helpful to the patient and the family.

5. Ask the patient to be seated, if ambulatory.
   a. Ask the family to go to the lounge or lobby while the patient is being admitted.
   b. Introduce the patient to roommates, if any.
   c. As permitted, explain what will happen in the next hour.

6. Screen the unit by closing window curtains and privacy curtains to provide privacy (Figure 22-6).

7. Help the patient to undress and put on a hospital gown or nightclothes from home.

8. Check the patient's vital signs, weight, and height.

9. Help the patient get into bed. Adjust the side rails as needed.

10. If the patient is wearing any jewelry or has valuables:
    a. Make a list of personal property and ask the patient to sign it. This protects the facility and the patient. Inform the nurse if the patient is unable to sign.

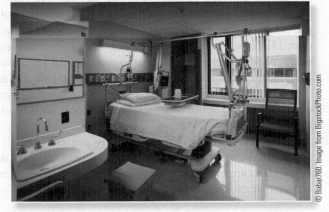

FIGURE 22-5 Obtain and set up needed items and special equipment prior to the patient's arrival.

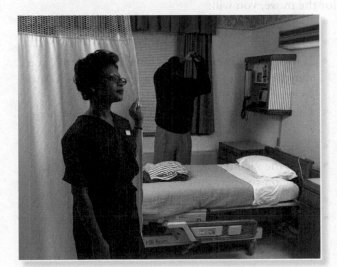

FIGURE 22-6 Provide privacy so the patient can undress.

(continues)

PROCEDURE **46** CONTINUED

b. Also ask the relatives to sign the list and take the valuables home. Alternatively, after checking and signing, give the valuables to the nurse to put in the hospital safe.

11. If a urine specimen is necessary, tell the patient.

   a. Put on gloves and assist the patient as necessary.

   b. Allow the patient to use the bathroom, if ambulatory, or offer the bedpan or urinal.

12. Pour the patient's specimen from the bedpan or urinal into the specimen bottle. Apply the cap. Remove and discard gloves. Be sure to label the specimen correctly (see Chapter 45).

13. An admission form may be completed at this time. Vital information includes:

   – Observations.

   – Vital signs (TPR, BP, height, weight).

   – Known allergies.

   – Medications being taken.

   – Food preferences and dislikes.

14. If admission is to a long-term care facility, label clothing and complete the personal belongings inventory form.

15. Orient the patient to the unit by explaining:

   – Visiting hours.

   – How to operate the bed and light switches, as appropriate.

   – Standard hospital regulations.

   – Any questions about facility routines.

   – When meals and refreshments are provided.

16. Carry out ending procedure actions.

🔓 Safety **ALERT**

Never leave the patient, the records, or medications unattended.

After the new unit has been notified and prepared for the move, you will:

- Tell the patient what you are doing.
- Gather the patient's belongings.
- If the patient is expected to return to the unit, you may be asked to gather only a few belongings, such as glasses, dentures, and toiletries.
- Get the patient's medicines, chart, and other personal information from the nurse.
- Assist in the physical transfer.
- Give the records and medications directly to the nurse on the new unit.
- Give the patient the call light.
- Make sure the patient is safe and comfortable in the new environment before you return to your own unit.

DISCHARGE

In recent years, health care costs have increased steadily. A government initiative, *diagnosis-related groups (DRGs)*, was introduced to control hospital costs. Under this initiative, hospitals are paid a specific amount of money for the care of an individual who has a particular condition or disease that is covered by a DRG.

If the hospital can provide the needed care and discharge the patient early, the hospital saves money and may keep the difference between actual expenses and the DRG-allotted payment. If the patient requires a longer hospital stay than is stipulated by the DRGs and the costs are higher, the hospital absorbs the additional cost. DRGs were developed for patients who are covered under Medicare, but they are used today by all insurance companies to determine how many hospital days they will pay for. This has resulted in sicker patients being discharged from acute care facilities sooner than is medically appropriate.

Following hospitalization, many patients are discharged to subacute units, long-term acute care hospitals, long-term care facilities for further care, or home to finish recuperation.

PROCEDURE **47** TRANSFERRING THE PATIENT

1. Find out which unit the patient will be transferred to. Check to see that it is ready.

2. Learn from the nurse in charge the method of transfer. Get the necessary vehicle (wheelchair, stretcher, or patient's own bed).

3. Check to see if any equipment is to be transferred with the patient.

4. Carry out initial procedure actions.

5. Explain to the patient what you are doing.

6. Gather all the patient's belongings.

    a. Place disposables in a bag to transport with you.

    b. Check against personal property list.

7. Assist the patient to put on robe and slippers, if permitted. Assist the patient into wheelchair or stretcher, as directed. The entire bed is often used to transport the patient. Make sure the side rails are up during transport.

8. Obtain from the nurse:

    – Patient's chart

    – Nursing care plan

    – Medications

    – Bag

9. Transport the patient and their belongings to the new unit (Figure 22-7). Use all precautions related to safe transport.

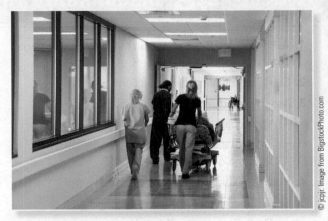

FIGURE 22-7 The nursing assistant is transporting the patient via stretcher.

10. Give any transferred medications, the nursing care plan, and the chart to the nurse in charge.

11. Introduce the patient to staff. Proceed to the patient's room.

12. Assist staff in helping the patient into bed. Assist in putting away the patient's belongings and helping the patient to get settled.

13. Before leaving the unit, carry out ending procedure actions.

The discharge procedure is usually simple if the patient is going to another facility. The social worker and nurse relay information to the receiving facility. The patient and the patient's belongings are sent to the new facility. Discharge to the patient's home is more complicated and requires a number of actions that make up *discharge planning* (see Chapter 34).

The Discharge Process

The **discharge**, or authorized release, of a patient requires a written order from the physician. If a patient indicates an intention to leave without an order, report it to the nurse immediately. The nurse will then make the necessary arrangements. Health care facilities have special policies that must be followed in these cases.

Spare the patient from fatigue and delay during a routine discharge (see Procedure 48). Assist the patient by:

• Checking with the nurse to make sure that the physician has written a discharge order.

• Gathering the patient's belongings and assisting in packing, if necessary.

• Carefully checking the closet and bedside table. Disposable equipment is often sent home with the patient. Make sure that the equipment is clean.

• Checking the patient's belongings against the personal inventory record or clothing list; have the patient sign the receipt.

• Checking with the nurse for any medications or other treatment-related equipment that should be sent home with the patient.

• Verifying that the patient has received discharge instructions from the nurse, physician, and/or discharge coordinator.

• Escorting the patient to the door of the facility. Never allow a patient to leave the health care facility unassisted. The patient is the staff's responsibility until they have left the building.

EXPAND YOUR SKILLS

PROCEDURE 48 DISCHARGING THE PATIENT

1. Ask the nurse if the physician has written discharge orders.

2. Carry out initial procedure actions.

3. Assemble equipment:
   - Wheelchair
   - Cart to transport items
   - List of belongings

4. Help the patient to dress, if necessary.

5. Collect the patient's personal belongings.
   a. Pack, if necessary. Most facilities allow patients to take their disposable utensils (such as a washbasin and urinal) home. If this is the policy of your facility, collect and bag the items the person plans to bring home.
   b. Check valuables against the admission list.
   c. Make sure that all of the patient's belongings have been removed from the closet and bedside stand.
   d. Check to see if medications or other equipment are to be sent home with the patient.
   e. Verify that the patient has received discharge instructions from the nurse, physician, and/or discharge coordinator.

6. Tell the patient or a member of the family how to collect valuables from the facility safe, if applicable.

7. Help the patient into a wheelchair.

8. Take the patient to the discharge entrance of the facility.
   a. Help the patient to transfer safely into the awaiting vehicle.
   b. Be gracious as you say goodbye.

9. Return the wheelchair.

10. Return to the patient unit.
    a. Strip the bed and dispose of linens.
    b. Clean and replace equipment, as appropriate.

11. Wash your hands.

12. Record the discharge in accordance with facility policy. Include:
    - Time
    - Method of transport
    - Patient's reaction
    - Signature

13. Report completion of task to the nurse.

REVIEW

A. True/False

Mark the following true or false by circling T or F.

1. T F When transferring a patient, leave the person in the room and return immediately to your own unit.

2. T F Use all precautions related to safe transport when admitting or discharging a patient.

3. T F You do not need to waste time introducing a new patient to others, because staff working on the unit are responsible for this.

4. T F It is acceptable to allow patients to leave a health care facility at any time.

5. T F After discharge, the patient's unit is stripped, cleaned, and restocked.

6. T F The patient's unit should be prepared as soon as you are notified that there will be an admission.

7. T F During a transfer, the patient's medications remain on the original unit.

8. T F Measuring the patient's height and weight is part of admission procedures.

9. T F The discharge order is written by the physician.

10. T F You should observe the patient carefully during the admission procedure.

B. Multiple Choice

Select the best answer for each of the following.

11. The assistant can do much to help facilitate admission procedures by:
  a. preparing equipment after the patient arrives on the unit.
  b. letting the nurse make all the observations.
  c. giving attention to all admission procedure details.
  d. recognizing that admission is more stressful for the staff than the patient.

12. When dealing with the newly admitted patient's family, you should:
  a. treat them with courtesy and consideration.
  b. send them home.
  c. let the nurse deal with them.
  d. allow them to stay at the patient's bedside at all times.

13. Part of admission procedures include:
  a. securing a stool specimen.
  b. obtaining a sputum specimen.
  c. rushing to prove you are efficient.
  d. measuring vital signs.

14. Valuables that accompany the patient to their unit should be:
  a. taken away.
  b. listed and signed for.
  c. left in the bedside stand.
  d. tucked under the pillow for safety.

15. When a patient is transferred, you should always include their:
  a. personal belongings.
  b. bed.
  c. pillow.
  d. blood pressure cuffs.

16. A risk assessment:
  a. requires a physician's order.
  b. measures the patient's strength.
  c. contributes to the nursing process.
  d. has no effect on the care plan.

17. When a patient is admitted to the facility, their family is likely to feel:
  a. happy to be rid of the person.
  b. mad at the doctor for admitting them.
  c. angry that they have to pay the bill.
  d. relieved that staff is caring for them.

18. The person who usually admits new patients to the facility is the:
  a. nurse.
  b. nursing assistant.
  c. doctor.
  d. supervisor.

19. DRG is the abbreviation for:
  a. diagnosis-related group.
  b. Division of Research Grants
  c. drug response guideline.
  d. data receiver group.

20. The purpose of the DRG is to:
  a. direct research.
  b. evaluate patient satisfaction.
  c. develop new drugs.
  d. save money.

21. When a patient is discharged:
  a. the washbasin and bedpan are washed and reused.
  b. the patient can take the washbasin and bedpan home.
  c. the washbasin and bedpan are thrown away.
  d. the nurse decides what to do with the washbasin and bedpan.

C. Nursing Assistant Challenge

Mrs. Leon is being admitted because her emphysema is making it very difficult for her to breathe. She is accompanied by her husband, and both are obviously nervous. The next morning, her condition worsens. She is moved to the intensive respiratory care unit. Answer the following questions yes or no.

22. _____ The anxiety of the patient and family is not natural.

23. _____ You should answer questions about facility routines during admission to your unit.

24. _____ When Mrs. Leon is transferred to the intensive respiratory care unit, take all of her personal articles with her.

25. _____ You should turn Mrs. Leon's oxygen up to at least 6 liters to assist with her breathing.

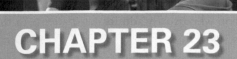

OBJECTIVES

After completing this chapter, you will be able to:

23.1 Spell and define terms.

23.2 List the different types of beds and their uses.

23.3 Describe how to operate each type of bed.

23.4 Explain how to properly handle clean and soiled linens.

23.5 Demonstrate the following procedures:
- Procedure 49: Making a Closed Bed (Expand Your Skills)
- Procedure 50: Making an Occupied Bed

VOCABULARY

Learn the meaning and the correct spelling of the following words and phrases:

box (square) corner	electric bed	low bed	open bed
closed bed	gatch bed	mitered corner	toe pleat

INTRODUCTION

The room, especially the bed, is the patient's home while they are in the health care facility. A well-made bed offers both comfort and safety. It is an extremely important contribution to the well-being of the patient.

OPERATION AND USES OF BEDS IN HEALTH CARE FACILITIES

The types of beds and the methods used to operate them may vary in different health care facilities, but the basic principles of bedmaking are the same. The most common beds are the:

- **Gatch bed**—a hospital bed in which the head, foot, and bed height are adjusted with manual crank handles at the foot of the bed (Figure 23-1). Hospitals have eliminated these beds. Some long-term care facilities continue to use them, and they are in the homes of many persons receiving home care. Refer to Chapter 14 for additional information.
- **Electric bed**—a bed similar to the gatch bed, in that the height can be raised or lowered and the knee and head areas can be adjusted. However, it is operated electrically (Figure 23-2). You will be using this bed most often.
- **Low bed**—a bed commonly used for persons who are at risk of falls, for whom use of side rails is not desirable. The bed frame is four to six inches from the floor to the top of the frame deck. These beds reduce the risk of injury if the patient falls from the bed. Some facilities place pads on the floor next to the bed to further reduce the risk of injury (Figure 23-3).

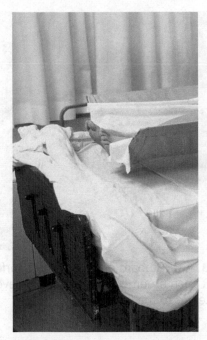

FIGURE 23-1 A gatch bed is operated manually by turning a handle at the foot of the bed. The bed cannot be moved independently by the patient.

Working with Low Beds

Low beds are wonderful tools for reducing patient injuries, but the nursing assistant must use good body mechanics and common sense to prevent back injuries when lifting, moving, and caring for patients, and when making beds. Some low beds have high–low features, but many are stationary, which increases

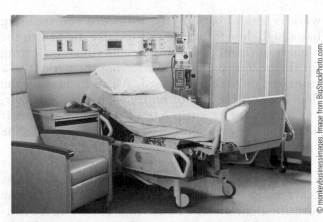

FIGURE 23-2 This is an example of a common hospital bed.

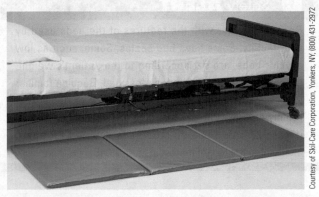

FIGURE 23-3 Low beds are often used for patients who are at high risk for falls.

GUIDELINES 23-1 Guidelines for Low Beds

- Caring for and making the low bed is very similar to making a regular hospital bed. However, certain adaptations must be made to reduce your risk of injury. You should:
  - Mentally plan and prepare yourself for the procedure.
  - Organize your work well to reduce the total number of motions required to complete the task.
  - Make sure you have everything you need before entering the room.
  - Elevate the bed, if possible.
  - Place linens and other needed items on a chair or within close reach in order of use.
  - Use good body mechanics.
  - Maintain a neutral posture and bend from the hip joints and legs, not the waist. Avoid twisting.

- You may squat, sit, or kneel on the plastic mat next to the bed if doing so is easier for you and helps keep your spine straight. Feel free to cover the area you kneel on with an underpad or sheet. Discard it when you have finished.

- Slowly remove the bed linens several pieces at a time. Avoid trying to remove all the linen in one bundle. The weight of the linen and how it affects your posture and increases the risk of back injury.

- Make one side of the bed at a time. This is faster, is more efficient, and conserves energy.

- Use a fitted bottom sheet to reduce the number of movements necessary for making the bed, thereby lowering the risk of back strain.

workers' risk of back injury. If the bed you are using has a high–low feature, use it to raise the bed to the highest horizontal working height whenever caring for the bedfast patient, transferring the patient to a stretcher, or making the bed. A pad or mat on the floor reduces the risk of injury when a patient falls, but it can also be a trip hazard. Fold it and store it under the bed or according to facility policy when the patient is out of bed.

Move slowly and carefully when working near a floor mat. Avoid entering the room in the dark. Leave a night light or the bathroom light on. You may turn the light on when entering, but try to be considerate of sleeping patients. Do not use the bright exam lights that shine directly over the bed and in a

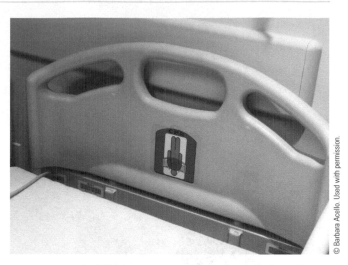

FIGURE 23-4B A CPR board provides a firm surface for doing CPR in an emergency. Some beds have this board fastened to the bed frame.

> ### 🔓 Safety **ALERT**
>
> Become familiar with the features of the beds used by your facility. Some have bed scales. Some, such as low air loss beds, are set according to the patient's weight. CPR is not effective in a low air loss bed. Become familiar with the location of the emergency switch or ribbon that rapidly deflates the air pillows to enable staff to do CPR (Figure 23-4A). Some electric beds have a CPR board attached to the foot of the bed (Figure 23-4B).

patient's face. Squat or kneel on the floor mat when caring for the patient to reduce back strain caused by bending at the waist. To prevent back injuries, use good body mechanics, a transfer belt, or a ceiling or mechanical lift when assisting patients into and out of low beds. The care plan will provide patient-specific instructions. Avoid bending at the waist when moving the patient.

Specialty Beds

Other types of beds are available for the treatment of patients with multiple or advanced pressure ulcers, flaps, grafts, burns, and intractable pain. Low air loss beds are commonly used for persons who have serious skin conditions. Special respiratory beds are available to turn

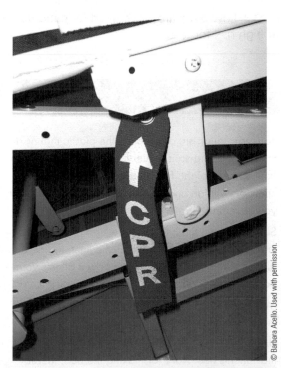

FIGURE 23-4A Become familiar with the location of the CPR ribbon on the low air loss beds used in the facility.

> ### ⚠ OSHA **ALERT**
>
> Elevating the bed to a working height that is comfortable for you takes a minute, but it is one of the most important things you can do to protect your back. Stay on one side of the bed until it is completely made before moving to the other side. This helps organize your time and conserves energy. Avoid moving quickly. Studies have shown that rapid motion increases the risk of injury. To reduce stress on your lower back, remove soiled linens a few pieces at a time, rather than in a large bundle all at once. Keep your spine straight and use good body mechanics. Make beds with a partner, if possible.

GUIDELINES 23-2 Guidelines for Handling Linens and Making the Bed

Handling Linens

1. Wash hands and use gloves if necessary; other personal protective equipment may also be required.

2. Laundry hampers should be separated from clean linen carts in the hallway by at least one room.

3. Keep the clean linen cart covered; replace the cover after removing required linens.

4. Take only the linens you need into the patient's room. Some facilities require staff to place clean linens in plastic bags as soon as they remove them from the linen cart. The bags are used for transporting the linens to the patient's room, and then used for removing soiled linens from the room.

5. Never return unused linens to the clean linen cart. Once they have been removed and carried into a room, they are contaminated. If they are not used, place them in the soiled laundry hamper.

6. Place linens that touch the floor in the laundry hamper; these are considered dirty and must not be used.

7. Avoid contact between the linens and your uniform (for both clean and soiled linens).

8. When removing soiled linens from the bed, fold or roll the linens toward the center to keep the soiled areas on the inside.

9. Never shake bed linens, because microbes will be released into the air.

10. Never place soiled linens on environmental surfaces in the room, such as the overbed table, chair, or floor.

11. Fill laundry hampers no more than two-thirds full. Keep the lid of the hamper on tightly at all times, except when depositing items.

12. Some facilities place small laundry hampers in patient rooms for use with biohazardous linens. Others do not permit laundry hampers or barrels to be taken into patient rooms. Soiled linens may be placed in a plastic bag or a pillowcase in the room.

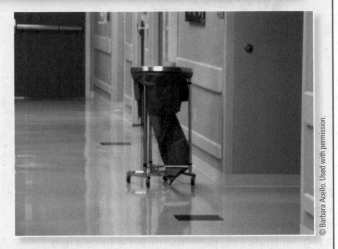

FIGURE 23-5 Most facilities place soiled linens in hampers in the hallway.

Make a cuff at the top of the bag or open end of the pillowcase and place the cuff over the back of a chair. When the bag or case is two-thirds full, secure the top and place it in the hamper in the hallway (Figure 23-5).

13. Return laundry hampers or barrels to the utility room or other holding area after use, or as directed by facility policy.

Making the Bed

1. Use proper body mechanics at all times to prevent back injury.

2. Work on one side of the bed at a time to complete removal of soiled linens and placement of clean linens.

3. Make sure the bottom sheet and draw sheet (if used) are smooth and unwrinkled (wrinkles in bed linens can lead to discomfort and skin breakdown, especially for patients who must remain in bed).

4. Follow the care plan for positioning the head and foot of the bed, the number of pillows to be used, and the use of pillows for positioning.

persons with lung problems. Bariatric beds are used for persons with obesity (Chapter 31).

A low air loss bed (Figure 23-6) provides pressure relief for patients with serious skin problems. This type of mattress is designed to keep the patient cooler and drier than other types of beds. Low air loss beds reduce pressure on the skin, and reduce friction and shearing, which contribute to skin breakdown. These beds use a system of air-filled pillows in which inflation pressure can be adjusted so the characteristics

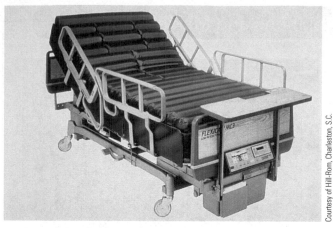

FIGURE 23-6 The low-air-loss bed is used for pressure ulcer prevention and treatment. Although these specialty beds exert less pressure on the skin than a regular mattress, patients must be turned and repositioned frequently to prevent skin breakdown.

 Safety **ALERT**

Incidences of serious injury and death have occurred when a patient's neck or other body parts became trapped between the mattress and side rails. The risk of injury is especially high when inflatable mattresses and low air loss beds are used, because these mattresses are easily compressed. Monitor patients carefully. Remember that gaps can be created by movement, compression of the mattress, and other factors such as the patient's weight and position.

of the support surface are matched to those of the body being supported. The pillows can be inflated and deflated to adjust the level of pressure relief. The design of the bed allows slight air escape upon movement, which reduces pressure.

 Safety **ALERT**

Be alert when removing bed linens. Look carefully for items that are a potential source of injury to yourself or the patient, such as lancets and needles. Make sure the patient's personal items are not accidentally sent to the laundry with the bed linens. It is not unusual to find a patient's glasses, hearing aids, or dentures in the bed linens. These items are expensive and will not survive a trip through the washer and dryer.

Patients using a low air loss or other pressure-relieving bed must still be turned and positioned regularly to prevent skin breakdown, which can occur despite the pressure-reducing mattress. Avoid tucking the bottom sheet in tightly, as this increases pressure within the bed. Some facilities use these beds with special nylon covers only, without sheets. The synthetic cover reduces friction and shearing. These covers are similar to fitted bottom sheets, but they are thicker. They require special handling and air-drying in the laundry, so your facility will have several for each bed. Check to make sure that an extra cover is available before routinely changing the bed. Follow the care plan and facility policies.

Special paper bed protectors are used with the low air loss bed. The air cannot flow through the thick cloth soaker pads (reusable bed protectors) used in most facilities.

Correct operation of any bed or equipment is important for patient safety. Always seek help and instruction from the nurse when using any specialized bed. Never try to operate any bed or other equipment with a patient in it without first practicing and gaining security and skill in the procedures. Although different types of hospital beds may be similar in design, the operating instructions vary. For safety, always follow the manufacturer's directions.

GUIDELINES 23-3 Guidelines for Low Air Loss Beds

- Check the mattress, side rails, and bed frame daily for potential areas of entrapment.

- Remember that the patient's weight, movement, or position can cause gaps and compress the mattress, increasing the risk for entrapment of body parts.

- Make sure the side rails fit correctly, do not move back and forth when pulled, and are the correct distance from the head and foot of the bed.

- Ensure that the size of the bed comfortably accommodates the patient's body size, height, and weight.

- Be sure that the bed is not over- or underinflated.

- Use adjunctive devices to keep patients safe, such as bed bolsters, guards, and pads. Position these devices to eliminate gaps between the rails and mattress.

BEDMAKING

Change bed linens promptly when soiled. Routinely change bed linens:

- Daily in the acute care facility.
- Two or three times a week (usually on shower days) and when soiled in long-term care facilities.

Residents in long-term care facilities may prefer to use their own pillows, blankets, and spreads.

Supplies for Bedmaking

You will need to gather supplies before making a bed. The supplies will vary slightly, depending on your facility's policies and the type of bedmaking procedure you will be using. Gather and stack linens in the order of use, so that the item used first is on top and the item used last is on the bottom. Bring only needed linens to the room. If linens are not used, they must be washed before they are returned to the unit's linen supply for use by another patient.

To do a complete linen change, you will need:

- *Mattress pad*, if used by the facility. A mattress pad is a heavy, quilted cotton pad. Mattress pads may be either flat or fitted to the mattress. A flat pad may have diagonal pieces of elastic across the corners to slip over the mattress to hold the pad in place. The purpose is to protect the mattress from spills, secretions, and excretions. Some facilities do not use mattress pads because the bed mattresses are covered with plastic or rubber, which protects the mattress. However, some patients become very hot and sweat profusely when lying on a plastic mattress that is covered only with a thin sheet. The sheet stays damp, which is uncomfortable for the patient and promotes skin breakdown. If heat and sweating are a problem for a patient, you can cover the mattress with one or two folded cotton bath blankets, and then apply the sheet.
- *Two sheets*. In some facilities, two large flat sheets are used to make each bed. Many facilities use a flat sheet on top and a fitted sheet on bottom. The fitted sheet makes it easier to make the bed, and the bottom sheet does not slip or wrinkle as much with patient movement. If you must use a flat sheet to cover the mattress, make sure to tuck it in tightly. Check the sheet frequently for bedfast patients, and straighten or tighten it as often as needed for patient comfort. The top sheet is always a regular twin-bed-size flat sheet.
- *Linen draw sheet*, or half-sheet, if used by the facility. These may also be called *lift sheets* or *turn sheets*. In most facilities, these are used only if the patient must be manually moved by staff.
- *Incontinence pad, underpad, soaker pad*, or *bed protector*. The pads may also be called by their brand name,

such as Chux or Depends. These items are soft, highly absorbent paper and plastic or heavy cloth pads. They are usually large (about 30 to 36 inches square). Bed protectors are used in the care of patients who are incontinent, use the bedpan or urinal when in bed, or have heavy drainage from a wound or surgical site. The reusable cotton pads are sometimes used in place of a lifting sheet. This practice is not permitted in some facilities due to the risk of injury.* Follow your facility's policy. The paper bed protectors are not suitable for moving patients. If the pad becomes wet or soiled, the pad is the only item that must be changed, which is easier for the patient, more efficient for staff, and more economical for the facility.

- *Pillow and pillowcase*. Hospitals use various types of pillows. Many are disposable, and are sent home with the patient or discarded. Some are reusable. Reusable pillows are usually covered with a plastic pillow protector. The pillow is always covered with a cloth pillowcase. Patients who require special positioning will need several pillows to prop and support various areas of the body for alignment and comfort.
- *Bath blanket*. A bath blanket is a soft flannel or cotton blanket that is used for modesty and warmth during procedures in which the patient's body is exposed. It is usually folded and stored in the closet or bedside stand when not in use.
- *Regular blanket*. A thermal cotton blanket is applied to the bed for patient comfort and warmth.
- *Bedspread*. A bedspread may be used for a decorative touch and to give the room a neat appearance.

Some facilities use other special items, such as foam mattress overlays and pressure-reducing pads or mattresses, which reduce friction and shearing and provide extra padding to decrease the risk of skin breakdown. These are issued only to patients who are at high risk of skin breakdown. Many foam pads lose their fire-retardant protection if they are washed and dried, so facilities use bed protectors to protect them. They are usually covered with a flat linen sheet. Each layer reduces the protective properties of the overlay. The mattress is covered with a separate sheet.

Occasionally, facilities use other items, such as bed boards, to meet special patient needs. Bed boards are placed between the mattress and bed frame to offer extra-firm support to the patient's back. These are more common in home care. Bed cradles (see Chapter 15) may be used to keep the weight of the linen off the patient's skin. A footboard (see Chapter 15) may also be applied to the foot of the bed for patients who have special positioning needs or are at risk for contractures.

Soaker Pads Are Not Repositioning Aids. Retrieved October 13, 2019, from https://www.worksafenb.ca/hazard-alerts/en/soaker-pads-are-not-repositioning-aids.html

Clinical Information **ALERT**

Some people associate bedbugs with unsanitary living conditions. However, bedbugs have been found in very clean hospitals and hotels. The bugs adapt well to any environment where they can obtain a blood meal. They can live up to a year without eating. Watch for signs of bedbugs, such as small red or black dots on the bed linens and clothing, egg cases, and tiny shed skins. Look in cracks and crevices near the mattress and bed frame. Pay close attention to the area under the mattress seams. Bedbugs can also hide behind headboards and behind the molding or baseboard of the walls. Although they tend to live around beds, they may also hide in furniture, such as sofas and upholstered chairs.

Closed Bed

The **closed bed** is made following discharge of a patient and after the unit is cleaned (terminal cleaning). It remains closed until a new patient is admitted. Details are important. Follow the same procedure when making an unoccupied bed, but open the bed at the end of the procedure, immediately before the patient is ready to occupy it. (Refer to Procedures 49 and 50.)

The Unoccupied Bed

Beds are often made while patients are up in a shower or chair. Follow the procedure for making a closed bed but then fan-fold the top bedding three-fourths of the way down. This "opens" the bed and makes it easier for the person to get into it.

EXPAND YOUR SKILLS

PROCEDURE **49**   MAKING A CLOSED BED

NOTE

This procedure describes both the mitered corner and the square corner, which are very similar. Your instructor will advise you as to which method to use. Follow your facility's policies for making beds.

1. Wash your hands and assemble equipment:
- 2 pillowcases
- Pillow
- Spread
- Blankets, as needed
- 2 large sheets (90" × 108") (substitute one fitted sheet, if used)
- Cotton draw sheet or half-sheet (if used)
- Mattress pad and cover, if used

NOTE

A cotton half-sheet (draw sheet) is not necessary unless it is used for moving or turning the patient. Most facilities use fitted bottom sheets. In this case, use a fitted sheet in place of one of the large sheets.

2. Elevate the bed to a comfortable working height in the horizontal position. Lock the wheels so the bed will not roll. Place a chair at the side of the bed.

3. Arrange the linens on the chair in the order in which they are to be used.

4. Grasp the mattress handles (or the edge of the mattress, if no handles are present) and position the mattress to the head of the bed.

5. If used, place a mattress cover on the mattress. Adjust it so that it is smooth. You will work entirely from one side of the bed until that side is completed. Then go to the other side of the bed. This conserves time and energy.

6. Place the mattress pad even with the top of the mattress and unfold it.

7. Place the bottom sheet on the bed and unfold it, seam side down and wide hem at the top. Position the small hem at the foot of the mattress (Figure 23-7A). The

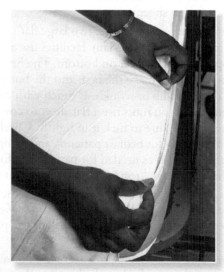

FIGURE 23-7A Place the flat bottom sheet even with the end of the mattress at the foot of the bed.

(continues)

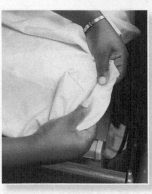
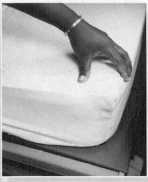

FIGURE 23-7B If a fitted bottom sheet is used, pull and smooth it around the corner.

center fold should be at the center of the bed. If a fitted bottom sheet is used, fit it smoothly around one corner (Figure 23-7B).

8. Tuck 12 to 18 inches of sheet smoothly over the top of the mattress (Figures 23-8A to C).

9. Make a **mitered corner** (Figure 23-9). The square corner, preferred by some facilities, is made in a way similar to the mitered corner. Mitered and square corners are commonly called *hospital corners*.

10. Tuck in the sheet on one side, keeping the sheet straight. Work from the head to the foot of the bed. If using a fitted sheet, adjust it over the head and bottom ends of the mattress.

11. Place the draw sheet (if used) with upper edge about 14 inches from the head of the mattress and tuck under one side (Figure 23-10). This sheet should cover the area from above the patient's lower shoulders to the mid-thigh. The extra space reduces the risk of pressure ulcers. The extra space is maintained on both sides.

12. Unfold and place the top sheet on the bed, seam up, top hem even with the upper edge of the mattress and the center fold in the center of the bed.

13. Spread the blanket over the top sheet and foot of the mattress. Keep the blanket centered (Figure 23-11).

14. Make a **toe pleat** by folding the top sheet over two to three inches at the end of the bed (Figure 23-12). The toe pleat provides extra space and keeps the sheet from pulling the feet downward. This is more comfortable for the patient and reduces the risk of contractures.

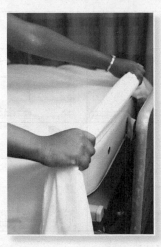

FIGURE 23-8A Gather about 12 to 18 inches of the top sheet at the bottom of the bed.

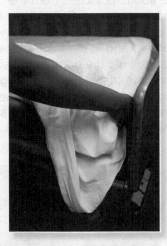

FIGURE 23-8B Face the foot of the bed and lift the mattress with your near hand.

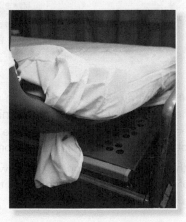

FIGURE 23-8C Bring the sheet smoothly over the end of the mattress with your opposite hand.

(continues)

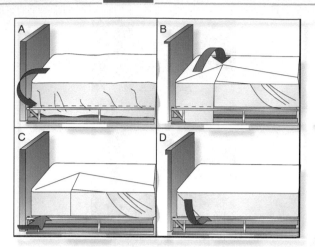

FIGURE 23-9 Making a mitered corner. A. The sheet is hanging loose at the side of the bed. B. Pick up the sheet about 12 inches from the head of the bed to form a triangle. C. Tuck the sheet in at the head of the bed. Pick up the triangle and place your other hand at the edge of the bed near the head to hold the edge of the sheet in place. D. Bring the triangle over the edge of the mattress and tuck it smoothly under the mattress. Tuck in the rest of the sheet along the side of the mattress. Make sure the sheet is wrinkle-free.

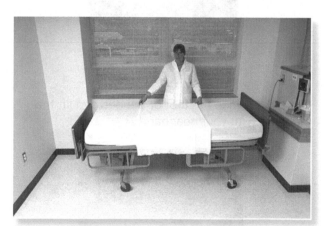

FIGURE 23-10 The draw sheet is placed on top of the bottom sheet and may be used as a turning sheet.

15. Tuck the top sheet and blanket under the mattress at the foot of the bed as far as the center only.

16. Place the spread with its top hem even with the head of the mattress. Unfold the spread to the foot of the bed.

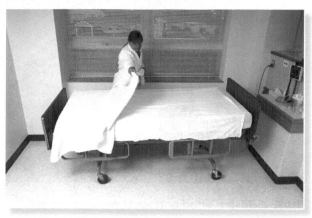

FIGURE 23-11 Place the blanket and spread over the top sheet.

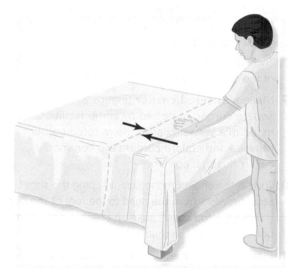

FIGURE 23-12 The toe pleat provides space for movement of the feet. For bedfast patients, the extra space reduces the risk of contractures and pressure ulcers. The extra space is much more comfortable for all patients.

17. Tuck the spread under the mattress at the foot of the bed and make a **box (square) corner** (Figures 23-13A to 23-13E). Sometimes the spread may be placed directly on top of the sheet. Rather than tucking the sheet, blanket, and/or spread under the end of the mattress separately and forming separate corners, tuck all of the covers under the mattress at the same time and form one corner.

18. Go to the other side of the bed. Fan-fold the top covers to the center of the bed so you can work with the lower sheets and pad.

(continues)

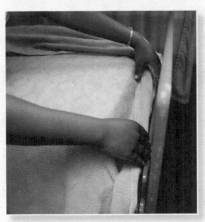

FIGURE 23-13A Gather the top sheet and bedspread together. Smooth evenly over the end of the mattress.

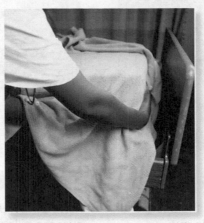

FIGURE 23-13B Tuck the sheet and spread under the mattress together.

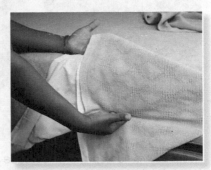

FIGURE 23-13C Continue as with the procedure for a mitered corner.

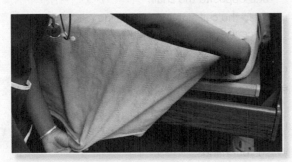

FIGURE 23-13D Slide your finger to the end to make a smooth edge.

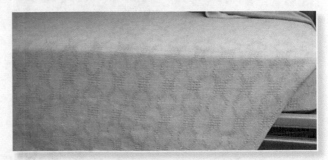

FIGURE 23-13E The completed top bedding. Repeat the procedure on the other side of the bed.

19. Tuck the bottom sheet under the head of the mattress and miter the corner. Working from top to bottom, smooth out all wrinkles and tighten these sheets as much as possible to provide comfort. (Adjust a fitted bottom sheet smoothly and securely around the mattress corners.)

20. Grasp the draw sheet (if used) and tuck it tightly under the mattress.

21. Tuck in the top sheet, blanket, and spread at the foot of the bed and make a square corner.

22. Fold the top sheet back over the blanket, making an eight-inch cuff.

23. Bring the top of the spread to the head of the mattress and cover the sheet and blanket.

24. Insert the pillow into a pillowcase:

    a. Place your hands in the clean case, freeing the corners.

    b. Grasp the center of the end seam with a hand outside the case and turn the case back over your hand (Figure 23-14A).

    c. Grasp the pillow through the case at the center of one end. Pull the case over the pillow with your free hand (Figures 23-14B and 23-14C). (Do not allow the pillow to touch your uniform.)

    d. Adjust the corners of the pillow to fit in the corners of the case.

25. Place the pillow at the head of the bed with the open end away from the door.

26. Lower the bed to the lowest horizontal position.

27. Arrange the room as follows:

    a. Replace the bedside table parallel to the bed. Place the chair in its assigned location.

(continues)

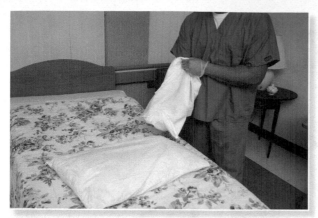

FIGURE 23-14A Grasp the pillowcase at the seam and fold it back and over your wrist, inside out.

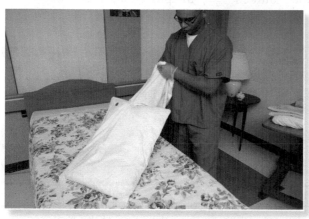

FIGURE 23-14B Grab the end of the pillow in the center with your pillowcase-covered hand.

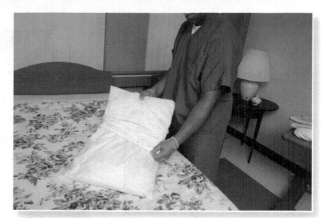

FIGURE 23-14C Unfold and smooth the pillowcase over the pillow.

b. Place the overbed table over the foot of the bed opposite the chair.

c. Snap the call signal into the side rail, or place the signal cord within easy reach of the patient.

d. Leave the side rails down.

e. Check for possible hazards and items that are out of place.

28. Leave the unit neat and tidy.

29. Wash your hands.

30. Report completion of the task to the nurse.

ICON KEY:

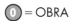 = OBRA   = PPE

 Clinical Information **ALERT**

Wear gloves when removing bed linens that are wet or soiled. Place the soiled linens in a plastic bag or linen hamper. Avoid contaminating environmental surfaces with gloves that have handled soiled linens. Remove one glove, if necessary. Follow facility policy for disinfecting the mattress. Allow it to dry. Discard your gloves and wash your hands. It is not necessary to wear gloves when you are handling clean linens. Cracks in the mattress are a potential source of odors and contamination. Report cracks in the mattress to the proper person in your facility.

The Open Bed

An **open bed** is like a sign saying "welcome" to a new patient. It indicates that the nursing assistant has prepared the unit for the patient's arrival. Residents in long-term care facilities are not sick, and are out of bed most of the day. Do not open the bed unless the resident will be going to bed soon.

The Occupied Bed

Unless the patient is permitted out of bed by physician's order, the bed is made with the patient in it (see Procedure 50). Bedmaking usually follows the bed bath, while the patient is covered with a bath blanket. It may, however, be done anytime it would add to the comfort of the patient.

Safety **ALERT**

Never turn your back on the patient or leave the bedside when the bed is in the high position and the side rails are down.

The Surgical Bed

The surgical bed provides a safe, warm environment to receive the postsurgical patient. It must be made in such a way that movement from stretcher to bed can be done with maximum safety and minimum effort. For this reason, the bed should be left open and at stretcher height.

All equipment needed to monitor vital signs and to supervise recovery should be in place and ready for use.

You should also keep alert for the patient's return so you can help make a safe transfer from stretcher to bed.

Modern surgical techniques have shortened the time many patients stay in an acute care facility after surgery. Patients are often admitted on the morning of surgery to special units, have the surgery performed, return to these same units immediately after surgery, and are discharged the same day to recuperate at home. These units are called *ambulatory, short-term,* or *day surgery units.* To prepare a postsurgical bed in one of these units:

- Tighten the bottom linen.
- Fan-fold the top linen to the side of the bed.
- Raise the bed to stretcher height and lock the wheels.
- Place the equipment to check vital signs and emesis basin by the recovery bed, according to facility policy. Bring a small box of tissues to the room in case they are needed to manage post operative secretions.

 PROCEDURE 50 MAKING AN OCCUPIED BED

1. Carry out initial procedure actions.

2. Assemble the equipment needed:
   – Disposable gloves (if linens are soiled with blood, body fluids, secretions, or excretions, or if this is your facility policy)
   – Cotton draw sheet or turning sheet for selected patients
   – 2 large flat sheets (or one large flat sheet and one fitted bottom sheet)
   – 2 pillowcases
   – Laundry hamper or plastic bag

3. Place the bedside chair at the foot of the bed.

4. Arrange the clean linens on the chair in the order in which they are to be used.

5. The bed should be flat, with the wheels locked, unless otherwise indicated. Raise the bed to a comfortable horizontal working height. Lower the side rails on your side of the bed.

6. If the bed linens are soiled with blood or other body fluids or if this is your facility's policy, wash your hands and put on disposable gloves.

7. Loosen the bedclothes on your side by lifting the edge of the mattress with one hand and drawing the bedclothes out with the other. Never shake the linens. This spreads germs.

8. Put the side rails up and go to the opposite side of the bed.

9. Remove the top covers except for the top sheet, one at a time.

 NOTE

Carefully look for and remove foreign articles (such as patient care equipment, eyeglasses, dentures, items of food, or eating utensils).

10. Place the clean sheet or bath blanket over the top sheet. Have the patient hold the top edge of the clean sheet if able. If the patient is unable to help, tuck the sheet beneath the patient's shoulder.

11. Slide the soiled top sheet out, from top to bottom. Put it in a hamper or plastic bag.

12. Ask the patient to move to the side of the bed toward you. Assist if necessary. Move one pillow with the patient and remove the other pillow. Pull up the side rail. (Alternatively, you may ask the patient to turn toward the opposite side of the bed, holding onto the raised side rail.)

13. Go to the other side of the bed. Fan-fold or roll the soiled draw sheet (if used), and bottom sheet close to the patient (Figure 23-15).

14. Straighten the mattress pad (if used). Place a clean sheet on the bed so that the narrow hem comes to the edge of the mattress at the foot. The seamed side of the hem is toward the bed. The lengthwise center fold of the sheet is at the center of the bed. Fan-fold or roll the opposite side of the sheet close to the patient (Figure 23-16).

(continues)

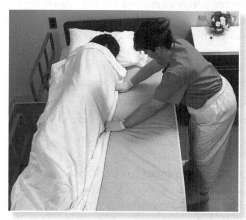

FIGURE 23-15 Fan-fold the bottom linens to the center of the bed, as close to the patient as possible. Change gloves before handling clean linen.

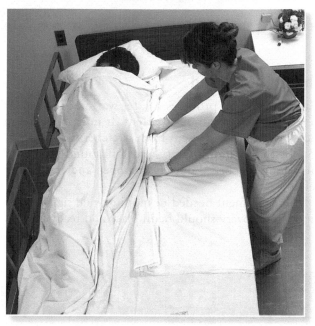

FIGURE 23-17 Fan-fold or roll the clean draw sheet and tuck it under the soiled linens.

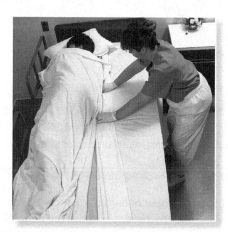

FIGURE 23-16 Fan-fold or roll the clean bottom sheet and tuck it under the soiled linens.

15. Tuck the top of the sheet under the head of the mattress.

16. Make a mitered corner.

17. Tuck the side of the sheet under the mattress, working toward the foot of the bed.

18. Position a fresh draw sheet, if used. Tuck it under the mattress (Figure 23-17).

19. Ask or assist the patient to roll toward you, over the linen in the center of the bed. Move the pillow with the patient.

20. Raise the side rail. Test for security.

21. Go to the other side of the bed. Lower the side rail. Remove the soiled linens by rolling the edges inward. *Keep soiled linens away from your uniform.* Placed soiled linens in the hamper or plastic bag. (Raise the side rails if leaving the bedside.)

22. Remove and discard gloves. Apply clean gloves, if necessary. Do not handle clean linens with soiled gloves.

23. Pull the clean bottom sheet into place. Tuck it under the mattress at the head of the bed. Make a mitered corner.

24. Pull gently to eliminate wrinkles. Then tuck the side of the sheet under the mattress, working from top to bottom.

25. Pull the draw sheet smoothly into place. Tuck it firmly under the mattress (Figure 23-18).

26. Place the top sheet over the patient. Remove the bath blanket underneath.

(continues)

PROCEDURE **50** CONTINUED

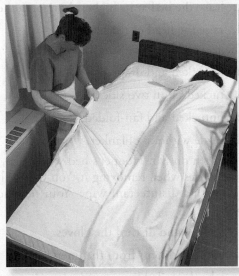

FIGURE 23-18 Unfold or unroll the bottom sheet and draw sheet. Grasp each piece and pull tightly. Tuck them in.

ICON KEY:
 **O** = OBRA   **P** = PPE

27. Complete the bed as an unoccupied bed. To reduce pressure on toes, make a toe pleat or grasp the top bedding over the toes and pull straight up. Some patients prefer not to have the blanket and top sheet or spread tucked in.

28. Assist the patient to turn onto their back. Place a clean pillowcase on the pillow that is not being used. Replace that pillow. Change the other pillowcase.

29. Carry out ending procedure actions.

REVIEW

A. True/False

Mark the following true or false by circling T or F.

1. T F   The patient is most comfortable in a closed bed.

2. T F   The low bed is used to avoid patient injury from falls.

3. T F   You should not attempt to operate a bed until you have had supervised practice and are approved to use it.

4. T F   The closed bed is made after terminal cleaning is finished.

5. T F   Bottom bed linens can be loosely tucked as long as there are no wrinkles when you have finished.

6. T F   A mitered corner is tucked in, forming a triangle.

7. T F   Shaking linens as you change the bed spreads germs.

8. T F   The open bed is like a sign saying "welcome."

9. T F   Before making an occupied bed, adjust the mattress to the head of the bed.

10. T F   The side rails opposite you must be up as you make an occupied bed.

B. Multiple Choice

Select the best answer for each of the following.

11. When removing soiled linens from the bed, you should:

    a. remove a piece at a time.

    b. roll the soiled linens inward.

    c. place them on the table or chair.

    d. pile them in the corner of the room.

12. When making an unoccupied bed:

    a. make the bottom, then the top.

    b. begin at the foot and work upward.

    c. make one entire side at a time.

    d. move back and forth from side to side.

13. Before making an unoccupied bed:
    a. elevate it to a comfortable working height.
    b. position the bed at the lowest horizontal height.
    c. raise the head of the bed.
    d. raise the side rails on the opposite side.

14. When collecting supplies to make the bed:
    a. cover clean linens with a pillowcase.
    b. carry clean linens close to your body.
    c. wear gloves when handling linens.
    d. stack the linens in order of use.

15. Sheets should be smoothly tucked in over the head of the mattress:
    a. 5 to 7 inches.
    b. 12 to 18 inches.
    c. 20 to 24 inches.
    d. 26 to 30 inches.

16. If a draw sheet or lift sheet is used, it should be placed so that it covers the area under the patient's:
    a. head and shoulders.
    b. heels and lower legs.
    c. buttocks only.
    d. shoulders to buttocks.

17. When placing the case on the pillow:
    a. tuck it under your chin.
    b. lay the pillow on the chair.
    c. pull the case over while grasping the pillow with the opposite hand.
    d. lay the pillow on the bedside stand.

18. When opening a closed bed:
    a. fan-fold top bedding to the foot.
    b. loosen all top bedding.
    c. leave the bed at its highest horizontal height.
    d. raise the head of the bed.

19. The top bedding on a surgical bed is:
    a. untucked and draped.
    b. tucked in on two sides.
    c. untucked and fan-folded.
    d. made without a blanket.

20. The linen on Mr. Hooper's bed was soiled, so you wore gloves when removing it. You wiped the mattress with a disinfectant wipe. Your next action is to:
    a. remove and discard the gloves.
    b. get clean linens from the linen cart.
    c. take the soiled linens to the laundry.
    d. begin putting clean linens on the bed.

C. Nursing Assistant Challenge

21. You are assigned to make a closed bed. You have washed your hands and assembled the following equipment: pillow, blanket, spread, and mattress pad. What else will you need?

    _____

    _____

    _____

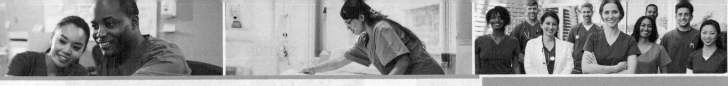

Patient Bathing

CHAPTER 24

OBJECTIVES

After completing this chapter, you will be able to:

24.1 Spell and define terms.

24.2 Describe the safety precautions for patient bathing.

24.3 List the purposes of bathing patients.

24.4 State the value of whirlpool baths.

24.5 Demonstrate the following procedures:
- Procedure 51: Assisting with the Tub Bath or Shower
- Procedure 52: Bed Bath
- Procedure 53: Changing the Patient's Gown

- Procedure 54: Waterless Bed Bath
- Procedure 55: Partial Bath (Expand Your Skills)
- Procedure 56: Female Perineal Care
- Procedure 57: Male Perineal Care
- Procedure 58: Hand and Fingernail Care
- Procedure 59: Foot and Toenail Care
- Procedure 60: Bed Shampoo (Expand Your Skills)
- Procedure 61: Dressing and Undressing the Patient

VOCABULARY

Learn the meaning and the correct spelling of the following words and phrases:

axilla	genitalia	perineum
bag bath	perineal care (peri care)	waterless bathing

INTRODUCTION

A daily bath is as important for the patient as it is for you. Some people become withdrawn and others are upset because they fear that they smell if they do not have a daily bath. They may not verbalize it, but they avoid contact with others. Following the bath, the patient feels relaxed, clean, and refreshed. A bath with warm water and mild soap:

- Removes dirt and perspiration
- Increases circulation
- Provides the patient with mild exercise
- Provides an opportunity for close observation

You as the caregiver are able to see firsthand how the patient's condition is improving, declining, or changing in any way. Your observations are valuable aids to accurate nursing assessments.

With the physician's permission, the patient may be allowed to take regular tub baths or showers. Some patients will be bathed in bed. Bathing may be performed as:

- A tub bath
- A shower bath
- A complete bed bath
- A partial bed bath
- A self-sponge bath or waterless bath
- A whirlpool bath
- Perineal care

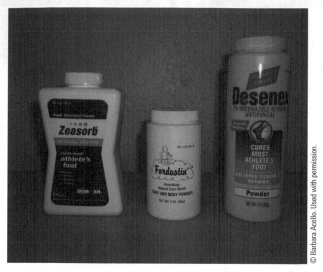

© Barbara Acello. Used with permission.

FIGURE 24-1 Some facilities stock Fordustin (Sween powder), a corn starch powder. Others issue antifungal powders such as Desenex in the admission kits for bariatric patients. Remember that yeast thrives in warm, moist, dark areas such as skin folds.

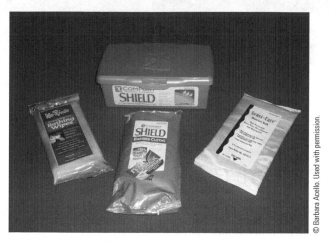

© Barbara Acello. Used with permission.

FIGURE 24-2 Waterless bathing is comfortable, convenient, and more economical than other methods of bathing because it saves time. These products contain a no-rinse cleanser and do not contain soap, so they are gentle on the skin. Comfort Shield is used only for peri care and contains a silicone barrier to protect the skin. Use these items once and then discard them in the trash. They are not flushable.

During bathing, special attention should be given to skin areas that touch each other, including:

- Between the legs
- Under the arms
- Under the breasts
- Under the scrotum
- Between the buttocks
- Around the anus
- For people who are obese, under folds of skin

Gently sponge and pat these areas dry. The skin is often fragile and may tear easily, especially in persons who are obese and elderly. Follow facility policy for the use of talcum powder or corn starch. Some facilities provide absorbent corn starch–based powders or antifungal powders such as Desenex (miconazole 2%) in the admission kit (Figure 24-1).

A partial bath cleans the hands, face, back, axillae, buttocks, and genitals. It is very refreshing. Many patients will be able to help with bathing. Whenever possible, encourage patients to do so.

Waterless Bath

Some facilities are taking a new approach to bathing called **waterless bathing**. It may also be called a **bag bath**. The only equipment needed is a package of premoistened disposable washcloths (Figure 24-2). Each package contains washcloths moistened with a special no-rinse cleansing solution that evaporates quickly

so that drying is not necessary. Eight washcloths are supplied so that separate parts of the body (face, arms, legs, torso, and genitalia) can be washed. Smaller kits are available for partial baths and perineal care. The washcloths can be warmed in the microwave or special product warmer. Monitor for hot spots if a microwave is used. Independent patients may also use these for bathing when in bed.

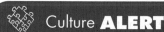

Culture **ALERT**

In the United States, we promote self-care in patient care and treatment. However, in some cultures, family members are expected to care for the patient. Some patients may expect certain people to be involved in their care. They may also feel that certain people are obligated to visit.

The waterless bathing system has several advantages:
- It is faster and more economical for the facility; each bath takes approximately 8 to 10 minutes.
- It is less fatiguing for the patient.
- It conserves moisture, reduces drying, and is gentler to skin than using soaps.
- It creates less friction, because the cloths are softer than regular washcloths and towels, and drying is eliminated.

Infection Control ALERT

Waterless bathing products are designed to be used for one bath. Select a small kit for partial baths and perineal care. The package may be resealed if not all of the cloths are used, but it should be dated and discarded within 48 hours, or according to your facility's infection control guidelines. Avoid flushing used cloths down the toilet. You may want to use a small plastic bag at the bedside for cloth disposal.

The following precautions are used when bathing patients with the waterless bathing system:

- The washcloths may be used at room temperature, but many facilities heat them for comfort.
- Peel the label back or open the package before heating to avoid bursting in the microwave.
- Follow the manufacturer's directions for heating the package. One minute or less is usually sufficient to warm the contents to a comfortable temperature.
- The cloths in the package are for single use only.
- Discard unused cloths within 48 hours of opening the package, or immediately if they are dry.

Whirlpool Bath

The most stimulating form of bathing for patients is a therapeutic bath that is given in a whirlpool tub (Figure 24-3). The whirlpool bath benefits patients because:

- The temperature of the water is regulated to a constant temperature and does not get cold.
- The movement of the water stimulates circulation.
- Warm circulating water is relaxing and invigorating.
- It provides the value of whirlpool activity with cleansing.

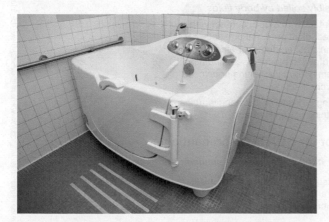

FIGURE 24-3 A whirlpool bath is very relaxing for patients. Today's tubs are ergonomically designed to reduce the risk of nursing assistant injury.

Care of the hair, teeth, and nails usually follows the bath procedure, but may be carried out as independent procedures. Range-of-motion exercises also frequently are done after bathing.

PATIENT BATHING

Follow the guidelines and the procedures for bathing carefully to ensure patient comfort and safety.

Culture ALERT

A patient may prefer to receive personal care from someone of the same sex. Honor these requests, whenever possible, and do not be offended that the request was made. In some cultures, a male cannot even be in the same room with a female unless she is covered from head to foot.

Culture ALERT

Learn ways of showing respect in the patient's culture, such as how to address the patient and how to address privacy concerns, including touching the body or wearing certain articles of clothing. Work on building a relationship of trust with each patient.

Safety Measures for Special Treatments

Patients receiving special treatments include, for example, patients who are receiving an intravenous (IV) transfusion, have drainage tubes, or are receiving oxygen. These patients can be bathed, but they need special care.

As you bathe and move the patient, be careful that you:

- Select the correct gloves (if any) for the procedure (Figure 24-4).
- Do not put stress on any tubes.
- Never lower an IV container below the level of the infusion site.
- Never raise a drainage tube above the drainage site.
- Never raise a catheter bag above the level of the bladder.

Infection Control **ALERT**

Follow your facility's policy for use of gloves. In many facilities, gloves are worn for all patient contact. This is not necessary. When bathing patients, remove the gloves and put on a clean pair immediately before and after contact with mucous membranes and nonintact skin. Do not cross-contaminate body sites by wearing the same pair of gloves for the entire procedure. For example, change gloves immediately after perineal care and anytime the gloves become soiled. Avoid contaminating the environment and clean items with used gloves.

 Safety **ALERT**

Make sure a chair is available next to the tub or shower in case the patient needs to sit quickly. Turn the hot water on last and off first to prevent injury.

The Glove Pyramid – to aid decision making on when to wear (and not wear) gloves

Gloves must be worn according to **STANDARD** and **CONTACT PRECAUTIONS**. The pyramid details some clinical examples in which gloves are not indicated, and others in which examination or sterile gloves are indicated. Hand hygiene should be performed when appropriate regardless of indications for glove use.

STERILE GLOVES INDICATED

Any surgical procedure; vaginal delivery; invasive radiological procedures; performing vascular access and procedures (central lines); preparing total parenteral nutrition and chemotherapeutic agents

EXAMINATION GLOVES INDICATED IN CLINICAL SITUATIONS

Potential for touching blood, secretions, excretions, other body fluids, and items visibly soiled by body fluids

DIRECT PATIENT EXPOSURE: Contact with blood; contact with mucous membrane and with nonintact skin; potential presence of highly infectious and dangerous organisms; epidemic or emergency situations; IV insertion and removal; drawing blood; discontinuation of venous line; pelvic and vaginal examination; suctioning nonclosed systems of endotrcheal tubes

INDIRECT PATIENT EXPOSURE: Emptying emesis basins; handling/cleaning instruments; handling waste; cleaning up spills of body fluids

GLOVES NOT INDICATED (except for CONTACT precautions)

No potential for exposure to blood or other body fluids, or contaminated environment

DIRECT PATIENT EXPOSURE: Taking blood pressure, temperature, and pulse; performing SC and IM injections; bathing and dressing the patient; transporting the patient; caring for eyes and ears (without secretions); any vascular line manipulation in absence of blood leakage

INDIRECT PATIENT EXPOSURE: Using the telephone; writing in the patient's chart; giving oral medications; distributing or collecting patients' dietary trays; removing and replacing linens for the patient's bed; placing noninvasive ventilation equipment and oxygen cannula; moving the patient's furniture

FIGURE 24-4 The glove pyramid provides guidance as to when and when not to wear gloves.

GUIDELINES 24-1 Guidelines for Giving a Whirlpool Bath

- Check with the nurse before giving a whirlpool bath to a patient with an infection, surgical incision, or pressure ulcer.

- Check with the nurse before giving a whirlpool bath if the patient is combative or disoriented. The noise from the whirlpool may worsen agitation.

- Disinfect the whirlpool tub immediately before and after each use.

- The water temperature in the whirlpool tub should not exceed 100°F because the temperature remains constant. (Use common sense; if the water is steaming, it is probably too hot. Check the water temperature with a thermometer.)

- Never leave a patient alone in the whirlpool tub, even for a minute.

- Always fasten the safety belt when moving a patient into or out of a whirlpool tub with a hydraulic lift seat. Keep the safety belt fastened throughout the procedure.

- The patient may be frightened when using the hydraulic lift. Explain the procedure and reassure the patient.

- Drape the patient's genital area with a bath towel for modesty during the whirlpool bath. Provide a dry towel after the bath.

- Use low-suds or no-suds products that are made for whirlpool use.

- Never pour liquid soap or shampoo into the whirlpool tub. A tiny bit of liquid soap will result in an abundance of suds. If you have a suds problem, rub a bar of soap against the walls of the tub to reduce the bubbles.

- The whirlpool activity provides a cleansing action. However, if you will be assisting the patient with bathing, apply the principles of standard precautions.

- Drape a towel over the shoulders when removing the patient from the tub. Wrap the person with a bath blanket for warmth and modesty as soon as they are out of the water.

- The jets in whirlpool tubs have the potential to harbor dangerous pathogens. Follow facility procedures for cleaning and disinfecting the tub. Follow directions and run the disinfectant through the tub for the correct amount of time.

- Raise the lift seat out of the soapy water and rinse it with warm water.

 ## Communication **ALERT**

The right glove for a task may be no glove at all. Touch is a means of communication. People need to be touched. Wearing gloves for all patient contact is offensive. Wear gloves only if you may encounter open lesions, blood, secretions, excretions, or other body fluids. Gloves are not needed for touching intact skin.

 ## Safety **ALERT**

Never leave a patient alone in the tub or shower. Use the call signal in the bathing area if emergency help is needed.

GUIDELINES 24-2 Guidelines for Patient Bathing

- Wear disposable gloves if this is facility policy or there may be contact with open lesions, mucous membranes, secretions, excretions, blood, or other body fluids.

- Make sure the shower or tub is cleaned before and after each use.

- Check that all safety aids, such as shower chairs and tub seats/benches, are in good repair and proper working order.

- Transport patients to and from the tub room and carry out the bathing procedure as efficiently as possible.

(continues)

GUIDELINES 24-2 Guidelines for Patient Bathing (continued)

- Cover the patient's body during transport.
- Do not lock the bathroom door.
- Remain in the room if a patient falls or feels faint during bathing. Use the emergency call signal to summon help.
- Use good body mechanics to protect yourself and the patient.
- Note that the nonskid strips in the tub and shower prevent slipping.
- Note that handrails secured to the walls help prevent falls as the patient transfers into and out of the tub.
- Assist the patient in all transfer activity related to the bath. Be sure to have enough help.
- Note that the shower chair prevents patient stress and fatigue, and reduces the risk of falls. Secure the wheels so the chair does not move during transfers.
- Wipe up all water on the floor immediately.
- Keep the room comfortably warm and free from drafts.

- Cover the patient with towels and cotton bath blankets for warmth and modesty. Avoid exposing the patient's body unnecessarily.
- Drape the patient's genital area with a bath towel during a tub bath or shower. Provide a dry towel after bathing.
- The water should not exceed 105°F. Check the temperature with a bath thermometer.
- Observe the patient's skin for any changes or problems. Report anything unusual.
- Dispense liquid soap into a small cup and carry it to the tub or bedside. Pour the liquid soap onto the washcloth as needed. Do not put it directly into the bath water.
- Label each patient's soap with their name. Use it for that patient only.
- Once a washcloth or towel has been used below the waist, put it in the hamper. Avoid using it above the waist.
- Hang the handheld shower spray on the hook when not in use. Do not let it hang down or touch the floor, which is always considered dirty.

PROCEDURE 51 ASSISTING WITH THE TUB BATH OR SHOWER

1. Carry out initial procedure actions.
2. Assemble equipment:
   - Disposable gloves
   - Liquid soap
   - Washcloth
   - 2–3 bath towels
   - Bath blanket
   - Lotion, if desired
   - Deodorant
   - Chair or stool beside shower or tub or bath or shower chair, as needed
   - Patient's gown, robe, and slippers
   - Bath mat
3. Take the supplies to the bathroom. Clean the tub and prepare the room for the patient.
4. Fill the tub half full of water that does not exceed 105°F or adjust the shower flow. If a bath thermometer is not

available, test the water with your wrist or elbow. It should feel comfortably warm.

5. Help the patient undress and put on a robe and slippers. Escort to the bathroom. Cover the nonambulatory patient when going to or from the bath or shower (Figure 24-5).
6. Help the patient undress.
7. Position a shower chair in the tub or shower, if needed.
8. Cover the bottom of the tub and the shower floor with a nonskid surface for safety. Then assist the patient into the tub or shower.
9. Encourage the patient to wash their body. Assist as needed.
10. Apply the principles of standard precautions if you are assisting.
11. Wash the patient's back. Observe the skin for signs of redness or breaks. (See Chapter 38 for information on observing and caring for skin problems.)

(continues)

PROCEDURE 51 CONTINUED

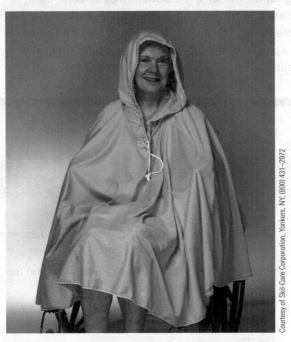

Courtesy of Skil-Care Corporation, Yonkers, NY, (800) 431-2972

FIGURE 24-5 Keep the patient warm and covered when transporting to and from the shower room.

12. The patient may wash the **genitalia** (external reproductive organs), if able.

   - If the patient is unable to wash the genitalia, put on gloves and provide perineal care (peri care).
   - Wash the genitalia last and dispose of the washcloth and towel in the laundry hamper. Change your gloves and get fresh linens if further bathing is needed.

---

13. If the patient shows any signs of weakness:
   - Get help. Use the call signal.
   - Remove the plug and let the water drain.
   - Turn off the shower.
   - Allow the patient to rest until feeling better before attempting to assist the person out of the tub or shower.
   - Keep the patient covered with a bath blanket to avoid chilling.

14. If you will be washing the patient's hair:
   - Ask the patient to hold a dry washcloth over the eyes.
   - Wet the hair.
   - Use a small amount of shampoo to lather hair.
   - Massage scalp gently.
   - Rinse hair with warm water.
   - Repeat lathering, massaging, and rinsing, if necessary.
   - Towel hair dry. You may dry it with a hair dryer after the person is dry and dressed.

15. Hold the bath blanket around the patient as they step out of the tub.

16. Assist the patient to dry off, apply deodorant, and dress.

17. Escort the patient back to their unit. Return personal supplies.

18. Carry out ending procedure actions.

19. Return to the bath or shower room. Put on gloves and clean and disinfect the tub, shower chair, and handrails.

20. Discard soiled bath linens.

21. Wash your hands.

⚖ NOTE

Draping the patient during bathing and personal care procedures is important, even if the room is completely private. Keeping the person covered provides a sense of dignity, reduces feelings of vulnerability, keeps the person warm, and protects modesty and self-esteem.

✚ Clinical Information **ALERT**

Good personal hygiene provides comfort, confidence, and a sense of well-being. Treat your patients with respect and be sensitive to their needs. Body odor is caused by the multiplication of bacteria in the presence of sweat and body secretions. Odor is common in the feet, groin, armpits, genitals, pubic hair and other hair, umbilicus (belly button), anus, and behind the ears. Body odor can be influenced by heredity, diet, gender, health, disease, and medication. Do not make the patient feel uncomfortable if they have an odor.

Difficult Situations

Bathing can be very upsetting for patients with Alzheimer's disease and other types of dementia. The patient may perceive being disrobed and having the body handled as a form of sexual assault. Early signs of distress are increased motor activity and a change in tone of voice. As the agitation worsens, the patient may scream, fight, and act out. Bathing becomes a source of stress for both the patient and the nursing assistant. This behavior is the person's way of telling you that this method of bathing is not acceptable. The person is asking you to find a less upsetting method. Consider a bag bath or towel bath, or doing a partial bath. Consult the nurse. Bathing should never upset a patient. Being flexible and considerate improves patients' quality of life, reduces stress, and saves time for the nursing assistant.

PROCEDURE **52**   **BED BATH**

 NOTE

Wear disposable gloves and apply the principles of standard precautions.

1. Carry out initial procedure actions.
2. Assemble equipment:
   - Disposable gloves
   - Bed linens
   - Bath blanket
   - Laundry bag or hamper
   - Bath basin
   - Bath thermometer
   - Soap and soap dish, or liquid soap
   - Washcloths
   - Face towels
   - Bath towels
   - Hospital gown/patient's nightclothes
   - Lotion
   - Equipment for oral hygiene: toothbrush, toothpaste, mouthwash, or items for denture care
   - Emery board, and orangewood stick (if needed)
   - Deodorant
   - Brush and comb
   - Bedpan and cover or urinal
   - Laundry hamper or plastic bag(s) for linen and disposables
3. Close the windows and door to prevent chilling.
4. Close the privacy curtain.
5. Put clean towels and linens on a chair in the order of use. Place a laundry hamper or bag nearby.

6. Offer the bedpan or urinal. Apply gloves, and assist as needed. Change your gloves before continuing.
7. Lower the head of the bed and the side rails on the side where you are working.
8. Loosen the top bedclothes. Remove and fold the blanket and spread and place them over the back of the chair.
9. Place a bath blanket over the top sheet and remove the sheet by sliding it out from under the bath blanket. Place the sheet in the laundry hamper.
10. Leave one pillow under the patient's head. Place the other pillow on a chair.
11. Remove the patient's nightwear and place it in the laundry hamper.
12. Fill a bath basin two-thirds full with water that does not exceed 105°F. Use a bath thermometer, if available, to check the temperature.
13. Assist the patient to move to the side of the bed nearest you.
14. Fold a face towel over the upper edge of the bath blanket to keep the blanket dry. Apply gloves, if needed.
15. Use a bath mitt (Figure 24-6A) or make a mitt by folding a washcloth around your hand (Figure 24-6B).
    a. Wet the washcloth.
    b. Wash the patient's eyes, using separate corners of the cloth for each eye.
    c. Wipe from inside to outside corner (Figure 24-7).
    d. Do not use soap near the eyes.
    e. After you have washed the eyes, remove and discard gloves.
    f. Do not use soap on the face unless the patient requests it.

(continues)

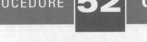

PROCEDURE **52** CONTINUED

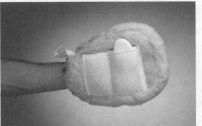

32370-24-06a1.tif Courtesy of Skil-Care Corporation,

FIGURE 24-6A A reusable bath mitt has a pocket for the soap and is very gentle to the skin.

16. Rinse the washcloth and apply soap if the patient desires. Squeeze out excess water. Do not leave soap in the water.

17. Wash and rinse the patient's face, ears, and neck well. Pat dry with a face towel.

18. Expose the patient's far arm. Place a bath towel under the arm to protect the bed.

   a. Wash, rinse, and pat the arm and hand dry.

   b. Wash and dry the **axilla** (armpit).

   c. Repeat on the near arm.

   d. Apply deodorant.

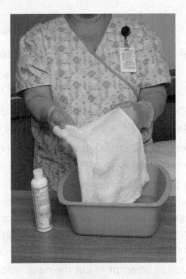

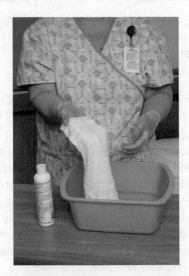

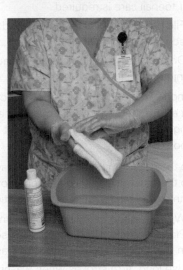

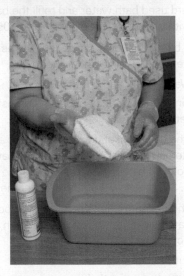

FIGURE 24-6B Use a washcloth to make a mitt over the hand. The mitt keeps the washcloth from dripping and retains more heat than a single layer.

(continues)

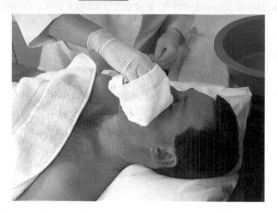

FIGURE 24-7 Avoid soap in the eye area. Wipe from the inner corner to the outer corner. Turn the washcloth before moving to the other eye.

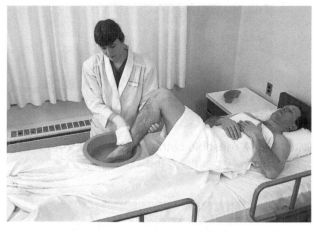

FIGURE 24-8 Support the leg and place the foot in the basin.

19. Care for hands and nails as necessary. Check with the nurse first to see if there are any special instructions.

   a. Place the patient's hands in a basin of water. Wash, rinse, and dry each hand carefully. Push cuticle (base of fingernails) down gently with a towel while wiping the fingers. Be sure to dry between fingers.

   b. Clean under the nails with an orangewood stick and/or shape the nails with an emery board, if needed. Be careful not to file nails too close. Do not cut nails if the person has diabetes. Inform the nurse if attention is needed.

20. Discard used bath water and refill the basin two-thirds full with water that does not exceed 105°F.

21. Put a bath towel over the patient's chest. Fold the blanket to the waist. Under the towel:

   a. Wash, rinse, and pat the chest dry.

   b. Rinse and dry folds under the breasts of a female patient carefully.

22. Fold the bath blanket down to the pubic area (location of external genitalia). Wash, rinse, and pat the abdomen dry. Fold the bath blanket up to cover the abdomen and chest. Slide the towel out from under the bath blanket.

23. Ask the patient to flex the far knee, if possible. Fold the bath blanket up to expose the thigh, leg, and foot. Protect the bed with a bath towel.

   a. Put the bath basin on the towel.

   b. Place the patient's foot in the basin (Figure 24-8).

   c. Wash and rinse the leg and foot.

   d. When moving the patient's leg, support it properly.

24. Lift the leg and move the basin to the other side of the bed. Dry the leg and foot. Dry well between toes.

25. Repeat for the other leg and foot. Remove the basin before drying the leg and foot.

26. Care for toenails as necessary. Check with the nurse for any special instructions. Apply lotion to the feet of a patient who has dry skin. Do not apply lotion between the toes, as this keeps the area moist and promotes fungal growth.

   a. Do not attempt to cut the nails. Inform the nurse if toenail care is required.

   b. File nails straight across, if needed. Do not round edges.

   c. Do not push back the cuticle, because it is easily injured and infected.

27. Change water and check for the correct temperature with a bath thermometer. (It may be necessary to change the water before this point if it becomes cold or too soapy.)

28. Help the patient to turn on the side away from you. Help them to move toward the center of the bed. Place a bath towel lengthwise next to the patient's back.

   a. Wash, rinse, and dry neck, back, and buttocks. Place washcloth and any towels used in this step in the hamper/laundry bag after washing buttocks.

   b. Use long, firm strokes when washing the back.

29. Give a backrub (see Chapter 25).

30. Help the patient to turn on the back.

(continues)

PROCEDURE **52** CONTINUED

31. Place a towel under the buttocks and upper legs. Change the water and check for the correct temperature. Place a washcloth, soap, basin, and bath towel within convenient reach of the patient. Have the patient complete the bath by washing the genitalia. Assist if necessary. You must take responsibility for the procedure if the patient has difficulty. Many times patients are reluctant to acknowledge the need for help. Apply gloves if assisting. Place washcloth and any towels used in this step in the hamper/laundry bag after washing the genitalia.

    a. For a female patient, wash from front to back, drying carefully.

    a. For a male patient, carefully wash and dry the penis, scrotum, and groin area. If the patient is not circumcised, gently push the foreskin back and carefully wash and dry the penis. Gently pull the foreskin down to its original position.

32. Remove and discard gloves.

ICON KEY:

 = OBRA = PPE

33. Carry out range-of-motion exercises as ordered (see Chapter 41 for Procedure 87).

34. Cover the pillow with a towel. Comb or brush the patient's hair. Provide oral hygiene (see Chapter 25).

35. Discard towels and washcloth in the laundry hamper.

36. Provide a clean gown. The patient may wear their own nightclothes, as preferred. Assist with dressing, as needed.

37. Clean and replace equipment.

38. Put clean washcloth and towels in the bedside stand.

39. Change the bed linens, following the procedure for making an occupied bed. Replace soiled nightclothes and discard soiled linens in a laundry hamper.

40. Remove and discard gloves. Wash your hands.

41. Raise the siderails, if required.

42. Carry out ending procedure actions.

PROCEDURE **53** CHANGING THE PATIENT'S GOWN

 NOTE

Wear disposable gloves if the patient has draining wounds; has nonintact skin; or if contact with mucous membranes, blood, secretions, excretions, or other body fluids is likely.

1. Carry out initial procedure actions.

2. Assemble equipment:
   – Disposable gloves
   – Bath blanket
   – Clean gown
   – Laundry bag or hamper

3. Place a bath blanket over the top sheet. Hold the bath blanket with the left hand, while pulling the sheet

down under it with the right hand. This prevents the patient from being exposed.

4. Loosen the gown from around the patient's neck.

5. Slip the gown down the arms.

6. Make sure the patient is covered by the bath blanket.

 NOTE

Use this procedure only when a patient does not have an IV infusion running through a pump. When a pump is used, the patient may wear a gown that snaps at the shoulder so the gown can be removed without interfering with the IV bag and/or tubing. If the patient is wearing a gown without snaps, call the nurse if the gown is to be changed. Never disconnect the tubing from the pump.

(continues)

PROCEDURE **53** CONTINUED

7. For a patient wearing a regular gown (nonsnap):

   a. Remove the gown from the arm without the IV and bring the gown across the patient's chest to the other arm.

   b. Place a clean gown over the patient's chest to avoid exposure.

   c. Gather the gown material in one hand so there is no pull or pressure on the IV line, and slowly draw the gown over the tips of the patient's fingers.

   d. With your free hand, lift the IV bag off the standard and slip the gown over the bag of fluid, removing the gown from the patient's body. *Always keep the bag of fluid above the level of the patient's arm.*

   e. Take the sleeve of a clean gown and slip it over the bag of fluid, over the tubing, and up the patient's arm (Figure 24-9).

   f. Replace the bag of fluid on the IV standard.

   g. Remove the soiled gown and place it at the end of the bed. Finish putting the clean gown on the patient's other arm. Secure the neck ties.

   h. Place the soiled gown in a laundry hamper.

   i. Make sure the IV is dripping at the required rate and that the tubing is not kinked or twisted.

8. If the patient has a weak or paralyzed arm:

   a. Untie the gown and remove the back from underneath the patient.

   b. Remove the gown from the stronger arm first.

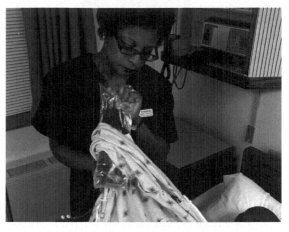

FIGURE 24-9 With your free hand, lift the IV off the standard and slip the gown over the bag of fluid.

   c. Bring the gown across the patient's chest and slide it down over the weak arm.

   d. Gently lift the patient's weak arm and pull the gown over the hand.

   e. To put a clean gown on the person, reverse the procedure by putting the gown on the weaker arm first.

9. Pull the sheet up over the bath blanket. Remove the bath blanket.

10. Carry out ending procedure actions.

ICON KEY:

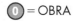 = OBRA

PROCEDURE **54** WATERLESS BED BATH

1. Carry out initial procedure actions.

2. Assemble equipment:
   - Disposable gloves
   - Bed linens
   - Bath blanket
   - Laundry bag or hamper
   - Hospital gown/patient's nightclothes

   - Bath towel
   - Lotion for backrub
   - Waterless bathing product, heated according to facility policy or patient wishes. Warm the package according to the manufacturer's directions.
   - Basin of warm water for soaking patient's hands (optional)
   - Comb, brush

(continues)

– Bedpan or urinal with cover, as needed

– Supplies for oral hygiene, as needed

– Supplies for nail care, as needed

– Small plastic bag to discard used bathing cloths

3. Close the windows and door to the room.

4. Pull the privacy curtain. Place clean supplies on the overbed table.

5. Offer the bedpan or urinal. Put on gloves if you will be assisting with this procedure.

6. Lower the head of the bed and the side rails on the side where you will be working.

7. Loosen the top bedclothes. Remove and fold the blanket and spread and place bedclothes and blanket over the back of the chair.

8. Place a bath blanket over the top sheet and remove the sheet by sliding it out from under the bath blanket. Place the sheet in the laundry hamper.

9. Leave one pillow under the patient's head. Place the other pillow on the chair.

10. Remove the gown (see Procedure 53) and place it in the laundry hamper.

11. Assist the patient to move to the side of the bed near you.

12. Open the waterless bathing product. (If you heated the package, check the cloths for hot spots.) Remove one cloth and cleanse the patient's face and neck. (The no-rinse solution on these cloths can safely be used around the eyes.)

13. Place a towel over the patient's chest. Fold the bath blanket down to the waist. Reach under the towel to cleanse the chest.

14. Fold the bath blanket down to the pubic area. Reach under the towel to wash the abdomen. Replace the bath blanket over the abdomen and chest. Slide the towel out from under the bath blanket. Discard the used cloth.

15. Uncover the far arm. Remove another cloth from the package and wash the arm and hand. Wash the axilla. Apply deodorant. Discard the used cloth. Cover the arm with the bath blanket.

16. Uncover the near arm. Remove a new cloth from the package. Wash the arm, hand, and axilla. Apply deodorant. Discard the used cloth in the plastic bag. Cover the patient with the bath blanket.

17. Provide nail care as needed.

18. Ask the patient to flex the far leg, if possible. Fold the bath blanket up to expose the thigh, leg, and foot. Remove a new cloth from the package. Cleanse the thigh, leg, and foot. Be sure the area between the toes is left dry. Discard the used cloth in the plastic bag. Cover the thigh, leg, and foot with the bath blanket.

19. Repeat step 18 with the near thigh, leg, and foot.

20. Make sure the side rails on the opposite side of the bed are up. Help the patient turn onto the side away from you.

21. Remove a new cloth from the package. Draw the bath blanket back to expose the back. Wash the back and buttocks. Discard the used cloth in the plastic bag. You may give a backrub at this time. Cover the patient with the bath blanket.

22. Assist the patient to turn onto the back. Remove a new cloth from the package. Hand the patient the cloth and instruct them to wash the genitalia. Assist if necessary. (Wear gloves if you will be assisting.) Discard gloves and the used cloth in the plastic bag.

23. Wash your hands.

24. Assist the patient to put on a clean gown.

25. Cover the pillow with a towel. Comb or brush the patient's hair. Assist with oral hygiene, if needed.

26. Change the bed linens, following the procedure for making an occupied bed (see Procedure 50). Put soiled linen in a plastic bag or linen hamper.

27. Carry out ending procedure actions.

ICON KEY:

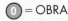 = OBRA   = PPE

Towel Bath

The towel bath procedure has become popular in long-term care facilities for bathing persons with dementia who become agitated with the tub or shower bath. Also consider the bathing environment. Eliminate clutter and remove unnecessary equipment. Keep the room calm and relaxing. A darkened room, with soothing music playing softly, works well. Products with a pleasant aroma are helpful. Some facilities have kits of aromatherapy items to create a spalike atmosphere (Figure 24-10).

Use a no-rinse skin cleanser. Two washcloths, two hand towels, one large towel, and two bath blankets are usually needed. Completely cover the patient with a bath blanket; if possible, prewarm the blanket. Coordinate with another nursing assistant to bring additional warm blankets, if necessary.

Prepare the bathing kit in advance, and bring it to the room in a large plastic bag so it is ready to use. With the person covered with the bath blanket, undress them gradually. Apply warm, moist towels prepared with skin cleanser, one at a time, over a large area of the body. Rather than using an established sequence or routine, begin the bath in an area of the body that is least distressing to the specific patient, such as the feet and lower legs. Use each prepared towel to simultaneously massage and cleanse the skin. Rinsing and drying are not necessary because a no-rinse product is used. The skin usually dries quickly when the towel is removed. Speak in a calm, soothing manner. Avoid rushing. Keep the person covered throughout the procedure. Use warm bath blankets and towels to keep the person comfortably warm.

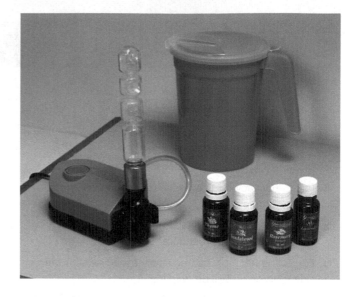

FIGURE 24-10 Aromatherapy is an ancient practice that uses fragrances to produce a reaction in the body. Certain scents are believed to change brain waves, breathing rates, and mood, among other things

The goal of this type of bath is to keep the person clean and odor-free, while avoiding a potentially upsetting situation. A variety of techniques can be used to personalize the procedure and make it as pleasurable as possible. This type of bath is more creative than normal bathing routines, but it is not more work and is not more time-consuming.

Difficult Situations

Bathing patients who have dementia requires the use of many nursing assistant skills, including communication, problem solving, and creativity. Strive to make the bath pleasant and comforting, dignified, patient-centered, and based on the person's individual needs instead of being a routine ritual of practice.

EXPAND YOUR SKILLS

PROCEDURE **55** **PARTIAL BATH**

1. Carry out initial procedure actions.

2. Assemble equipment:
   - Disposable gloves
   - Bed linens
   - Bath blanket
   - Bath thermometer
   - Soap and soap dish or liquid soap
   - Washcloth
   - Face towel
   - Bath towel
   - Gown and robe
   - Laundry bag or hamper
   - Bath basin
   - Lotion
   - Equipment for oral hygiene
   - Nail brush, emery board, and orangewood stick
   - Brush, comb, and deodorant
   - Bedpan or urinal and cover
   - Paper towels or protector
   - Plastic bag(s), if needed

> ### ✐ NOTE
> A package of premoistened washcloths can be substituted for the basin of water, soap, washcloth, and towel if a waterless bath system is available. Use a small plastic bag to discard cloths.

3. Close windows and door and pull the privacy curtain to prevent chilling the patient.

4. Put the towels and linen on the chair in the order of use. Make sure a laundry hamper is available.

5. Put on disposable gloves.

6. Offer the bedpan or urinal (see Chapter 25). Empty and clean it before proceeding with the bath. Remove and discard gloves. Wash your hands.

7. Elevate the head of the bed, if permitted, to a comfortable position.

8. Loosen the top bedclothes. Remove and fold the blanket and spread and place them over the back of the chair. Place a bath blanket over the top sheet. Remove the top sheet by sliding it out from under the bath blanket.

9. Leave one pillow under the patient's head. Place the other pillow on the chair.

10. Assist the patient to remove the gown. Place the gown in the laundry hamper. Make sure the patient is covered with a bath blanket.

11. Place paper towels or a bed protector on the overbed table.

12. Fill a bath basin two-thirds full with water that does not exceed 105°F. Place the basin on the overbed table.

13. Push the overbed table comfortably close to the patient.

14. Place towels, washcloth, and soap on the overbed table within easy reach.

15. Instruct the patient to wash as much as they are able and tell them that you will return to complete the bath.

16. Place the call bell within easy reach. Ask the patient to signal when ready.

17. Wash hands and leave the unit.

18. Wash hands and return to the unit when the patient signals. Put on a new pair of gloves.

19. Change the bath water. Complete bathing of any areas the patient could not reach. Make sure the face, hands, axillae, buttocks, back, and genitals are washed and dried.

20. Remove and discard gloves.

21. Wash your hands.

22. Give a backrub with lotion.

23. Assist the patient in applying deodorant and a fresh gown.

24. Cover the pillow with a towel. Comb or brush the patient's hair. Assist with oral hygiene, if needed (see Chapter 25).

25. Clean and replace equipment.

26. Put a clean washcloth and towels in the bedside stand.

27. Change the bed linens, following the procedure for making an occupied bed (Procedure 50). Put soiled linens in the laundry hamper.

28. Carry out ending procedure actions.

ICON KEY:

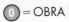 = OBRA   = PPE

Perineal Care

The **perineum** is an area between the legs. In females, it is the area between the vagina and the anus. In males, it is the area between the scrotum and the anus.

Perineal care may be performed as part of general bathing or as a separate procedure, as needed. **Perineal care (peri care)** involves washing the area including the genitals and anus (see Procedures 56 and 57). Always wear gloves and use standard precautions when caring for the perineal area.

 NOTE

If the patient has been incontinent, remove the wet pad or linen and replace with a dry pad before beginning perineal care. Clean excess stool off with toilet tissue before beginning.

 Communication **ALERT**

Patients who need assistance with perineal care and those who are incontinent may feel guilty and embarrassed. Avoid showing disgust. Be sensitive to the patient's feelings. Communicate with the patient tactfully. Use proper terms when referring to body parts and excretions.

 Infection Control **ALERT**

Providing perineal care is one of the most important procedures you will perform as a nursing assistant. Always apply the principles of standard precautions. Remember that there are mucous membranes in the genital area. If you are wearing gloves, change them before beginning care. Change them again during the procedure if they become contaminated with stool. Using proper technique is critical because of the high risk of contamination and infection. Avoid scrubbing back and forth. Always wipe from clean to dirty with a single wipe, then turn or discard the cloth. Guidelines for female perineal care vary depending on the institution. In some facilities, you will be instructed to clean the center first, then each side. In others, you will clean the sides of the genitalia first, then the center. Discard your gloves properly and avoid contaminating environmental surfaces with your used gloves.

Clinical Information **ALERT**

Excretions cause skin damage (similar to a rash or chemical burn) and skin breakdown. The damage to the skin worsens with the length of exposure.

PROCEDURE **56** FEMALE PERINEAL CARE

 NOTE

The guidelines and sequence for this procedure vary slightly from state to state, and from one facility to the next. Your instructor will inform you if the sequence in your state or facility differs from the procedure listed here. Know and follow the required sequence for policies in your state and facility.

1. Carry out initial procedure actions.
2. Assemble equipment:
   - Disposable gloves
   - Bath blanket or top sheet
   - Bedpan and cover
   - Liquid soap
   - Basin
   - Bed protector
   - Washcloth(s) and towel(s)
   - Plastic bag(s), if needed to discard linen or trash
   - Laundry barrel or hamper
3. Lower the siderails on the side where you will be working. Be sure the opposite siderails are up and secure.
4. Remove the bedspread and blanket. Fold and place them on the back of the chair.
5. Position the patient on her back. Cover her with a bath blanket and fan-fold the sheet to the foot of the bed.

(continues)

PROCEDURE **56** CONTINUED   O   P

6. Put on disposable gloves. Fill a basin with water that does not exceed 105°F.

7. Ask the patient to raise her hips while you place a bed protector underneath her.

8. Offer the bedpan to the patient.

   a. If used and the patient is on intake and output, record the amount.

   b. Empty and clean the bedpan before continuing with the procedure.

   c. Remove and discard gloves.

   d. Wash your hands and put on a new pair of gloves.

9. Position the bath blanket so that only the area between the legs is exposed.

10. Ask the patient to separate her legs and flex her knees.

 NOTE

If the patient is unable to spread her legs and flex her knees, turn the patient on her side with the legs flexed. This position provides easy access to the perineal area.

11. Wet the washcloth, make a mitt, and apply a small amount of liquid soap. You may also use a commercial mitt if the patient prefers (Figure 24-6).

 NOTE

Heavy soap application may be difficult to rinse off completely. Soap residue is irritating.

12. Separate the labia with one gloved hand. Keep the labia separated as much as possible during the procedure. Avoid placing your fingers on an area after washing it. Turn the washcloth so you are using a clean section each time you move to a new area. Use a fresh washcloth, if necessary. You may need several washcloths to perform the procedure without contamination. (Some facilities require an additional clean washcloth for rinsing; the used cloth is not put back into the basin of water.)

   a. With the other gloved hand, wash the center of the labia, using a single downward stroke from top to bottom.

   b. Turn the washcloth to a clean area.

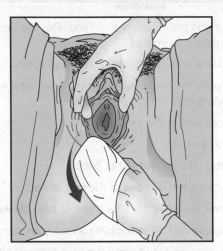

FIGURE 24-11 Spread the labia with one hand. With the washcloth in the other hand, start in the front and stroke downward along the outer labia.

   c. Wash the far side of the labia, using a single downward stroke from top to bottom (Figure 24-11).

   d. Turn the washcloth to a clean area.

   e. Wash the near labia, using a single downward stroke from top to bottom.

   f. Continue to alternate from side to side, working outward to the thighs, using the same technique. Turn the washcloth, or use a new washcloth, so that a fresh section is used to cleanse each area.

   g. If a urinary catheter is present, wash, rinse, and dry the perineal area surrounding the urinary meatus and catheter. Change the washcloth. Beginning at the urinary meatus, wash down the catheter approximately three to four inches. Use a single downward stroke. Do not rub back and forth. Rinse and dry in the same direction. Hold the catheter firmly to avoid pulling and traction. After washing the catheter, continue with perineal care.

   h. Rinse the area from top to bottom with the washcloth. Avoid rubbing back and forth. Rinse in the same sequence as the area was washed, beginning in the center and moving outward from side to side. Turn the washcloth so a clean surface is used for each downward stroke.

   i. Gently pat the area dry with a towel. Avoid rubbing back and forth. Dry in the same sequence as the area was washed and rinsed, beginning in the center and moving out ward from side to side. Position the towel so a clean surface is used for each downward stroke.

(continues)

PROCEDURE **56** CONTINUED

13. Turn the patient away from you. Flex the upper leg slightly, if permitted.

14. Make a mitt, wet it, and apply soap lightly.

15. Expose the anal area. Wash the area, stroking from perineum to coccyx (front to back).

16. Rinse well in the same manner.

17. Dry carefully.

18. Return the patient to her back.

19. Remove and dispose of the bed protector.

20. Cover the patient with a sheet or bath blanket.

21. Remove and discard gloves. Wash your hands.

22. Remove, fold, and store the bath blanket. Alternatively, if it is soiled or wet, put it in the soiled laundry hamper.

23. Replace the top covers, tuck them under the mattress, and make mitered corners. (Some patients prefer that the top covers not be tucked in.)

24. Put up the side rails, if required.

25. Put on gloves. Empty the water from the basin. Clean equipment.

26. Remove and discard gloves. Wash your hands.

27. Carry out ending procedure actions.

Clinical Information **ALERT**

Be gentle when cleansing patients after incontinent episodes. Scrubbing produces extra friction. The excretions are irritating to the skin, and vigorous scrubbing is abrasive, furthering the risk of infection and skin breakdown.

ICON KEY:
 = OBRA   = PPE

PROCEDURE **57** MALE PERINEAL CARE

NOTE

The guidelines and sequence for this procedure vary slightly from state to state, and from one facility to the next. Your instructor will inform you if the sequence in your state or facility differs from the procedure listed here. Know and follow the required sequence for policies in your state and facility.

1. Carry out initial procedure actions.

2. Assemble equipment:
   – Disposable gloves
   – Bath blanket
   – Urinal and cover or bedpan and cover
   – Soap, washcloth(s), and towel(s)
   – Washbasin
   – Plastic bag(s)
   – Bed protector or bath towel
   – Laundry hamper

3. Fill a basin with warm water that does not exceed 105°F.

4. Lower the side rail on the side where you will be working.

5. Fan-fold the blanket and spread to the foot of the bed. Remove, fold, and place them on the back of the chair.

6. Cover the patient with a bath blanket and fan-fold the sheet to the foot of the bed.

7. Put on disposable gloves.

8. Place a bed protector under the patient's buttocks.

(continues)

PROCEDURE **57** CONTINUED

9. Offer the bedpan or urinal.

   a. If used and the patient is on intake and output, record the amount.

   b. Empty and clean the bedpan or urinal before continuing with the procedure.

   c. Remove and discard gloves.

   d. Wash your hands and put on a new pair of gloves.

> **NOTE**
>
> If the patient is unable to spread their legs and flex the knees, turning them on their side with the legs flexed provides easy access to the perineal area.

10. Have the patient flex and separate his knees.

11. Draw the bath blanket upward to expose the perineal area only.

12. Make a mitt with a washcloth, wet it, and apply a small amount of soap.

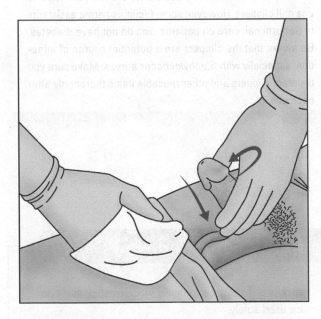

FIGURE 24-12A Grasp the penis gently with one hand. With the other, wipe in a circular motion, beginning with the urinary meatus and working outward over the glans (head of the penis). Continue to wash down the penis and the rest of the perineal area, including the scrotum, using downward strokes and working outward to the thighs.

> **NOTE**
>
> Heavy soap application may be difficult to rinse off completely. Soap residue is irritating.

13. Grasp the penis gently with one hand and wash. Begin at the meatus and wash in a circular motion (Figure 24-12A). If a urinary catheter is present, hold the tubing securely to one side and support it against the leg to avoid unnecessary movement or traction on the catheter. Keep the tubing and drainage bag below the level of the bladder.

14. If the patient is not circumcised, draw the foreskin back (Figure 24-12B). Be sure the entire penis is washed. Rinse thoroughly.

15. Continue to wash down the penis and the rest of the perineal area, including the scrotum, using downward strokes and working outward to the thighs. Lift the scrotum and wash the perineum. If a urinary catheter is present, wash, rinse, and dry the perineal area surrounding the urinary meatus and catheter. Change the washcloth. Beginning at the urinary meatus, wash down the catheter approximately three to four inches. Use a single downward stroke. Do not rub back and forth. Rinse and dry in the same direction. Hold the catheter firmly to avoid pulling and traction. After washing the catheter, continue with perineal care.

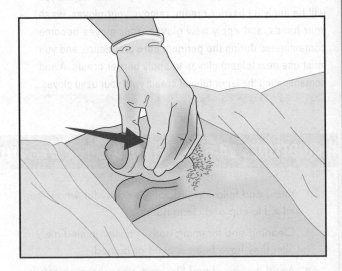

FIGURE 24-12B If the patient is not circumcised, gently push the foreskin back so the glans can be washed. Once the penis is washed and dried, return the foreskin to its normal position.

(continues)

PROCEDURE **57** **CONTINUED**

16. Rinse the washcloth and remake a mitt. Rinse the urethral and perineal areas well, working in the same direction until the entire area is clean and soap-free.

17. Dry the washed area with a towel. Reposition the foreskin if necessary.

18. Turn the patient away from you. Flex his upper leg slightly.

19. Make a mitt, wet it, and apply soap lightly.

20. Expose the anal area. Wash the area, stroking from perineum to coccyx.

21. Rinse well in the same manner.

22. Dry carefully.

23. Return the patient to his back.

24. Remove and dispose of the bed protector.

25. Cover the patient with a sheet.

26. Remove and discard gloves. Wash your hands.

27. Remove, fold, and store the bath blanket. Alternatively, if it is soiled or wet, put it in the soiled laundry hamper.

28. Replace the top covers, tuck them under the mattress, and make mitered corners. (Some patients prefer that the top covers not be tucked in.)

29. Put up the siderails, if required.

30. Put on gloves. Empty the water from the basin. Clean equipment.

31. Remove and discard gloves. Wash your hands.

32. Carry out ending procedure actions.

ICON KEY:

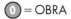 = OBRA   = PPE

 Infection Control **ALERT**

When giving perineal care, always wash from the most clean area to the least clean. Turn the cloth frequently and rinse well. After giving perineal care, avoid using the same washcloth, towel, and gloves elsewhere on the body. If further bathing or touching is necessary, apply new gloves and use different linens. Some patients may have orders for barrier cream or another product following perineal care. If you will be applying barrier cream, remove your gloves, wash your hands, and apply new gloves. Your gloves become contaminated during the perineal care procedure, and you must use new (clean) gloves to apply barrier cream. Avoid contaminating the jar or tube of cream with your used gloves.

Infection Control **ALERT**

In many facilities, nursing assistants are not permitted to use nail clippers. However, some facilities permit assistants to perform nail care on patients who do not have diabetes. Be aware that the clippers are a potential source of infection, especially with *Staphylococcus aureus*. Make sure you disinfect clippers and other reusable items thoroughly after each use.

GUIDELINES 24-3 Guidelines for Providing Hand, Foot, and Nail Care

- Know and follow your facility's policy for who is permitted to clip and clean nails.
- Cleaning and trimming nails is easier immediately after they have been soaked or bathed.
- Avoid the use of nail files and other sharp objects for cleaning nails. An orange (also called orangewood)

stick is a disposable pointed wooden stick that can be used safely.

- If your facility allows you to clip fingernails, use clippers, not scissors.
- When trimming nails, be very careful not to accidentally clip or damage the skin surrounding the nails.

(continues)

GUIDELINES 24-3 Guidelines for Providing Hand, Foot, and Nail Care (continued)

- Notify the nurse if you observe any abnormalities, such as redness, cracking, or signs of infection, by the fingernails or toenails.
- Clip fingernails straight across, then round at the edges with an emery board.
- Push the cuticles back with a washcloth or the dull end of the orange stick.
- After washing the feet, dry well between each toe and inspect for red or cracked areas. Moisture promotes fungal growth and skin breakdown, which can lead to more serious complications.

- Apply lotion to the hands or feet if the skin is dry. Avoid the area between the toes.

 NOTE

Many facilities do not permit nursing assistants to clip nails. Use clippers only if you are permitted to do so according to state law and facility policies.

PROCEDURE **58** **HAND AND FINGERNAIL CARE**

 NOTE

Check with the nurse and nursing care plan to learn if this procedure is permitted for the patient or if it is to be modified based on the patient's condition.

This procedure can be carried out independently or can be modified and added to the bath procedure.

1. Carry out initial procedure actions.

2. Assemble equipment:
   - Basin
   - Bath thermometer
   - Liquid soap
   - Bath towel and washcloth
   - Lotion
   - Plastic protector
   - Nail clippers, if permitted
   - Emery board
   - Orangewood stick
   - Nail polish (optional)

3. Elevate the head of the bed, if permitted, and adjust the overbed table in front of the patient. Alternatively, if the patient is allowed out of bed, assist the patient to transfer to a chair and position the overbed table waist-high across the patient's lap.

4. Place a plastic protector on the overbed table.

5. Fill a basin with warm water that does not exceed 105°F, using the bath thermometer to test temperature. Add soap. Place the basin on the overbed table.

6. Instruct the patient to put hands in the basin and soak for approximately five minutes. Place a towel over the basin to help retain heat. Add warm water if necessary. Remove the patient's hands before adding water.

7. Wash the patient's hands. Push cuticles back gently with a washcloth or an orangewood stick (Figure 24-13). (A cream may be used to soften the cuticles first.) Use a soft brush or orangewood stick to clean under nails. (Check with the nurse before using an orangewood stick on a patient with diabetes.) Rinse hands.

8. Dry the patient's hands with a towel. Remember to dry between the fingers.

9. Use nail clippers to cut fingernails straight across, if permitted.
   - Do not cut below the tips of the fingers.
   - Keep nail clippings on the protector to be discarded.

10. Shape and smooth the fingernails with an emery board. Apply polish to nails if the patient desires.

(continues)

PROCEDURE **58** CONTINUED

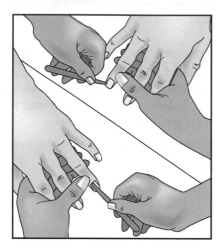

FIGURE 24-13 Gently push the cuticles back with a washcloth or orange stick, if permitted.

ICON KEY:
 = OBRA

11. Pour a small amount of lotion in your palms and gently smooth it on the patient's hands.

12. Empty the basin of water. Clean and store equipment.

13. Return the overbed table to the foot of the bed. If the patient has been sitting up for the procedure, assist to return to bed.

14. Carry out ending procedure actions.

PROCEDURE **59** FOOT AND TOENAIL CARE

1. Carry out each beginning procedure action.
2. Assemble equipment:
   - Basin
   - Soap
   - Bath mat, if available
   - Bath thermometer, if used
   - Lotion
   - Nail brush
   - Disposable bed protector
   - Paper towels/towel
   - Bath towel and washcloth
   - Orangewood stick
3. If permitted, assist the person out of bed and into chair.
4. Place bath mat, towel, bed protector, or paper towels on floor in front of the person. Fill basin with warm water (105°F). Put basin on barrier.
5. Remove slippers and allow the person to place feet in water. Cover with bath towel to help retain heat.

6. Soak feet approximately 10 minutes. Add warm water as necessary. Lift feet from water while warm water is being added.

7. At end of soak period, wash feet with soap.

8. Rinse and pat dry. Note any abnormalities such as corns or calluses.

9. Remove basin, covering feet with towel.

10. Use orangewood stick to gently clean toenails. If nails are long and need to be cut, inform the nurse. Follow facility policy.

11. Pour lotion into palms of hands. Hold hands together to warm lotion and apply gently to feet. Do not apply lotion between toes. Wipe off excess lotion using a towel.

12. Assist the person with socks or stockings and shoes if ambulatory. Otherwise, return the person to bed.

13. Make the person comfortable.

14. Gather equipment, clean, and store according to facility policy. Leave unit neat.

15. Carry out each procedure completion action.

Clinical Information ALERT

In some facilities, a doctor's order is needed for a shampoo. If permitted, the hair can be washed in the tub or shower. Offer the patient a washcloth or towel to hold over the face while hair is being washed and rinsed. Hair must be washed in bed for patients who are on complete bedrest. Some facilities use dry chemical shampoos that are brushed out. No-rinse shampoos are also available for patients who are bedfast.

Difficult Situations

Like bathing, washing the hair of a patient who is cognitively impaired under running water can cause of great stress and distress. Consider washing the hair using a bed shampoo tray, an inflatable shampoo basin, a no-rinse shampoo, a shampoo cap, or a dry shampoo product. Follow the instructions on the care plan. Select the product that is least upsetting to the patient.

EXPAND YOUR SKILLS

PROCEDURE 60 BED SHAMPOO

1. Carry out initial procedure actions.

2. Assemble equipment needed:
   - Shampoo tray
   - Shampoo
   - Large empty basin
   - Washcloths
   - 3 bath towels
   - Bath blanket
   - Pitcher of water (that does not exceed 105°F)
   - Safety pin
   - 2 bed protectors
   - Waterproof covering for pillow
   - Large bucket to collect used water
   - Hair dryer, if available (portable)
   - Hairbrush and comb
   - Small empty pitcher or cup
   - Larger pitcher of water (that does not exceed 105°F)—use if additional water is needed

3. Place a large empty basin on the floor under the drain of the shampoo tray.

4. Arrange on the bedside stand, within easy reach.
   Large pitcher of water (that does not exceed 105°F)
   - Washcloth
   - 2 bath towels
   - Shampoo
   - Small pitcher of water (that does not exceed 105°F)

5. Replace the top bedding with a bath blanket.

6. Ask the patient to move to the side of the bed nearest you. Assist as needed.

7. Replace the pillowcase with a waterproof covering.

8. Cover the head of the bed with a bed protector. Be sure it goes well under the patient's shoulders.

9. Loosen neck ties of the gown.

10. Place a towel under the patient's head and shoulders. Brush hair free of tangles.

11. Bring the towel down around the patient's neck and shoulders and pin it. Position the pillow under the shoulders so that the patient's head is tilted slightly backward.

12. Raise the bed to high horizontal position.

13. Raise the patient's head and position the shampoo tray so that the drain is over the edge of the bed directly above the basin.

14. Give the patient a washcloth to cover the eyes (Figure 24-14).

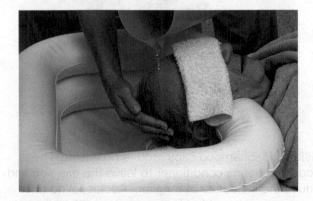

FIGURE 24-14 When shampooing hair in bed, cover the patient's eyes with a washcloth to prevent soap from getting in the eyes.

(continues)

PROCEDURE **60** CONTINUED

15. Recheck the temperature of the water in the basin.

16. Using the small pitcher, pour a small amount of water over the hair until it is thoroughly wet. Use one hand to help direct the flow away from the face and ears.

17. Apply a small amount of shampoo, working up a lather. Work from scalp to hair ends.

18. Massage the scalp with your fingertips. Do not use your fingernails.

19. Rinse thoroughly, pouring from hairline to hair tips. Direct the flow into the drain. Use water from the pitcher if needed, but be sure to check the water temperature before use.

20. Repeat lathering and rinsing (steps 17–19).

21. Lift the patient's head. Remove the tray and bed protector. Adjust the pillow and slip a dry bath towel underneath the head.

22. Place the tray on the basin. Wrap hair in a towel. Be sure to dry face, neck, and ears as needed.

23. Dry hair with the towel. If available and not otherwise contraindicated, a portable hair dryer may be used to complete the drying process. Brushing the hair as you blow-dry helps the hair to dry. Be sure to keep the dryer moving and not too close to the hair.

24. Comb hair appropriately. Remove the protective pillow cover. Replace with a cloth cover.

25. Lower the bed to a comfortable working position.

26. Replace the bedding and remove the bath blanket.

27. Help the patient assume a comfortable position. Lower the bed to the lowest horizontal position. Leave the call bell within reach.

28. Allow the patient to rest undisturbed. The length of this procedure may tire the patient.

29. Empty the water from the collection basin.

30. Carry out ending procedure actions.

ICON KEY:
 = OBRA

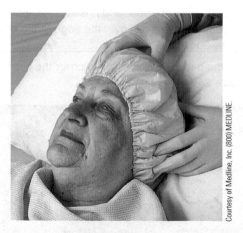

FIGURE 24-15 Shampoo caps require no rinsing. The product contains conditioner to leave the hair soft and reduce the incidence of tangling. Additional no-rinse shampoo can be added for longer hair or if additional liquid is needed.

 Safety **ALERT**

Do not use a hair dryer if oxygen is in use in the room.

The Waterless Shampoo

Various waterless preparations are available for washing the hair of patients whose hair cannot be shampooed by other methods. Shampoo caps (Figure 24-15) are a popular alternative for patients who are bedfast. These are most comfortable if they are warmed in a microwave for 30 seconds or less, or in the product warmer. If a microwave is used, feel the outside of the cap by pressing the various areas against your forearm to make sure there are no hot spots. Place the cap on the patient's head, and then massage and rub gently with the fingertips for one to two minutes for short hair and four to five minutes for long hair. After this time, remove the cap; towel-dry and comb the hair. Shampoo caps reduce tangling and do not leave residue like some dry chemical products.

DRESSING A PATIENT

Patients in hospitals generally wear hospital gowns because they are in bed most of the time. However, some may prefer to wear their own nightgowns or pajamas and will need assistance in dressing. Patients in rehabilitation units and those who participate in some special programs may be up and fully dressed each day. You may also need to assist patients to dress when they are discharged from the hospital. It is usually easier to help people dress while they are still in bed.

GUIDELINES 24-4 Guidelines for Dressing and Undressing Patients

The patient who requires help in dressing may wish to sit in a chair with clothing placed nearby. You can help by:

- Allowing the patient to choose the clothing to be put on.
- Encouraging the patient to participate in the dressing or undressing procedure as much as they are able.
- Being prepared to assist with shoes and stockings, even for patients who can do much for themselves.

Bending over to adjust shoes and stockings can result in dizziness and loss of balance.

- Putting clothing on the affected or weakest side first if the patient has difficulty moving one side or is paralyzed.
- Removing clothing from the unaffected or strongest side first if the patient has difficulty moving one side or is paralyzed.

PROCEDURE 61 DRESSING AND UNDRESSING THE PATIENT

1. Carry out initial procedure actions.

2. Select appropriate clothing and arrange in order of application. Encourage the patient to participate in the selection process.

3. Cover the patient with a bath blanket and fan-fold top bedclothes to the foot of the bed.

4. Elevate the head of the bed to sitting position.

5. Assist the patient to a comfortable sitting position.

6. Remove nightclothes, keeping the patient covered with the bath blanket. Remove from strong side first and then from weaker side. Place nightclothes in a laundry hamper or fold them to be taken home.

7. To assist a female patient with a bra, slip the straps over the patient's hands (weak side first), move the straps up her arms, and position them on her shoulders. Adjust the breasts in the cups. Then hook the bra in back (assist the patient to lean forward so the bra can be fastened).

8. For an undershirt, or any garment that slips on over the head:

   a. Gather the undershirt and place it over the patient's head (Figure 24-16A).

   b. Grasp the patient's hand and guide it through the armhole by reaching into the armhole from the outside.

   c. Repeat the procedure with the opposite arm.

   d. Assist the patient to lean forward, and adjust the undershirt so it is smooth over the upper body.

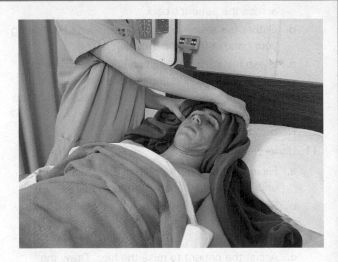

FIGURE 24-16A Gather the garment and pull it over the patient's head.

NOTE

A garment must be large enough or made of stretchy fabric for this procedure.

9. Alternate the procedure for slipover garments:

   a. Place the garment front side down on the patient's lap, with the bottom opening facing the patient.

   b. Put the patient's hands into the bottom of the garment and, one at a time, into the sleeve holes.

(continues)

c. Pull the sleeves up as far as possible on the patient's arms and pull the hands through at the wrist if it is a long-sleeved garment. The garment should now be high on the patient's chest.

d. Gather up the back of the garment with your hand and slip the garment over the patient's head.

e. Smooth the garment down and position it comfortably about the patient's body. Adjust sleeves and shoulders as needed.

10. Shirts or dresses that fasten in the front:

a. Insert your hand through the sleeve of the garment and grasp the patient's hand. Draw the sleeve over your hand and the patient's.

b. Adjust the sleeve at the shoulder.

c. Assist the patient to sit forward. Arrange clothing across the patient's back.

d. Gather the sleeve on the opposite side by slipping your hand in from the outside.

e. Grasp the patient's wrist and pull the sleeve of the garment over your hand and the patient's hand. Draw the sleeve upward and adjust it at the shoulder.

f. Button, zip, or snap the garment.

11. Underwear or pants:

a. Facing the foot of the bed, gather the patient's undergarment from waist to leg hole.

b. Slip the garment over one foot at a time (Figure 24-16B). Pull the garment up the legs as high as possible.

c. Assist the patient to raise the hips. Draw the garment over the buttocks and up to the waist. If patient cannot raise the buttocks, assist the patient to roll first to one side, as you pull up the garment, and then the other side. Adjust the garment until comfortable.

d. Fasten the garment, if required.

12. Socks or knee-high (or thigh-high) stockings:

a. Roll a sock or stocking with heel in back and place it over the toes.

b. Draw the sock up over the foot and adjust until smooth. Pull stockings smoothly up to knee or thigh.

c. Repeat for other foot.

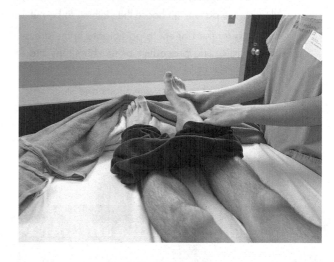

FIGURE 24-16B Slip pants over feet and lower legs.

13. Pantyhose:

a. Gather pantyhose and adjust over toes and feet. Draw up legs as high as possible.

b. Draw over hips as described in step 11c. Adjust until comfortable at waist.

14. Shoes:

a. Open laces of shoes completely so the foot can easily slip into the shoe. Slip shoe on, using a shoehorn if necessary.

b. Be sure the shoe is fastened securely (Velcro tabs or ties). If the shoes tie, be sure that the ends of the shoelaces do not drag on the floor. Fasten the shoes so they are tight enough to prevent them from slipping off the patient's feet but not so tight that circulation is impaired.

c. Be sure that shoes are appropriate to the floor surface.

15. To undress, reverse order of steps.

16. Carry out ending procedure actions

ICON KEY:
⓪ = OBRA

REVIEW

A. True/False

Mark the following true or false by circling T or F.

1. T F The nursing assistant should carefully observe the patient during the bath procedure.

2. T F Perineal care is not given to men.

3. T F Range-of-motion exercises are often performed during the bath.

4. T F Patients receiving special treatments such as oxygen, tube feeding, or IV fluids may be bathed.

5. T F During the bed bath, only the part being bathed should be exposed.

6. T F Patients should be encouraged to use hand rails when getting into and out of the bathtub.

7. T F Traction may be applied to drainage tubes as long as they are not disconnected.

8. T F The tub need not be cleaned between patients because soap from bathing keeps it clean.

9. T F Movement during the bathing procedure provides mild exercise.

10. T F Gloves should be worn when bathing the patient.

B. Matching

Match the words in Column II with the descriptions in Column I.

Column I

11. _____ external reproductive organs
12. _____ area at base of nails
13. _____ area under the arms

Column II

a. axillae
b. genitalia
c. cuticle

C. Multiple Choice

Select the best answer for each of the following.

14. The temperature of the whirlpool is a constant:
    a. 105°F.
    b. 78°F.
    c. 97°F.
    d. 86°F.

15. When providing perineal care to a female patient:
    a. wash from the front to the back.
    b. wash the genitals from side to side.
    c. wipe from back to front.
    d. scrub back and forth vigorously.

16. Bath water temperature that does not exceed:
    a. 105°F.
    b. 90°F.
    c. 80°F.
    d. 120°F.

17. When giving hand and nail care, soak the hands for approximately:
    a. 1 hour.
    b. ½ hour.
    c. 20 minutes.
    d. 5 minutes.

18. When a patient takes a bath, the bathroom door should:
    a. not be locked.
    b. be left wide open for emergency access.
    c. be locked for privacy.
    d. be left partially open.

D. Nursing Assistant Challenge

Mr. Rodriguez is taking a shower before going home. He had bowel surgery four days ago. Answer the following about his care by selecting the correct word.

19. The person responsible for the cleanliness of the shower is the _____.
    (nurse) (nursing assistant)

20. The patient _____ be assisted into and out of the shower.
    (should not) (should)

21. You can protect the patient from fatigue by _____ to the shower.
    (walking slowly) (transporting him by wheelchair)

22. If Mr. Rodriguez feels faint during his shower, you should turn the water _____.
    (to cold) (off)

23. To prevent chilling if Mr. Rodriguez feels weak, you should _____.
    (turn on the warm water) (wrap him in a bath blanket)

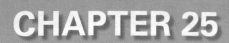

CHAPTER 25

General Comfort Measures

OBJECTIVES

After completing this chapter, you will be able to:

25.1 Spell and define terms.

25.2 Discuss the reasons for early morning and bed-time care.

25.3 Identify patients who require frequent oral hygiene.

25.4 List the purposes of oral hygiene.

25.5 Explain nursing assistant responsibilities related to a patient's dentures.

25.6 State the purpose of backrubs.

25.7 Describe safety precautions when shaving a patient.

25.8 Describe the importance of hair care.

25.9 Explain the use of comfort devices.

25.10 State the purpose of bed boards and list guidelines for their use.

25.11 Explain why regular elimination is essential to good health.

25.12 Demonstrate the following procedures:

- Procedure 62: Assisting with Routine Oral Hygiene
- Procedure 63: Assisting with Special Oral Hygiene—Dependent and Unconscious Patients
- Procedure 64: Assisting the Patient to Floss and Brush Teeth
- Procedure 65: Caring for Dentures
- Procedure 66: Providing Backrubs
- Procedure 67: Shaving a Male Patient (Expand Your Skills)
- Procedure 68: Providing Daily Hair Care
- Procedure 69: Giving and Receiving the Bedpan
- Procedure 70: Giving and Receiving the Urinal (Expand Your Skills)
- Procedure 71: Assisting with Use of the Bedside Commode (Expand Your Skills)

VOCABULARY

Learn the meaning and the correct spelling of the following words and phrases:

a.m. care	caries	footboard	oral hygiene
anticoagulant	dentures	foot drop	periodontal disease
bridging	feces	halitosis	p.m. care

INTRODUCTION

You can do many things for your patients that will add to their general comfort and feeling of well-being. This includes:

- Providing a.m. and p.m. care
- Giving oral hygiene care
- Giving backrubs
- Brushing hair
- Shaving
- Using pillows and special equipment to maintain comfortable positions

A.M. CARE AND P.M. CARE

Early morning (a.m.) care prepares the patient for a day of activities, and p.m. care prepares the patient for a night of rest. Each provides an opportunity for the patient to meet elimination needs and to be refreshed. The nursing assistant has an opportunity to closely observe the patient's condition and to interact supportively with the patient.

Early Morning (a.m.) Care

Early morning care, or a.m. care, helps to set the tone for the entire day. If the patient is refreshed and comfortable before eating breakfast, the day is off to a good start. The nursing assistant provides a.m. care by:

- Awakening the patient gently—never abruptly—by saying the patient's name. And if necessary, gently touching the arm.
- Organizing time so the person is awake and a.m. care has been completed before breakfast trays arrive on the unit.
- Giving the patient the opportunity to use the bathroom, if permitted, or to use the bedpan or urinal.
- Helping the patient to wash hands and face. The person may prefer to brush teeth before breakfast.
- *Not* awakening the patient early (for breakfast) if they are
  - Going to surgery
  - Having tests that prohibit eating

Bedtime (p.m) Care

The care given to the patient just before bedtime is similar to that given in the early morning. Bedtime care is called **p.m. care** (or *HS care*). The nursing assistant gives p.m. care:

- In a quiet, unrushed manner that will help prepare the patient for sleep
- Before medication for sleep is given by the nurse

Other routine procedures that may be carried out during a.m. and p.m. care include:

- Measuring vital signs.
- Giving a backrub.
- Providing mouth and hair care.
- Straightening the linen and lowering the head of the bed.
- Positioning the patient for comfort, as needed. A side-lying position is very comfortable when the patient is well supported in good alignment with pillows.

ORAL HYGIENE

Oral hygiene is care of the mouth and teeth (refer to Procedures 62 to 64).

- Routine oral hygiene (including brushing and flossing the teeth) should be performed at least three times a day.

 Infection Control ALERT

A clean mouth has about 100 million bacteria on the teeth, tongue, gums, and other surfaces. If the teeth are not regularly brushed, the bacteria can multiply quickly. They will move to other areas, including the pharynx, sinuses, larynx, and lungs. In patients with dysphagia (Chapter 26), small amounts of oral fluid are aspirated frequently and rapidly. Even healthy adults occasionally aspirate small amounts of saliva during deep sleep, increasing the risk of pneumonia. However, they usually do not get sick because they brush their teeth daily and have healthy immune systems. Poor oral care contributes to heart disease and other serious medical problems.

- Patients should be encouraged to do as much as possible for themselves.
- *Special oral hygiene* is the cleansing of the mouth of a patient who is helpless or unconscious, using commercially prepared lemon–glycerin swabs, sponge-tipped applicators, and other preparations.

Patients requiring more frequent oral hygiene include those who are:

- Unconscious
- Vomiting
- Experiencing a high temperature
- Receiving certain medications. It is the nurse's responsibility to identify the medications affecting oral hygiene
- Dehydrated
- Breathing through the mouth
- Receiving oxygen (Figure 25-1)
- Cannot eat or drink
- Receiving tube feeding
- Dying

Proper cleansing of the teeth and mouth helps:

- Prevent tooth decay (**caries**)
- Prevent periodontal disease
- Eliminate bad breath (**halitosis**)
- Contribute to the patient's comfort

Bacteria, mucus, and other particles in the mouth form *plaque*, a sticky substance that adheres to teeth. Brushing and flossing help get rid of plaque. If plaque is not removed, it hardens and forms tartar, which

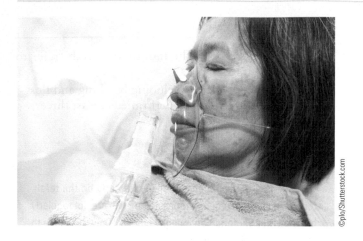

FIGURE 25-1 Oxygen is very drying to the mucous membranes.

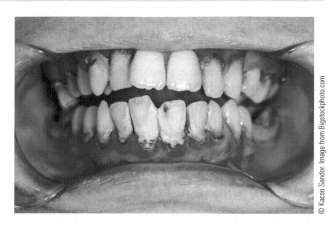

FIGURE 25-2 This person has very serious periodontal disease. The gums have pulled back and are bleeding. Tartar, plaque, and caries are present. Pockets of pus are visible in the gums.

must be removed by a dental professional. Damage occurs if plaque and tartar are not regularly removed from the teeth. Over time, **periodontal disease** develops (Figure 25-2). This is a potentially serious condition that damages the soft tissue and bone that support the teeth. In the worst cases, teeth are lost.

 Infection Control **ALERT**

Store the patient's toothbrush covered or away from other items, such as the hairbrush.

 Infection Control **ALERT**

Apply the principles of standard precautions when selecting protective equipment for assisting with dental procedures. Always wear gloves. If there is a chance of spraying or splashing of oral secretions, you will need a gown, gloves, mask, and face shield.

PROCEDURE **62** ASSISTING WITH ROUTINE ORAL HYGIENE

1. Carry out initial procedure actions.

2. Assemble equipment:
   - Disposable gloves and face mask
   - Goggles or face shield
   - Toothbrush
   - Toothpaste
   - Dental floss
   - Mouthwash solution in cup, if permitted
   - Emesis basin
   - Bath towel
   - Straw
   - Tissues
   - Cup of fresh water
   - Bed protector
   - Paper bag

3. Raise the head of the bed so that the patient may sit up, if their condition permits.

4. Lower the side rail (if used) on the side where you are working, and position the overbed table across the person's lap.

5. Cover the table with a bed protector and place equipment on the table.

6. Place a bath towel over the patient's gown and bedcovers.

7. Be prepared to help as the patient brushes and flosses teeth.

8. Pour water over the toothbrush and put toothpaste on the brush. Encourage the person to do as much as possible. Assist as needed.

9. Put on disposable gloves. A face mask and eye protection may be used.

(continues)

PROCEDURE **62** CONTINUED

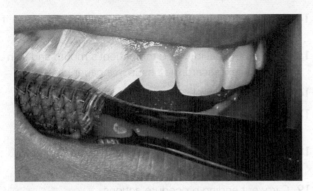

FIGURE 25-3A Place the head of the toothbrush beside the teeth, with the bristle tips at a 45° angle against the gumline. Move the brush back and forth in short strokes several times, using a gentle scrubbing motion. Brush the outer surfaces of each tooth, upper and lower, keeping the bristles angled against the gumline.

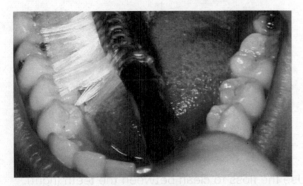

FIGURE 25-3B Use the same method on the inside surfaces of all the teeth, still using short back-and-forth strokes.

10. Brush teeth as follows:

   a. Insert the toothbrush into the mouth with bristles pointing downward (Figure 25-3A).

   b. Turn the toothbrush with bristles toward teeth (Figure 25-3B).

   c. Brush all tooth surfaces with a back-and-forth motion using short strokes (Figure 25-3C).

   d. Use the "toe" end of the brush to clean the inner surfaces of the front teeth, using a gentle up-and-down motion (Figure 25-3D).

   e. Brush the front of the tongue gently, if tolerated by the patient (Figure 25-3E). Avoid the back of the tongue, as touching this area may cause gagging and coughing.

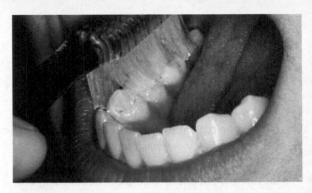

FIGURE 25-3C Gently scrub the chewing surfaces of the teeth.

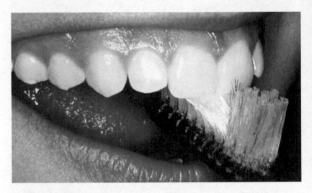

FIGURE 25-3D To clean the inside surfaces of the front teeth, tilt the brush vertically and make several gentle up-and-down strokes with the "toe" (front part) of the brush.

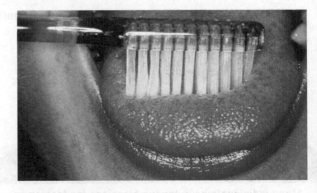

FIGURE 25-3E Brushing the patient's tongue will help freshen the breath and clean the mouth by removing bacteria.

11. Give the patient water in a cup to rinse the mouth. Use a straw, if necessary. Turn the patient's head to one side, with the emesis basin near the chin, for return of fluid.

(continues)

PROCEDURE **62** **CONTINUED**

12. Repeat steps 10 and 11 as necessary.

13. To floss the patient's teeth:

    a. Select a piece of dental floss about 12 inches long. Wrap the end of the floss around your middle fingers, leaving the center area free (Figure 25-4).

    b. Ask the patient to open their mouth. Gently insert the floss between each tooth down to, but not into, the gum line.

    c. Ask the patient to rinse their mouth using the emesis basin.

14. Offer the patient mouthwash. Dilute the mouthwash if the patient wishes.

15. Remove the basin. Wipe the patient's mouth and chin with tissue. Discard the tissue in a paper bag.

16. Remove the towel.

17. Rinse the toothbrush with water, cover, and store in top drawer of bedside stand or designated location.

18. Remove and discard gloves and mask. according to facility policy.

19. Carry out ending procedure actions.

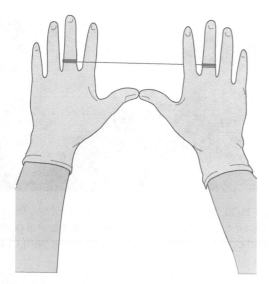

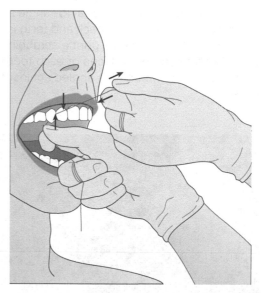

FIGURE 25-4 Wrap the floss around the middle fingers (left). Use the floss to clean between the teeth (right).

ICON KEY:

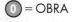 = OBRA   = PPE

 Culture **ALERT**

Many individuals have tongue piercings for fashion or cultural reasons (Figure 25-5). Many risks accompany this practice. Inform the nurse promptly if a patient with a tongue piercing has pain, bleeding, increased flow of saliva, swelling, or signs of infection in the mouth. Swelling of the tongue can become severe, closing off the airway.

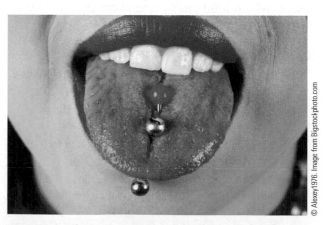

FIGURE 25-5 Serious complications can result from tongue piercings, including bleeding, airway obstruction, brain abscess, and death. Report complications to the nurse promptly.

DENTURES

Some patients have full sets of dentures. Other patients have partial plates that are removable, but attach by small metal clips to existing teeth. Partial plates should be given the same care as full dentures. **Dentures** are artificial teeth that are removable (Figure 25-6A). They must be cleaned. The patient may feel embarrassed about wearing dentures and may dislike being seen after the dentures have been removed. Always provide privacy when dentures are to be removed and cleaned (see Procedure 65). Some people have dental implants (Figure 25-6B). Most are permanent, but some are removable.

 Infection Control **ALERT**

Overall health is affected by a clean mouth. Studies have shown that providing thorough, regular oral hygiene reduces the risk of infection in elderly persons and those with a weakened immune system. Avoid sponge swabs if there is a risk that the patient may bite off or swallow the tip. Lemon–glycerin swabs are drying and should not be used frequently. The patient may complain of feeling thirsty after they are used. Mint-flavored sponge swabs are refreshing. The physician may order an artificial saliva product to increase patient comfort.

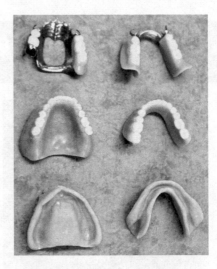

FIGURE 25-6A Assortment of dental appliances.

Denture Care

Denture care includes:

- Cleaning dentures daily under cool running water. Avoid hot water when caring for dentures
- Handling dentures carefully to prevent damage

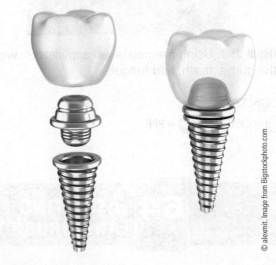

FIGURE 25-6B Dental implant.

© alexmit. Image from Bigstockphoto.com

PROCEDURE 63 ASSISTING WITH SPECIAL ORAL HYGIENE— Ⓞ Ⓟ DEPENDENT AND UNCONSCIOUS PATIENTS

 NOTE

Special oral hygiene is provided when the patient cannot actively participate in such care.

1. Carry out initial procedure actions.

2. Assemble equipment:
   - Disposable gloves
   - Sponge-tipped applicators or lemon–glycerin applicators
   - Emesis basin
   - 2 bath towels
   - Plastic bag
   - Premoistened applicators
   - Cotton swabs
   - Tissues
   - Tongue depressor
   - Water-based lubricant for lips
   - Laundry hamper

3. Put on gloves.

4. Cover pillow with a towel. If the patient is able to sit up, elevate the head of the bed. If the patient is unable or not permitted to sit up, turn the patient's

(continues)

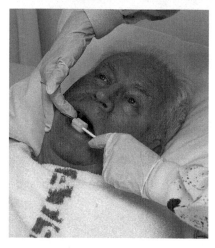

FIGURE 25-7 Using premoistened applicators, wipe the gums, teeth, and tongue.

ICON KEY:

 = OBRA   = PPE

head to one side and slightly forward so any excess fluid will not run down the throat. Cover the patient's upper chest with a towel. Place an emesis basin under the patient's chin.

5. Gently pull down on the chin to open the mouth, or open the mouth gently with a tongue depressor.

6. Using moistened sponge-tipped applicators, wipe gums, teeth, tongue, and the inside of the mouth (Figure 25-7).

7. Discard used applicators in a plastic bag.

8. Using clean cotton swabs, apply lubricant to the patient's lips. Place used swabs in a plastic bag.

9. Remove towels. Clean and replace equipment.

10. Remove and discard gloves. Wash your hands.

11. Carry out ending procedure actions.

PROCEDURE **64** ASSISTING THE PATIENT TO FLOSS AND BRUSH TEETH

1. Carry out initial procedure actions.

2. Assemble equipment:
   - Disposable gloves
   - Emesis basin
   - Toothbrush
   - Toothpaste
   - Dental floss
   - Glass of cool water
   - Straw
   - Mouthwash (if permitted)
   - Hand towel
   - Bed protector
   - Plastic bag
   - Laundry hamper

3. Elevate the head of the bed. Help the patient into a comfortable position.

4. Lower the side rails on the side where you are working, and position the overbed table across the patient's lap.

5. Cover the table with a bed protector.

6. Place the emesis basin and a glass of water on the overbed table.

7. Place a towel across the patient's chest.

8. Be prepared to assist, if needed. Remind the patient to clean the tongue and gums. Apply gloves and use standard precautions if you will be assisting.

9. After the patient has flossed and brushed teeth:
   a. Push the overbed table to the foot of the bed.
   b. Remove the emesis basin, clean it, and replace it.
   c. Rinse toothbrush.
   d. Remove the towels and put them with the soiled linens.
   e. Remove and discard gloves. Wash your hands.

10. Carry out ending procedure actions.

ICON KEY:

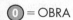 = OBRA   = PPE

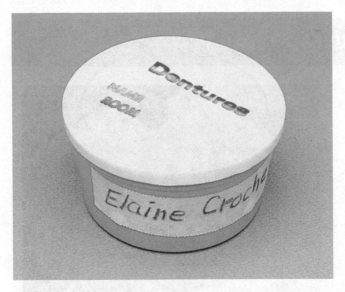

FIGURE 25-8 Dentures are stored in a cup of fresh water that is labeled with the patient's name.

- Storing dentures in a container in a safe place when they are out of the patient's mouth, such as in the drawer of the bedside stand. Label the denture cup with the patient's name (Figure 25-8)
- Brushing dentures daily. Soaking dentures in solution does not eliminate the need for daily brushing
- Changing the soaking solution and washing the denture cup daily. Rinse well. Store dry when not in use
- Rinsing dentures well before brushing under running water. Do not rinse them in standing water in the sink
- Brushing the tissues and gums in the mouth daily, even if the patient has no teeth. Use a soft-bristled brush to clean the mouth. This improves circulation and removes tartar and oral debris
- Cleaning and checking the patient's mouth for signs of irritation
- Checking the patient's lips for cracking and dryness
- Applying cream, petroleum jelly, or glycerin to lips to avoid excessive dryness

Age-Appropriate Care **ALERT**

Elderly patients may experience dry mouth and reduced saliva production. This is often a side effect of medications. Related complaints are burning or sore throat, difficulty in swallowing, hoarseness, and dry nasal passages. Saliva helps break down food for digestion and neutralizes acids in the mouth. Artificial saliva and medicated oral rinses may be ordered. The dentist may recommend sugar-free gum or candy to increase saliva production. Inform the nurse if the patient complains of a dry mouth.

Safety **ALERT**

Remove dentures from a comatose patient to prevent accidental airway obstruction by the denture. Remove dentures from patients preoperatively to prevent potential damage to the dentures and accidental airway obstruction in surgery.

Age-Appropriate Care **ALERT**

Dentures are made to fit tightly in the patient's mouth. Natural aging changes in the bones and gums may cause the shape of the patient's mouth to change over time. If dentures are loose or ill-fitting, chances are that this is because of aging-related changes to the mouth. Loose dentures can cause sores in the mouth, make eating difficult, and—in the worst case scenario—cause choking. Denture adhesive may be used temporarily, but is not a solution for ill-fitting dentures. If used, about three dots of adhesive per denture should be enough for most people. If a patient regularly needs more than this, the dentures may have to be refitted, and the person will need to be referred to a dentist. Inform the nurse if the patient's dentures hurt or do not fit correctly.

If you must place items such as the toothbrush, toothpaste, or dentures on the bathroom counter, put them on a clean paper towel. Never place them in the sink or on an unprotected countertop.

BACKRUBS

When properly given, backrubs can be:
- Stimulating to the patient's circulation
- A major aid in preventing skin breakdown (*pressure injuries*).
- Soothing and relaxing
- Refreshing

Keep your nails short to prevent injuring the patient. The backrub procedure provides a good opportunity for you to observe the condition of the patient's skin. Report all observations to the nurse. Look for:
- Reddened areas that do not blanch (whiten) when pressed
- Raw areas of skin
- Condition of skin over bony prominences

Unless contraindicated, the backrub is given:
- Routinely as part of the bed bath or partial bath
- Following use of the bedpan
- When changing the position of the helpless patient
- At bedtime
- When it could be a comfort to the patient

PROCEDURE **65** **CARING FOR DENTURES**

1. Carry out initial procedure actions.

2. Assemble equipment:
   - Disposable gloves
   - Tissues
   - Emesis basin
   - Tongue depressor
   - Toothbrush or denture brush (Figure 25-9)
   - Denture toothpaste or powder
   - Mouthwash, if permitted
   - Cup of water
   - Straw
   - Gauze squares
   - Applicators
   - Denture cup
   - Plastic bag

3. Apply disposable gloves.

4. Allow the patient to clean the dentures if they are able to do so. If the patient cannot, give a tissue to the patient and ask them to remove the dentures. Assist if necessary.

   a. To remove upper dentures, grasp the dentures firmly, ease them downward and then forward, and remove them from the mouth (Figure 25-10).

   b. To remove lower dentures, grasp the dentures firmly, ease them upward and then forward, and remove them from the mouth.

5. Place the dentures in a denture cup padded with gauze squares. Take them to the bathroom or utility room.

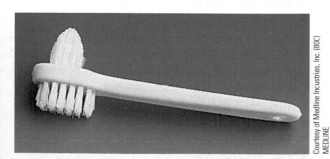

Courtesy of Medline Industries, Inc. (80C)
MEDLINE

FIGURE 25-9 The denture brush has a smaller head than a toothbrush. The back side has a tuft of bristles that works well for cleaning between teeth and in areas that are otherwise difficult to clean.

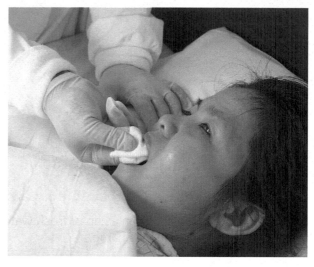

FIGURE 25-10 Grasp the upper dentures firmly with gauze-covered fingers to prevent slipping. Ease down and forward to remove.

6. Place a paper towel or washcloth in the bottom of the basin to protect the dentures. Fill the sink half full with cool water. The combination of water and towel protect the dentures from chipping or breaking if they are accidentally dropped in the sink.

7. Dentures may be soaked in a solution with a cleansing tablet before brushing, if desired.

8. Wet the dentures by rinsing under cool water.

9. Put toothpaste or tooth powder on a brush. Dentures are not as strong as regular teeth. Use a product that is meant for denture care. Otherwise, the product may scratch the surface of the dentures. If this occurs, the denture cannot be repaired. Hold the dentures firmly and brush until all surfaces are clean (Figure 25-11).

10. Rinse the dentures thoroughly under cool running water. Never use hot water. Rinse the denture cup.

11. Place fresh gauze squares in the denture cup with clean, cool water unless instructed otherwise.

12. Place the dentures in the gauze-lined cup and take them to the bedside.

13. Assist the patient to rinse their mouth with mouthwash, if permitted. Otherwise, use water. Hold the mouth open gently with a wooden tongue depressor. Clean the gums and tongue with applicators moistened with mouthwash, or use sponge-tipped applicators.

(continues)

PROCEDURE **65** CONTINUED

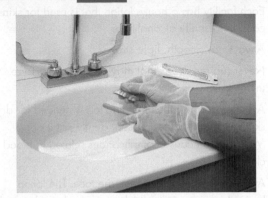

FIGURE 25-11 Brush dentures until all surfaces are clean.

ICON KEY:

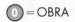 = OBRA = PPE

NOTE

Carefully observe and report the condition of the teeth, mouth, tongue, lips, and dentures.

14. Use a paper towel or gauze to hand wet dentures to the patient. If the patient is able, they can remove the dentures from the cup. Insert if necessary, upper denture first.
15. Clean and replace equipment.
16. Remove and discard gloves.
17. Carry out ending procedure actions.

DAILY SHAVING

Daily shaving is part of the routine self-care of most men. It should not be neglected in a health care facility. When patients cannot shave themselves, shaving is your responsibility.

Infection Control **ALERT**

Use only denture toothpaste or powder for brushing dentures. Regular toothpaste contains abrasives that scratch the surface of the denture, causing it to accumulate plaque and bacteria over time.

OSHA **ALERT**

When giving a backrub, elevate the bed to a comfortable height for you. Stand with one foot slightly ahead of the other, with knees bent slightly. Use your arm and shoulder muscles to massage the back. Rock back and forth, using the strong muscles in your legs. Avoid bending from the waist.

Safety **ALERT**

Health care workers have known for years that if swallowed, denture cleaning tablets can cause serious injury to a confused or pediatric patient. The fizzing, foaming action of the tablet causes burns of the mucous membranes in the mouth, throat, esophagus, and stomach. In 2005, new information was published about the ingestion and systemic absorption of denture adhesive paste. Zinc is used in the paste as a bonding agent and odor blocker. It is not always listed on the label. There is a risk of zinc toxicity with ingestion of denture paste if swallowed. Keep all denture cleaners and paste preparations out of the hands of those who are confused, as well as others (such as a patient who is having suicidal ideations) who may ingest them.

Difficult Situations

For many years, backrubs were an almost sacred, routine part of nursing care. Over time, we have become much more dependent on technology. When we are busy or staffing is short, it seems as if there is no time to give backrubs. Yet, calming the agitated patient who cannot sleep is time-consuming; the pregnant mother with a backache may use the call signal frequently; the patient with spasticity just cannot get into a comfortable position.

You may find that taking a few minutes to give a backrub will save you a great deal of time in caring for your patients. A good backrub is comforting and relaxing. Agitated patients often calm down. Uncomfortable patients become more comfortable and demand less attention. Do not omit this important part of nursing care that pays such large dividends in patient comfort and satisfaction. In the long run, it may even make your job easier.

Long, smooth strokes are relaxing. Short, circular strokes tend to be more stimulating. Avoid massaging red areas over bony prominences.

GUIDELINES 25-1 Guidelines for Applying Lotion to the Patient's Skin

- Massaging the patient's skin is comforting and refreshing. It stimulates circulation and helps prevent skin breakdown.

- Warm the lotion in a basin of warm water or the palm of your hand.

- Refer to the care plan to see if massage is indicated.

- Applying lotion immediately after the bath helps hold moisture in the skin.

- Patients who are elderly and those with very dry, fragile skin will benefit from an application of lotion several times a day to keep skin supple and more resistant to injury.

- Each facility has a house lotion that is used for skin care. It is usually alcohol-free.

- Always use smooth, light strokes.

- Never rub red areas that may be stage I pressure injuries.

- Avoid massaging the legs. If lotion is needed for dry skin or for some other reason, gently pat it on. Massage can cause complications related to blood clots.

- Avoid putting lotion between the toes. The lotion keeps the area moist, which promotes fungal growth.

PROCEDURE 66 PROVIDING BACKRUBS

1. Carry out initial procedure actions.
2. Assemble equipment:
   - Disposable gloves
   - Basin of water (105°F)
   - Washcloth
   - Bath towel
   - Soap and lotion
3. Put up the far side rails.
4. Place the lotion container in a basin of water to warm.
5. Put on disposable gloves if the patient has open lesions.
6. Turn the patient on the side with the back toward you.
7. Expose and wash the back; dry carefully. This step is not necessary if the backrub is given after a bath.
8. Pour a small amount of lotion into one hand and warm it in the palm of your hand. Cold lotion may be very uncomfortable for the patient.
9. Apply the lotion to the patient's skin and rub with gentle but firm strokes. Give special attention to all bony prominences. Do not rub red areas. Report these to the nurse, if noted.
10. Review the strokes in Figure 25-12. Begin at the base of the spine:
    - With long, soothing strokes, rub up the center of the back, around the shoulders, and down the sides of the back and buttocks.
    - Repeat the previous step four times, using long, soothing upward strokes and a circular motion on the downstroke.

    - Repeat, but on the downward stroke rub in small circular motions with the palm of your hand. Include areas over the coccyx (base of the spine).
    - Repeat long, soothing strokes on muscles for three to five minutes.
    - Dry the area well.
    - If redness on bony prominences is noted, notify the nurse. Straighten and tighten the bottom sheet and draw sheet.
11. Change the patient's gown, if necessary.
12. Remove and discard gloves if used. Wash your hands.
13. Replace equipment.
14. Carry out ending procedure actions.

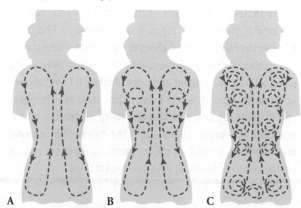

FIGURE 25-12 Strokes to be used during the backrub: A. soothing strokes; B. circular movement; C. passive movement.

Infection Control **ALERT**

Shaving may be done with an electric razor that is the patient's personal property. Such a razor is used for one patient only and cleaned according to manufacturer's directions after use by brushing the heads with a small brush designed for this purpose. Remove all hair from the shaver head. Some battery-operated electric razors must be recharged periodically. Electric razors are expensive. Handle the razor carefully and avoid dropping it. Wearing gloves is not necessary when an electric razor is used.

Age-Appropriate Care **ALERT**

Elderly women may grow facial hair as a result of hormonal changes during aging. Coarse hair is common on the chin. Body hair thins and becomes sparse. Most women prefer to have facial hair removed. Most also remove hair from the legs and underarms. Honor the patient's preferences. Know your facility's policy for removing facial hair from female patients. Check with the nurse before shaving a female because it may cause the hair to become thicker and coarser. Some facilities use depilatories (chemical products that remove hair).

⚠ OSHA **ALERT**

Because of the high risk of contact with blood, always wear gloves when shaving patients with a nonelectric razor. Discard the razor in a puncture-resistant (sharps) container.

Older women have an increase in the growth and coarseness of hairs on the chin and upper lip. Many women find this distressing. Tweezers can be used to remove some of the hairs, but having the hairs removed professionally is a more permanent method. Some women may require a daily shave. In some facilities nursing assistants are not permitted to shave female patients' faces. Check the policy of your facility.

DAILY HAIR CARE

Daily care of the hair, for both male and female patients, is usually done after the patient's bath.

Comb and brush the hair each morning. Tangles can be loosened by sectioning the hair with a comb or brush and then working with one section at a time. Grasp the hair near the scalp to reduce pulling (Figure 25-14). Start combing or brushing tangles out starting at the ends and working toward the scalp. Braiding long hair after brushing can help reduce tangles. Tangles can be reduced in dry, wiry hair by using conditioner and keeping the hair short or in braids.

NOTE

Avoid braiding a patient's hair tightly, because it can be uncomfortable. Secure the braids with hair ties. Avoid rubber bands, if possible. If the hair is very tangled, applying a small amount of alcohol or oil to the tangle will make it easier to remove.

Brushing the hair:
- Stimulates circulation of the scalp
- Refreshes the patient
- Removes dust and lint
- Helps to keep the hair shiny and attractive

Wash the patient's hair at the frequency specified by the care plan.

Procedure 68 assumes that the patient is a female. Hair care for a male is very similar, however, so the procedure can easily be adapted.

GUIDELINES 25-2 Guidelines for Safety in Shaving

- Use the patient's own shaving equipment if possible. For safety, use an electric razor or rotary razor.
- Check with the nurse before shaving a person who is taking **anticoagulants** (medications that thin the blood and increase the risk of bleeding).
- Consult the nurse before shaving a person who is using oxygen. Never use an electric razor with such a patient.
- The patient may use a preshave or aftershave product as desired. Keep these products out of the hands of patients who may swallow them.

EXPAND YOUR SKILLS

PROCEDURE 67　SHAVING A MALE PATIENT　

1. Carry out initial procedure actions.
2. Assemble equipment:
   - Disposable gloves
   - Electric shaver or safety razor
   - Shaving lather or preshave lotion (for electric razor)
   - Basin of water (105°F)
   - Face towels
   - Mirror
   - Washcloth
   - Aftershave lotion
   - Plastic bag
   - Facial tissues
3. Raise the head of the bed. Place equipment on the overbed table.
4. Put on gloves.
5. Place one face towel across the patient's chest and one under his head.
6. Moisten face and apply lather (or preshave lotion).
7. Starting in front of one ear:
   a. Hold skin taut and bring razor down over cheek toward chin (Figure 25-13).
   b. Repeat until lather on cheek is removed and area has been shaved. Rinse frequently.
   c. Repeat on the other cheek.
   d. Use firm, short strokes. Shave in the direction of hair growth.
   e. Rinse razor frequently.
8. Ask the patient to tighten his upper lip. Shave from the nose to the upper lip in short downward strokes.
9. Ask the patient to tighten his chin. Shave the chin in downward strokes.
10. Assist the patient to tip his head back.
11. Lather the neck area and stroke up toward the chin. Rinse and repeat until all lather is removed.
12. Wash the patient's face and neck and dry thoroughly.
13. Apply aftershave lotion if desired.
14. If the skin is nicked, apply a small piece of tissue and hold pressure directly over the area with your gloved hand. Then apply an antiseptic and bandage. Notify the nurse.
15. Clean and replace equipment. Discard disposable razor in the sharps container. Remove the head of electric razor. Use a razor brush to remove clippings. Store the razor in the top drawer of the nightstand, away from the toothbrush.
16. Remove and discard gloves.
17. Carry out ending procedure actions.

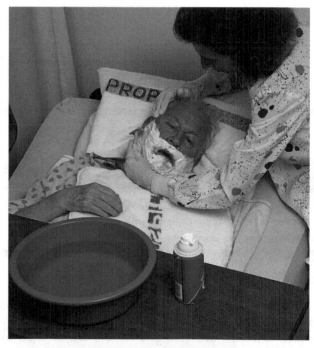

FIGURE 25-13 Shaving is part of the daily routine for most men. Hold the skin taut while using downward strokes.

ICON KEY:
 – OBRA　 = PPE

Patients may have different hair care needs. Asking the patient or family how to care for the hair is not offensive; they are experts at it. They also know which products work and which do not. Asking for their advice shows that you care about meeting the patient's needs.

COMFORT DEVICES

The physician, nurse, or physical therapist orders comfort devices such as bed cradles, footboards, and pillows (see Chapter 15) to relieve pressure on specific areas or to help maintain body position.

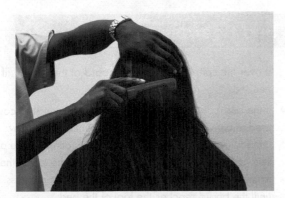

FIGURE 25-14 To remove tangles, divide the hair into sections. Work with one section at a time. Hold the hair near the scalp to reduce pulling. Start combing at the end of the hair, working up toward the scalp.

Difficult Situations

Hair is important to many people's self-esteem and appearance. Some diseases and medications cause hair loss (Figure 25-15). Some cause changes to the volume and texture of hair. Some medications cause hair to become dry and brittle. Patients who have problems with their hair may become anxious or angry because the appearance of the hair affects their self-esteem. If the patient is experiencing problems with hair, treat it gently. Brush the hair to remove tangles before washing. Use products such as baby shampoo and conditioner. Use tepid water. Pat the hair dry rather than rubbing it with a towel. Do not brush wet hair. Use a wide-toothed comb or pick to style wet hair gently. Avoid rubber bands, which may worsen the problem. Assist the patient to wear a scarf or turban, if desired.

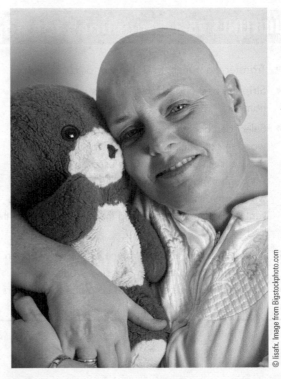

FIGURE 25-15 This patient has lost her hair because of chemotherapy for breast cancer.

Bed Boards

Bed boards are used to make the mattress firm, and are occasionally ordered for persons with back problems. They are placed under the mattress. A physician's order is needed to apply them to the bed.

Bed Cradle

A bed cradle (see Chapter 15) prevents the weight of the bedclothes from falling on a specific part of the body. It

PROCEDURE **68** **PROVIDING DAILY HAIR CARE**

1. Carry out initial procedure actions.

2. Assemble equipment:
   - Towel
   - Comb and brush

3. Ask the patient to move to the side of the bed nearest you; or the patient may sit in a chair if permitted. If the patient is sitting up, put a towel around their shoulders.

4. Cover the pillow with a towel.

5. Part or section the hair and comb with one hand between the scalp and the ends of the hair.

6. Brush carefully and thoroughly.

7. Have the patient turn so that you can comb and brush the hair on the back of their head. If the hair is tangled, work section by section to remove the tangles, beginning near the ends and working toward the scalp.

8. Complete brushing and arrange the hair attractively. Braid long hair to prevent repeated tangling. Allow the patient to choose the style, if able.

9. Clean and replace equipment.

10. Carry out ending procedure actions.

ICON KEY:

 = OBRA

GUIDELINES 25-3 Guidelines for Applying Bed Boards

- Transfer the patient to a stretcher or chair.
- Strip the bed and place the linens in a laundry hamper.
- Select bed boards that are hinged or made from wooden slats similar to straw or wooden window shades, such as those that are used on a sun porch. Although it may seem as if a solid piece of plywood would serve the same purpose, the wood would prevent the patient from elevating the head and foot of the bed.
- If the bed board is a multipiece or hinged wooden frame, lift the mattress on one side while another worker slides the bed board into place and centers it over the springs. Unfold the board at the hinges, if needed.
- If the bed board is made from many wooden slats covered in canvas, it will be rolled up similar to a straw window shade. Lift the top end of the mattress while a second worker centers the bed board at the top of the frame. Unroll the bed board while lifting the mattress until the board reaches the foot of the bed.
- Check to be sure the bed board or slats do not protrude from the sides, top, or bottom of the bed, as they may cause injury.
- Make the bed with clean linens and assist the patient to return to bed.

can be used therapeutically or as a comfort device. It can be used:

- Over fractured limbs
- When there are burns
- To prevent skin lesions
- Over widespread skin conditions, such as psoriasis or eczema
- To prevent contractures of the feet
- Over a wet cast until it dries

Coverings that maintain some degree of warmth within the cradle may also be needed to keep the patient comfortable. Be sure to position the limbs in good alignment within the cradle.

Footboard or Footrest

The **footboard** or *footrest* is a device placed between the mattress and bed to keep the feet at right angles to the legs (natural standing position) (see Chapter 15). A footboard is always padded. It is used to prevent a type of contracture called **foot drop**. In foot drop, the leg's calf muscle tends to tighten, causing the toes to point downward (Figure 25-16). Foot drop may happen when the patient must remain in bed over a long period of time. Even a brief period in bed can cause a degree of foot drop that makes walking difficult when the patient does get out of bed.

If a footboard is not available, a pillow folded lengthwise may be placed against the foot of the bed to serve the same purpose. Some facilities use special tennis shoes or soft boots (see Chapter 15) to prevent foot drop in patients who are at risk because they are bedfast.

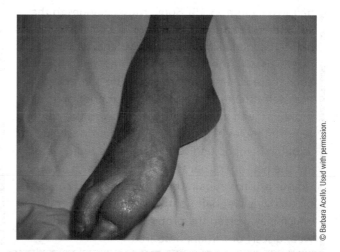

FIGURE 25-16 This patient has foot drop, as evidenced by the toes resting on the bed instead of pointing up toward the ceiling.

Pillows and Bath Blankets

Pillows can be used as comfort devices and to maintain alignment when properly arranged. For directions on positioning the patient in good alignment, refer to Chapter 15.

The trochanter roll helps prevent external rotation of the hip (Figure 25-17A). Trochanter rolls should be used routinely to help prevent deformities in patients who are bedfast. Unless a specific medical condition, such as a hip fracture, is present, no special order is needed.

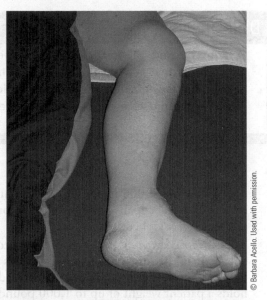

FIGURE 25-17A External rotation of the hip. The toes point to the side instead of the ceiling.

A trochanter roll or support can be made as follows:

1. Fold a bath blanket lengthwise in thirds.
2. Position the patient in the center of the folded bath blanket. The blanket should extend from mid-thigh to above the waist.

3. Roll each side of the blanket under and toward the patient until the blanket roll is firmly against the patient. Then tuck the roll inward toward the bed and patient to maintain the patient's position (Figure 25-17B).

Pillows are also used to relieve pressure in such a way that spaces are left for specific areas. This technique is called **bridging**. Bridging elevates an area of the body off the surface of the bed. It is useful for patients with healing pressure injuries.

Bridging is commonly used for the sacrum, hips, heels, and ankles. No special equipment is necessary. Facilities may use a combination of pillows, foam props, and bath blankets to support an area.

ELIMINATION NEEDS

Regular, periodic elimination of body wastes is essential for maintaining health. Patients who are confined to bed must rely on you to help them with this physical task (see Procedures 69 to 71). You should know that:

- The patient must regularly empty the bladder by urinating (voiding).
- A urinal (duct or bottle) is used by male patients when they need to urinate. A bedpan is used by female patients to void when they are confined to bed.
- A regular bowel movement (which is the discharge of solid waste from the body; see Chapter 44) is also important to a patient's health.

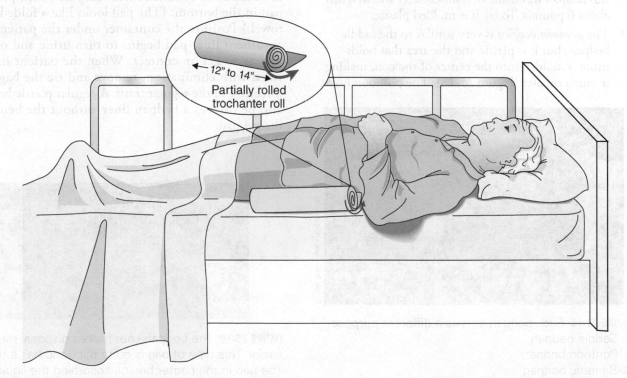

12" to 14"
Partially rolled
trochanter roll

FIGURE 25-17B The trochanter roll should extend from the hip to just above the knee. Partially rolled trochanter roll.

- The solid waste produced by the patient is called **feces** or *stool*.
- Both male and female patients use a bedpan for solid waste elimination when confined to bed.
- Many patients are somewhat sensitive about using a bedpan or urinal.
- Personal hygiene is exceedingly important when carrying out these procedures properly.
- Bedpans are very uncomfortable.
- Pushing with sufficient force to empty the rectum is very difficult when lying on the back. Elevating the head as much as possible is helpful.

Keep these four important points in mind. You must:

- Wear disposable gloves.
- Wash your hands immediately before and after the procedure. This will help prevent the transmission of any disease to others and to yourself.
- Provide privacy for the patient. Obtain the proper type of bedpan according to patient needs.
- As soon as possible, answer the light indicating that the patient is finished.

Bedpans

Four types of bedpans are commonly used in health care facilities to meet patients' needs.

- The *saddle bedpan* is the oldest design (Figure 25-18). The inside is hollow and holds a large amount of liquid (about 1,500 mL) without spilling. At one time this bedpan was made of stainless steel and weighed about 6 pounds. Today it is molded plastic.
- The *pontoon bedpan* is very similar to the saddle bedpan, but it is plastic and the area that holds urine is molded into the center of the pan, making it much smaller (Figure 25-18). The pontoon holds

Difficult Situations

A light dusting of powder on the edges of the bedpan that contact the patient's skin will reduce friction, making the bedpan easier to insert and remove, especially if the patient is obese.

only 800 mL to 1,000 mL of liquid without spilling. These two bedpans (saddle and pontoon) are also called *regular* bedpans.

- The *bariatric bedpan* is probably the most comfortable bedpan. Because of this, some facilities use this type of bedpan exclusively. The bariatric bedpan holds a patient weight of up to 1,000 pounds and will hold about 1,500 mL of liquid. Position the flat side of the bedpan under the coccyx.
- The *fracture bedpan* (Figure 25-18) is used for patients who cannot elevate the pelvic area, such as those with a hip or pelvic fracture. It is positioned under the perineum, with the handle on the end closest to the knees. It holds only about 500 mL of liquid without spilling.

Bedpan and Commode Liners

Bedpan liners (Figure 25-19) are popular in home health care, but are also used in some facilities. Cover the bedpan or commode with the liner, then place the pad in the bottom. (The pad looks like a folded paper towel.) Position the container under the patient. The absorbent liner pad begins to turn urine and organic matter to gel on contact. When the patient has finished with elimination, remove and tie the bag, then discard it in the regular trash. A regular plastic bag may also be used as a bedpan liner without the benefit of the gel pad.

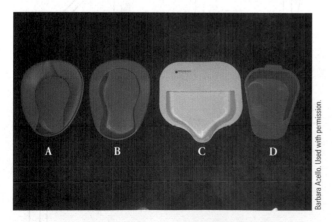

FIGURE 25-18 Each bedpan serves a different purpose.
A. Saddle bedpan
B. Pontoon bedpan
C. Bariatric bedpan
D. Fracture bedpan

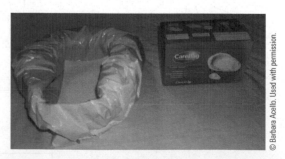

FIGURE 25-19 The bedpan liner makes disposal much easier. This type of bag is quite thick and has a tie top. The pad in the center begins absorbing the liquid and turning it to gel right away.

Make sure that bedpans and urinals are labeled with the patients' names for patients in rooms with two or more beds. After cleaning the bedpan or urinal, store it properly in the bedside stand or according to facility policy. Do not leave uncovered bedpans and urinals on the floor or in the bathroom.

One-Glove Technique

The one-glove technique prevents environmental contamination when carrying bedpans, urinals, and other contaminated items. Cover the item before carrying it to the bathroom or into the hallway. Remove the glove from one hand and hold it in the palm of your gloved hand. Use the gloved hand to carry the contaminated item. Use the ungloved hand to open doors and turn on faucets. By using this method, you avoid contaminating the environment with your gloves.

PROCEDURE **69**   **GIVING AND RECEIVING THE BEDPAN**

1. Carry out initial procedure actions.

2. Assemble equipment:
   - Disposable gloves
   - Bedpan and cover
   - Basin
   - Washcloth
   - Bath blanket
   - Paper towels/bed protector
   - Toilet tissue
   - Soap
   - Towel
   - Plastic bag

3. Lower the head of the bed, if necessary.

4. Put on gloves.

5. Take the bedpan and toilet tissue from the bedside stand.
   - Place a protector on the chair. Place the bedpan on it.
   - Never place a bedpan on the bedside stand or overbed table.
   - Put the remainder of the articles on the bedside table.

6. Place the bedpan cover at the foot of the bed.

   Never carry or allow a used bedpan to sit uncovered. If a bedpan cover is not available, cover the bedpan with a towel, bed protector, newspaper, plastic or paper bag, or paper towels (Figure 25-20). This is more sanitary and markedly reduces odors in the room.

7. Cover the patient with a bath blanket. Fold the top bedcovers back at a right angle. Raise the patient's gown. If the patient is thin or has a pressure sore, consult the nurse for the appropriate action.

8. Ask the patient to flex the knees and rest weight on the heels, if able.

9. Help the patient to raise the buttocks by:
   - Putting one hand under the small of the patient's back and lifting gently and slowly with that hand.
   - With the other hand, place the bedpan under the patient's hips.

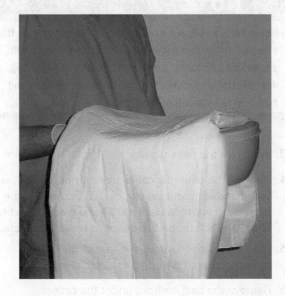

FIGURE 25-20 This bedpan is covered with a bed protector.

(continues)

PROCEDURE **69** CONTINUED   **O**   **P**

– The pan may also be placed by rolling the patient to one side, positioning the bedpan against the buttocks, and rolling the patient back onto the pan (Figure 25-21A). Check to be sure the bedpan is positioned properly.

– Alternatively, if a trapeze is in place over the bed, place the bedpan under the patient as the patient uses the trapeze to help lift the hips (Figure 25-21B).

– The patient's buttocks should rest on the rounded shelf of the regular bedpan.

– The narrow end should face the foot of the bed. If a fracture pan is being used, the narrow end is positioned under the patient's buttocks, with the handle end facing the foot of the bed.

– Place the flat end of the bariatric bedpan under the coccyx.

10. Replace the top bedcovers. Raise the head of the bed to a comfortable height. Remove gloves and dispose of them properly.

11. Make sure the toilet paper and signal cord are within easy reach of the patient. Leave the patient alone unless contraindicated in the nursing care plan.

12. Wash your hands.

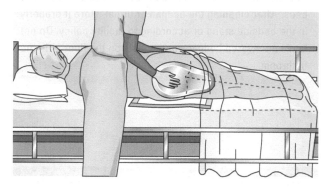

FIGURE 25-21A Roll the patient away from you. Provide support by placing one hand on the hip. Position the bedpan with the other hand, and then roll the patient back onto the bedpan.

> ✒️ **NOTE**
>
> Never carry or allow a used bedpan to sit uncovered. If a bedpan cover is not available, cover the bedpan with a towel, bed protector, newspaper, plastic or paper bag, or paper towels (Figure 25-20). This is more sanitary and markedly reduces odors in the room.

13. Watch for the patient's signal.

14. Answer the patient's call signal immediately. Wash your hands and put on disposable gloves. Fill the basin with warm water (105°F) and place it next to soap, washcloth, and towel on the overbed table.

15. Fold the top bedcovers back so that the patient remains covered only with the bath blanket.

16. Remove the bedpan from under the patient.

– Ask the patient to flex the knees and rest weight on the heels. Place one hand under the small

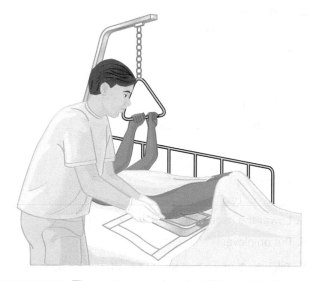

FIGURE 25-21B The patient assists by lifting with the trapeze as the bedpan is being placed. Support the small of the patient's back with one hand as the patient pulls up on the trapeze.

of the back and lift gently to help raise the buttocks off the bedpan. Remove the bedpan with the other hand. Cover it and place it on the chair.

– If the patient is unable to raise the buttocks, roll the patient off the pan to the side and remove the pan. Lift and move carefully. Hold the pan firmly with one hand (Figure 25-21C).

– Assist with peri care as needed.

(continues)

17. If the bed protector is wet, change it. Provide perineal care.

- Discard used toilet tissue in the bedpan unless a specimen is to be collected.

- Cover the bedpan again.

- Cleanse the patient with warm water and soap, if necessary.

18. Replace the bedclothes, changing linens as necessary.

19. Cover the patient with top bedding and remove the bath blanket.

20. Assist the patient to wash hands and freshen up after the procedure. An antiseptic hand rub or alcohol product may be used, if desired.

21. Cover the bedpan and take it to the bathroom or utility room and observe its contents. Some facilities use bedpans with self-fitting lids (Figure 25-21D).

22. Measure the urine, if required. Empty the bedpan. (Do not empty if you observe anything unusual (such as blood). Save the contents for the nurse's inspection; see Chapter 45.)

23. Turn on the faucet, using a paper towel. Rinse the bedpan with cold water and disinfectant. Rinse, dry, and return the bedpan to storage in the patient's bedside stand.

24. Remove gloves and dispose of them properly. Wash your hands.

25. Carry out ending procedure actions.

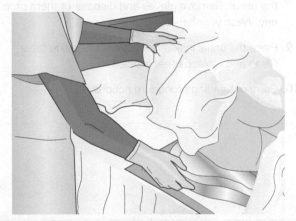

FIGURE 25-21C Hold the bedpan securely while the patient turns to the side.

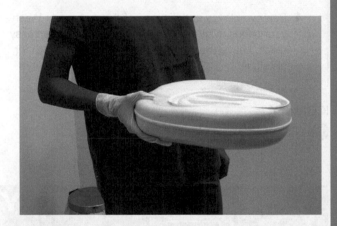

FIGURE 25-21D Always cover the full bedpan. This bedpan has a disposable lid that fits securely.

ICON KEY:

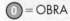 = OBRA   = PPE

EXPAND YOUR SKILLS

PROCEDURE **70**   GIVING AND RECEIVING THE URINAL

1. Carry out initial procedure actions.

2. Assemble equipment:

- Urinal (Figure 25-22)
- Basin
- Soap

- Washcloth
- Towel
- Disposable gloves

3. Put on gloves. Lift the top bedcovers and place the urinal under the covers so the patient can grasp the

(continues)

PROCEDURE 70 CONTINUED

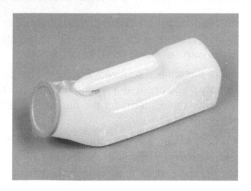

FIGURE 25-22 A male urinal with a snap-on lid.

handle. Instruct the patient to place his penis in the urinal opening. If he cannot do this, you must position the urinal and place the penis in the opening.

4. Remove gloves and dispose of them properly. Wash your hands. Make sure the signal cord is within easy reach. Leave the patient alone if possible. Watch for his signal.

5. Answer the signal promptly. Put on gloves. Ask the patient to hand the urinal to you. Cover it.

6. Rearrange the bedclothes if necessary. Fill a basin with warm water (105°F), and place it next to soap, washcloth, and towel so the patient can wash and dry his hands.

7. Take the urinal to the bathroom or utility room and observe the contents. Measure, if required. Do not empty the urinal if you observe anything unusual (such as blood). Save the contents of the urinal for the nurse's inspection (see Chapter 45).

8. Empty the urinal. Rinse the urinal with cold water and clean it with warm soapy water. Rinse, dry, and cover the urinal. Remove gloves and dispose of them properly. Wash your hands.

9. Place the urinal inside the patient's bedside table. Clean and replace other articles.

10. Carry out ending procedure actions.

ICON KEY:

 = PPE

EXPAND YOUR SKILLS

PROCEDURE 71 ASSISTING WITH USE OF THE BEDSIDE COMMODE

1. Carry out initial procedure actions.

2. Assemble equipment:
   - Disposable gloves
   - Portable commode
   - Toilet tissue
   - Basin
   - Washcloth
   - Soap
   - Towel
   - Bath blanket

3. Position the commode beside the bed, facing the head. Lock the commode wheels and open the lid. Be sure a receptacle is in place under the seat.

4. If the bed and side rails are elevated, lower the side rails nearest you and lower the bed to the lowest horizontal position. Lock bed wheels.

5. Put on gloves.

6. Assist the patient to a sitting position. Swing the patient's legs over the edge of the bed.

(continues)

7. Assist the patient to put on a robe and slippers. Assist the patient to stand. If needed, use a transfer belt.

8. Support the patient with hands on either side of the chest. Remember to use proper body mechanics. Pivot the patient and lower their to the commode.

9. Cover the patient's legs with a bath blanket.

10. Leave the call bell and toilet tissue within reach.

11. Remove and discard gloves.

12. When the patient signals, return promptly. Wash your hands and put on gloves. Fill a basin with water at 105°F. Bring the basin to the bedside along with soap, a towel, and a washcloth.

13. Remove the bath blanket. Assist the patient to stand.

14. Cleanse the anus and perineum if the patient is unable to do so.

15. Allow the patient to wash and dry their hands. Remove and discard gloves. Wash your hands.

16. Assist the patient to return to bed. Adjust bedding and pillows for comfort.

17. Leave the signal cord within easy reach.

18. Put on gloves.

19. Remove the receptacle from the commode and cover it. Close the commode lid.

20. Take the receptacle to the bathroom. Note its contents and measure if required.

21. Empty and clean the receptacle per facility policy. Replace it in the commode. Remove and dispose of gloves properly.

22. Put the commode in its proper place.

23. Carry out ending procedure actions.

ICON KEY:
 O = OBRA   **P** = PPE

REVIEW

A. True/False

Mark the following true or false by circling T or F.

1. T F   Store dentures in an antiseptic solution.

2. T F   Backrubs should be routinely given as part of the bath procedure.

3. T F   A padded footboard is one method of preventing foot drop.

4. T F   Routine oral hygiene should be carried out one or more times daily.

5. T F   Proper oral hygiene helps prevent tooth decay.

6. T F   Store the denture cup on the back of the sink.

7. T F   Patients who have no teeth and no dentures require regular oral hygiene.

8. T F   When giving p.m. care, tighten the bottom sheet and straighten the top linens.

9. T F   Wear gloves when giving oral care.

10. T F   The patient who is unconscious needs no oral care because they are not eating.

B. Matching

Choose the correct word(s) from Column II to match the phrases in Column I.

Column I

11. _____ bad breath

12. _____ mouth care

13. _____ tooth cavities

14. _____ means of relieving pressure

15. _____ artificial teeth

Column II

a. oral hygiene

b. caries

c. dentures

d. bridging

e. halitosis

f. foot drop

C. Completion

Complete the statements by writing the correct word from the following list.

arm   name

breakfast   p.m. care

down   removed

early a.m. care   surgery

hand

16. After p.m. care, the bed should be left with the backrest _____.

17. _____ should be completed before sleep medication is given.

18. The best way to awaken a patient is to place your _____ on the patient's arm and say their _____.

19. Patients are not wakened early if they are going to have _____.

20. Early morning care awakens the patient before _____.

D. Multiple Choice

Select the best answer for each of the following.

21. Which of the following patients should be given special mouth care?

   a. One who can brush their own teeth

   b. One who is drinking water ad lib

   c. One who has a broken leg

   d. One who has a nasogastric tube

22. To warm lotion before giving a backrub:

   a. hold it under running water.

   b. soak it in a basin of warm water.

   c. let the patient hold the bottle for a few minutes.

   d. microwave the bottle for 15 seconds.

23. The best way to support a patient in a side-lying position is to:

   a. use a footboard to keep the feet aligned.

   b. place a pillow doubled under the head.

   c. place two pillows lengthwise between the legs.

   d. double a pillow lengthwise behind the back.

24. The best technique for toothbrushing includes:

   a. inserting the toothbrush with the bristles down.

   b. scrubbing the outer surface well and avoiding the sensitive inner surface.

   c. inserting the toothbrush with bristles facing the teeth.

   d. brushing the teeth in a downward motion only.

25. Backrubs are given:

   a. routinely as a comfort measure.

   b. before use of the bedpan.

   c. routinely every two hours.

   d. only for patients with red areas.

26. Mrs. Menendez will be admitted to your unit from the emergency department with congestive heart failure. The doctor has ordered bedrest. The patient weighs 473 pounds. She is very weak and needs a bed bath. She has bowel and bladder control and requires assistance with elimination. Intake and output have been ordered. When you set up the unit, you will bring:

   a. emesis basin, washbasin, bariatric bedpan.

   b. commode, washbasin, urinal.

   c. pontoon bedpan, emesis basin, washbasin.

   d. washbasin, fracture bedpan, emesis basin.

27. The fracture bedpan:

   a. holds about 1,000 mL.

   b. is used when a specimen is needed.

   c. is used for persons who cannot elevate the hips.

   d. is positioned with the handle under the coccyx.

28. Bed boards are used:

   a. to reduce the risk of skin breakdown.

   b. for patients with back problems.

   c. when the mattress is worn out.

   d. to reduce the risk of entrapment in rails.

29. Mr. Hernandez has tremors of the hands and cannot shave himself. He has heavy growth of facial hair. The assignment sheet lists "daily shave" as a nursing assistant responsibility. You should:

   a. Set up equipment so the patient can shave himself.

   b. Shave the patient as part of his ADL care.

   c. Ask the patient's wife to shave him when she visits.

   d. Ask Mr. Hernandez if he prefers to grow a beard.

30. The nurse asks you to shave Mr. Hernandez with a disposable razor. You will:

   a. shave in the direction opposite that of hair growth.

   b. use upward strokes when shaving the chin.

   c. hold skin taut and use short, firm downward strokes.

   d. wipe the razor with a tissue when it fills with hair.

31. The patient's hair is very tangled. The nursing assistant should:

   a. Section the hair. Using a comb, work from top to bottom.

   b. Cut the tangle as close to the scalp as possible with scissors.

   c. Coat the hair with shampoo and let it soak for 30 minutes.

   d. Applying alcohol or oil to the tangled area makes it easier to remove.

32. Daily haircare is important for:

   a. maintaining self-esteem.

   b. absorbing medication.

   c. preventing dandruff.

   d. reducing itching

33. Feces is:

   a. elimination from the urinary tract.

   b. a liquid substance from the bladder.

   c. a solid waste that may also be called stool.

   d. undigested food from the stomach.

34. When a patient is bedfast, solid waste elimination is usually done by using a/an:

   a. toilet

   b. urinal

   c. catheter

   d. bedpan

35. Foot Drop

   a. is a goal for bedfast patients.

   b. makes walking much easier.

   c. occurs when if the leg is straight.

   d. is a type of contracture.

E. Nursing Assistant Challenge

Your patient, Mrs. Ubanan, has a history of heavy smoking and breathes through her mouth. She has plastic dentures and her care plan indicates that she needs assistance with denture care. Complete the following statements regarding this patient.

36. State two reasons special oral hygiene has been ordered for Mrs. Ubanan.

   a. _____

   b. _____

37. Where are the dentures stored when not in use?

   _____

38. Should the dentures be stored dry or wet?

   _____

39. Should you wear gloves when removing her dentures?

   _____

40. Will you clean the dentures in cool or hot water?

   _____

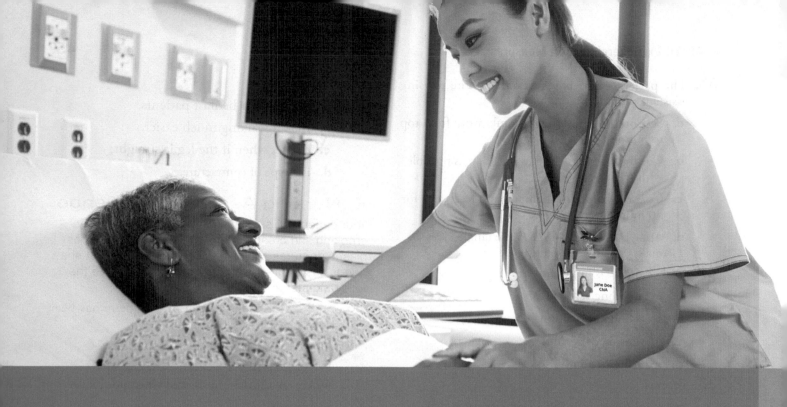

SECTION 8

Principles of Nutrition and Fluid Balance

CHAPTER 26
Nutritional Needs and Diet Modifications

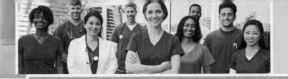

Nutritional Needs and Diet Modifications

OBJECTIVES

After completing this chapter, you will be able to:

26.1 Spell and define terms.

26.2 Define normal nutrition.

26.3 List the essential nutrients.

26.4 Name the food groups and list the foods included in each group.

26.5 Identify the basic facility diets and describe each.

26.6 State the purposes of the following diets:
- Clear liquid
- Full liquid
- Soft
- Mechanically altered

26.7 State the purpose of calorie counts and food intake studies.

26.8 Define dysphagia and explain the risks of this condition.

26.9 Describe general care for the patient with dysphagia and swallowing problems.

26.10 State the purposes of therapeutic diets.

26.11 List types of alternative nutrition.

26.12 Describe the nursing assistant actions when patients are unable to drink fluids independently.

26.13 Demonstrate the following procedures:
- Procedure 72: Assisting the Patient Who Can Feed Self
- Procedure 73: Feeding the Dependent Patient
- Procedure 74: Abdominal Thrusts—Heimlich Maneuver

VOCABULARY

Learn the meaning and the correct spelling of the following words and phrases:

amino acids
aspiration
carbohydrates
cellulose
clear liquid diet
consistent carbohydrate
(CHO) diet
defecation
dehydration
diaphoresis
digestion
diuresis
dysphagia

edema
emesis
enteral feeding
essential nutrients
exchange list
excrete
fats
fluid balance
force fluids
full liquid diet
gastroesophageal
reflux disease
(GERD)

gastrostomy feeding
graduate
Heimlich maneuver
intake and output
(I&O)
intravenous infusion (IV)
jejunostomy tube
(J-tube)
mechanically altered
mechanical soft
minerals
nasogastric feeding
(NG feeding)

nourishments
nutrients
nutrition
percutaneous
endoscopic
gastrostomy (PEG)
protein
pureed diet
push fluids
soft diet
supplement
therapeutic diets
vitamins

INTRODUCTION

Nutrition is the entire process by which the body takes in food for growth and repair and uses it to maintain health. The signs of good nutrition include:

- Shiny hair
- Clear skin and eyes
- A well-developed body
- An alert expression
- A pleasant disposition
- Healthy sleep patterns
- Appropriate appetite
- Regular bowel habits
- Body weight appropriate to height

NORMAL NUTRITION

The mouth is the beginning of the digestive tract. **Digestion** is the process of breaking down foods into simple substances that can be used by the body cells for nourishment. These substances are called **essential nutrients**.

To be well nourished, we must eat foods that:

- Supply heat and energy
- Build and repair body tissue
- Regulate body functions

These foods are called **nutrients**. The six nutrients essential to good health are:

- Proteins
- Carbohydrates
- Fats
- Minerals
- Vitamins
- Water

Protein

Protein is an essential nutrient that is present in every body cell. It is the only nutrient that can make new cells and rebuild tissue. The foods that contain the greatest amount of protein come from animals. They include:

- Meat
- Poultry
- Fish
- Eggs
- Milk
- Cheese

Proteins are made of small building blocks called **amino acids**. The body can manufacture some of the necessary amino acids, but not all of them.

- *Complete proteins* are proteins that contain all the amino acids the body cannot manufacture. Examples of foods that provide complete proteins are meat, fish, eggs, and poultry
- *Incomplete proteins*, though still important, do not contain all the essential amino acids. Essential amino acids are those that must be obtained through foods. Examples of foods that provide incomplete proteins are corn, soybeans, peas, beans and nuts

Carbohydrates and Fats

Carbohydrates and **fats** are called energy foods because the body uses them to produce heat and energy. When a person eats more energy foods than the body needs, the remainder is stored as fat. Foods that contain the greatest amount of carbohydrates come from plants (Figure 26-1). They include:

- Fruits
- Vegetables
- Foods that are made from grains, such as breads, cereals, and pasta products

Carbohydrate foods also supply the body with fiber or roughage (**cellulose**), which is important in maintaining bowel regularity. Fiber is an important part of a healthy diet. Eating a high-fiber diet reduces the risk of heart disease, stroke, type 2 diabetes, diverticulosis, and hemorrhoids. A high-fiber diet also helps digestion and prevents and treats constipation and diarrhea. Fiber is found in plants, fruits, vegetables, nuts, beans, and grains.

Fats come from both plants and animals. Examples of foods that are rich in fat include:

- Oils, lard, and shortening
- Pork

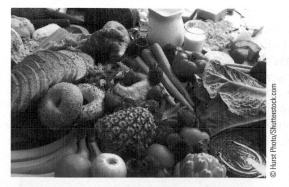

FIGURE 26-1 Fruits, vegetables, grains, and some dairy products are good sources of carbohydrates.

- Butter
- Nuts
- Egg yolk
- Cheese
- Some meats, especially processed meats such as sausage
- Some fish
- Dried coconut
- Dark chocolate
- Whipped cream
- Ice cream

Vitamins and Minerals

Vitamins and minerals are present in a wide variety of foods. The best way to be sure that you are getting enough vitamins and minerals is to include a variety of foods in your daily diet.

Vitamins are substances that regulate body processes. They help to:

- Build strong teeth and bones
- Promote growth
- Aid normal body functioning
- Strengthen resistance to disease

You probably know the vitamins by their letter names:

- Vitamin A
- B-complex vitamins
- Vitamin C
- Vitamin D
- Vitamin E
- Vitamin K

Fat-soluble vitamins do not dissolve easily in water. They can be stored in the body. Vitamins A, D, E, and K are fat-soluble vitamins.

Vitamins B and C are water soluble. Water-soluble vitamins dissolve in water, so they can be lost in the cooking process. In general, these vitamins are not stored in large amounts in the body. Deficiencies in water-soluble vitamins are more common.

Minerals help to build body tissues, especially the bones and teeth. They also regulate the chemistry of body fluids such as the blood and digestive juices. Minerals needed in the daily diet include:

- Calcium
- Potassium
- Iron
- Phosphorus
- Iodine
- Copper

THE FIVE FOOD GROUPS

Foods are sorted into food groups to help you eat a balanced diet. We must eat from five main food groups each day to stay healthy. These groups are:

- Grain
- Fruits
- Vegetables
- Dairy
- Protein

Dietary Guidelines for Americans

More than one-third of U.S. adults (35.7%) are obese. Approximately 17 percent (or 12.5 million) of children and adolescents aged 2 to 19 years are obese (see Chapter 31). The *2015–2020 Dietary Guidelines for Americans (DGA)* provide the foundation for federal dietary guidance. Published in December 2015 by the U.S. Department of Health and Human Services and U.S. Department of Agriculture, they are available at https://health.gov/dietaryguidelines/2015/guidelines/.

MyPlate

A dinner plate is the visual symbol that illustrates the five food groups in a place setting (Figure 26-2). MyPlate follows the federal government's *2015–2020 Dietary Guidelines for Americans (DGA)*. Dietary suggestions listed in Figure 26-2 summarize these guidelines. Use the plate to plan meals.

Grains Group

Foods in this group include bread, cereal, rice, tortillas, and pasta.

- This is the food group that you should eat most often.
- At least half the grains you eat each day should be whole grains (look for the name "whole" on the ingredients list). Whole grains contain the entire grain kernel.

Vegetables Group

Eat a variety of green vegetables such as leafy lettuces and spinach, broccoli, and cabbage. Add orange vegetables such as carrots and sweet potatoes. Dry beans and peas may be included in this group as long as they are not being used as a meat substitute.

- Vegetable juice is also part of this group.

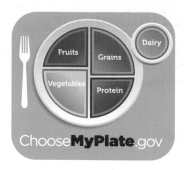

Courtesy of the USDA

Balancing Calories
- Enjoy your food, but balance your calories so you do not overeat.
- Avoid oversized portions.

Foods to Increase
- Make half your plate fruits and vegetables.
- Make at least half your grains whole grains.
- Switch to fat-free or low-fat (1%) milk.

Foods to Reduce
- Compare sodium in foods like soup, bread, and frozen meals—and choose the foods with lower numbers.
- Drink water instead of sugary drinks.

FIGURE 26-2 My Plate Food Guide.

- Vegetables may be raw, cooked, canned, frozen, dried, dehydrated, whole, cut up, or mashed.
- The portion size of vegetables should be slightly larger than the fruit portion.

Fruits Group

Choose whole fruits whenever possible, and eat a variety of fruits.

- Choose fresh, frozen, canned, or dry fruit
- 100 percent fruit juice is part of this group.

Milk (Dairy) Group

Use low-fat or fat-free products whenever possible. If you cannot consume milk because of lactose intolerance, choose lactose-free products and other foods that are rich in calcium.

- Cheese, yogurt, and milk-based desserts are included in this group.
- Foods such as cream, butter, and cream cheese are low in calcium and are not part of this group.

Meat and Beans Group

Vary the protein in your diet to include beef, pork, fish, chicken, tofu, soy, veggie burgers, beans, peas, nuts, and seeds. Select lean cuts of meat whenever possible to limit the amount of saturated (animal) fats in your diet. Avoid fried food if possible.

- Meat may be baked, grilled, roasted, or broiled.
- Fish, nuts, and seeds contain healthy oils, so select these instead of meat and poultry whenever possible. Become familiar with fish that has a low mercury content. Follow local and U.S. Food and Drug Administration (FDA) recommendations for fish and seafood intake.

Essential Nutrients

Oils

Oils are not a food group, but they provide essential nutrients. Oils are fats that are liquid at room temperature; they come from many different plants and fish. Some are used mainly as flavorings, such as walnut oil and sesame oil. Many are used in cooking and food preparation. Foods such as nuts, olives, and avocados are naturally high in oil.

Limit solid fats such as butter, margarine, and shortening. Avoid saturated fats and trans fats. Select the healthy fats found in fish, nuts, and vegetable oils.

Water

Water is an essential nutrient that is necessary for all cellular functions in the body. A person can live only a few days without water. An adequate intake of fluids is required to replace fluids lost through urine, stool, sweat, and evaporation through skin. The normal adult intake of fluids should be two to three quarts a day. Offering liquids to patients frequently is important for the following reasons:

- Some patients are not able to drink liquids without your help.
- Elderly patients often have a decreased sense of thirst.
- Adequate fluid intake is necessary to prevent urinary problems and constipation.

Some people will have medical conditions in which fluids are restricted. Follow your assignment and the care plan.

Use the ideas in Figure 26-3 to make food choices for a healthy lifestyle.

BASIC FACILITY DIETS

The food you serve to patients in the health care facility will be prepared by the dietary department. This food includes the essential nutrients. The way in which it is prepared and its consistency will depend on the individual patient's condition and needs. Sometimes very strict dietary control is needed.

10 tips
Nutrition Education Series

choose MyPlate
10 tips to a great plate

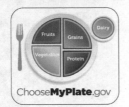
ChooseMyPlate.gov

Making food choices for a healthy lifestyle can be as simple as using these 10 Tips.
Use the ideas in this list to *balance your calories*, to choose foods to *eat more often*, and to cut back on foods to *eat less often*.

1 balance calories
Find out how many calories YOU need for a day as a first step in managing your weight. Go to www.ChooseMyPlate.gov to find your calorie level. Being physically active also helps you balance calories.

2 enjoy your food, but eat less
Take the time to fully enjoy your food as you eat it. Eating too fast or when your attention is elsewhere may lead to eating too many calories. Pay attention to hunger and fullness cues before, during, and after meals. Use them to recognize when to eat and when you've had enough.

3 avoid oversized portions
Use a smaller plate, bowl, and glass. Portion out foods before you eat. When eating out, choose a smaller size option, share a dish, or take home part of your meal.

4 foods to eat more often
Eat more vegetables, fruits, whole grains, and fat-free or 1% milk and dairy products. These foods have the nutrients you need for health—including potassium, calcium, vitamin D, and fiber. Make them the basis for meals and snacks.

5 make half your plate fruits and vegetables
Choose red, orange, and dark-green vegetables like tomatoes, sweet potatoes, and broccoli, along with other vegetables for your meals. Add fruit to meals as part of main or side dishes or as dessert.

6 switch to fat-free or low-fat (1%) milk
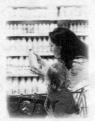
They have the same amount of calcium and other essential nutrients as whole milk, but fewer calories and less saturated fat.

7 make half your grains whole grains
To eat more whole grains, substitute a whole-grain product for a refined product—such as eating whole-wheat bread instead of white bread or brown rice instead of white rice.

8 foods to eat less often
Cut back on foods high in solid fats, added sugars, and salt. They include cakes, cookies, ice cream, candies, sweetened drinks, pizza, and fatty meats like ribs, sausages, bacon, and hot dogs. Use these foods as occasional treats, not everyday foods.

9 compare sodium in foods
Use the Nutrition Facts label to choose lower sodium versions of foods like soup, bread, and frozen meals. Select canned foods labeled "low sodium," "reduced sodium," or "no salt added."
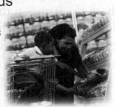

10 drink water instead of sugary drinks
Cut calories by drinking water or unsweetened beverages. Soda, energy drinks, and sports drinks are a major source of added sugar, and calories, in American diets.

USDA
Center for Nutrition Policy and Promotion

Go to www.ChooseMyPlate.gov for more information.

DG TipSheet No. 1
June 2011
USDA is an equal opportunity provider and employer.

Courtesy of the USDA

FIGURE 26-3 Ten tips for creating an ideal MyPlate.

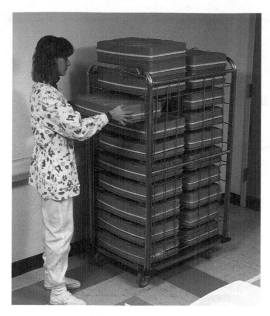

FIGURE 26-4A Patient diets are prepared in the dietary department and transported to the units in containers that maintain the temperature.

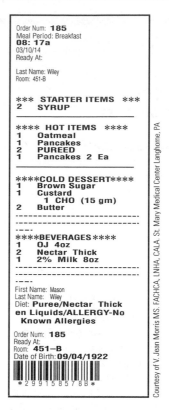

```
Order Num: 185
Meal Period: Breakfast
08: 17a
03/10/14
Ready At:

Last Name: Wiley
Room: 451-B


***  STARTER ITEMS   ***
 2    SYRUP
_____

****  HOT ITEMS  ****
 1    Oatmeal
 1    Pancakes
 2    PUREED
 1    Pancakes 2 Ea


****COLD DESSERT****
 1    Brown Sugar
 1    Custard
         1 CHO (15 gm)
 2    Butter
--------------------------
--------------------------
----
****BEVERAGES****
 1    OJ 4oz
 2    Nectar Thick
 1    2% Milk 8oz

--------------------------
----
First Name: Mason
Last Name:  Wiley
Diet: Puree/Nectar Thick
en Liquids/ALLERGY-No
   Known Allergies

Order Num: 185
Ready At:
Room: 451-B
Date of Birth: 09/04/1922
```

Courtesy of V. Jean Morris MS, FACHCA, LNHA, CALA, St. Mary Medical Center Langhorne, PA

FIGURE 26-4B The diet slip is on the tray to make sure the right diet gets to the correct person. Note the bar code at the bottom. This is scanned and the patient's wristband is scanned. Both should match.

The trays are usually delivered to the patient units in large food containers (Figure 26-4A). Each tray is labeled with the patient's name and type of diet. You will:

- Prepare the patient for the meal.
- Check the diet slip (Figure 26-4B) or tray card against the patient's name and armband.
- Check the items on the tray to make sure they are allowed on that patient's diet.
- Serve the tray to the patient.
- Assist with feeding as necessary.

Health care facilities have many types of diets. Four common diets are:

- Regular or house, sometimes called a general diet
- Full liquid
- Clear liquid
- Soft

Following surgery, a *progressive* diet is served: Foods progress from liquids and foods that are easy to digest to solid, regular food items:

1. Ice chips/sips of water
2. Clear liquids
3. Full liquids
4. Soft diet
5. Regular diet

In addition, the dietary department prepares special or **therapeutic** (treatment) **diets**. Therapeutic diets are described later in this chapter.

Regular Diet

The regular or general diet is a normal diet based on the five food groups. The regular diet:

- Includes a great variety of foods
- Excludes only very rich foods: pastries, heavy cakes, fried foods, and highly seasoned foods, which might be difficult for inactive people to digest.
- Has a lower caloric count, because an inactive person does not require as many calories as an active person.

In many health care facilities, patients may select foods from a menu.

Liquid Diets

Clear Liquid Diet

A **clear liquid diet** (Figure 26-5) is a temporary diet because it is nutritionally inadequate. It is made up primarily of water and carbohydrates for energy. Feedings are given every two, three, or four hours as prescribed by the physician. It replaces fluids that may have been lost by vomiting or diarrhea. When a clear liquid food item is held up to the light, you can see through it. The clear

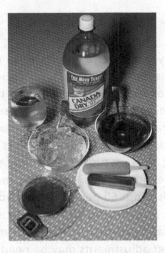

FIGURE 26-5 Items on a clear liquid diet include only liquids you can see through.

liquid diet consists of liquids that do not irritate, cause gas formation, or encourage bowel movements (**defecation**).

Foods allowed on the clear liquid diet include:

- Tea or coffee with sugar but without cream
- Strained fruit or vegetable juice with gelatin (occasionally)
- Fat-free meat broths
- Ginger ale (usually), 7Up, Coke, strained grape or apple juice
- Gelatin
- Popsicles
- Ice chips, refrigerated, and frozen liquids also fit into this category.

Full Liquid Diet

The **full liquid diet** does supply nourishment and may be used for longer periods of time than the clear liquid diet but is also considered a temporary diet because it is not nutritionally complete. Six to eight ounces are usually given every two to three hours.

The full liquid diet is given to:

- Some patients with acute infections
- Patients with conditions involving the digestive tract

In addition to all of the foods allowed on the clear liquid diet, the full liquid diet includes following:

- Strained cereal, such as cream of wheat or rice, blenderized soup, or potatoes pureed in soup
- Strained soups and milk-based soups
- Sherbet
- Gelatin
- Eggnog
- Malted milk

- Milk and cream
- Plain ice cream
- Strained vegetables and fruit juices
- Junket
- Solids that liquefy at room temperature
- Yogurt

Soft Diet

The **soft diet** usually follows the full liquid diet. Although this diet nourishes the body, between-meal feedings are sometimes given to increase the calorie count. Foods allowed on the soft diet are:

- Low residue, which are almost completely used by the body.
- Mildly flavored, slightly seasoned, or unseasoned
- Prepared in a form that is easy to digest

The diet includes liquids and semisolid foods that have a soft texture. It is given to patients who:

- Have infections and fevers
- Have minor difficulty swallowing
- Have conditions involving the digestive tract
- Are on a progressive postoperative dietary regime

The following foods are usually allowed on the soft diet:

- Soups
- Cream cheese and cottage cheese
- Crackers, toast
- Fish
- White meat of chicken or turkey (boiled or stewed)
- Fruit juices
- Cooked fruit (sieved)
- Tea, coffee
- Milk, cream, butter
- Cooked cereals
- Eggs (not fried)
- Beef and lamb (scraped or finely ground)
- Cooked vegetables (mashed or sieved)
- Angel food or sponge cake
- Small amounts of sugar
- Gelatin, custard
- Pudding
- Plain ice cream

Foods to be avoided include:

- Coarse cereals
- Spices
- Gas-forming foods (e.g., onions, cabbage, beans)
- Rich pastries and desserts
- Foods high in roughage/fiber

Hospital food is the subject of many jokes. For example, after having a bad meal in a restaurant, a person may comment that they had better food at the hospital. Food is the issue most often complained about by hospital patients and their families. Some studies have shown that up to a third of the food served each day is not touched. Medical and nutritional professionals recognize that good-tasting, culturally appropriate food served at the correct temperature is well accepted by patients. Patients begin to feel better, and hospitals save money by wasting less food. Many facilities are now providing more diverse food. Some provide food on demand via room service (Figure 26-6A). Some have professional chefs who plan and prepare restaurant-quality food. Some serve all fresh or organic food. Many serve fresh vegetables exclusively (rather than canned, frozen, etc.) (Figure 26-6B). These changes were made in response to patient dissatisfaction with food.

- Fried foods
- Raw fruits and vegetables
- Corn
- Pork (except bacon)

SPECIAL DIETS

Special diets are planned to meet specific patient needs. Patients may require special diets because of religious preferences or health needs.

Religious Restrictions

Religious practice requires changes in diet for some patients. For example, persons of the Orthodox Jewish faith follow strict food laws:

- There are strict prohibitions against shellfish and nonkosher meats such as pork.
- Certain fishes, such as tuna and salmon, are permitted.
- Foods may not be prepared with utensils that have been used for nonkosher food preparation.
- There are strict rules regarding the sequence in which milk products and meat may be consumed.

Some other faith restrictions are summarized in Table 26-1.

For many years, calorie counts were used when ordering the diet for patients with diabetes. Today, more relaxed diets are used to control blood sugar without being overly restrictive. These are often called *liberal or liberalized* diets. For example, the no concentrated sweets diet restricts sources of free sugar; heavy syrups in fruit; and cakes, pies, and sweetened desserts. The recommended diabetic diet is about 60 percent carbohydrate, 20 to 30 percent protein, and 20 to 30 percent fat. The dietitian may make individual adjustments for each patient. Diet adjustments may be needed for children, adolescents, patients who are metabolically stressed, geriatric patients, and pregnant women. Several other newer meal systems also focus on counting carbohydrates instead of calories.

Therapeutic Diets

Standard diets can be changed to conform to special dietary requirements. For example, a patient with ill-fitting dentures and heart disease may have an order for a low-sodium, mechanical soft diet. Therapeutic diets are prepared to address the patient's health problems. Common therapeutic diets include the diabetic diet, sodium-restricted diet, and low-fat diet.

The Diabetic Diet

Diet is an integral part of the therapy for patients with diabetes mellitus. The diet is nutritionally adequate. It provides enough energy in the form of calories for a 24-hour period. Sometimes a proper diet is all that is needed to control the disease. Usually, however, the food intake is balanced by the administration of insulin or oral hypoglycemic drugs.

Accurately evaluating and reporting the patient's intake is important because foods and liquids have a major impact on diabetes management. Illness increases the need for insulin because the liver releases more glucose in response to the stress. Dehydration is a serious problem for patients with diabetes. This can occur when the person does not consume enough fluids. Insulin administration may depend on your observations.

Some physicians prescribe a very carefully balanced diet and insulin to maintain the blood sugar (glucose) within normal limits. All foods must be measured, and repeated injections of insulin may be required. Other physicians are much more liberal in their approach. They permit an unmeasured diet, limiting only sugar and high-sugar foods. This diet is known as a *no concentrated sweets diet*. It may be balanced by insulin or drugs that lower blood sugar.

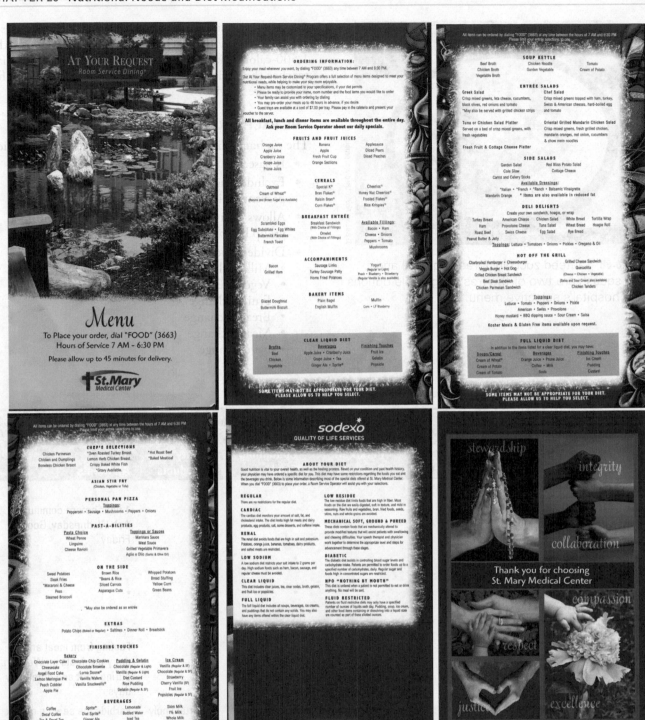

FIGURE 26-6A Patients at this hospital select their meals from a broad assortment of nutritious food items. The menu provides an overview of each therapeutic diet to help patients understand their diet order.

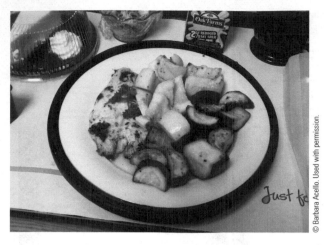

© Barbara Acello. Used with permission.

FIGURE 26-6B Sauteed zucchini (green squash) and yellow squash are two of the fresh vegetable options on this hospital's selective menu.

Many physicians prescribe American Dietetic Association diets with specific calorie levels, such as the 1,500-calorie diet or the 1,800-calorie diet. The dietitian teaches the patient about the diet and is a resource for health care providers.

THE EXCHANGE LIST

The **exchange list** method of balancing the diabetic diet:

- Is based on standard household measurements
- Excludes sugar and high-sugar-content foods, to prevent rapid swings in blood sugar
- Allows equivalent exchanges to be made within a group but not from group to group
- Divides foods into six groups:
  - Milk exchange
  - Vegetable exchange: Group A, Group B
  - Fruit exchange
  - Bread exchange
  - Meat exchange
  - Fat exchange

TABLE 26-1 Religious Dietary Practices

					Restricted Food		
Faith	**Coffee**	**Tea**	**Alcohol**	**Pork/Pork Products**	**Caffeine-Containing Foods**	**Dairy Products**	**All Meats**
Christian Science	•	•	•				
Roman Catholic							1 hour before communion, Ash Wednesday, Good Friday
Latter Day Saints (Mormon)	•	•	•		•		
Seventh Day Adventist	•	•	•	•	•		•
Some Baptist	•	•	•				
Greek Orthodox (on fast days)						•	Fasting from meat and dairy products on Wed./Fri. during Lent and other holy days
Jewish Orthodox				• Also shellfish		Certain holy days	Forbids the serving of milk and milk products with meat; regulates food preparation; forbids cooking on the Sabbath
Muslim, Islamic		•		•			Fasting during Ramadan during day, feasting at night
Hindu							Some are vegetarians
Buddhist							Meat must be blessed and killed in special ways; some sects are vegetarians

CONSISTENT CARBOHYDRATES

Control of blood sugar forms the basis of treatment for diabetes mellitus. When blood sugar is elevated, the person is at risk for complications, including infection and slower healing. Many patients come to the hospital with elevated blood sugar. In some situations the blood sugar increases in the hospital. Calorie-level diabetic diets are no longer recommended for patients during hospitalization. Instead, the American Diabetes Association (ADA) recommends that a **consistent carbohydrate (CHO) diet** be served to persons with diabetes. Currently, it does not endorse any meal plan or percentages of nutrients as it has done in the past.

The consistent carbohydrate diabetes meal plan is ordered to provide nutrient-rich carbohydrates and maintain a consistent carbohydrate content each day. Calories are not counted. The diet also focuses on maintaining fat levels. The patient receives about 50 percent of the calories from carbohydrates, 20 percent from protein, and 30 percent from fat. This diet is based on the belief that restricting regular food items increases the risk of malnutrition and does not improve blood sugar control. However, the food supply is not unlimited. The person is served three meals a day. The portion sizes are based on the dietitian's recommendations. The diet is modified in special situations such as surgery, but consistent carbohydrate levels are maintained.

Sodium-Restricted Diet

Sodium-restricted diets may be ordered for patients with chronic renal failure and cardiovascular disease. Sodium-restricted diets are some of the most difficult diets to follow. The average American consumes two to six grams of sodium in food each day. Table salt is a major source of sodium in the diet.

Processing may add significant amounts of sodium to foods, and this is considered when planning and selecting foods for the sodium-restricted diet. It is important to read the labels for the contents of all commercially prepared foods.

Some foods that naturally contain large amounts of sodium may be restricted for this diet. They include:

- Pork, ham, and bacon
- Breads
- Potato chips, pretzels, nuts, and similar snacks
- Saltine crackers
- Salad dressing, soy sauce, and other sauces
- Bouillon cubes, gravies, other soups, and broths
- Pop (soda) containing sodium
- Pickles and other pickled foods
- Cheese
- Processed meats such as salami, cold cuts, and sausage
- Canned foods such as vegetables and soups

Some foods are naturally low in sodium, and thus can be used more liberally. They include:

- Some cereals, such as shredded wheat
- Vegetables
- Fruits

Calorie-Restricted Diet

Calorie-restricted diets are prescribed for patients who are overweight. These diets are planned to meet general nutritional needs. They take into consideration the patient's activity and energy output, general nutritional state, and weight goal. As long as activity remains constant, a person must take in approximately 500 calories a day less than usual to lose one pound. The dietitian tries to create a realistic balance between fats, proteins, and carbohydrates.

Some physicians use a factor of 10 calories multiplied by the desired weight in calculating the daily calorie requirements. For example:

- Desired weight 120 lb × 10 = 1,200 calories per day
- Desired weight 160 lb × 10 = 1,600 calories per day

Low-Fat/Low-Cholesterol Diet

Low-fat/low-cholesterol diets are prescribed for patients who suffer from vascular, heart, liver, or gallbladder disease, and for those who have difficulty with fat metabolism. Fats are limited and calories are balanced by increasing proteins and carbohydrates. Foods are baked, roasted, or broiled, and the skin is removed from chicken. Low-fat foods include:

- Low-fat cottage cheese (no other type of cottage cheese allowed)
- Skim milk, buttermilk, and yogurt
- Lean meats, fish, and chicken
- Vegetables and fruits
- Jams, jellies, and ices
- Cereals, pasta, bread, potatoes, and rice
- Carbonated beverages, tea, and coffee

Mechanically Altered Diets

Any diet may be **mechanically altered**. This means that the consistency and texture are modified to make the food easier to chew and swallow. The **mechanical soft** diet (Figure 26-7) is commonly served to patients who have no teeth, or those with serious dental problems. Meats and hard foods are ground to the consistency of hamburger. Soft items, such as bread, are not ground. The **pureed diet** (Figure 26-8) is blended with gravy or liquid until it is the consistency of pudding. This diet is

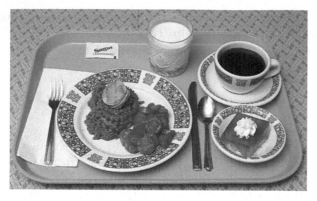

FIGURE 26-7 The mechanical soft diet is blenderized so foods are the consistency of hamburger. Soft foods, such as bread and cooked carrots, are easily chewed and are not blended.

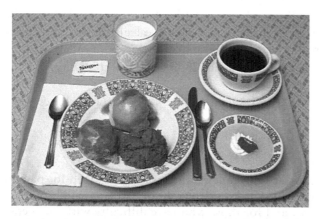

FIGURE 26-8 The pureed diet is given to patients who have difficulty swallowing. The consistency of the food should be firm enough to support a plastic spoon in an upright position. Attention is given to attractive appearance so food is not runny and does not resemble baby food.

used for patients who have difficulty swallowing. Pureed foods should not be watery. Properly pureed food items will support a plastic spoon in the upright position.

Nutritional problems to observe and report are listed in Table 26-2.

SUPPLEMENTS AND NOURISHMENTS

Many patients receive a nutritional **supplement** or between-meal nourishments. Supplements are ordered by the physician and have a definite therapeutic value. Patients who have wounds may receive supplements high in protein to facilitate healing. Supplements are also given to persons who have experienced weight loss and those who need additional calories to meet a medical need.

TABLE 26-2 Nutritional Problems to Observe and Report

- Increase or decrease in food (caloric) intake
- Increase or decrease in body weight
- Diabetic patients who do not eat all their food, or who eat more than allowed on diet
- Patients on restricted diets who do not adhere to their diet
- Refusal to accept meal, supplement, snack
- Refusal to accept food substitute for meat or vegetable
- Meal intake of less than 50% (or 75%, according to facility policy)
- Difficulty chewing or swallowing, coughing, choking
- Distracted or wanders at meals, needs to be refocused
- Requires prompting or hands-on assistance to feed 60% or more of the time. Specify when assistance is required, the type of assistance provided, and for what reason.

Special supplements are used to treat patients with specific medical needs, such as pediatric patients as well as those with renal failure, diabetes, chronic obstructive pulmonary disease, or HIV. These supplements may be liquid or in any form that is easy to eat and digest, such as pudding. It is essential that the patient consume the entire serving.

Nutritional supplements:

- Are ordered by the physician or dietitian. In some facilities, they are given without an order.
- Are given for a specific therapeutic purpose. They are not nutritionally complete, and are not a replacement for meals. They are given to make up for a nutritional deficiency, strengthen the patient, or promote healing.
- Come in a variety of preparations and flavors to promote patient acceptance
- Usually taste best when served cold
- Contain approximately 170–250 calories per container
- Are usually lactose free, and higher in sodium and protein than most tube-feeding formulas
- Are flavored and are used for oral nutrition. They are not recommended for tube feedings, and tube-feeding formulas are not recommended for nutritional supplementation.
- Are very filling, and should not be given with meals or immediately before mealtime
- Are expensive and should not be wasted!

In most facilities, the nursing assistant must document on a flow sheet the percentage of the product the patient consumed.

Nourishments are substantial food items given to patients to meet medical needs and increase nutrient intake. They are often planned and ordered by the facility dietitian and include foods such as:

- Sandwiches
- Instant breakfast
- Milkshakes

- Pudding
- Whole or chocolate milk
- Yogurt
- Cottage cheese
- Ice cream or sherbet
- Liquid milk-type products, such as Great Shake and Shake Up

Nourishments are usually given between meals to provide needed nutrients or prevent hunger. Between-meal nourishments are usually served:

- Midmorning—between 9:30 and 10:00 a.m.
- Midafternoon—between 2:30 and 3:00 p.m.
- At bedtime—between 8:00 and 10:00 p.m.

Snacks may be planned and regularly given, or unplanned upon patient request to prevent or eliminate hunger between meals. Snacks that may be served include:

- Milk
- Juices
- Gelatin
- Custard
- Ice cream
- Sherbet
- High-protein drinks
- Fruits
- Cookies
- Graham crackers

Serving snacks, nourishments, and supplements is an important nursing assistant responsibility. To serve nourishments:

- Wash your hands.
- Check the nourishment list for each patient for any limitations or special dietary instructions.

Difficult Situations

Liquid nutritional supplements are very filling, which is why they are usually served between meals, not with meals. Most patients prefer them cold. If the beverage is warm, the patient may not accept it. Because some of these products are milk based, serving them warm can also be an infection control hazard. When serving supplements and nourishments, make sure the patient is able to consume the beverage independently. Do not just set it on the table and walk out. Pour the beverage into a cup or provide a straw, according to patient preference. Assist the patient, if needed. Inform the nurse if the patient expresses a preference or dislike for a certain product or flavor.

- Allow patients to choose from the available nourishments whenever possible.
- Assist patients who are dependent.
- Provide straws and napkins as needed.
- Remember to pick up wrappers and packages. Return used glasses and dishes to the proper area.
- Document the patient's intake.
- Record on intake and output (I&O) sheet if required.

CALORIE COUNTS AND FOOD INTAKE STUDIES

The physician or dietitian may order food intake studies for patients with special nutritional needs. The patient's food intake is carefully recorded for a period of time, usually three days. The dietitian analyzes the information for nutritional adequacy and number of calories consumed. They will use the information to plan the diet.

If a food intake study is ordered, a food documentation form (Figure 26-9) is prepared and placed in a designated location. The study usually begins with the breakfast meal on the day after the physician writes the order. Some facilities post a sign in the room or on the door to remind staff and visitors that a study is in progress. In some facilities, each food item is weighed or measured. At the end of each meal, you will accurately record the patient's food intake on the form. Facility policies vary on how food intake is documented, but this is usually done by recording an accurate percentage of each individual meal item consumed. You will also accurately document intake of all snacks, liquid nutritional beverages, and food items brought from home by visitors.

Return the form to the dietitian or dietetic technician at the end of the study period. They use the information to calculate the amount of protein, carbohydrates, fat, and calories the patient consumed each day. In some facilities, nutrient, vitamin, and mineral intake are also calculated. The dietitian uses this information to adjust the patient's diet and nutritional plan of care. The physician may order extra vitamin or mineral supplements. Completing a food intake or calorie count study requires a team effort, good communication, and accurate documentation.

DYSPHAGIA

Swallowing is something we do automatically, like breathing. Most people swallow about 600 times each day. Swallowing is a coordinated effort involving about 50 pairs of muscles and nerves. Although it seems easy, swallowing is

Diet _____

CALORIE/PROTEIN SUMMARY

PATIENT _____　　ROOM # _____

DAY 1					DAY 2					DAY 3				
DATE ___ / ___ / ___					DATE ___ / ___ / ___					DATE ___ / ___ / ___				
	% 0–25	% 25–50	% 50–75	% 75–100		% 0–25	% 25–50	% 50–75	% 75–100		% 0–25	% 25–50	% 50–75	% 75–100
Breakfast					**Breakfast**					**Breakfast**				
Meat					Meat					Meat				
Milk					Milk					Milk				
Fruit					Fruit					Fruit				
Starch					Starch					Starch				
Fat					Fat					Fat				
Other					Other					Other				
AM Supp.					AM Supp.					AM Supp.				
Noon Meal					**Noon Meal**					**Noon Meal**				
Meat					Meat					Meat				
Milk					Milk					Milk				
Juice					Juice					Juice				
Starch					Starch					Starch				
Vegetable					Vegetable					Vegetable				
Bread					Bread					Bread				
Fat					Fat					Fat				
Dessert					Dessert					Dessert				
Other					Other					Other				
PM Supp.					PM Supp.					PM Supp.				
Evening Meal					**Evening Meal**					**Evening Meal**				
Meat					Meat					Meat				
Milk					Milk					Milk				
Juice					Juice					Juice				
Starch					Starch					Starch				
Vegetable					Vegetable					Vegetable				
Bread					Bread					Bread				
Fat					Fat					Fat				
Dessert					Dessert					Dessert				
Other					Other					Other				
PM Supp.					PM Supp.					PM Supp.				
Total Kcal					**Total Kcal**					**Total Kcal**				
Total Pro					**Total Pro**					**Total Pro**				
Avg. for 3 days Kcal:							**Avg. Protein for 3 days:**							

PLEASE RETURN COMPLETED FORM TO NUTRITION CARE MANAGER

FIGURE 26-9 The calorie count provides an accurate picture of the patient's calorie and nutrient intake over a three-day period. The registered dietitian analyzes the information and uses it to make adjustments in the patient's diet and nutritional plan of care.

a complex process. Some patients have **dysphagia**, or difficulty swallowing food and liquids. People with dysphagia also have difficulty swallowing saliva. The swallowing problem can lead to the patient literally breathing saliva, food, or liquid into the lungs. For these people, swallowing can be a nightmare of choking, gagging, and spitting up food.

Approximately 53 to 74 percent of long-term care facility residents have this condition. This condition may also occur in persons who have:

- Had a stroke
- Neurological diseases
- Cancer of the head, neck, or esophagus

- Undergone radiation therapy to the head or neck
- Dementia

People who take medications that cause sedation or reduce saliva production are also at risk of dysphagia. Signs and symptoms of dysphagia are:

- Taking a long time before beginning to swallow
- Swallowing three or four times with each bite of food
- Frequent throat clearing or coughing
- Lack of a gag reflex or weak cough
- Difficulty controlling liquids and secretions in the mouth
- Wet, gurgling voice
- Refusing to eat, spitting food out, or pocketing food in cheeks
- Unintentional weight loss
- Tightness in the throat or chest
- Feeling as if food is sticking in the esophagus or sternal area

Notify the nurse if the patient has any of these signs or symptoms. Patients with dysphagia are at high risk of developing malnutrition, dehydration, aspiration, and pneumonia. Consultation with a speech-language pathologist and diagnostic tests for dysphagia may be necessary.

Dysphagia is treated with swallowing exercises, practice of proper swallowing techniques, and alteration of the consistency of food and beverages. The dietitian works closely with the speech-language pathologist to ensure that the food is the proper consistency to meet the patient's needs and reduce the risk of aspiration. The goal is to keep the food's look, taste, and consistency as close to normal as possible, considering the patient's safety needs.

One important key to safe swallowing is to keep food moist. Dry food is hard to chew and swallow. Adding sauces and gravies will moisten food and help hold it together. This helps the person who has trouble forming a ball of food on the tongue. Adding sauces and condiments as allowed makes the food more flavorful and appealing. Adults may be resistant to eating pureed food because it resembles baby food. Molds and special methods of preparation are used to enhance the appearance of pureed foods.

Monitor the patient's food and fluid intake accurately. The physician may order frequent weight monitoring. The speech therapist will order special approaches to eating and drinking to prevent aspiration and ensure good intake.

People with dysphagia have much more difficulty swallowing liquids than swallowing solid food. This is because liquids are harder for the tongue to manage during swallowing. The tongue must hold the liquid up near the roof of the mouth so it can be swallowed all at once.

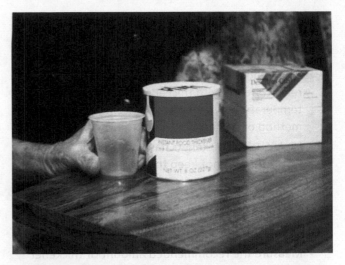

FIGURE 26-10 Food thickener is used to change the texture and consistency of liquids to prevent choking and aspiration.

This is more difficult than managing a ball of food with the tongue. Because of this, some patients limit fluids for fear of choking. This often results in dehydration.

The speech professional may recommend using food thickeners (Figure 26-10) to slow the movement of fluid through the esophagus. *Thickeners* are nonprescription products that are mixed into beverages and some foods. The consistency of the liquid depends on the amount of product added. Add exactly the amount that has been ordered. Thickeners do not change the taste of food or liquids, but they may change the intensity, making it taste stronger. Prethickened liquids are also used in some facilities.

The care plan will specify the type and amount of thickener to use to achieve the necessary texture. For example, the therapist may recommend that liquids be mixed to the thickness that is safe for the person to drink, such as:

- *Thin.* Examples: water, coffee, apple juice
- *Nectar-thick.* Examples: cold tomato juice, buttermilk
- *Honey-like.* Example: honey
- *Pudding-thick* (also called spoon-thick). Example: a thick milkshake, drinkable yogurt

Follow the speech therapist's instructions and plan of care for positioning and feeding.

GASTROESOPHAGEAL REFLUX DISEASE

Gastroesophageal reflux disease (GERD) is another condition that interferes with a person's meal intake. GERD is a backflow of stomach contents into the esophagus. It may be described as having "heartburn," which is painful and irritating. Over time, the acids in the stomach cause erosion of the walls of the esophagus.

Many people have occasional heartburn. People with GERD have this problem much of the time. Treatment involves elevating the head of the bed, modifying one's lifestyle, and eliminating irritating food and beverages. Sleeping on the side is also effective for some people.

FLUID BALANCE

Fluid balance is the balance between liquid intake and liquid output. Because two-thirds of the body's weight is water, there must be a balance between the amount of fluid taken in and the amount lost under normal conditions. This balance usually takes care of itself.

The metric system is used for fluid measurements: milliliters (mL) or cubic centimeters (cc). A mL and a cc are the same amount. Table 26-3 compares U.S. customary and metric measurements.

Intake

Most adults take in approximately 2.5 to 3 quarts (2,500 to 3,000 mL) of fluid daily:

- In liquids such as water, tea, and soft drinks

TABLE 26-3 Comparison of U.S. Customary and Metric Measurements

U.S. Customary Units	Metric Units
1 ounce	30 mL
1 pint	500 mL
1 quart	1,000 mL (1 liter)
1 gallon	4,000 mL
2.2 pounds	1 kilogram (kg)
1 inch	2.5 centimeters (cm)
1 foot	30 cm

- In foods such as fruits and vegetables
- Artificially, such as by intravenous infusions or tube feeding

A minimum of 1,300 mL of liquid is needed every 24 hours to maintain kidney function. Kidney damage will occur if daily intake is consistently less than this. Provide extra fluids whenever possible, especially in hot and humid weather.

Excessive fluid retention is called **edema**. Inadequate fluid intake results in **dehydration**, or the lack of sufficient fluid in body tissues. Some disease conditions may change the amount of fluids the patient is allowed to have.

Output

Typical output equals about 2.5 quarts (2,500 mL) daily in the form of:

- Urine, 1.5 quarts (1,500 mL)
- Perspiration
- Moisture from the lungs
- Moisture from the bowel

Excessive fluid loss results in dehydration. This usually occurs due to:

- Diarrhea
- Vomiting
- Excessive urine output (**diuresis**)
- Excessive perspiration (**diaphoresis**)
- Wound drainage or blood loss

Recording Intake and Output

An accurate recording of **intake and output (I&O)**, or fluid taken in and eliminated by the body, is basic to the care of many patients. Intake and output records are kept when ordered by the physician and when patients:

- Are dehydrated or at high risk for dehydration
- Receive intravenous infusions
- Have recently had surgery
- Have a urinary catheter
- Are perspiring profusely or vomiting
- Have specific diagnoses, such as congestive heart failure or renal disease, that require accurate monitoring of I&O

Fluid intake may have to be encouraged in some patients. This situation is called **push fluids** or **force fluids**. In some situations (as in kidney disease), fluid intake may have to be restricted. Fluid restriction requires a physician's order. You will find information regarding whether to push or restrict fluids on the patient's care plan.

Fluid intake and output is calculated by measuring and recording the fluids the patient takes in and the fluids the patient **excretes** (eliminates from the body) (Table 26-4). Because the fluids taken in by the patient cannot actually be measured, an estimate is made and recorded. This is done by:

- Knowing what the liquid container holds when full.
- Estimating how much is gone from the container (what the patient drank), such as one-third of a glass of juice or half of a cup of coffee.
- Converting this to mL. *Example:* A water glass holds 240 mL when filled. The patient drinks ¾ of the glass of water. ¾ × 240 = 180 mL. Intake for the glass of water is recorded as 180 mL. Fluids that are calculated and recorded include all liquids, such as water, juice, soda, coffee, tea, milk, and soup. Also included are foods that melt at room temperature, such as ice cream, sherbet, and gelatin.

TABLE 26-4 Computing Intake and Output

Intake	
IV	1,500 mL
By mouth	2,000 mL
Total	*3,500 mL*
Output	
Urine	1,500 mL
Vomitus	500 mL
Drainage	600 mL
Total	*2,600 mL*

NOTE

Sizes of containers vary. Learn the fluid content of the containers used at your facility. Remember that there are 30 mL per ounce (240 mL ÷ 30 mL = 8 oz).

- Coffee/tea cup, 8 oz = 240 mL
- Water carafe, 16 oz = 480 mL
- Foam cup, 8 oz = 240 mL
- Water glass, 8 oz = 240 mL
- Soup bowl, 6 oz = 180 mL
- Jello, 1 serving = 120 mL
- Ice chips, full 4 oz glass = 120 mL

NOTE

Containers may vary from one facility to the next. Each facility should have a chart that tells you what each size of glass, cup, and bowl holds when full.

Record each type of fluid separately, such as fluids taken by mouth, through intravenous infusion, or through gastric feeding. (The nurse will record intake from an IV and tube feeding.) Total the figures at the end of each 8- or 12-hour shift and the end of 24 hours (Figure 26-11).

Fluid output amount is obtained by measuring all fluids excreted from the body. This includes urine; **emesis** (vomitus); and drainage from body cavities, such as gastric drainage. A container called a **graduate** is marked in mL or cc (Figure 26-12). Pour the substance into the graduate to determine the amount of output. Record each type of excretion separately.

NOTE

Apply standard precautions when measuring any body excretion. Wear gloves when measuring all forms of output.

Observations of fluid balance problems to make and report are listed in Table 26-5.

CHANGING WATER

Water is essential to life, so provide fresh water regularly. Check the care plan to see if a patient is allowed ice or tap water. Some patients will have a doctor's order for no ice because of a medical problem. The care plan will also note whether fluids are to be encouraged. The physician may order a specific quantity of fluids the patient should consume each day. Encourage patients to take 6 to 8 glasses of fluids every 24 hours, unless the patient

Date Amount	Time	Method of Adm.	Solution	Intake Amounts Rec'd	Time	Output Urine Amount	Others Kind	Others Amount
7/16	0700	PO	water	120 mL		500 mL		
	0830	PO	coffee	240 mL				
			or.jce	120 mL				
	1030	PO	cran.jce	120 mL				
	1100					300 mL		
	1230	PO	tea	240 mL				
	1400	PO	water	150 mL				
Shift Totals	1500			990 mL		800 mL		
	1530	PO	gelatin	120 mL				
	1700	PO	tea	120 mL				
			soup	180 mL				
	2000					512 mL		
	2045						vomitus	500 mL
	2205						vomitus	90 mL
Shift Totals	2300			420 mL		512 mL		590 mL
	2345						vomitus	80 mL
	0130	IV	D/W	500 mL				
	0315					400 mL		
Shift Totals	0700			500 mL		400 mL		80 mL
24-Hour Totals				1,910 mL		1,712 mL		670 mL
								vomitus

FIGURE 26-11 Sample intake and output record.

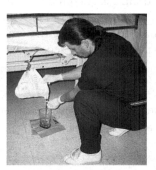

FIGURE 26-12 The principles of standard precautions are used to collect urine in a graduated pitcher for accurate measurement. The amount is documented as output on the intake and output record.

TABLE 26-5 Observations of Fluid Balance Problems to Make and Report

- Fluid intake or output too high
- Fluid intake or output too low
- Patients with fluid restrictions exceeding limitations
- Fluid intake and output not reasonably balanced
- Accepts or refuses water, if offered
- Prefers a certain liquid instead of water
- Difficulty swallowing liquids, coughing, choking
- Signs of dehydration, including low fluid intake; low output of dark urine with strong odor; weight loss; dry skin; dry mucous membranes of the lips, mouth, tongue, eyes; drowsiness; confusion
- Edema; obvious fluid in tissues, particularly face, fingers, legs, ankles, feet

is NPO (nothing by mouth) or has a doctor's order to restrict fluid to a specified amount. Give special attention to patients who are confused, patients who may not be able to reach a source of water, and elderly persons.

Forcing fluids is an old term that is not quite accurate. Patients should never be forced to consume water or other beverages. When "force fluids" is ordered, encourage the patient to drink each time you are in the room. Offer to assist, if necessary. Some patients will not drink water. Find out what beverages the patient likes, and provide these, whenever possible.

Infection Control **ALERT**

Avoid contaminating the ice machine, ice chest, or ice scoop when filling pitchers and passing fresh drinking water. Keep the ice scoop covered when not in use. Note that the handle is contaminated and should not touch the clean ice supply. Avoid filling the pitcher over the source of clean ice. (If ice hits the rim of the pitcher and drops back into the clean ice supply, the whole supply is contaminated.) Do not allow the scoop to touch the pitcher. Always keep water pitchers covered at the bedside. If more than one patient shares the room, make sure each pitcher and cup is labeled with a single patient's name. To reduce the potential for infection, some facilities are now giving patients a bottle or large disposable cup of water each shift and upon request, rather than filling a carafe. If ice is requested, staff provides it in a plastic bag or disposable cup with a lid.

Clinical Information **ALERT**

Accurately document each patient's meal intake. This is especially important for patients who have weight loss, have diabetes, are on calorie counts, or are on special diets. Many professionals depend on the accuracy of documented information. If you have trouble understanding percentages, work with your instructor until you master the information.

Providing fresh water is one way to encourage the patient to increase intake of fluids. The procedure for providing fresh water varies greatly.

- In some hospitals, the water pitcher and glass are replaced with a new disposable set each time water is provided.
- In others, the pitcher and glass are washed, refilled, and returned to the patient's bedside table.
- Some facilities serve water in a disposable container.

FOOD ACCEPTANCE

Making mealtime special is an important responsibility. Having friendly staff who show sincere concern for patient welfare helps create a comfortable atmosphere at meals. If patients are satisfied with the quality of food and food service, they tend to view everything else in a positive light. Complaints do not necessarily reflect poor-quality food. They may reflect personal problems or dissatisfaction with care.

- Make the environment as pleasant as possible. Remove unpleasant sights and smells. Clear and wipe the overbed table before serving food trays.
- Provide supplies for patients to wash hands
- Be sure patients have dentures, glasses, and hearing aid, if used.
- Make sure patients are positioned correctly. Ensure that they can reach the food. Make adjustments, if necessary.

The human sensory response to food is complicated. The brain coordinates signals of smell and taste with sight, temperature, and texture. Sensory disorders have many causes, including normal aging, various diseases, deficiencies of certain vitamins and minerals, certain medications, cigarette smoking, and wearing dentures. Sensory problems are very difficult to overcome. Sensory problems may affect:

- Temperature
- Smell
- Taste
- Hearing and vision
- Touch
- Texture

The presentation and attractiveness of food are especially important for patients whose smell, taste, and texture sensations are impaired. They may not be able to smell the food. Always check food temperature. All patients are at risk of burns if food is too hot. Patients with abnormal temperature sensations are at greater risk than others. The facility dietitian and occupational, physical, and speech therapists will work with the patient to help resolve sensory problems.

Many patients look forward to meals. However, we know that certain common problems cause patient complaints and decreased food intake. Common complaints about food service are:

- Inability to make choices or select food
- Unappetizing appearance of food
- Lack of seasoning
- Dislike of food served
- Food temperatures not maintained; hot food too cold or cold food too warm
- Not getting enough to eat

PREVENTION OF FOODBORNE ILLNESS

Hot foods and beverages must be served hot, and cold foods and beverages must be served cold. Food tastes best when it is served at the proper temperature. Imagine how a scrambled egg or bowl of chicken noodle soup tastes when it is ice cold, or a popsicle or ice cream tastes when it is warm. Food acceptance is only one concern. The potential for foodborne infection is a much more serious problem. Many of the pathogens implicated in "food poisoning" (foodborne illness) have the potential to cause serious illness and death. Foodborne illness is often spread through the common-vehicle method of contamination. This type of infection occurs when Listeria, Salmonella, and other pathogens contaminate a food source. Common examples are delicatessen salads and lunch meats. This can cause a serious community infection. This is the type of infection that plagues cruise ships, hospitals, and others. (Chapter 12). Wash your hands well before serving meal trays. If you stop to assist a patient, wash your hands again before continuing to distribute trays.

In addition to proper sanitation and food preparation in the kitchen, nursing personnel have an important responsibility for ensuring that patients' trays are served and dependent patients are fed when food is the proper temperature. The temperature danger zone is fairly narrow (Figure 26-13). Foods served in the danger zone are potentially hazardous and have an increased risk for

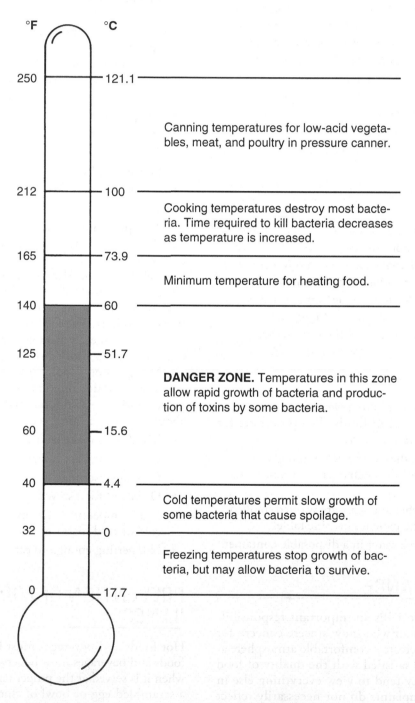

FIGURE 26-13 Temperatures of food for control of pathogens. The danger zone is very close to the average serving temperature, so the temperature of food trays must be carefully maintained. Food should be served promptly upon arrival on the unit.

pathogen growth. Hot foods must be served at 140°F or above, and cold foods must be 40°F or below. You may be surprised to learn that hot foods are often 140°F to 150°F when they are delivered to your unit. Serve trays promptly, because the food cools quickly.

FEEDING THE PATIENT

Eating should be an enjoyable experience. (See Procedures 72 and 73.) Prepare the patient for the meal tray before it arrives by:

- Offering the bedpan or helping the patient to the bathroom
- Assisting the patient to wash hands and face
- Assisting with oral hygiene, if needed
- Raising the head of the bed or assisting the patient out of bed and into a chair, as permitted
- Adjusting the in-bed patient's position with pillows
- Clearing away anything that is unpleasant, such as the emesis basin and bedpan
- Clearing the overbed table
- Encouraging the patient to do as much as possible

When you have served the tray and after you have washed your hands, assist the patient as needed by:

- Being unhurried and pleasant
- Opening prepackaged items
- Cutting meat

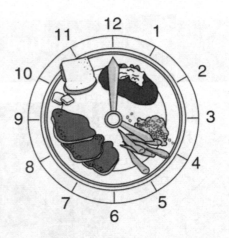

FIGURE 26-14 Describe the location of each food item compared with the positions on the face of a clock.

- Pouring liquids
- Buttering bread
- Explaining the arrangement of the tray as if items were on the face of a clock (Figure 26-14) if the patient cannot see

There are times when you will be responsible for the entire feeding procedure.

> 🔨 **NOTE**
>
> Carry some extra straws with you during mealtimes. It can save you steps.

PROCEDURE **72** **ASSISTING THE PATIENT WHO CAN FEED SELF**

1. Carry out initial procedure actions.
2. Assemble equipment:
   - Bedpan/urinal
   - Disposable gloves
   - Basin of warm water
   - Towel
   - Soap
   - Washcloth
   - Oral hygiene items
   - Tray of food
3. Offer the bedpan/urinal. Use standard precautions when assisting with elimination.
4. If permitted, elevate the head of the bed or assist the patient out of bed.

5. Provide a washcloth to wash the patient's hands and face.
6. Assist with oral hygiene or dentures.
7. Remove and discard personal protective equipment.
8. Clear the overbed table and position it in front of the patient. Remove unpleasant items.
9. Wash your hands. Obtain the meal tray from the food cart.
10. Check the diet against the dietary card or paper diet slip with the patient's identification band (Figure 26-15).
11. Place the tray on the overbed table and arrange food in a convenient manner.

(continues)

PROCEDURE **72** CONTINUED

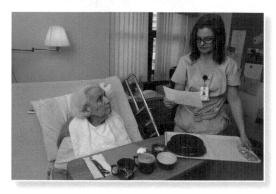

FIGURE 26-15 Check the patient's identification band against the diet slip or tray card.

ICON KEY:

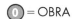 = OBRA

12. Assist in food preparation as needed. Encourage the patient to do as much as possible.

13. Remove the tray as soon as the patient is finished.

14. Record fluids on the intake record, if necessary. Record food intake.

15. Push the overbed table out of the way.

16. Carry out ending procedure actions.

PROCEDURE **73** FEEDING THE DEPENDENT PATIENT

1. Carry out initial procedure actions.
2. Assemble equipment:
   - Disposable gloves
   - Basin
   - Soap
   - Towel
   - Washcloth
   - Clothing protector
   - Oral hygiene items
3. Offer the bedpan or urinal. Follow standard precautions.
4. Provide oral hygiene, if desired.
5. Remove unnecessary articles from the overbed table.
6. Elevate the head of the bed with the patient's head bent slightly forward.
7. Place a towel or clothing protector under the patient's chin (Figure 26-16A). Avoid calling this item a bib, which is demeaning to adults.
8. Obtain the meal tray. Check the diet against the patient's identification band and dietary card or paper diet slip.

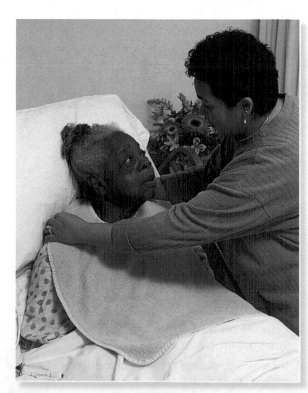

FIGURE 26-16A Place a towel or clothing (garment) protector over the patient. Avoid calling this item a bib.

(continues)

PROCEDURE **73** CONTINUED

9. Place the tray on the overbed table.

10. Butter bread and cut meat. Do not pour a hot beverage until the patient is ready for it.

11. Use different drinking straws for each fluid, or use a cup. Thick fluids are more easily controlled by using a straw. Use adaptive devices as indicated on the care plan.

12. Sit down while you are feeding the patient, so that you are at eye level, if possible. If the person is in bed, you may have to stand due to the distance.

13. Holding the spoon at a right angle:
    – Give solid foods from the point of the spoon (Figure 26-16B).
    – Alternate solids and liquids.
    – Ask the patient in what order she would like the food.
    – Describe or show the patient what kind of food you are giving.
    – If the patient has had a stroke, direct food to the unaffected side and check for food stored in the affected side. Watch the patient's throat to check for swallowing.
    – Test hot foods by dropping a small amount on the inside of your wrist before feeding them to the patient (Figure 26-16C).
    – Never blow on the patient's food to cool it.

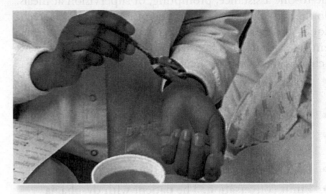

FIGURE 20-16C Check the temperature of food and beverages by placing a drop or small amount on the wrist or forearm.

    – Never taste the patient's food.
    – Do not hurry the meal.

14. Allow the patient to assist to the extent that she is able (Figure 26-16D).

15. Use a napkin to wipe the patient's mouth as often as necessary.

16. Remove the tray as soon as the patient is finished. Record the percentage of food eaten. Record fluid intake if the person has an order for I&O.

17. Carry out ending procedure actions.

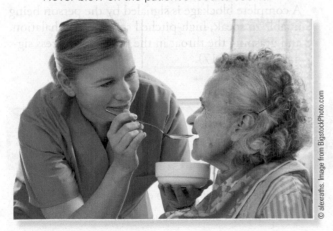
© alexraths. Image from BigstockPhoto.com

FIGURE 20-16B Stand close to the patient when feeding from the tip of a spoon.

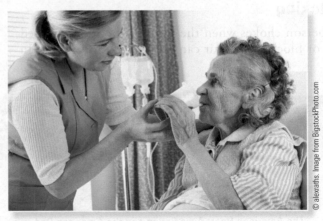
© alexraths. Image from BigstockPhoto.com

FIGURE 20-16D Encourage the patient to participate or assist by holding the cup or utensil.

ICON KEY:

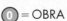 = OBRA

Mealtime Assistance for Patients Who Have Swallowing Problems

Patients who have difficulty swallowing may require one-to-one assistance, prompting, or supervision at meals. On the care plan, the speech therapist will list special techniques and positions for improving swallowing and preventing aspiration. The therapist may work closely with each staff member who may feed the patient. In general:

- Before serving food or beverages, make sure the patient is fully awake and alert
- Position the patient as upright as possible
- Position the patient facing forward, with the neck flexed forward slightly
- Reduce distractions during the meal
- Limit conversation. The patient with dysphagia should not try to carry on a conversation while eating. Focus the patient on eating
- Prompt or feed the patient slowly, offering small bites. Remind the patient to chew the food well

The speech-language pathologist may order other special positions and exercises, depending on the patient's medical condition and needs. The care plan will provide additional directions, such as reminding the patient to tuck the chin in when swallowing. In some types of dysphagia, this changes the position of the airway, further reducing the risk of aspiration. In other types, this technique increases the risk. Because dysphagia care is highly individualized, many staff members must work as a team to ensure that the patient's nutritional needs are safely met.

Choking

A person chokes when the throat is occluded (closed up or blocked) and air cannot get into the airway. In

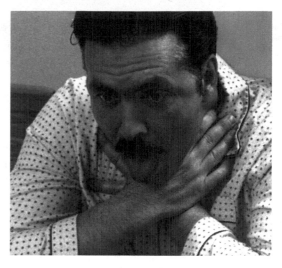

FIGURE 26-17 The universal distress signal for choking is one or both hands about the throat. This patient has a red face and is obviously in distress.

this situation, you must take quick, decisive action. In a feeding situation, food blocks the airway, but air passages may also be blocked by the tongue, dentures, or another foreign body in the back of the throat. Tilting the head back may open the airway by allowing the tongue to move forward so some air can pass.

- If the person can speak and is coughing vigorously, do not intervene. Stay close by and encourage coughing. Follow your facility's procedure for calling for backup help.
- A complete blockage is signaled by the person being unable to speak, high-pitched sounds on inhalation, and grasping the throat in the universal distress signal (Figure 26-17).

PROCEDURE 74 ABDOMINAL THRUSTS—HEIMLICH MANEUVER

 NOTE

The American Heart Association and the American Red Cross both offer courses in first aid and CPR in communities across the country. The information in this book is not intended to take the place of an approved course. Use these guidelines as a quick reference or refresher. Perform chest compressions and CPR *only* if you have completed an approved course taught by an approved instructor.

1. Ask the person if they are choking.
2. If the person starts to cough, wait.
3. If the person cannot speak, cough, or breathe—but is conscious—apply abdominal thrusts (**Heimlich maneuver**) until the foreign body is expelled.
   a. Stand behind the victim and wrap your arms around the waist.
   b. Clench your fist, keeping the thumb straight (Figure 26-18A).

(continues)

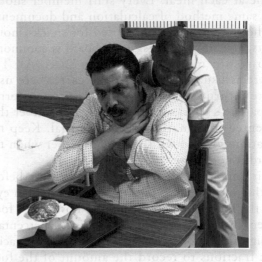

FIGURE 26-18B Grasp the clenched fist with the opposite hand. Avoid pressing against the patient's ribs with the forearms.

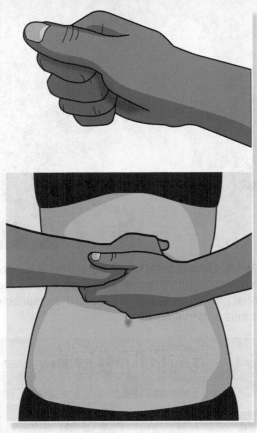

FIGURE 26-18A Clench the fist, keeping the thumb straight

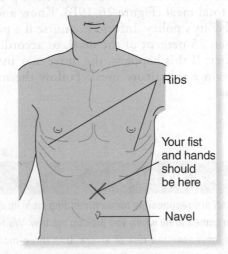

FIGURE 26-18C Thrust forcefully, inward and upward, with the thumb side of the fist just above the navel.

c. Place your fist, thumb side in, against the victim's abdomen slightly above the navel and below the tip of the xiphoid process.

d. Grasp your clenched fist with your opposite hand (Figure 26-18B).

e. Avoid pressing on the patient's ribs with your forearms.

f. Thrust forcefully with the thumb side of your fist against the midline of the victim's abdomen, slightly above his navel, inward and upward (Figure 26-18C). Be sure you are below the tip of the sternum (xiphoid process). Deliver each thrust with the intention of freeing the obstruction.

4. Keep thrusting if the object is not dislodged. If the person begins to cough forcefully, wait.

5. Activate the EMS system.

6. Continue the Heimlich maneuver until the obstruction is expelled or the victim becomes unconscious. If the victim becomes unconscious, place the victim in supine position.

Alternative Action: Chest thrusts are used when pressure to the abdomen would be harmful or impossible. Chest thrusts are used if the choking person is in late pregnancy or if the victim is so large you are unable to get your arms around them. Follow steps 1 and 2, then stand behind the victim, place arms directly under the victim's armpits, and around the chest. Place the thumb side of your fist in the middle of the breastbone (avoid the ribs and the tip of the breastbone). Grab your fist with your other hand and perform thrusts until the foreign body is expelled or the victim becomes unconscious.

DOCUMENTING MEAL INTAKE

Each facility has a policy and procedure for documenting and recording the amount of food patients consume at each meal. Every staff member should use the same method of calculation and documentation. The system may also be used for snacks, nourishments, and supplements. A clipboard is commonly used to record meal intake (Figure 26-19A). The clipboard is usually on top of the cart where used trays are returned. The information is transferred to the patient's chart after the meal. Remember that documented information is confidential. Keep the information covered with a piece of paper when the clipboard is not in use.

Wait until the patient has finished eating before calculating meal intake. This involves more than eyeballing the food tray and estimating how much food was eaten. Instead, you must document the percentage of the significant food items on the tray. Some facilities use fractions to record the amount of the food consumed. Some write "good," "fair," or "poor." Some facilities record the percentage of each individual food item. Others estimate and document a percentage of the total meal (Figure 26-19B). Know and follow your facility's policy. Inform the nurse if a patient eats less than 75 percent of the meal, or according to facility policy. If this happens, the nurse may instruct you to obtain a substitute meal. Follow the nurse's instructions.

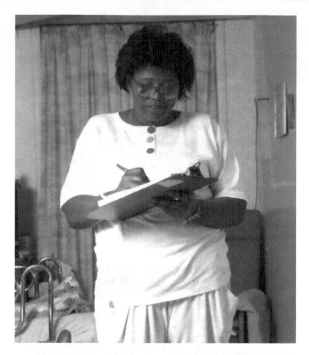

FIGURE 26-19A Documentation of meal intake is one means of monitoring the patient's response to the nutritional plan of care, and preventing undesirable weight loss and malnutrition.

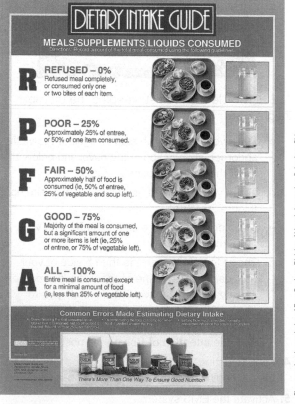

FIGURE 26-19B Accurate documentation of meal intake is an important nursing assistant responsibility. Inaccurate documentation of meal intake can cause patient harm.

⚖ Legal **ALERT**

Facility staff are responsible for documenting meal intake. Document immediately when you pick up the tray. Waiting until later increases the risk of errors. One three-month study showed that facility staff overestimated meal intake 22 percent of the time. Another found only 44 percent agreement between the nursing assistants' documentation and actual meal intake. These results are statistically significant, and inaccurate documentation exposes staff to great legal exposure if the patient has a negative outcome. Be sure your documentation of meal intake is accurate.*

---

*Hammer-Castellanos, V., & Andrews, Y. N. (2002). Inherent flaws in a method of estimating meal intake commonly used in long-term care facilities. *Journal of the American Dietetic Association, 102,* 826–830; Simmons, S. F., & Reuben, D. (2000). Nutritional intake monitoring for nursing home residents: A comparison of staff documentation, direct observation, and photography methods. *Journal of the American Geriatric Society, 48,* 209–213.

ALTERNATIVE NUTRITION

There may be situations in which the patient is unable to take in food in the usual way. This may occur if the patient:

- Is unconscious
- Has a disease of the digestive tract
- Has persistent vomiting and cannot hold down food
- Is unable to swallow without aspiration (choking)

Aspiration is a very serious condition in which food, water, gastric contents, or other objects enter the trachea and lungs. It is usually accidental, such as when the patient "swallows down the wrong tube" or accidentally inhales food or fluids. If you suspect that a patient has aspirated, inform the nurse promptly.

To maintain life, the body must meet its requirements for daily essential nutrients. This may be done by administration of total parenteral nutrition (TPN) (also called hyperalimentation), which is a form of **intravenous infusion (IV)**, or by **enteral feedings** (tubes inserted into the digestive tract).

Total Parenteral Nutrition

Total parenteral nutrition (TPN) is a technique in which high-density (concentrated) nutrients are introduced into a large blood vessel, such as the subclavian vein. This method of feeding is used for patients with diseases of the digestive tract. Caring for patients with TPN is discussed in Chapter 36.

Enteral Feedings

Enteral feedings may be administered by a tube that is:

- Inserted through the nose and into the stomach (**nasogastric feeding (NG feeding)**) (Figure 26-20A)

- Inserted directly through the abdominal skin and into the stomach (**gastrostomy feeding**) (Figure 26-20B)

The **jejunostomy tube (J-tube)** (Figure 26-20C) is a long, small-bore tube that is threaded through the GI tract until the tip reaches the small intestine. Occasionally, you may see a J-tube that has been placed through the nose (nasojejunostomy), but these are less common. The most common J-tube is surgically inserted through an incision in the abdominal skin. This is a long-term tube. Jejunostomy tubes are used for patients who do not have a stomach, and those in whom recurrent formula aspiration is a problem.

Many different types of tubes may be used for enteral feedings. The nurse or physician inserts the feeding tube. Some tubes are placed surgically, such as the gastrostomy (Figure 26-21A) and **percutaneous endoscopic gastrostomy (PEG)** tube. The physician surgically inserts a PEG tube by threading the tube through the patient's mouth and into the stomach and then pulling the tube out through an incision in the patient's abdomen. The operative site for tubes that have been surgically placed is

 Infection Control ALERT

People often believe that those who are fed by tube need less oral care. In fact, the reverse is true. *All patients need regular oral care.* Poor oral health is a contributing factor to poor nutrition, pain, weight loss, decreased quality of life, and serious illnesses such as diabetes and hypertension, as well as increased risk of stroke, heart disease, and pneumonia.

 Safety ALERT

Most patients receiving tube feedings are NPO, but some are also permitted to have food or liquids orally. Verify the orders for that patient before giving food or fluids. The head of the bed must be elevated at all times when a tube feeding is being administered, to prevent accidental aspiration of formula into the lungs. Monitor for signs of respiratory distress. The patient will begin coughing, choking, gurgling, or they will become cyanotic if formula is aspirated into the lungs. If any of these occur, call the nurse immediately. While providing routine care, monitor the skin on the hips and buttocks frequently, as the patient's feeding position increases pressure and the risk of skin breakdown. Move the patient in bed with an assistant. Elevating the head of the bed also increases the risk of skin damage from friction and shearing.

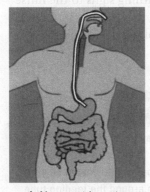 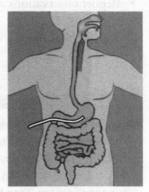

A. Nasogastric route   B. Gastrostomy route

FIGURE 26-20A Common methods of enteral feeding: A. nasogastric (NG) tube; B. gastrostomy tube.

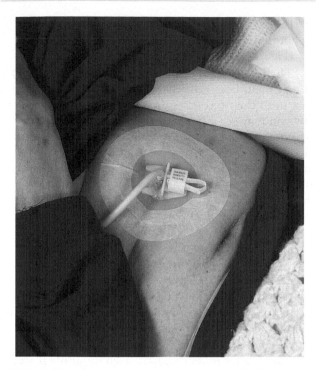

FIGURE 26-21A Gastrostomy tubes are surgically inserted through the abdominal skin into the stomach. This type of tube is used when long-term tube feeding is anticipated.

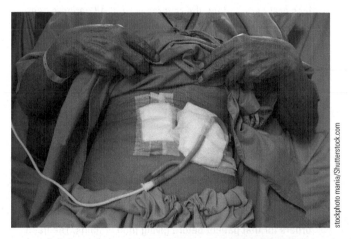

FIGURE 26-21B Enteral feedings are administered through a mechanical pump. This patient is receiving a feeding through a gastrostomy tube.

covered with a dressing for the first few weeks. Once the insertion site has healed, the area is usually left uncovered. Specially prepared solutions containing all the required nutrients are given through the tube. Feedings may be administered intermittently or may run continuously. In either case, the container of solution is hung from an IV (intravenous) pole and may be attached to a device that automatically controls the administration (Figure 26-21B). Water is also given through the tube.

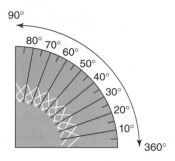

FIGURE 26-22 Elevate the head of the bed at least 30° to 45°, or as specified on the care plan, during feeding and for at least an hour after the feeding is completed. Monitor the skin on the hips and buttocks because this position increases pressure.

When caring for the patient who is receiving tube feedings, you need to:

- Keep the head of the bed elevated at least 30° to 45° (Figure 26-22) during feeding and for 60 minutes after feeding.
- Check the taping of tubes. If tape is loose, pulls, or is causing skin irritation, inform the nurse.
- Follow the nurse's instructions and care plan for care of the skin around the feeding tube
- Move these patients carefully and position them to avoid tension or traction on the tube.
- Report any retching, nausea, or vomiting immediately.
- Check the tubing for kinks. Be sure the patient is not lying on the tubing.
- Provide frequent mouth care. Patients with an NG tube will also need nasal care.
- Give the patient something to hold if they are pulling on the feeding tube; notify the nurse promptly.
- Turn the patient on the side if coughing or choking.
- Report observations and warning signs to the nurse promptly.
- Notify the nurse if a controlling device alarm sounds.

🔒 Safety **ALERT**

Know the location of the tube at all times and avoid pulling on it. Take care when moving the patient to avoid accidentally dislodging or moving the tube, which can cause serious complications. Keep the skin around the feeding tube clean and dry. If the patient has a nasogastric tube, it may be clipped to the gown or clothing to prevent pulling.

Tube Feeding Complications

Tube feedings are common treatments. Persons receiving tube feedings are also at nutritional risk. Their medical needs sometimes change, and tube-feeding formula and fluid orders must be adjusted to keep up with their bodies' demands. Signs and symptoms of tube-feeding complications to make and report are:

- Nausea
- Vomiting
- Diarrhea
- Swollen stomach
- Constipation
- Excessive flatus or cramping
- Pain, redness, heat, swelling, crusting, or fluid oozing from the site where the feeding tube enters the body
- Cough
- Wet breathing
- Feeling that something is caught in the throat
- Complaints of dryness or discomfort in the mouth or throat
- Pulling at or removing the feeding tube

Infection Control ALERT

Reflux is the regurgitation of stomach contents back into the esophagus. When this occurs, the stomach contents can be aspirated into the trachea. If the person is NPO, they will also have a dry mouth and fewer automatic swallows. This is common in persons who are fed by tube, as well as those who consume food by mouth. The aspiration causes a burning pain, and the patient may complain of an acid taste. Pneumonia may develop if the fluid enters the lungs. Because of this, proper positioning is very important.

Accepting tube-feeding formula can be difficult for the patient. Notify the nurse so they can adjust the rate and strength of the formula to meet the patient's needs. In some patients, the formula causes diarrhea. Inform the nurse if the patient's bowel activity increases, or if the patient experiences multiple loose or liquid stools. Keep the perineum clean and dry, and wash the patient well after each bowel activity.

REVIEW

A. True/False

Mark the following true or false by circling T or F.

1. T F Vitamins are nutrients that help regulate body activities.
2. T F The exchange list is used by patients on low-salt diets.
3. T F Fats are one of the six essential nutrients.
4. T F Ice cream would be served to a patient on a clear liquid diet.
5. T F Labels of canned foods must be checked when planning their use in low-sodium diets.
6. T F A gastrostomy tube introduces nutrients directly into the stomach.
7. T F Foods with carbohydrates are used to make new body cells and build tissues.
8. T F Green leafy vegetables are a good source of calcium, iron, and B vitamins.
9. T F Complete protein foods like poultry contain all of the essential amino acids.

10. T F A person can live for about a week without water.
11. T F Foods such as nuts, olives, and avocados are naturally high in oil.
12. T F Oils and fats are a food group.
13. T F Adequate fluids are needed to prevent constipation.
14. T F It is a good idea to provide nutritional supplements on the meal tray so they are not overlooked.
15. T F Most people swallow about 200 times each day.
16. T F Adult males should take in about two liters of fluid each day.
17. T F Adult females should take in about one liter of fluid each day.
18. T F Cellulose is harmful if ingested.

B. Matching

Match the correct term from Column II with the words and phrases in Column I.

Column I

19. _____ difficulty swallowing

20. _____ roughage

21. _____ encourage liquid intake

22. _____ regurgitation of stomach contents back into the esophagus

23. _____ all the processes involved in taking in food and building and repairing the body

24. _____ an essential nutrient

25. _____ treatment-related

26. _____ calcium

Column II

a. therapeutic

b. mineral

c. dysphagia

d. water

e. force fluids

f. cellulose

g. reflux

h. gastrostomy

i. nutrition

C. Multiple Choice

Select the best answer for each of the following.

27. Feeding the patient through a nasogastric tube is known as a(n):
    a. intravenous infusion.
    b. gastrostomy feeding.
    c. enteral feeding.
    d. hyperalimentation.

28. Which of the following is a water-soluble vitamin?
    a. vitamin C
    b. vitamin E
    c. vitamin A
    d. vitamin D

29. An example of a fat-soluble vitamin is:
    a. vitamin C.
    b. vitamin B-complex.
    c. vitamin D.
    d. vitamin N.

30. Water is a(n):
    a. vitamin.
    b. essential nutrient.
    c. mineral.
    d. discretionary calorie.

31. Which of the following is part of the meat group?
    a. Whole grains
    b. Rice
    c. Fish
    d. Butter

32. Foods naturally high in sodium include:
    a. milk.
    b. cereals.
    c. cold cuts, such as salami.
    d. fruits.

33. Supplemental nourishments might include:
    a. hot fudge sundaes.
    b. mashed potatoes.
    c. candy bars.
    d. high-protein drinks.

34. Nutritional supplements are:
    a. given for a specific therapeutic purpose.
    b. withheld if the patient has a fluid restriction.
    c. given on request when a patient is hungry.
    d. high in sugar, protein, and lactose.

35. It is especially important to report to the nurse that the patient only ate two-thirds of their meal when the patient is on a:
    a. low-salt diet.
    b. calorie-restricted diet.
    c. diabetic diet.
    d. house diet.

36. The consistent-carbohydrate meal plan:
    a. ensures that the patient consumes 50 percent of their calories from protein.
    b. focuses on maintaining equal parts of food from all food groups.
    c. is a high-fiber diet that is served to persons with constipation.
    d. permits regular food as long as carbohydrates are the same each day.

D. Nursing Assistant Challenge

Mrs. Gole is one of your assigned patients. She is 72 years old, is on a regular dysphagia diet, and is a member of the Seventh Day Adventist Church. She also has Parkinson disease with tremors of her hands and has trouble swallowing. Mrs. Gole sometimes eats food brought in by family and friends that is not on the ordered diet. Consider Mrs. Gole's care as you answer the following questions.

37. Discuss safety issues that you need to think about when Mrs. Gole is eating.

_____

_____

38. Are there conflicts between the ordered diet and the dietary restrictions of her church? If so, what are the conflicts and how might they be resolved?

_____

39. Do you anticipate that Mrs. Gole will have any problems feeding herself? If so, what are those problems, and what can you do to help her eat independently?

_____

_____

40. Discuss the issues of residents' or patients' rights that may arise because of the conflict between the patient's desire to eat foods different from what the physician has prescribed.

_____

_____

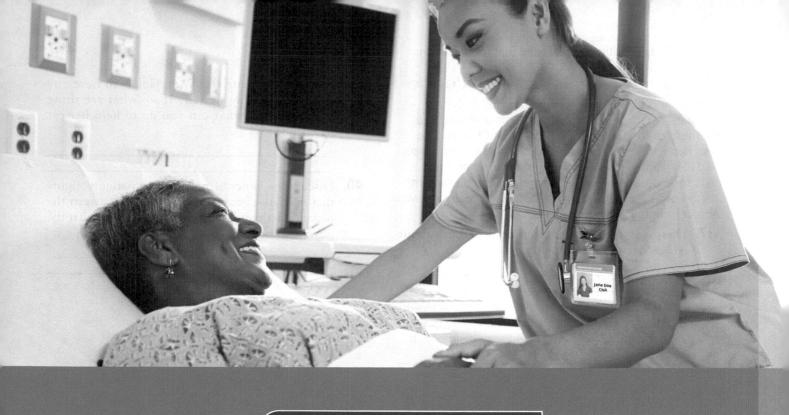

SECTION 9

Special Care Procedures

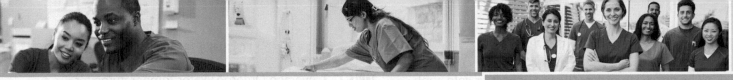

Warm and Cold Applications

CHAPTER 27

OBJECTIVES

After completing this chapter, you will be able to:

27.1 Spell and define terms.

27.2 List the physical conditions requiring the use of heat and cold.

27.3 Name types of heat and cold applications.

27.4 Describe the effects of local cold applications.

27.5 Describe the effects of local heat applications.

27.6 List safety concerns related to application of heat and cold.

27.8 Demonstrate the following procedures:
- Procedure 75: Applying an Ice Bag or Gel Pack (Expand Your Skills)
- Procedure 76: Applying a Disposable Cold Pack (Expand Your Skills)
- Procedure 77: Giving a Sitz Bath (Expand Your Skills)

VOCABULARY

Learn the meaning and the correct spelling of the following words and phrases:

Aquamatic K-Pad (aquathermia pad)	hemorrhage	hypothermia–hyperthermia blanket (aquathermia blanket)	thermal blanket
cold pack	hot water bottle		vasoconstriction
core body temperature	hyperpyrexia		vasodilation
diathermy	hyperthermia	ice bag	warm soak
	hypothermia	sitz bath	wet compress

INTRODUCTION

Heat and cold applications are used only when there are written orders from the physician, and only for a specific length of time. Some facilities allow only professional personnel to apply heat and cold. In others, nursing assistants who have been specially trained may provide heat and cold treatments under the supervision of the nurse. Be sure you know and follow the policy of your facility and are adequately prepared and *supervised*.

 Safety **ALERT**

Some states prohibit nursing assistants from applying heat or cold in any setting. Some prohibit heat and cold applications in a home health setting.

THERAPY WITH HEAT AND COLD

A localized application supplies heat or cold to a specific area. For example, a hot water bottle on an abscess is a local application. A generalized application provides heat or cold to the whole body. A hypothermia blanket is a generalized application.

The physician orders the use of heat or cold applications to:

- Relieve pain
- Combat local infection
- Relieve or reduce swelling or inflammation
- Control bleeding (**hemorrhage**)
- Reduce body temperature
  Local applications of heat and cold are made with:
- Ice bags
- Hot water bottles
- Electronically operated Aquamatic K-Pads (aquathermia pads). K-Pads come in many shapes and sizes. They are used to apply heat. By using an attachment, they can also be used for cooling.
- Prepackaged, single-use chemical packs for the application of heat and cold. A single hit on the surface activates the contents, providing a controlled temperature.
- Gel packs that can be cooled or heated as needed.

General heat or cold treatments are done with thermal mattresses known as **hypothermia–hyperthermia blankets (aquathermia blanket)**. These are widely used to:

- Lower body temperature when there is fever
- Elevate body temperature in cases of hypothermia

Applications of warm and cold may be either dry or moist. Moisture makes both heat and cold more penetrating. Therefore, moist heat or moist cold is more likely to cause injury. Protect and closely monitor the patient when moist treatments are used. Be sure you know:

- The exact method to be used
- The correct temperature and placement
- The proper length of time the warm or cold application is to be performed.
- How often the area being treated is to be checked.

Table 27-1 lists moist and dry applications.

Table 27-2 lists the average temperatures ordered for heat and cold applications.

TABLE 27-1 Moist and Dry Applications

Dry	Moist
Hypothermia blanket	Soaks
Aquathermia pad	Compresses
Commercial warm or cold pack (chemical or gel)	Packs
Ice bag	Tub bath
Hot water bottle	Sitz bath

TABLE 27-2 Average Ordered Water Temperatures for Hydrotherapy Treatments and Procedures

Hot: 100°F to 105°F

Warm: 95°F to 105°F (this is the range used for hydrotherapy treatments)

Tepid: 80°F to 95°F

Cool: 65°F to 80°F

Cold: 45°F to 65°F

- Never set the whirlpool for higher than 100°F without first checking with the nurse. (The whirlpool is preset to maintain a constant temperature of 97°F. Because it maintains a constant water temperature, you should not have to adjust it.)
- These guidelines may also be appropriate for other heat treatments; follow the nurse's instructions.

🔓 Safety **ALERT**

Each state has laws governing the water temperature in patient care areas of the facility. These vary slightly from one state to the next, but in most, water temperature in patient care units and bathing areas should not exceed 120°F. Although the maintenance department monitors water temperatures throughout the building daily, the regulators sometimes fail, sending very hot water into the facility. However, water in bath and shower areas must be warm enough to bathe patients comfortably. Comfortable temperature for most people is 95°F to 105°F. Report water in bathing areas that does not warm up enough for comfortable bathing. Also report steaming water, or water that feels hot to touch at any faucet in a patient care area. Use a bath thermometer to check water temperatures before patient care whenever possible. If a thermometer is unavailable, check the temperature on the inside of your forearm, wrist, or elbow.

Commercial Preparations

Easy-to-use commercial warm and cold packs are available for dry applications. One type of pack is activated by a single hit or blow to the pack before application. The kind of pack is discarded after one use. Reusable packs are also available, but infection control issues make them less desirable.

USE OF COLD APPLICATIONS

Cold applications are given only with a physician's order. The application of cold:

- Constricts or decreases the size of blood vessels (**vasoconstriction**) and reduces swelling
- Decreases sensitivity to pain
- Reduces temperature
- Slows inflammation
- Reduces itching

Cautions

Remember that moisture intensifies the effect of cold just as it does heat. Use caution when applying moist cold.

- Excessive cold can damage body tissues.
- Report color changes such as *blanching* (turning white) or *cyanosis* (becoming bluish).
- Report feelings of numbness or discomfort experienced by the patient.
- Stop the cold treatment if the patient starts to shiver. Cover the patient with a blanket and report immediately to the nurse. (See Procedures 75 and 76.)

GUIDELINES 27-1 Guidelines for Warm and Cold Treatments

You must be very watchful when applying cold or warm treatments. When assigned to this task, keep in mind:

- The age and condition of the patient. Give extra care to:
  - Young children.
  - Persons who are elderly.
  - Patients with cognitive impairment.
  - Patients who are uncooperative.
  - Patients who are unconscious.
  - Patients who are paralyzed.
  - Patients with tissue damage.
  - Patients with poor circulation.
- Apply the principles of standard precautions if your hands will contact blood, moist body fluids (except sweat), secretions, excretions, nonintact skin, or mucous membranes.
- Consult the nurse for directions if the patient has a dressing covering the area to be treated
- Check the temperature of liquid solutions with a thermometer (Figure 27-1). You may need to add more liquid during the treatment to maintain the temperature. Avoid pouring hot or cold liquid directly over the patient.
- Remove all metal jewelry, buttons, or zippers that could conduct heat or cold and thereby injure the skin.
- Avoid using heat treatments with temperatures over 105°F. Temperatures higher than this can cause burns, particularly in infants and elderly persons.
- Avoid using heat in the first 48 hours after an injury.
- Follow all safety rules to prevent spills and falls.
- Use an approved heating pad. A regular household heating pad must not be used.
- Check patients frequently, because sensitivity to heat varies from person to person.

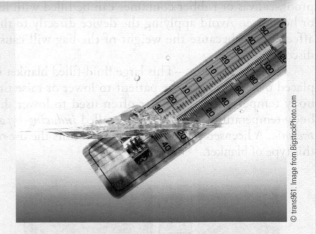

FIGURE 27-1 A bath thermometer is used to measure the temperature of bath water. The temperature should not exceed 105°F

- Do not apply heat to the head or abdomen.
- Check the skin under the application every 10 minutes, or as instructed. If it appears red, or a dark area appears, stop the treatment and notify the nurse. Stop a cold application and notify the nurse if the skin appears cyanotic, pale, white, or bright red; if the patient complains of numbness or is shivering. Cover the patient with a blanket.
- Be sure all appliances are covered with cloth. Rubber or plastic should never touch the patient's skin.
- Do not leave a heat or cold application in place longer than 20 minutes. Follow the care plan and the nurse's instructions.
- Pat the skin dry and make the patient comfortable after the treatment. Clean and store used equipment. Remove and discard gloves. Wash your hands. Inform the nurse that the procedure was completed and the patient's reaction.

Dry Heat and Cold Applications

There are several methods for applying therapeutic heat and cold (Figure 27-2). Pay careful attention to the application to prevent injury.

Disposable heat pack or **cold pack**—This single-use commercial pack contains chemicals and can be stored until needed. Reusable commercial gel packs are also available for both warm and cold applications. The pack remains effective for approximately 15 to 30 minutes. Do not hold a chemical pack in front of your face when squeezing or striking to activate it. If the pack leaks or bursts, the chemicals inside the pack may splash. Check the area being treated every 10 minutes. Discard the chemical pack after one use. Do not attempt to reheat or refreeze it.

Ice bag or **hot water bottle**—This reusable, waterproof, canvas or rubber container can be filled with ice or hot water. Avoid applying the device directly to the affected area because the weight of the bag will cause discomfort.

Thermal blanket—This large fluid-filled blanket is placed over or around the patient to lower or raise the body temperature. It is most often used to lower the body temperature. This process is called *inducing hypothermia*. A licensed professional also monitors the use of this type of blanket.

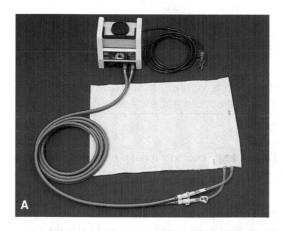

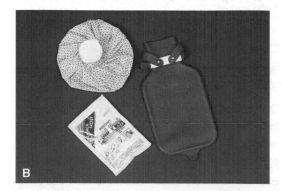

FIGURE 27-2 Types of heat and cold applications: A. An aquathermia pad B. Items used for heat or cold treatments.

Clinical Information **ALERT**

A partially filled bottle or application is flexible and molds to the patient's body easily. The weight of a full bottle may cause pain to an injured area. Make sure the patient can tolerate the weight of the application without increasing or causing pain. A partially filled bottle with the air expelled stays warm longer. Extra air in the bottle cools hot water. You can tie the application to the treatment area with roller gauze to hold it in place.

Safety **ALERT**

Cold therapy should not be used for patients who have:

- Deep vein thrombosis.
- Peripheral vascular disease.
- Open wound(s).
- Skin sensation impairment.
- Severe cognitive impairment.
- Cold intolerance or cold allergy.
- Medical conditions such as rheumatoid arthritis and Reynaud's phenomenon.

Moist Cold Applications

Wet compresses are moistened with a solution and placed on the affected area. A syringe may be used to add water to the compresses to keep them moist. Compresses can be kept cold by covering them with an ice bag. Make sure the patient can tolerate the weight of the ice bag without increased pain. Reposition the protective covering each time the pad is removed and replaced.

Follow facility policy and the patient's care plan for:

- Method of applying the treatment
- Length of time the treatment is to be applied.
- How often the patient is to be checked for condition of the skin in the treatment area and general response to the treatment.
- Signs that treatment should be discontinued.

USE OF WARM APPLICATIONS

Warm applications are ordered to:

- Relieve muscle spasms
- Reduce pain
- Reduce inflammation
- Promote healing

- Combat local infection
- Increase circulation
- Improve mobility before exercise periods
- Relax the patient

The value of heat treatments (**diathermy**) is that heat dilates or increases the size of blood vessels (**vasodilation**). This brings more blood to the area to promote healing. Warmth is very soothing when there is pain.

Safety ALERT

The heat application should feel comfortably warm to the patient, not uncomfortably hot. Cover the application with cloth. Touch a pack or pad to your forearm to check the temperature before applying it. If the patient complains of burning, remove the application and consult the nurse.

EXPAND YOUR SKILLS

PROCEDURE 75 APPLYING AN ICE BAG OR GEL PACK

1. Assemble equipment:
   - Ice bag or gel pack
   - Cover (usually flannel, cotton, a towel, or a cover specified by your facility)
   - Paper towels
   - Spoon or similar utensil
   - Ice cubes or crushed ice

2. Prepare the ice bag or gel pack as follows:
   a. Fill the ice bag with cold water and check for leaks.
   b. Empty the bag.
   c. Rinse ice cubes (if used) in water to remove sharp edges. Using crushed ice makes the bag more flexible and comfortable for the patient.
   d. Fill the ice bag half full, using an ice scoop, paper cup, or large spoon (Figure 27-3A). Avoid making ice bags too heavy. Do not allow the scoop to touch the ice bag.
   e. To remove air from the ice bag:
      - Rest the ice bag flat on a paper towel on a flat surface.
      - Put the top in place, but do not tighten it.
      - Press the bag until the air is removed (Figure 27-3B).
   f. Fasten the top securely.
   g. Test for leakage.
   h. Wipe the ice bag dry with paper towels. Place it in a cloth cover.

NOTE

As an alternative, a gel pack stored in the freezer can be used for cold applications. These packs can be refrozen and reused for the same person.

3. Take the equipment to the bedside on a tray. Carry out initial procedure actions.

4. Apply the ice bag to the affected part.

5. Refill the ice bag before all the ice has melted.

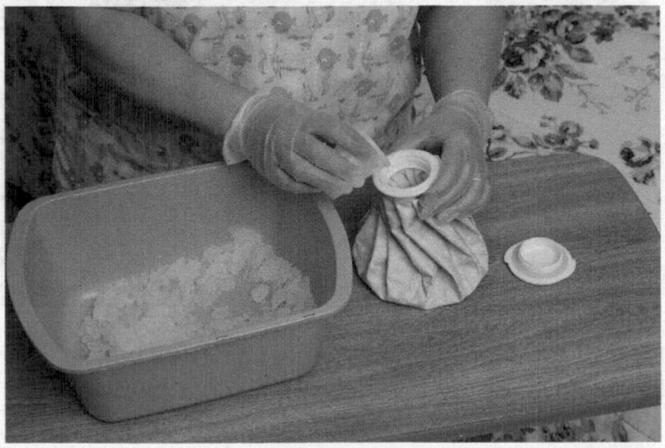

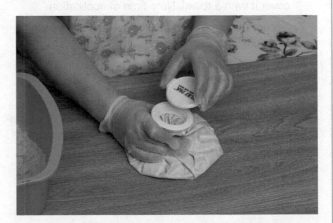

FIGURE 27-3A Fill the ice bag half full.

FIGURE 27-3B Place the ice bag on a flat surface, and then press firmly to remove air.

(continues)

PROCEDURE **75** CONTINUED

6. Check the skin area under the application every 10 minutes, or as instructed. Remove the treatment and report to the nurse immediately if skin is cyanotic or white, or if the patient reports that the skin is numb.

7. Continue the cold application for the amount of time specified. If the patient feels cold, cover with a blanket, but do not cover the area being treated.

8. Carry out ending procedure actions.

9. When the treatment is complete, wash the bag or gel pack with soap and water. Rinse and dry it completely, and then close the top. Wipe the bag with a disinfectant if this is your facility's policy. Leave air in the ice bag to prevent the sides from sticking together.

10. If a reusable gel cold pack is used, wash it thoroughly with soap and water or wipe with a disinfectant. Return the pack to the refrigerator. Discard a disposable pack.

EXPAND YOUR SKILLS

PROCEDURE **76** APPLYING A DISPOSABLE COLD PACK

1. Carry out initial procedure actions.

2. Assemble equipment:
- Disposable commercial cold pack
- Cloth covering (flannel, a towel, a warm water bag cover, or another cover specified by the facility)
- Tape or rolls of gauze

3. Expose the area to be treated. Note the condition of the area.

4. Place the cold pack in a cloth covering (Figure 27-4).

5. Strike or squeeze the cold pack to activate chemicals. (Follow the manufacturer's instructions.)

6. Place the covered cold pack on the proper area and cover it with a towel. Note time of application.

7. Secure the cover with tape or gauze, if necessary, to hold it in place.

8. Leave the patient in a comfortable position, with the signal cord within easy reach.

9. Return to the bedside every 10 minutes, or as instructed. Check the area being treated for discoloration or numbness. If any adverse signs or symptoms occur, notify the nurse.

10. If no adverse signs or symptoms occur, remove the pack after 20 minutes, or the length of time given in your instructions. Note the condition of the area.

11. Remove the pack from the cover and discard the pack.

12. Put the cover in a laundry hamper.

13. Carry out ending procedure actions.

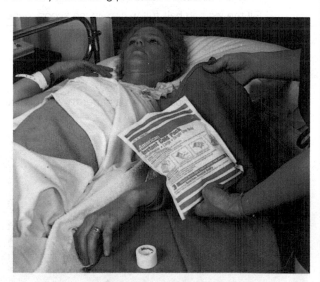

FIGURE 27-4 Cover the disposable cold pack with a flannel cover or towel before applying it to the patient.

Cautions

Follow these precautions when working with patients:

- Carefully monitor heat applications.
- Moisture intensifies the effect of warmth. Use extra caution.
- Never allow a patient to lie on a constant heat unit, because heat may be trapped and build up to dangerous levels.
- The temperature of a constant heat unit should be between 95°F and 100°F.
- Use a bath thermometer to check solution temperatures.
- Remove the body part being soaked before adding warm solution.
- Protect areas not being treated from excessive exposure.
- Warmth can cause blood vessels in the head to dilate, resulting in headache.
- Rubber or plastic should never touch the patient's skin. Be sure all appliances are covered with cloth.

Dry Warm Applications

The **Aquamatic K-Pad (aquathermia pad)** is commonly used to provide dry warmth. It consists of a plastic pad with fluid-filled coils and a control unit that maintains a constant temperature.

A reservoir in the control unit supplies distilled water to the pad. Place the control unit on the bedside stand and plug it into an electrical outlet. In most facilities, the temperature is preset at 95°F to 100°F.

> **NOTE**
>
> When setting up the K-Pad for the first time, check the pad for leaks. Tip it back and forth several times to eliminate air pockets, which cause hot spots. Make sure the control unit is higher than the patient so that water will run into the pad by gravity. Make sure the tubing is free of kinks.

Moist Warm Applications

Moist warm treatments include:

- **Warm soaks**—The patient, or the part of the patient's body that is being treated, is immersed in a tub filled with water at a specific temperature, usually 105°F.
- **Wet compresses**—The same precautions apply to warm compresses as to cold compresses. They may

Safety ALERT

Heat therapy should not be used for patients who have:

- Acute inflammation
- Dermatitis
- Deep vein thrombosis
- Peripheral vascular disease
- Open wound(s)
- Recent soft tissue injuries in which swelling or bleeding would be increased by heat.
- Skin sensation impairment and paralysis
- Severe cognitive impairment
- Acute edema
- Rash
- Infection
- Hemophilia

Use with caution and careful monitoring if the patient is very young or very old. Some physicians also recommend avoiding heat with women during pregnancy. Check with the nurse before applying a heat application.

be kept wet with a syringe and warm by covering them with an Aquamatic K-Pad.

Sitz Bath

A **sitz bath** is a method of bathing in which only the perineal area is immersed in a special tub or disposable basin. It is usually done to relieve discomfort following childbirth, perineal surgery, or rectal surgery. Immersing the perineum in warm water is relaxing and enhances healing by reducing inflammation, stimulating circulation, and promoting wound healing. The water temperature must be constant.

Some older hospitals have permanent sitz bathtubs (Figure 27-5A). If you use this type of unit, make sure to clean and disinfect it well. Some use portable chairs that are similar to commode chairs (Figure 27-5B). Most newer facilities use a portable (disposable) sitz bath kit (Figure 27-5C). The kit contains a plastic basin that fits over the toilet and an irrigation bag with tubing and clamp. It is issued to the patient and presents a lower infection control risk than shared units. It is sent home or discarded upon discharge. An individual unit such as this is the best type to use for infection control purposes.

Drape the patient's lower body with a bath blanket during the bath (Figure 27-6), and keep them warm throughout the procedure. Dress the patient promptly after the sitz bath to maintain body heat.

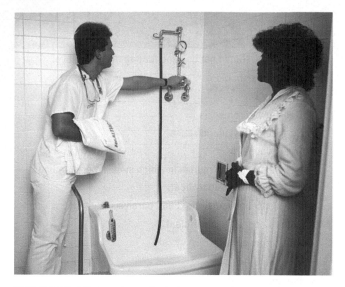

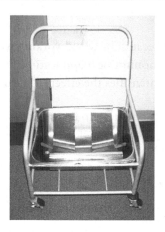

FIGURE 27-5B A stand-alone sitz bath chair.

FIGURE 27-5A Some hospitals have stationary sitz bathtubs in areas of frequent use, such as obstetrics and surgical units.

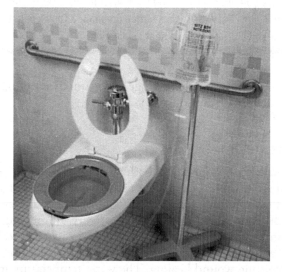

FIGURE 27-5C A portable sitz bath tub is placed under the base of the toilet after the seat is lifted. Many hospitals prefer this type of sitz bath because it is for single patient use and may be taken home for continued therapy after hospital discharge.

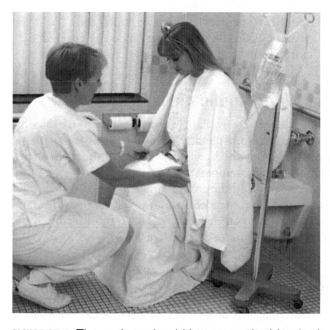

FIGURE 27-6 The patient should be covered with a bath blanket after being seated on the sitz bath. This will prevent chilling.

EXPAND YOUR SKILLS

PROCEDURE **77** GIVING A SITZ BATH

1 Carry out initial procedure actions.

2 Assemble equipment:
- Disposable exam gloves
- Permanent sitz tub, portable sitz tub, or bathtub
- 2–3 bath towels
- 2 bath blankets
- Floor bath mat
- Rubber bath mat
- Bath thermometer
- Gown

(continues)

- Footstool, if needed

- Overbed table

- Pitcher, if needed to refill irrigation bag

- IV standard (if needed, to hold irrigation bag)

- Dressings

- Supplies to disinfect tub, as needed

- Plastic bag for used supplies

3 Clean and disinfect the tub. Rinse thoroughly.

4 Instruct the patient to void before beginning this procedure.

5 Remove dressings and/or peri pad, if used. If a dressing adheres to a wound, soak it off in the tub. Discard these items in a plastic bag and place the bag in biohazardous trash.

6 Fill the sitz tub or bathtub one-third to one-half full, so that the water will cover the perineum, or will reach the patient's umbilicus if a permanent sitz tub is used. Use hot water, 105°F to 110°F, or as instructed by the nurse. (The water will cool before the patient uses it; if the patient will be using it immediately, the temperature should not exceed 105°F.)

7 Check the water temperature with a bath thermometer.

8 If you are using a disposable kit, fill the basin to the designated line.

9 Place the basin under the commode seat.

10 Close the plastic clamp on the irrigation tubing.

11 Fill the irrigation bag with 105°F to 110°F water. (The water will cool before use.)

12 Hang the solution bag from the towel bar, hook, or an IV standard.

13 Insert the irrigation tubing through the entry hole near the front of the plastic bowl.

14 Pull the tubing inside the bowl.

15 Secure the tubing by snapping it into the channel in the center bottom of the bowl.

16 Make sure the small hole at the end of the tube faces up.

17 Assist the patient to sit on the seat. If the patient's legs do not reach the floor, support them on a footstool.

18 Cover the patient's shoulders and lap with a bath blanket.

19 Position a folded towel behind the lower back to reduce discomfort.

20 Offer to place the overbed table in front of the patient, if desired, to provide additional support and comfort.

21 Open the clamp to begin the flow of solution. Show the patient how to regulate the flow.

22 Follow your instructions for remaining in the room during the procedure.

23 Frequently monitor the patient's color and condition. If the patient becomes dizzy or weak, check the pulse and blood pressure promptly. Use the call signal to get help. Return the patient to bed using a wheelchair.

24 Refill the irrigation bag when necessary.

25 After the prescribed time (usually 15 to 20 minutes), clamp the tubing.

26 Assist the patient to stand. Encourage them to use the handrails. Monitor closely for dizziness, weakness, faintness, or nausea.

27 Assist the patient to dry, if necessary.

28 Apply a clean dressing or peri pad, if necessary.

29 Assist the patient to dress and return to their room.

30 Cleanse and disinfect the sitz tub.

31 Store the disposable tub for reuse by the same patient.

32 Carry out ending procedure actions.

ABNORMALITIES IN TEMPERATURE REGULATION

Human survival depends on the person's ability to maintain a stable body temperature between 97°F and 100°F. Normally, the nervous system controls the body's response to heat and cold, and regulates temperature automatically to keep the body at normal operating temperature. Extreme environmental conditions and various medical problems will disrupt normal body response.

Hypothermia

When heat loss exceeds heat production, the nervous system will trigger certain involuntary responses, such as shivering, to restore the balance. If the cold stress is great and the person's system is overwhelmed, body temperature decreases. **Hypothermia** is a lowering of core body temperature to 95°F or below. Very young and very old persons are at high risk for this condition. **Core body temperature** is the normal operating temperature of the body center, or *core*. This temperature value reflects the temperature in deep structures of the body such as the liver. The severity of hypothermia is determined by the degree to which core temperature is lowered. Rectal temperatures are taken when hypothermia is suspected or diagnosed.

🔓 Safety ALERT

Persons who are elderly are at higher risk of developing hypothermia than are younger individuals. Inform the nurse if an elderly patient has a temperature of 96°F or below. Monitor the person closely and watch for signs and symptoms of infection. Instead of running a fever, many elderly persons become hypothermic with sepsis (overwhelming infection). Identifying and treating this serious condition promptly is essential.

Indications of hypothermia to report include:
- Drop in body temperature
- Poor coordination and confusion
- Slurred speech
- Decreased respiratory and heart rates

Untreated, the hypothermic patient's condition worsens, with dehydration, liver and kidney failure, and death. In the early stages of hypothermia, pulse, respirations, and blood pressure may rise. The vital signs decrease as the body temperature drops.

Nursing Assistant Actions

- Report observations to the nurse
- Check the environmental temperature and adjust it
- Provide external warmth with a sweater or blanket
- Reduce drafts with screens or curtains
- If permitted, give something warm to drink
- Check vital signs

Heat-Related Illness

Abnormally high body temperature is called **hyperpyrexia** or **hyperthermia**. It occurs when the rectal temperature is 104°F or above. When environmental temperature exceeds body temperature or the humidity is high, the body retains heat, increasing body temperature. Certain medical problems can also cause severe temperature elevation. When the patient has a fever, the normal mechanisms causing thirst are reduced. The body sweats to cool off. Aging and many chronic diseases further reduce the effectiveness of sweating in cooling the body. Untreated, high body temperature is a very serious condition that leads to brain damage and death. Very high temperatures are treated aggressively.

Indications of hyperthermia to report include:
- Elevated body temperature
- Hot, flushed skin
- Faintness
- Headache
- Nausea
- Convulsions

Fever (*pyrexia*) occurs when core body temperature rises to at least 101°F (rectally). Fever is often associated with infections, injury, surgery, and serious trauma. Indications of fever are the same as those for general hyperthermia.

Nursing Assistant Actions

- Report observations to the nurse
- Check the environmental temperature and adjust it
- Reduce external warmth. Cover the patient with only a gown or sheet
- If permitted, give a cooling drink
- Carry out cooling procedures as ordered. For example, give cooling baths or enemas
- Check vital signs frequently

TEMPERATURE CONTROL MEASURES

Excessively high or low body temperatures are treated in acute care facilities by placing hypothermia–hyperthermia blankets (Figure 27-7) over and under the patient. These blankets are units filled with water. The blankets may be called thermal blankets or *aquathermia blankets*. *Aqua* is the Latin term for *water*. The temperature of the water can be adjusted higher or lower depending on whether the patient's body temperature is to be raised or lowered.

Using the Aquathermia Blanket

The aquathermia blanket is operated either manually or automatically. For manual operation, the licensed nurse will set the blanket to a predetermined temperature. The blanket maintains this temperature regardless of changes in the patient's body temperature. When the unit is set

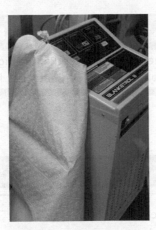

FIGURE 27-6A Thermal blanket.

for automatic operation, it monitors the patient's temperature through a rectal, skin, or esophageal probe that is secured to the body. The blanket temperature changes according to the patient's temperature. The goal is to maintain the patient's body temperature. An alarm will sound for abnormal temperature variations. Before using the blanket, check it for cracks, tears, or leaks in the system. Do not use it if there are cracks or an electrical malfunction.

The patient should wear a hospital gown when using the aquathermia blanket. Use a gown with tie closures. Snaps, pins, or other metal may cause injury to the skin. Before beginning the procedure, check and record the patient's baseline vital signs as a basis for comparison.

One or two aquathermia blankets may be used. The nurse may instruct you to place one under the patient and to cover them with the other. The blankets must be covered with a disposable cover, sheet, or bath blanket to absorb perspiration and prevent complications. Avoid using pins to secure covers on the blanket. These can puncture the unit or injure the patient's skin by creating hot or cold spots. Use tape or Velcro fasteners, if necessary, to attach a cover to the unit.

🔒 Safety **ALERT**

Always read the instructions before using a hypothermia–hyperthermia blanket. Some units are manually operated. This means that the blanket will maintain the preset temperature regardless of the patient's temperature. You will have to adjust the temperature setting manually. Make sure you are familiar with the directions for the unit you are using.

Set up and preheat or precool the blanket before applying it to the patient. Connect the blanket to the control unit by plugging in the tubing. The nurse will set the blanket for automatic or manual operation. They will also set the desired body temperature or blanket temperature and instruct you as to what temperature values are being used. Turn the device on, and then add distilled water to the reservoir. Position the controls at the foot of the bed. After the blanket has reached the designated temperature, apply it to the patient. If the patient will be lying on a blanket, place a pillow or folded bath blanket under the patient's head.

The patient's head should not contact the blanket directly. The combination of heat or cold and the surface of the blanket promotes skin breakdown on the back of the head. The nurse may instruct you to apply lanolin or another designated product to the skin in exposed areas that contact the blanket directly. You may wrap the patient's hands and feet to prevent chilling, if desired.

Complications

Immediately notify the nurse if you observe any of these complications:

- Changes in skin color
- Cyanosis of the lips or nail beds
- Sudden changes in body temperature
- Marked changes in pulse, respirations, or blood pressure
- Respiratory distress
- Pain
- Changes in sensation
- Edema
- Shivering and chills
- Urinary output below 50 mL/hour

Discontinuing Blanket Use

The nurse will inform you when to discontinue use of the blanket. Follow the manufacturer's directions for the type of blanket you are using. Turn the unit off. (Some types must remain plugged in for 30 to 60 minutes to

---

🔒 Safety **ALERT**

The nurse will instruct you on how often to monitor vital signs when an aquathermia blanket is being used. The patient's temperature and the blanket temperature are usually monitored and documented every 15 to 30 minutes. Inform the nurse immediately if the patient's temperature drops more than 1°F in 15 minutes. Continued temperature monitoring is necessary after the blanket is removed because the patient's temperature can continue to drop as much as 5°F after the procedure ends.

---

dry condensation inside the unit.) Dry the patient's skin and assist them into a dry gown. Position the patient in a comfortable position. Remove the aquathermia blanket from the bed after the designated time. Continue checking vital signs and intake and output every 30 minutes for the first 2 hours, then hourly or as directed by the nurse.

Age-Appropriate Care ALERT

In children, temperatures tend to rise higher than in adults. This puts children at greater risk for seizures.

REVIEW

A. True/False

Mark the following true or false by circling T or F.

1. T F Heat and cold treatments should be supervised by the nurse.

2. T F Do not apply heat to the abdomen if a patient has a diagnosis of possible appendicitis.

3. T F The temperature of a warm soak solution should be approximately 100°F.

4. T F Special blankets used to alter the patient's temperature are called infrared blankets.

5. T F A patient who is unconscious must receive special attention during a heat treatment.

6. T F In hyperthermia, core body temperature is reduced to below 95°F.

7. T F Heat is frequently applied to the head to reduce temperature quickly.

8. T F When charting an application of cold, always include the length of time of the application.

9. T F Aquamatic K-Pads are usually set at 115°F.

10. T F Hypothermia may be a sign of severe infection in an elderly person.

11. T F An elderly person is hypothermic when the body temperature is below 97°F.

B. Multiple Choice

Select the best answer for each of the following.

12. Heat affects the body by:
    a. causing blood vessel constriction.
    b. increasing blood supply to the area.
    c. reducing oxygen in tissues.
    d. increasing white blood cells.

13. Special care with heat and cold treatments must be taken when the patient is:
    a. alert and oriented.
    b. very young.

c. cooperative.
d. ambulatory.

14. Dry cold is provided by:
    a. compresses.
    b. sitz baths.
    c. ice caps.
    d. soaks.

15. Cold affects the body by:
    a. reducing pain sensations.
    b. stimulating life processes.
    c. promoting inflammation.
    d. promoting healing.

16. Moist cold is applied with:
    a. ice bags.
    b. ice caps.
    c. ice collars.
    d. cold soaks.

17. When applying heat and cold treatments, the nursing assistant should:
    a. always remain in the room for the duration of the treatment.
    b. check the temperature of the solution with an elbow.
    c. monitor the skin under the application every 30 minutes.
    d. remove jewelry, buttons, or zippers that may conduct heat or cold.

18. When caring for a patient who is using an aquathermia blanket, the nursing assistant should:
    a. regulate blanket temperature at least every 15 minutes.
    b. give the patient plenty of iced liquids to drink to reduce fever.
    c. monitor the patient for cyanosis or changes in vital signs.
    d. turn the patient at least every two hours.

C. Matching

Choose the correct word from Column II to match each description in Column I.

Column I

19. _____ excessive blood loss

20. _____ increase in size of blood vessel

21. _____ heat treatment

22. _____ decrease in size of blood vessel

23. _____ used to lower body temperature

Column II

a. diathermy

b. vasoconstriction

c. vasodilation

d. hypothermia blanket

e. hemorrhage

D. Nursing Assistant Challenge

Peggy, who is 17 years of age, was admitted to your unit from the emergency department. She fractured an ankle and will require internal repair with screws and wire. You will care for her prior to surgery. The physician has ordered an ice bag for her ankle, and her leg is to be elevated. Answer the following questions.

24. What are two reasons for applying the ice bag?
    _____
    _____

25. How full should the ice bag be filled?
    _____
    _____

26. Why should ice cubes be rinsed?
    _____
    _____

27. How should metal caps be positioned when the ice bag is placed on the patient?
    _____
    _____

28. When should the ice bag be refilled?
    _____
    _____

29. How is the ice bag held in place?
    _____
    _____

30. What important observation should be reported immediately to the nurse?
    _____
    _____

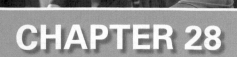

CHAPTER 28

Assisting with the Physical Examination

OBJECTIVES

After completing this chapter, you will be able to:

28.1 Spell and define terms.

28.2 Describe the responsibilities of the nursing assistant during the physical examination.

28.3 Name the various positions for physical examinations.

28.4 Drape the patient for the various positions.

28.5 Name the basic instruments necessary for physical examinations.

VOCABULARY

Learn the meaning and the correct spelling of the following words and phrases:

dorsal lithotomy position   dorsal recumbent position   knee–chest position   Trendelenburg position

INTRODUCTION

Physical examinations are done in the physician's office, in clinics, after the patient's admission to a facility, and in the patient's home. Remember to carry out each initial procedure action and ending procedure action as you assist.

The physical examination helps the primary care provider:

- Evaluate the patient's current status.
- Establish a diagnosis.
- Determine the patient's progress and response to therapy.

Nursing physical assessments will be performed by the nurse in the facility after the patient is admitted. The nurse uses this information to establish a nursing diagnosis.

Both of these assessments are carried out in a similar manner. The responsibilities of the nursing assistant include:

- Providing for the comfort and privacy of the patient
- Trying to anticipate the examiner's needs
- Draping and positioning patients
- Using proper body mechanics and exposing only the part of the patient being examined
- Preparing equipment that might be needed
- Reassuring the patient
- Caring for and labeling specimens
- Handing equipment as needed
- Cleaning equipment after use
- Adjusting lighting
- Remaining available during the examination
- Assisting the patient after the examination

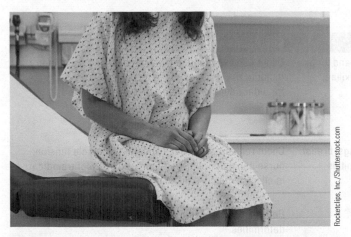

FIGURE 28-1 A disposable gown is commonly used for a physical examination.

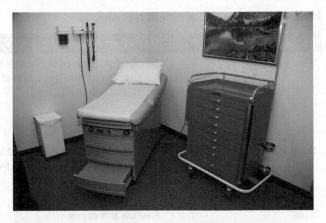

FIGURE 28-2 Each facility has specific examination tables. These tables can be raised or lowered in sections and may have stirrups and shoulder braces to assist with patient positioning.

You are not expected to assess the patient. Keep the person's body covered and ensure modesty and dignity are protected. Assessment is the responsibility of the nurse or physician. You will be expected to assist the patient and examiner and ensure that necessary supplies are available. The examination is typically done in a treatment room, examination room, or clinic setting that has the necessary equipment and supplies available. In this setting, disposable items are commonly used, such as disposable:

- Gown (Figure 28-1)
- Drapes or sheets
- Instruments and equipment

The gowns are usually "one size fits all," but they may not fit larger patients. Regular cloth gowns are usually available. The disposable gown and drapes are paper. Caution the patient to handle them gently because they tear easily. Discard them when the examination is complete.

TIPS

- Adjust the room temperature for comfort and make sure the room is free of drafts. Cover the examination table with a clean sheet or disposable paper. Use another clean sheet or blanket to cover the patient. Remember that their body should not be unnecessarily exposed. Instruct the patient to empty the bladder before beginning.

POSITIONING THE PATIENT

When the physical examination takes place on an examination table, extra attention must be given to safety (Figure 28-2). The examination table may be raised or lowered in sections and stirrups and shoulder braces

applied to assist in positioning. Be sure you know how to properly operate the examination table before positioning a patient on it. The physical examination positions are shown in Table 28-1.

Modifications

Some of the positions discussed here may be modified and used for other purposes. For example, they might be used to change the position of a patient who is confined to bed, or to perform specific procedures. Pillows must be used to support a patient who is to be kept in position for a period of time. Remember, the patient who feels covered and comfortable will be able to cooperate more fully. Providing privacy for the patient is an important task.

Dorsal Recumbent Position

The **dorsal recumbent position** is the basic examination position.

- Assist the patient to be flat on the back, with knees flexed and slightly separated. The feet should be flat on the bed or table.
- Place a small pillow under the patient's head.
- Loosen the gown at the neck.
- Cover the patient with a sheet.

Supine or Horizontal Recumbent Position

- Assist the patient to lie flat on the back. The legs are extended and slightly separated.
- Place a pillow under the patient's head.
- Cover the patient with a sheet.
- Loosen the gown at the neck.

TABLE 28-1 Physical Examination Positions

Position	Body Part Assessed	Key Points and Contraindications
Sitting	Head, neck, back, posterior thorax and lungs, anterior thorax and lungs, breast, axillae, heart, and extremities	Client can expand lungs; nurse can inspect symmetry. Institute risk precautions (e.g., falls) for older adults and clients who are debilitated.
Supine	Head, neck, anterior thorax and lungs, breast, axillae, heart, abdomen, and extremities	Client relaxed; decreases abdominal muscle tension; nurse can palpate all peripheral pulses. Contraindicated in clients with cardiopulmonary alterations.
Sims'	Rectum and vagina	Relaxes rectal muscles. Painful for clients with joint deformities.
Prone	Posterior thorax and lungs, hip	Assessment of hip extension. Contraindicated in clients with cardiopulmonary alterations.
Knee–chest	Rectum	Maximal rectal exposure. Contraindicated in clients with respiratory alterations.
Lithotomy	Female genitalia, rectum, and genital tract	Maximal genitalia exposure; embarrassing and uncomfortable for client. Contraindicated in clients with joint disorders.

Knee–Chest Position

The **knee–chest position** may be used to examine the rectal or vaginal areas and to relieve pain following childbirth. The patient may feel very self-conscious when using this position. It is also a difficult position to maintain, so never leave the patient alone. Place the patient in a prone position until the examiner is ready.

- Draping may be done with one or two sheets.
- Place a small pillow under the patient's head.
- Assist the patient to turn and lie on the abdomen with head turned to one side.
- Have the patient flex the arms and bring them up on either side of the head.
- Assist the patient to flex the knees and draw them up as far as possible toward the chest.

Prone Position

This position is used to examine the patient's back.
- Assist the patient to lie on the abdomen with head turned to one side.
- Place a small pillow under the patient's head.

- Arms may be extended at the patient's side or flexed and brought up on either side of the head.
- One sheet is used for draping.

Sims' Position

This position is used for vaginal and rectal procedures, including enema administration.

- Assist the patient to turn on the left side, with the head turned to the same side and resting on a small pillow.
- Position the left arm extended behind the body.
- Flex the right arm and position it in front of the patient.
- The left leg is slightly bent and the right leg is sharply flexed.
- One drape is usually adequate.

Semi-Fowler's Position

This is a common position for head and neck examinations of the in-bed patient.

- Assist the patient to a semisitting position with the backrest elevated at a 45° angle to the bed.
- The knees are supported in a slightly flexed position
- The arms rest at the sides.
- One drape is usually enough.

Trendelenburg Position

The **Trendelenburg position** encourages circulation to the patient's heart and brain. It is used in some facilities when the patient is in shock, or to prevent shock. The determination to use this position is made by a licensed nurse, not a nursing assistant. It is not a comfortable position to maintain. It may be more difficult for the patient to breathe because the weight of the lower body is resting on the diaphragm and lungs.

- Assist the patient to lie flat on the back with the head lower than the rest of the body.
- If possible, the lower half of the bed or table is tilted so the legs are slightly flexed (Figure 28-3A). In an emergency, the entire bed frame may be supported on blocks, tilting the bed to a 45° angle. Some hospital beds, stretchers, and examination tables have a switch that enables the user to position the device in the Trendelenburg position quickly in emergencies.
- Beds that are electrically powered may be adjusted to this position.
- Shoulder braces may be needed to prevent the patient from slipping.
- One drape is usually sufficient.

There are several other variations of the Trendelenburg position. Of these, Figure 28-3B shows the most common. Another variation may be used for some emergencies and surgical procedures. You will need to know the nature of

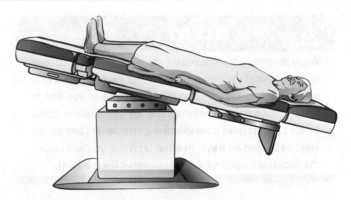

FIGURE 28-3B This is a variation of the Trendelenburg position that is used for some treatments and procedures. Support is needed to prevent the patient from sliding toward the head of the bed.

Clinical Information **ALERT**

A modification of the Trendelenburg position is taught as an initial treatment for hypotension, and to prevent shock in emergency situations. When you are instructed to use the Trendelenburg position for this purpose, you will elevate the patient's legs so they are higher than the heart. If possible, the feet are elevated so they are higher than the head, with the patient in a 30° to 45° head-down angle. The underlying principle is that in an emergency, this position will help shunt blood and oxygen from the legs to the vital structures of the heart and the brain. However, despite being a time-honored ritual and an accepted treatment since World War I, evidence to date does not support the use of this position for the treatment of shock, and limited data suggest it may be harmful. This is an area of clinical practice in which research has been and is being done, but much additional research is needed.

the examination or procedure being done to know which Trendelenburg position to use. Never use the head-down Trendelenburg position for a patient with shortness of breath, dyspnea on exertion, or a known or suspected head injury.

Safety **ALERT**

Remember that it is difficult for the person to breathe in this position. When the legs are up, pressure is increased on the abdomen and torso, interfering with breathing. Use the position for the least amount of time possible.

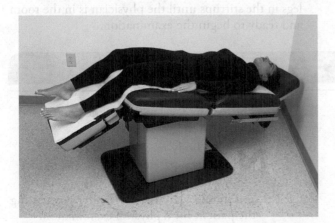

FIGURE 28-3A The Trendelenburg position. Note the addition of the head support on the table.

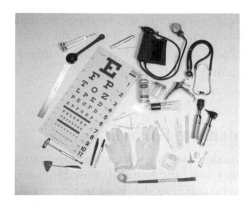

FIGURE 28-4 Equipment and supplies for the physical examination.

EQUIPMENT AND SUPPLIES

The equipment used is determined by the type of exam being done. Obtain disposable items, whenever possible. Always provide gloves of the size needed by the examiner. Several pairs (2 or more) will be needed for each person. In general:

- examiner gown (s)
- 2 goggles or face shield for staff in room, additional eye protection if needed for patient
- patient gown (s)
- stethoscope
- alcohol sponges
- sphygmomanometer (blood pressure cuff)
- paper and pens
- gauze sponges (4 × 4)
- disinfectant products as needed (wipes or spray with paper towels)
- disposable drape or sheet
- bath blanket
- tongue depressors (tongue blades)
- 6 inch wooden applicators
- supply items for the exam, such as a speculum for a Pap smear
- otoscope, ophthalmoscope, other instruments if needed and not mounted on wall

Having extra supplies and PPE is always a good idea. This way you will have immediate replacements in the event of contamination or loss. Check with the nurse or with the procedure manual to be sure you have everything you need to assist with the examination.

Dorsal Lithotomy Position

The **dorsal lithotomy position** is frequently used for the pelvic examination of female patients. This is a difficult examination for most women, so make sure your draping makes the patient feel covered.

- Make sure the patient voids before the examination. Check to see if you must collect a urinalysis.
- Position the patient on their back.
- Separate and flex the knees.
- Usually this position is achieved by placing the feet in stirrups.
- One or two drapes may be used to cover the patient. The draping may be similar to draping for the knee–chest position.
- This position can be difficult and uncomfortable for the patient to maintain. Do not place the patient's legs in the stirrups until the physician is in the room and ready to begin the examination.

REVIEW

A. True/False

Mark the following true or false by circling T or F.

1. T F The physical examination helps the physician establish a nursing assessment.
2. T F A patient who feels covered is able to cooperate more fully.
3. T F Positions used for the physical examination can be used only for that purpose.
4. T F The nursing assistant performs the actual physical exam.
5. T F The feet are level with the knees in the Trendelenburg position.
6. T F Use good body mechanics when positioning a patient for a physical examination.
7. T F You should leave the room after positioning the patient for a physical examination.
8. T F Draping and positioning the patient are two of the nursing assistant's responsibilities during the physical examination.

9. T F   Lighting may have to be adjusted during the examination.

10. T F   The semi-Fowler's position encourages blood flow to the head and heart.

B. Multiple Choice

Select the best answer for each of the following.

11. The basic examination position is:

a. Sims'.

b. dorsal recumbent.

c. dorsal lithotomy.

d. Trendelenburg.

12. Stirrups are used in which position?

a. Dorsal lithotomy

b. Semi-Fowler's

c. Sims'

d. Trendelenburg

13. The person in the prone position is lying on the:

a. left side.

b. back.

c. right side.

d. abdomen.

14. A person in the Sims' position is on the:

a. left side.

b. back.

c. right side.

d. abdomen.

15. The semi-Fowler's position is commonly used for:

a. genital and rectal examination.

b. head and neck examination.

c. back and buttocks examination.

d. abdomen and back examination.

16. The Trendelenburg position may be ordered to treat:

a. rectal bleeding.

b. shock.

c. high blood pressure.

d. stroke.

17. The dorsal lithotomy position is used for:

a. vaginal (pelvic) examination.

b. head and neck examination.

c. back and buttocks examination.

d. abdomen and back examination.

18. All of these are used in a nursing physical assessment *except*:

a. stethoscope.

b. sphygmomanometer.

c. thermometer.

d. scalpel.

C. Matching

Choose the correct word from Column II to match the word or phrase in Column I.

Column I

19. _____ variation in position

20. _____ how a patient is placed

21. _____ fearful

22. _____ covering

Column II

a. apprehensive

b. drape

c. modification

d. position

D. Nursing Assistant Challenge

Robert Ubek is to have a physical examination in the doctor's office. He is 88 years of age and appears very nervous. He tells you that he is afraid he has prostate cancer. You are to assist the doctor. Complete the following statements using words from the following list.

anticipate
dorsal recumbent
drape
off
on
reassure

23. One of your responsibilities will be to _____ the patient.

24. Because of Mr. Ubek's age, you will be especially careful in assisting him to get _____ and _____ the table.

25. You can help him feel more comfortable if you _____ him properly.

26. You can help the examination go more smoothly if you _____ the examiner's needs.

27. You will position Mr. Ubek in the _____ position to begin the examination.

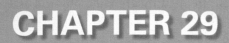

CHAPTER 29

The Surgical Patient

OBJECTIVES

After completing this chapter, you will be able to:

29.1 Spell and define terms.

29.2 Describe the concerns of patients who are about to have surgery.

29.3 List the various types of anesthesia.

29.4 Describe how to shave the area to be operated on.

29.5 Explain how to prepare the patient's unit for the patient's return from the operating room.

29.6 Explain how to give routine postoperative care when the patient returns to the room.

29.7 Describe the care and observations for surgical drains.

29.8 Assist the patient with deep breathing and coughing.

29.9 Apply elasticized stockings or bandages and pneumatic sleeves.

29.10 Demonstrate the following procedures:

- Procedure 78: Assisting the Patient to Deep Breathe and Cough (Expand Your Skills)
- Procedure 79: Applying Elasticized Stockings
- Procedure 80: Applying an Elastic Bandage (Expand Your Skills)
- Procedure 81: Assisting the Patient to Dangle (Expand Your Skills)

VOCABULARY

Learn the meaning and the correct spelling of the following words and phrases:

ambulation	disruption	NPO	pulmonary embolism
anesthesia	distention	operative	recovery room
anti-embolism hose	drainage	orifice	sequential compression
aspirate	dressings	perioperative	therapy
atelectasis	embolus	perioperative hypothermia	singultus
bandages	general anesthetic	postanesthesia care unit	spinal anesthesia
binders	hypoxia	(PACU)	stable
dangling	local anesthetic	postoperative	surgical bed
deep vein thrombosis (DVT)	Montgomery straps	preoperative	TED hose
depilatory	nosocomial	prosthesis	thrombophlebitis
			vertigo

INTRODUCTION

Patients facing any surgical procedure tend to be fearful. Remember that these patients require great emotional as well as physical support (Figure 29-1), from the time the patient is admitted through the discharge.

Patients are concerned with:

- Disfigurement
- Pain
- Loss of control as they undergo anesthesia
- What serious conditions might be found.
- Length and cost of recovery
- Possibility of death

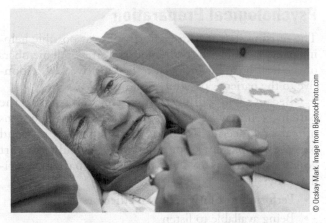

© Ocskay Mark. Image from Bigstock Photo.com

FIGURE 29-1 An older patient being comforted before surgery.

Surgery is often associated with anxiety, pain, and discomfort. For this reason, medications are given before, during, and after surgery.

PAIN PERCEPTION

When a person feels pain sensations, the:

- Pain receptors record the sensation.
- Sensation is sent by the spinal nerves to the spinal cord and then to the brain.
- Sensation is received and interpreted in the brain.

Before surgery, the patient is given medication to promote relaxation. During surgery, anesthetics are given to prevent pain (Figure 29-2). After surgery, medications are given to reduce discomfort.

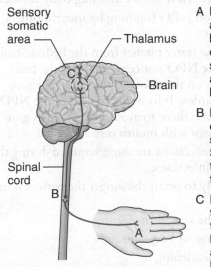

Sensory somatic area — Thalamus

C — Brain

Spinal cord

A Pain messages are picked up by free nerve endings in the skin. Local anesthetic blocks this.

B Message is carried into the spinal cord. Spinal anesthetic blocks this.

C Message is then carried to the cortex of the brain. General anesthetic blocks this.

FIGURE 29-2 Anesthetics will block pain impulses at points A, B, or C.

ANESTHESIA

In addition to preventing pain, **anesthesia** is also given to relax muscles and to induce forgetfulness. The anesthetic agent (drug) and method of administration used are determined by the location and type of surgery, the length of time needed for surgery, and the patient's physical condition.

There are two main types of anesthetics:

- **General anesthetics**—These induce the patient to become unconscious.
- **Local anesthetics**—These induce loss of feeling in a specific area.

General Anesthetics

General anesthetics block reception of pain in the brain. They are usually given in one of two ways:

- *Inhalation*—Inhaled anesthetics are likely to make the patient secrete more mucus and to experience nausea.
  - After surgery, monitor the patient to be sure the respiratory tract is clear.
  - There is a real danger that the patient may **aspirate** (inhale) vomitus into the respiratory tract.
- *Intravenous*—Drugs are introduced directly into the veins.
  - These drugs act rapidly.
  - The patient quickly loses consciousness.
  - IV anesthetics are often used with other types of anesthesia for short operations.

Local Anesthetics

Local anesthetics act by:

- Blocking pain receptors in the operative area. Drugs that are injected around the operative area stop the sensation of pain only in that area. The patient remains awake but free from pain during the operation.
- **Spinal anesthesia** blocks transmission of the pain sensation at the level of the spinal cord.
  - A drug injected into the spinal canal prevents feeling in any point below the level of the injection.
  - The patient remains awake.
  - This type of anesthesia is commonly used for abdominal surgery because it produces good relaxation of the muscles.
  - After getting this type of anesthetic, the patient is unable to feel or move the legs for a period of time. If not prepared ahead of time, the patient may be frightened by this experience.

SURGICAL CARE

Care of the **perioperative** (surgical) patient can be divided into three parts:

- **Preoperative** (before surgery)
- **Operative** (in the operating room)
- **Postoperative** (after surgery)

PREOPERATIVE CARE

Preoperative care begins when surgery is planned by the physician with the patient. Your responsibilities begin when the patient is admitted to the facility. You may answer general questions that the patient asks but refer specific questions about the surgery, its possible outcome, and anesthesia to the nurse. Although it is the responsibility of the physician and nurse to answer questions and give explanations, it is helpful if you are aware of the information that has been given.

Teaching

Time spent with the patient in the preoperative period is very helpful. Patients who are prepared are able to cooperate more successfully in their recovery. Ideally, this time occurs shortly after the patient's admission. Sometimes much of the information is given in the doctor's office or clinic.

During the preoperative period, the nurse will determine the patient's specific needs. The nurse also does preoperative teaching. The other staff members support this effort.

- Tests, medications, and preoperative procedures are explained.
- Questions regarding the postoperative period are answered.
- The patient is taught and given an opportunity to practice postoperative exercises, such as leg exercises and respiratory exercises.
- The patient and staff discuss the events of the preoperative period, and what the patient may experience while being taken to the operating room and being given anesthesia.
- The recovery period is outlined and the purpose of special procedures or equipment, such as tubes or intravenous fluid lines, that may be used after surgery is explained.
- Play therapy may be used to explain to children.
- Every effort is made to teach ways of decreasing discomfort and to assure the patient that pain relief will be available.
- Planning for the discharge period begins now.

Psychological Preparation

The nursing staff spends as much time as possible helping patients deal with their emotional stress. All members of the health care team need to be sensitive and responsive to the patient's psychological needs.

Because you will be in frequent contact with the patient, you may be the first person to recognize signs of fear or concern. Listen to what the patient says and observe the patient's body language carefully. Report your observations to the nurse. Build patient confidence by:

- Performing your work in an efficient, calm manner
- Being available to listen
- Explaining what you plan to do before carrying out any procedure
- Encouraging the patient to participate in their own care as much as possible. This helps the patient feel that they still has a measure of control over their life.
- Immediately transmitting requests for clergy visits

Physical Preparation

The Evening Before Surgery

If the patient is in the facility the evening before surgery, part of the surgical preparation may be done then. It usually includes:

- Bath or shower with surgical soap
- Enema
- Surgical prep (shaving of the operative site, if ordered)
- Special tests
- Medication to ensure a good night's rest, when indicated
- Insertion of special tubes for draining body cavities
- Being placed on **NPO** (nothing by mouth) orders after midnight
- Removal of the water pitcher from the bedside table and having the NPO notice posted over the bed, bedside stand, on the door, on the patient's chart, and on the Kardex. Inform the patient of the NPO status and advise them to avoid items such as gum and mints. Assist with mouth care as needed

Nosocomial infections are those acquired during the facility stay. Such infections:

- Are more likely to occur the longer the patient is in the facility
- Add days to the stay in the facility
- Increase the cost of hospitalization
- Can be life-threatening

To decrease costs and the potential for nosocomial infections, patients are often admitted on the morning of surgery and are sometimes discharged on the day of surgery or the day after. In this instance, much of the preoperative care must be done at home or immediately upon admission. This is called *outpatient* or *short-term surgery*.

Patients who remain at home until they are admitted for surgery usually have laboratory testing done on an outpatient basis before surgery. The patient is advised not to eat or drink anything after midnight on the evening before the scheduled surgery. They may be instructed to shower with a special antiseptic soap before coming to the hospital early in the morning, on the day of surgery. After admission, you may be assigned to complete the skin preparation. The patient then goes right to surgery.

Many surgeries are performed on an outpatient basis. The patient goes home, or returns to a long term care or subacute care facility, after they have recovered from the anesthesia. If the patient experiences complications, they will be admitted to the hospital. Many patients are first admitted to the nursing unit after surgery, so they are not familiar with the staff, and may need information about what to expect postoperatively.

When the patient is admitted before surgery, preoperative teaching is done on the nursing unit the evening before surgery. Because most patients are not admitted until after surgery, patient teaching may be done later. Patient teaching is also done in the physician's office before surgery. The office may mail instructions to the patient before hospital admission. Some physicians hold informational classes. Some provide information and instructions on their website. Personnel in the operating room may also do some patient teaching, but you must reinforce it on the nursing unit. You will be assisting the nurse in teaching the patient how to move and turn, cough and deep breathe, do foot and leg exercises, manage pain, and handle other aspects of care.

The Surgical Prep Area

Skin preparation before surgery may or may not include hair removal. There is a trend away from removing the hair unless its thickness will interfere with the surgery. In fact, some studies have shown more infections among shaved patients compared with unshaved patients.

If shaving is ordered, it must be done according to facility procedure in a well-lighted area. The area to be washed and shaved will be larger than the surgical incision area (Figure 29-3). In some cases, a **depilatory** (hair-removing) cream will be ordered for use the night before surgery. If a depilatory is to be used, check the skin for sensitivity. Apply a small amount to the skin of the forearm and wait 10 minutes. If redness occurs, do not continue, but report to the nurse.

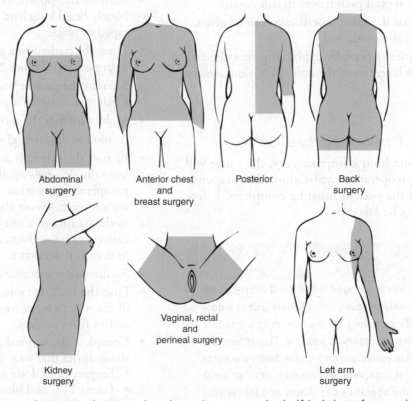

Abdominal surgery

Anterior chest and breast surgery

Posterior

Back surgery

Kidney surgery

Vaginal, rectal and perineal surgery

Left arm surgery

FIGURE 29-3 The shading indicates the areas that may be shaped preoperatively if hair interferes with the surgical procedure.

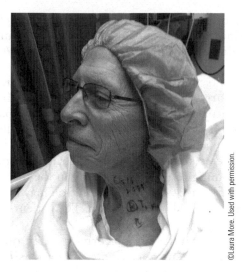

FIGURE 29-4 A patient ready for surgery will have a cap over the head. The neck markings indicate the correct operative site. The eyeglasses will be removed before being transported to the operating room.

Skin preparation may be performed by:

- A special surgical prep team
- Operating room (OR) staff in the OR
- Nursing staff in the patient's unit or preoperative holding area just prior to surgery
  To prepare the surgical area by shaving:
- Make sure you know exactly what area is to be shaved. Most hospitals have routine prep areas.
- Do not shave the neck or face of a female patient. If in doubt, check with the nurse.
- Never shave the eyebrows.
- Be aware that the preparations for cranial surgery are usually performed after the patient has been medicated and taken to the operating room. Doctors have special preferences in this regard.
- Remember that if a spinal anesthesia is to be given, the back may also be shaved.

Calm the patient's fears by explaining that the area prepared is much larger than the actual incision area, to prevent infection.

Immediate Preoperative Care

Approximately one hour before surgery, the nurse will give the patient preoperative medication. Your responsibilities regarding the patient must be completed before this time. You may be asked to:

- Take and record vital signs (see Section 6).
- Take care of valuables according to hospital policy. Remove dentures and any other **prosthesis** (artificial body part or device), such as an artificial leg, hearing aid, or eyeglasses. See that they are safely marked with the patient's name and stored appropriately.
- Remove nail polish, makeup, hairpins, and jewelry. Neatly braid long hair. Plain wedding bands may be taped in place.
- Dress the patient in a gown and cover the hair with a surgical cap (Figure 29-4).
- See that the patient voids and measure the urine. Drain the catheter, if present, and record.
- Make sure that the room is quiet and comfortable.
  As soon as the nurse gives the preoperative medication:
- Be sure the side rails are in place for safety. Always keep the side rails up after the patient receives the preoperative injection. Make sure the call signal is within reach. Never allow a patient to get up and go to the bathroom alone after the preoperative medication has been given. Assist with using the bedpan or urinal, if necessary.
- Remove all unnecessary equipment.
- Push the bedside table, overbed table, and chair out of the way to make room for the stretcher when it arrives from surgery.
- Complete the surgical checklist by checking off those duties that were assigned to you:
  - Surgery prep done and charted, if required
  - Latest TPR and blood pressure charted
  - Identification band on patient
  - Fingernail polish and makeup removed

- Metallic objects removed (wedding ring may be taped)
- Dentures removed
- Other prostheses removed (such as artificial limb or eye, wigs, and hairpieces)
- Glasses or contact lenses removed
- Bath blanket and head cap in place
- Bed in high position and side rails up after preop medication is given
- Patient has voided

- Note the time your patient leaves for surgery.
- Follow facility policy regarding visitors. Sometimes they are allowed to wait quietly with the patient. Sometimes they should be directed to the visitors' waiting room.
- Elevate the bed to stretcher height when the transporter arrives to take the patient to surgery.

The nurse and surgical attendant will check the patient's identification and surgical checklist before moving the patient. A staff member accompanies the patient to the doors of the operating room. You will probably be asked to assist in transferring the patient from the bed to the stretcher and, after surgery, from the stretcher to the bed. Review Procedures 24 and 25 in Chapter 16.

DURING THE OPERATIVE PERIOD

Prepare the room for the patient's return while the patient is in the operating room.

- Prepare the room and make the surgical bed (Chapter 23). The **surgical bed** is also called a *postop bed* or *recovery bed*.
- Remove everything from the top of the bedside stand except an emesis basin, tissues, tongue depressors, equipment to check vital signs, and a pen and small pad to record vital signs
- Check with your team leader for any special equipment, such as oxygen, IV poles, suction, or drainage bags that might be needed when the patient returns.
- Watch for your patient's return from surgery.
- Follow facility policy regarding the location of visitors and family during surgery. They are sometimes permitted to wait in the patient's room. In most cases, they are directed to a special waiting area.

POSTOPERATIVE CARE

During the immediate postoperative period, the patient recovers from anesthesia. The patient is moved to a special care area called the **postanesthesia care unit (PACU)** for close monitoring. The PACU is located next to the operating room and is sometimes called the **recovery room** (Figure 29-5).

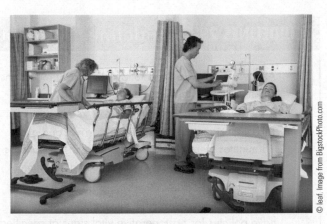

FIGURE 29-5 Patients recover after surgery in the postanesthesia care unit (PACU). Staff monitor the patients and transfer to a hospital room or discharge from the unit when completely recovered and medically stable.

When the patient's condition is stabilized, the patient is returned to the unit. Upon the patient's return from the PACU, you should:

- Identify the patient.
- Assist in the transfer from stretcher to bed (see Chapter 16).
- Never leave the unconscious patient alone at any time.
- Check with the nurse for any special instructions.
- Realize that the patient may be drowsy for several hours after return.
- Notify the nurse if the patient's temperature is below 97°F.
- Have an extra blanket available—many patients complain of feeling cold upon return.

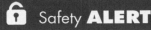 Safety **ALERT**

Patients receive many drugs when they are in surgery. Many of these can alter the person's mental status. The drugs are excreted from the body slowly. The patient may sleep soundly upon return to the unit. Keep the side rails up and follow all safety precautions until the patient is fully awake and the nurse instructs you that side rails are no longer necessary. Do not leave liquids at the bedside until the nurse instructs you that it is safe to do so. Check on the patient regularly.

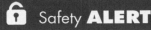 Safety **ALERT**

Anesthesia reduces body temperature. Keep the patient warm. If the patient's temperature is below 97°F, inform the nurse promptly.

GUIDELINES 29-1 Guidelines for Postoperative Care

- Always wear gloves and follow standard precautions when contact with blood, body fluids, mucous membranes, or nonintact skin is likely.

- Take vital signs upon the patient's arrival and every 15 minutes thereafter for four readings. The patient's temperature may not always be taken at this time.

- When taking postoperative vital signs, count pulse and respirations for one full minute. Most facilities have policies for postoperative vital signs at specified frequencies that decrease if the vital signs are **stable** (approximately the same), such as:
  - Every 15 minutes for 1 hour.
  - If stable, every 30 minutes for 1 hour.
  - If stable, every hour for 2 hours.
  - If stable, every 4 hours for 24 hours.

- Always follow the protocol for vital signs used by your facility. The nurse may alter the vital sign schedule if the patient's condition warrants. The physician may also order vital signs at a specifically designated frequency. Monitor the patient's level of consciousness (drowsy, unresponsive, alert) each time you check the vital signs.

- Ask the patient if they are having pain each time you check the vital signs. If so, inform the nurse.

- Check dressings for amount and type of any drainage. Inform the nurse if blood or other drainage leaks through the dressings. The nurse may reinforce them as necessary.

- Check IV solution for flow rate.

- Encourage the patient to breathe deeply, cough, and move in bed. Reposition the patient every 2 hours or more often if needed for comfort.

- Turn the patient's head to one side and support it if they are vomiting. Have an emesis basin ready, as well as tissues and a wet washcloth. If the patient is conscious, assist them to rinse the mouth after vomiting. Note the type and amount of vomitus and record on the output worksheet. Notify the nurse.

- Check the pulses distal to the operative site. Inform the nurse if the pulse is weak or cannot be felt.

- If the patient was given a spinal anesthetic:
  - Turn them frequently and maintain proper alignment.
  - Remember that the patient will be unable to move independently until sensation and motor functions return. Reassure the patient.
  - Some physicians require that the patient remain flat on the back and without a pillow for 8 to 12 hours following spinal anesthesia, to avoid headaches.
  - Report complaints of a headache promptly.

- Be sure all drainage tubes have been connected (the nurse will usually attend to this). If a tube is clamped shut, check with the nurse.

- Measure and record the first postoperative voiding. Inform the nurse.

- Report any complaints of pain to the nurse.

🔓 Safety **ALERT**

Some patients are very sensitive and will not let anyone see them unless their dentures are in the mouth. Monitor postoperative patients to be sure they have not inserted their dentures before they are fully awake. Remove dentures from an unconscious or comatose patient to prevent accidental airway obstruction by the dentures.

Carefully observe the patient for complications. Potential problems and complications and appropriate nursing assistant actions are summarized in Table 29-1.

General observations to make and report regarding complications are listed in Table 29-2.

SURGICAL WOUNDS WITH DRAINS

Patients often return from surgery with a variety of tubes and drains in place.

- Some tubes may deliver materials into the patient. Examples are oxygen tubes and intravenous tubes

- Other tubes may have been placed in the patient to provide **drainage** from wounds or body cavities. Examples are drains in the incision and urinary catheters

Drains remove fluids that have collected below the skin. The drain exits the skin through a small incision and may be sutured in place. Some drains are hollow, and empty directly to the outside of the body. Others are connected to closed containers that must be emptied.

TABLE 29-1 Postoperative Complications and Nursing Assistant Actions

Possible Discomfort	Report	What You Can Do*
Thirst	Patient complaints of dryness of lips, mouth, and skin	Carefully check I&O. Give ice chips or increase fluid intake by mouth with permission. Monitor IV if ordered. Give mouth care. Assist patient with rinsing mouth. Check BP and pulse. Watch for signs of shock and hemorrhage.
Singultus (hiccups)—intermittent spasms of the diaphragm	Incidence of hiccups	Allow the patient to rest; hiccups can be tiring. Support the incisional area. Assist the patient to breathe into a paper bag.
Pain	Location, intensity, type	Change position. Apply warmth if instructed. Monitor carefully for and report effects of medication given by nurse. Assist with nursing comfort measures such as supportive positioning with pillows.
Distention (accumulation of gas in bowel)	Distention of abdomen, complaints of pain	Increase mobility. Insert a rectal tube if instructed and permitted.
Nausea, vomiting	Nausea, character of vomitus	Keep an emesis basin at the bedside. Monitor IV fluids, which are substituted for oral fluids. Give mouth care. Limit fluids by mouth. Encourage the patient to breathe deeply.
Urinary retention	Amount and time of first voiding. Distention, restlessness, imbalance between I&O	Monitor I&O carefully. Check for distention.
Hemorrhage (excessive blood loss)	Fall in blood pressure; cold, moist skin; weak, rapid pulse; restlessness; pallor/cyanosis; condition of dressing; thirst	Report immediately to nurse. Keep the patient quiet. Monitor bleeding. Monitor vital signs and pulse oximeter.
Shock	Fall in blood pressure; weak, rapid pulse; cold, moist skin; pallor	Report immediately to nurse. Keep the patient quiet. Monitor ordered oxygen. Monitor vital signs and pulse oximeter. Be prepared to follow additional instructions.
Hypoxia (lack of oxygen)	Restlessness, dyspnea, crowing sounds with respirations, pounding pulse, perspiring	Report immediately to nurse. Monitor oxygen, if ordered. Monitor vital signs and pulse oximeter.
Atelectasis (decreased or absent air in all or part of a lung, resulting in loss of lung volume and inability to expand lung fully)	Dyspnea; cyanosis/pallor	Report immediately to nurse. Monitor oxygen, if ordered. Monitor vital signs and pulse oximeter.
Wound infection	Increased pain in incisional area; fever; chills, anorexia, increased drainage on dressing	Be observant. Report findings promptly to nurse. Check dressing.
Wound **disruption** (separation of wound edges)	Pinkish drainage; complaints by the patient that they "feel open," "broken," "given away"	Report immediately to nurse. Keep the patient quiet. Support incisional area.
Pulmonary embolism	Anxiety, difficulty breathing; feelings of "heaviness in chest," cyanosis, chest pain	Keep the patient quiet. Report immediately to nurse. Elevate head of bed. Monitor oxygen. Monitor vital signs and pulse oximeter. Prepare to transfer to the intensive care unit (ICU).

*In all cases, be prepared to follow the nurse's additional instructions.

TABLE 29-2 General Observations of Complications to Make and Report

- Decreased responsiveness or unresponsiveness
- Change in the level of responsiveness
- Increased restlessness accompanied by complaints of thirst
- Changes in blood pressure
- Weak, rapid, or irregular pulse
- Changes in temperature
- Changes in respiratory rate
- Difficulty breathing; labored or noisy respirations
- Nausea or vomiting
- Complaints of pain
- Increased drainage, wet or saturated dressings
- Active bleeding
- Coughing or choking

TABLE 29-3 Drain Observations to Report to the Nurse

- Drain is not intact or patent
- Drain appears blocked, dislodged, or kinked
- Surrounding skin appears abnormal (erosion, red, hot, swollen, macerated)
- Drainage is eroding surrounding, healthy skin
- Drainage is purulent, cloudy, or foul smelling
- Drainage color changes or appears abnormal
- Amount of drainage decreases markedly or stops entirely
- Amount of drainage increases markedly
- Patient has fever, tachycardia, hypotension
- Urinary output decreases

Care of the device varies with physician orders and the type of drain used. Wound drains are considered sterile. If you are permitted to care for them, use sterile technique. The drain is a portal of entry through which pathogens can enter the body. Always apply standard precautions principles.

Drainage Outlets

Drains are used to remove body fluids such as blood, pus, serous drainage, or gastric contents before or after surgery. The drainage outlet may be a:

- Catheter
- T-tube
- Jackson-Pratt (J-P) or Hemovac drain
- Penrose drain
- Cigarette drain
  Follow these special precautions:
- Wear gloves if contact with drainage from the tube is likely.
- Learn the type, purpose, and location of each tube.
- Check drainage for character and amount.
- Check for obstructions to the tube system.
- Check flow rate of infusions from intravenous lines.
- Keep **orifices** (body openings) clear of secretions and discharge.
- Never disconnect tubes or raise drainage bottles above the level of the drainage site.
- Never lower infusion or irrigation bottles below the level of the infusion site.
- Never put stress on the tubes when moving the patient or giving care.
- Monitor levels of infusions and report to the nurse before they run out.
- Report any signs of leakage or disconnected tubes immediately.

- Report pain, discoloration, or swelling at sites of drainage and infusion.
- Check with the nurse before changing or reinforcing a dressing.
- Use sterile technique whenever you manipulate or empty a tube or drain or change a dressing. Be sure this is a permitted nursing assistant procedure in your facility. You will find additional, advanced procedures in Chapter 36.
- Never assume responsibility for chest drainage or attempt to empty chest bottles. Chest bottles and irrigations require the nurse's or physician's attention.

Observations to make and report for patients with drains are listed in Table 29-3.

Dressings and Bandages

Dressings are gauze, film, or other synthetic substances that cover a wound, ulcer, or injury. Some dressings have an adhesive backing. Some are affixed with tape. **Bandages** are fabric, gauze, net, or elasticized materials that are wrapped around a body part to hold dressings securely in place.

Bandages are available in different sizes and shapes. Gauze bandages are the most common. Elastic bandages reduce edema and support injured body parts. Avoid wrapping bandages so tightly that they restrict circulation. Monitor bandages regularly to ensure that circulation is adequate. Inform the nurse if wound drainage seeps through the bandage.

Montgomery straps (Figure 29-6) are long strips of adhesive attached to the skin on either side of the wound to hold dressings in place. They are used for wounds that require regular dressing changes. The straps eliminate the need for adhesive tape to hold bandages in place, making them much less traumatic to the skin because the straps are not removed unless they are soiled. The straps are tied to hold the dressing securely. **Binders** (Figures 29-7A and 29-7B) may also be used to hold dressings in place.

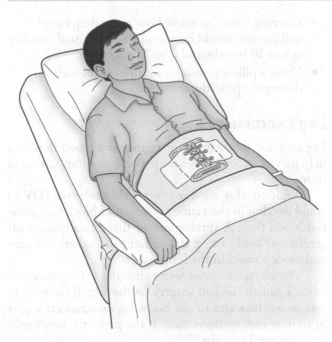

FIGURE 29-6 Montgomery straps hold dressings securely in place so they can be observed, changed, and reinforced without tape. This is much less traumatic for the patient.

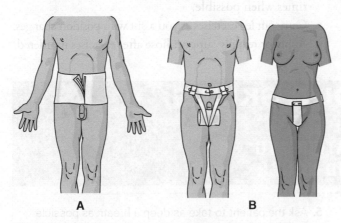

A   B

FIGURE 29-7 A. Various surgical binders support the body part and hold dressings in place. B. Male and female T-binders.

Perioperative Hypothermia

During the perioperative period, many factors interfere with the patient's normal temperature-regulating mechanisms. The blood vessels constrict. **Perioperative hypothermia** develops because anesthesia and some sedative drugs disrupt the internal ability to regulate temperature. Normally, we shiver when we are cold. The drugs promote heat loss by reducing the shivering response and preventing blood vessel constriction. Underlying factors such as age, chronic disease, and body size also affect temperature regulation.

The operating room is kept very cool because cooler temperature reduces oxygen requirements. Open body cavities and administration of blood and IV fluids further contribute to temperature loss. In the first 30 minutes after being given general anesthesia, body temperature usually decreases. The American Association of Nurse Anesthetists (AANA) recommends continuous temperature monitoring on pediatric patients receiving general anesthesia and, when indicated, on all other patients. Some experts recommend checking the temperature at 15- to 30-minute intervals while the patient is in the operating room.

The body cannot return to normal temperature until the concentration of anesthetic in the brain decreases and the normal temperature-regulating responses are triggered and can take over. Pain further decreases the effectiveness of these responses. Return to normal temperature may take two to five hours, depending on the degree of hypothermia and the patient's age. Perioperative outcomes are better if the patient does not become hypothermic.

To maintain patient temperature during and after surgery, the hyperthermia–hypothermia blanket may be used. The circulating water is a very effective warming mechanism. The blankets may be used under or over the patient but are most effective when positioned over the patient's body. If the patient is cold, but not hypothermic, wrapping them with several warm bath blankets is a good comfort measure that will help maintain body heat.

POSTOPERATIVE EXERCISES

When the patient has responded sufficiently and vital signs are stable, they may be refreshed by:

- Washing the hands and face
- Changing the linens
- Being given a light backrub

The patient is now ready to participate more actively in recovery by doing exercises taught in the preoperative period, including:

- Deep breathing and coughing
- Leg exercises

🔓 Safety **ALERT**

Although we routinely encourage postoperative patients to cough and deep breathe, there are a few exceptions you must be aware of. Avoid this procedure with patients who have had eye, nose, or neurologic surgery. Coughing and deep breathing will increase pressure, causing complications. Check with the nurse if you are unsure of what action to take.

Deep Breathing and Coughing

Deep breathing and coughing help clear the air passages and help prevent respiratory complications such as pneumonia and **atelectasis** (collapse of the alveolar air sacs). Coughing and taking very deep breaths may be uncomfortable when the patient has a new incision and feels fatigued (see Procedure 78). You can best assist the patient by:

- Explaining the value of the exercise and carrying out the procedures
- Checking with the nurse to see if pain medication is to be administered before the exercise. If so, wait 45 minutes after the medication has been given before carrying out the exercise.

⚠ OSHA **ALERT**

Apply the principles of standard precautions when assisting with coughing and deep breathing procedures. If the patient is expelling loose secretions, select and wear appropriate protective equipment, including gloves, gown, mask, and face shield. Show the patient how to contain secretions in a tissue and how to discard used tissues in a plastic bag. Assist the patient with handwashing after the activity.

- Learning from the nurse how many deep breaths and coughs should be attempted. The usual number is 5 to 10 breaths and 2 to 3 coughs.
- Using a pillow or binder to support the incision during the procedure

Leg Exercises

Leg exercises following surgery improve blood flow and help prevent blood clots, another serious complication of immobility.

A blood clot or **deep vein thrombosis (DVT)** could develop in the venous system and block the essential blood flow. A small piece of thrombus broken off (**embolus**) could travel throughout the vascular system and block a vessel in the lungs.

The physician must write an order for leg exercises when a patient has had surgery on the legs. If the surgery was on another area of the body, leg exercises are a part of routine postoperative care. If the patient is very weak, you may need to assist.

- Encourage leg exercises; be sure the patient does them as specified on the care plan.
- As a rule, each exercise should be done three to five times at least every one or two hours, and at other times when possible.
- Carry out leg exercises as you assist with position changes.
- Apply or reapply support hose after exercises if ordered.

EXPAND YOUR SKILLS

PROCEDURE **78** ASSISTING THE PATIENT TO DEEP BREATHE AND COUGH

1. Carry out initial procedure actions.

2. Assemble equipment:
- Disposable gloves
- A pillowcase-covered pillow or abdominal binder, if ordered
- Tissues
- Emesis basin

3. Elevate the head of the bed and assist the patient to assume a comfortable semi-Fowler's position.

4. Have the patient place their hands on either side of his rib cage or over the operative site (Figure 29-8A). A pillow over the operative site can be used to support an incision during respiratory exercises.

5. Ask the patient to take as deep a breath as possible and hold it for three to five seconds; then exhale slowly through pursed lips.

6. Repeat this exercise about five times unless the patient seems too tired. If so, stop the procedure and report to the nurse.

7. Place the pillow across the incision line as a brace. Have the patient hold the pillow on either side or have the patient interlace fingers across the incision to act as a brace (Figure 29-8B).

8. Pass tissues to the patient and instruct them to take a deep breath and cough forcefully twice with the mouth open, collecting any secretions that are brought up in the tissues.

(continues)

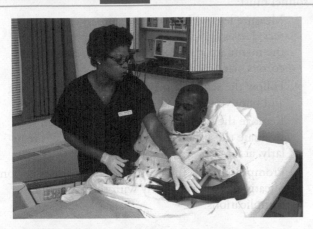

FIGURE 29-8A Remind, encourage, and assist the patient to perform deep breathing exercises.

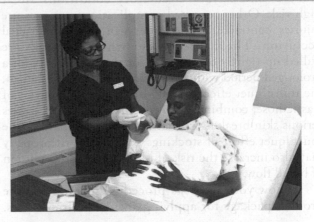

FIGURE 29-8B A pillow helps support the abdomen and splints the incision during deep breathing and coughing.

9. Put on disposable gloves to handle the tissues.

10. Dispose of tissues in an emesis basin.

11. Assist the patient to assume a new comfortable position.

12. Clean the emesis basin.

13. Remove and discard gloves.

14. Carry out ending procedure actions.

15. Report to the nurse on the number of times the patient performed each exercise, how the patient

tolerated the exercise, and the type and amount of any sputum coughed up.

- Be sure the patient does not become overly fatigued.
- Encourage the patient to cough and clear the respiratory passages.
- Report to your team leader if the patient seems overly fatigued during the procedure.
- Carefully observe and report any unusual responses such as pain, dizziness, or throat and airway irritation.

Elasticized Stockings

Elasticized stockings, called **TED hose** or **anti-embolism hose**, extend from the ankle or foot to calf or mid-thigh. They may also be called *graduated compression stockings (GCS)*, which refers to the graduation of pressure. Sometimes they are referred to by the brand name, such as TED or Jobst hose. The stockings are tightest at the ankle, and become looser as they move up the leg. They are often applied during the preoperative and postoperative periods to support the veins of the legs and reduce the incidence of **thrombophlebitis**, which is inflammation of the veins that can lead to blood clots.

Apply the stockings smoothly and evenly before the patient gets out of bed. Several different types of anti-embolism hose are used. Some have closed toes, but most have an opening on the top or the bottom of the

foot, just proximal to the toes. Check the heel placement on the stocking. By using the heel as a landmark, you will see where to position the hole in the stocking.

Preventing Complications

A physician's order is needed for the application of special sleeves. The ordering physician will specify if knee-high or thigh-high hose should be used. Anti-embolism sleeves is available in various grades of pressure, ranging from 8 through 46 mm Hg. Become familiar with the criteria used by your facility to establish what constitutes light, medium, and firm compression. Make sure you apply the correct sleeves, according to the original order and facility policies.

The risk of complications from anti-embolism sleeves is low. However, they are not risk-free. The greatest risk is a reduction in blood flow from pressure. This leads to decreased oxygen in the tissues and increases the potential for blood clots. Patients with diabetes and certain circulatory conditions are at high risk. Other reported complications are pressure injuries, contractures of the toes, gangrene, and arterial occlusion. These often occur when the socks are pulled up tightly on the foot, or the patient sits for a prolonged period without moving. Sometimes, though, the tourniquet effect created by bunched-up layers of elastic hose, combined with swelling of the leg, causes serious skin breakdown that requires amputation. The tourniquet effect of stockings that do not fit properly may also increase the risk of blood clots and occlusion of blood flow.

Follow your facility's procedure manual and the product package for applying anti-embolism sleeves.

Never guess at the size. Always use a tape measure to ensure that the size is accurate. Ill-fitting sleeves is the most common cause of complications, so nursing personnel must:

- Measure legs with a tape measure to ensure correct sleeves fit. Compare the measurements with the manufacturer's size chart, and then select the correct size.
- Follow the schedule on the care plan for applying and removing the sleeves.
- Remove the sleeves for patient bathing each day. Evaluate the appearance of the feet and legs regularly, at least several times each day.
- Promptly inform the nurse of abnormalities or complications. Intervene early with the occurrence of complications.

GUIDELINES 29-2 Guidelines for Applying Anti-Embolism Stockings

- The care plan will specify the wearing schedule for the stockings, according to physician orders and facility policies. For most patients, the sleeves is applied during the day and removed at bedtime.

- It is best to apply the stockings before the patient gets out of bed in the morning. Elevating the legs for 20 to 30 minutes before applying the sleeves will reduce swelling and make hose easier to apply.

- Make sure the legs are dry before attempting to apply the sleeves. An adaptive device is used in some facilities to make them easier to apply. If this is not available, the nurse may permit you to dust the legs lightly with baby powder, which will make the hose easier to apply. Avoid using baby powder if the patient has respiratory difficulties, a rash, or dressings on the legs.

- Never apply the sleeves over open areas, fractures, or deformities. If the patient has an open or abnormal skin area, fracture, or deformity on the legs or feet, inform the nurse.

- Make sure the stockings are applied smoothly, with no wrinkles.

- Check the stockings every few hours to be sure the tops have not rolled or turned down. Keep the fabric straight.

- Monitor circulation in the patient's toes every two to four hours, or as specified on the care plan. Note color, sensation, swelling, temperature, and ability to move. Report abnormalities to the nurse. Document that you have done regular skin and circulation checks.

- Anti-embolism stockings must be hand-washed and drip-dried. The stockings are damaged by the commercial washers and dryers used in health care facilities. Because of this, your facility may issue two pairs to each patient.

- To preserve the life of the stockings, avoid contact with lotions, ointments, or oils containing lanolin or petroleum products. These products deteriorate the elastic.

PROCEDURE **79** APPLYING ELASTICIZED STOCKINGS

1. Carry out initial procedure actions.

2. Assemble equipment:
   - Elasticized stockings of proper length and size

3. Always apply stockings when the patient is lying down. Expose one leg at a time.

4. Grasp the stocking with both hands at the top and roll it toward the toe end.

5. Adjust the stocking over the patient's toes, positioning the opening at the base of the toes (unless the toes are to be covered) (Figure 29-9A). Raised seams (if any) should be on the outside.

6. Apply the stocking to the leg by rolling it upward toward the torso.

7. Apply the stocking evenly and smoothly and avoid wrinkles (Figure 29-9B).

8. Repeat the procedure on the opposite leg.

9. Carry out ending procedure actions.

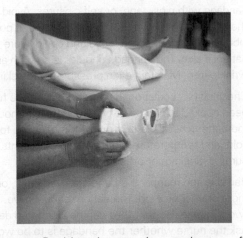

FIGURE 29-9A Position the opening on the top of the foot, at the base of the toes.

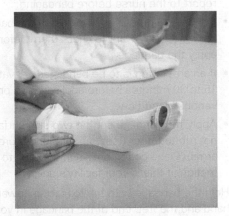

FIGURE 29-9B Draw the stocking up smoothly

Elastic Bandage

An elasticized bandage (Ace bandage) may be used to keep dressings in place, especially on an extremity or on the head. You may need to remove and reapply the bandage once or twice on your shift. Elastic bandages are also used on nonsurgical patients, to promote venous blood flow in the legs; and for injuries of the musculoskeletal system, to reduce swelling. Elastic bandages come in two-inch to six-inch widths and in four-foot and six-foot lengths (Figure 29-10). Check with the nurse for the appropriate size bandage.

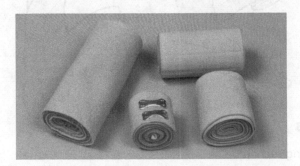

FIGURE 29-10 Elastic bandages are available in a variety of widths.

EXPAND YOUR SKILLS

PROCEDURE **80** APPLYING AN ELASTIC BANDAGE

1. Carry out initial procedure actions.

2. Assemble equipment:
   - Appropriate size bandage (check for cleanliness).
   - Tape, pins, or self-closures that come with bandage; some have a Velcro closure. Avoid clips.

3. Check the area to be bandaged.
   - If there are lesions or signs of skin breakdown, report to the nurse before bandaging.
   - If there are dressings underneath the bandage, the nurse may want to check them before you apply the bandage.
   - If an arm or leg is to be bandaged, elevate it for 15 to 30 minutes before application to promote venous blood flow.
   - Apply the bandage so that two skin surfaces do not rub together (toes, fingers, under breasts and arms). Place cotton between the toes to prevent friction, if this is your facility's policy.

4. Hold the bandage with the roll facing upward in one hand and the free end of the bandage in your other hand (Figure 29-11A).
   a. Hold the roll close to the part being bandaged so that pressure is even.
   b. When bandaging an extremity, always wrap from the distal (far) area to the proximal (near) area (Figure 29-11B).
   c. Unroll the bandage as you wrap the body part. Never unroll the entire bandage at once.

5. Use appropriate bandaging technique (Figure 29-11C). Overlap each layer of bandage by one-half the width of the strip.

6. When finished rolling (Figure 29-11D), secure the bandage with pins, tape, or self-closures. Avoid using the clips that may come with the bandage, if possible. They tend to come loose and could injure the patient's skin. The bandage should be smooth and wrinkle-free. Maintain even pressure on the skin.

7. Check distal circulation just after the bandage has been applied and once or twice every eight hours thereafter (check the skin under the bandage for color and temperature; note patient complaints of burning, tingling, or other discomfort).

8. Remove and reapply the bandage every shift, or more often if needed. The patient should have two bandages so that they can be laundered daily. Ask the nurse whether the bandage is to be worn continuously or only at specified times.

9. Carry out ending procedure actions.

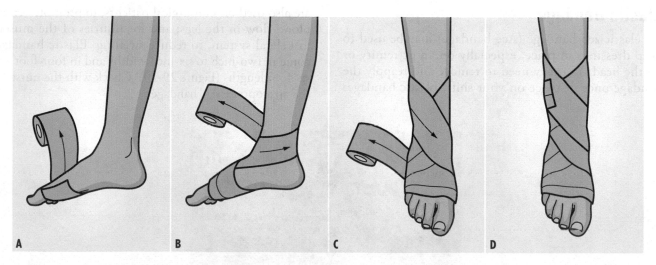

FIGURE 29-11 Bandage-wrapping technique.

Sequential Compression Therapy

Deep vein thrombosis and **pulmonary embolism** (a blood clot in the lungs) are serious postoperative complications. Approximately 10 percent of all patients with DVT die from pulmonary embolism. Most have no symptoms until they develop the pulmonary embolism. The femoral vein, the large blood vessel in the groin, is particularly susceptible to clot formation. Because of the high risk and serious consequences associated with blood clots, the physician may order **sequential compression therapy** to reduce the risk. Sequential compression therapy massages the legs using a milking, wavelike motion.

Pneumatic sleeves (Figure 29-12) is also called *sequential compression sleeves.* This device prevents blood clots by mechanically massaging the legs. Pneumatic sleeves inflates and deflates rhythmically to produce the massaging motion. It is contraindicated in patients with lower leg ulcers, blood clots, massive edema, deformities, infected or broken skin, or arterial disease. Shiny, hairless skin is an indication of arterial problems. If you observe any hard nodules, red areas, or warm areas on the patient's lower legs, inform the nurse before applying pneumatic sleeves.

Measuring and Connecting the Sleeves

Before beginning this procedure, you must determine the proper size sleeves for the patient. Do this by measuring the circumference of the patient's upper thigh with a tape measure when they are in bed. Hold the measure snugly against the leg and note the circumference. Compare the measurement with the sizing chart, and select the proper size sleeves.

Familiarize yourself with the sleeves and compression controller if you have not used them before. Open the package and lay the hose on a flat surface. Open them completely, with the cotton lining facing up. Inside you will notice markings for the ankle and knee.

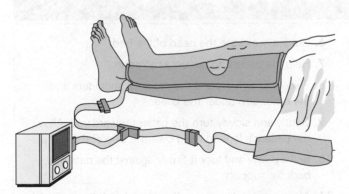

FIGURE 29-12 Pneumatic compression device sleeves are applied on the legs and are used to prevent blood pooling in the legs.

When you apply the garment to the patient's leg, line it up exactly with these landmarks. Next, familiarize yourself with the compression controller. The device may have a cooling adjustment. It is turned off during routine use. Follow your facility's policy and the nurse's instructions for activating this feature. The controller also has arrows to adjust the pressure inside the hose. It should be set at 35 to 55 mm Hg. The unit may automatically set at 45 mm Hg, the midway point. The nurse will set the unit or instruct you on the setting to use.

Both legs of the sleeves must be connected to the controller for the unit to operate. Position the arrows on the hose opposite the arrows on the tubing. Push the ends together firmly until you hear a clicking sound. If the patient will be using only one sleeve, such as when they have a cast on one leg, leave the unused sleeve in the sealed plastic bag. Cut a small hole in the bag and connect the tubing.

Applying Pneumatic Sleeves

Before applying the sleeves, palpate the pedal (Figure 29-13A) and posterior tibial pulses (Figure 29-13B). In most facilities, staff mark the location of these pulses with a marker, making a small "X" on the patient's skin. Compare the movement, sensation, and color in both feet. Consult the nurse if you note abnormalities. The nurse will assess the patient's legs and check for contraindications. Follow the nurse's instructions.

Pneumatic sleeves may be applied over anti-embolism hose, but both the sleeves and the anti-embolism hose must be smooth and wrinkle-free to reduce the risk of skin breakdown. The device is used 24 hours a day, when the patient is lying down, until the patient is completely ambulatory. It may be removed for bathing, ambulation, and any other time the person is out of bed, then reapplied immediately. The nurse may instruct the patient to perform certain leg exercises while the device is being used.

Caring for the Patient Who Is Using Pneumatic Sleeves

The compression controller has a visual display that identifies the chamber being inflated. When the chambers decompress, the unit will say "vent." Make sure the audible alarm is turned on, and check that the key has been removed. If the alarm sounds, the panel will display a message code. A card in a slot in the top of the unit will display the numerical message code with the nature of the problem. Follow the directions on the card to correct the problem, or ask the nurse for instructions. The hose deflates automatically when the alarm sounds.

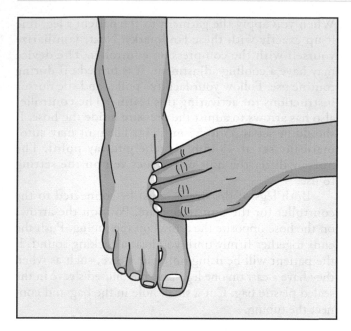

FIGURE 29-13A To locate the dorsalis pedis (pedal) pulse, draw an imaginary line from the ankle to the area between the great toe and second toe.

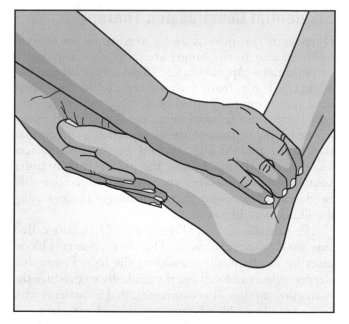

FIGURE 29-13B To locate the posterior tibial pulse, place the fingers in the groove between the Achilles tendon and the tibia. Move the fingers in slightly, toward the tibia.

Turn the power off and remove the hose every four hours. Disconnect the sleeves from the tubing by releasing the latches on each side of the connectors, and then pulling the connectors apart. Observe the skin under the device, and provide skin care as ordered. Avoid massaging the legs. Massage may dislodge a blood clot, which will quickly migrate to the lungs. Inform the nurse when you will be removing the device so that they can assess the patient's legs.

Use of the hose will be discontinued when the patient is fully ambulatory. The unit is not disposable.

Clean and store the controller device after use, or return it to central supply.

Documentation

Follow your facility's policy for documenting use of the pneumatic compression device. You may be asked to document the procedure, pulses in the feet, skin color, the patient's response, and the settings, including use of the alarm and cooling settings.

EXPAND YOUR SKILLS

PROCEDURE 81 ASSISTING THE PATIENT TO DANGLE

1. Carry out initial procedure actions.
2. Assemble equipment:
   • Bath blanket
   • Pillow
3. Check the pulse.
4. Lower the side rails nearest to you. Lock the bed at the lowest position.
5. Drape the patient with a bath blanket and fan-fold the top bedcovers to the foot of the bed.

6. Gradually elevate the head of the bed.
7. Help the patient to put on a bathrobe.
8. Place one arm around the patient's shoulders and the other arm under the knees.
9. Gently and slowly turn the patient toward you. Allow the patient's legs to hang over the side of the bed.
10. Roll a pillow and tuck it firmly against the patient's back for support.
11. After putting slippers on the patient, ask the patient to swing the legs over the side of the bed.

(continues)

PROCEDURE **81** CONTINUED

12. Have the patient dangle as long as ordered.
    - If the patient becomes dizzy or feels faint, help them lie down.
    - Report to the supervising nurse immediately.
13. Check the patient's pulse.
14. Rearrange the pillow at the head of the bed. Remove the patient's bathrobe and slippers.

15. Place one arm around the patient's shoulders and the other arm under the knees. Gently and slowly swing the patient's legs onto the bed.
16. Check the patient's pulse. Lower the head of the bed and raise the side rails.
17. Carry out ending procedure actions. Remember to wash your hands, report completion of your task, and document the time dangled (duration), pulse, and the patient's reaction.

ICON KEY:

 = OBRA

Initial Ambulation

Some time after surgery, a patient is permitted to sit up with the legs over the edge of the bed. This position is called **dangling**.

- Watch carefully for signs of fatigue or dizziness (**vertigo**)
- Assist the patient to assume the position slowly

The first **ambulation** (walk) is usually short. The patient usually dangles for a short time before ambulating. Dangling and ambulation are important parts of postoperative care because they stimulate circulation and help prevent the formation of blood clots (thrombi). (Refer to Procedure 81.)

The patient may need assistance the first few times they stand up to ambulate. Based on the patient's size, be sure you have an assistant available to help you. The

anesthesia and medications administered before, during, and after surgery may affect the patient's balance, endurance, and strength. You may have to move drainage tubes or an intravenous feeding with the patient. In any event, know where the tubes are at all times so they are not accidentally pulled out.

🔒 Safety **ALERT**

Remain next to the patient during the first dangling and ambulation. For patient safety, do not turn your back or leave the bedside. These precautions will probably not be necessary as the patient recovers and gains strength. Use common sense and follow the care plan and the nurse's instructions.

GUIDELINES 29-3 Guidelines for Assisting the Patient in Initial Ambulation

- Check with the nurse to see if a transfer belt can be used.
- Assist the patient to sit on the edge of the bed with the bed in low position.
- Assist the patient to put on footwear appropriate to the floor surface. Never allow a patient to ambulate with bare feet or socks.

- Take the patient's pulse before and after standing. If there is a difference of more than 10 points, return the patient to bed and inform the nurse.
- If the patient becomes dizzy or faint, return the patient to bed and inform the nurse.
- Walk with the patient, as instructed in Chapter 17.

REVIEW

A. True/False

Mark the following true or false by circling T or F.

1. T F Patients receiving local anesthetics lose consciousness during the surgery.

2. T F When spinal anesthetics are used, patients may lose feeling and movement in the legs.

3. T F Preoperative teaching has little effect on the patient's postoperative recovery.

4. T F You help build patient confidence when you explain what you plan to do when carrying out procedures.

5. T F Skin preparation involves shaving an area larger than the size of the incision.

6. T F The nursing assistant has no responsibilities related to the patient while the patient is in surgery.

7. T F Patients should be dangled without incident before initial ambulation.

8. T F Patients who are unconscious following surgery should not be left alone.

9. T F Nosocomial infections affect the cost and length of hospital stay.

10. T F Patients facing surgery are often filled with apprehension and fear.

B. Matching

Choose the correct word or phrase from Column II to match each item in Column I.

Column I

11. _____ inflammation of a vein leading to clot formation

12. _____ period before surgery

13. _____ medicine given to prevent pain

14. _____ hospital-acquired

15. _____ opening

16. _____ walking

17. _____ dizziness

18. _____ loss of lung volume; inability to expand lung fully

19. _____ blood clot

20. _____ unit where immediate postoperative care is given

Column II

a. ambulation

b. orifice

c. nosocomial

d. PACU

e. umbilicus

f. vertigo

g. anesthesia

h. preoperative

i. aspiration

j. embolism

k. atelectasis

l. thrombophlebitis

C. Multiple Choice

Select the best answer for each of the following.

21. When assisting a patient with coughing and deep breathing exercises, teach them to:
    a. inhale through the nose.
    b. inhale through the mouth.
    c. exhale through the nose.
    d. take 20 breaths in a row.

22. The main purpose of coughing and deep breathing exercises is to prevent:
    a. pneumonia.
    b. dizziness.
    c. pain.
    d. anxiety.

23. The main purpose of pneumatic compression sleeves is to prevent:
    a. edema.
    b. pneumonia.
    c. blood clots.
    d. pain.

24. Pneumatic compression sleeves is contraindicated:
    a. in patients who have had abdominal surgery.
    b. if the patient is using oxygen.
    c. if a rash or open area is present.
    d. for patients with a cast on one leg.

25. Check the postoperative patient's vital signs every:

   a. 5 minutes for the first hour, then every 15 minutes for 4 hours.

   b. 15 minutes for an hour, then every 30 minutes for an hour.

   c. 30 minutes for 4 hours, then every 8 hours for 72 hours.

   d. 60 minutes for 4 hours, then every 4 hours for 16 hours.

26. Wound drains are:

   a. clean.

   b. contaminated.

   c. sterile.

   d. pathogenic.

27. Hypoxia is:

   a. inadequate oxygen.

   b. cold body temperature.

   c. an allergic reaction.

   d. a normal response.

28. Pulmonary embolism is:

   a. not a serious condition.

   b. a blood clot in the leg.

   c. a complication of edema.

   d. a blood clot in the lungs.

D. Nursing Assistant Challenge

Mr. Dovetski is a 47-year-old patient on the surgical unit. He has had abdominal surgery. When he arrives on the unit after surgery, you note that he has a Foley catheter, an intravenous feeding running, dressings on the abdominal incision, and elastic stockings. Think about what procedures you will include in your care of Mr. Dovetski.

29. How often will you take his vital signs? Which procedures are included in vital signs? What are the "normal" ranges for each vital sign for a person of this age? If there are changes in the vital signs, these changes may be indications of what complications?

_____

_____

_____

30. What observations will you make regarding the Foley catheter? Why do you think he has the catheter in place?

_____

_____

_____

31. What observations will you make regarding the intravenous feeding? Why do you think the physician ordered IV feeding?

_____

_____

_____

32. You know you will need to have Mr. Dovetski perform coughing and deep breathing exercises. Why is this important? How can you help him do the exercises with the least discomfort?

_____

_____

33. Why do you think he has elastic stockings on? How often should you take the stockings off and reapply them? What do you need to remember when putting the stockings back on?

_____

_____

_____

34. How will you report any complaints of pain?

_____

_____

_____

35. How will you check for bleeding from the incision?

_____

_____

_____

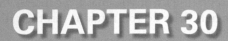

CHAPTER 30

Caring for the Emotionally Stressed Patient

OBJECTIVES

After completing this chapter, you will be able to:

30.1 Spell and define terms.

30.2 Explain mental health and the process of adaptations.

30.3 Describe bipolar affective disorder, schizoaffective disorder, seasonal affective disorder, borderline personality disorder, and depression.

30.4 Give an overview of anorexia nervosa and bulimia nervosa.

30.5 Explain how physical and mental health are related.

30.6 Define and discuss substance abuse.

30.7 Describe the care of persons who are in withdrawal.

30.8 Identify common defense mechanisms.

30.9 Describe ways to help patients cope with stressful situations.

30.10 Define and discuss mental illness.

30.11 Describe the care of persons with adaptive and maladaptive behavior.

30.12 Describe methods of caring for the demanding patient.

30.13 List at least 10 guidelines for dealing with a violent individual.

30.14 Describe bullying behavior and triggers.

30.15 List steps to prevent being the target of a bully.

VOCABULARY

Learn the meaning and the correct spelling of the following words and phrases:

adaptation
affective disorders
agitation
alcoholism
anorexia nervosa
anxiety
anxiety disorder
bipolar affective disorder
borderline personality disorder (BPD)
bulimia nervosa
bullying

compulsion
coping
defense mechanisms
delirium tremens (DTs)
delusions
denial
depression
disorientation
eating disorders
enabling
hypochondriasis
maladaptive behavior

mental illness
obsession
obsessive-compulsive disorder (OCD)
panic disorder
paranoia
phobia
posttraumatic stress disorder (PTSD)
projection
psychosis
reaction formation

repression
schizoaffective disorder
seasonal affective disorder (SAD)
stressors
substance abuse
suicide
suicide precautions
suppression

INTRODUCTION

There are varying degrees and differing aspects of health. A person who is in poor physical health may be mentally healthy. A person with good mental health is self-reliant, able to make decisions, and able to live an effective, productive life (Figure 30-1).

532

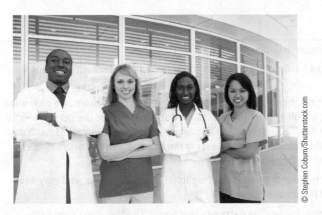

FIGURE 30-1 People who are mentally and physically healthy are happy, productive workers.

Culture **ALERT**

Patients from various cultures have different views about how disabling certain conditions are. In some cultures, mental illness is considered shameful, a punishment from a higher power, a curse from an enemy, or the result of a supernatural force (Figure 30-2). Some may not tell anyone outside the family of a relative with a mental illness. Some may fear that the mental problem is contagious, or that others will develop a similar problem.

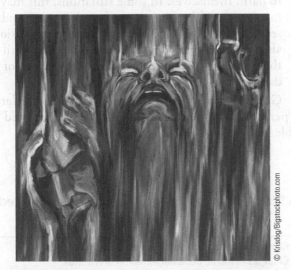

FIGURE 30-2 Some cultures believe that mental illness is a curse or punishment from a deity or evil higher power.

In contrast, a person with good physical health may not be able to cope with and adapt to changes. This limits the person's ability to participate successfully in society.

MENTAL HEALTH

Mental health means exhibiting behaviors that reflect a person's **adaptation** or adjustment to the multiple stresses of life. Stresses or **stressors** are situations, feelings, or conditions that cause a person to be anxious about their physical or emotional well-being. Good mental health leads to positive adaptations. Poor mental health is demonstrated by maladaptive behaviors (behaviors that harm the person or their adjustment).

Physical and mental health are interrelated. Physical illness is often preceded by stressful life situations. Ill health causes emotional stress. It is easy to understand that each of these factors contributes to the total health pattern of each person.

Ways of **coping** with (handling) stressful situations (Figure 30-3) are learned early in life. As people grow, they find the behaviors that work best for them. They learn to use those behaviors to reduce stress and protect self-esteem. These coping patterns become part of the individual's habitual responses, becoming more and more obvious as the person ages.

ANXIETY DISORDERS

Anxiety is fear, apprehension, or a sense of impending danger. It is often marked by vague physical symptoms, such as tension, restlessness, and rapid heart rate. An **anxiety disorder** is one of a group of recognized mental illnesses involving anxiety reactions in response to stress. These are listed in Table 30-1.

AFFECTIVE DISORDERS

Affective disorders are a group of mental disorders characterized by a disturbance in mood. They may also be called *mood disorders* and are usually marked by a

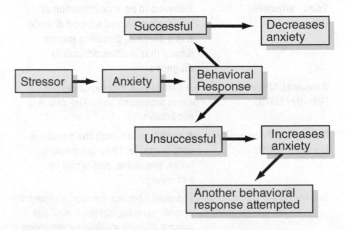

FIGURE 30-3 Each individual has ways of coping with stress.

TABLE 30-1 Anxiety Disorders

Generalized anxiety	The most common anxiety disorder; a common trigger of agitation.
Panic Disorder	Condition in which a person has panic attacks, or bouts of overwhelming fear with no specific cause or basis.
Obsessive-Compulsive Disorder (OCD)	An anxiety disorder in which the patient has recurrent obsessions or compulsions. An **obsession** is a frequently occurring idea, impulse, or thought that does not make sense. The person cannot suppress it. A **compulsion** is a purposeful, repetitive behavior that is done many times each day. This is called repeated ritualistic activity, such as washing the hands hundreds of times each day. The person cannot control the behavior.
Posttraumatic Stress Disorder (PTSD)	Common in survivors of major trauma; the person has nightmares or flashbacks, and may have trouble with normal emotional responses.
Phobia	An unfounded, recurring fear that causes the person to feel panic. The fear can range from mildly annoying to severely disabling.
Agitation	Inappropriate verbal, vocal, or motor activity due to causes other than disorientation or real need.

profound and persistent sadness. Common affective disorders are listed in Table 30-2.

Nursing Care of a Patient with the Potential for Suicide

Never assume that a suicide attempt is a means of getting the attention of staff or family. At least 15 percent of people who try to commit suicide do it again.

Be aware that the suicide rate is higher in acute medical units than it is on psychiatric units. Most of the suicides occur while the patient is under the supervision of a health care provider, who either misses or ignores the clues. Suicide attempts may occur either when the patient is successfully recovering or is getting worse. It is the responsibility of all staff members to observe patients carefully and immediately report any signs of **depression** and/or suicide. You should:

- Implement **suicide precautions** according to your facility's policies and procedures. These are checks and practices a facility follows if a patient states that they no longer wish to live and intend to harm themselves. In some situations, this may involve modifying the physical environment and securing the assistance of mental health professionals. The facility maintains these procedures until the patient is discharged or believed to be out of danger.

General observations to make and report related to persons with mental health problems are listed in Table 30-3.

TABLE 30-2 Affective Disorders

Bipolar Affective Disorder (may also be called *manic depression*)	A condition in which the person has marked mood swings, ranging from elation (also called *mania*) to severe depression.
Schizoaffective Disorder	Believed to be a combination of schizophrenia and a mood disorder. It is a chronic, disabling mental illness that is often difficult to diagnose.
Seasonal Affective Disorder (SAD)	A depression that recurs at the same time each year. The cause is not known.
Borderline Personality Disorder (BPD)	A condition in which the person is very unstable. They are manipulative, impulsive, and prone to self-injury.
Depression	The most common functional disorder in older persons, but seen in all age groups. May be masked by symptoms of physical illness.

TABLE 30-3 Observations to Make and Report Related to Mental Health Problems

- Change in consciousness, awareness, or alertness
- Changes in mood, behavior, or emotional status
- Changes in orientation to person, place, time, season
- Change in communication
- Changes in memory
- Excessive drowsiness
- Changes in ability to respond verbally or nonverbally
- Sleepiness for no apparent reason
- Sudden onset of mental confusion
- Threats of suicide or harm to self or others
- Signs or symptoms of illness or infection
- Has been very depressed, but suddenly is happy and cheerful

GUIDELINES 30-1 Guidelines for Managing the Patient Who Is Anxious or Agitated

- Do not argue with or confront the person.
- Make the environment safe.
- Monitor the person's activities. They are at risk for injury.
- Make sure each patient wears an identification bracelet.
- Keep a recent photo in case the patient wanders off.
- Always know what the person is wearing, to help in identification in case they wander away.
- Notify the nurse promptly if you cannot find the patient.
- Engage the patient in short-term activities. Realize that the patient's attention span is short. Thus, the patient needs rewards for short-term activities.

- Assign the patient brief tasks or engage the person in games, walks, and other activities that enhance self-esteem.
- Use bean-bag seats and rocking chairs in the long-term care facility or the patient's home.
- Watch for injuries.
- Engage the patient in conversation.
- Avoid arguing with the person; enter their reality.
- Prevent the patient from becoming exhausted.
- Check the feet of wanderers for signs of pressure and injury.

GUIDELINES 30-2 Guidelines for Assisting the Patient Who Is Depressed

- Be honest, supportive, and caring.
- Be a good listener. Encourage the person to express feelings. Avoid passing judgment or criticizing what the person feels. Avoid interrupting or changing the subject.
- Give positive feedback on the person's strengths and successes.
- Acknowledge the person's feelings.
- Avoid comments like "Cheer up. Things could be worse."
- Encourage physical activity to the extent possible. Exercise reduces stress.
- Encourage the person to laugh regularly. Laughter is therapeutic and reduces stress. Turn on a funny television program or tell a joke.
- Monitor the person's appetite and report over- or undereating to the nurse.
- Reinforce the person's self-concept by emphasizing their value to society and helping them use their support systems.
- Encourage and allow the person to make decisions over daily routines and activities. Give them as much control as possible.
- Do not act sympathetic. This validates the person's poor self-image and depressed feelings.
- Make sure physical supports, such as eyeglasses and hearing aids, are clean and in place to help the person remain oriented and focus on reality.

- Report complaints so that problems may be identified, assessed by the nurse, and corrected rather than be attributed to the depression.
- Provide the person with activities within their limitations.
- Use simple language and speak slowly when giving instructions.
- Monitor elimination carefully; constipation is common.
- Provide fluids frequently, because the patient who is depressed may be too preoccupied to drink.
- Be alert to the potential for **suicide** (the taking of one's own life). Watch for and report:
  - Change in mood or behavior such as deepening depression or suddenly seeming happy and calm.
  - Withdrawal or secretiveness.
  - Repeated, prolonged, or sporadic refusal of food, care, medications, or fluids.
  - Hoarding medications.
  - Sudden decision to donate body parts to a medical school.
  - Sudden interest or disinterest in religion.
  - Purchase of a gun, razor blades, or other harmful items and hiding them.
  - Statements such as "I just want out" or "I want to end it all."
  - Increased use of alcohol and drugs.
  - Deep preoccupation with something that cannot be explained.

GUIDELINES 30-3 Guidelines for Suicide Precautions

When a person is on suicide precautions, you should:

- Be observant for clues to suicide attempts, and report them to the nurse.
- Be consistent in approaches and care.
- Emphasize the positive aspects of the person's life.
- Give the patient hope while being realistic.
- Work to restore the person's self-esteem, self-worth, and self-respect.

- Help the patient find a support network within the family, religious groups, and self-help groups.
- Make the person feel accepted as a unique, valued person.
- Never ignore the person's statements or threats about suicide.

EATING DISORDERS

Eating disorders are a group of conditions in which the person has disturbances in appetite or food intake. The two most common eating disorders are **anorexia nervosa** (Figure 30-4) and **bulimia nervosa**. These conditions can occur in both males and females. Summary descriptions appear in Table 30-4.

Eating disorders are common in persons with **borderline personality disorder**. The conditions often overlap and are difficult to identify. People with eating disorders are very secretive about it, so family members and close friends are often unaware of the problem until weight loss is so profound that it cannot be ignored. Serious medical problems can occur, as well as depression, moodiness, and low self-esteem. The electrolyte imbalance and starvation caused by these conditions can lead to death.

SUBSTANCE ABUSE

Substance abuse is characterized by the use of one or more substances (such as alcohol or drugs) to alter mood or behavior, resulting in impairment and poor judgment. Over time, the behavior strains finances, causes irresponsibility, makes the user unable to fulfill social or occupational obligations, and interferes with the person's ability to function normally.

Drug abuse can involve use of illegal (street) drugs or misuse of prescription drugs without proper physician knowledge or oversight. Drugs of abuse (Figure 30-5A)

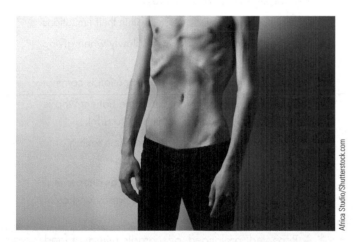

FIGURE 30-4 A patient who is seriously underweight may have an eating disorder.

TABLE 30-4 Common Eating Disorders

Anorexia nervosa	Condition in which the person views their body as fat and limits food intake through diet, exercise, purging, and taking laxatives and diuretics.
Bulimia nervosa	Condition in which the person binge-eats huge amounts, then vomits (*purges*), or takes laxatives and diuretics to undo the binge.

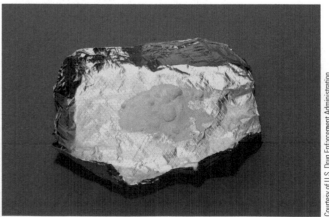

FIGURE 30-5A Methamphetamine powder wrapped in foil.

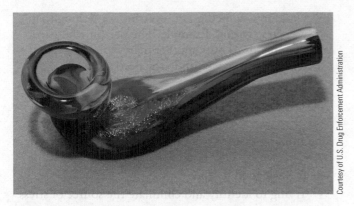

FIGURE 30-5B A pipe for smoking methamphetamine.

are swallowed, chewed, inhaled, injected, or smoked (Figure 30-5B). Some definitions of substance abuse also include use of anabolic steroids (body-building drugs), tobacco, and overeating, but the discussion in this book is confined to alcohol and drug use. Use of narcotic pain medications is not discussed here. Marijuana is discussed only as it applies to nontherapeutic use.

Drug Abuse

Many individual drugs can be abused. Abusers may use a single drug or a combination of drugs.

Alcoholism

Alcohol is a drug and **alcoholism** is a disease. Alcohol slows brain activity and alters alertness, judgment, coordination, and reaction time. Some people use it as a means of coping with stress.

The National Institute for Alcohol Abuse reports that two-thirds of the senior population use alcohol. Fifteen percent of them become alcoholics. Because of its effects on both brain and body, alcohol increases the risk of falls and accidents, particularly in the senior population.

Alcohol can affect the body in unusual ways. It can make some diseases and cardiovascular conditions difficult to diagnose. It can mask pain that might otherwise serve as a warning sign of heart attack and other problems.

The drug alcohol mixes unfavorably with many other drugs (Table 30-5). It causes some drugs to metabolize more rapidly, producing exaggerated responses.

Persons who are withdrawing from alcohol may have **delirium tremens (DTs)**. The DTs are serious withdrawal symptoms seen in persons who stop drinking alcohol suddenly after a long period of alcohol dependence. The condition usually begins 48 to 96 hours after the person takes the last drink. These symptoms can

Courtesy of U.S. Drug Enforcement Administration

TABLE 30-5 Common Alcohol–Drug Interactions

Drug Taken by Patient	Effects to Report
Narcotics, narcotic analgesics	Increased central nervous system (CNS) depression with acute intoxication
Salicylates	Gastrointestinal bleeding
Sedatives and psychotropic drugs	Increased CNS depression with acute intoxication
Barbiturates	Decreased sedative effect after chronic alcohol abuse
Chloral hydrate	Prolonged hypnotic effects
Chlordiazepoxide (Librium, Librax)	Increased CNS depression
Chlorpromazine (Thorazine)	Increased CNS depression
Diazepam (Valium)	Increased CNS depression
Oxazepam (Serax)	Increased CNS depression
Antihistamines	Increased CNS depression
Antabuse	Flushing, vomiting, excessive sweating, hyperventilation, confusion, and drowsiness
Xanax and similar drugs (benzodiazepines)	Increased CNS depression, behavior changes, intoxication
Ritalin, Adderall	Blocks the depressant effect, turning off warning signs that the person is drinking too much. This leads to alcohol poisoning.
Soma compound, Flexeril, muscle relaxants	Increased CNS depression, impaired judgment, thinking, impaired psychomotor skills, decreased coordination

become life-threatening and require immediate treatment. Common signs and symptoms of DTs are:

- Severe confusion
- Tremors
- Hallucinations
- Overactivity of the nervous system
- Seizures
- Hypotension

The alcoholic in withdrawal feels depressed and defensive. They need to identify the stressors that stimulate their desire for alcohol and find new ways of coping. This process takes professional skill, but you can:

- Not allow the alcoholic to manipulate you.
- Listen with empathy.
- Reflect the person's ideas and thoughts.
- Be sure alcohol is not available; this includes items containing alcohol, such as mouthwash.
- Be consistent in maintaining the limits that have been set.

DEFENSE MECHANISMS

The inability to cope with stress threatens self-esteem, causing the person to act in protective ways. These actions are called **defense mechanisms**. Everyone uses defense mechanisms from time to time. Most people use a combination of defenses. People are usually unaware that they are behaving defensively. The behavior becomes harmful only when it is the major means of coping with stress and the person avoids recognizing and responding to reality with effective problem-solving methods. The defense mechanisms reduce the stress, but the problem is not resolved. Such a person needs counseling from a trained mental health provider.

Some common defense mechanisms include:

- **Repression**—the involuntary exclusion from awareness of a painful or conflict-creating thought, memory, feeling, or impulse.

- **Suppression**—a mechanism that differs from repression in that the person is aware of the unacceptable feelings and thoughts but deliberately refuses to acknowledge them.

- **Projection**—a person's own unacceptable feelings and thoughts are attributed to others. The person blames others for their own shortcomings.

- **Denial**—blocking out painful or anxiety-producing events or feelings. This is one of the most common defenses against the stress of diagnosis and illness.

- **Reaction formation**—a person using this defense mechanism represses the reality of a situation and then behaves in a manner that is the exact opposite of their real feelings

Other adaptive behaviors include:

- Displacement—substituting an object or person for another and behaving as if it were the original object or person. Example: Being angry with the nursing assistant because a patient is annoying.

- Identification—behaving like another person whom one holds as an ideal. Example: Speaking to co-workers with the same tone the supervisor uses with you.

- Compensation—excelling in one area to make up for feelings of failure in another. Example: The nursing assistant overachieves in the skill area because their ability to read written directions is poor.

- Conversion—offering a socially acceptable reason to avoid an unpleasant situation. Example: The nursing assistant calls saying they cannot report for duty because they have the flu, when they are really just tired from staying up too late.

- Fantasy—the use of imagination to solve problems. Example: The supervisor criticizes the nursing assistant, who then daydreams of a time when they are the head of nursing and can fire the supervisor.

- Undoing—a method of reversing something that was done wrong. Example: The person who used their hands to hurt another may wash their hands repeatedly to try to undo the deed

ASSISTING PATIENTS TO COPE

The nursing assistant can help patients cope and adapt by:

- Being a good listener
- Trying to identify and eliminate the source of stress
- Being sensitive to body language that may give clues to the source of stress
- Treating the person with respect, recognizing them as a unique individual
- Trying to understand the person's point of view without passing judgment
- Showing that you are dependable and that you respect the patient's privacy and feelings
- Never arguing or debating with a patient, even when you know they are wrong
- Being supportive (Figure 30-6)

Remember that illness, age, and separation from family and home are major stress factors.

Difficult Situations

Patients with coping and behavior problems usually have a behavior management care plan that lists steps to follow when certain problems are exhibited. Implement the plan in the order listed as soon as the behavior starts. Modify your behavior in response to the patient's behavior by monitoring how the patient responds to you, then adjusting your approach.

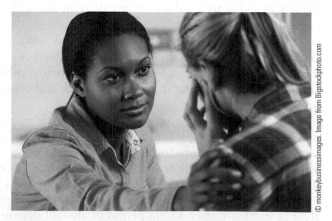

FIGURE 30-6 Demonstrate caring and support to all patients.

THE DEMANDING PATIENT

In every nursing care situation, you will meet patients who are very demanding. This can be a difficult experience for everyone if it is not handled correctly.

Being demanding is a coping behavior that some patients use when they are frustrated. Persons who are very demanding usually feel as if they have lost control. To be successful in caring for these patients, the nursing assistant must:

- Reassure the patient that you understand the complaint or problem and will report it to the appropriate person.
- Remain neutral if the complaints are about other workers. If complaints are about your care, listen, but do not argue or become defensive.
- Attempt to determine the causes of unjustified complaints and correct them, if possible.
- Try to identify the triggers of the demanding behavior.
- Show that you care, but control your emotions.
- Support the patient, be a good listener, and be sensitive to the patient's body language.
- Provide opportunities that allow the patient to regain some control.
- Encourage the patient to make simple decisions about daily routines and activities.
- Be consistent in the manner of care.
- Do not take the patient's demands personally.
- Stop and check on the patient without being asked.
- Keep your promises.
- Report observations to the nurse with suggestions for changes in the care plan.

MALADAPTIVE BEHAVIORS

Mental illness or **maladaptive behavior** occurs when behaviors and responses disrupt the person's ability to function smoothly within the family, environment, or community.

Avoid labeling anyone as mentally ill. Even when an official diagnosis of mental illness has been made, avoid stereotyping the person. Remember that stereotypes are often associated with *myths* (false beliefs). It is far better to view the person as an individual who is demonstrating poor behavioral responses.

Be aware that sometimes signs and symptoms such as fatigue, loss of appetite, insomnia, and pain may reflect either physical or emotional stress. Note and report any unusual behavior or symptoms. Be objective. Do not make judgments about your findings. Blaming and judging a patient is not helpful.

Remember also that confusion, disorientation, and aggressive behavior may only be temporary responses to a fever, drug interaction, or a full bladder. Continuation of such behavior may be the result of organic brain changes.

Psychosis

Psychosis is a serious condition that appears in a number of different mental disorders, including substance abuse, mood disorders, and personality disorders. Occasionally it is triggered by a medical condition. The person loses contact with reality, hallucinates, and has delusions that seem real. Their behavior may be inappropriate and their communication incoherent. Psychosis is a defining feature of schizophrenia and other severe mental disorders.

Hypochondriasis

The patient suffering from **hypochondriasis** imagines or magnifies each physical ailment. Some authorities feel that hypochondriasis is an expression of depression and is one way these individuals reduce stress. These patients need reassurance and understanding but should not be encouraged to focus on or believe in their supposed illnesses. However, the staff must be careful not to overlook real illness when it occurs, just because they have become used to hearing the patient complain. Nursing assistants should report all complaints and never make a judgment that a patient is a hypochondriac.

Paranoia

Paranoia is another extreme maladaptive response to stress. It is characterized by a heightened, false sense of self-importance and delusions of being persecuted. **Delusions** are false beliefs about oneself, other people, and events. People with paranoia believe that everyone is against them. When treating the patient with paranoia, you should:

- Find ways to reduce the patient's feelings of insecurity and misunderstanding.
- Keep the person as involved as possible in reality activities.
- Report and document observed responses to medication and psychotherapy.
- Monitor nutrition and fluid balance—these patients often refuse to eat or drink for fear of poisoning.
- Observe sleep patterns—the person may be fearful of being harmed while sleeping.
- Be direct and honest in all interactions.
- Not support any misconceptions or delusions that the person exhibits.
- Never argue with anyone who has delusions; it can trigger a serious confrontation.

Assessing the Patient's Behavior

A licensed professional will do an initial assessment of the patient's mental and emotional state. You contribute to the nursing process by making careful and sensitive objective observations. Report:

- Physical responses related to eating, personal hygiene, sleeping, participation in activities, or any strange or unusual behaviors
- Emotional responses related to interactions between the patient and yourself or between the patient and other patients, emotional outbursts, or inappropriate responses
- Patient behavior as it relates to judgment and affects memory, orientation, and comprehension

Disruptive Behavior

Disruptive behaviors cause the staff to immediately stop or change what they are doing in order to control a situation. The patient may be verbally and physically aggressive. Although some nondisruptive behaviors may be irritating, they do not create a need for immediate staff intervention. Disruptive behavior creates a potential safety risk for staff and patients. Observations of disruptive behavior to make and report are listed in Table 30-6.

Disorientation (Disordered Consciousness)

Disorientation is a condition in which a person shows a lack of reality awareness with regard to time, person,

TABLE 30-6 Disruptive Behavior Observations to Make and Report

- No behavior problems exhibited.
- Requires immediate staff intervention one to four days per month, but not weekly.
- Requires immediate staff intervention one to six days per week.
- Requires staff intervention once a day or more.
- Patient is verbally aggressive or uses abusive language (such as swearing, threatening, baiting/provoking, or yelling). Document and describe behavior, staff response, and frequency.
- Patient is physically aggressive, combative, or assaultive to self or others (such as by hitting self or others, throwing objects at others). Document and describe behavior, staff response, and frequency.
- Other disruptive acts, such as inappropriate undressing, stealing, smearing feces, destruction of property, wandering, sexually displaying self, or refusing treatment. (Do not include nonphysical behavior such as withdrawal, paranoia, etc.) Document and describe behavior, staff response, and frequency.

Difficult Situations

Reward patients for positive behavior. Behavior that is rewarded is usually repeated. The goal is to show the patient a healthy way of directing energy. Verbal praise, positive feedback, and other signs of approval are rewards. Nonverbal rewards such as a hug, smile, or pat on the back may also be used, when appropriate. Snacks and privileges are sometimes used as rewards.

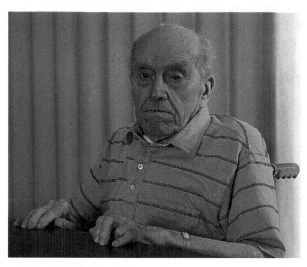

FIGURE 30-7 Orientation is being aware of the dimensions of person, place, and time. Disorientation occurs when awareness is lost in one or all of the dimensions and occurs in reverse order. Disorientation to time will be lost first, followed by place. The last dimension to be lost is orientation to person.

or place (Figure 30-7). It may be mild or severe, temporary or prolonged. Report patient behavior, actions, and responses. The disoriented person has impaired:

- Judgment, including safety judgment
- Memory
- Comprehension (understanding)
- Orientation to time, place, or person

Nursing Assistant Responsibilities

Persons with disorientation cannot be responsible for their actions and cannot protect themselves. The patient's

 Safety **ALERT**

Protecting patients from harm is the most important nursing responsibility.

sensory problems (delusions or hallucinations) may put others at risk. Be objective in observing and reporting behavior problems. Gather as much information as possible, including who, what, when, why, and how.

Enabling

Enabling behavior is reacting to a patient in a manner that shields the person from the consequences of their actions. Enabling behavior differs from helping behavior in that it allows the person to be irresponsible. By respecting professional boundaries, you will avoid helping others inappropriately. Enabling behavior with patients creates dependency rather than moving the person toward independence and good mental health. Methods of enabling patients that you should avoid include:

- Protecting the patient from the natural consequences of their behavior
- Keeping secrets about a patient's behavior
- Making excuses for a patient's behavior
- Taking steps to get a patient out of personal trouble

- Blaming others for the patient's behavior
- Seeing the patient's problems as a result of something else
- Giving money to patients
- Attempting to control patients' lives and activities
- Doing things for the patient that they should do themselves.

Strive to keep your behavior in the zone of helpfulness to avoid crossing professional boundaries and enabling patients.

VIOLENCE IN THE WORKPLACE

Episodes of workplace violence are increasing in our society. Serious violence has occurred in hospitals and nursing homes in both rural and urban communities. OSHA has developed guidelines for preventing violence in the health care facility, and many employers use these guidelines.

Workplace violence is any physical assault, threatening behavior, or verbal abuse that occurs in the workplace.

GUIDELINES 30-4 Guidelines for Assisting Patients Who Have Behavior Problems

- Follow the care plan.
- Control your own responses and reactions.
- Use good communication and listening skills.
- Avoid lying to the patient.
- Avoid making promises you cannot keep.
- Avoid discussing facility or staff problems with the patient.
- If the patient complains, inform the nurse; avoid becoming defensive.
- Protect the safety of the patient and others.
- If the care plan tells you how to respond to a specific behavior, apply the approaches when the behavior starts. Do not wait until the patient loses control.
- Practice empathy.
- Attempt to learn the cause of the behavior. Communicate with other team members.
- Remove the cause (or trigger) of the behavior, if known.

- Let others know if you discover an approach that works.
- Modify your behavior in response to the patient's behavior.
- Watch the patient's response to your approaches. Adjust your approach, equipment, routine, and other care, if necessary.
- Discuss family, friends, or other pleasant information with patients. This provides a source of strength, comfort, and support.
- Meet the patient's physical needs.
- Give patients as much control as possible. Offer choices in care and routines. Encourage them to direct their own care.
- Be patient. Control your reaction to the patient. Make sure your body language does not send the wrong message.
- Be happy. Smile. Make sure your body language sends a positive message. Positive behavior is contagious.

The workplace includes, but is not limited to, the facility's buildings and the surrounding perimeters, including parking lots, field locations, clients' homes, and traveling to and from work assignments. Workplace violence includes:

- Beatings
- Stabbings
- Suicides and attempted suicides
- Shootings
- Rapes
- Psychological traumas
- Threats or obscene telephone calls
- Intimidation
- Verbal or physical harassment
- Being followed, sworn at, or shouted at
- Drug holdups
- Robbery

Violence in the workplace can be committed by strangers, spouses, patients, family members, co-workers, or personal acquaintances. The potential for fatal violence is increased by the prevalence of handguns and other weapons in society at large. Some of the potential causes of health care facility violence are:

- Use of hospitals by the criminal justice system for criminal holds and the care of individuals who are disturbed and violent
- Patients with acute and chronic mental illness
- Poor judgment and loss of inhibition due to abuse of alcohol, street drugs, or illicit use of prescription drugs
- The availability of controlled substances in the facility, making it a likely target of robbery
- The increasing number of gangs and gang members in many communities
- Unrestricted movement of the public in health care facilities
- Distraught family members and other individuals who become angry and frustrated
- Low staffing levels, particularly during meals and at other times when staff is busy caring for patients and unable to observe activity in the hallways
- Poorly lit parking lots, garages, and ramps
- Lack of staff awareness of risk factors

GUIDELINES 30-5 Guidelines for Violence Prevention

Follow all facility policies and procedures involving safety and security. Other things you can do to prevent potential incidents are:

- Attend classes to learn how to recognize and manage escalating aggression.
- Attend classes on cultural diversity and sensitivity training on racial and ethnic issues and differences.
- Keep secure areas locked. Avoid propping locked doors and windows open. Never disable a door alarm.
- Do not leave keys unattended. Never share security alarm codes.
- Close shades or curtains at night.
- Report assaults or threats of assaults to the nurse immediately.
- Avoid wearing scarves, necklaces, earrings, and other jewelry that could cause injury if you are attacked.
- Do not carry valuables or large sums of cash to work.
- Avoid remote, dark areas when you are alone.

- Report burned-out lights and locks that are not working.
- Exercise caution in elevators, stairwells, and unfamiliar areas. Immediately leave the area if you believe that a hazard exists.
- Use the "buddy system" if personal safety may be threatened.
- Do not let a potentially aggressive person come between you and an exit.
- Keep your head up, look ahead, and be aware of your surroundings.
- If your facility has security personnel, request that they escort you in dark or potentially dangerous areas. If no security personnel are on duty, ask other staff members to accompany you.
- Park in well-lighted areas. Always lock your car after parking. Look in the car before getting in, and then lock the doors after you get in. Do not roll windows down to speak with individuals who approach your car.
- Report suspicious individuals or other potential safety hazards to the proper person. Never approach a suspicious person by yourself.

GUIDELINES 30-6 Guidelines for Dealing with an Individual Who Is Violent

- Remain calm and avoid raising your voice, which may further agitate the person.
- Speak slowly, softly, and clearly.
- Call for help, if possible, or send someone to get help.
- Move away from heavy or sharp objects that may be used as weapons.
- Monitor your body language and avoid movements that could be challenging, such as placing your hands on your hips, moving toward the person, pointing your finger, or staring directly at the person. However, focus your attention on the person so you know what they are doing at all times.
- Position yourself at right angles to the person. Avoid standing directly in front of them. Maintain a distance of three to six feet.
- Position yourself so that an exit is accessible. Never let the person come between you and the exit.
- Avoid making sudden movements.

- Listen to what the person is saying. Encourage the person to talk, and communicate that you genuinely care and will try to help. Acknowledge that you understand that they are upset. Break big problems into smaller, manageable ones.
- Avoid arguing and defensive statements. Accept criticism in a positive way. Ask clarifying questions.
- Ask the person to leave and return when they are calmer.
- Ask questions to help regain control of the conversation.
- Avoid challenging, bargaining, or making promises you cannot keep.
- Describe the consequences of abusive behavior.
- Avoid touching an angry person.
- If a weapon is involved, ask the person to place it in a neutral location while you continue talking. Avoid trying to disarm the person, which may put you in danger.

- Failure to use safety precautions, such as locking doors and reporting suspicious individuals
- Marital and relationship problems
- Domestic discord in the home that continues when one party comes to the facility intending to harm others

BULLYING

Bullying is repeated behavior that makes fun of, embarrasses, scares, threatens, belittles, degrades, offends, scares, or insults another person. Bullying is repetitious. It is not one-time bad behavior. The person initiating the behavior is called a *bully*. The person being bullied is the *target*. Bullies select new, shy, weak, or timid targets. In health care, the bully seeks to control others and is often in a real or imagined position of power.

An old Japanese proverb is: "The nail that sticks up gets hammered down." This is true in terms of bullying. Bullies target anyone who is different, such as a person from a different race or culture; a worker who is short, tall, large, or small; a person who is from a different economic class; a person with a disability; or someone with a different sexual preference. However, any minor difference might be targeted. Although the behavior may be

illegal, workers often look the other direction because bullying is difficult to manage.

Bullying is a common workplace behavior. Bullies have accomplices about a third of the time. They form groups that exclude the target, which makes standing up to the bully much more difficult. However, bullies are lazy and often back down if the target resists their efforts. Challenge the bully. Maintain eye contact. Don't look down.

Bullying behaviors vary. They may be subtle or obvious. Common behaviors are:

- Being rude or impolite
- Acting arrogant or superior
- Displaying frightening or aggressive facial expressions such as glaring, staring, or grimacing (Figure 30-8)
- Hostile body language, such as making obscene gestures, pointing, shaking a fist, slamming doors, or throwing items
- Making cruel or insulting personal remarks
- Ignoring or belittling the target
- Shunning or purposefully excluding another worker
- Starting rumors or gossip
- Withholding needed information or intentionally making it difficult for the target to do their job

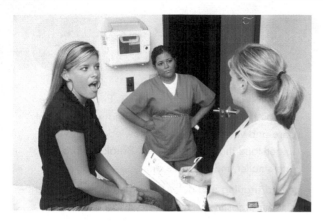

FIGURE 30-8 A bully may appear mad and demonstrate aggressive or menacing behavior. Aggressive facial expressions are frightening.

- Shifting the workload so the target gets most of the work
- Questioning the target's skill, qualifications, judgment, or ability to do the job
- Giving the target the most unpleasant jobs

Bullying is a violent behavior that is more common in health care than other professions. It can have serious negative effects on patient care as well as the morale of both targets and witnesses.

Bullying Triggers

Examples of triggers that can make a health care worker a potential target for bullying include:

- Receiving special attention from managers or those in power
- Being newly hired or recently graduated
- Poor staffing
- Receiving a promotion, award, or benefit that others believe is undeserved
- Jealousy of a worker's ability or appearance
- Problems working with team members

Prevention

You are much more likely to recognize bullying behaviors in others than you are in yourself. To prevent bullying, you should:

- Call people by name. Failing to use someone's name can be a sign of disrespect or contempt.
- Help others when asked. Help even when they don't ask, if possible. Refusing to help, hiding, or pretending to be too busy to help are forms of bullying.
- Do your share of the work.
- Don't talk behind others' backs.
- Avoid asking inappropriate questions about personal matters or teasing others about personal issues.
- Show respect for others. Use good manners. Be polite, kind, and sincere.
- Recognize the contributions of others.
- Avoid pointing fingers and blaming others.
- Be willing to admit and correct your mistakes.
- Treat everyone the same.
- Bullying is never acceptable. If you see bullying, say something! By remaining silent, you are acknowledging that bullying is okay.

REVIEW

A. True/False

Mark the following true or false by circling T or F.

1. T F   Mental health refers to the adaptations a person makes to the multiple stressors of life.
2. T F   Stressors are the physical and emotional problems that a person encounters throughout life.
3. T F   Defense mechanisms are used only by mentally unhealthy persons.
4. T F   If you know that the patient is wrong about something they are saying, it is proper to tactfully debate the issue with the patient.
5. T F   The best way to handle a demanding patient is by trying to determine the factors underlying the patient's distress.
6. T F   Panic attacks are isolated events that seldom recur.
7. T F   The use of alcohol impairs mental alertness, judgment, reaction time, and physical coordination.
8. T F   It is dangerous for a person to drink alcohol while taking other medications.
9. T F   Alcohol is a drug.
10. T F   An intoxicated person could choke on food.
11. T F   Alcoholics have a poor chance for recovery.
12. T F   Maladaptive behaviors reflect the failure of usual defense mechanisms.
13. T F   Depression is the least common of the functional disorders in older people.

14. T F Obsessive-compulsive disorder is an affective disorder.

15. T F The onset of symptoms in posttraumatic stress disorder may be delayed for months to years after the event.

16. T F Phobias are seldom serious or disabling.

17. T F Mania is a period of elation.

18. T F If a patient threatens suicide, you need not be concerned.

19. T F At least 15 percent of those who attempt suicide will do it again.

20. T F Only licensed staff are responsible for guarding against suicide attempts.

21. T F Suicides are attempted only by patients in psychiatric institutions.

22. T F The patient who is agitated may ask the same question repeatedly.

23. T F Agitation is a significant problem for the elderly, their families, and facility staff.

24. T F Paranoia is a maladaptive response that usually requires medication and psychotherapy.

25. T F Individuals who are paranoid believe that others are out to get them.

B. Matching

Choose the correct word from Column II to match each description in Column I.

Column I

26. _____ shielding a patient from the consequences of behavior

27. _____ blocking out painful or anxiety-producing events or feelings

28. _____ lack of awareness of reality

29. _____ handling stressful situations

30. _____ attributing one's own failing to another

31. _____ excelling in one area to make up for feelings of failure in another

Column II

a. projection

b. denial

c. compensation

d. enabling

e. coping

f. disorientation

C. Multiple Choice

Select the best answer for each of the following.

32. The patient tells you that their doctor says they have AIDS, but they know that isn't possible. They most likely is using the defense mechanism of:

a. repression.

b. displacement.

c. projection.

d. denial.

33. The best way to enhance a patient's capability to cope with an unpleasant situation that has developed with another patient is to:

a. tell them to ignore it.

b. let them know they can talk to you safely.

c. tell them everyone has problems; their aren't so important.

d. suggest they discuss it with their clergyperson.

34. A patient who refuses to eat or drink because they are convinced that they are being poisoned is suffering from:

a. paranoia.

b. depression.

c. agitation.

d. disorientation.

35. A patient is depressed. You can best help them by:

a. pitying them.

b. keeping them from interacting with others.

c. agreeing that they probably deserve the way they feel.

d. stressing their continued value to society.

36. The best way to help a patient remain oriented to reality is to:

a. keep eyeglasses in the bedside stand so they will not be broken.

b. isolate the patient.

c. place a clock and calendar nearby.

d. explain things in detail.

37. Enabling behavior:

a. is used when caring for patients who require total care.

b. involves orienting patients to person, place, and time.

c. is used to help patients relieve stress.

d. shields an individual from the consequences of their actions.

38. Purging behavior is:

   a. self-induced vomiting.

   b. refusing to eat.

   c. exercising vigorously.

   d. a form of substance abuse.

39. People who abuse substances use alcohol or drugs to:

   a. relieve chronic pain.

   b. alter their mood.

   c. get back at family members.

   d. treat medical problems under physician supervision.

40. Bullying:

   a. is one-time bad behavior.

   b. is a form of health care violence.

   c. is not common in nursing.

   d. does not affect patient care.

41. Psychosis:

   a. is not serious.

   b. causes depression.

   c. does not affect behavior.

   d. causes hallucinations.

42. Disruptive behaviors:

   a. are irritating but harmless.

   b. cause staff to respond immediately.

   c. can safely be ignored.

   d. are not dangerous.

43. Reaction formation is:

   a. the use of imagination to solve problems.

   b. behaving in manner opposite to one's true feelings.

   c. reversing something wrong that was done.

   d. substituting one object or person for another.

44. When dealing with an individual who is potentially violent, the nursing assistant should:

   a. speak loudly and clearly.

   b. maintain a distance of two feet.

   c. listen to what the person is saying.

   d. attempt to touch the person gently.

D. Nursing Assistant Challenge

You are assigned to care for Mr. Simonson, who was recently diagnosed with diabetes. He is learning how to administer his insulin, how to plan his diet, and how to test his blood sugar. He has been very quiet and keeps his eyes closed most of the time, although he is not sleeping. One day as you enter the room, he screams at you to get out and then picks up his water pitcher and throws it. Think about what you learned in this chapter about human behavior as you consider these questions.

45. What examples of nonverbal communication is Mr. Simonson displaying?

   _____

   _____

46. Do you think he is using defense mechanisms to cope with his diagnosis? If so, which ones?

   _____

   _____

47. If Mr. Simonson displays this kind of behavior again, what would be an appropriate response from the nursing staff?

   _____

   _____

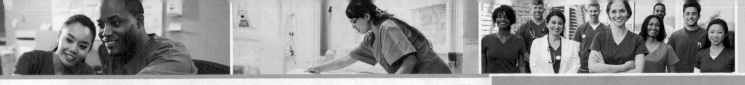

Caring for the Bariatric Patient

CHAPTER 31

OBJECTIVES

After completing this chapter, you will be able to:

31.1 Spell and define terms.

31.2 Define overweight, obesity, and morbid obesity, and explain how these conditions differ from each other.

31.3 Explain why weight affects life span (longevity) and health.

31.4 Define comorbidities and explain how they affect a person's health.

31.5 Briefly state how obesity affects the cardiovascular and respiratory systems.

31.6 Explain how stereotyping and discrimination affect persons with obesity.

31.7 List some team members and their responsibilities in the care of the bariatric patient.

31.8 Explain why environmental modifications are needed for bariatric patient care.

31.9 Describe observations to make and methods of meeting bariatric patients' ADL needs.

31.10 List precautions to take when moving and positioning bariatric patients.

31.11 List at least five complications of immobility in bariatric patients.

31.12 Describe nursing assistant responsibilities in the postoperative care of patients who have had bariatric surgery.

VOCABULARY

Learn the meaning and the correct spelling of the following words and phrases:

advocate	gastric bypass	morbid obesity	stenosis
bariatrics	hyperventilation	obesity	stricture
bariatric surgery	ideal body weight (IBW)	overweight	trapeze
body mass index (BMI)	minimally invasive	panniculus	
comorbidities	surgery	reflux	

INTRODUCTION

Being **overweight** (Figure 31-1) is a condition in which a person weighs more than they should, according to standards based on height and bone (frame) size. A person who is overweight has a body weight greater than is considered desirable or medically advisable.

The disease of obesity is a complex condition with multiple causes—and it is very misunderstood. A popular myth is that obese people eat an enormous amount of food and lack willpower. This is untrue. Genetics plays an important role in the distribution of body fat, metabolism, and regulation of the appetite. In fact, heredity may account for up to 70 percent of all weight problems. Some experts believe that the hormones used to fatten meat supply animals are also affecting the humans who consume the meat. The definition of **obesity** varies, but it is usually considered being overweight by 20 to 30 percent of the ideal body weight. Environmental factors are also very important. Obesity negatively affects every system of the body and increases patient risk for many other serious medical conditions and diseases. Untreated, it results in a shorter life span.

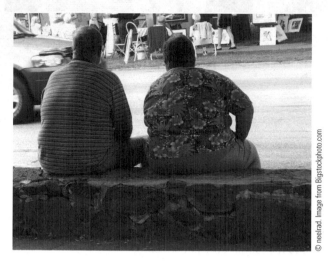

FIGURE 31-1 Obesity is a very misunderstood condition, in which the person is 20% to 30% above ideal body weight. Heredity may account for up to 70% of all weight problems.

Clinical Information ALERT

Obesity is a disease that has become a serious, major health problem in the United States, accounting for thousands of deaths each year. A variety of procedures may be done to address the health issues of overweight, obese, and morbidly obese individuals. In 2004, approximately 140,000 bariatric surgeries were done. In 2017, there were 228,000 bariatric surgeries done.

Clinical Information ALERT

A panel of medical experts determined that Americans die sooner and have higher rates of disease than people in 16 other high-income countries. Conditions in which people in the United States ranked poorly were cardiovascular disease, diabetes, and obesity. The United States had the highest number of overweight and obese children, with 35.9 percent of girls and 35 percent of boys ages 5 to 17 being overweight or obese, according to 2018 information.

Americans age 20 and older have a high rate of diabetes and the highest average body mass index of the countries studied. Persons older than age 50 are more likely to die of cardiovascular disease than people in other countries. Other factors that contribute to poor outcomes are limited access to medical care due to lack of health insurance, a shortage of doctors, and lack of exercise. The United States is used as an example to show why obesity and related health problems must be prevented to avoid similar outcomes in other countries.

Sources: American Society for Medicine and Bariatric Surgery (ASMBS). (2018, June). Estimate of bariatric surgery numbers, 2011–2018. https://asmbs.org /resource-categories/estimate-of-bariatric-surgery-numbers

---

Obesity is a chronic condition that is a factor in 5 of the 10 leading causes of death. Besides the health risks, person who is obese often experiences emotional problems, including depression, low self-esteem, social isolation, anxiety, substance abuse, and eating disorders (see Chapter 30). Experts believe that society's treatment of and response to persons who are obese increases their risk for emotional problems.

Persons with obesity experience discrimination and prejudice in social and employment situations. Activities of daily living are difficult. The person who is obese often has limited access to public facilities. It is not unusual for a person who is obese to experience difficulty in forming and maintaining personal relationships. Many are victims of physical and psychological abuse. When they are hospitalized, they know that their size makes it hard for staff to care for them, and they may be admitted to your unit with feelings of shame, embarrassment, and fear.

Bariatrics is a relatively new field of medicine that focuses on the treatment and control of obesity, as well as medical conditions and diseases associated with obesity. Bariatric patients have many highly specialized needs. Treatment may be medical, surgical, or both. Some hospitals and long-term care facilities have special bariatric treatment units. Others integrate bariatric patients into the general population. Regardless of the setting, as a nursing assistant you are likely to encounter bariatric patients, and must know how to care for them correctly.

Caring for bariatric patients presents many challenges and risks, both physical and emotional. Care that is routine for normal-size patients may be done differently for the bariatric population. This includes many activities of daily living (ADLs) and nursing assistant tasks, such as bathing, transfers, mobility, and patient transport. Simple activities such as standing up, sitting down, and walking to the bathroom can be strenuous or painful for the patient. Certain aspects of care can be frustrating or humiliating for bariatric patients. For example, the patient may not be able to put on shoes and socks. Some facilities do not have scales to accommodate persons who weigh more than 350 pounds.

To obtain an accurate weight, some patients have been taken to the laundry, loading dock, or maintenance department, where a freight scale was used to weigh them. Think carefully about the patients' feelings before performing an action like this. Using a freight scale to weigh a patient is a tremendous assault on dignity and self-esteem.

WEIGHT AND BODY MASS INDEX

Ideal weight is a concept developed from life insurance statistics related to life span (longevity) and health. The registered dietitian calculates the **ideal body weight (IBW)** for each patient based on a mathematical formula that considers the person's height, age, sex, build, activity, medical condition, and need for nutrients.

Body mass index (BMI) is also a consideration. BMI is a mathematical calculation used to determine whether a person is at a healthy normal weight, is overweight, or is obese. Table 31-1 lists BMI and categories of body mass. *Ideal weight* is having a BMI that is less than 25. Obesity is a BMI of 27–40. **Morbid obesity** (Figure 31-2) usually qualifies for surgical treatment. Patients who are morbidly obese have a BMI of 41 or higher and are 100 pounds or more over their ideal body weight.

Comorbidities

Being overweight or obese increases the risk for many health conditions, including chronic pain, arthritis and joint pain, sleep apnea, high cholesterol, hypertension, diabetes, heart disease, and stroke. These conditions are called comorbidities. **Comorbidities** are diseases and medical conditions that are either caused by or contributed to by morbid obesity. Comorbidities are listed and sorted by system in Table 31-2. Besides creating risk factors and medical management problems, comorbidities lower the weight threshold for surgical treatment. Medical problems are often compounded by mental

TABLE 31-1 Classification of Weight/Body Mass Index

BMI	Category
Less than 18.5	Underweight
18.5 to 24.9	Normal
25 to 26.9	Overweight
27 to 30	Mild obesity
31 to 35	Moderate obesity
36 to 40	Severe obesity
41 to 45	Morbid obesity
Greater than 50	Super obesity

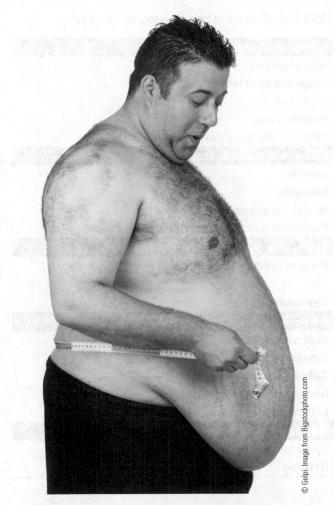

© Gelpi. Image from Bigstockphoto.com

FIGURE 31-2 Patients with morbid obesity qualify for bariatric surgery, but medical problems must be stabilized first. Most have a BMI of 40 or higher and are 100 pounds or more over ideal body weight. A 60-inch tape measure may not be long enough to measure the waist.

health problems. Weight loss often improves or eliminates many comorbid conditions.

Some bariatric patients will be admitted for weigh-loss surgery. Some will be admitted for management of complications of comorbidities. These patients tend to wait a long time before going to the doctor or emergency department, because getting out of the house is very difficult. They are often very ill and unstable upon admission.

Patients with some comorbidities may need stabilization and management of comorbid conditions before bariatric surgery can be done safely. For example, patients may have severe sleep apnea, uncontrolled high blood pressure, or abnormally high blood sugar. Stabilizing the comorbid conditions will reduce the risk of perioperative complications. This could take a long time, depending on the nature of the comorbid problem. However, this

TABLE 31-2 Comorbidities Related to Obesity

Cardiovascular System	Genitourinary System (*continued*)
Atherosclerosis	Infertility
Congestive heart failure	Polycystic ovarian disease
Hypertension	Urinary stress incontinence
Varicose veins	Glomerulosclerosis and renal failure
Venous insufficiency and stasis	**Musculoskeletal System**
Integumentary System	Bone demineralization
Cellulitis	Carpal tunnel syndrome
Dermatitis	Low back pain
Necrotizing skin infections	Osteoarthritis
Panniculitis (painful nodules under the skin)	**Neurological and Psychiatric Conditions**
Endocrine System, Metabolic Disorders	Depression
Diabetes mellitus	Idiopathic intracranial hypertension
Gout	Stroke
Hyperlipidemia	**Ophthalmologic**
Gastrointestinal System	Cataracts
Abdominal wall hernia	Glaucoma
Fatty liver	**Respiratory System**
Gallbladder disease	Asthma
Gastroesophageal reflux disease	Obesity hypoventilation syndrome
Irritable bowel syndrome	Pulmonary hypertension
Genitourinary System	Sleep apnea
Dysmenorrhea	
Hirsutism	

Difficult Situations

The cardinal sign of sleep apnea is excessive day-time sleepiness. The patient may fall asleep at inappropriate times. Drowsiness interferes with the ability to concentrate and to perform complex tasks, such as operating machinery or driving. Other signs and symptoms include mood swings, personality changes, and irritability. If you observe patients with excessive sleepiness, snoring, or other signs of sleep apnea, inform the nurse.

initial management is essential to successful anesthesia and surgery, as well as stable postoperative recovery.

Malignancies

Persons with obesity are also at increased risk for cancer. Cancers believed to be related to obesity are:
- Breast cancer
- Colorectal cancer
- Endometrial cancer
- Gallbladder cancer
- Ovarian cancer
- Pancreatic cancer
- Prostate cancer
- Uterine cancer

EFFECTS OF OBESITY ON THE CARDIOVASCULAR AND RESPIRATORY SYSTEMS

Obesity places a great strain on the heart and lungs (Figures 31-3A and 31-3B). The strain of supplying oxygenated blood to the tissues increases the work of the heart. Adipose (fat) tissue is poorly nourished and less resistant to injury than other tissues. Postoperatively, wound healing will depend on nutrients and oxygen, which are supplied by the circulatory system.

The respiratory system takes in oxygen and delivers it to body cells. Effective oxygen saturation of body parts depends on the volume of each ventilation, how well the oxygen is taken into the bloodstream, and how

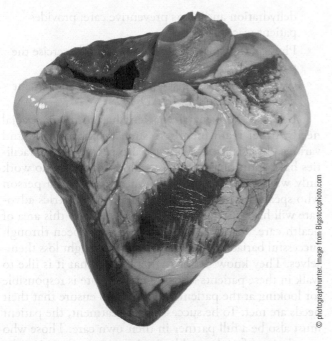

© photographhunter. Image from Bigstockphoto.com

FIGURE 31-3A The heart is much less efficient when it is enlarged and covered with fat.

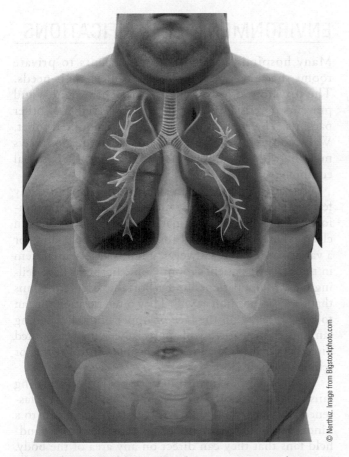

© Nerthuz. Image from Bigstockphoto.com

FIGURE 31-3B Morbid obesity places a great strain on normal lungs.

well saturated the blood is with oxygen when it moves through the system. Many obese patients hyperventilate because of the weight of the chest and the inability of the diaphragm to descend during inhalation. Normally, the descending diaphragm provides space for the lungs to fill with air. In a person who is obese, the weight of the abdominal tissue prevents the diaphragm from descending fully. This inhibits chest expansion. **Hyperventilation** is breathing abnormally fast and deep, resulting in excessive amounts of oxygen in the lungs and reduced carbon dioxide levels in the bloodstream. The decrease in lung capacity and function results in inadequate oxygenation of the body and its tissues. Wound healing is also affected by lack of oxygen.

Some bariatric patients routinely use supplemental oxygen (Chapter 39). Others use BiPap and CPAP devices (Chapter 39) for ventilatory assistance when in bed, because gravity plus the weight of the chest and abdomen further inhibit ventilation. A special mask may be needed. Monitor the fit of the mask. It may cause pain, redness, or skin breakdown on the nose if it is too tight. The patient may be more comfortable in the semi-Fowler's position when the mask is being used. Wash the mask in soap and water each morning, or whenever the patient takes it off.

STEREOTYPING AND DISCRIMINATION

Being overweight brings many challenges. Overweight people often feel deep emotional pain caused by insensitivity and stereotyping by the public at large. Discrimination is a great obstacle for them. Making assumptions about others who are different from ourselves can be automatic, and assumptions about obese

Difficult Situations

All patients have a right to considerate, respectful care. Patients do not choose to be overweight. Most bariatric surgery patients have tried every diet and exercise program available, without lasting success. Repeated diet failures negatively affect their self-esteem. These patients experience rejection and discrimination as part of everyday life. Imagine how that feels! Avoid passing judgment on patients because of their size and weight. Monitor your facial expressions and body language to avoid sending a negative message to the patient. Recognize that obesity is a chronic medical problem, like diabetes and congestive heart failure. Always treat patients with consideration, dignity, and respect.

individuals are common. Avoid passing judgment on patients. Be careful with remarks and body language that may be interpreted as insensitive, prejudicial, or discriminatory.

Bariatric patients may feel isolated or shunned by everyone. They may isolate themselves to protect against hurt feelings. The care plan will list approaches to build trust and rapport with the patient. Show empathy. Try to put yourself in the patient's shoes and understand how they feel. Be very compassionate. If you regularly work with bariatric patients, your facility will provide classes on sensitivity, or you may wish to take a continuing education class on sensitivity training.

INTERDISCIPLINARY TEAM APPROACH TO CARE

A team effort is truly needed to provide care and ensure that bariatric patients' many needs are met. Here is an example of team members and their responsibilities for patients needing medical management or bariatric surgery:

- Licensed nurses—assess the patient; plan, deliver, and supervise direct care; provide patient teaching.
- Nursing assistants—provide direct personal care to meet the patient's ADL needs.
- Social service and/or mental health workers—care for emotional and psychosocial needs; coordinate services needed after discharge.
- Pastoral workers—care for spiritual and religious needs.
- Attending physician and/or internal medicine specialist—prescribes the medical plan of care.
- Bariatric surgeon—performs bariatric surgery, if planned for that patient.
- Anesthesiologist—delivers anesthesia; plans and supervises postoperative pain management.
- Bariatric nurse (a nurse with additional education and experience in care of bariatric patients)—oversees all nursing care and coordinates the care plan.
- Infection control nurse—addresses prevention and treatment of perioperative infection.
- Wound, ostomy, and continence (WOC) nurse—determines skin care plan for wound healing and prevention of new skin breakdown.
- Respiratory care practitioner (respiratory therapist)—manages postoperative ventilation needs; cares for comorbid conditions, such as sleep apnea.
- Dietitian—writes dietary plan of care; supervises menu; addresses risk of malnutrition and

dehydration and plans preventive care; provides patient teaching.
- Physical therapist—helps mobilize and exercise the patient.
- Occupational therapist—works to help the patient become independent in ADLs.

Because the bariatric patient has so many special needs, other team members such as pharmacists and various physician specialists are also needed. Some facilities have additional specialists and advocates who work only with bariatric patients. An **advocate** is a person who speaks on behalf of the patient. A bariatrics advocate will have special knowledge and skill in this area of health care. Many of these workers have been through successful bariatric surgery and massive weight loss themselves. They know better than anyone what it is like to walk in these patients' shoes. The advocate is responsible for looking at the patient as a whole to ensure that their needs are met. To be successful in treatment, the patient must also be a full partner in their own care. Those who are admitted for planned bariatric surgery often view the procedure with both fear and optimism. They often view this day as an important event, like a wedding anniversary; many consider it the first day of the rest of their lives.

ENVIRONMENTAL MODIFICATIONS

Many hospitals admit bariatric patients to private rooms that have been modified to meet their needs. The private room upholds the patient's dignity and prevents potential infringement on the rights of other patients. The room must have a floor-mounted toilet. Wall-mounted toilets should not be used. Doorways must be wide enough to move beds and other special equipment in and out.

Bariatric patients often sweat profusely, and many feel as if they are chronically short of breath. The discomfort of these conditions is markedly relieved by using an electric fan. Most hospital rooms do not have fans, for a variety of reasons. However, a fan is an essential item in the bariatric patient's room. Some hospitals have ceiling fans. Many patients prefer portable oscillating fans that they can position at will. They often position the fan to blow directly on the face or upper body. If a ceiling fan is used, the patient will appreciate having it mounted directly over the bed with an accessible control switch or remote control.

Some facilities furnish battery-operated oscillating fans that the person can position at will. They are fastened to the overbed table with a large clip similar to a binder clip. Some patients use battery-operated handheld fans that they can direct on any area of the body. The patient can position the fans to blow directly on the face or upper body to facilitate breathing and improve

Clinical Information ALERT

The care of medical and surgical bariatric patients differs in many ways from the care of adults with no weight problems. Avoid assuming that bariatric patients are just larger versions of the normal adult. Bariatric patients have many problems not seen in adults of normal weight, including internal fluid shifts and a change in the body's center of gravity. They have a higher risk of blood clots from immobility. Many have fragile skin and many skin-related problems. The increased weight of the chest may make it difficult to breathe, and the patient may need to use oxygen regularly (Figure 31-4). Breathing is even more difficult when the patient is lying down. The extra body tissue causes many to feel hot most of the time, and the patient may want to wear only lightweight clothing. Some have mental and emotional issues related to their weight.

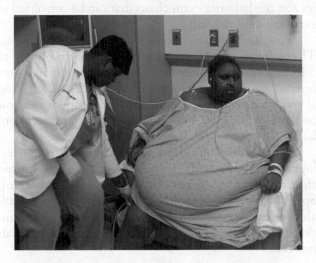

FIGURE 31-4 The weight of the chest can make breathing difficult and the patient may need supplemental oxygen.

comfort. The fan is sent home or discarded when the person is discharged.

Specialized Equipment and Supplies

Some hospitals have bariatric units that are fully supplied with the equipment needed for patient care. If the hospital does not have dedicated bariatric beds, the nurse manager must anticipate patient needs and gather essential items promptly. Emergency or unplanned admissions can be challenging if the facility does not maintain a regular stock of basic items needed for bariatric care. Regular hospital furniture (including toilets) is designed to safely hold patients who weigh 350 pounds or less. Having a wall-mounted toilet break and fall off under a bariatric patient's weight would be emotionally traumatic and likely to cause a serious physical injury.

The patient who is obese may be unable to fit into a regular hospital bed or sit in a regular chair. Even if the patient is able to fit into the bed or chair, getting stuck is a real possibility. There is not enough space to turn the patient. In addition, regular furnishings may be unsafe and break under the patient's weight. Learning the weight limits of regular equipment and furniture is important. Many items that are marked "large size" may still be unsafe for a bariatric patient. Specially manufactured bariatric items are often necessary. Check the specific weight limits of equipment before using it. Many facilities mark this information directly on the back or underside of the equipment, where it is not visible to the public. Others use specially colored stickers, with abbreviations such as EC (expanded capacity, or extra capacity), to denote bariatric-safe equipment. Bariatric furnishings reduce the risk of injury to patients and workers, and increase patient comfort.

The Bed

The bed is the most important piece of equipment in the hospital room. It is literally the center of the hospital patient's universe. From your classes, you know that most daily activities are modified so they can be done when the patient is in bed. Because of concern for patient safety and comfort and the risk of staff injury, special bariatric beds (Figure 31-5A) have been developed that

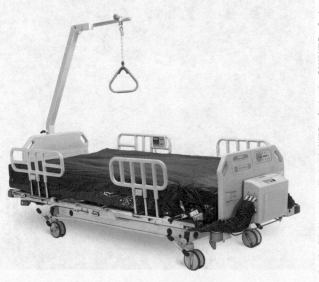

FIGURE 31-5A The Excel Care bed is manufactured for the care of bariatric patients. The trapeze is an accessory for the bed.

will safely support patients who are morbidly obese, and allow enough space for turning. Become familiar with the bed you are using. Most have an electronic high–low function, but the bed may not elevate as high as a regular hospital bed. The side rails on these beds have been strengthened so patients can safely pull on them for moving and positioning support. When a patient is in a regular hospital bed, they must go through a number of twists, turns, and pivots when getting out of bed to stand or transfer. These maneuvers can be awkward for the nursing assistant who is moving a bariatric patient, further increasing the risk of injury because of the positions and repetitive motions.

Special bariatric beds enable staff to move the bed from the flat position into the sitting position. After the patient is seated, the footboard can be removed so the patient can take a step and walk out of the bottom of the bed. Most beds of this type can also be used as a transport vehicle, so that the patient need not transfer to a stretcher or wheelchair. Keep the wheels locked when the bed is not in motion. An additional safeguard is to position the bed against the wall on one side, with the brakes locked, for staff-assisted transfers or for patients who are able to transfer at will. Bariatric wheelchairs (Figure 31-5B) and walkers can be used when the patient is up, if needed.

Some hospitals use bottom sheets made of Gore-Tex or nylon, which have a surface that feels slippery. The fabric reduces friction and shear when moving the patient. Another benefit is that the fabric wicks moisture (perspiration) away from the skin. Some experts also

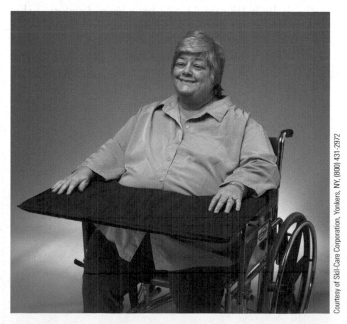

Courtesy of Skil-Care Corporation, Yonkers, NY, (800) 431-2972

FIGURE 31-5B A large person may need a larger wheelchair to prevent skin breakdown. The tray is used for support and may be removed at will, so it is not a restraint.

recommend using these sheets to ease transfers, such as when moving the patient from the bed to a chair positioned against the bed. Various effective techniques have been developed in which caregivers pull on the sheet or special device instead of the patient. This reduces the risk of discomfort and injury to the patient as well as the nursing assistant.

Depending on the type of bed used, an overbed or ceiling-mounted **trapeze** (refer to Figure 31-5A) may also be used to assist the patient with independent bed mobility. The trapeze is also useful when bringing the patient to a standing position for ambulation. A trapeze (see Chapter 41) is a triangular frame that hangs on a chain from the ceiling or base support attached to the bed. Several types of trapeze setups are usually available in every hospital. Special bariatric beds that convert to a chair position have a special trapeze that can be attached to the unit. A regular trapeze defeats the purpose of the conversion bed, because the bed cannot be changed to the sitting position with the trapeze in place. Most hospital clinics, some physician offices, and many wound clinics also use bariatric exam chairs that can be converted to exam tables, if needed.

Low beds are also available for bariatric patients. These have a deck height of approximately 6 to 8 inches. Although they do have an electronic high–low feature, most cannot be elevated above 22 to 26 inches. If you are providing personal care for a patient in a low bed, follow the guidelines in Chapter 23 to protect your back.

Your facility may also have pressure-reducing overlays for bariatric beds. Regular foam overlays are too thin to be of much benefit to the bariatric patient. Special bariatric low air loss beds and overlays are available for bedfast bariatric patients and those with serious skin breakdown. (The bed in Figure 31-5A is a low air loss bed.)

Bedside Chairs

Many of the bariatric patient's visitors will also be large. Chairs in the patient's room should have expanded capacity for the patient and visitors. Chairs the size of loveseats and chairs without arms give the best fit, although the lack of arms will make standing difficult for some people (Figure 31-6).

Mechanical Lift

The mechanical lift you normally use may not support the bariatric patient's weight. The hydraulic mechanical lift is normally safe for persons who weigh about 350 pounds or less. A special high-capacity lift is necessary to safely transfer bariatric patients. Some facilities mount a ceiling lift (Figure 31-7) in each dedicated bariatric room. The lift moves on a track in the ceiling so

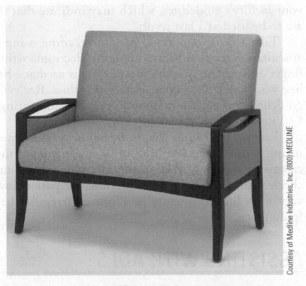

Courtesy of Medline Industries, Inc. (800) MEDLINE

FIGURE 31-6 The furniture in the patient's room is also oversized to accommodate large-size family and friends.

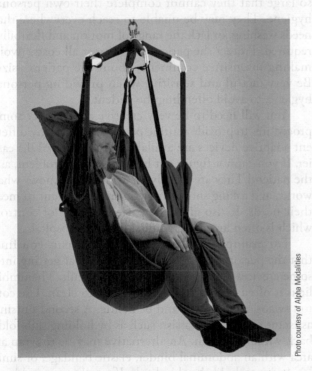

Photo courtesy of Alpha Modalities

FIGURE 31-7 Some facilities have a sling suspended from a ceiling-mounted hoist that slides on a track to move from one location to another. A switch in the hoist releases a cord to lower the sling to seat the patient in the bed or chair.

you can safely slide the sling suspending the patient from bed to chair. After the patient is centered over the chair, the sling is lowered to seat the patient. The sling remains in place. Some slings have a hole cut into the bottom so the lift can be used to lower the patient over the toilet or commode.

Although these mechanical lifts are designed to be used by one person, having two or more caregivers is necessary for safety when moving a bariatric patient. When lowering the patient over a chair or commode, one person must hold the seat in place because there is a risk of tipping when the sling is lowered.

Gowns

Regular hospital gowns do not fit bariatric patients. Extra-large, or "ample" size gowns are needed, and are stocked by most hospitals. If there are none on your unit, check the perioperative department. If no large-size gown is available, use two regular gowns, with one on backward. However, this may an assault on the patient's dignity that should be avoided, if possible.

Toileting and Bathing

Double-size bedside commodes, shower chairs or benches, wheelchairs, and stretchers are also necessary. Regular equipment cannot support more than 300 pounds. Some equipment will not even support that much.

Scales

A number of scale options have become available for weighing bariatric patients without offending their dignity. Hospitals may purchase standing and chair or wheelchair scales that will accommodate patients who weigh less than 1,000 pounds. (Review the information in Chapter 21 on obtaining weights using mechanical lifts.) Your facility may have a scale attachment for the mechanical lift. If so, check the weight limit. Some of these have only a 350-pound capacity. Some of the mechanical lifts used for bedfast patients also have a scale attachment. If your facility has a bed-size mechanical lift, check the weight limits for the scale attachment. Some will accommodate up to 650 pounds. Bed lifts that have scales with a capacity of more than 600 pounds are hard to find. Many bariatric beds have built-in scales, but this feature must be requested when the bed is ordered. The best option is to use a scale that is built into the bed when it is manufactured.

ANTICIPATING PATIENT CARE NEEDS

Try to anticipate needs in advance when you are assigned to care for a bariatric patient. You may have to request equipment from central supply. Make sure you have necessary supplies available, such as a hospital gown and a blood pressure cuff. Try to plan care, and inform the nurse if you will need additional items that are not routinely stocked on the unit. Because of the special nature of bariatric care, you should plan to spend more time doing tasks that you can do quickly for most adult patients. Expect bariatric patients to need more time than the average medical or surgical patient. On a bariatric unit, your assignment will be adjusted to allow enough time to provide conscientious patient care.

Patient Transport

Conduct a dry run before transporting a patient to another area of the facility. Make sure the transport vehicle will make the turns, as well as fit through doors, elevators, and other areas; and that both the patient and extra equipment (such as an IV pole with a pump) will fit. Have another assistant accompany you to assist with pushing on ramps and inclines to prevent a runaway stretcher or wheelchair on a downward slope. Alert the receiving department of the patient's special needs. They may also have to make special preparations and obtain extra help to care for the patient.

Taking Blood Pressure

Regular blood pressure cuffs are too small for bariatric patients and will give inaccurate readings. A large, extra-large or thigh-size cuff may be necessary. Occasionally, even these will not solve the problem. The upper arm is triangular in shape, with the wide part closest to the shoulder and the narrow part near the elbow. Sometimes no blood pressure cuffs will fit securely when wrapped and will slip off. If this occurs, the care plan will identify how to take the blood pressure. Some facilities use a regular-size manual or electronic cuff on the forearm to take blood pressure. Occasionally, the lower leg is used. The accuracy of these methods has been questioned,[1] so be sure your facility accepts values taken in these areas.

Some facilities use digital blood pressure units that register the blood pressure in an artery in the wrist[2] or finger for patients who need frequent or continuous blood pressure monitoring. The wrist blood pressure device may also be used. To obtain the reading, you just press a button. The finger blood pressure device clips on or slips over the finger. Pushing a button will enable you to obtain a digital reading. However, these devices are not always as accurate as a regular sphygmomanometer. Make sure to use them according to your facility's guidelines, which may indicate that they are to be used as a last resort.

Take at least one blood pressure reading using the auscultation method before using the electronic wrist or finger device. The auscultation reading is used as a baseline with which to compare electronic values. Review the guidelines for electronic blood pressure monitoring in Chapter 20.

Patients for whom electronic blood pressure monitoring is not acceptable should be made known to all caregivers and identified on the care plan. If in doubt, check with the nurse for instructions for patients with very high blood pressure or rapid or irregular heart (pulse) rates.

ASSISTING WITH ADLS

Some patients may refuse an offer of help with personal care because they are embarrassed by their inabilities or ashamed of their bodies. However, some patients are so large that they cannot complete their own personal hygiene. They may be unable to reach everywhere that needs washing, or lack the range of motion and flexibility required. Protect the patient's dignity at all costs. Avoid making insensitive comments about the patient's size. Be very tactful and sensitive when providing personal hygiene, to avoid offending the patient.

You will need to be very creative and modify some procedures to provide routine personal care. Many different adaptive devices are available for making ADLs easier. If you cannot figure out how to solve a problem, ask the patient! They are usually an expert who knows what works, and asking shows that you sincerely want to meet their needs. It also gives the patient a sense of control, which is often lost upon admission to the hospital.

For example, when bathing the patient, you find that the person has so much extra skin that getting into some crevices and skin folds is very difficult. The umbilicus is often deep, making it difficult to clean. Use cotton swabs, if necessary, and be gentle. A second nursing assistant may need to assist, such as by holding skin folds back while you wash. An alternative may be to wrap an area with an abdominal binder, elastic bandage, or similar device to hold the skin back. If you have a problem, ask the nurse to assist.

[1]Schell, K., Lyons, D., Bradley, E., et al. (2006, March). Clinical comparison of automatic, noninvasive measurements of blood pressure in the forearm and upper arm with the patient supine or with the head of the bed raised 45 degrees: A follow-up study. *American Journal of Critical Care, 15*(2), 196–205.

[2]Palatini, P., Longo, D., Toffanin, G., et al. (2004, April). Wrist blood pressure overestimates blood pressure measured at the upper arm. *Blood Pressure Monitoring, 9*(2), 77–81.

Difficult Situations

The special care needed by bariatric patients can be time-consuming. Plan your daily schedule and routines. Organize your work to make the best use of your time and allow enough time to meet patients' highly individual needs.

Difficult Situations

Bariatric patients have many skin folds (see Figure 31-8). Keeping them very clean and dry is essential because of the excess skin and moisture that gets trapped there. However, if the skin is very sensitive, a washcloth and towel will be very irritating. Rubbing firmly may even cause purpura or tear fragile skin. Most facilities stock disposable washcloths that have a softer texture than terrycloth (Figure 31-9A). Using a disposable washcloth and gently patting skin dry with a flannel bath blanket may be easier on the skin. A soft, clean, white cotton sock (such as a tube sock) is also effective. You can put it over your hand to wash and rinse the skin, or use a dry sock for padding. The padding absorbs the moisture that further increases skin irritation. A fleece mitt is also a good alternative to a washcloth with a rough surface (Figure 31-9B). A hair dryer on the cool setting is helpful for drying sensitive skin. Improvising care in this manner will become second nature to you as you gain experience working with bariatric patients.

FIGURE 31-9A The disposable washcloth is soft and not as irritating as a terrycloth washcloth. Be sure to dry skin folds well.

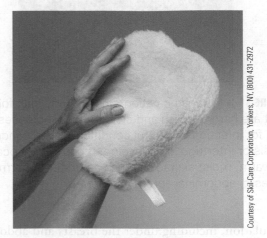

FIGURE 31-9B The fleece bath mitt is very gentle to the skin.

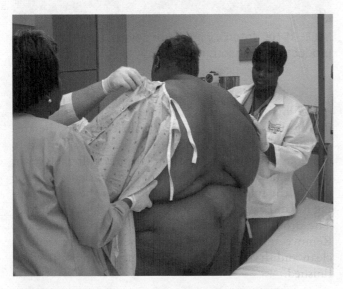

FIGURE 31-8 Large patients have many skin folds. They are usually surgically removed after massive weight loss. This is a medically necessary surgery. Complications will develop over time if the loose skin is left hanging.

Skin Care

The skin is the largest organ of the body, and the bariatric patient has much extra skin. Usually, it has been stretched and is fragile and easily injured. You know that the skin is very sensitive to the effects of moisture, pressure, friction, and shear force. Pressure injuries normally develop over bony prominences. The soft tissue is easily damaged by external pressure applied over the surface of the skeletal structure. Common areas of pressure injury development are the back of the ears and head, sacrum and coccyx, hips, heels, and any other area where high, prolonged external pressure exists. The buttocks are at high risk because patients tend to sit for long periods without moving or shifting their weight. A pressure-relieving cushion is much more comfortable to sit on and helps protect the skin. The hips are also a high-risk area because of the pressure from sitting for long periods in a chair or wheelchair that is too small or narrow.

Red, Weepy Skin Areas

Check the skin folds each time you reposition the patient to make sure they do not have an odor and are not red, "weeping" (overly moist), itchy, or painful. This problem can develop in any moist skin area with a lack of air

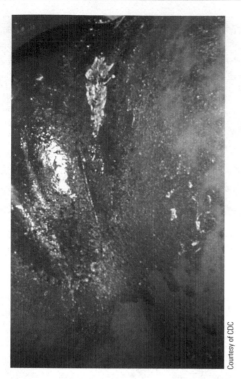

FIGURE 31-10A Bariatric patients have many skin folds that are hard to reach and clean, which increases the risk for infection. A painful condition, called candidiasis or intertrigo, can develop. It commonly occurs in warm, moist skin folds, such as under the arms, breasts, abdominal apron, and groin.

Courtesy of CDC

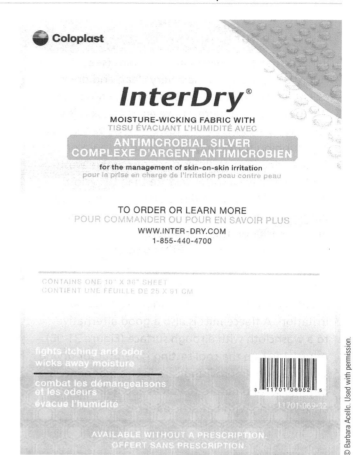

FIGURE 31-10B InterDry is one of several treatment products that absorb moisture.

© Barbara Acello. Used with permission.

circulation, including under the breasts and abdominal apron (panniculus and skin folds, armpits, thighs, and groin). Excessive moisture from perspiration thrive in the warm, moist, dark environment with skin-on-skin friction.

Carefully check the skin folds behind the neck if the patient is unconscious or using ventilator support. These areas tend to become wet from sputum and saliva, and the patient's position produces constant pressure, placing them at risk of both yeast infection and pressure injuries. Reposition the head manually each time the patient is turned. Otherwise, it tends to say in the same position. Reposition the pillow when you move the head.

If necessary, a flannel bath blanket can be cut, folded, and placed in the skin folds. A better alternative is to obtain a supply of flannel receiving blankets, such as those used in the newborn nursery, and fold and place them between the skin folds to absorb moisture. Avoid the temptation to use rough-textured washcloths and towels in these fragile skin areas. Wash the skin with mild soap or baby shampoo if it has an odor, or is damp or sticky. Be gentle and pat dry.

Commercial products are also available to wick moisture and keep skin folds dry (Figure 31-10B). Some contain silver, which reduces the itching, pain, and odor caused by bacteria, fungi, and yeast. After washing and drying the skin, cut a length of fabric that fits the area and provides a two-inch border outside the skin fold to promote moisture evaporation. Position a single layer in the skin fold, making sure that one edge reaches into the base of the fold. Smooth the fabric over the skin, keeping it flat. Leave at least two inches outside the skin fold. The product can remain in place for up to five days. Remove and replace it if it becomes wet. If it remains clean and dry, remove it for bathing and reuse it when finished.

Other Skin Problems

Make sure that the various lines and tubes are not tunneled into, trapped between, or pressing on the patient's skin. This is also a problem that is seldom seen in adults of normal size. Elevate the heels off the surface of the bed, or use a bariatric product that relieves pressure on the heels (Figure 31-11). The heels are also a very high-pressure, high-risk area. Remember, fleece and sock-type heel protectors prevent friction and shearing, but do not relieve pressure.

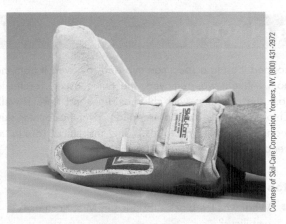

Courtesy of Skil-Care Corporation, Yonkers, NY, (800) 431-2972

FIGURE 31-11 The heel float eliminates all pressure from the heels. It is available in both regular and bariatric sizes.

Dressing the Patient

Because some bariatric patients feel warm and perspire, they may want to remain in a hospital gown or light pajamas all day. Some may prefer to wear nothing and be covered only with a sheet. Make sure the patient is fully covered if they have visitors or must leave the room. Other clothing that is comfortable and easy to put on includes:

- Large T-shirts
- Loose, open-neck shirts that are not tucked into pants
- Caftans or ponchos for females instead of blouses
- Cotton house dresses or muu-muus
- Sweatshirts and sweatpants
- Boxer shorts and boxer briefs instead of brief-style underwear
- Sports bras instead of regular brassieres
- Overalls and coveralls
- Pants with an elastic waist instead of a button and zipper
- Slip-on shoes, shoes that have Velcro fasteners, bedroom slippers, or thong sandals
- Suspenders instead of belts

Nutrition and Hydration

Obese patients often have nutritional problems. Surprisingly, many are malnourished, with a protein deficiency. For many, carbohydrates are dietary staples. This may be a financial issue. High-carbohydrate items stop hunger pangs and often cost less than foods with higher nutrient value. The dietitian will evaluate the patient and make dietary recommendations. The physician will write a diet order. Occasionally, a patient will have signs or symptoms of an eating disorder, such as binging and purging.

Bariatric patients are at high risk for type 2 diabetes. Many patients' blood sugar must be controlled with insulin injections. Oral medications do not provide adequate control for all patients with type 2 diabetes. Type 2 diabetes used to be considered an adult-onset condition, but young obese teens are increasingly being diagnosed with this condition. Blood sugar monitoring will be ordered. You should monitor for and report any signs and symptoms of diabetic problems, such as thirst, fatigue, weakness, increased urination, or dehydration. Patients who are bedfast may have difficulty feeding themselves because of their size or position, or because they cannot use the overbed table. Assist the patient, if necessary.

Elimination

You will probably be assigned to do intake and output (I&O) monitoring. The patient will require a large amount of fluid to support body needs. Many bariatric patients perspire excessively and eliminate a large amount of fluid through the skin. Be sure to inform the nurse if excessive perspiration is a problem. Fluids may be restricted if the patient has a comorbid condition, such as congestive heart failure. Tachycardia and decreased urinary output are early signs of dehydration, followed by a decrease in blood pressure. Inform the nurse promptly if the patient shows any of these signs.

In many facilities, the bariatric patient is catheterized to monitor fluid balance. Because of the patient's size, you may wish to perform perineal care with the patient in the side-lying position instead of on the back. Getting a condom catheter to stay in place on a male patient who is obese is difficult. An indwelling catheter may be a better option. Because of the patient's size, the catheter may appear short, and it may be difficult to attach to drainage tubing or secure to the thigh. Even more important, there is a high risk that the catheter will be pulled out during patient movement. Attaching extension tubing between the indwelling catheter and the drainage-bag tubing may be necessary. The patient is also at high risk for developing pressure injuries in skin folds where a catheter or other device has burrowed into the skin surface. This may also be a problem if items, packaging, and supplies are accidentally dropped in the bed.

Patients may need assistance cleaning themselves after toileting. If the patient uses the bathroom or commode and is able to stand, one nursing assistant can stand in front of the patient to provide instruction and support while a second assistant cleans the perineum and rectum.

MOVING THE BARIATRIC PATIENT

Bariatric patients have many individual needs and many types of equipment are used in patient care. One staff person should never lift or move more than 35 pounds of

CRITICAL THINKING IN ACTION

Use the nursing process and critical thinking skills to analyze the best methods of caring for this patient. (See the answers at the end of this chapter.)

Mrs. Kosmacek was an obese patient on the fourth floor of the John and Ethel Rosenbaum Memorial Hospital. Her care plan noted that she gets short of breath with activity, so the nursing assistant must give her a bed bath each day.

Loretta, a CNA, was bathing Mrs. Kosmacek when she noticed a black area on the umbilicus. It would not come off by rubbing with a washcloth and liquid soap. Mrs. Kosmacek said she did not know what it was and did not know it was there. She seemed very embarrassed.

Loretta got some cotton-tipped applicators and asked another nursing assistant to help. Loretta tried to clean the umbilicus with an applicator while the other assistant held the loose skin to keep it from moving. Still no luck. Mrs. Kosmacek began complaining that the procedure hurt.

Stop and think: What is the next nursing assistant action would you take?

Loretta stopped the procedure and asked the nurse (Johanna) to assess the patient. The nurse noted that Loretta had loosened a solid substance with the applicators. She could see that the substance was protruding slightly from the umbilicus, but she could not grasp it to pull it out.

Johanna asked Loretta to stretch the skin. Johanna pushed the object up with a wooden applicator while Loretta stretched as instructed. Finally, Johanna grasped the black item with a Kelly (see Chapter 36, Figure 36-12) and pulled it out in one piece, putting it on a piece of gauze. It looked like an upside down triangle ▼, although it soon fell apart. The umbilicus looked a little pink and irritated. It was not open or bleeding.

The substance looked like thick, fuzzy black felt. It was approximately ¾ inch wide and 1 inch deep. Johanna

scooped it up in a specimen cup and removed it from the room. After it was removed, the nurse asked Loretta to wash the umbilicus with chlorhexidine and rinse it well. (Chlorhexidine is a nonprescription, over-the-counter skin cleanser that kills microbes.) She instructed Loretta to "keep her eyes on it."

Stop and think:

- What was the black substance in Mrs. Kosmacek's umbilicus?
- Why didn't Mrs. Kosmacek notice the substance?
- Were Loretta's actions appropriate when she noticed a black area on the umbilicus?
- Is washing intact skin with chlorhexidine within the scope of nursing assistant practice?
- Johanna instructed Loretta to "keep her eyes on" the area. What does this mean? If Loretta does not know, how should she find out? What should she look for?

Loretta had two days off and was assigned to care for Mrs. Kosmacek on the day she returned to work. She noticed that the patient's umbilicus looked like a small slit. There were no negative effects from the procedure. Johanna congratulated her on a job well done and thanked her for paying close attention to her patient, making careful observations, using good judgment in getting help, and assisting with the procedure. Loretta was overjoyed with the compliments! She asked what the substance was. Johanna told her that it was just an accumulation of dirt and old skin cells that had been packed into a small, deep umbilicus for a long period of time.

Answers appear at the end of this chapter.

---

body weight without extra help or a mechanical device.[3] A variety of devices have been developed to make procedures as easy as possible for the patient and the nursing assistant.

Another concern about equipment designed for lifting and moving is its ability to support the patient's weight adequately, to reduce the risk of injury for both the patient and the nursing assistant. Explaining positioning and moving techniques beyond the general principles of patient care is impossible. This is a subject for which an entire book is necessary. Your facility will

teach you its policies and procedures and how to use its special equipment. Even when a device is used, two or more nursing assistants are often needed for procedures that involve moving the patient, as well as for personal hygiene.

The HoverMatt Air Transfer System

The HoverMatt Air Transfer System (Figure 31-12) is commonly used for lifting, moving, and transferring bariatric patients. The device improves patient comfort and helps reduce the risk of injury to nursing assistants. The HoverMatt Air Transfer System may be used for moving patients of any size. There is no weight limit. Patients feel

[3]Waters, T. R. (2007, August). When is it safe to manually lift a patient? *American Journal of Nursing, 107*(8), 53–58; quiz 59.

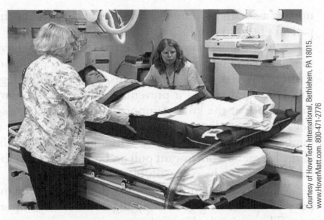

Courtesy of HoverTech International, Bethlehem, PA 18015. www.HoverMatt.com. 800-471-2776

FIGURE 31-12 The HoverMatt Air Transfer System reduces friction, so it feels as if only about 10% of the patient's weight is being moved.

more secure when they are moved in this manner, and use of this equipment eliminates the need to pull on the person's body. Larger mattresses are available for patients with greater body mass.

The HoverMatt Air Transfer System is inflated quickly (in about 5 seconds) by connecting a separate air supply unit. When the mattress is inflated, air escapes from tiny holes on the underside. The escape of air acts as a lubricant, reducing friction during transfers. Because the friction is reduced, nursing assistants are moving only about 10 percent of the patient's actual weight. A 400-pound patient seems to weigh only 40 pounds when the HoverMatt Air Transfer System is used. A two-person transfer is done for most bariatric patients, so each worker is moving about 20 pounds, thus reducing the risk of injury. When you have finished the transfer, unplug the air supply. The mattress deflates on its own within 15 to 20 seconds.

The HoverMatt Air Transfer System cradles the patient when it is inflated, so they feel secure and is less likely to roll off. Nevertheless, reassure the patient and never leave them alone when the mattress is inflated. Many facilities apply this mattress to the bed at the time of admission, so it is quickly available when the patient needs lifting and moving assistance. If the patient slides down in bed, the HoverMatt Air Transfer System slides as well. Inflating the mattress and using the handles on the sides is all that is necessary to move the patient up in bed.

Moving the Patient: Bed Mobility

Review the guidelines for moving patients in Chapters 15 through 17 of this book. Apply the principles of good body mechanics for yourself and the patient. Lifting and moving present a high risk of injury to the patient and the nursing assistant. Bedfast patients must be turned every two hours or more often, even if a special therapeutic, low air loss, rotational, or turning mattress is used. If the patient turns themselves, check the position to ensure that they are turning often enough.

Bariatric patients who are able to move themselves tend to use their body weight to aid in movement. For example, when turning from side to side, they tug and pull on the side rail until they reach a point where only a little more effort will result in a comfortable position. In making this final turn, tubes such as a catheter, IV, or electrode monitoring wires may be pulled and the traction may result in tube removal. Make sure that all tubes are firmly secured, and monitor them for proper placement each time you are in the room.

Because the patient uses their arms for bed mobility, try to avoid devices that limit movement of the hands and arms. For example, having an IV in the left arm and an electronic blood pressure monitor on the right arm acts as a method of restraint and will restrict the patient's ability to move about in bed. Accessories such as a bed ladder will help facilitate movement. The ladder is attached to the bed frame, and the patient pulls on it to rise to an upright position. If this device is not available, tying a sheet or rope to a secure spot on the frame at the end of the bed may help.

Manual Patient Handling Devices

Many bariatric patients prefer to keep the bed in the high Fowler's position (Chapter 15), which relieves pressure on the chest and helps maximize respiratory efficiency. However, patients in this position often slip down in bed. Elevating the knee of the bed slightly will reduce strain and help prevent downward sliding. If the patient complains of back pain when the head is elevated, elevating the knee of the bed may not provide sufficient relief. A commercial knee elevator (Chapter 15) or pillows under the knees will relieve pressure on the back.

The TLC Pad (Figure 31-13) and other similar patient-handling devices can be used for moving patients up in the bed or chair, and from side to side in bed. A regular-size patient can often be moved by a single caregiver. Two to four workers may be necessary to move a bariatric patient up in bed or chair using this type of device. The handles make the job easier, and using a sturdy lifting device reduces the risk of injury.

Some bariatric beds have an adjustable length feature at the foot end, which makes slipping down in bed less of a problem than it is in a regular bed. The nurse may instruct you to position the patient's head slightly downward, in a modified Trendelenburg position (see Chapter 28), before turning and repositioning the bedfast patient. (This increases the risk of respiratory complications, so use the position only under the direction and supervision of the nurse.) A full Trendelenburg position places the head downward 60°. For this procedure, lowering the head 20° to 30° is sufficient. Using the

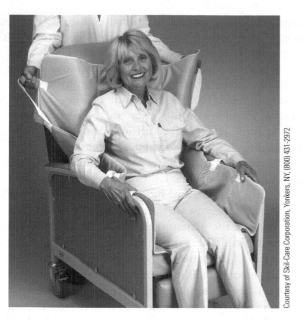

FIGURE 31-13 The TLC Pad is used for moving patients up in the bed or chair, and from side to side in bed. A regular-size patient can be moved by a single caregiver. Two to four workers may be necessary to move the bariatric patient up in a bed or chair.

Trendelenburg position when moving the patient up in bed makes the job easier and reduces the risk of injury because gravity will assist you. A Gore-Tex or nylon sheet or lifting device will also make this job easier.

> **NOTE**
>
> Always check with the nurse before using the Trendelenburg position. Avoid leaving the patient in this position for more than a few minutes.

Return the bed to the flat position as soon as possible, and then proceed with skin care and use pillows and props to support the body. Some bariatric beds have inflatable air bolsters on each side. These provide an adjunct for positioning and support, and can be inflated and deflated at will. This feature is also useful when moving the bed through narrow spaces and doorways.

Moving the patient by tugging on their body increases the risk of injury to patient and staff. If staff will be moving the patient in bed, use a lifting device made for this purpose. A draw sheet, two draw sheets, or a full-size sheet may also be used. Supporting the patient's body during positioning reduces the effects of gravity, making the move easier for both patient and staff. Four to six people may be needed to reposition a total-care patient safely. One person lifts the head. Second and third nursing assistants are positioned on each side, and a lift sheet or other device is also used. Another

nursing assistant positioned at the foot of the bed lifts the patient's heels to eliminate friction and shearing.

When the patient is on their side, you may have to support the upper leg on pillows. The extra support reduces the risk of skin problems caused by the legs rubbing together, and it prevents pressure on the bony prominence at the knee. Supporting the upper leg also does much to relieve pain in the pelvis, hip joint, and lumbar–sacral area of the spine. Unsupported, the weight of the leg exerts a downward pull on both the hip and the spine, which can be very painful.

When moving and positioning the patient, remember that maintaining good body alignment is very important. The patient's skin and extremities are heavy and will not move on their own. You will have to move their body parts manually. Some hospitals have an arrangement of slings and pulleys for moving the arms and legs (Figure 31-14). Encourage the patient to assist by pulling on the rope to which the sling is attached.

Moving the Patient: Transfers and Ambulation

Some bariatric patients can walk for short distances. Some will use a walker for support. Others use mobility scooters. Some will need help or use a mechanical device to come to a standing position (Figure 31-15), and others require assistance with transfers. The care plan will list instructions for mobilizing each patient. Some patients will be able to ambulate in their rooms with minimal assistance and support. The gait of an obese patient is

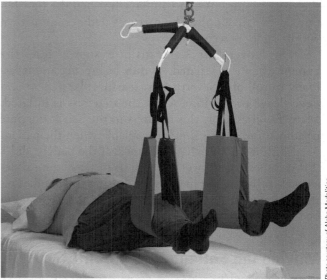

FIGURE 31-14 Various lifts, slings, and pulleys may be used to move the patient's extremities. Legs can be elevated to relieve edema and pressure from the heels by using a ceiling-mounted hoist to hold them in place.

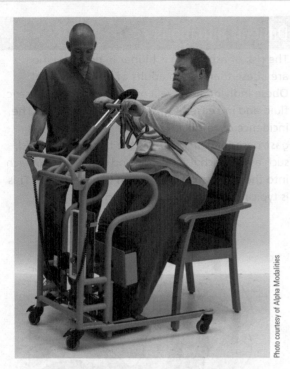

Photo courtesy of Alpha Modalities

FIGURE 31-15 Many different devices are available to make moving the patient easier for staff and less traumatic for the patient.

usually wide based, with the legs spread quite far apart. This helps the patient balance and the wide stance accommodates the width of the legs. The arms may be held out, slightly away from the body, and swing forward with each step to help propel the person forward. The patient may arch the back slightly to counterbalance the weight of the abdomen.

A long (72-inch) gait/transfer belt may be used for transfers and ambulation (Chapter 16). Ask two or three assistants to help. The transfer belt should not be used if the patient has recently had abdominal surgery or other contraindications are present (Chapter 16). Check with the nurse if you are unsure. Avoid doubling a gait belt, if possible. If a long belt is not available and you must join two regular belts, make sure to lock the buckles down securely. Position both buckles close to your hands so you can see their position. If they begin to slip, even slowly, stop the procedure.

Some hospitals use only plastic-type belts because of infection control issues. The buckles on these slip more readily, and they are not as gentle to the skin as cloth and canvas belts. Avoid connecting two plastic belts to make a single long belt. The buckles may not hold. Your hospital may furnish a 72-inch cloth or canvas belt for each bariatric patient; often it is left in the room. (The patient takes the belt home or it is discarded upon discharge.)

When using any type of gait/transfer belt with a patient who is obese, avoid placing it over bare skin.

Make sure the belt and buckle do not penetrate, rub, or cut into the skin folds, causing injury. The nurse may instruct you to apply an abdominal binder before moving the patient so that the abdomen does not interfere with safe patient handling and movement. The fatty apron of abdominal skin is called the **panniculus**. This is a dense flap of hanging fatty skin. It is usually seen in the abdomen of a person who has recently lost a significant amount of weight. Patients often like the feeling of support the binder provides.

Moving the patient is a high-risk procedure for the nursing assistant and patient alike. Whether moving the patient in bed or a chair, you will need adequate help. Five or six caregivers may be needed. In addition to being at high risk for falls, patients are at risk for skin tears and abrasions. The nursing assistants are at risk for neck, shoulder, and back injuries, as well as other musculoskeletal injuries. Injury can occur even if a mechanical device is used. Instruct the patient to push themselves to a standing position with the arms. Avoid straining or pulling on the patient to assist, especially under the arms. You will not be able to pull them up. Because of the highly individualized needs of the bariatric patient, the care plan will list instructions for moving. In many cases, a special mechanical lift is used to stand or transfer the patient.

Falls

If a standing patient starts to fall to the floor, you may instinctively try to hold them up or break the fall. Trying to do so will cause injury. Do all you can to prevent injury, but avoid trying to stabilize or brace the falling patient. For example, quickly push items out of the way that could cause injury to the patient. Try to protect the patient's head. When standing or ambulating the patient for the first time, have plenty of help. Monitor the patient for dizziness or weakness. If they experience these problems, stop the procedure and return the patient to the supine position. It is best to have a walker, an arm chair, or a wheelchair turned backward in position in front of the patient. Have one assistant on each side to hold and stabilize the device. If the patient starts to fall, they may be able to stop the fall by using the arms and holding the walker or chair.

If the patient falls to the floor, a team will be required to get them up. Several methods are used, depending on how much assistance the patient can provide. The HoverJack Air Patient Lift (Figure 31-16) operates in a manner similar to the HoverMatt Air Transfer System. The HoverJack Air Patient Lift is used to lift a patient in a supine position from the floor to bed or stretcher. In addition to using the HoverJack Air Patient Lift for bariatric patients, the device is helpful and effective for any patient who falls, especially those with fractures and

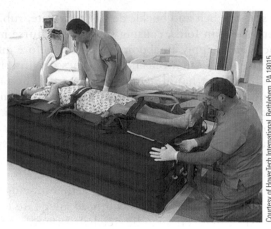

FIGURE 31-16 The HoverJack Air Patient Lift effortlessly moves the patient from the floor to a bed or stretcher. By placing the HoverMatt on top, the patient is easily transferred back to bed.

other injuries. By placing the HoverMatt Air Transfer System on top, the patient is easily lifted from the floor and transferred back to bed.

A dependent patient may be rolled onto a bariatric sling made of nylon or canvas (Figure 31-17), or a heavy blanket. The patient is lifted only enough for a team member to slide a backboard or other solid lifting device underneath. The backboard (or other device) is used for moving the patient. If the patient is able to assist, a strong chair may be positioned against their back, then turned upright, or a team can lift the patient's arms and legs while another person slides a chair under them. These are potentially dangerous maneuvers for caregivers. Do not move a patient who is obese and dependent until you have enough staff to accomplish the task, as well as proper instruction, supervision, and adaptive mobility devices.

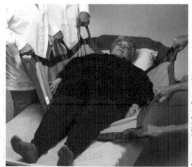

FIGURE 31-17 A patient who is dependent may be moved by rolling onto a bariatric sling made of nylon or canvas.

Difficult Situations

The risk of aspiration is higher in persons who are obese than it is in adults of normal weight. Obese individuals have a greater volume of gastric fluid and increased intra-abdominal pressure. The incidence of reflux is higher. **Reflux** (also called *gastroesophageal reflux*) is the backflow of fluid, such as stomach juices and food, from the stomach into the esophagus and mouth (Figure 31-18). This is typically the cause of heartburn.

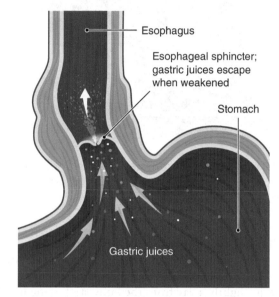

FIGURE 31-18 *Gastroesophageal reflux* (acid reflux) occurs when gastric juices and food backflow into the esophagus and mouth.

COMPLICATIONS OF IMMOBILITY

Bariatric patients are at very high risk of complications when they are immobile. Even new postoperative patients are ambulated or gotten out of bed within 24 hours after surgery, whenever possible. Because of the risk of complications, some facilities strive to ambulate the patient within 2 hours after returning to the unit from surgery, and then every 2 hours while awake. Patients who are unconscious or bedfast are at high risk of developing:

- Pneumonia
- Atelectasis
- Deep vein thrombosis (DVT; blood clots in the legs)
- Pulmonary embolism (PE; a blood clot in the lungs)
- Pressure injuries
- Yeast infections in the skin folds

TABLE 31-3 Observations to Make and Report Related to the Care of Bariatric Patients

- Skin problems, rashes, red areas in skin folds
- Open areas
- Weeping skin
- Nonhealing wounds
- Pain
- Apathy or signs of depression
- Binging, purging, and other behaviors in dietary regulation
- Excessive thirst
- Unexplained weakness
- Increased urination
- Hypoventilation (shallow breathing)
- Respiratory distress
- Unexplained hypoxia (pulse oximeter values below 90; see Chapter 39)
- Rapid respirations
- Complaint of chest pain or discomfort
- Dyspnea
- Sleep apnea
- Complaints of heartburn or esophageal reflux
- Change in leg color, sensation, swelling, or temperature
- Change in patient's ability to move legs
- Signs of fatigue, becoming quieter, lethargy, progressive sleepiness

Observations to make and report related to the care of bariatric patients are listed in Table 31-3.

BARIATRIC SURGERY

Bariatric surgery is surgery on the stomach and/or intestines to help the patient with morbid or super obesity lose weight. Many different procedures may be done, depending on patient needs and doctor preference. Surgery is used as a treatment for weight loss for persons with a body mass index greater than 40. It is sometimes used as a treatment for people with a BMI between 35 and 40 who have health problems and potentially serious comorbidities, such as heart disease or type 2 diabetes.

Patients do not suddenly wake up one day, decide to have surgery, and schedule the procedure for the following day or week. The patient's BMI is only one of many considerations. The patient must have a thorough medical workup first. Medical instabilities and comorbidities may have to be treated and stabilized. The insurer, Medicare, or Medicaid must preapprove the procedure. It is never done on young children, and is seldom done on teenagers who are still growing. A few surgical centers will do bariatric surgery on teens as young as 15 or 16, if they meet the criteria established by the professionals at the facility. To be approved for bariatric surgery, most insurers require adult patients to:

- Be committed to making eating and lifestyle changes

- Have severe obesity (BMI over 35 with one or more comorbidities *or* have a BMI of 40 or higher with or without comorbidities
- Have made numerous attempts at weight loss through diet and exercise

A person who is obese is at very high risk for complications of surgery and anesthesia. Because of this, patients may be required to lose weight by dieting before the physician will perform the operation. Due to the risks involved, most physicians set age and weight limits for the procedure, such as 18 to 60 years of age weighing no more than 500 pounds. Persons exceeding the surgeon's upper weight limit must diet by more conventional methods to meet the surgical weight criteria.

Goals and Objectives of Bariatric Surgery

Electing to have bariatric surgery is a major, life-altering decision. It is usually done after the patient has tried and failed at numerous diet and exercise programs. The physician has informed the patient that without weight loss, their life is at risk. Persons who elect to have bariatric surgery face many difficult problems and challenges. This surgery is much more than a painless, will-free approach to weight loss. As a full partner on the team, the patient makes a great investment in recovery and lifestyle changes. The surgery changes patients' lives completely. Their diet and manner of eating change forever. They must replace their clothing every few weeks as their body size decreases. When they reach their goal weight, they have an abundance of extra, stretched-out skin, which may require additional surgery. If the skin is not removed, the various fungal infections and skin problems related to friction will persist.

The goals of bariatric surgery are for the patient to achieve permanent weight loss and reduce the risk factors associated with the many comorbidities of obesity. The surgery is recognized as the only successful, permanent method for treating morbid obesity. Although some people lose weight by using nonsurgical methods, many regain the weight and often more. Few people are able to successfully maintain the weight loss achieved with diet and exercise alone.

Surgical Procedure

Bariatric surgery has been evolving since the 1950s. Some procedures are minimally invasive. A **minimally invasive surgery** is any surgical procedure that does not require a large incision. It can be done by entering the body through a small cut or incision in the skin, or through a body cavity or other anatomical opening. The surgeon uses miniature scopes and instruments to visualize and repair the organs on the inside of the body. All of the accepted bariatric surgery techniques can be done by using a minimally invasive (also called *laparoscopic*) technique. There are both advantages and disadvantages to this method. Whether to use a minimally invasive or fully invasive procedure, in which the abdomen is opened, is determined by the surgeon, based on the patient's condition and needs. The minimally invasive technique is commonly used.

Potential Complications

Patients who have minimally invasive bariatric surgery usually go home after the procedure, and can return to work and normal activities soon after surgery. However, certain risks are associated with this surgery. Some patients who anticipate immediate discharge must be admitted to the hospital because of complications. In fact, the rate of complications is higher than for other surgeries. However, living with morbid or super obesity is believed to be much more life threatening than the potential for perioperative problems.

Patients who undergo bariatric surgery have an approximately 40 percent chance of developing complications within six months. In many surgical procedures, complications occur in the immediate postoperative period, while the patient is still in the hospital, or within a few weeks of surgery. The surgeon will continue to follow the postoperative bariatric patient closely for at least a year. Because this is somewhat different from the usual postoperative course, the surgeon will look for complications if a patient has a problem any time during the first year.

Deep Vein Thrombosis

A blood clot can develop anywhere in the circulatory system, but the deep veins of the legs are most commonly affected. This condition is called deep vein thrombosis (DVT) (see Chapter 29). A DVT most commonly develops in the legs, thighs, or pelvis. The blood clot has the potential for blocking blood flow to the extremity below the level of the clot, causing a change in skin color to gray or blue. In yellow- and dark-skinned persons, the skin under the toenails will appear cyanotic. A DVT may have no signs and symptoms at all, but usually the patient will have an abnormality in one leg, but not the other. A DVT usually causes swelling and redness. The most common sign is swelling in one leg, but not the other. The area will feel tender to the touch and warmer than the same area on the other leg. The patient may have a low-grade fever; lose their appetite; and feel sick, weak, or fatigued. They may not associate these symptoms with a problem in the leg. The patient may complain of:

- Pain in the affected leg
- A heavy feeling in the leg
- Inability to use the leg normally

- Enlargement of veins about the ankle
- Edema in one leg but not the other

Pulmonary Embolus

A moving blood clot is called an *embolus* (*emboli* is plural). The embolus is usually part of another clot that has broken off, instead of a new clot formation. An embolus can block small blood vessels, such as those in the lungs. A pulmonary embolus (PE) (see Chapter 29) is a clot that travels to the lungs and becomes lodged in the small blood vessels. Pulmonary embolus is a serious, potentially life-threatening condition that is a leading cause of perioperative death. Signs and symptoms are chest pain, cyanosis, shortness of breath, rapid pulse, and coughing up blood. The presence of these symptoms is a medical emergency. Immediately call the nurse and follow their instructions.

Prevention of DVT

Common nursing measures to prevent DVT are anti-embolism hosiery, sequential compression hosiery, coughing and deep breathing, incentive spirometer, and leg exercises. Medications are usually given.

Other Complications

The most common complications (in 20% of patients) are vomiting, reflux, and diarrhea. About 10 to 12 percent of bariatric surgery patients develop problems from the surgical joining of the stomach and the intestine. Problems in this area usually involve leaking or strictures. A **stricture** is the narrowing of a passageway in the body, which is often caused by inflammation or scar tissue. This condition is also called **stenosis**. Approximately 7 percent of complications are abdominal hernias. A lower percentage of patients develop an infection or pneumonia after surgery.

Surgical Procedures

Three categories of surgical procedures are used for bariatric surgery. The category and specific type of surgical procedure selected are individualized to the patient's needs. The surgeon also makes the decision on whether to do an invasive or noninvasive procedure. The **gastric bypass** (Figure 31-19) is the most common of the six surgical techniques that are widely accepted. In this procedure, the stomach is made smaller and is connected directly to the small intestine, reducing calorie absorption. The surgeon creates a two-inch-long pouch at the top of the patient's stomach. The surgeon attaches a portion of small intestine to the stomach pouch. After the surgery, the patient can eat or drink only a small

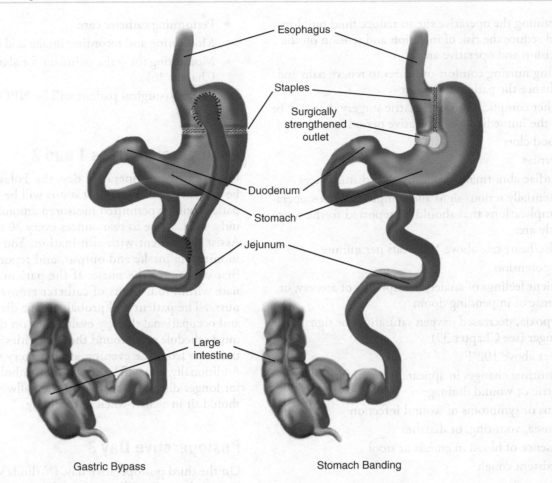

FIGURE 31-19 The gastric bypass and stomach banding are common bariatric surgeries.

amount. The food will quickly pass through the stomach and digestive tract. Because of this, fewer calories are absorbed.

Other common procedures are:

- Gastric banding—a reversible procedure in which an adjustable band is placed around the stomach to restrict food consumption
- Sleeve gastrectomy—a procedure in which the stomach is divided vertically, which reduces the space available for food intake

Revision surgeries are occasionally done for persons who have not achieved the desired weight loss.

Postoperative Care

Gastric leaks are a very serious potential complication. Leaks often occur when a staple fails. This causes the stomach contents to leak internally, creating a serious or fatal infection. *Postoperative care is targeted to reduce pressure and strain on both the internal and external staples.* For example, splinting the abdomen with a pillow during deep breathing and coughing reduces pressure on the staples. The patient may use a nasogastric (NG) tube after

surgery to reduce the strain on staples caused by vomiting. If an NG tube is present, the patient will be NPO (nothing by mouth) and will have an IV. A Foley catheter will be present that was placed during surgery. You will be expected to carefully monitor intake and output. Each bariatric surgery has procedure-specific postoperative instructions. Other postoperative care includes:

- Using the incentive spirometer and coughing and deep breathing. Teach the patient to firmly support the abdomen with pillows to reduce tension on the skin from coughing
- Applying an abdominal binder (see Chapter 29). The binder should be fastened gently and released slowly. Make sure the tape over the incision does not stick to the binder. If it does, inform the nurse. Accidentally pulling the tape off when removing the binder will cause skin damage and potentially damage the operative site
- Preventing constipation, which causes abdominal pressure. Inform the nurse if the patient complains of constipation or is straining to have a bowel movement

- Draining the operative site to reduce fluid buildup and reduce the risk of infection and tension on the incision and operative area
- Using nursing comfort measures to relieve pain and enhance the patient's comfort

Other complications of bariatric surgery that may be seen in the immediate postoperative period are:

- Blood clots
- Hernias
- Cardiac abnormalities and rhythm disturbances

Potentially serious signs and symptoms of postoperative complications that should be reported to the nurse promptly are:

- Pulse/heart rate above 100 beats per minute
- Hypotension
- Patient feelings of anxiety, complaints of anxiety, or a sense of impending doom
- Hypoxia, decreased oxygen saturation, or signs of air hunger (see Chapter 39)
- Fever above 102°F
- Abnormal changes in appearance or volume of gastric or wound drainage
- Signs or symptoms of wound infection
- Nausea, vomiting, or diarrhea
- Presence of blood in emesis or stool
- Persistent cough

Postoperative Care on the Night After Surgery

Routine postoperative care given on the evening after surgery will probably include remote telemetry monitoring. The patient may be receiving supplemental oxygen through a cannula. Procedures the nursing assistant may be responsible for include:

- Monitoring vital signs according to postoperative routine, then hourly or as instructed by the nurse
- Applying or caring for an abdominal binder
- Applying ice packs to the incision
- Checking the dressing over the incision and draining hourly, or as instructed
- Encouraging use of the incentive spirometer at least 10 times every hour
- Assisting with coughing and deep breathing
- Applying anti-embolism hosiery; performing circulation checks of feet every two to four hours
- Applying sequential compression devices, as ordered
- Getting the patient up in a chair with assistance one or more times

- Performing catheter care
- Monitoring and recording intake and output
- Monitoring the pulse oximeter for alarms (see Chapter 36)

The postsurgical patient will be NPO except for ice chips.

Postoperative Days 1 and 2

On the first postoperative day, the Foley catheter will be discontinued. The NPO status will be lifted, and the patient will be permitted measured amounts of clear liquids, such as one to two ounces every 30 to 60 minutes. Assist the patient with elimination. You will continue monitoring intake and output, and report the patient's first voiding to the nurse. If the patient does not urinate within four hours of catheter removal, inform the nurse. The patient will probably have dietary, physical, and occupational therapy evaluations on this day, so you must schedule care around these activities. Nursing assistant care from the evening after surgery will continue. Additionally, you will be assigned to ambulate the patient for longer distances, such as in the hallway. The patient should sit in a chair when not walking.

Postoperative Day 3

On the third postoperative day, IV fluids will be discontinued, but you will continue I&O monitoring. The patient's diet will advance to full liquid, low-carbohydrate items to see how they tolerate them. Stable patients are often discharged on the third day unless complications develop.

Discharge Instructions

The dietitian or registered nurse will teach the patient about the postoperative diet. The patient is instructed to advance food intake gradually every few days, as tolerated. In this case, *advancing* means adding new food items, not increasing portion size. The patient's stomach will hold only a few ounces, and overfilling it risks rupturing a staple and causing a leak. On the fifth and sixth postoperative days, the diet will advance to pureed foods, including baby foods, applesauce, and blended soft foods. The patient needs to drink frequently to prevent dehydration.

On the sixth and seventh days, the diet progresses to soft foods, including all of the pureed items taken previously, all allowed liquids, and soft foods, such as baked white fish without bones, imitation crab meat, hot dogs, canned fruits, and overcooked vegetables. Hard meats, such as steak, pork, and chicken, are not allowed. During the second and third weeks, the patient begins a regular food trial. This trial includes all items eaten previously plus red meat, chicken, and well-cooked vegetables. The patient is permitted to try only one new item at a time. By adding one new regular food per day, 14 new items will have been added by the end of this period.

ONGOING CARE AND SUPPORT

At home, the patient should be as active as possible, walking up to one mile a day by the appointment for the first postoperative office visit. The patient should continue wearing the abdominal binder when active. The patient must avoid heavy lifting until released by the physician. If a minimally invasive procedure was done, the patient should be able to return to work in a week. If an invasive procedure was done, they should plan to return to work after about six weeks. The patient must keep a food diary with exact amounts and portion sizes of everything they eat and drink for the first month after surgery. The surgeon will evaluate this record to determine whether the patient's protein intake was adequate. This is very important to prevent malnutrition.

The commitment to the bariatric surgery patient does not end when the immediate perioperative period is complete. The surgeon and others continue to follow the patient's progress. Support groups are available for preoperative and postoperative patients. These are very important to patients' long-term weight-loss success. As you can see, an effective bariatric program encompasses many aspects besides the surgical intervention. Other key components are nutritional support, psychological support, and availability of health care professionals to help with any complications the patient may experience.

The care of the bariatric patient is not technically or cognitively difficult. Nevertheless, it is physically demanding, and must be done according to directions to prevent injury to patients and staff. Paying close attention to detail and working as a member of a team are keys to successful care of bariatric patients. Bariatric surgery is a positive, health-promoting, life-sustaining intervention. Nursing assistants are essential members of the bariatric team. The care you give is vital to a quality outcome in the patients' care and quality of life. When a shapely, attractive patient returns to your unit to thank the staff, you will feel pride in yourself, your team, and your former patient that is well beyond expectation.

REVIEW

A. True/False

Mark the following true or false by circling T or F.

1. T F Approximately 25 percent of adults in the United States are overweight.

2. T F Genetics and environment affect a person's weight.

3. T F Persons with mild to moderate obesity qualify for bariatric surgery if they have one comorbidity.

4. T F Comorbidities are genetic, environmental, and other problems that cause or contribute to obesity.

5. T F Obesity places a great strain on the heart and lungs.

6. T F Bariatric patients are just larger versions of normal-size adults.

7. T F When taking the blood pressure of a bariatric patient, a large, extra-large, or thigh-size cuff may be necessary.

8. T F Bariatric patients cannot develop an eating disorder.

9. T F Wall-mounted toilets should not be used for patients who weigh more than 500 pounds.

10. T F Patients who are obese do not develop malnutrition.

B. Matching

Choose the correct phrase from Column II to match the terms in Column I.

Column I

11. _____ minimally invasive surgery
12. _____ panniculus
13. _____ ideal body weight
14. _____ advocate
15. _____ gastric bypass
16. _____ bariatrics
17. _____ overweight
18. _____ comorbidities
19. _____ reflux
20. _____ hyperventilation

Column II

a. most common bariatric surgery, in which the patient is left with a two-inch-long stomach pouch

b. diseases and conditions that are caused by or contributed to by morbid obesity

c. a condition in which a person weighs more than they should, considering their height and bone size

d. breathing abnormally fast and deep

e. surgical procedure that is done through a scope and does not require a large incision

f. mathematical formula related to life span or longevity and health

g. backflow of stomach juices and food from the stomach into the esophagus and mouth

h. field of medicine that treats obesity and diseases associated with obesity

i. a large hanging flap of abdominal skin

j. a person who speaks on behalf of the patient

C. Multiple Choice

Select the best answer for each of the following.

21. Early signs of dehydration in the bariatric patient include:

   a. fever, high blood pressure, and edema.

   b. bradycardia and increased urination.

   c. decreased urinary output and tachycardia.

   d. diarrhea, edema, and tachycardia.

22. Bariatric patients who complain of feeling hot may obtain relief from:

   a. the assistant removing the patient's clothes and top sheet, then closing the door.

   b. an electric fan that the patient can position and control.

   c. folding a newspaper to create a handheld fan.

   d. bathing in ice water.

23. One staff person should never lift or move more than:

   a. 5 pounds of body weight without extra help or a mechanical device.

   b. 35 pounds of body weight without extra help or a mechanical device.

   c. 65 pounds of body weight without extra help or a mechanical device.

   d. 90 pounds of body weight without extra help or a mechanical device.

24. When moving the bariatric patient up in bed, initially position the bed in the:

   a. Trendelenburg position.

   b. semi-Fowler's position.

   c. lithotomy position.

   d. Sims' position.

25. If a standing bariatric patient starts to fall to the floor, you should:

   a. protect the patient's head, if possible.

   b. grab the patient under the arms.

   c. hold the patient up however you can.

   d. run for extra help.

26. The goals of bariatric surgery include:

   a. removing the large abdominal panniculus.

   b. temporarily reducing the size of the stomach until the patient loses at least 100 pounds.

   c. removing extra fat by using liposuction and cutting away massive areas of skin.

   d. helping the patient achieve permanent weight loss and reduce the risks of comorbidities.

27. A minimally invasive surgery is:

   a. one in which the patient is under anesthesia for an hour or less.

   b. commonly done by using spinal anesthesia and IV sedation.

   c. done through a scope after making a small incision.

   d. done by making a large incision through which to enter the body cavity.

28. After bariatric surgery, the patient should be assisted or reminded to:

   a. cough forcefully every 15 minutes.

   b. use the incentive spirometer 10 times every 4 hours.

   c. cough and deep breathe 10 times every shift.

   d. use the incentive spirometer 10 times every hour.

29. During the evening after bariatric surgery, the patient should be:

   a. given two ounces of water every four hours.

   b. NPO except for ice chips.

   c. served a clear liquid diet.

   d. encouraged to eat to gain strength.

30. During the evening after bariatric surgery, the patient should be:

    a. kept on bed rest for at least 12 hours.

    b. ambulated in the hall at least every two hours.

    c. gotten up in the chair one or more times.

    d. given a hot water bottle for incisional pain.

31. A moving blood clot is called a(n):

    a. pulmonism.

    b. deep vein thrombosis.

    c. embolus.

    d. orifice.

32. Of the sites listed, the most common site for a DVT is the:

    a. brain.

    b. leg.

    c. arm.

    d. lung.

33. Signs and symptoms of DVT include all of these *except*:

    a. pain in the affected part.

    b. a heavy feeling in the affected part.

    c. an inability to move the affected part normally.

    d. edema on both sides of the body.

D. Nursing Assistant Challenge

You are assigned to care for Mrs. Esmerelda Gonsalves, a 31-year-old female who has been admitted to room 306 on your unit. She is scheduled for bariatric surgery tomorrow. Mrs. Gonsalves tells you that she has gradually been gaining weight since she was a child. She tells you she tried every diet she could find and nothing worked for her. She gets teary-eyed and tells you that surgery is her last hope for a normal life. Her height on admission was 68 inches and her weight was 423 pounds. This calculates to a body mass index of 64.5. Her comorbidities include type 2 diabetes, sleep apnea, osteoarthritis of the lumbar spine and knees, and symptoms of depression.

34. The thigh blood pressure cuff slips down every time you apply it, so you have not finished taking Mrs. Gonsalves's admission vital signs. There is no electronic vital signs monitor on the unit. What action will you take?

_____

_____

35. You finally get the cuff to stay on the patient's arm, so you take a manual blood pressure. Your reading is 266/178. The patient has no history of hypertension. What action will you take?

_____

_____

36. The nurse informs you that the blood pressure cuff you used is broken. You cannot find another cuff that will stay on the patient's arm without slipping. What will you do?

_____

_____

37. After putting Mrs. Gonsalves to bed, you note that she has a large abdominal panniculus. Under the panniculus, the skin is bright red, with weeping and irritation. The patient tells you this is a chronic problem, which is painful for her. Is it necessary to notify the nurse? What else should you do to help this patient?

_____

_____

38. No special preoperative orders have been written. The nurse informs you to teach the patient about the routine care you will be giving after surgery. What will you tell this patient?

_____

_____

ANSWERS TO "CRITICAL THINKING IN ACTION"

Stop and think:

- What was the black substance in Mrs. Kosmacek's umbilicus?

  – Dirt from not being washed

- Why didn't Mrs. Kosmacek notice the substance?

  – Mrs. Kosmacek was a bariatric patient. She probably could not see the umbilicus without pulling the skin or using a mirror. People usually do not do these things.

- Were Loretta's actions appropriate when she noticed a black area on the umbilicus?

  – Yes

- Is washing intact skin with chlorhexidine within the scope of nursing assistant practice?

  – Yes. This is an over-the-counter product and a task the nurse instructed the assistant to do.

She should not wash an area with a medicated product unless it is facility policy or she has been given a direct order to do so.

- Johanna instructed Loretta to "keep her eyes on" the area. What does this mean?

  – Watch it when she is on duty to make sure there are no negative changes. Check it after her days off to be sure there are no negative changes. In general, she should watch for improvement in the area. If it deteriorates, she should notify the nurse.

- If Loretta does not know what it means to "keep her eyes on" the area, how should she find out? What should she look for?

  – Loretta should ask the nurse to clarify what she means and check the care plan. She should also check the facility assignment sheet to see if anything pertains to the area.

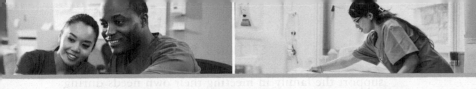
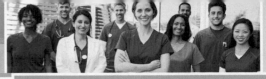

Death and Dying

CHAPTER 32

OBJECTIVES

After completing this chapter, you will be able to:

32.1 Spell and define terms.

32.2 Discuss the five stages of grief.

32.3 Describe differences in how people handle the process of death and dying.

32.4 Describe the spiritual preparations for death practiced by various religions.

32.5 State the purpose of the Patient Self-Determination Act.

32.6 Discuss Physician Orders for Life-Sustaining Treatment (POLST).

32.7 Describe the nursing assistant's responsibilities for providing supportive care.

32.8 Describe the hospice philosophy and method of care.

32.9 List the signs of approaching death.

32.10 Demonstrate the following procedure:

- Procedure 82: Giving Postmortem Care (Expand Your Skills)

VOCABULARY

Learn the meaning and the correct spelling of the following words and phrases:

acceptance
advance directive
anger
autopsy
bargaining
cardiac arrest
cardiopulmonary
  resuscitation (CPR)

critical list
denial
depression
DNR
durable power of attorney
  for health care
harvested
hospice care

life-sustaining treatment
living will
moribund
no-code order
Physician Orders for
  Life-Sustaining
  Treatment (POLST)
postmortem

postmortem care
rigor mortis
Sacrament of the Sick
supportive care
terminal

INTRODUCTION

Death is the final stage of life. It may come suddenly, without warning, or it may follow a long period of illness. It sometimes strikes the young, but it always awaits the old. Death represents the final journey in the continuum of life. As a nursing assistant, you will be providing care throughout the period of dying and into the after-death (**post-mortem**) period. Accepting the idea that death is the natural result of the life process may help you respond to your patient's needs more generously.

The concept of death and dying is handled differently by different people (Figure 32-1). There are many reactions to the diagnosis of a **terminal** (life-ending) illness:

- Some patients may have had time to prepare psychologically for their deaths. They may accept or be resigned to the inevitable.
- Some may actually look forward to relief from the pain and emotional burden of a long illness and await death calmly.
- Some may be fearful or angry and demonstrate moods that swing from outright denial to depression.
- Others may reach out, trying to verbalize feelings and thoughts of an uncertain future.
- In others, despair and anxiety may give way to moments of active hostility or periods of searching, groping questions.

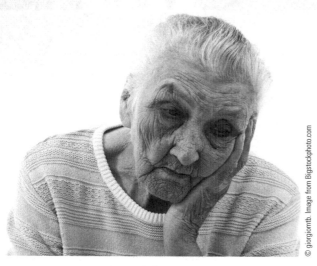

FIGURE 32-1 Each person handles death differently.

Communication **ALERT**

Health care workers may feel helpless when caring for a dying patient. Remember that active listening is a means of therapeutic communication. Listening to a patient's concerns shows honest and caring regard for the patient. Using touch can also communicate caring and acceptance. When you are at a loss for words, consider these other means of showing the patient that you care.

None of the reaction states are predictable, and no patient falls into one rigid pattern or another. You must accept each patient's behavior with understanding, interpret the patient's very real need for family support, and support the family in meeting their own needs during this adjustment period.

FIVE STAGES OF GRIEF

Dr. Elisabeth Kübler-Ross identified five stages of grief that usually occur in the dying patient: denial, anger, bargaining, depression, and acceptance (Table 32-1). If there is adequate time and support, some patients may be able to move psychologically through each stage to a point of acceptance of their illness and death.

Denial begins when the person becomes aware that they are going to die. They may not accept this information as truth, and may instead deny it. Making long-range plans that are not likely to be fulfilled may indicate that the patient is in the denial stage. Most people with a terminal illness must go through denial before they are eventually able to reach acceptance. This is a necessary and therapeutic stage. Other people should not try to convince the patient of their diagnosis or argue with the person. If denial begins to interfere with the person's adjustment, then professional counseling may be needed.

Anger comes when the patient is no longer able to deny the fact that they are going to die. The patient may blame those around them, including those who are giving care, for their illness. Added stresses, however small, are likely to upset the patient who is in the anger stage (Figure 32-2). Statements such as "It's all your fault. I should never have come to this hospital" are typical of a patient in the anger stage. Remember, if the patient expresses anger, they are angry about the diagnosis, not with you personally. Remain calm and avoid saying anything that may make them angrier. If you think the

TABLE 32-1 Emotional Responses to Dying

Stages of Grief	Response of the Nursing Assistant
Denial	Reflect the patient's statements, but try not to confirm or deny the fact that the patient is dying. **Example:** *"The lab tests can't be right—I don't have cancer." "It must have been difficult for you to learn the results of your tests."*
Anger	Understand the source of the patient's anger. Provide understanding and support. Listen. Try to meet reasonable needs and demands quickly. **Example:** *"This food is terrible—not fit to eat." "Let me see if I can find something that would appeal to you more."*
Bargaining	If it is possible to meet the patient's requests, do so. Listen attentively. **Example:** *"If only God will spare me this, I'll go to church every week." "Would you like a visit from your clergyperson?"*
Depression	Avoid clichés that dismiss the patient's depression ("It could be worse—you could be in more pain"). Be caring and supportive. Let the patient know that it is all right to be depressed. **Example:** *"There just isn't any sense in going on." "I understand you are feeling very depressed."*
Acceptance	Do not assume that because the patient has accepted death, they are unafraid, or that they do not need emotional support. Listen attentively and be supportive and caring. **Example:** *"I feel so alone." "I am here with you. Would you like to talk?"*
Releasing pain and grief	Honor the person who has died. Remember them with love. Look for meaning to transform loss and bring peace and hope to yourself and your family.

In 2019, with permission of the Kübler-Ross family, David Kessler wrote a book adding a sixth stage to the grieving process, describing how to find meaning after a loss. He notes that pain is inevitable, but suffering is optional.

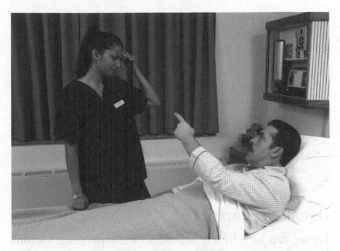

FIGURE 32-2 Patients may demonstrate feelings of frustration and anger.

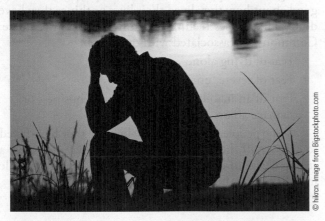

FIGURE 32-3 Depression is a normal part of the grieving process.

patient is angry about something other than the diagnosis, inform the nurse.

Bargaining is the stage in the grief process in which the patient attempts to gain more time to live. The patient may ask to be allowed to go home to finish a task before they die. Trying to make private "deals" with God or their higher power is also common. For example, "If you will let me live another two months, I promise I will try to be a better person." Bargaining frequently involves an important event that the patient has been looking forward to, such as a child's wedding or the birth of a grandchild. The patient in this stage is basically saying, "I know I'm going to die and I'm ready to die, but not just yet." This may be done in private and not stated verbally.

Depression is the fourth stage identified in the grief process. During this stage, the patient comes to a full realization that they will die soon (Figure 32-3). They are saddened by the thought that they will no longer be with family and friends, and by the fact that they may not have accomplished some goals that they had set for themselves. The patient may also express regrets

about not having gone somewhere or done something: "I always promised my wife that we would go to Europe and now we'll never go."

Acceptance is the stage during which a patient understands and accepts the fact that they are going to die (Figure 32-4). During this stage, they may try to complete unfinished business. Having accepted their eventual death, they may also try to help those around them to deal with it, especially family members.

Not all patients progress through these stages in sequential order. Nor does movement from one stage to the next mean that the previous stage will be completely left behind. Patients sometimes move back and forth between stages several times before completely resolving one stage and moving on to the next. The staff must be aware of the possible psychological positions and be able to identify the patient's current reactions. For example, a patient who displays anger one day may be full of optimism and denial the next.

Communication ALERT

The grieving process begins immediately when someone is diagnosed with a life-threatening or terminal illness. Mourning before someone dies is called *anticipatory grief*. Part of this process involves grieving for past, present, and future losses. Patients and families grieve for their former way of life, recognizing that returning to it will be impossible. Roles and responsibilities within the family change. Illness may change the patient's body image. Friends and family may begin to separate themselves from the dying person. This is one way they deal with loss, but it may make the patient feel isolated. Losses are many. Some are very private and personal. Each loss triggers the grieving process, causing feelings of isolation, abandonment, anger, and depression.

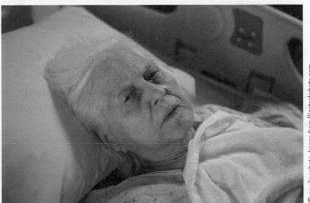

FIGURE 32-4 A patient may understand that the end of life is near and calmly wait for death.

Denial frequently comes first, followed by anger and despair. Frustrated by feelings of helplessness, the person lashes out at those who are nearby. If each of these stages is expressed with some degree of success, the person is then able to move on to a level of grieving, for themselves and for loved ones. When all five stages have been passed, it is believed that the patient is better able to accept the termination of life. If there is adequate time and support, many patients can be helped to reach a more accepting frame of mind.

The family and staff move through these same stages, but not necessarily at the same time. It is particularly difficult when the patient is at one stage and the family is at another stage.

Some experts believe that grief triggers the fight-or-flight mechanism, similar to when someone is chasing you. It causes the body to be in a state of alarm. These experts believe that some grieving people will not eat because the body is prioritizing survival. This is one of the reasons that postfuneral meals are part of the death ritual in many cultures. Providing food for the surviving family is a means of offering emotional support. The belief is that survivors need nourishment to replace the nutrients that have been depleted by caregiving and bereavement.

PREPARATION FOR DEATH

The knowledge of impending death comes to the patient directly from the physician or indirectly from the staff. A diagnosis of terminal illness is very difficult to conceal from the patient. The staff may, without realizing it, reveal the information by:

- Exhibiting false cheerfulness
- Being evasive
- Making fewer visits to the patient's room
- Spending less time with the patient

You must realize that most patients who are terminally ill do eventually come to accept that death is part of their near future. Keep the following in mind:

- Each patient reacts to this understanding in a unique way.
- How many feelings the patient wishes to share and with whom are very personal decisions.
- You should be available to listen, but do not force the issue.

Upon being told of the terminal diagnosis, the patient may proceed through several stages of emotional adjustment. Initially, the:

- Patient may react to the situation by denying the truth.
- Patient may refuse all opportunities to discuss their illness with the staff or with family.

- Patient may request private meetings with the person designated as the durable power of attorney healthcare. The patient may modify or add a living will.
- Patient may review and/or modify banking, insurance, and life insurance records.
- Patient's interpersonal relationships with family and staff may become greatly strained.
- Patient may become defeated and full of despair, actively expressing a loss of hope.

Common Fears

Dying can be a lonely business. We experience various losses throughout life, but when a person is dying, they are losing everything—family, friends, pets, and belongings. It is natural to be afraid of the unknown, regardless of religious and spiritual beliefs. Some people do not feel good about how they lived their lives or things they have done. This causes feelings of guilt, grief, and remorse. Common fears associated with dying are:

- Fear of dying alone
- Fear of severe, unrelieved pain
- Fear of an inability to finish personal business or manage affairs

Some people feel incomplete because they have failed to achieve all they wanted to do. They may also have a strong desire to do something that is no longer possible in light of their imminent death.

Reactions of Others

In a long-term care facility or other residential setting, other residents and staff will also be upset about a terminal diagnosis or death of a resident. The age group in long-term care experiences many losses of friends and family to death. Each loss reminds residents that they are in the twilight years at the end of life. They must also cope with their own pain and grief. The nursing assistant will provide support and help others cope. In the residential care setting, others will:

- Be sad and grieve the loss of a good friend
- Reminisce about the person who died
- Want to know how the person died (if they were alone, in pain, etc.)

Encourage others to express their feelings and talk about their sadness, loss, anger, and fear. This helps the grieving person come to grips with their own feelings. Be honest and answer questions as completely as possible, without violating confidentiality.

THE PATIENT SELF-DETERMINATION ACT

The Patient Self-Determination Act of 1990 requires health care providers to supply written information about state laws regarding advance directives. An **advance directive** is a document that is put into effect if the patient later becomes unable to make decisions. All health care providers, including hospitals, long-term care facilities, and home health care agencies, must have policies and procedures covering these issues. The patient must be informed of the right to execute an advance directive before or at the time of admission. The patient may choose to execute an advance directive at any time during the stay. Likewise, the patient may choose not to execute an advance directive.

Decisions often must be made when a patient is terminally or critically ill. These decisions involve provision of supportive care or life-sustaining treatment. The Patient Self-Determination Act was passed to assure patients and their families that their wishes will be followed. **Supportive care** means that the patient's life will not be artificially prolonged but that the patient will be kept comfortable physically, mentally, and emotionally. Supportive care includes:

- Oxygen to ease breathing if the patient needs it
- Food and fluids that the patient can consume by mouth
- Medications for pain, nausea, anxiety, or other physical or emotional discomforts
- The continuation of physical care such as grooming and hygiene, cleanliness, positioning, and range-of-motion exercises
- Staff's caring and emotional support

All patients deserve supportive care, but for patients who are terminally or critically ill, supportive care means the absence of life-sustaining treatment. **Life-sustaining treatment** means giving medications and treatments for the purpose of maintaining life (Figure 32-5). Life-sustaining treatments include all of the items listed under supportive care and may also include:

- Being placed on a ventilator to maintain breathing
- Receiving **cardiopulmonary resuscitation (CPR)** if **cardiac arrest** occurs (the heart and lungs stop functioning)
- Artificial nutrition through a feeding tube or hyper-alimentation device
- Blood transfusions
- Surgery
- Radiation therapy
- Chemotherapy
- Other treatments that will maintain life

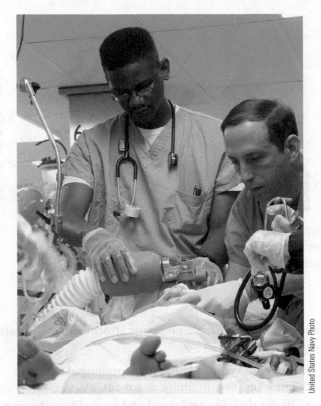

United States Navy Photo

FIGURE 32-5 Emergency care includes sustaining life with machines and drugs.

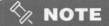

NOTE

Radiation therapy and chemotherapy may also be given to relieve pain, not to extend life.

There are basically two types of advance directives: the living will and the durable power of attorney for health care. A **living will** is a request that death not be artificially postponed if the patient has an incurable, irreversible injury, disease, or illness that the physician judges to be a terminal condition. A living will must be witnessed by two other individuals who do not stand to benefit because of the person's death.

A **durable power of attorney for health care** is a directive that assigns someone else the responsibility for making medical decisions for the patient if the patient becomes unable to do so themselves. In most states it must be signed by the *agent* (the person given the durable power of attorney) and by the *principal* (the person appointing the agent). The person designated as the agent may also be called the *proxy* or *health care proxy*. This document also must be signed by one or more adult

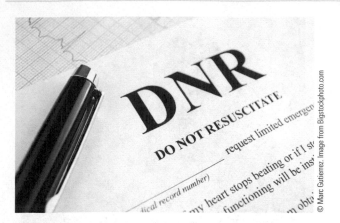

FIGURE 32-6 When a DNR order is written, no extraordinary measures are taken to save the patient's life.

witnesses. The durable power of attorney may indicate whether the person:

- Does not want their life to be prolonged and does not want life-sustaining treatment
- Wants their life prolonged and wants life-sustaining treatment to be provided unless the physician believes they are in an irreversible coma
- Wants their life to be prolonged to the greatest extent possible without regard to their condition

A durable power of attorney is one way to ensure that the wishes and rights of an individual will be followed and protected when the person is no longer able to make decisions. The health care proxy must make decisions in keeping with the patient's wishes. As a nursing assistant, you must be aware of the patient's status for supportive care or life-sustaining treatment. The person on supportive care will have a **no-code order** or **DNR** (do not resuscitate) order. This means that no extraordinary means, such as CPR to resuscitate the person, will be used to prevent death (Figure 32-6). This allows a person to die peacefully with maximum dignity. A no-code decision is reached after discussion by the patient with their family and physician. Once made, the no-code decision is entered in the patient's chart. All staff members are made aware of the decision, but it is kept confidential. If the patient changes their mind, the order in the chart is changed.

Witnessing Advance Directives

The nursing assistant must become familiar with facility policies and state laws for witnessing advance directives. In many states, persons who care for the patient are not permitted to witness advance directives. In most states, caregivers cannot legally be appointed to be the agent (medical decision maker) for a patient unless they are related by blood or marriage.

Withdrawing or Modifying Advance Directives

Patients may withdraw or modify their advance directives at any time. For example, a patient's advance directive states that they wants full life support if their heart and breathing stop. The patient later finds out that they have cancer, and wants only supportive care at the end of life. If a patient informs you of changes that affect the advance directive, notify the nurse promptly.

Legal ALERT

Note that both patients in the following examples are at the hospital to have procedures done. Please assume that both have valid living wills specifying no heroic measures. Neither patient has a DNR order.

Health care workers sometimes become confused about the meaning of a living will in which the patient specifies that no heroic procedures are to be undertaken if the patient is in a terminal, irreversible condition. If the patient is not known to be in a terminal condition, resuscitation will be done. For example, a 32-year-old patient in good health enters the hospital for a diagnostic procedure that involves the injection of contrast material into the veins. The patient has an allergic reaction to the contrast material and suffers a cardiac arrest. In this case, *CPR would be done*, because the patient is not known to be in a terminal condition.

In another instance, an elderly patient enters the hospital for insertion of a central intravenous catheter to be used for pain management as part of terminal care for cancer. The patient is known to have inoperable cancer, as documented by two or more physicians. The patient experiences a complication during the procedure and has a cardiac arrest. In this case, the provisions of the living will would be observed, and *CPR would not be done*. In some hospitals, CPR would be done on this patient unless a signed DNR order is in the chart. Become familiar with your facility's policies for situations such as this.

The person designated as the agent in a durable power of attorney for health care should be familiar with the patient's wishes. The authority for making decisions takes effect only if the patient becomes physically or mentally unable to speak for themselves. If the patient subsequently regains the ability to make decisions, the power of attorney and the agent's power are inactivated. Your facility will have a procedure for securing another person, usually a relative, to make decisions on the patient's behalf if they have not designated a durable power of attorney for health care. The durable power of attorney for health care covers only health care decisions, and only for the period of time during which the patient is unable to make decisions. It does not cover management of finances or other areas of the patient's life.

Legal ALERT

Your facility may have designations for different levels of emergency care, ranging from comfort care to full advanced life support. Become familiar with the criteria for these levels. Many facilities have ethics committees made up of professionals from many disciplines. The committee meets to review some difficult care situations.

PHYSICIAN ORDERS FOR LIFE-SUSTAINING TREATMENT

Physician Orders for Life-Sustaining Treatment (POLST) is a standardized medical order form that specifies the types of life-sustaining treatment a seriously ill patient does or does not want. Once the POLST is signed by the patient and physician, it becomes part of the medical orders. It is transferred with the patient from one health care setting to the next. POLST is a valid medical order that can be used immediately, whenever needed. This differs from an advance directive, which states the patient's wishes, but requires additional physician orders in each different care setting. The advance directive is not actionable without these orders.

THE ROLE OF THE NURSING ASSISTANT

As a nursing assistant, you spend much time with the patient. You have a unique opportunity to be a source of strength and comfort. You must behave in a way that instills confidence in both the patient and the patient's family. Developing the proper attitude and approach for this type of situation is not easy. It will come with experience. There are some things to keep in mind:

- Your response should be consistent. It should be guided by the patient's attitude and the care plan.
- You must be open and receptive, because the terminal patient's attitude may change from day to day.
- Make sure you inform the nurse of incidents related to the patient that reflect moods and needs.
- Remember that each person's idea of death and the hereafter differs. You must be open to patients' ideas and not force your own upon them.
- Your own feelings about death and dying influence your ability to care for the dying patient. Honestly explore your feelings by talking about them with others until you can resolve any conflicts you may have. Your acceptance of death as a natural occurrence will enable you to meet patient needs in a realistic manner.

- Give your best and most careful nursing care, with special attention to comfort measures such as mouth care and fluid intake.
- You should be quietly empathetic and carry out your duties in a calm, efficient way.

Culture ALERT

The medical system and views about death and dying in the United States are based on Western values, which often differ greatly from those of other cultures. Cultural beliefs and values run deep and usually cannot be changed. People from other cultures have many views about care of the dying person. Many believe the family should care for the patient. Some cultures maintain that the patient should die at home, believing the spirit remains at the place of death and is comforted by the grieving of loved ones. Some cultures do not want life-saving measures. They may not want the family told of the terminal nature of their illness, but want to be told themselves. With some, this is to ensure that their financial affairs are in order. Some want the family close, but may prefer that someone other than family take care of them. Others are often concerned with dying a dignified death. Some people want to be buried in the ground within 24 hours of death. Some want to be involved; others do not.

When a patient's condition is critical, the physician will place the patient's name on the official **critical list**. Then the family and the chaplain will be notified.

Providing for Spiritual Needs

Many people find spiritual faith to be a source of great comfort during difficult times.

- Some religions have specific rituals that are carried out when a person is very ill or dying (see Table 32-2). Your role is to cooperate with the patient, family, and clergyperson so that these rituals may be performed in a dignified, caring manner (Figure 32-7A).
- When a Catholic patient is ill, a priest may be called for the **Sacrament of the Sick** (Figure 32-7B). It is preferable that the family be present and leave the room only while the confession is heard. Practicing Catholics and their families consider it a privilege to have the opportunity for confession. Many patients recover completely, but this hope should not prevent reception of this sacrament if this is the patient's wish.

TABLE 32-2 Beliefs and Practices Related to Dying and Death for Major Religions

Religion	Autopsy	Organ Donation	Beliefs and Practices
Judaism (Orthodox)	Only in special circumstances	With consultation of rabbi	• Visits to the dying are a religious duty. • Witness must be present if death occurs, to protect family and commit soul to God. • Torah and Psalms may be read and prayers recited. • Conversation is kept to a minimum. • Someone should be with the body after death until burial, usually within 24 hours. • Body must not be touched 8 to 30 minutes after death. • Medical personnel should not touch or wash body unless death occurs on Jewish Sabbath; then care may be given by staff wearing gloves. • Water is removed from the room. • Mirrors may be covered at family's request. • Jewish practices and beliefs can be very different from family to family. Asking the patient or family members about their practices is probably best. Asking is not offensive, and shows that you care about and respect the patient's and family's wishes.
Hinduism	Permitted	Permitted	• Priest ties thread around neck or wrist of deceased and pours water in the mouth. • Only family and friends touch body.
Buddhism	Personal preference	Permitted	• Buddhist priest is present at death. • Last rites are chanted at the bedside.
Islam (Muslim)	Only for medical or legal reasons	Not permitted	• Before death, read Koran and pray. • Patient confesses sins and asks forgiveness of family. • Only family touches or washes body. • After death, turn the head towards the right shoulder.
Roman Catholic	Permitted	Permitted	• Sacrament of the Sick administered to ill patients, to patients in imminent danger, or shortly after death.
Christian Scientist	Unlikely	Not permitted	• No ritual is performed before or after death.
Church of Christ	Permitted	Permitted	• No ritual is performed before or after death.
Jehovah's Witness	Only if required by law	Not permitted	• No ritual is performed before or after death.
Baptist	Permitted	Permitted	• Clergy ministers through counseling and prayers.
Episcopalian	Permitted	Permitted	• Last rites are optional.
Lutheran	Permitted	Permitted	• Last rites are optional.
Eastern Orthodox Christian	Not encouraged	Not encouraged	• Last rites are mandatory and are given by ordained priest.

• Other religions do not have specific practices, but patients of those religions may spend time in prayer (Figure 32-7C). Allow the patient and family privacy, but let them know you are close by if you are needed.

• Some patients may have no formal religious affiliation. This does not mean they do not have spiritual needs. They may request the services of a clergyperson and not know who to call on. Relay this request to the nurse, because most health care facilities have chaplains to provide these services.

• Some patients do not believe in any higher spiritual being. This is their right and no one should try to change their minds.

• Always respect the beliefs or nonbeliefs of any patient. Treat all religious items, such as holy books, medals, and rosaries, with respect.

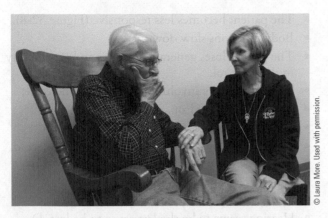

FIGURE 32-7A A pastor may be contacted to provide prayer and support. Provide privacy but be available if needed.

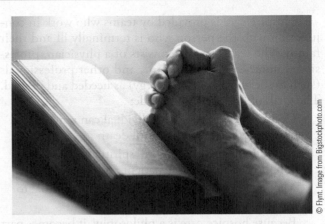

FIGURE 32-7C Personal religious practices are very comforting.

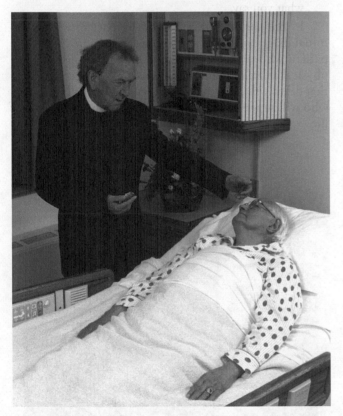

FIGURE 32-7B The Sacrament of the Sick may be administered to Roman Catholics who are gravely ill.

- Spiritual reading of the patient's faith, if requested, may be of some spiritual help through this crisis. Be courteous and provide privacy when the patient's clergyperson visits.

Be aware that dying is a lonely business, a journey each person must finish alone. Until the final moment comes, privacy, but not total solitude, should be the guiding rule.

It is important to remember the family and other loved ones when a patient is dying. Check the policies of your health care facility and assist in the following actions:

- Allow the family to be with the patient as they desire.
- Allow the family to assist with some of the care, if they wish to do so and the patient does not object; for example, moistening the patient's lips or giving a backrub.
- Inform the family where they can get a cup of coffee or a meal.
- Show the family where they can use their phones in private.
- If a family member stays during the night, offer a pillow and blanket. Some facilities provide recliners or cots for family members.
- Avoid being judgmental of family members. Remember that each person grieves in their own way. The emotions that others see are not necessarily an accurate indication of what the individual is feeling.

HOSPICE CARE

Hospice care has evolved around the philosophy that death is a natural process that should neither be hastened nor delayed and that the dying person should be kept comfortable. **Hospice care:**

- Is provided to people who are terminally ill with a life expectancy of six months or less
- Is provided in special hospice facilities, hospitals, long-term care facilities, and patients' homes
- Involves direct physical care when needed
- Is largely carried out by a home health assistant or a nursing assistant under the direction of professional health care providers
- Supports both the family and the patient
- Offers follow-up bereavement counseling to help survivors accept the death of a loved one
- Is a program in which volunteers play an important role, making regular personal visits to the patient and family

Hospice care is provided by teams who work in conjunction with the person who is terminally ill and their family. The team usually consists of a physician, professional nurse, nursing assistant, and other professionals (such as social workers and clergy) as needed and desired. The goals of hospice care include:

- Controlling pain so the individual can remain an active participant in life until death
- Coordinating psychological, spiritual, and social support services for the patient and the family
- Making legal and financial counseling available to the patient and family

Because hospice care is a philosophy, it becomes part of the guide for your actions when caring for the terminally ill. Hospice care is provided as you give your usual care. There are some things to keep in mind, however:

- Report pain immediately and give close attention to comfort measures.
- Encourage the patient to carry out as much self-care as possible.
- Be readily available to listen. Spend as much time with the patient as possible and desired by the patient.
- Get to know the family and be supportive of them.
- Give the same care you would if a terminal diagnosis had not been made.
- Carry out all activities with dignity and respect.

Sometimes hospice care may seem to go against everything you have been taught. For example, a patient has bone cancer that is very painful. The patient is expected to die within a few days. Pain management may involve the use of oral, intramuscular, or intravenous drug therapy. Despite high doses of drugs, nurses are having trouble controlling the pain. Moving the patient worsens the pain, so the care plan instructs you to leave the patient on their back, rather than turning them every two hours. You know the patient has skin breakdown that will worsen if they are not turned. However, you must follow the care plan and *not turn* the patient. This shows respect for the patient's needs and supports the quality of their final hours of life. It is not within the nursing assistant's scope of practice to advise patients or families regarding the treatment being given. Refer all questions to the nurse.

You will find additional information on hospice care and nursing assistant certification through the National Association for Home Care and Hospice (NAHC). See also Chapter 35.

PHYSICAL CHANGES AS DEATH APPROACHES

As death approaches, there are notable physical changes. As these changes occur, report them immediately to the nurse.

- The patient becomes less responsive (Figure 32-8).
- Body functions slow down.
- The patient loses general voluntary and involuntary muscle control.
- The patient may involuntarily void and defecate.
- The jaw tends to drop.
- Breathing becomes irregular and shallow.
- Circulation slows and the extremities become cold. The pulse becomes rapid and progressively weaker.
- Skin pales.
- The eyes stare and do not respond to light.
- Hearing seems to be the last sense to be lost. Do not assume that because death is approaching, the patient can no longer hear. You must be careful what you say.

In the period before death, the patient with a terminal diagnosis needs and receives the same care as the patient who is expected to recover. Attention is paid to physical as well as emotional needs. As it becomes clear that death will occur very soon, you should call the nurse, who will supervise the care during the final moments of life.

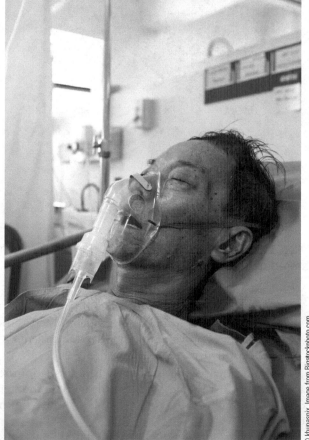

FIGURE 32-8 Dying is a lonely, solitary event.

Signs of Death

After death, changes continue to take place in the body. These changes are called **moribund** (dying) changes.

- Pupils become permanently dilated.
- There is no pulse or respiration.
- Heat is gradually lost from the body.
- The patient may urinate, defecate, or release flatus.
- Blood pools in the lowest areas of the body, giving a purplish discoloration to those areas.
- Within 2 to 4 hours, body rigidity, called **rigor mortis**, develops.
- Unless embalmed within 24 hours, there is indication of progressive protein breakdown.
- When circulation stops, the body begins to pull blood into the lowest areas of the body. This process can begin within 20 minutes of death. Over time, this will result in a stained appearance on the back of the body if the patient is in the supine position. To reduce the risk of staining about the head and neck, elevate the head of the bed 30°, in the semi-Fowler's position. Some facilities do not use ties in the morgue pack to position the body. Follow your facility's policies. If used, tie them loosely. If the ties are too tight, they may also cause permanent marks on the body.

POSTMORTEM CARE

The patient's body should be treated with respect at all times. After death occurs, the limbs should be straightened and the head elevated on a pillow. The body should be cleaned by gently washing it with warm water. Discharges must be washed off and wiped away.

Care of the body after death is called **postmortem care** (Figure 32-9). This may be your responsibility. You may find it easier if you ask a coworker to assist.

- Use gloves when giving postmortem care. The body may continue to be infectious following death. Because of this, funeral directors are entitled to information they seek about the patient's medical condition. Information is not withheld because of HIPAA rules.
- Treat the body with the same dignity you would a living person.
- Some facilities prefer to have the patient left alone until mortuary staff arrives. Your responsibility will be only to prepare the body for viewing by the family.
- Check your facility's procedure manual before proceeding with postmortem care.

The contents of morgue kits vary (Figure 32-10), but they usually include:

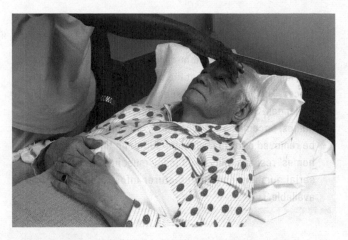

FIGURE 32-9 Postmortem care is given after death occurs.

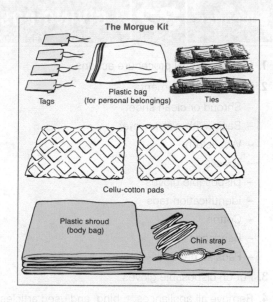

FIGURE 32-10 Supplies needed for postmortem care.

- A shroud of some kind (paper or cloth)
- A clean gown
- Tags used to identify the body
- Gauze squares for padding
- Safety pins

One procedure for postmortem care is described in Procedure 82.

ORGAN DONATIONS

Some people desire to share their organs with others after death. They use an organ donor card or designation that is part of the driver's license. The card specifies if particular organs or the whole body is being donated. At times,

Clinical Information **ALERT**

Patients with implanted medical devices are given special identification cards at the time the device is surgically placed. The body may need special preparation if cremation is planned. Some older artificial joints, implanted medication pumps, pacemakers, defibrillators, and other devices must be removed prior to cremation. Although this is the funeral homes' responsibility, the facility must inform them of any serial numbers and manufacturer information they have available.

because of a special need, the patient's family is asked for permission so that certain body organs may be removed and saved or removed and **harvested** (reused). Such a request is made by the physician or the nurse, never by the nursing assistant.

If the patient or family inform you of their wishes related to organ donation, notify the nurse promptly.

EXPAND YOUR SKILLS

PROCEDURE **82** GIVING POSTMORTEM CARE

1. Carry out initial procedure actions.

2. Assemble equipment:
   - Shroud or clean sheet
   - Basin with warm water
   - Washcloth
   - Towels
   - Disposable gloves
   - Identification tags
   - Cotton
   - Bandages
   - Pads as needed

3. Put on disposable gloves.

4. Remove all appliances, tubing, and used articles, if instructed to do so.

5. Work quickly and quietly; maintain an attitude of respect.

6. With the bed flat, place the body on the back, with head and shoulders elevated on a pillow.

   a. Close the eyes by grasping the eyelashes, gently pulling the eyelids down, and holding shut for a few seconds.

   b. Replace dentures in the patient's mouth, if used, or clean the dentures and place them in a denture cup. Make sure they are sent to the funeral home with the body. Replace an artificial eye, if used.

   c. Secure the jaw with a chin strap or light bandaging.

   d. Pad beneath the bandage. Handle the body gently, as tight bandaging or undue pressure from your hands may leave marks.

   e. Straighten the arms and legs and place the arms at the sides.

7. Bathe as necessary. Remove any soiled dressings and replace with clean ones. Groom hair.

8. Place a disposable pad underneath the buttocks. **If the family is to view the body:**

   a. Put a clean hospital gown on the patient.

   b. Cover the body to the shoulders with a sheet.

   c. Remove disposable gloves and wash your hands.

   d. Make sure the room is neat.

   e. Adjust the lights to a subdued level.

   f. Provide chairs for the family.

   g. Allow the family to visit in private.

9. Return to the patient's room after the family leaves. Wash your hands and put on disposable gloves.

10. Collect all belongings and make a list. Wrap them properly and label them. Valuables remain in the hospital safe until they are signed for by a relative.

11. Fill out the identification cards or tags in the morgue kit and attach them as follows:

    a. Place one card on the right ankle or right great toe.

    b. Attach one card to the bag with the patient's valuables.

12. Put the shroud on the patient and attach an identification card or tag to the outside.

13. Transport the body to the morgue.

    a. Call an elevator to the floor and keep it empty.

(continues)

PROCEDURE 82 CONTINUED

b. Close patient corridor doors.

c. Empty the corridor.

d. With an assistant, place the body on a gurney.

e. Keep the patient supine, with a rubber head elevator under the neck.

f. Cover the body with a sheet.

g. Remove disposable gloves and discard according to facility policy. Wash your hands.

h. Take the body to the morgue, if this is facility policy. Many facilities leave the body in the room until the funeral home arrives.

i. Attach one identification card or tag to the morgue compartment.

ICON KEY:

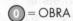 = OBRA   = PPE

POSTMORTEM EXAMINATION (AUTOPSY)

In certain situations, the law requires a medical postmortem examination or **autopsy** of the body. At other times, the family and physician may desire such an examination to understand the reasons for the patient's death. It is possible that information learned from the examination can be used to protect other family members. As in the case of organ donations, however, requesting family permission for an autopsy is not part of the nursing assistant's responsibilities. The nursing assistant is responsible for being supportive of the family and the decisions that have been made.

REVIEW

A. True/False

Mark the following true or false by circling T or F.

1. T F   All people respond to a terminal diagnosis in the same way.

2. T F   Hearing is the first sense to be lost in the dying patient.

3. T F   Death is the final stage of life.

4. T F   The nursing assistant should call the physician when the patient dies.

5. T F   Sometimes the staff unintentionally allow others to learn of a terminal diagnosis through their behavior.

6. T F   The dying patient receives the same complete care that would be given to someone who is expected to recover.

7. T F   Pain relief is one of the main goals of hospice care.

8. T F   Permanent dilation of the pupils is a moribund sign.

9. T F   Hospice-type care is only possible in the acute care facility.

10. T F   The dying person needs a great deal of understanding and realistic support.

B. Matching

Choose the correct word from Column II to match each phrase or statement in Column I.

Column I

11. _____ refusal to accept reality

12. _____ after death

13. _____ covering for the body after death

14. _____ stiffening of the body after death

15. _____ dying

Column II

a. moribund

b. rigor mortis

c. denial

d. hospice

e. postmortem

f. shroud

g. anger

C. Multiple Choice

Select the best answer for each of the following.

16. Organs from a dead person may be:

a. harvested without permission.

b. obtained on an as-needed basis.

c. donated with permission of the family at the time of death.

d. donated only if listed in the patient's will.

17. Postmortem examinations:

a. are not done in hospitals.

b. may provide valuable information.

c. are arranged by the nursing assistant.

d. are forbidden by law.

18. As death approaches, changes include:

a. constriction of the pupils.

b. muscle spasms.

c. slowing of circulation.

d. skin developing a yellow hue.

19. Moribund changes include:

a. permanent pupil constriction.

b. increased body heat.

c. increased pulse and respirations.

d. blood pooling in the lower body.

20. A no-code order in a patient's chart means:

a. start CPR immediately.

b. do not resuscitate.

c. begin postmortem care at once.

d. call the family if the patient seems in danger of dying.

21. POLST is:

a. a DNR order.

b. a legal medical order.

c. a power of attorney.

d. not a legal document.

D. Nursing Assistant Challenge

Mrs. Goldstein is a patient in the hospital where you work. She was diagnosed with cancer of the ovaries two years ago. She has been at home but is admitted periodically for chemotherapy. You have taken care of her each time she has been in the hospital. The first time was right after Mrs. Goldstein was diagnosed. She seemed happy and made frequent comments like, "I'm glad I don't have cancer." The last time she was a patient, she refused to follow the suggestions of the nursing staff, but did allow her chemotherapy to be administered. When her family visited, she was irritated and hostile toward them. This time, she is agreeable with the staff on all matters and seems genuinely happy to see her family. She has told you that if she can live to see her granddaughter get married in two months, she will become a volunteer at the hospital so she can help other patients. She is not receiving chemotherapy anymore because the cancer is in an advanced stage. She is hospitalized for pain management now but plans to go home for hospice care. Consider these questions about Mrs. Goldstein.

22. Do you think she is preparing for her death?

_____

_____

23. How would you describe the stages of dying she has been experiencing?

_____

_____

24. What response is appropriate to her comments about the wedding?

_____

_____

25. Do you think hospice care will benefit Mrs. Goldstein? Give reasons for your answer.

_____

_____

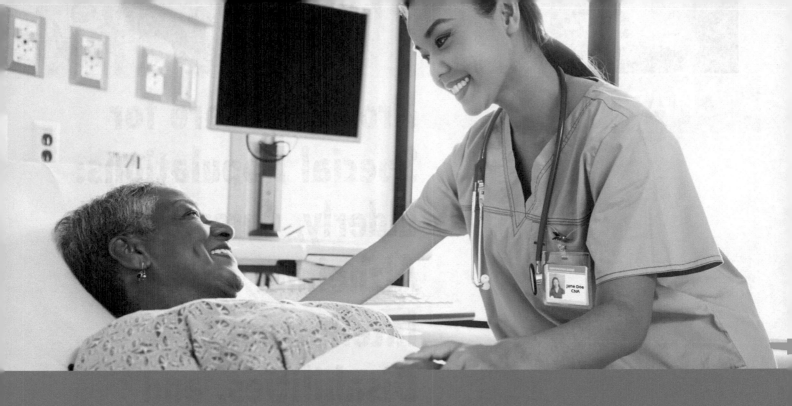

SECTION 10
Other Health Care Settings

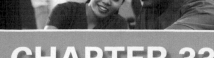

Providing Care for Special Populations: Elderly, Chronically Ill, Alzheimer Disease, Intellectual Disabilities, and Developmental Disabilities

OBJECTIVES

After completing this chapter, you will be able to:

33.1 Spell and define terms.

33.2 Describe the services provided by the various types of long-term care facilities.

33.3 Discuss how culture change is transforming long-term care services.

33.4 Identify the expected changes of aging.

33.5 Identify residents who are at risk for malnutrition and dehydration.

33.6 List measures to promote sufficient intake.

33.7 Discuss how to meet the hygiene and grooming needs of long-term care residents.

33.8 Give an overview of at least eight diseases that cause dementia.

33.9 Briefly describe each of the three main stages of Alzheimer disease

33.10 Explain how delirium differs from dementia.

33.11 List potential signs and symptoms of delirium to report.

33.12 Describe the nursing assistant's care for persons with cognitive impairment, disorientation, dementia, and wandering.

33.13 State the purpose of animal-assisted therapy, music therapy, reality orientation, reminiscing, and validation therapy.

33.14 List three criteria that must be present for a developmental disability diagnosis.

33.15 Define intellectual disability.

33.16 Discuss the care of persons with intellectual and other common developmental disabilities.

33.17 State the difference between a congenital developmental disability and an acquired developmental disability, and give examples of each.

33.18 Describe the nursing assistant's care and communication guidelines for persons with developmental disabilities.

VOCABULARY

Learn the meaning and the correct spelling of the following words and phrases:

acquired	debilitating	eloping	pigmentation
Alzheimer disease	delirium	flatulence	reality orientation
animal-assisted therapy	delusion	hand-over-hand technique	rectal prolapse
assisted living facility (ALF)	dementia	intellectual disability (ID)	reminiscing
autism	developmental disability (DD)	intermediate care facility (ICF)	respite care
catastrophic reaction	disorientation	long-term care (LTC)	skilled nursing facility (SNF)
cerebral palsy (CP)	diverticula	morbidity	sundowning
chronologic	diverticulitis	mortality	validation therapy
congenital	diverticulosis	music therapy	
culture change	Down syndrome	pica	

⊹ Clinical Information **ALERT**

Two people in the world celebrate their 60th birthday every second. Japan has the highest concentration of people age 60 and older. Forty-seven percent of males and twenty-four percent of females over age 60 are still in the workforce. Sixty-five percent of people over age 60 live in less developed countries. In some countries, more than 90 percent of people over age 60 continue to work. Harlan David Sanders (Colonel Sanders) founded Kentucky Fried Chicken at the age of 65.

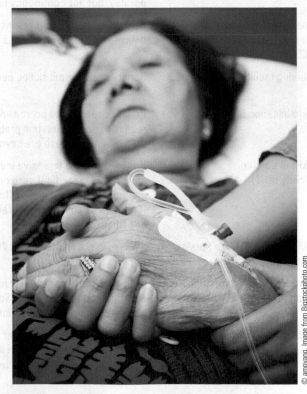

FIGURE 33-1 People of all ages need continuing health care, but most of those in the long-term care facility are elderly.

INTRODUCTION

Many individuals require continuing health care (Figure 33-1). Most of these are elderly. As people age, their risk of acquiring a chronic disease increases. A young person may also require continuing care for a chronic illness or severe injury. Persons of any age who are chronically ill or severely injured may require **long-term care (LTC)**. This care is provided either in the person's home or in a long-term care facility (LTCF). This chapter gives information about working in a long-term care facility. You will learn about home care in Chapters 34 and 35.

Nursing assistants are valuable members of the health care team in long-term care facilities (Figure 33-2). The skills you use in acute care facilities are also used in long-term care facilities. There are some changes in the application of these skills because of the differences between long-term and acute care.

TYPES OF LONG-TERM CARE FACILITIES

Many types of facilities provide ongoing health care for persons with chronic medical problems. The services provided by these facilities are summarized in Table 33-1.

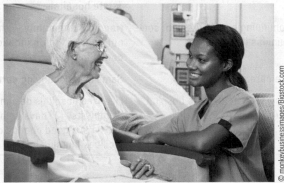

FIGURE 33-2 Nursing assistants are valuable caregivers in long-term care facilities.

TABLE 33-1 Facilities That Provide Long-Term Care

Type of Facility	Description
Board and care homes	A group living arrangement providing assistance with ADLs. For persons who need supervision and minimal assistance with personal care.
Assisted living facility (ALF)	Provides daily supervision and assistance with activities of daily living. Monitors the activities of residents to ensure their health, safety, and well-being. Does not provide medical or nursing care.
Group homes	Homelike settings providing care to persons of all ages who are mentally ill, intellectually disabled, or developmentally disabled. They teach residents to be as independent as possible. Most group homes have four to six residents with a live-in, 24-hour caregiver. (Four is ideal.) These homes are usually three- or four-bedroom houses in neighborhoods in the community.
Intermediate care facility (ICF)	Cares for persons with stable chronic conditions who cannot live independently, but do not need constant care. Provides supportive care and nursing supervision under medical direction 24 hours per day, but not continuous nursing care. This level of care is not available in some states.
Intermediate care facility for the intellectual disability (ICF-MR)	Facilities that care for persons who are intellectually or developmentally disabled. They teach residents to be as independent as possible.
Nursing facility (NF)	Services range from skilled nursing care, rehabilitation services, and assistance with ADLs, to supervision.
Rehabilitation facility	Provides services to persons needing long-term rehabilitation for complex conditions, such as those related to nervous system problems. (Facilities are also available for substance abuse, alcohol, and drug treatment; these are beyond the scope of this book.)
Skilled nursing facility (SNF)	Provide the most intensive level of care on the residential care continuum. Residents are stable but have complex medical care or rehabilitation needs. Some are chronically ill and cannot live independently. Some facilities offer **respite care** (temporary or periodic care) or hospice services (Chapters 32 and 35). Some facilities specialize in a certain type of care, such as rehabilitation or pediatrics.
Skilled unit or Skilled nursing unit (SNU)	Same as a skilled nursing facility. This is a licensed long-term care facility located in a hospital.
State school or state-supported living center (SSLC)	Long-term residential facility for persons with intellectual disability (mental retardation) that is operated by a state government. Some state schools also have recreational and employment facilities. Most are approved intermediate care facilities for persons who are mentally retarded.
Subacute care facilities	Facilities that provide a higher level of care than a SNF and bridge the gap between the acute care hospital and the chronic care setting. Subacute care units may also be located in some hospitals and long-term care facilities. However, they hold a license separate from the rest of the facility.
Psychiatric hospitals	Long-term chronic care hospitals for persons who are medically stable but too mentally ill to live in the community. Some also care for persons who have acutely unstable psychiatric conditions. Some residents may have been adjudicated mentally ill by the court and sent to the psychiatric facility instead of prison. Many of these facilities are state owned and operated and are called "state hospitals."
Continuing care retirement communities (CCRC)	Housing community with a continuum of care ranging from independent living through skilled nursing, based on individual need. Residents can move back and forth between levels within the community.
Life care community	Same as a continuing care retirement community.
Long-term acute care hospital (LTACH or LTAC)	Licensed hospitals designed for patients who need long-term services and are expected to have a lengthy stay (25 days or more). The patient must have a medically complex condition, need acute care, and have a good chance of improvement. The level of care is higher than provided in long-term care facilities (nursing homes) or subacute care facilities.

Long-term care facilities used to be called *nursing homes*. The long-term care facilities of today bear little resemblance to the nursing homes of the past. Some long-term care facilities provide general care for any chronic condition. Some specialize in the care of people with a specific diagnosis or unusual care needs. Others provide only specialized services, such as ventilator care or rehabilitation. Some are licensed to care only for children. The majority care for adults with a variety of diagnoses and problems.

CULTURE CHANGE

Culture change is the name of a national movement that promotes the transformation of long-term care facilities and other services for older adults. Culture-change facilities practice person-directed care. In this model of care, residents are treated with respect and allowed to direct their own care. The trend toward this type of care began in the early 1990s. Facilities believe that older persons can continue to grow and develop rather than decline. One goal is to transform the typical clinical facility environment into a comfortable, homelike community. Most such facilities are restraint free.

In addition to improving the quality of the residents' lives, most culture-change facilities have improved staff satisfaction and have much lower turnover than traditional facilities. Many have self-managed work teams. In some, unit staff provides all services for residents, including nursing and personal care, meal preparation, laundry, collecting specimens for laboratory testing, light housekeeping, and activities. Most of these facilities have many plants. They allow animal visitors and usually have facility pets.

PAYING FOR LONG-TERM CARE SERVICES

One important issue facing our country today is the financing of long-term health care. Few hospital insurance policies cover expenses of a resident in a long-term care facility. The average annual cost for a private long-term care facility in the United States increases about 3 to 4 percent each year. The average costs in 2018 were[1]:

- Semiprivate room, long-term care facility—$89,297
- Private room, long-term care facility—$100,375
- Assisted living facility—$48,000
- Home health aide—$50,336
- Homemaker home services—$48,048
- Adult day care—$18,720

[1]Genworth 2018 Cost of Care Survey, conducted by CareScout, September 2018. https://www.genworth.com/aging-and-you/finances/cost-of-care.html

The four primary sources of long-term care funding are:
- Private pay from personal funds
  - People who pay for care from private funds may find that their money is soon used up.
- Long-term care insurance
  - The cost of premiums is prohibitive for many people.
  - Many policies use Medicare criteria to determine eligibility for coverage. Most people do not meet the criteria, so the policies they have paid for will not cover the cost of routine long-term care.
- Medicaid
  - This is a government reimbursement system through which the federal government issues money to the states. The states determine how to distribute the money to health care facilities to care for people who do not have enough money to pay for their care.
- Medicare
  - Another government program that partially pays for health care for persons over the age of 65 and those who are permanently disabled. There is a co-payment from days 21 to 100. The co-payment may be paid privately by the patient, by a long-term care insurance policy, a private supplemental insurance policy, or Medicaid. The standard Medicare Part B monthly premium for 2019 was $135.50. Medicare beneficiaries can buy into the Part D drug plan for varying amounts. This decreases the cost of prescription drugs.
  - Medicare covers only limited long-term care expenses for up to 100 days. It pays only for skilled care according to a rigid set of criteria, and many people do not qualify.
  - Medicaid and Medicare funds are available only to facilities that participate in the Medicaid and Medicare programs and have met their requirements. Some facilities do not qualify, and some do not accept government funding.

LEGISLATION AFFECTING LONG-TERM CARE

The Nursing Home Reform Act is federal legislation that has mandated improvements in the quality of long-term care. This legislation is the result of the Omnibus Budget Reconciliation Act of 1987 (OBRA). These rules require facilities to assist residents to attain and maintain the highest possible level of mental, physical, and psychosocial well-being given in their individual situation. Care must be provided in a homelike environment.

Much OBRA content affects nursing assistants directly or indirectly. Chapter 2 of this book provides information about working as a nursing assistant in long-term care facilities and OBRA resident care requirements.

ROLE OF THE NURSING ASSISTANT IN A LONG-TERM CARE FACILITY

The nursing assistant carries out procedures under the direct supervision of a nurse. Basic physical care and special procedures are done to help residents reach their maximum degree of well-being.

The long-term caregiver is a very special person who works in an important area of health care. Nursing assistants provide approximately 75 to 80 percent of the care in long-term care facilities. Because of this close contact, they come to know the residents well and know if a resident's condition or behavior is different from usual. They are the eyes and ears of the nurses, who depend on the assistants to report important changes, findings, and observations.

Nursing is both an art and a science. Committed career nursing assistants are skilled in both. The science is doing your job in the way you were taught. Each step of the procedures you do has a scientific rationale that is supported by nursing research. However, a robot could be programmed to be an efficient caregiver. This is why the art of nursing is so important. Being caring and compassionate with the people you care for is the art. There are many demands on your time (see Chapter 2). Take a deep breath and avoid becoming overwhelmed. Never get so busy with technical tasks that you forget the caring and compassion. This is as important, or even more important, than the science, because it humanizes the care you give. Using the nursing process and providing patient-focused care are ways of applying the science. As you gain experience, you will find ways of balancing the art and science so you are organized and efficient, while also being caring and compassionate. This is the essence of nursing assistant care.

EFFECTS OF AGING

Many residents in the long-term facility are advanced in age and have one or more chronic, somewhat **debilitating** (weakening) conditions. Some are mentally alert. Others are confused and disoriented.

Aging is a natural, progressive process that begins at birth and extends to death. Every resident will exhibit some aging characteristics. Do not expect every resident to exhibit the same characteristics at the same **chronologic** (year) age.

Physical Changes in Aging

Some investigators believe that we are born with a biological time clock. This clock is programmed for a specific life span, barring accidents and disease. As we move toward old age, changes that have been taking place gradually become more evident. For example, elderly persons store less fluid in body tissue and are at risk for dehydration. However, change occurs in every body system. Examples are listed in Table 33-2. They do not occur at the same rate in each system.

TABLE 33-2 Physical Changes of Aging

Body System	Physical Changes
Integumentary (Figure 33-3A)	• Graying or loss of **pigmentation** (color) is usual in the hair. The color changes as pigment is lost. • Hair becomes thinner. • Baldness and receding hair line in some people (this is probably genetic). • Amount of hair may be reduced in both males and females, and texture becomes coarser in other areas such as eyebrows and face. • Decreased oil makes the hair dull and lifeless. • Skin dries, becomes less elastic; wrinkles develop. • Skin is fragile and tears easily. • Bruises easily (senile purpura common). • Reduced blood flow in vessels that nourish the skin results in delayed healing. • Fingernails and toenails thicken. • Sweat glands do not excrete perspiration as readily. • Oil glands do not secrete as much oil. • Increased sensitivity to cold. • Skin discolorations (age spots) become more common. • Blood supply to the feet and legs is reduced, increasing the risk of injury and ulcers, and sensations of cold.

(continues)

TABLE 33-2 *(continued)*

Body System	Physical Changes
Nervous	• Tasks involving speed, balance, coordination, and fine motor activities take longer because of slowed transmission of nerve impulses. • Balance and coordination problems result from deterioration in the nerve terminals that provide information to the brain about body movement and position. • Temperature regulation is less effective. • Deep sleep is shortened; the person awakens more during the night and may need rest periods during the day. • Brain cells are lost, but intelligence remains intact unless disease is present. • Decreased sensitivity of nerve receptors in skin (heat, cold, pain, pressure). • Risk of injury increases because of decreased ability to feel pressure and temperature changes. • Decreased blood flow to the brain, which may result in mental confusion and memory loss.
Sensory	• More difficult to see close objects. • Night vision may decrease. • Cataracts (clouding of the lens of the eye) are more common. • Dryness and itching of the eyes may result from decreased secretion of fluids. • Side vision and depth perception diminish. • Hearing ability diminishes in most elderly persons. • Smell receptors and taste buds become less sensitive, so foods have less taste.
Musculoskeletal	• Loss of elasticity of muscles and decrease in size of muscle mass result in reduced strength, flexibility, endurance, muscle tone, and delayed reaction time. • Slower movements. • Bones lose minerals, become brittle, and break more easily; arthritis and osteoporosis are common (Figure 33-3B). • Spine becomes less stable and flexible, increasing the risk of injury. • Posture may become slumped because of weakness in back muscles (Figure 33-3C). • Degenerative changes in the joints result in limited movement, stiffness, and pain.
Respiratory	• Lung capacity decreases as a result of muscular rigidity in the lungs. • Coughing is less effective; this results in pooling of secretions and fluid in the lungs, increasing the risk of infection and choking. • Shortness of breath on exertion, as a result of aging changes in the lungs. • Gas exchange in the lungs is less effective, resulting in decreased oxygenation.
Urinary	• Kidneys decrease in size. • Urine production is less efficient. • Bladder capacity decreases, increasing the frequency of urination. • Kidney function increases at rest, causing increased urination at night. • Bladder muscles weaken, causing leaking of urine or inability to empty the bladder completely; complete emptying of bladder becomes more difficult. • Enlargement of the prostate gland in the male, causing frequency of urination, dribbling, urinary obstruction, and urinary retention.
Digestive	• Saliva production in the mouth decreases, causing difficulty with swallowing and digestion of starches, and increasing risk of tooth decay. • Taste buds on the tongue decrease, beginning with sweet and salt; changes in taste buds may result in appetite changes and increase in condiment use. • Gag reflex is less effective, increasing the risk of choking and aspiration. • Movement of food into the stomach through the esophagus is slower. • Food in the stomach is digested more slowly, so food remains there longer before moving to the small intestine. • Flatulence increases. • Indigestion and slower absorption of fat result from a decrease in digestive enzymes. • Food movement through the large intestine is slower, resulting in constipation.
Cardiovascular	• Heart rate slows, causing a slower pulse and less efficient circulation. This results in decreased energy and a slower response, causing the individual to tire easily. • Blood vessels lose elasticity and develop calcium deposits, causing vessels to narrow. • Blood pressure increases because of changes to the blood vessel walls. • Heart rate takes longer to return to normal after exercise. • Veins enlarge, causing blood vessels close to the skin surface to become more prominent. • Heart may not pump as efficiently, leading to decreased cardiac output and circulation.
Endocrine	• Decrease in levels of estrogen, progesterone. • Hot flashes, nervous feelings. • Higher levels of parathormone and thyroid-stimulating hormone. • Delayed release of insulin, increasing blood sugar level; incidence of diabetes increases greatly with age. • Metabolism rate and body functions slow, reducing the amount of calories needed for the body to function normally. This increases the risk of overweight and obesity. • Reduced function of secretory and endocrine cells and reduced nerve sensitivity.

(continues)

TABLE 33-2 *(continued)*

Body System	Physical Changes
Reproductive	*Females:* • Fewer female hormones are produced. • Ovulation and menstrual cycle cease. • Vaginal walls become thinner and drier. • Vagina becomes shorter and narrower. • Breast tissue decreases and the muscles supporting the breasts weaken. *Males:* • Scrotum less firm. • Prostate gland may enlarge. • Male hormones (testosterone) begin to decrease at about age 50 at the rate of approximately 1% per year. • As hormone production decreases, testes become smaller and sperm count is lower. • More time required for an erection, but sexual activity is possible and the person is able to father children.

OSTEOPOROSIS

NORMAL BONE   OSTEOPOROSIS

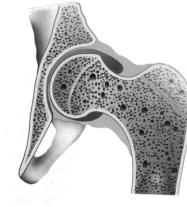

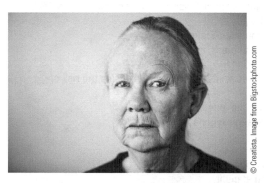

FIGURE 33-3A This patient's skin and hair show marked signs of aging.

FIGURE 33-3B A typical bone compared with a bone with osteoporosis.

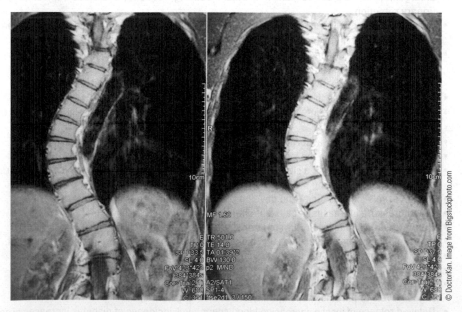

FIGURE 33-3C Spinal deformities can develop as a result of immobility and osteoporosis. These X-rays show an S-curve scoliosis.

SPIRITUAL NEEDS

Long-term care facility residents often have many spiritual needs. Finding a way to meet these needs is very important to residents' well-being. Many depend on spirituality and religion to help them cope with the many losses they experience, such as the loss of:

- Home, belongings, and beloved pets
- Independence
- Loved ones, including friends and family members, through separation and death
- Health, physical, and/or mental ability

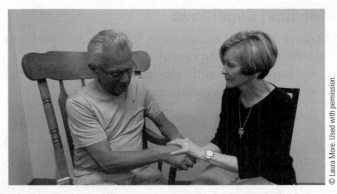

FIGURE 33-4 This man is receiving comfort and support from a visitor.

© Laura More. Used with permission.

Clinical Information ALERT

Women get more wrinkles than men because most men have a thicker dermis that remains elastic longer than a female's dermis.

Age-Appropriate Care ALERT

Consider other factors that may affect care. For example, an older person may lose vitality and assume that certain problems such as a change in condition or an increase in pain are a normal part of aging and not mention them. The person may not report the problem out of fear of what the change means, including loss of independence, worsening condition, or even death.

Age-Appropriate Care ALERT

You may find that caring for elderly individuals is time-consuming. Aging changes may cause a person to move more slowly than they did previously. Do not complete tasks that residents can do themselves, just for the sake of saving time. Test a person's ability to do a task instead of assuming that they cannot do it. Follow the care plan. Be patient and encourage independence.

- Have a support system or mechanism for dealing with loss or coping with problems.
- Have a constructive way of managing and expressing anger and doubt.
- Forgive others and be forgiven.
- Be thankful for what they have.
- Conduct a life review.
- Prepare for their own death.

NUTRITIONAL NEEDS

Find out what each loss means to the resident, and try to help them come to terms with (cope with) these losses.

Residents have the spiritual need to:

- Love and be loved unconditionally.
- Help or serve others.
- Maintain and validate their relationship with their higher power.
- Feel that they have a daily relationship with their higher power.
- Engage in spiritual or religious behaviors and activities (Figure 33-4).
- Have purpose, meaning, and hope in their daily lives.
- Transcend their circumstances.
- Have continuity in their lives.
- Maintain personal dignity, a sense of worth, and self-esteem.

The diet for older persons should:

- Be culturally and generationally appropriate.
- Be well balanced and nutritionally adequate.
- Be easy to chew and digest.
- Prevent malnutrition and provide sufficient fluid to prevent dehydration.
- Contain decreased amounts of refined sugars, fats, and cholesterol.
- Have adequate proteins and vitamins to provide for the best bodily function and repair.
- Contain many complex carbohydrates (found in fruits, vegetables, and grains). These foods are also good sources of vitamins and minerals, which tend to be deficient in the elderly person's diet.
- Have adequate fiber.

Medical Conditions

Because of loss of muscle tone, four intestinal problems are commonly seen in the elderly patient:

- **Constipation**—difficulty in eliminating solid waste
- **Flatulence**—gas production

 Clinical Information **ALERT**

The brain consumes more energy than any other organ in the body, or about one-fifth of the total calories we take in.

Clinical Information **ALERT**

Aspiration, dehydration, and constipation are potentially serious conditions that are often unrecognized. The symptoms are subtle, and some elderly individuals cannot communicate their discomfort.

- **Diverticulosis**—small pockets (**diverticula**) of weakened intestinal wall
- **Rectal prolapse**—occurs when a large portion of the rectum protrudes from the body; in the early stages, the rectum may intermittently protrude and retract, but over time the rectum will protrude permanently; inform the nurse promptly if a section of intestine protrudes from the anus

Dietary adjustments can help reduce these problems:

- Soft bulk foods, such as whole-grain cereals and fruits and vegetables, are helpful in overcoming constipation.
- To prevent **diverticulitis**, which is an inflammation of the diverticula, avoid skins and seeds.

- Persons with a prolapsed rectum are helped by reducing the need to strain during bowel movements. Encourage high-fiber foods and fluids. Surgery is often necessary to reattach and secure the rectum.

The presentation and service of food are important in stimulating appetites. Keep in mind the following:

- Several smaller meals seem to be more easily tolerated than three large meals.
- Encourage residents to feed themselves, whenever possible. Cut the food into bite-sized pieces and encourage the resident to eat finger foods independently. Suggest adaptive devices that you think will be helpful.
- Fruit and vegetable juices, eggnog, and soups provide both nourishment and fluids.

Types of Meal Service

Facilities use a variety of methods to serve meals. Some of these overlap. For example, home-style seating may be used with buffet or restaurant dining. Examples are given in Table 33-3.

Malnutrition

In the United States, eating is a social activity. Most people do not eat as well if they are alone. Residents in long-term care facilities eat in community dining areas. Meals are often the highlight of the day. Sitting at a table with compatible persons and having the ability to select food helps improve meal intake and prevent weight loss. Malnutrition is a problem for some elderly persons. It can and does occur in long-term care facility residents, despite the fact that a balanced diet is served and nutritional supplements are available. Factors that contribute to lack of appetite and poor nutritional intake include:

TABLE 33-3 Meal Service

Type of Meal Service	Description
Home style	Small tables that seat four to eight residents, tablecloths and table decorations, china, and stainless steel flatware. Residents usually select one of two entrees at lunch and dinner.
Family style	Providing food in serving bowls on the table, enabling residents to serve themselves like they did at home.
Buffet	Allowing residents to select hot and cold food items from a temperature-controlled buffet. Staff assist as needed.
Selective buffet	Same as buffet, but a chef cooks the main course at the buffet to the residents' specifications.
Restaurant style	Residents receive written menus with choices. Residents are shown a tray displaying the food choices available. Residents are verbally told the available food choices.
Room service	Residents order food as desired and food is served in the person's room.
Tray service	Food is prepared and served on trays in the resident's room or a dining room.
Traditional	Dining-room tables are served one table at a time. Usually there are no menu choices, but substitutes are available for meat and vegetables.

- Decreased activity
- Inadequate teeth
- Ill-fitting dentures
- Decreased saliva
- Diminished smell and taste
- Poor oral hygiene
- Eating alone

The incidence of malnutrition ranges from 23 to 85 percent of residents, making it one of the most serious problems that facilities face. Persons with malnutrition are at high risk for negative outcomes and have an increased **mortality**. This means that they have a greater risk of

death than others in the same population. The American Dietetic Association (ADA) reports that malnutrition has a negative effect on both the quality and length of life. It may come as a surprise to learn that most residents with evidence of malnutrition are on restricted diets. It appears that the very diets that were ordered to treat medical conditions may actually discourage nutrient intake.

Meals and Quality of Life

Meal service and satisfaction with food have a great impact on quality of life and quality of care. Evidence-based research published in 2013 revealed that older individuals with chronic conditions obtain little to no benefit from diets that limit sugar and sodium (salt). Tube feedings, pureed diets, and thickened liquids also have questionable benefits. The Centers for Medicare & Medicaid Services (CMS) published dietary standards recommending that most residents be served a regular diet. Only a small number of residents need restricted diets. Most long-term care professional groups support this recommendation. As a result, most facilities are serving a regular diet to as many residents as medically possible. Most offer residents a selective menu (Figure 33-5).

✚ Clinical Information **ALERT**

Nursing assistants are responsible for recording each resident's meal intake. Studies have shown that meal intake is often overestimated. Practice the method used by your facility for recording food intake and be sure your documentation is accurate.

Breakfast Week 1 Monday (Circle Selections):

Scrambled Egg, Pancakes with Syrup, French Toast with Syrup,
Blueberry Muffin, Bran Muffin, Sausage, Bacon

Cereal:		Fruit or Juice:		Beverage:	
Oatmeal	Corn Flakes	Chilled Fruit	Orange Juice	Decaf Coffee	Whole Milk
Grits	Rice Krispies	Fresh Fruit	Cranberry Juice	Hot Tea	2% Milk
Cheerios	Raisin Bran	Banana	Apple Juice		Skim Milk

Week 1 Noon Meal Monday Chef Specials (Circle Selection):

Meatloaf with Mashed Potatoes, with Mixed Vegetables, and a Dinner Roll
OR
Cottage Cheese Fruit Plate with a Muffin and Chicken Noodle Soup

Dessert:	Beverages:		Other Request:
Apple Cobbler	Decaf Coffee	Ice Tea	
	Hot Tea	Lemonade	

Week 1 Evening Meal Monday Chef Specials (Circle Selection):

Roasted Turkey Breast with Cornbread Dressing, Baby Carrots, and a Dinner Roll
OR
Fish Fillet Sandwich with Coleslaw, Potato Chips

Dessert:	Beverages:		Other Request:
Vanilla Pudding	Decaf Coffee	Ice Tea	
	Hot Tea	Lemonade	

Courtesy of Laura L. Fowler, LNHA, Kingston Nursing Center, Conway, S.C.

FIGURE 33-5 Example of a long-term care facility selective menu.

This is a positive and well-accepted change that came about as a result of the culture-change movement. Before that time, all residents received the same food items and there were no choices.

Nursing Assistant Actions Regarding Nutrition

Mealtime is a very busy time in the long-term care facility. Make sure each resident gets the correct tray containing the correct food items. The dietary department will place the complete menu or a smaller diet slip on the tray that lists the resident's name, type of diet, and other important information (Figure 33-6). Check this before serving the tray to be sure the tray goes to the correct person, and that the resident can have the food items on the tray. Prepare the tray as needed before leaving the room. Circulate on the unit or in the dining room to monitor and assist as needed. Do not get so busy that you overlook residents who are having difficulty or who are not eating. Residents who are at greatest risk of malnutrition and unplanned, undesirable unintentional weight loss are those who:

> **Clinical Information ALERT**
>
> Poor nutrition is associated with infections, pressure injuries, poor healing, anemia, low blood pressure, confusion, and hip fractures. Poor nutrition results in weakness, fatigue, and depression. Compared with well-nourished residents, persons who are hospitalized have a five-fold increase in mortality in the hospital.

A.

Resident:
Allergies

Diet: LIMIT CONC SWEETS PUREE DIET
* If puree diet-consistency should be: REGULAR PUREE

Liquid Consistency: NECTAR
Adaptive Device:

Special Instructions

Breakfast Drinks: TEA, JUICE, WATER
Lunch Drinks: JUICE, WATER
Dinner Drinks: JUICE, WATER

Likes: Whole wheat bread, bacon, cereal and milk, pancakes.
Dislikes: Eggs, rye bread, tomato juice.

B.

SUPPER

INSTRUCTIONS: Guest Tray

Room: Albany NY   3/10/2020

DIET: Regular, Nectar Thick Liq

BEVERAGES: N/A

No Photo Available

Food Likes	Food Dislikes

REG

C.

2991585788

First Name:
Last Name: Lopez
Diet: **Puree/Nectar Thicken Liquids/ALLERGY-No Known Allergies**

Order Num: **185**
Ready At:
Room: **444-A**
Date of Birth: **02/28/1922**

*** **STARTER ITEMS** ***
2 SYRUP

**** **HOT ITEMS** ****
2 Pancakes
2 PUREED

****COLD DESSERT****
1 Brown Sugar
1 Pudding
    1 CHO (15 gm)
2 Butter

****BEVERAGES****
1 OJ 4oz
2 Nectar Thick
1 2% Milk 8oz

Order Num: **185**   Last Name: Lopez
Meal Period: Breakfast   Room: 444-A
08: 17a
03/10/20
Ready At:

A. Courtesy of George Colbert, LNHA, Citizens Memorial Healthcare Facility, Bolivar, MO
B. Courtesy of Laura L. Fowler, LNHA, Kingston Nursing Center, Conway, S.C.)
C. Courtesy of V. Jean Morris MS, FACHCA, LNHA, CALA, St. Mary Medical Center Langhorne, PA

FIGURE 33-6 (A) Example of a long-term care facility diet slip. (B) Example of a long-term care facility diet slip. (C) Example of a hospital diet slip.

- Need help eating and drinking.
- Eat less than half their meals and/or planned snacks.
- Have mouth pain.
- Have no dentures, or have dentures that do not fit correctly.
- Have difficulty chewing or swallowing.
- Have difficulty getting utensils or glasses to the mouth.
- Cough or choke while eating.
- Are sad, have crying spells, or are withdrawn from others.
- Are confused, wander, or pace.
- Dislike the food.
- Have diabetes, lung disease, cancer, HIV, dementia, or other chronic diseases.

Create a pleasant, positive dining atmosphere to increase food intake and prevent weight loss and malnutrition. Be aware of each resident's self-feeding ability and changes in eating patterns. Report your observations and changes in residents' conditions and appetite to the nurse. You should also:

- Provide oral care before meals.
- Position residents correctly for feeding.
- Honor food preferences, likes, and dislikes.
- Offer substitutes according to facility policy.
- Serve meals promptly so foods are at the proper temperature; check foods by dropping a small amount on your wrist.
- Offer a variety of foods and beverages.
- Help residents who are having trouble feeding themselves.
- Provide adaptive utensils and dishes, as ordered.
- Provide condiments and sauces such as ketchup that are permitted on the resident's diet.
- Notify the nurse if a resident has difficulty feeding themselves, eating, or using utensils.
- Prompt and encourage residents to eat.
- Allow enough time for residents to finish eating; avoid rushing.
- Reheat cold food items, if necessary.
- Ask what's wrong if a resident's appetite decreases, or they seem sad.
- Accurately record the resident's intake at each meal.
- Assist and prompt residents to consume planned, ordered snacks and supplements.

Generational Meal Service

Facilities have traditionally cared for two generations at a time. Presently, most long-term care facility residents are members of the GI generation and the veteran generation (see Chapter 9). Members of the baby boom generation are also entering long-term care facilities. Dining service is one of the biggest challenges facilities face. In addition to sanitation, maintaining proper food temperature, and serving many meals at the same time, the dietary department must serve food that meets medical needs, is culturally appropriate, and is acceptable to two generations with different food preferences. The entrance of the baby boomers has made the job much more difficult because their food preferences are very different from those of older generations. For example, members of the GI and veteran generations are usually happy when the facility serves a casserole and canned vegetables. Baby boomers typically prefer ethnic food such as tacos or stir-fry with fresh or frozen vegetables.

According to studies done by the food industry, items with strong flavors are the most popular.[2] For example, more hot salsa is sold than mild and medium varieties. Foods that are considered sensory irritants, such as habanero, jalapeño, black pepper, horseradish, ginger, and cinnamon, are also very popular. Experts in the food industry believe the reason for increased use is because baby boomers are developing a reduced sense of taste and smell as a result of the normal aging process. Unlike previous generations, the nation's 80 million baby boomers tend to have broad appetites, a full set of teeth, and the spending power to shape the entire food industry. Some other potential reasons are the easy availability of hot, spicy, strong, salty, sweet, sour, high-flavor, and full-flavor products. Many baby boomers have used these items throughout their lifetime and refuse to eat bland facility food. All of the items listed are permitted on a regular diet. Provide them if a resident requests them. Check with the nurse if you believe there is a potential problem with an item.

PREVENTING INFECTIONS IN RESIDENTS

Section 4 provides instruction on infection control procedures. Effective and frequent handwashing or use of alcohol-based hand rubs is the best method of preventing the spread of disease from resident to resident, staff person to resident, or resident to staff person. Use standard precautions for all residents. Isolation will be ordered for residents with known or suspected infections.

Elderly persons are at high risk for infection because:

- Aging changes reduce the ability of the immune system to protect the person; resistance is further reduced when a person has chronic health problems.
- The skin becomes much more fragile; infection can develop rapidly if it is broken.

[2]Pfeiffer, S. (2007, October 7). Some like it hot. *Boston Globe*. Retrieved from http://www.boston.com/news/globe/ideas/articles/2007/10/07/some_like_it_hot/

- The bladder empties less efficiently; urine left in the bladder promotes infection.
- Reduced ability to cough up secretions makes it hard to get rid of bacteria in the lungs.
- The person may not eat well or consume enough fluids.
- Signs of infection are harder to identify in older persons; the resident may be sick for some time before someone recognizes that there is a problem.
- Persons who are elderly do not always have a fever with an infection. Their normal temperature may be a few degrees less than that of a younger person, so the "normal" temperature in a younger adult may represent a fever in an older person.
- Older persons may have a low temperature, such as 96°F or below, when they have a serious infection; the problem goes unrecognized because of the low temperature.
- Elderly persons do not readily show signs of inflammation; signs may be delayed or missing entirely.
- Older persons may not have an increase in white blood cell count; this is a common sign of infection in younger adults.
- Persons with communication problems cannot tell you that they are ill; they cannot describe their symptoms.
- Residents may not be able to communicate feelings of pain, nausea, or signs of infection.

You can help prevent infection by:

- Assisting residents to consume enough food and fluids.
- Promoting activity by following positioning schedules and orders for range-of-motion exercises and ambulation. Activity increases circulation and reduces the risk of skin breakdown. It also improves breathing, thus decreasing the risk of respiratory infections.
- Assisting with ADLs, such as regular bathing, oral care, and regular toileting. Use proper technique when providing perineal care.
- Providing catheter care as directed on the care plan. Avoid opening the closed drainage system, and use aseptic technique when emptying the drainage bag.
- Observing residents carefully and reporting any unusual signs or changes. Changes in the urine, incontinence, and confusion in people who are usually alert may be signs of infection. A change in behavior or worsening of confusion may indicate an infection in persons with dementia. Residents with infections have an increased risk of falls.

👪 Age-Appropriate Care ALERT

New-onset or worsening confusion often signals illness, infection, or a reaction to medication or anesthesia. A change in mental status is a very important observation. Early mental changes may be subtle, and the nursing assistant is in the best position to detect them. Monitor residents carefully for signs of new and worsening confusion, and notify the nurse.

👪 Age-Appropriate Care ALERT

Remember that incontinence is a medical problem, not a normal change related to aging. Loss of bladder control affects the resident's dignity and self-esteem. Make every effort to assist elderly residents with toileting and maintaining normal bowel and bladder function.

- Using proper technique when collecting specimens to check for infection.

Fighting infection is everyone's responsibility. You can do your part by washing your hands and applying standard precautions.

🦠 Infection Control ALERT

Facilities are required to have an infection control nurse and to make regular infection control rounds of nursing units, patient/resident rooms, and work areas such as the utility room and linen room. Facilities may purchase check sheets for rounds, or develop their own so the checks are consistent.

GENERAL HYGIENE

Cleanliness of the skin is essential, but a full daily bath for the older person is neither necessary nor advisable. In fact, many elderly persons are reluctant to bathe daily. Hygiene also includes observations of the eyes, ears, and nose, as well as care of the hands and feet, hair, facial hair, and mouth. Infection-related precautions, isolation techniques, and all principles of medical asepsis are essential in health care facilities. Help new employees to acquire these skills, and assist residents to maintain good personal hygiene.

Partial Baths

Although a daily bath is unnecessary, frequent sponging of specific areas is necessary. The face, hands, underarms, perineum, and other body creases need regular cleaning and care. Use standard precautions when cleaning the eyes and genital area.

Keep skin areas that touch free from perspiration. Do not allow them to rub together. Skin breakdown and infection are possible whenever moisture, perspiration, urine, or feces are present. Gently wash and dry local areas.

Total Baths

Bed baths clean the skin, but they are a rather passive activity for the resident. A tub or shower bath is desirable two or three times a week to stimulate the resident.

Hand and Foot Care

Fingernails and toenails become thickened and brittle with age. They may split because of decreased peripheral circulation. Clean fingernails regularly during morning care. Do not overlook them. Residents should never have dirty fingernails.

Provide regular foot care, including:

- Careful washing and drying of the feet. Problems tend to develop in warm, moist/damp, dark areas between and behind the toes (Figure 33-7A).
- Close inspection for any abnormalities (Figure 33-7B).
- Application of olive oil, lanolin, cocoa butter, hand cream, or lotion to dry, scaly skin, but not between the toes.
- Application of a very light dusting of powder to perspiring feet.
- Provision of slippers or shoes that fit well and are in good repair. Caution residents not to stand or ambulate with bare feet or wearing only stockings.

> ### ⚖ NOTE
> Follow facility policy regarding nail and foot care for residents who have diabetes.

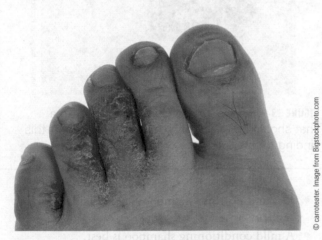

FIGURE 33-7A Athlete's foot (*tinea pedis*) is the most common type of fungal infection. Although less common, the same fungus may also grow on the heels, palms, and between the fingers. It is easily spread by both direct and indirect contact. The fungus thrives in warm, moist, dark areas.

© carrotteater. Image from Bigstockphoto.com

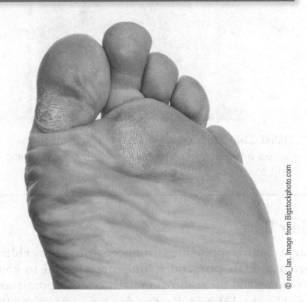

FIGURE 33-7B A *callus* is a thick, hard, tough area that has been exposed to repeated friction, pressure, or irritation. Although not harmful, they may be painful and some may become ulcerated and infected.

© rob_lan. Image from Bigstockphoto.com

GUIDELINES 33-1 Guidelines for Bathing the Elderly Person

- Some soaps are very drying. Superfatted soaps and lotion soaps are less irritating.
- Handle residents gently. The skin is easily damaged and takes a long time to heal because of aging changes and reduced circulation.

- Pat the resident's skin dry.
- Apply lotion to dry areas. Avoid bath oils, which make the bathtub slippery.
- Applying lotion and skin moisturizer immediately after the bath helps to seal moisture into the skin.

(continues)

GUIDELINES 33-1 Guidelines for Bathing the Elderly Person (continued)

- Consider general safety factors and the resident's physical limitations before giving a tub or shower bath (Figure 33-8). Check the placement of handrails and availability of tub and shower seats or hydraulic lifts. Be sure you know how to use the hydraulic lift in a whirlpool tub before trying to use it with a resident.

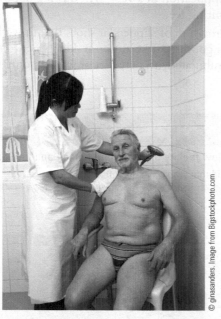

FIGURE 33-8 Most residents are showered three times a week. This resident is wearing a bathing suit for modesty purposes.

- Inspect the resident's skin over bony prominences for signs of skin breakdown, including redness, warmth, and ischemic pallor.
- Report any change in skin color; size of any lesion, open area, bruise, injury, and so on; or texture. All skin lesions are suspect. Cancer of the skin, often seen in elderly persons, has an excellent cure rate (93%) when treated early, because the cells grow slowly and tend not to spread. However, some skin cancers are malignant and rapidly fatal. The lesions are usually painless (Figure 33-9). Report skin changes promptly.

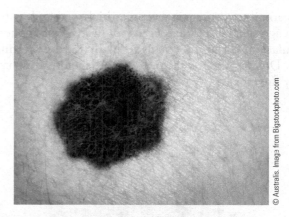

FIGURE 33-9 This is a potentially cancerous area that should be checked by a physician. Report this finding to the nurse.

Hair Care

An attractive appearance is important to many elderly persons. Hair care and styling are essential to good grooming and the resident's overall personal appearance.

- Hair should be styled and neatly arranged (Figure 33-10).
- Hair is usually washed when the resident is showered unless the person goes to the beauty shop weekly. Check the care plan for information.

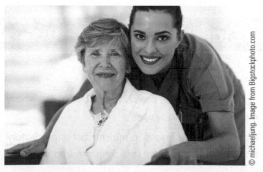

FIGURE 33-10 An attractive appearance is important to people of all ages.

- Dry and no-rinse shampoos are available for residents who are bedfast.
- A mild conditioning shampoo is best.
- A dryer will dry the hair quickly, decreasing the chance of chilling. Remove oxygen tanks and turn off piped-in oxygen in the resident's room whenever a hair dryer will be used. Hair dryers cannot be used in the beauty shop if a resident is using oxygen.
- Keep the resident out of drafts while the hair is being washed and dried.
- Hair care may be provided by a beautician or barber, if available, or by a family member or nursing assistant.

Facial Hair

Elderly women tend to have an increase in the growth and coarseness of the hair on the chin and upper lips. This hair can be removed:

- With tweezers
- By shaving

- With a *depilatory* (a chemical that removes hair)
- By waxing by a qualified person

Ask the resident's preference or consult the nurse.

Age-Appropriate Care ALERT

Style residents' hair in age-appropriate styles. Avoid juvenile hairstyles and accessories, which can be demeaning.

Shave elderly men regularly, usually daily. Provide the setup so they can shave themselves, if able.

Mouth Care

The condition of the teeth affects the older person's total health. Hygienic routines and observations are your responsibility when an individual is no longer able to do these things for themselves. See Chapter 25 for care procedures.

Residents with no teeth or dentures still need regular mouth care.

- Check the mouth and gums routinely for signs of irritation. Clean the mouth and gums with a soft brush.
- A commercial mouthwash, a warm wash of saline solution, or a warm baking soda solution should be used before and after meals.
- Wiping with moistened sponge-tip applicators between meals is very refreshing.
- Regularly check lips for excessive dryness or cracking.
- Creams, petroleum jelly, or lip balm applied to the lips can prevent cracking from developing into deep sores and infections.

Natural Teeth

Poor oral hygiene can result in loss of appetite and weight. In addition, the germs in the mouth can cause infection elsewhere in the body. This is one of the primary reasons for good toothbrushing and oral hygiene. Teeth should be brushed regularly, even if some teeth are missing. Residents should have regular dental checkups and cleanings.

Dentures

Clean dentures (false teeth) daily (see Procedure 65 in Chapter 25). Inspect dentures for cracks, rough edges, and broken teeth. Dentures should be marked with the resident's initials on the sides, near the back of the plate. Never engrave the top. This is usually done with a denture engraving kit. Follow product instructions.

Eyes, Ears, and Nose

Check the eyes, ears, and nose daily for signs of irritation, redness, drainage, or excessive dryness of the skin that could lead to breaks and fissures. Observations of this nature should be part of routine care.

MENTAL CHANGES ASSOCIATED WITH AGING AND DISEASE

Mental decline is not a normal part of aging, but the risk of mental deterioration increases with age. Mental decline may be the result of physical (organic) or emotional causes, or a combination of both. Periods of mental confusion are often temporary. They may be due to unusual stress, such as an infection; sudden injury, such as a fracture; or transfer to an unfamiliar environment. In some situations, the changes may signify a progressive deterioration of mental abilities. The term **dementia** refers to any disorder of the brain that causes deficits in thinking, memory, and judgment.

CARING FOR PERSONS WITH DEMENTIA

You will care for many persons with dementia. Dementia is not a disease in itself, but is a group of symptoms seen in a number of different diseases. Dementia is permanent and progresses slowly, over a long period of time.

Alzheimer's disease is the most common form of dementia. Other types of dementia are listed in Table 33-4. The term *dementia* is used here when referring to symptoms, behavior, and nursing actions that are appropriate for people with any dementia. The term *Alzheimer's* is used when the information is specific to that dementia.

Alzheimer Disease

Alzheimer disease (AD) can begin during middle age, but is more common in older persons. It has been called a "slow death of the mind." The cause is not known. The disease affects people of all races, levels of intelligence, and education. It is progressive and cannot be cured. In the past, the term *senility* was used to describe these signs and symptoms. We know now that it is a disease of the brain cells and is not part of normal aging.

Clinical Information ALERT

Approximately 40 percent of persons with severe Alzheimer disease experience significant weight loss. Several promising studies have shown that these individuals eat and drink more when food is served on brightly colored dishes, such as the bright colors of some disposable plastic plates and cups.

TABLE 33-4 Description of Major Forms of Dementia

Disease	Features	Course
Alzheimer's disease (*senile dementia* is an older term for this condition; some professionals call this disorder "senile dementia of the Alzheimer's type" [SDAT])	The most common type of dementia. Lack of certain chemicals in the brain causes neurofibrillary tangles and neuritic plaques. The person has progressive memory loss, behavioral changes, poor judgment, and loss of ability for abstract thinking. Eventually may cause loss of speech, loss of self-care ability, and apathy.	Onset age: 60–80. Slowly progressive and irreversible. Most people die within 4 to 6 years after diagnosis, but the illness can last from 3 to 20 years.
Vascular dementia (also called *multi-infarct dementia*)	Interference with blood circulation in brain cells due to arteriosclerosis or atherosclerosis. Many different areas of the brain die due to lack of oxygen. The most common form of dementia after Alzheimer's disease. Believed to be caused by a series of strokes. Each stroke involves a progressive mental decline. (For additional information, see Chapter 43.)	Onset age: 55–70. Outcome depends on rate of damage to brain cells. People who have had a stroke have a ninefold greater risk of dementia compared with people who have not had a stroke. About 1 in 4 people who have had a stroke develop signs of dementia within 1 year.
Mixed dementia	Several types of mixed dementia have been identified: Alzheimer's protein deposits and blood vessel problems from vascular dementia are both present. Alzheimer's changes and Lewy bodies may both be present. Occasionally, brain changes linked to Alzheimer's disease, vascular dementia, and Lewy body dementia are present at one time.	Much more research is needed. Unfortunately, this cannot be done on living individuals. It appears that mixed dementia may be more common than previously realized. Signs and symptoms are determined by the affected area in the brain and the types of brain changes involved.
Lewy body dementia (DLB or LBD)	Gets its name from the round nerve cell deposits found in the brain after death. These are different from Alzheimer's deposits. Agitation, delusions, and problems with speech are early symptoms. Involves a progressive mental decline, fluctuations in alertness and attention span, drowsiness, staring into space for long periods, and visual hallucinations. The person develops motor symptoms similar to those of Parkinson's disease (Chapter 43).	Tends to develop later in life than other types of dementia; usually between ages 68 and 80.
Normal pressure hydrocephalus	Caused by pressure from buildup of cerebrospinal fluid in the ventricles of the brain. Symptoms include memory loss, difficulty thinking and reasoning, incontinence, and difficulty walking.	Some cases can be corrected with surgical implantation of a shunt in the brain to drain excess fluid. No nonsurgical treatments have been effective. Additional research needed.
AIDS dementia complex (ADC)	HIV-1 virus.	Symptoms sometimes precede diagnosis of AIDS. Cognitive, motor, and behavioral problems in persons with advanced AIDS. Not as common as previously because of the availability of anti-retroviral drugs.
Frontotemporal dementia (Pick's disease)	Accounts for about 5% of all dementias. Caused by damage to the frontal and temporal lobes of the brain, resulting in marked changes in behavior, personality, and/or speech. Similar to Alzheimer's in that it deposits Pick bodies in areas of damage. Behaviors vary from socially inappropriate to listless and apathetic.	Can occur in people as young as 20, but usually begins between ages 40 and 60; the average age at which it begins is 54. A brain biopsy is the only test that can confirm the diagnosis. Rapidly worsens, causing total disability early in the course of the disease. Usually causes death within 2–10 years, usually from infection or organ failure.
Huntington's disease	Inherited from either parent who has a gene for the disease. Causes a progressive mental decline. (For additional information, see Chapter 43.)	Onset age: 25–45. Average duration: 15 years.

(continues)

TABLE 33-4 *(continued)*

Disease	Features	Course
Parkinson's disease	Deficiency of chemical (dopamine) in brain. Causes a progressive mental decline in some persons. Signs of dementia include memory loss, distractibility, slowed thinking, disorientation, confusion, moodiness, and lack of motivation. (For additional information, see Chapter 43.)	Involves approximately 20% of people with Parkinson's, usually those who develop the condition after age of 70. There is usually a delay of 10–15 years from the Parkinson's diagnosis until the onset of dementia. This condition is also caused by Lewy bodies, but they are in a different area of the brain than in Lewy body dementia.
Tertiary syphilis	Untreated syphilis causes neurological problems. The spirochete (bacteria) causes brain damage. The internal organs are also affected. At this stage, the person cannot be cured.	Usually occurs 15–20 years after primary infection, but can occur as early as 1 year in some people. Although the person is highly symptomatic, the condition is not contagious and standard precautions are used.
Creutzfeldt-Jakob disease	A rare and incurable disorder that causes changes in the brain. Thought to be viral in origin for many years, it is now believed to be caused by prions. Harmless and infectious prions are nearly identical, but the infectious form has a folded appearance and structure.	Onset age: 50–60. Rapidly progressive. About 90% of persons die within 1 year.
Prion diseases	The existence of prions was discovered only fairly recently. *Prion* is an abbreviation for *proteinaceous infectious particle*. Prions may be ingested through infected food, such as meat. This is an area in which research must be done to identify factors that influence prion infectivity and determine how they cause brain damage. Researchers are also trying to identify risk factors for the condition and determine when in life the disease appears.	Usual onset age: 50–60. Rapidly progressive and incurable.

Despite having a healthy appearance, persons with Alzheimer's have changes in the structure and function of the brain, which becomes smaller overall. If an autopsy is performed after death, areas resembling spider webs, called *neuritic plaques* and *neurofibrillary tangles*, are seen in the brain. In the past, the presence of these areas was the only way to confirm an Alzheimer's diagnosis. In 2014, researchers announced the development of a blood test that can identify whether a person will develop the disease many years before symptoms appear. This information gives the person time to get their affairs in order. Research continues to determine whether the information gained from this test may be used to identify methods of prevention or a cure.

Alzheimer disease has three broad stages, with symptoms becoming progressively worse. Staging helps predict the course of the disease and enables the person and family to make plans. However, the stages overlap and it is sometimes difficult to accurately stage a person. The three primary stages have been further divided into seven categories (Table 33-5). However, there are many individual variables, and the disease varies markedly from person to person. The symptoms progress in a general way, related to the underlying nerve cell degeneration that distinguishes the condition. Damage begins with cells used for memory and learning, and gradually spreads to brain cells that control behavior, thinking, and judgment. The best-learned skills tend to remain the longest. An English teacher, for example, may maintain verbal or written skills longer than another person.

However, once a skill is lost, it is lost forever. As the disease progresses, the ability to speak declines and the ability to walk is lost. In late stages, the physical ability needed for daily life skills, such as eating, drinking, coordination, and voluntary movement, is also affected.

Stage I: Mild Dementia

During the first stage, most people remain at home if they have a supportive family to provide assistance. They are physically capable and can manage activities of daily living with supervision.

Characteristics of stage I include:

- Short-term memory loss.
- Personality changes with loss of spontaneity and indifference.
- Decreased ability to concentrate and shortened attention span.
- Disorientation to time and space.
- Poor judgment.
- Lack of safety awareness.
- Carelessness in actions and appearance (Figure 33-11).
- Anxiety, depression, and agitation.
- Delusions of persecution—the person thinks that others are conspiring to harm them.
- Enough alertness to recognize that they have a memory problem; may fabricate stories and make excuses to cover for memory loss.

TABLE 33-5 Brief Overview—Seven Stages of Alzheimer's Disease

Stage		Characteristics
Stage 1	No impairment (normal function)	No memory problems; no evidence or symptoms of dementia.
Stage 2	Very mild decline (may be normal age-related changes or early signs of AD)	Person has memory lapses but no symptoms of dementia can be detected.
Stage 3	Mild decline (early-stage AD can be diagnosed in some, but not all)	People begin to notice problems, such as inability to come up with the right word or name and forgetting material that was just read; losing things.
Stage 4	Moderate decline (mild or early-stage AD)	Forgetfulness of recent events; difficulty doing mental arithmetic and doing complex tasks.
Stage 5	Moderately severe decline (moderate or mid-stage AD)	Noticeable gaps in memory and thinking; needs help with day-to-day activities; may be unable to recall address and telephone number.
Stage 6	Severe decline (moderately severe or mid-stage AD)	Memory continues to worsen; personality changes may take place; person needs extensive help with daily activities.
Stage 7	Very severe decline (severe or late-stage AD)	Loss of ability to respond to environment, to carry on a conversation, and, eventually, to control movement. May still say words or phrases.

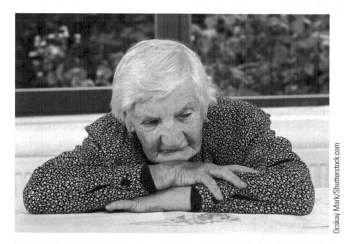

Ocskay Mark/Shutterstock.com

FIGURE 33-11 This resident shows signs of indifference and confusion.

Stage II: Moderate Dementia

Symptoms of this stage are:

- Increased short-term memory loss and deterioration of memory for remote events.
- Complete disorientation.
- Wandering and pacing.
- **Sundowning**, which is confusion and restlessness that occur during the late afternoon, evening, or night.
- Sensory/perceptual changes. The person is unable to recognize and use common objects, such as eating utensils, combs, and pencils. They cannot distinguish between right and left, up and down, hot and cold.
- *Perseveration phenomena*, which refers to repeated actions. Examples are repeating the same word or

phrase, such as "Hooch McGooch, Sylvester Jester, Totes McGoat, Ace McFace, and Kill the bill." Lip-licking, chewing even though the mouth is empty, and finger-tapping are also perseveration behaviors.

- Problems walking.
- Problems with speech, reading, writing.
- Incontinence of bowel and bladder.
- Catastrophic reactions, hallucinations, and **delusions**. A **catastrophic reaction** is the response of a person with dementia to overwhelming stimuli.

Most people with Alzheimer's are admitted to long-term care facilities during the second stage. Although they are healthy physically, they require constant care. Most families do not have the emotional resources and physical energy to cope. Wandering and poor safety judgments are usually the problems that cause the family to seek outside care. Nevertheless, admission is often traumatic for families. Remember that families are vital members of the interdisciplinary team. They can provide staff with insights about the person and how to deal with problems.

Stage III: Severe Dementia

The person in stage III:

- Is totally dependent
- Is verbally unresponsive
- May have seizures
- May refuse to eat and drink
- May refuse bathing
- May resist and refuse care

GUIDELINES 33-2 Guidelines for Activities of Daily Living for Persons with Dementia

- Encourage and allow the person to do as much as possible.
  - Give only one short, simple direction at a time.
  - Use the **hand-over-hand technique** for personal care and eating by placing the person's hand around an object, then guiding the desired activity by placing your hand on top. Refer to the restorative techniques in Chapter 48.
- Observe the person's physical condition. People with dementia are usually unaware of signs of illness.
- Assist the person to maintain a dignified, attractive appearance.
- Monitor food and fluid intake.
  - Encourage and provide sufficient fluids to prevent dehydration.
  - Offer the person a drink each time you enter the room.
  - Some persons do not like water, but will drink fruit juice, soda, or sugarless beverages. Provide fluids that the person likes and will consume readily.
  - Too many foods at once are confusing.
  - Placing one food at a time in front of the person may improve food acceptance.
  - Avoid plastic utensils that can break in the person's mouth.
  - Provide nutritious finger foods when the person is unable to use utensils.

- Avoid pureed foods for as long as possible.
- Check food temperature. If the person is a slow eater, you may have to reheat the food.
- Prepare foods for eating as needed by buttering bread, cutting meat, removing wrappers, and opening cartons and packages.
- Check the person's mouth after eating for food. "Squirreling" food (hoarding food in the cheeks) can lead to aspiration.
- Weigh the patient regularly to identify patterns of weight gain or loss.
- Keep the dining area quiet and calm.
- Persons with dementia eventually lose bowel and bladder continence. Taking them to the bathroom on a regular schedule helps them stay dry and maintains dignity. Monitor their behavior for body language and hints that they may need to use the bathroom.
- Persons with dementia need activities geared to their abilities.
  - Avoid large groups or competitive activities.
  - In later stages, use sensory stimulation with quiet music, soft touching, and calm talk.
  - Holding puppies or kittens (pet therapy) brings pleasure to persons who are severely impaired.
- Provide daily exercise according to the plan of care and the persons' habits and abilities.

In this stage, the ability to speak and swallow are lost, and the person is totally dependent. Caregivers must be compassionate, be calm, and have a sense of humor. When you are caring for persons with dementia, remember to:

- Protect the person from physical injury.
- Encourage independence for as long as possible.
- Support dignity and self-esteem.
- Maintain nutrition and hydration for as long as possible. Follow the care plan and speech therapist's recommendations to prevent choking and aspiration.

To meet these goals, the care must be:

- Consistent
- Structured with a flexible routine
- Given in an environment that is calm, quiet, and simple

It is helpful to:

- Make eye contact.
- Monitor your body language. Persons with dementia get clues from your body language. When this occurs, the person's behavior tends to reflect the mood of the staff (Figure 33-12).
- Be accepting of the person without being judgmental or critical.
- Use touch appropriately. However, avoid startling the person. Make sure they know you are approaching. Do not try to touch the person if they are agitated. Surprising the person with unexpected body contact can trigger a catastrophic reaction. This is the disorganized response of a person with dementia. It is triggered by the person's inability to cope with the situation. They may scream, yell, cry, or become violent. This may be the

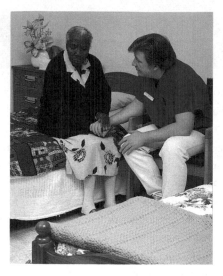

FIGURE 33-12 Residents with dementia are in tune with the body language of the caregiver.

only way the person can communicate their high level of frustration with the activity or situation.

- Avoid using logic, reasoning, or lengthy explanations.
- Remember that when the ability to speak is lost, communication occurs through nonverbal means. Biting, scratching, and kicking may be the only way the person can express displeasure.
- Watch facial expressions and body language for clues to feelings and moods.
- Learn what triggers agitation or anger. Work on preventing those situations.
- Use diversion and distraction. For example, calmly take the person by the hand and walk together or direct the person's attention to another activity. These techniques work well because of the shortened attention span.
- Realize that people with dementia are not responsible for what they do or say. They do not want to act this way but are unable to control or change the behavior. They lose the ability to control their impulses.
- Avoid confrontations and always allow them to keep their dignity.
- Remember that no one really knows what is happening in the minds of people with dementia.

SPECIAL PROBLEMS

Persons with dementia present several special problems to caregivers. Though each person is unique, techniques have been developed to deal with common problems.

Problems with Bathing

Resistance to bathing is common in persons with dementia. The person may have forgotten the purpose of bathing, or resist removing clothing. They may misinterpret your assistance as a sexual assault. Staff may label this behavior "uncooperative," "combative," or "aggressive" when in fact the person is just using normal defense mechanisms. Describe the behavior without labeling the person. The behavior may worsen if you ignore requests to stop the activity. Try to view the procedure from the patient's perspective. Observe and listen to the verbal and nonverbal clues.

If a person steadfastly refuses a bath, consider whether it is really necessary to bathe them in this way at this time. Return and try again later, or consult the nurse. Try to avoid agitating the person further. Consider a different method of bathing, such as using a towel bath or bag bath (see Chapter 24). Modify the environment so it is comfortable and pleasurable, and be flexible in your approach to and communication with the person.

Prepare the tub room before attempting to bathe the person with dementia. Your best approach is to be sure the room is warm, quiet, and private. Eliminate equipment noises as much as possible, such as from the whirlpool, heater, or running water. Sound tends to echo in shower and tub rooms, causing agitation. Residents who have forgotten the purpose of bathing may be afraid of water. Distracting the resident by encouraging them to sing an old song with you or playing pleasant music may help. (You may also use a special battery-operated shower radio, or a regular radio if the plug is kept away from sources of water.)

Persons in the early stages of Alzheimer's disease may also be sensitive and less cooperative with an unfamiliar nursing assistant. Wrapping a towel or bath blanket around the shoulders and pinning or clipping it securely may help with modesty problems. Leave it in place during the bath. Dementia causes problems with sensation, so bathing may be uncomfortable. A person with Alzheimer's may not be able to identify the warm, comfortable sensation. Say something like, "This feels good." Bathing is a complex task involving many steps. Explain what you are going to do and what you want the person to do, one step at a time. Avoid giving too many directions at once, which may overwhelm the person and trigger a catastrophic reaction. Taking a bath may simply be too overwhelming for the person. Washing the hair may also be frightening. Use the person's responses to guide your actions. Washing the hair in the sink or an inflatable basin, using a shampoo cap, or using a no-rinse product (see Chapter 24) may be much less traumatic.

Follow the bathing instructions on the care plan. The behavior is the person's only means of communicating the panic they feel. Modify your behavior and care according to the person's responses to the procedure. Be slow, calm, and reassuring. Share successful approaches with the nurse and other team members so these approaches can be added to the care plan.

Dressing Problems

Some persons with dementia are resistant to dressing or changing clothes. As with bathing, they may view your assistance as a form of sexual assault. Others remove their clothing after they are dressed. Keep the morning routine consistent and familiar. Avoid interruptions, which cause the person to forget what they are supposed to be doing. Make sure the room is warm and private. Ask the person to select clothing by giving them the choice between two outfits. If making decisions overwhelms them, select the clothes yourself. Select clothes that are color-coordinated and appropriate for the person's age and the season. Lay out clothing in the order in which it will be put on. Break the task down into simple, manageable steps and give the person easy instructions, one step at a time. Assist if needed. Allow the person to do as much for themselves as possible, but intervene promptly if they start to become frustrated. Understand the person's need for privacy and unwillingness to disrobe in front of you. Be sensitive to grooming issues and encourage the person to comb hair, shave, or wear cosmetics and jewelry. Praise the person and compliment their appearance.

Disrobing

Sometimes persons who are mentally confused disrobe (remove clothing) in public areas. Some individuals who are bedfast remove the covers many times each day, exposing themselves to anyone who looks in the door. This sight is offensive to adults, and can be traumatic to a young child who is visiting. It is your responsibility to keep all residents covered so their bodies are not exposed. This may be a difficult task. As with all other behavior problems, look for a cause. Some reasons for disrobing are:

- Boredom
- Need to use the bathroom
- Being tired and ready for bed
- Uncomfortable clothing
- Very warm room temperature

Evaluate the situation and common triggers. Sometimes there is no apparent cause, but rule out all logical triggers before arriving at this conclusion. Identifying and eliminating the trigger will stop the behavior.

You cannot put a person's clothing on backward to keep them from disrobing. Ask the nurse to contact the appropriate person to obtain clothing that fastens in back and is difficult to remove. Consult the care plan

and nurse about other approaches to use. Tying a sheet to the back of a bed or chair is a restraint, but wrapping it around the person's body and tying it in back may be effective. If the sheet does not limit the person's movement or access to their own body, it is not a restraint. Monitor the person who disrobes frequently and do your best to keep them covered.

Sexual Behavior

Sexuality is a basic need in all humans. It does not diminish with age (Figure 33-13). It involves much more than physical sexual activity. Sexual expression may be physical or psychological. Maintaining an attractive appearance is one way of expressing one's sexuality. Some people may touch certain areas of their bodies because doing so results in pleasurable sensations. Many health care workers feel that masturbation is inappropriate. However, masturbation is satisfying to the person and is not harmful. It is acceptable as long as it is done in a private area. Always knock before entering a person's room and wait for a response before entering. If you enter a room and find the person masturbating, provide privacy and leave the room.

If you enter a room and find two consenting adults engaged in a sexual act, provide privacy and leave. Adults have a legal right to do whatever is pleasing to them, as long as it is not medically contraindicated and both partners are mentally capable of consent. Do not pass judgment on the person's choice of partner or methods of sexual expression.

Facility staff is responsible for protecting persons who are physically or mentally vulnerable to unwanted sexual contact. Sexual contact with unwilling, alert persons who are physically unable to defend themselves, or with confused persons who cannot give full informed consent, is *sexual abuse*. Sexual abuse is a violation of the person's rights and is a felony-level crime. No health care worker, resident, patient, visitor, or other person may sexually abuse others. If sexual abuse occurs, the police

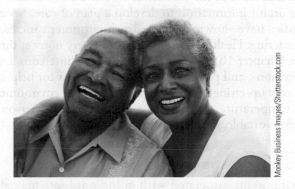

FIGURE 33-13 Maintaining an attractive appearance is part of sexuality and is important throughout life.

will be notified. Report anyone who sexually harasses or abuses another person to the nurse, manager, or other appropriate person.

Sometimes individuals make unwanted sexual advances toward the nursing assistant. The person's desire for sexuality is normal, but the choice of partner is not. Evaluate the situation to determine whether the person is misinterpreting your use of touch. If a person makes sexual advances, do not ridicule or belittle them. Be patient, understanding, and matter-of-fact. Tactfully inform the person that the behavior is not acceptable. Follow your facility's policy for reporting sexual advances.

Wandering and Pacing

Persons with Alzheimer's may wander or pace for hours at a time. A person may repeatedly try to leave the facility. No one knows why this occurs. The person may not know where they are, but they know they do not want to be there. They are seeking a state of mind, not a physical location. Ask the person their intended destination. They may tell you they are going to work. Another may say they are going home to cook dinner for the children. Avoid arguing or providing reality orientation, which will agitate the person. Instead, talk about the person's activities, work, meal preparation, or cooking. Make comments such as "That must be very interesting work" or "You must be a very good cook." Ask the person about their former work routines. Ask what the person likes to cook, how they prepared their favorite recipe, what foods are family favorites, and other related questions. This restores the state of mind the person seeks, reducing stress and the risk of **eloping** (wandering away from the facility).

Wandering Triggers

Many different things trigger wandering behavior. The facility may keep a log to help identify a person's wandering triggers. On the log, you will record information such as the person's behavior, staff on duty, and temperature and noise in the environment. The nurse will use this important information to develop a plan of care. Several studies have shown that a noisy environment increases wandering. Health care facilities can be very noisy at times (see Chapter 10). Loud talking, using the intercom, loud televisions, and persons yelling or calling out for help can be very upsetting to wanderers. Hot or cold environmental temperature may also be a problem. If the person is uncomfortable, they may wander to escape.

Nursing Assistant Approaches

Seeing items associated with going outdoors may also trigger wandering. Remove purses, hats, coats, shoes, or other outerwear from sight. Allow the person to wander and pace in a safe area. Using restraints increases anxiety and frustration, worsening the problem. Walk with the person and circle back. Adapt the environment so it is safe and secure. Keeping the person's stress as low as possible is important because if they feel overwhelmed, they may elope or have a catastrophic reaction. As a rule, try to meet the person's needs for hunger, thirst, and elimination. If you meet the need, the wandering will often cease.

Thinking is a very complex process. If someone tells you *not to think* of a purple dog, you will think of it, then have to "unthink" it. Unthinking is very difficult or impossible, especially for a person who is cognitively impaired. Avoid saying, "Don't go outside" or "Don't go in that room," because that will cause the person to think about doing exactly what you told them not to. A better approach is to say, "Stay inside," or "Stay here." Communication is best if it is simple, is concrete, and does not require abstract thinking or unthinking.

Avoid forcing your own agenda on the person, which will cause agitation and worsen the behavior. Instead, use gentle persuasion. Avoid making too many demands during ADLs and direct care. Keep instructions simple and brief. As the person completes one task, give them another. Be patient, calm, and reassuring. Tell them that they are in the right place and safe, and that you will help them. Compliment them for their successes, even if they are small. The person will probably not remember the compliment, but will feel good about themselves. They will be more cooperative and less likely to act out or wander.

There is no single effective approach for all wandering behavior. Use the approaches listed here and see if they work. If you discover an effective approach, inform the nurse so they can add it to the care plan. Remember that identifying and modifying the person's agenda, feelings, and unmet needs will usually modify or stop the problem behavior. Effective management is individualized to the person and is often the result of trial and error. As a rule, try to meet the person's needs for hunger, thirst, and elimination first. Consider whether they are having pain, and inform the nurse. Try distraction, such as by providing a magazine, newspaper, book, or picture album. Take the person to activities that they enjoy (Figure 33-14). If you meet the need, the wandering will likely cease.

Remember that persons who wander will burn extra calories and are at risk for weight loss. Some are so busy wandering they will not sit long enough to eat a meal. Give them finger foods and walk with them, if necessary. Follow the plan of care to ensure that the person takes in enough nutrients.

Persons who wander may become physically exhausted. They have forgotten how to sit down and may need reminders. Special reclining chairs and beanbag-type chairs may be used to enable persons to rest, but they are restraints if the person cannot readily get up.

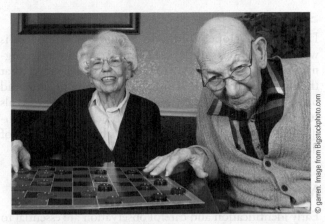

FIGURE 33-14 Find out the activities the resident enjoys. If a game or activity is too challenging, find something simpler. Watch for signs that the resident is becoming overwhelmed.

The care plan will specify the method to use. If you find another effective method, inform the nurse so they can add it to the care plan.

Agitation, Anxiety, and Catastrophic Reactions

An increase in physical activity, such as pacing or perseveration behaviors, is a sign of agitation and anxiety. A catastrophic reaction will likely occur if appropriate interventions are not implemented promptly. You may note any or all of the following warning signs:

- Increased physical activity
- Increased talking or mumbling
- Explosive behavior with physical violence

When agitation or a catastrophic reaction occurs:

- Do not use physical restraints or force to subdue the person. This increases agitation and can result in injury to the person or staff.
- Avoid having several staff persons approach the person at the same time. This is frightening and the person may react violently.
- Use a soft, calm voice. Do not try to reason with the person. Using touch may or may not be appropriate. Some persons respond to smooth stroking of the arms or back with lotion. Others may strike out if they are already agitated.
- If the person is violent, maintain a safe distance so you are not injured.

Sundowning

Sundowning is increased confusion, restlessness, and wandering during the late afternoon, evening, or night. It is sometimes prevented by avoiding too much activity before bedtime and by establishing a consistent bedtime routine. The person should eat the evening meal at least two hours before bedtime. Avoid caffeine in the late afternoon and evening. Provide a light bedtime snack that is easily chewed and digested. Take the person to the bathroom before putting them in bed for the night. Check the lighting. Shadows and reflections are disturbing. If the person awakens during the night, repeat the bedtime routine. If this is ineffective and the person does not remain in bed, try a recliner or Alzheimer's chair.

Pillaging and Hoarding

Pillaging means rummaging through property and taking others' belongings. *Hoarding* is acquiring numerous unnecessary items. These events do not present a major problem unless a resident collects items from others' rooms or hides things, making them difficult to find. This person usually believes they are in their own home, and they can explore and take whatever they want because everything in the "house" belongs to them. Some residents take items needed by other residents. For example, a resident acquires five sets of dentures. The dentures are needed by other residents. With luck, they are marked so you can disinfect them and return them to the correct resident. The person has very poor safety awareness and is at high risk of injury from entering housekeeping closets and service areas, and ingesting chemicals or becoming injured by sharp objects. Others may harm the resident, such as by hitting them, because they believe they are stealing their belongings.

Check the room daily for stale food and items belonging to other residents. Keep the person's hands busy. Activities like folding washcloths, "fiddling" with keys on a ring, clipping coupons (using safety scissors), using an activity apron, or sorting junk mail may help. Provide a dresser, nightstand, suitcase, or box in the hallway with items that they can safely rummage through. Distract the person with pictures (Figure 33-15A) or an activity such as a sensory stimulator, which is available in many different formats and patterns (Figure 33-15B).

Disorientation (Disordered Consciousness)

Disorientation is a condition in which a person shows a lack of reality awareness with regard to time, person, or place. It may be mild or severe, temporary or prolonged. The disoriented person has impaired judgment, memory, and understanding.

Delirium

Delirium is an acute state of confusion caused by reversible medical problems. It is often hard to tell whether a

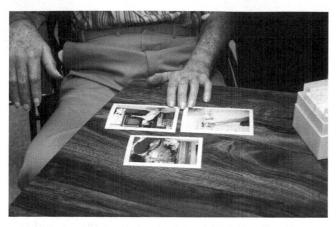

FIGURE 33-15A Residents with dementia retain long-term memory even though short-term memory is lost. Looking at family pictures is an excellent way to reminisce.

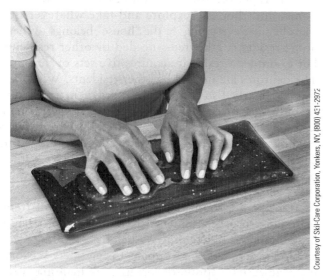

Courtesy of Skil-Care Corporation, Yonkers, NY, (800) 431-2972

FIGURE 33-15B Making designs on one of the many types of sensory stimulator pads is a fun activity!

person is disoriented, has delirium, or both. Delirium is common in elderly persons as a result of medical problems such as infection and dehydration. Anesthesia, some medications, and uncorrected vision or hearing problems may cause the person to misinterpret the environment correctly. Delirium goes away when the physical and mental triggers of the problem are identified and eliminated. This can be confusing, because delirium often has multiple causes. All must be treated before the mental status returns to baseline. The return to baseline mental status may not be immediate.

Delirium is a very serious condition. Unrecognized and untreated, the mortality rate is high, particularly in persons with chronic disease, mental problems, or dementia. This is unfortunate, because delirium can be reversed if promptly identified and treated.

Signs and Symptoms of Delirium

Delirium develops rapidly. In most cases, the onset is within a few hours or days. Delirium may not be recognized until the person is critically ill. Staff believes that the individual became ill suddenly, because of the rapid onset of mental changes, but a closer look often reveals subtle changes in the individual's physical or mental condition over the course of several days before the onset of delirium. *Any change in mental status is significant.*

Nursing Assistant Responsibilities

Early identification and careful observation are essential to preventing more serious problems. You will become familiar with each person's usual or normal condition. Monitor changes carefully, and report them to the nurse promptly. Avoid changes in routines and the environment.

People with disorientation and delirium are not responsible for their actions, and cannot protect themselves. The person's sensory problems (delusions or hallucinations) may put others at risk. *Protecting the people you care for is the most important nursing responsibility.*

Table 33-6 lists observations to make of specific behaviors, such as wandering, yelling, or disrobing. Table 33-7 lists general observations to make of persons with cognitive impairment. Sudden onset of these problems suggests illness. Further nursing assessment is needed. Report your observations to the nurse.

TABLE 33-6 Behavior Observations to Make and Report

Always report abnormal behavior to the nurse, even if you believe the behavior is "normal for the person."
Does the behavior involve another person (resident, visitor, staff)? How are these individuals alike? Does the behavior occur whenever a patient or staff member is in close proximity to the patient? If so, can you identify why the person is acting out?
What? Describe the behavior. Is the behavior predictable? What were the triggers? What were the circumstances in which the behavior occurred?
Where? Did/does the behavior occur in one specific area? What were the environmental conditions? Was it light, dark, hot, cold, noisy, quiet?
When? What is the time of day? Does the behavior occur at predictable times or in predictable situations, such as during bathing? When the person is tired, when the person awakens, and so on?
How do others respond to the person's behavior? Does the resident avoid someone? If so, is there a reason? How does the person manage or prevent the behavior?
Is there a pattern or clue to the behavior? Can you identify signals that the behavior is about to begin? Does the person need to use the restroom? How do they respond to toileting?

TABLE 33-7 Observations to Make and Report Related to Persons with Cognitive Impairment

Change in consciousness, awareness, or alertness
Changes in orientation to person, place, time, season
Changes in memory
Increasing agitation
Excessive drowsiness; sleepiness for no apparent reason
Changes in ability to respond verbally or nonverbally
Sudden inability to follow instructions
Inability to understand what is being said
Recent fall (witnessed or unwitnessed)
Sudden loss of ability to communicate
Sudden-onset wandering, worsening of wandering, or trying to leave facility
Refusal of food or fluids
New-onset incontinence or change in usual pattern of incontinence
Changes in usual mood or affect
Rapid worsening of confusion
Loss of ability to recognize familiar persons
Sudden onset of mental confusion (or worsening confusion)
Abnormal vital signs
Signs or symptoms of illness or infection

In addition to other abnormalities, the nurse should assess these problems further:

Significant change in nature or pattern of usual behavior
Sudden or persistent decline in function (i.e., ability to perform an ADL)
New onset of resistance to care
Abrupt onset or progression of significant agitation or combative behavior
New-onset violent/destructive behaviors directed at self or others

CARE PLAN APPROACHES FOR COGNITIVE IMPAIRMENT

The care plan may instruct you to use reality orientation, reminiscing, or validation to calm the person, orient them, or make them feel good about themselves. Persons with dementia are often unable to remember family members and others. They may not know where they are, the time, or the weather. They become agitated and upset. Reality orientation, validation, reminiscing, and other forms of therapy help them recognize and understand their surroundings. Rather than correcting wrong information, viewing pictures and discussing the past comforts the person.

Use reality orientation activities (such as shown in Figure 33-15A) to assist persons who are disoriented. **Reality orientation** involves making the individual aware of person, place, and time by visual reminders, activities, and verbal cues. This approach reduces agitation in some individuals, but increases agitation in others. Follow the care plan and the nurse's instructions. Avoid arguing with the person if their interpretation of reality is not accurate.

You may see *reminiscing* listed on the care plans of some individuals. **Reminiscing** (remembering past experiences) is a natural activity for people of all ages. We reminisce when we see old friends or get together with families. Listening to reminiscence will help you understand the person better. Reminiscence:

- Is an appropriate activity for individuals with dementia if long-term memory is still intact.
- May serve as a life review. This is a developmental task of old age. Review of past life experience helps older persons work through unresolved problems and find peace of mind.
- Helps people adapt to old age and maintain self-esteem.

Validation therapy is a technique that helps maintain dignity by acknowledging the person's memories and feelings. It involves encouraging individuals to express their feelings, and reassuring the person that the feelings are worthwhile. Using validation involves encouraging individuals to express emotions, and then assuring them that their feelings are okay. Validation helps:

- Maintain identity and dignity.
- People with dementia who are disoriented feel good about themselves.
- People acknowledge feelings and memories.
- People who are disoriented express feelings despite their disorientation.

Your facility will teach you how to provide reality orientation, reminiscing, and validation therapy if you will be using these techniques when giving care.

You may also wish to review the information on managing behavior problems, problems sleeping, aggression, yelling and calling out, sexual behavior problems, wandering, reality orientation, reminiscence, and validation therapy.

Music Therapy

Music therapy is an allied health service similar to occupational therapy and physical therapy. Although it is an enjoyable activity, it is not strictly for fun and games. Music therapy consists of using music therapeutically to address physical, psychological, cognitive, and social functioning. Music therapy is used successfully with people of all ages and many types of disabilities.

Music therapy dates back to ancient Greece. In that culture, music was part of medical treatment. Think about the effect music has on your own life. Children learn the alphabet by singing the letters. We listen to "oldies" and remember events from our past. We remember the words to songs we have not heard in many years.

Restorative music therapy is used for relieving stress. It can be a planned, formal activity or a spontaneous, informal activity. Singing with a person during bathing

Difficult Situations

The Velveteen Rabbit is a children's story that was copyrighted in 1922. This is a conversation between two stuffed animals:

"What is REAL?" asked the Rabbit one day, when they were lying side by side near the nursery fender, before Nana came to tidy the room. "Does it mean having things that buzz inside you and a stick-out handle?"

"REAL isn't how you are made," said the Skin Horse. "It's a thing that happens to you. When a child loves you for a long, long time, not just to play with, but REALLY loves you, then you become REAL."

"Does it hurt?" asked the Rabbit.

"Sometimes," said the Skin Horse, for he was always truthful. "When you are REAL you don't mind being hurt."

"Does it happen all at once, like being wound up," he asked, "or bit by bit?"

"It doesn't happen all at once, like being wound up," said the Skin Horse. "You become. It takes a long time. ... Generally, by the time you are REAL, most of your hair has been loved off, and your eyes drop out and you get loose in the joints and very shabby. But these things don't matter at all, because once you are REAL you can't be ugly, except to people who don't understand."[3]

There is a lesson for all health care workers in this old children's story. The persons entrusted to your care may be "loose in the joints" and "shabby in appearance," but they have shaped the communities and the world in which we live. Many have families and others who love and value them just as they are: shabby, balding, hard of hearing, slow, confused, even combative. They are worth your investment, even if they don't always appreciate it. They are *real*.

[3]Williams, M. (1922). *The Velveteen Rabbit.* New York. Doubleday & Company, Inc. Retrieved September 28, 2014, from http://www.gutenberg .org/files/11757/11757-h/11757-h.htm . (In public domain).

and range-of-motion exercises can be therapeutic and fun for both the individual and the nursing assistant. Studies have shown that engaging with music has various mental and physical benefits, including:

- Increased metabolism
- Increased muscle flexibility
- Improved circulation

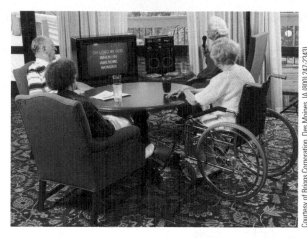

FIGURE 33-16 A teleprompter is one way for residents to participate in an activity by singing along with the words.

- Increased lung capacity and improved respirations
- Improved memory, which contributes to reminiscing and satisfaction
- Improved mood and emotional states
- A feeling of a sense of control over life
- Increased self-awareness
- Reduced anxiety
- Stimulation
- Opportunities to interact socially with others

Sometimes music therapy is part of a planned exercise program. Playing music during exercise helps make the activity more fun. Music motivates the participants, and singing and clapping relieve stress and anxiety. Music teleprompters make it easier for everyone to participate even if they do not know the words (Figure 33-16). For relaxation therapy, a telephone or other digital device and headset may be used.

The activities department may present music activities for other purposes. A professional music therapist may visit the facility regularly to work with designated individuals. Regardless of whether music is used formally as a form of therapy or informally for recreation, most people respond well to it. Engaging with music is a pleasurable activity that maintains or improves physical, mental, social, and emotional functioning. The sensory and intellectual stimulation of music helps maintain quality of life.

Animal-Assisted Therapy

Animal-assisted therapy is also called *pet therapy*. Pets are used in many different ways in the health care environment. Formal programs are developed in which the handler and health care provider consult on specific goals and plan how to accomplish them. With informal pet therapy, an animal visits periodically. Visiting with animals can reduce feelings of loneliness and depression. Some people become more active and responsive because of visits from pets. The pet may make it easier for the person to talk and express thoughts, feelings, and memories. Stroking a dog or cat may reduce a person's blood pressure, and encourages good range of motion of the hands and arms. Animals used in pet therapy must have a health certificate. Some formal groups offer special certifications to pets and handlers based on the experience of the animal–human team and complexity of the working environment. Dogs are commonly used for pet therapy, but other types of animals may be used as well.

INTELLECTUAL DISABILITY AND DEVELOPMENTAL DISABILITY

You may care for persons who have been diagnosed with an *intellectual disability* or a *developmental disability*. Although these are permanent medical conditions, persons with these types of disabilities usually live in the community. Many do not need facility care.

Persons with Developmental Disabilities

Some individuals have a **developmental disability (DD)**. This condition first occurs in the developmental period, which is before the age of 22. Developmental disabilities are conditions that change or delay the normal development of one or more of the following activities:

- Language
- Speech
- Learning
- Self-help
- Mobility
- Independent living

A developmental disability is a permanent condition that interferes with physical or mental development. The person may have a physical impairment, mental impairment, or a combination of both. The condition may be **congenital**, meaning the person is born with the condition, or **acquired**, indicating that the disability was not present at birth but developed before the age of 22 (Figure 33-17). For example, a child with a traumatic brain injury from an auto accident at age 7 would be considered to have a developmental disability (Figure 33-18). Examples are listed in Table 33-8.

Some persons with developmental disabilities have below-average intelligence, but many are of typical intelligence or above. Common forms of developmental disability are:

- Intellectual disability
- Cerebral palsy
- Epilepsy and other seizure disorders
- Autism
- Other organic conditions

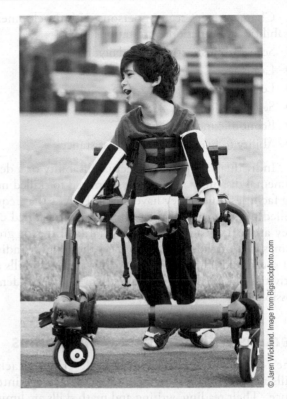

FIGURE 33-17 Cerebral palsy is a developmental disability caused by lack of oxygen at birth.

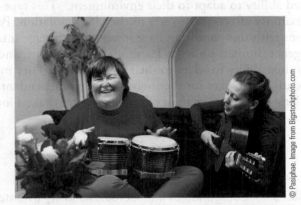

FIGURE 33-18 Music therapy is beneficial for those with all types of physical and developmental disabilities.

TABLE 33-8 Congenital and Acquired Developmental Disabilities

Congenital	Acquired
Fetal alcohol syndrome, maternal drug use	Trauma at birth
Maternal infection during pregnancy	Head injury, traumatic brain injury, shaken baby syndrome, child abuse
Poor maternal nutrition	Near-drowning
Genetic conditions	Poisoning
Lack of oxygen	Malignancy

Characteristics seen in persons with developmental disabilities are functional limitations in:

- Some or most activities of daily living
- Language
- Learning ability
- Self-direction
- Economic independence
- Ability to live alone without assistance

Individuals with an intellectual disability or a developmental disability may not be admitted to skilled nursing facilities unless they have medical needs that require skilled nursing care. If they do not require skilled care, they are usually admitted to special facilities or group homes that provide services to meet their highly individual social and emotional needs, and teach life skills and activities of daily living to make them as independent as possible.

Persons with Intellectual Disabilities

The term **intellectual disability** describes a lack of skills needed for daily living and below-average intelligence. Their reading, writing and math skills are limited. This condition was previously called mental retardation. These people are socially immature and have limited ability to adapt to their environment. This type of disability affects 2% to 3% of the US population. Persons with this condition have lower-than-average intelligence, limited ability to learn, social immaturity, and a limited ability to adapt to their environment. They may be unable to care for themselves or live independently. Many can learn new things, but learning may take a long time. There may be some things the person cannot learn. Those who are severely retarded are usually cared for at home or in a special facility for persons with similar problems. Epilepsy is more common in this population than it is in the general public. Intellectual disability (ID) is divided into five general categories based on cognitive ability, as shown in Table 33-9.

The current trend in health care is to place higher-functioning individuals in homelike group settings in the community, where four to six individuals live together with a caregiver. Over time, they learn skills that help them to function at their maximum potential. Although persons with an intellectual disability require lifelong care, many can feed, bathe, and dress themselves. Some are very high functioning and can go to work, use public transportation, and do many of the things that adults with typical mental function do each day.

> ### ✚ Clinical Information **ALERT**
>
> At the time of this writing, terminology describing this condition is in a state of flux. The term intellectual disability has been used for many years, but it has become a negative stereotype. President Obama signed *Rosa's Law* in October 2010. This law changed the label for the condition to *intellectual disability (ID)*, although the official definition of the disorder remains the same. Health care workers are slow to adopt new terminology, and it is likely that you will hear both terms for quite some time.

TABLE 33-9 Categories of Intellectual Disability (Mental Retardation)

Category	IQ	Percent of Population	Characteristics
Borderline intellectual functioning	70–84	Not known	Technically a cognitive impairment. Below-average cognitive ability, but deficit not as severe as mental retardation (intellectual disability). Abstract thinking limited. Prefers concrete thinking. Most can function independently, hold a job, and live alone.
Mild	50–69	75% to 90% of all cases	May have no unusual physical signs. Slow in all areas. Can learn reading and math up to sixth-grade level. Can conform in social situations.
Moderate	35–49	About 10% to 25% of all cases	Noticeable delays, especially in speech. Can learn simple health, hygiene, and self-care.
Severe	21–34	About 10% to 25% of all cases	Obvious delays. May walk late. Can learn repetitive activities and simple routines. Needs direction and close supervision.
Profound	Below 20	About 10% to 25% of all cases	Usually have congenital abnormalities. Marked delays in all areas. Not able to do self-care. May need attendant care.

Cerebral Palsy

Cerebral palsy (CP) is a motor control disorder caused by an injury or abnormality affecting the immature brain. It is also a developmental disorder. The injury occurs in the prenatal or postnatal period, or as a result of lack of oxygen during labor and delivery. The cause is not always known. CP is the most common condition associated with childhood disability. It is a stable condition that is not progressive.

Motor dysfunction is the hallmark of cerebral palsy. The type of motor disability depends on the location of the brain injury. The severity varies. Persons with CP can have impaired, average, or superior intellect. Other signs and symptoms are:

- Seizures
- Abnormal muscle tone, movement, and posture
- Spasticity (may have contractures due to abnormal muscle tone and spasms)
- Hearing impairments
- Visual impairments
- Intellectual disability
- Speech and language disorders
- Difficulty eating
- Growth disorders, developmental delays
- Gastroesophageal reflux (GERD)
- Nutritional deficiencies (due to poor feeding, reflux, and aspiration)
- Emotional and behavioral problems
- Contractures and deformities

Autism

Autism is a developmental disorder that appears during the first three years of life. It affects the person's ability to communicate and interact with others. There is a period of typical functioning after birth, followed by regression in function and progression of certain deficits. The person must display 6 of 12 specific symptoms for a diagnosis of autism to be made. Persons with autism often have verbal and nonverbal communication impairment, social impairment, and repetitive and ritualistic behavior. They sometimes dislike and resist change. Autism is more common in males. Approximately 70 to 75 percent of persons with autism have cognitive impairments.

Down Syndrome

Chromosomes are strands of DNA that transmit hereditary information. Most people are born with 46 chromosomes. Persons with Down syndrome have 47. **Down syndrome** is also called *trisomy 21* because in most cases the person has an extra copy of chromosome 21.

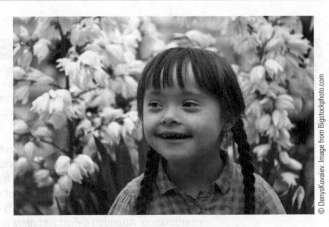

FIGURE 33-19 This little girl has facial characteristics associated with Down syndrome.

This congenital disorder occurs about once in every 1,000 births and is the most common cause of birth defects. There is a relationship between Down syndrome and women having children later in life. However, children with Down syndrome can also be born to younger mothers.

Persons with Down syndrome have a characteristic appearance (Figure 33-19). The head is smaller than is typical and is abnormally shaped. The inner corner of each eye is rounded instead of pointed. The eyes have a slight upward slant. You may see white spots on the iris. Most children with Down syndrome need glasses. Cataracts are common. The ears are small and sit low on the sides of the head. The nose is slightly flat. Physical development is often slow, and their stature is small. Down syndrome symptoms vary from person to person and can range from mild to severe.

Common problems include:

- Impulsive behavior
- Poor judgment
- Short attention span
- Slow learning
- Frustration and anger due to awareness of their limitations

Other Conditions

Other conditions that cause intellectual and developmental disabilities are listed in Table 33-10.

Caring for Persons with an Intellectual Disability or a Developmental Disability

Children and young adults with mental and physical problems often need the skills of an occupational therapist. Some need special teachers, but many go to regular schools. Those with highly special needs may have to go to a special school. Remember that some individuals

TABLE 33-10 Other Conditions That Cause Intellectual or Developmental Disabilities

Condition	Summary
Fetal alcohol syndrome	Fetal alcohol syndrome (FAS) develops when a pregnant woman drinks alcohol. The developing fetus also drinks and metabolizes alcohol more slowly than the mother, resulting in higher levels of alcohol concentration. In addition to intellectual disability, facial abnormalities may be present, such as small eyelid openings, short nose, and flat face. The person may have poor coordination, poor growth, hyperactive behavior, and developmental disabilities.
Fragile X	A genetic disorder caused by mutation in the RNA of the X-chromosome. It is the most commonly known cause of inherited developmental disability worldwide. Physical features are not always present, but if they are the affected child has prominent ears and a high forehead. The face becomes longer after puberty. Ear infections are common and there is an increased risk of epilepsy (seizures), squinting, hernia, and joint dislocations. Intellectual disability occurs in 80% of males and 65% of females. The person may have delays in speech, movement, and coordination. Attention deficit disorders and features of autism are common.
Hydrocephalus	Hydrocephalus has a number of causes that may be congenital or acquired. Loosely translated, *hydrocephalus* means "water on the brain." The extra fluid applies pressure, increasing the risk of brain damage. This section describes congenital hydrocephalus, which is present at birth and may be caused by problems during fetal development or genetic abnormalities. The head of an infant with this condition will expand markedly. Adults may develop normal pressure hydrocephalus, which will cause the person to have problems walking, impaired bladder control leading to urinary frequency and/or incontinence, progressive mental impairment, and dementia.
Spina bifida	Spina bifida is caused by the failure of the spine to close completely during the first month of pregnancy (Figure 33-20). Depending on the level of the lesion, the infant may be born with paralysis, hydrocephalus, learning disabilities, and/or swallowing problems. As you will recall, developmental disabilities are conditions that become apparent before age 22. These conditions are chronic and alter or delay development of normal life skills. Spina bifida meets these criteria, but persons with this condition are the least likely to have problems with speech and cognition. Some have a learning disability, but others are of normal intelligence. Persons with spina bifida are likely to be paraplegics with bowel and bladder incontinence. They may use wheelchairs or other ambulatory aids, depending on the severity of the injury. The prevalence of this condition is estimated to be approximately 1 in 2,000. However, the prevalence is higher in Kentucky due to folic acid deficiencies and hereditary factors.

with disabilities have typical or above-average intelligence. Respect their intelligence and allow them to direct their care. Treat them in an age-appropriate manner.

Total independence may not be possible. Some will need help with activities of daily living throughout their lives. Care is designed to promote the highest degree of independence possible, enhance self-esteem, and provide the highest quality of life possible. Nursing assistant care for the person with intellectual or developmental disability includes:

- Ensuring a safe environment and teaching safety
- Allowing the person to direct care, if able
- Encouraging the person to make choices
- Providing information in a slow, simple manner
- Promoting self-esteem
- Learning the person's interests
- Creating opportunities for success
- Building on and developing the person's strengths
- Being patient and repeating simple instructions when needed
- Assisting and supervising the person with activities of daily living
- Using praise and rewards liberally
- Smiling and showing support and affection (as appropriate)

Break large tasks into small pieces. Give specific instructions. A demonstration may be more effective than verbal instructions. Provide immediate feedback. Provide opportunities for practice (Figure 33-21). Recognize that you can make a difference in the person's life! Emphasize their strengths and interests. Create opportunities for success.

The Americans with Disabilities Act of 1990 was passed to improve access to health care, guaranteeing access to education, employment, transportation, and public services to persons with disabilities. Health care workers are responsible for protecting the rights of persons with physical, mental, and developmental disabilities.

Important Medical Issues

Four major health issues that are more common in people with developmental disabilities than in the general population are sometimes called the "fatal four" risks:

- Aspiration
- Dehydration
- Constipation
- Seizures

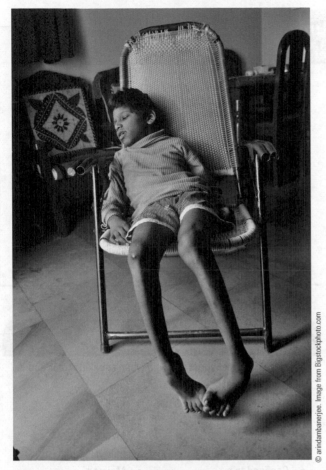

FIGURE 33-20 This child has cerebral palsy which has caused paralysis below the waist. There are contractures of both knees and deformities of the feet which limits the ability to wear shoes.

© arindambanerjee. Image from Bigstockphoto.com

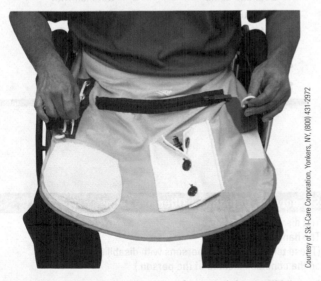

FIGURE 33-21 This is an example of an activity apron that teaches dressing skills with a zipper and buttons. This type of device is helpful to improve cognitive function, finger dexterity, and hand–eye coordination.

Courtesy of Ski I-Care Corporation, Yonkers, NY, (800) 431-2972

 Safety ALERT

Many persons with have seizures. These are unpredictable and occur suddenly. The person is at high risk of injury and aspiration.

All four conditions can lead to severe morbidity and even death. **Morbidity** is the incidence or rate at which an illness or abnormality occurs in a given population. The signs and symptoms of these problems may be hard to identify. Some individuals cannot communicate the problem. Careful monitoring and reporting are essential.

You will find additional information about communicating with persons who have mental health problems and other special needs in Chapters 7 and 30 of this book.

Pica

Some persons with developmental disabilities have a condition called **pica**, in which the person eats nonfood items. Although there are many theories about the cause of pica, the reason is not known. Many risks are associated with this practice, including:

- Aspiration and choking
- Poisoning
- Bowel perforation or obstruction
- Dental injuries
- Parasitic infection

Prevention is the best practice. Some persons are predictable and eat only certain items, but others eat random small items in the environment. Keep small nonfood and all potentially harmful and toxic items out of the room and out of reach. Carefully monitor the person and the environment. Follow the plan of care. Notify the nurse right away if you suspect that a person has swallowed a nonfood item.

Communication

Caring for persons with developmental disabilities is very similar to caring for persons with cognitive impairment and dementia. Some are very high functioning. Good communication skills are important. Many of these individuals thrive on acceptance and attention. Most are happy and loving. Treat them with dignity and respect. Help them express themselves and relieve stress. Let them make simple choices, but avoid overwhelming them with too many options. They usually respond well to consistent treatment. Use the

GUIDELINES 33-3 Guidelines for Communicating with Persons Who Have Developmental Disabilities

- Keep your words and sentences short and simple.
- Give clear, concise instructions.
- Do not "talk down" to the person. Treat adults as adults.
- Do not make assumptions and do not talk over a person. If you have a question, ask!
- Listen to what the person says. They probably know more than you think.
- People who have intellectual disability are very sensitive to the moods of others. If you are upset, they will

be too. If you are happy and relaxed, they will be too. Ask yourself how you look to them.
- If making decisions is upsetting to the person, limit choices to two.
- If you notice the person becoming frustrated, slow down. Do not push.
- Praise and compliment the person for even small accomplishments.
- Treat people who have developmental disabilities with the same respect that you would give others.

care plan to ensure consistent care. They like to help and feel like they are contributing. It is important to make them feel worthwhile. Avoid pressuring them to learn things or perform new tasks unless those things are on the care plan. They can learn, but it takes a long time and teaching requires great patience. They do not function well in high-pressure situations, and may not function well in large, loud, confusing groups unless someone is there to support them. They know if others are making fun of them, and feel hurt and rejection.

People-First Language

People with the conditions discussed in this chapter have *disabilities*. Nursing assistants must avoid stereotypes and use language that emphasizes the value, individuality, and capabilities of each person. People-first language focuses on the person rather than the disability. Think before you speak. The people-first language in Table 33-11 should be part of your vocabulary.

Communication ALERT

The following are words to *avoid* when speaking to or about persons with disabilities:

- Abnormal
- Afflicted
- Burden
- Cerebral palsied
- Confined to a wheelchair
- Courageous
- Cripple
- Crippled
- Deaf and dumb
- Deaf mute
- Defect
- Defective
- Deformity
- Diseased
- Epileptic
- Gimp
- Invalid
- Imbecile
- Maimed
- Moron
- Palsied
- Poor
- Spastic
- Stricken with
- Sufferer
- Suffers with
- Suffering
- Unfortunate
- Victim

TABLE 33-11 People-First Language

People-First Language	Stereotypes, Derogatory, Offensive Terms
Person with a disability (This focuses on the person, not the condition)	The disabled The handicapped (These terms categorize persons with disabilities and focus on the condition instead of the person.)
People with intellectual disability Person with cognitive impairment	Retard, MR The retarded Retarded people Slow, stupid, dumb

(continues)

TABLE 33-11 *(continued)*

People-First Language	Stereotypes, Derogatory, Offensive Terms
Person with Down syndrome	Mongoloid Mongol Down's kid
Person with autism	The autistic
Person with mental illness	The mentally ill, maniac, demented
Person with a learning disability	The learning disabled Suffers from a learning disability
Person with hearing loss Person who is Deaf Person who is hard of hearing	The deaf The hard of hearing
Person who is deaf and cannot speak Person with a speech disorder Person who uses a communication device Person who uses synthetic speech	Deaf and dumb Mute
Person with a visual impairment Person with blindness	The blind
Person who is deaf and blind	The deaf and blind (or deaf, dumb, and blind)
Person with epilepsy Person with seizure disorder	The epileptic Victim of epilepsy Has fits
Person with a mobility impairment Person who uses a wheelchair	Crippled, crip Confined to a wheelchair Gimp Wheelchair-bound
Person with quadriplegia Person with paraplegia Person with paralysis	Quadriplegic, quad Paraplegic The paralyzed
Person who is small	Dwarf Midget
Person with a congenital disability	They have a birth defect
Person *without* disabilities	Normal person Healthy person Typical kid
Older persons Elderly individuals	Old, old age The elderly Senior citizens
Person with	Victim of Suffers with/from
Person with an emotional instability Person with mental illness	Crazy, insane, nuts, psycho
Accessible bathrooms, buses, etc.	Handicap, handicapped bathrooms, buses, etc.
Reserved parking for people with disabilities	Handicapped parking
Long-term care facility Nursing facility	Nursing home Old folks' home Rest home

REVIEW

A. True/False

Mark the following true or false by circling T or F.

1. T F Cerebral palsy is a motor control disorder.

2. T F The current trend in health care is to place lower-functioning persons with intellectual disabilities in skilled nursing facilities.

3. T F Persons with cognitive impairment have poor safety judgment.

4. T F Older adults may not be aware of their need for fluids.

5. T F Prions are the most common cause of dementia.

6. T F Persons with a developmental disability have an intellectual disability.

7. T F Cognitive impairment is a normal change that comes with aging.

8. T F Intellectual disability develops before age 25.

9. T F Elderly persons need more calories than younger individuals do.

10. T F Traumatic brain injury is a congenital condition.

11. T F Elderly persons are not interested in spirituality.

12. T F Perseveration phenomena involves using vulgar words.

13. T F Fetal alcohol syndrome is an acquired developmental disability.

14. T F A catastrophic reaction always occurs in response to boredom.

15. T F Persons with stage III Alzheimer's usually have a good appetite.

16. T F Stroking a dog or cat can reduce a person's blood pressure.

17. T F Some persons with cerebral palsy have above-average intelligence.

18. T F New-onset or worsening confusion may be a sign of illness in an elderly person.

19. T F Infections are easily identified in elderly persons.

20. T F An intellectual disability is a developmental disability.

B. Multiple Choice

Select the one best answer for each of the following.

21. Residents in assisted living facilities:
  a. need 24-hour nursing care.
  b. require supervision with ADLs.
  c. need skilled rehabilitation.
  d. have mental health needs.

22. A resident with dementia tells you they are going home to prepare dinner for their children, and then proceeds to go toward the front door. Your best response is to walk with them and say:
  a. "Don't go outside. The children aren't hungry."
  b. "Your children live in another state."
  c. "Stay inside. What do you like to cook?"
  d. "Your children are spending the night at a friend's house."

23. Sensory changes that occur with aging include all of the following *except*:
  a. smell and taste buds become less sensitive.
  b. reduced tear production causes dry, itchy eyes.
  c. side vision and depth perception diminish.
  d. clouding of the lens of the eye is less common.

24. Dementia is:
  a. a symptom, not a disease.
  b. the result of mental illness.
  c. a temporary condition.
  d. a physical illness.

25. An example of the art of nursing is:
  a. efficiency and technical skill.
  b. accurate reporting.
  c. caring and compassion.
  d. good organization.

26. Alzheimer disease is:
  a. common in middle-aged adults.
  b. a progressive condition.
  c. a temporary genetic disorder.
  d. easily cured with medication.

27. A person in the first stage of Alzheimer disease:

    a. will not recognize their relatives.

    b. will have seizures and weight loss.

    c. will display perseveration phenomena.

    d. may try to cover up the memory loss.

28. A characteristic of the nursing assistant that is especially important while caring for older adults is:

    a. logical reasoning ability.

    b. kindness.

    c. technical skill.

    d. advanced certification.

29. A whirlpool bath:

    a. is soothing and refreshing to a person with Alzheimer disease.

    b. is the preferred method of bathing persons with dementia.

    c. may frighten some individuals with Alzheimer disease.

    d. will increase confusion because of the high water temperature.

30. When caring for a person who disrobes frequently:

    a. put the clothes on backward, making them hard to remove.

    b. turn the air conditioner up so the person is too cold to disrobe.

    c. evaluate the environmental temperature to see if it is too warm.

    d. tie a sheet to the rails to keep the person in bed to prevent exposure.

31. Residents who are at risk of dehydration:

    a. drink six cups of fluid each day.

    b. are always confused.

    c. have straw-colored urine.

    d. may have difficulty holding a cup.

32. The Americans with Disabilities Act of 1990:

    a. limits what health care workers can do.

    b. guarantees access to health care services.

    c. applies only to persons with physical disabilities.

    d. limits out-of-pocket expenses for health care.

33. A person with Alzheimer disease who wanders is probably:

    a. looking for a state of mind.

    b. trying to find their family.

    c. looking for their clothing.

    d. trying to go home.

34. Treat persons with developmental disabilities:

    a. in an age-appropriate manner.

    b. like infants and small children.

    c. by limiting the need for them to make decisions.

    d. by providing total care.

35. OBRA regulations:

    a. are guidelines that all hospitals follow.

    b. mandate "aging in place."

    c. require facilities to maintain or improve residents.

    d. do not apply to nursing assistants.

36. Delirium:

    a. is unavoidable in persons with dementia.

    b. is caused by acute illness and can be reversed.

    c. is a sign that a person's condition has improved.

    d. cannot be identified in persons with dementia.

37. A developmental disability first occurs before age:

    a. 2.

    b. 15.

    c. 21.

    d. 22.

38. Malnutrition:

    a. is a risk to residents of long-term care facilities.

    b. is a chronic condition in most elderly individuals.

    c. occurs in residents who skip occasional meals.

    d. only occurs in persons on medically restricted diets.

39. Pica is:

    a. a complication of Down syndrome.

    b. a developmental disability.

    c. a common form of autism.

    d. an urge to eat nonfood items.

40. Persons with Down syndrome have:

    a. deformed chromosomes.

    b. 47 chromosomes.

    c. a high forehead.

    d. long arms.

41. Validation therapy:

    a. reinforces the date and time.

    b. acknowledges the person's feelings.

    c. orients the person to reality.

    d. reinforces the person's delusions.

42. The "fatal four" risks to persons with developmental disability include:

    a. constipation.

    b. influenza.

    c. pneumonia.

    d. brain damage.

C. Completion

Complete the statements in items 43–53 by writing the correct word from the following list.

brain	inflammatory response
confusion	medical problem
diverticulitis	mental status
handwashing	nutrition
heart	support system
infection	

43. Residents need a _____ or mechanism for dealing with loss or coping with problems.

44. The _____ consumes more energy than any other organ in the body.

45. The _____ may not work as efficiently in aging.

46. To prevent _____, which is an inflammation of the bowel, avoid eating skins and seeds.

47. Poor _____ is associated with infections, pressure injuries, poor healing, anemia, low blood pressure, confusion, and hip fractures.

48. Effective and frequent _____ is the best method of preventing the spread of disease.

49. Aging changes cause older people to be at higher risk for _____.

50. Elderly persons do not readily develop signs of _____.

51. Changes in the urine, incontinence, and _____ in people who are not usually disoriented are often signs of infection.

52. A change in _____ is a very important observation.

53. Incontinence is a _____, not a normal change with aging.

D. Nursing Assistant Challenge

You are assigned to care for Mr. Wardlaw. He is in the second stage of Alzheimer disease, and keeps setting off the door alarm. He says he must go rewire his house so it does not burn down. Your unit is very busy. To make matters worse, you are short one nursing assistant, and you fear Mr. Wardlaw will elope.

54. What is your best immediate response to keep Mr. Wardlaw in the building?

_____

_____

55. Should restraints be used to keep this person safe?

_____

_____

56. How will you reduce Mr. Wardlaw's agitation?

_____

_____

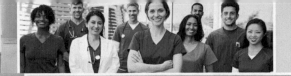

The Organization of Home Care: Trends in Health Care

OBJECTIVES

After completing this chapter, you will be able to:

34.1 Spell and define terms.

34.2 Briefly outline the history of home care.

34.3 Describe the types of nursing services that are provided in the home.

34.4 Describe the benefits of working in home care.

34.5 List the qualifications for working as a nursing assistant in home care.

34.6 Identify members of the home health team.

34.7 State the purpose of the case manager.

34.8 State the purpose of the Outcome and Assessment Information Set (OASIS).

34.9 List guidelines for avoiding liability while working as a home health assistant.

34.10 Describe the types of information a home health assistant must be able to document.

34.11 Identify several time management techniques.

34.12 List ways in which the home health assistant can work successfully with client's families.

VOCABULARY

Learn the meaning and the correct spelling of the following words and phrases:

case manager
client care records
custodial care

intermittent care
Outcome and Assessment
Information Set (OASIS)

skilled home health nursing care
time/travel records

INTRODUCTION

The health care of persons (*clients*) in their own homes is an age-old tradition. It was not until the middle of the twentieth century that there was a massive trend to move patient care out of the home and into the community health care facility. The late nineteenth century saw the growth of medical schools and the licensing of physicians. Schools of nursing soon followed. Hospital staffing slots were filled with students enrolled in these programs. Although the permissive laws of the early 1900s listed rules for nursing licensure, the laws did not restrict nursing practice. There were few legal restrictions on people who provided care in private homes. Almost anyone could hire out to provide such care. A few years later, laws were passed to control nurses' education. These laws specified what a nurse could and could not do. Anyone practicing nursing without a license could be held liable.

World War II brought with it:

- A gradual increase in the need for more technical care, as procedures and equipment became more complex.

- Introduction of antibiotics and better techniques of infection control. (Initially the supply of antibiotics was very limited and most were reserved for use in treating military service members.)

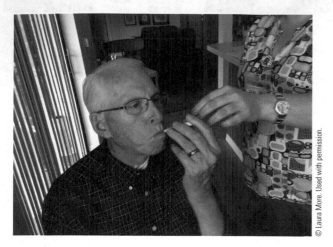

FIGURE 34-1 This client is recovering at home after surgery and is being assessed by a home health care nurse.

- Growth of a new type of worker (nursing assistant) to help provide nursing care.
- Construction of many new health care facilities.
- Hospital care of sick people.

Today, the pendulum has swung back once more toward treating only acutely ill people in hospitals and providing alternative care (such as home care, day care, or long-term care) for all others (Figure 34-1). Factors that foster this interest in home care include:

- Expensive high-technology treatments and equipments
- Introduction of diagnosis-related groups (DRGs), resulting in earlier discharge from hospitals
- Growing population of chronically ill people
- Difficulty finding and hiring licensed nurses
- The establishment of hospice care, enabling people with terminal illnesses to receive care at home during their last months of life
- The preference of the health care consumer to remain at home if possible

PROVIDERS OF HOME HEALTH CARE

Home health is one of the fastest-growing types of health care. Because of the increasing demand for home care, there are many different types of home care providers:

- Government-sponsored agencies controlled by city or county governments
- Private agencies; some are for profit and others are nonprofit
- Hospital-sponsored agencies
- Hospices

These providers employ several types of health care workers, including nurses, nursing assistants, therapists, and social workers. Nursing assistants may be called home health assistants, but the education program is the same for both in many states. There is no consistency in the classes that prepare workers for these positions. Each employer has personnel policies that regulate job descriptions, salaries, and benefits. The employer provides new employees with an orientation to the organization and to their responsibilities.

In addition to working in clients' homes, home care workers may also visit residents in assisted living facilities (ALFs). These facilities do not provide regular nursing services. Residents who become ill or injured may need temporary or short-term nursing care. Rather than moving them from the ALF to a facility that provides a higher level of care, home health care workers visit the resident to provide necessary services. Using home care workers in this manner promotes the aging in place philosophy of the ALF and enables residents to remain in a familiar environment while they recover.

TYPES OF HOME HEALTH CARE

Skilled home health nursing care is intermittent, medically necessary skilled care that is ordered by a physician and given by a nurse, physical therapist, occupational therapist, and/or speech-language pathologist. Care that can be given by nonprofessional staff is not considered skilled.

The skilled nursing service must be reasonable and necessary for the treatment of the illness or injury, individualized to the person, and meet accepted standards of care. It is given without regard to whether the illness or injury is acute, chronic, terminal, or expected to last a long time.

- Skilled home health nursing care is given to maintain or restore the person's maximum level of function and health. Recovery is desirable, but not required.
- Nursing care is not primarily for comfort or convenience.
- Home health care services are provided in lieu of a continued hospitalization, confinement in a skilled nursing facility (SNF), or receipt of outpatient services outside of the home.
- Skilled nursing home health care is appropriate for the active treatment of a condition, illness, disease, or injury to reduce the risk of complications.
- Hospice care (Chapters 32 and 35) may also be given in the home.

Custodial care involves providing services and supplies to assist a person with activities of daily living, such as bathing, eating, and mobility (Figure 34-2). It can be safely provided by persons who do not have the technical skills of a health care provider. It may also include routine activities such as using eye drops, using oxygen, and

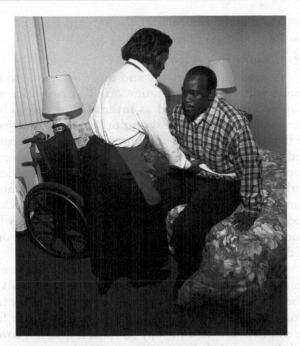

FIGURE 34-2 The home health care nursing assistant helps with activities of daily living, including bathing, eating, and ambulation.

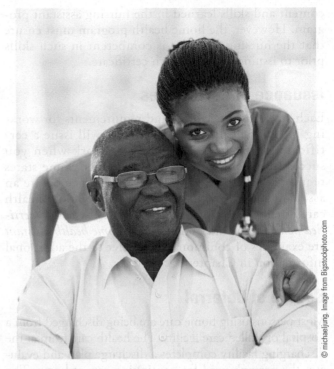

© michaeljung. Image from Bigstockphoto.com

FIGURE 34-3 Caring for the same client provides continuity and client satisfaction.

taking care of a colostomy or bladder catheter. State laws vary as to who can provide this care.

Some agencies provide homemaking, personal assistance, companion, and supportive care services to clients in their homes. The agency sends the worker to the home for a block of time. Most have a minimum number of hours for these services. Each agency sets its own qualifications for positions of this nature. As a rule, on-the-job training is all that is needed to work through a private agency. A companion may be required to complete a special class, testing, and certification if they plan to work for a state or federally funded facility or agency.

In most states, homemakers and companions cannot provide hands-on personal care. They assist with housekeeping, meal preparation, and transporting or accompanying clients to appointments. A few states permit homemakers, companions, and personal care assistants to help clients who have chronic and stable conditions with activities of daily living. In other states, only a qualified home health nursing assistant can provide this care.

BENEFITS OF WORKING IN HOME HEALTH CARE

Many career options are available to nursing assistants. One of these is working for an agency that provides home health care. There are advantages to working in such agencies:

- Satisfaction of giving complete care to one client at a time
- Satisfaction of caring for the same client over a period of time (Figure 34-3)

- Opportunity to work with greater independence and autonomy
- Part-time employment, if desired

The person working in home care must have dependable transportation to the homes of the clients. In small towns and rural areas, the worker needs to have a car to get from one client to the next. In larger cities, the worker may be able to use public transportation.

QUALIFICATIONS FOR WORKING AS A NURSING ASSISTANT IN HOME CARE

Each state sets its own requirements for nursing assistants working in home health care. There are no uniform national requirements other than the completion of a state-approved nursing assistant class. Home health–specific education requirements and the assistants' legal titles vary from state to state.

In some states, home health agencies and hospices are required to establish policies on employee qualifications and home health care education. The registered or certified home health nursing assistant may work independently in home health care if the assistant is competent in their responsibilities and successfully completes an approved competency evaluation. A certified nursing assistant must complete only the home health portion of the program. They are is not required to repeat the content and skills learned in the nursing assistant program. However, the home health program must ensure that the nursing assistant is competent in such skills prior to issuing a home health certificate.

Issuance of Certificates

Each state has procedures and requirements for working in home health care. Your state will issue a certificate giving you permission to work when you successfully complete the requirements. Some states require at least a year of facility experience before an assistant may work in home care. The home health care nursing assistant's title also varies by state. *Certified home health aide* and *registered home health assistant* are examples of common titles. Refer to the additional information in Chapter 35.

Source of Referral

Most persons using home care are being discharged from a hospital or skilled care facility. The health care team at the discharging facility completes a discharge plan and evaluates the person's need for continuing care at home. The physician must then write an order for home health care. The discharge planner at the hospital or long-term care facility provides the client and family with a list of agencies from which to choose a home care provider (Figure 34-4). (In some areas of the country, only one agency may be available.) The selected agency is given medical information about the client and then begins to plan care.

PAYMENT FOR HOME HEALTH CARE

Home health care may be paid for by:
- Medicare, for persons over 65 years of age or for those who have had a disability for two or more years. Most home health care is paid for under the Part A Medicare benefit.

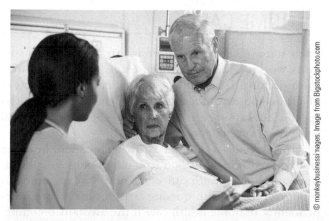

FIGURE 34-4 A patient and family may select an agency for home care before being discharged from the hospital.

- Medicaid (in some states).
- Private insurance companies.
- Client's personal funds.

Government programs and most insurance companies will only pay for home care if it is considered "skilled" and is provided as **intermittent care**. This means that the nursing assistant or other caregiver goes to the home, performs certain procedures or treatments, and then leaves. Clients who need a caregiver for several hours a day will probably have to pay for the services with their own money. Because this is very costly, most home care is given on an intermittent basis. Medicare does not pay for custodial care. This type of care may be paid for by some insurance policies, but most is paid out of the client's pocket.

Clients who are members of an HMO must use a home health agency that is affiliated with the HMO. The Medicare program and insurance companies pay for most home health care. However, Medicare pays only for intermittent care and therapy services; it does not cover full-time care. This is a maximum of 28 hours per week of skilled nursing and home health aide care combined. To qualify for payment, a home health agency must be approved by the Medicare program. This means that surveyors will regularly inspect the agency to ensure that it meets quality standards. The client's doctor must have approved the need for home health care, and must prepare a plan of care to be delivered in the client's home.

Medicare does not pay for home health aide care unless the client is also getting skilled care such as nursing or therapy. In special situations, skilled nursing and home health aide services can be provided for up to a combined total of 8 hours a day, 7 days a week, for several weeks. Likewise, the weekly limit for care may be increased to 35 hours, but these exceptions are for a limited, predictable period of time only. A reduced level of care may be provided (and paid for) after that.

The client must be homebound. A home can be a house or apartment, a relative's home, or an assisted living facility. Facilities that mainly provide skilled nursing or rehabilitation services do not qualify. Absences from home must be infrequent, or of short duration, or to get medical care. A client can be considered homebound even if they occasionally go to the barber or beauty shop or for a walk around the block or a short drive.

THE HOME HEALTH CARE TEAM

The home health care team consists of:
- The client (the person in need of care)
  - Are of various ages and need differing levels of nursing and physical care
  - May have chronic, progressive ailments

Clients receiving home care vary widely in age. They are not all elderly. Many are children with serious illnesses or disabilities. Some will need temporary care, but others will need lifetime care. The needs of some clients are complex, placing great demands on family caregivers. In many situations, hospice care is provided in the home. In this situation, the nursing assistant will help meet the end-of-life needs of the client and family. The scope of home health services ranges from assistance with ADLs to very complex therapy, wound care, infusion therapy, and chronic ambulatory peritoneal dialysis (CAPD).

Caregiving can be difficult for family members and loved ones. Having outside caregivers come to the home assists them to maintain the quality of their own lives, and gives them time to take care of their personal affairs.

- May be recovering from acute illness, surgery, or childbirth
- Needs assistance with activities of daily living
- Usually requires skilled service
- The client's family
- Various hospice workers
- The family
  - May act as alternate caregivers
  - May live in the client's home
  - May or may not be supportive of the client
- The nursing assistant
  - Provides direct client care (Figure 34-5)
  - Provides for the client's safety and comfort
  - Makes observations and reports them to the nurse
  - Documents observations and care that was given
- Supervising nurse or case manager
  - Completes periodic client assessments

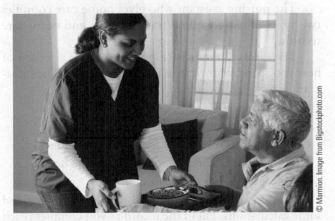

FIGURE 34-5 The home health assistant provides direct client care.

- Plans the care
- Teaches and supervises nursing assistants
- Coordinates care and members of the home care team
- Physician
  - Writes orders and acts as a consultant and guide
- Other specialists
  - Physical therapist
  - Occupational therapist
  - Speech therapist
  - Social worker
  - Dietitian

THE CASE MANAGER

The **case manager** is a registered nurse who coordinates the health care of each client. They use the nursing process to assess the client's health status, clinical needs, and treatment needs, and uses this information to plan, implement, coordinate, monitor, and evaluate care and the plan of care. The case manager schedules and coordinates nursing care with the services provided by other disciplines, and ensures that the level of care provided is appropriate.

Case managers help provide services as efficiently as possible. They work with the client and family to identify goals, needs, and resources. When the assessment is complete, the case manager and client will formulate a plan to meet these goals. The nurse will assist in finding resources and help the client connect with services. Occasionally the case manager advocates on behalf of a client to obtain other community services and help achieve a better quality of life. The case manager regularly communicates with the staff, client, and family to evaluate the plan of care and ensure that it is effective in meeting the client's goals. The case manager may also be responsible for providing health education, coaching, and treatment decision support, depending on client needs. They complete exhaustive paperwork on each client.

OUTCOME AND ASSESSMENT INFORMATION SET (OASIS)

The **Outcome and Assessment Information Set (OASIS)** is the Medicare data collection tool that the case manager must complete and transmit electronically to the government. The form is very time consuming to complete. However, it contains a great deal of information. It:

- Validates the client's need for skilled care
- Verifies that the agency has given quality care
- Measures client outcomes and promotes improved outcomes
- Serves as the foundation of the care plan
- Provides the basis for ongoing management

The Centers for Medicare & Medicaid Services (CMS) adopted the Home Health Care Initiative from the Institute of Medicine (IOM). The initiative is a model for quality care. The Home Health Care Initiative quality care domains are:

- Safety
- Effectiveness
- Client-centeredness
- Timeliness
- Efficiency
- Equity

They also promote:

- Better health by encouraging healthier lifestyles, increased physical activity, better nutrition, avoidance of behavioral risks, and widespread use of preventive care
- Lower costs by improving health, promoting preventive care, improving coordination of health care services, and reducing waste and inefficiencies

These efforts will reduce the national cost of health care and lower out-of-pocket expenses.

The Assessment Process

The case manager does an OASIS assessment of the client during the first visit. Other health care professionals assigned to the case also complete assessments. After the assessments are finished, the nurse and other team members:

- Identify the client's problems (Figure 34-6)
- Determine approaches to resolve the problems
- Establish goals for the client
- Evaluate the home situation for safety
- Determine the amount of time needed for each visit and the length of time the services may be required

The case manager discusses the plans with the client and develops the plan of care. They include the client's

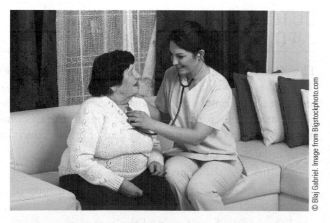

FIGURE 34-6 The nurse will assess the client on admission and initiate the plan of care with the client.

wishes as much as possible within the available payment plan. The case manager then develops the assignment for the nursing assistant. You may be assigned to care for several clients or a particular client for a:

- Specified number of hours daily
- Specified period two or three days per week
- Long-term period
- Brief period

The frequency of home health visits depends on physician orders and client needs. Although the case manager supervises and coordinates the care, visits, and schedule for their case load, some agencies have other nurses do many of the regular visits. This varies with agency policy and case load.

The doctor and home health agency personnel review the plan of care as often as necessary, but at least once every 62 days. Professional staff must notify the doctor promptly of any changes in condition that suggest a need to modify the plan of care.

LIABILITY AND THE NURSING ASSISTANT

You need to be aware of the responsibilities involved in home care and how to avoid legal problems associated with caregiving.

Recordkeeping

Be sure you know exactly what documentation you are expected to do, what types of records you should keep, and the forms you need to use. Many home health agencies use handheld tablets and electronic devices for documentation. Paper forms are seldom used anymore. All documentation must be accurate, complete, and up to date. Medicare and insurance companies frequently audit these records to decide whether to pay for the services.

The nursing assistant who gives home care compiles two types of records: time/travel records and client care records.

Time/travel records (Figure 34-7) are a record of how you spend your time in the client's home. The information recorded includes:

- Time of arrival
- Time of departure
- Length of time required for specific activities
- Travel time if working in more than one home
- Mileage or other transportation costs

Keeping a time/travel record requires accuracy and some calculations. Fill in the record as you complete each assignment. Do not wait until the end of the shift and then try to rely on your memory.

GUIDELINES 34-1 Guidelines for Avoiding Liability

- Be sure you are given a job description upon employment that lists your specific duties and responsibilities. In some areas, home health assistants are only allowed to do certain assigned tasks if they or the employing agency are working with an insurance company or Medicare. Auditors check the tasks assigned and confirm what is actually done in the client's home.

- Carry out procedures carefully and do them as you were taught.

- Notify your supervisor if you break something in a client's home.

- Always keep safety factors in mind and be on the lookout for possible hazards.

- Be familiar with the Client's Rights.

- Ask for assistance if you are assigned to do a procedure that you are not familiar with or have never performed before. Make sure the procedure is within the legal boundaries of nursing assistant practice.

- Follow the care plan. Do only those tasks that are assigned to you.

- Know how to contact the case manager for questions and issues related to the care of your client. Do not overstep your authority.

- Know how and when to contact emergency services for the client.

- Document your care and observations carefully and completely.

- Participate in care conferences with the other team members.

RIVERVIEW HOME HEALTH SERVICE
8987 Walkman Ave
Parkhurst, Nebraska
Time and Travel Log

CAREGIVER NAME Laura Siadto CNA   TITLE Home Health Assistant   EMPT. NO. 62718   DATE Aug. 29

CLIENT NAME/ADDRESS (Last, first)	SERVICE PROVIDED	VISIT CODE	NON-BILL CODE	TIME IN	TIME OUT	CLIENT CONTACT TIME	ODOMETER READING	MILES
Volheim, Eleonore	Bedbath, shampoo	4		8^{15}	9^{05}	50 min	From: 45,061 To: 45,068	7 miles
Jaronello, Sharri		1		9^{30}	9^{45}	15 min	From: 45,068 To: 45,083	15 miles
Doyle, Kindra	Enema, bedbath, amb	4		10^{10}	11^{30}	1 hr. 20 min.	From: 45,083 To: 46,001	18 miles
Hammond, Rachel	Ass't c colostomy cath care, bath, ROM	4		11^{50}	1^{20}	1 hr. 30 min.	From: 46,001 To: 46,017	16 miles
Minzey, Aimee		2		1^{30}	1^{35}	—	From: 46,017 To: 46,025	8 miles
Galloway, Rosa		5		1^{50}	2^{00}	10 min	From: 46,025 To: 46,028	3 miles
							From: To:	

Total Visits   6   Total Mileage   67   Parking Fees   —

Visit Code
1 IE Initial Eval & Rx   4 HC Home Care
2 FV Follow-up Visit   5 Hospital/Hospice
3 DV Discharge Visit   6 MC Maternal/Child

Supervising Nurse: Bruce Davenport R.N.

Nonbill Code
1. Refused Care
2. Patient Not Home
3. Non-Bill
4. Expired
5. Delivered Supplies

FIGURE 34-7 Example of a time/travel record.

Communication ALERT

Home health care workers spend many hours driving. Traveling 200 to 300 miles a day is not unusual in suburban and rural areas. Use your time productively by listening to audio books. These can be rented, purchased on CD, or downloaded in MP3 format. Some are free; many are inexpensive. You can also borrow them free from your public library. Reading for pleasure is something few people have time to do. Having books read to you when you are driving is enjoyable and makes the time go faster!

To compute mileage (round off to the nearest full mile):

- Record the car odometer reading before starting to your assignment.
- Record the odometer reading when you arrive at the client's home.
- Subtract the starting odometer reading from the arrival reading.
- Record this difference as the mileage.

For example, if the reading on your car odometer before starting was 45,061 and upon arrival at the client's home it is 45,068, the mileage should be recorded as 7 miles (45,068 − 45,061 = 7).

Client care records (Figure 34-8) are a record of:

- Care given, such as bathing, dressing, grooming, positioning, range-of-motion exercises, and ambulation
- Client responses to care
- Housekeeping tasks completed, if assigned to you by the case manager
- Observations:
  - Condition of skin
  - Vital signs
  - Elimination (bowel and urine)
  - Food and fluid intake
  - Appetite
  - Incidents such as client falls
  - Anything that indicates a change in the client's health status
  - Mental status: orientation, alertness, mood, and behavior

You may be expected to keep reports that cover a longer period of time. For example, you may need to keep a weekly or monthly record of daily blood sugar testing results for a client with diabetes. The physician may change the schedule of insulin based on your long-term report.

Agencies that use electronic documentation usually place your assignment and client care plan information so that you can access it on a handheld device. They require staff to transmit client care records to the office via a secure Internet connection soon after the visit. They also track your time in and out and the services you provide.

Legal ALERT

For your own protection and peace of mind, you should insure your vehicle. You should also check with your employer to find out about auto insurance if you are driving your own car to and from work, as well as to homes of various clients throughout the workday. You may be surprised to learn that the employer's insurance does not cover 100 percent of that time. For example, the policy does not cover you if you have an accident while traveling to or from work and your home. However, it may cover you if you have an accident during the course of your normal workday, when you are visiting clients' homes. Knowing exactly when your employer's insurance policy covers your automobile is important. You should also find out if you will be expected to transport clients in your personal vehicle. If so, investigate whether your insurance or the employer's insurance will cover the client if you are in an accident. Likewise, find out if you will be expected to drive the client's car. If so, you must learn whose insurance will be responsible in the event of an accident. Never drive the client in an uninsured vehicle. Do not drive the client's vehicle unless you are insured to do so.

Communication ALERT

In health care, things do not always go as planned. Be flexible. Although you plan your schedule each day, things happen. Your agency may call and ask you to see an extra person. A patient may take more time than usual. Delays will occur. Remain calm. Contact your patients and offer to reschedule. Be courteous of their time.

TIME MANAGEMENT

As a home health care assistant, you are responsible for planning your assignment and completing the client's care within a certain amount of time. You may have several clients to see during your shift. They will be expecting you at a specific time of day. You can take several actions to make the best use of your time:

- Be sure you have everything you will need for your assignments before you leave home. This might include a thermometer, watch with a second hand, stethoscope, blood pressure cuff, forms or a device for documenting, pen.
- Have a work plan in mind before you arrive at the client's home. For example, will you give the client a bath first or help them with their exercises first?
- Organize your supplies before you begin your assignment. Gather the linens, client clothing, and other items you will need.

RIVERVIEW HOME HEALTH SERVICE
8987 Walkman Ave
Parkhurst, Nebraska
Client Care Plan / Progress Notes

HOME HEALTH ASSISTANT   YOLANDA BROWN, CNA

CLIENT NAME   NICHOLAS FRENCH   CLIENT ID #   72824C

ADDRESS: 529 MAPLE AVE.   PARKHURST, NEBRASKA

ACTIVITY

0800	Arrived, Determined needs, planned activities Client seemed fatigued "Slept poorly". On nasal O_2 2.5L
0830	Circumoral pallor noted. Vital signs checked. Dyspneic on exertion.
0900	Put laundry into washing machine. Started breakfast. Client ate 1 sl. toast, 8 oz oatbran cereal / milk 6oz orange juice
0930	Prepared equipment for A.M. care – complete bath, shave and denture care.
1000	Asst to commode, soft brown formed stool.
1030	Made comfortable in easy chair. Reading newspaper. Nasal O_2 Cleaned kitchen including refrigerator
1100	Linen changed – dusted and dust mopped bedroom. Vacuumed living room.
1130	Prepared lunch.
1200	Client ate 1/2 chicken sandwich, 8 oz. tea, chocolate pudding, 8 oz. tomato soup.
1230	Client returned to bed for nap
1300	Cleaned lunch dishes and prepared salad, jello for evening meal
1330	Put washed laundry into dryer.
1400	Cleaned bathroom, washed kitchen floor
1430	Put bed linen into washer.
1500	Made out shopping list for A.M.
1530	Client awake. Assisted into living room. Watching T.V. Ordered O_2 tank replacement.
1600	Folded and put clean laundry away. Put washed linens in dryer.
1630	Client seems more rested. Color improved. Resp. easier. Notified supervisor of client's progress. Left client's home @ 3²⁵ P.M.

Y. Brown CNA

VITAL SIGNS	T	P	R	B/P
	97⁴	92	26	116/74
INTAKE	486 mL			
OUTPUT	730 mL			

SUP. SIGNATURE _____

FIGURE 34-8A Side 1 of the client care plan and nursing assistant record.

- Avoid being distracted by the family. You may need to discuss many things with the family, but you probably will not have time for lengthy conversations. If a family member asks you to do a task that makes you uncomfortable, call your supervisor for direction.
- Call your next client if you find you will be arriving later than expected.
- Avoid getting bogged down in tasks that you are not assigned to perform.

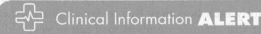
Clinical Information **ALERT**

Expect the unexpected and keep an open mind. Avoid judging people because of their environment. Accept that each person is different. Treat each client with respect and professionalism.

RIVERVIEW HOME HEALTH SERVICE
8987 Walkman Ave
Parkhurst, Nebraska
Client Care Plan / Progress Notes

WT. __146__ TEMP. __98__ BP __114/80__ P __70__ R __14__   MD CONTACT __C. Boylston__

HOMEBOUND DUE TO __Spinal Cord Injury – Paraplegia__   MEN. STATUS __Alert – Coherent__

PROBLEMS	INTERVENTIONS	TIME	PLAN	OUTCOME
① Potential altered	Maintain high-calorie, low-residue, high protein diet		Morning Care	Tol. Well
nutrition: less than	Reduce high calcium and gas-producing foods.	0700	Breakfast	ate entire meal
body requirements	Provide balanced meals and supplements morning and evening	0815	Commode	soft formed stool
		0900	Bath, Cath Care,	
		0945	ROM	
			up in wheelchair	Tolerated well
② Potential for disuse	Exercise to tolerance Avoid fatigue ROM	1030	6oz High Cal drink	
syndrome related to	Turn and reposition q 1 hr.	1045	Returned to Bed	
effects of immobility	Up in wheelchair B.I.D.	1130	Positioned on Rt. Side	
	Encourage self-care activities to tolerance		Positioned on Back	
③ Alteration in bowel	Stool Softener, Glycerine	1230	Lunch	½ tuna sand/tea
elimination: constipation	Suppositories, enemas, PRN.			
	Check for BM q 3 day		up in wheelchair	
		1330	Returned to Bed	
④ Potential for infection	Routine catheter care	1430	Positioned on left side	
related to indwelling	Change per routine schedule		Watching T.V.	
Foley catheter		1500		
⑤ Self-concept disturbance	Encourage verbalization of feelings and fears.			
related to effects of	Encourage independence. Be positive and reassuring.			
limitations				
DAILY SUMMARY				

Diet and supplements taken fairly well. Activity tolerated. Muscles soft but some tone. Soft formed stool.
Expressed frustration during transfers from bed to wheelchair. Enjoys reading and watching T.V.
Seems to be gaining some confidence in t ransfer activities.

Visit Date _____   Pt. Last Name,   Employee
Nursing Supervisor Report _____   First Initial __Mitchell, D.__   Signature __Ruthy Chek, CNA__

Joint Visit in Home _____   Patient's personal care and comfort measures by home assistant are:

Conference _____   superior _____ ; good _____ ; satisfactory _____ ; need improvement _____ ;

Services provided were appropriate _____ ; inappropriate _____ .

Comments

FIGURE 34-8B *(continued)* Side 2 of the image.

WORKING WITH FAMILIES

Clients may have a spouse or other family members who reside in the home. For other clients, their families may live elsewhere but stop in periodically. In some situations, family members may live so far away that they can seldom visit. Family members may call or visit while you are there, seeking information on the client's condition. It is best to let the client speak with them directly if possible. If the client cannot do this, then remember to be objective in your comments. If you do not know the answer to a question, be honest and say so rather than providing potentially incorrect information. Refer all medical questions to the physician or the case manager.

Remember that as a home health assistant, you are a guest of the family and client. You may be assigned to clients who have values and cultural beliefs that are vastly different from yours. It is not your role to try to change this. Report to your supervisor if you feel that family practices are harmful to the client's well-being and health. Families can be an excellent resource for you. They may be able to give you additional information about the client that will help you to give better care. This can avoid frustration for both you and the client. The family may also be able to tell you how they have cared for the client in the past.

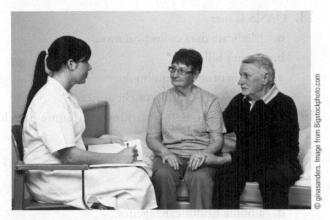

FIGURE 34-9 Demonstrate respect and hope when talking with home care clients.

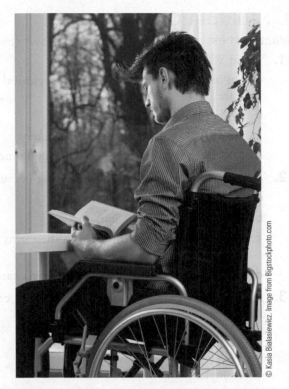

FIGURE 34-10 This home care client spends time reading and enjoying the tranquil environment outside of the home.

Tact and courtesy are important when communicating with the family. They may wish to be involved in the caregiving, but it is important that you complete the tasks to which you have been assigned. The family has a right to know the progress the client is making, but there may be some information that the client does not wish you to tell the family. You may need to discuss this issue with your supervisor. Families may feel overwhelmed and discouraged at times, particularly if the client has had a long illness. They need your support, so you must be realistic yet hopeful (Figure 34-9).

If you are spending an entire shift with the client, remember that you are getting paid to spend this time giving care. If all procedures are completed, take your cue from the client or family as to what activities you should complete for the rest of your tour of duty. Some clients may wish to be left alone to read (Figure 34-10) or watch television. Others may seek your companionship for visiting or playing cards. If you are working through the night, ask the client or family if you may read or do quiet

activities such as needlework while the client is sleeping. Family members may ask you to do something that is not part of your assignment. Whether you can meet their request depends on:

- The nature of the request
- The time involved in filling the request
- The policies of the home care agency
- Whether you are assigned to intermittent visits to the client or assigned to work a full shift

REVIEW

A. True/False

Mark the following true or false by circling T or F.

1. T F   World War I stimulated the enrollment of students in hospital-based nursing programs.

2. T F   Many new hospitals were built after World War II.

3. T F   Only nurses and nursing assistants are employed in home health care.

4. T F   The physician acts as care coordinator for the client's home care.

5. T F   Home health assistants are expected to provide direct client care.

6. T F   Documentation is an important responsibility of the home care assistant.

7. T F   The demand for home care has decreased within the past few years.

8. T F   The client may receive the services of a physical therapist.

9. T F   The home health care assistant may have the opportunity for part-time employment.

10. **T** F   The home health assistant is responsible for completing periodic assessments of the client.

B. Multiple Choice

Select the best answer for each of the following.

11. World War II brought about:
    a. an increase in the need for more technical care.
    b. widespread use of antibiotics.
    c. a limited supply of health care workers.
    d. construction of hundreds of nursing homes.

12. The demand for home care is increasing because:
    a. hospitals are overcrowded.
    b. there are fewer physicians.
    c. people prefer being cared for in their own homes.
    d. families always do some of the nursing care.

13. The person receiving home health care is called the:
    a. client.
    b. patient.
    c. resident.
    d. recipient.

14. Members of the home care team include:
    a. housekeepers.
    b. the family.
    c. laundry workers.
    d. gardeners.

15. Time management is important because:
    a. you can get home earlier.
    b. you may have more than one client to care for during your shift.
    c. the client may have other business to tend to.
    d. the agency will make more money if you work faster.

16. Home care assistants must be able to:
    a. know how to care for family pets.
    b. make accurate observations.
    c. manage the household bills.
    d. drive the client's car.

17. The case manager:
    a. is a social worker who coordinates the care of each client.
    b. uses the nursing process to meet the clients' care needs.
    c. does all of the assessments and directs other team members.
    d. coordinates the paperwork and is not involved in client care.

18. OASIS is the:
    a. Medicare data collection tool.
    b. client's bill.
    c. case manager's handbook.
    d. doctor's verification of client need.

19. The qualifications for working as a home health assistant are established by:
    a. the federal government.
    b. the school you attend.
    c. the state of residence.
    d. a home health care agency.

20. The home health assistant avoids liability by:
    a. documenting care and observations carefully.
    b. allowing family to determine care routines.
    c. informing the client to do what works best for you.
    d. using public transportation when going to work.

21. A home health assistant documents all of the following daily except:
    a. name of physician.
    b. care given to the client.
    c. name of family contact.
    d. information family gives you.

22. The home health assistant works best with client families by:
    a. organizing the household each day.
    b. being clear that you are in charge.
    c. acting as a guest in their home.
    d. telling them exactly what to do.

C. Nursing Assistant Challenge

23. You are almost finished with your nursing assistant course and are thinking about employment. You have been offered jobs at a home health agency and at a hospital and are having trouble making a decision. Your instructor advises you to think about both the advantages and disadvantages of working for each type of employer. Make a two-column list for each employer, labeling the columns "advantages" and "disadvantages." Fill in the columns for each.

_____ _____

_____ _____

_____ _____

_____ _____

_____ _____

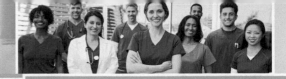

CHAPTER 35

The Nursing Assistant in Home Care

OBJECTIVES

After completing this chapter, you will be able to:

35.1 Spell and define terms.

35.2 Summarize the four levels of hospice care.

35.3 Define core values and explain why they are important.

35.4 Describe the characteristics that are especially important to the nursing assistant who provides home care.

35.5 List at least 10 methods of protecting your personal safety when working as a home care assistant in the community.

35.6 Describe the duties of the nursing assistant who works in the home setting.

35.7 Describe appropriate circumstances for assisting clients with medications and list the "Six Rights" of medication administration.

35.8 Describe the duties of the homemaker assistant.

35.9 Explain how to carry out home care activities needed to maintain a safe and clean environment.

VOCABULARY

Learn the meaning and the correct spelling of the following words and phrases:

core values
home health assistant

homemaker aide
homemaker assistant

respite care

THE HOME HEALTH CAREGIVER

In Chapter 34 you learned about the structure of home health care. In this chapter you will learn more about the responsibilities of the nursing assistant (home health assistant) who works in the client's home.

The nursing assistant is an important part of the health team in the acute hospital setting and in the long-term care facility. The nursing assistant is part of an equally important team that provides home care (Figure 35-1).

The nursing assistant may be called:

- **Home health assistant**, home health nursing assistant, home health care nursing assistant, or home health aide, whose primary role is to provide assistance with nursing care.
- **Homemaker assistant** or **homemaker aide** when the primary role is to do housekeeping chores. The homemaker assistant carries out general household tasks, prepares meals, and runs errands such as food shopping.

The nursing assistant providing health care services may be asked to carry out homemaker assistant duties in some cases.

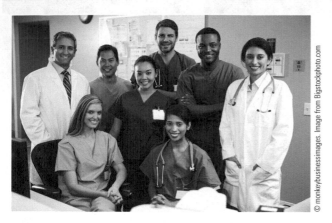

© monkeybusinessimages. Image from Bigstockphoto.com

FIGURE 35-1 The interdisciplinary home health care team.

Preparation and Qualifications

Home health care nursing assistants must meet the requirements set by the home state. These are not uniform. Each state has its own requirements for education and job preparation. Some states require completion of a specific home health curriculum. Others require a combination of certified nursing assistant education and on-the-job experience. Those who work for agencies that accept federal funds must receive a minimum of 75 hours of education. Some states require that the person have at least one year of facility experience before being allowed to work in a home without direct supervision.

Certificate programs enable students to meet state requirements. After successfully completing the program and passing a competency exam, the assistant can seek employment. Home health assistants must have a minimum of 16 hours of education before working with clients. As a rule, the assistant must work regularly in home health care to keep their certificate active. In most states, the certificate will expire if the assistant does not work for a period of 24 months.

Certification

Certification is a state-specific issue. Completing a certificate program in your state does not guarantee certification. Check with your state regulatory agency for additional information. Home health care nursing assistants can seek voluntary certification through the National Association for Home Care and Hospice (NAHC) by completing a minimum of 75 hours of education, passing a skills exam, and passing a written test. Passing the certification test may expand your opportunities and open doors. For information, refer to http://www.nahc.org/.

Other Levels of Care

Some states have several different levels of home care workers. The responsibilities vary with the level of education and experience. Workers can usually upgrade their skills from one level to the next, if desired. In some states, nursing assistants and others with similar education will qualify to work in home health by passing the home health competency exam. Some employers have additional requirements for employment, such as requiring CPR certification or a food handler's certificate.

HOSPICE CARE

The principles of hospice care were described in Chapter 32. Hospice care can be provided in various settings and is common in home health care. Medicare is the primary payer of hospice care in the United States. Medicare has four levels of hospice care. A person can be admitted to any level of care that meets their needs. If the person's condition and care needs change, they may be transferred between levels of care as often as necessary.

Routine Care

Most people are admitted to hospice at the routine home care level. If a person lives in a nursing facility, this level of care is called routine nursing home care. It includes:

- Nursing care—a nurse usually visits 1–3 times per week or more often, if needed
- Home health assistant services—a home health care nursing assistant visits two or three times per week, as needed.
- Social services, as needed.
- Physician services (vary with setting and need) —may include attending physician, following physician, hospice physician, medical director, and specialists.
- Counseling services (pastoral, spiritual, bereavement, and others as necessary).
- Dietitian consultation, if needed.
- Medications.
- Medical equipment.
- Medical supplies.
- Lab and diagnostic studies related to terminal diagnosis and medication management.
- Therapy services (physical, occupation, speech), if needed.
- Respiratory therapy services, if oxygen is needed.

Continuous Care

Continuous care may be given for a short period of time if the client cannot be readily managed. This is a higher level of care that is given on a short-term basis. A nurse or home health assistant will care for the client from 8 to 24 hours per day until problems are controlled. The need for this level of care is evaluated every 24 hours.

Inpatient Care

The qualifying criteria for continuous care are the same as those for inpatient care. The difference is that clients needing inpatient care are too unstable to be managed in the home. This situation must be managed through the hospice because clients who accept Medicare hospice care agree to give up their Part A medical benefits, which pay for hospital care. When coordinated through hospice, inpatient care can be given by hospice personnel in their own home, in a free-standing hospice, a hospital, or a long-term care facility. The need for this level of care is also evaluated every 24 hours. Once stabilized, the person is discharged back to the home.

Respite Care

Caring for a family member 24 hours a day is a difficult job. There are various models of respite care, depending on the situation. However, Medicare-approved **respite care** for a hospice recipient is short-term, time-limited, temporary care that enables an unpaid family member to take a break. It is given when the client's full-time family caregiver needs some personal time or temporarily cannot meet the client's needs. In this situation, the client may be transferred to an inpatient setting for up to a five-day period, then returned home.

Philosophy of Care

Hospice is a philosophy of care. It is not a location where one goes to die. Hospice care emphasizes comfort instead of cure. It enables clients to live out their remaining time with the support of loved ones and compassionate caregivers.

THE HOME HEALTH ASSISTANT AND THE NURSING PROCESS

You are part of the nursing process. During:

- *Assessment*, your observations and careful reporting can make a valuable contribution to the objective and subjective data from which the nursing analysis of the client's needs is made (Figure 35-2). Assessment is only done by an RN. Practical/vocational nurses and nursing assistants make important contributions to the assessment by noting:
  - Vital signs at each visit
  - The client's response to your care
  - The interactions between family members and friends that could cause the client to feel stressed
  - Support services that may be needed
  - Elimination, such as bowel activity and fluid intake and output
- *Planning*, you contribute as you actively provide information for care conferences (Figure 35-3).

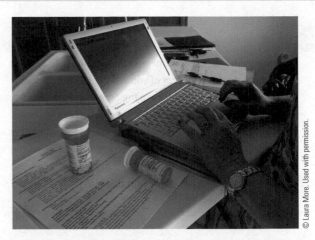

FIGURE 35-2 The home health nurse updates the client medical record and enters new information after every visit.

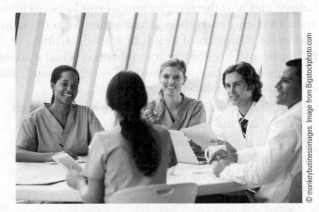

FIGURE 35-3 The home health nursing assistant contributes during care conferences.

- *Implementation*, you spend more time with clients than other workers, so you have an important responsibility for seeing that the plan of care is carried out.
  - Report any difficulties in carrying out the plan.
  - Develop ways of organizing your work to make the plan more efficient.
- *Evaluation*, you once more contribute to the nursing process when you share your observations about the success or lack of success of the care.
  - Be accurate and concise in your reporting.
  - Be honest in your appraisal of the client's progress and the point at which your services are no longer needed.

CORE VALUES

Core values are deeply held principles and beliefs that guide an organization's conduct. The core values of management and the employees shape the organization's

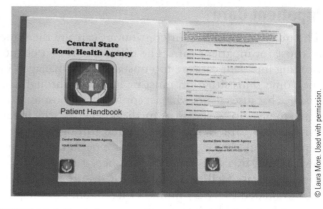

Clinical Information ALERT

Remember the importance of first impressions. The client and family's first impression of you will set the tone for your future working relationship. Take the time to introduce yourself and explain your responsibilities as a nursing assistant. Many people know what nurses are expected to do, but they are unsure of the nursing assistant's responsibilities on the health care team. Taking the time to introduce yourself and have a quick discussion about your role will help to begin a positive working relationship.

FIGURE 35-4 Each home care agency has information that is kept in a folder in the client's home. Documentation of vital signs and care provided during each visit is kept in the folder.

culture. The organization's mission statement usually summarizes its core values. Core values are guiding principles that form the basis of who you are, what you believe, and how the agency wants its employees to interact with clients and others. These values form the foundation for all aspects of health care, in all settings. They have a strong effect on client satisfaction. When working in home health care, you must know, understand, and demonstrate the following core values:

- An understanding of how the environment affects the client and their adjustment to care
- The dignity and worth of each client as an individual
- Respect for the diversity of individuals
- The ability to establish and maintain a therapeutic relationship that:
  - Encourages independence
  - Values and promotes autonomy and control.
  - Adjusts and adapts to the client's schedule, preferences, routines, and limits
  - Maintains privacy and confidentiality
  - Demonstrates caring and compassion
  - Understands the client's response to the plan of care

Most home health agencies leave a folder of information in each client's home (Figure 35-4). Documents that are kept in the folder usually include information about:

- The agency's mission statement
- The agency's scope of service
- The agency's nondiscrimination statement
- The client's rights and responsibilities
- Medicare
- Agency responsibilities
- How to contact the home health agency
- Medications
- Abuse and neglect
- HIPAA and privacy
- Safety and emergencies
- Advance directives

The agency may also include information it wants the client to know about managing their medical condition, directions for using special equipment, and how to prevent complications, such as how to prevent infection when a catheter is being used. Many agencies have their workers write their names and agency cell phone numbers on the cover of this folder so they are readily available and easy to find.

CHARACTERISTICS OF THE HOME CARE NURSING ASSISTANT AND HOMEMAKER ASSISTANT

The home care nursing assistant and homemaker assistant must have a full measure of the characteristics you have already come to associate with a successful facility-based assistant. However, some characteristics should be particularly strong in an assistant who works in clients' homes.

Remember that you will be working directly with the client and their personal possessions, without a supervising nurse constantly available. This means you must demonstrate:

- Honesty, as you handle the client's possessions and shopping money. Treat the possessions with care and respect. Keep an accurate record of all money spent and receipts received.
- Self-starter ability. You must know and carry out your assigned tasks promptly and efficiently without needing someone to remind or urge you.
- Self-discipline. Do not allow yourself to waste time on activities such as smoking, chatting with friends on the phone, texting, and drinking soda or coffee just because no supervisor is constantly checking on your progress.

- Accuracy and attention to details, so that each task is performed exactly as you were taught.
- Organization, so that you plan your activities to make the best use of your in-home time. Plan your activities around the client's schedule, not your own.
- Maturity, so that judgment can be exercised and assessments can be made properly.
- Ability to perform independently, making decisions within the limits of your responsibilities and the scope of the assignment.
- Insight that gives you the ability to see the client as a whole person who is an interactive member of a family unit and community.
- Observational skills. Be able to recognize and report abnormal signs and symptoms.
- Adaptability. Although you will need all the physical, emotional, and communication skills you learned and practiced in the clinical setting, you must be creative in adapting them to the home situation. For example, a cut-open plastic trash bag covered with a towel may be substituted for the bed protectors used in the hospital. Housekeeping chores may be performed as the client rests.
- Trustworthiness. A trustworthy person is dependable and can be relied upon to be at work on time when scheduled, do assigned tasks, keep their word, and keep client information confidential.
- Compassion, which means caring about and showing true concern for others.
- Good communication skills. Home health care nursing assistants must be able to communicate clearly with the client and family, case manager, and others. Communication may be nonverbal, verbal, and written.
- Cooperation.
- Responsibility.
- Good physical and mental health.
- Acceptance of clients and their home environments. Remember, your clients will be of all ethnic and religious groups and economic levels.

 Clinical Information **ALERT**

You will find that a smartphone or a global positioning system (GPS) unit are invaluable in helping you find unfamiliar addresses. If neither of these are available, keep a phone book in the car when you make home visits. In addition to telephone numbers and addresses, most phone books contain maps of the community, which may be helpful.

THE NURSING BAG

Most home health care workers carry a nursing bag stocked with the supplies they use routinely in client care. Your bag should be stocked with enough supplies to carry you through the day without having to replenish it. You will probably need it on every visit, and when special treatments or procedures are assigned. Use a tote bag, backpack, or other carrying case that helps you keep your supplies organized and easy to find. The fabric or outside of the bag should be washable or otherwise easy to clean. You should clean and restock your bag daily. Bring it in your house at night, or leave it in the clinical office. Never leave it in the car. This invites theft, and heat and cold extremes may damage some of your equipment and supplies. People see the bag and associate it with helping clients. Make it clear to anyone who inquires that the bag does not contain any medications or syringes. When leaving your car for a short period of time, store the bag out of sight and lock the doors.

Nursing Bag Supplies

As you gain experience, you will quickly customize your nursing bag to include items that you find necessary and convenient. Your agency may have a basic supply list. If not, consider your responsibilities and assignments, and pack a basic list of supplies to get started.

NOTE

Sometimes clients have very dry skin, or very dirty areas on the body, such as the feet. Shaving cream is inexpensive and very effective for cleaning and softening skin. Instead of rubbing fragile skin raw, apply a generous amount of shaving cream to the area. Wrap in warm, moist bath towels and let them rest for about 15 minutes. Remove the towels and gently remove the shaving cream. This will leave the skin soft and moist. A second application may be necessary, but this is not common. Your client will feel relaxed, pampered, and well cared for.

Some home health care nursing assistants carry inexpensive travel size personal care items, such as aromatherapy soap, lotion, and shampoo. Grooming and hygiene products of this nature are not required, but they are certainly a bonus for the client's self-esteem. If you encounter an unwanted source of products of this nature, collect them and give the items to clients who would appreciate them.

Some homes do not have running water. Alcohol-based hand cleaner is effective, but the CDC recommends washing hands with soap and water if the hands are visibly soiled. Some workers carry a gallon jug of water in the car for this purpose. Others use premoistened towelettes. In general, towelettes are not as effective for hand cleansing as alcohol gel or handwashing with soap and water. If an alternate method of handwashing must be used, you may want to find other facilities and wash your hands with soap and water as soon as possible after leaving the client's home.

Many agencies recommend placing your nursing bag on a barrier, such as a piece of newspaper, when you bring the bag into a home. Some workers carry disposable underpads ("blue pads"), newspaper, or a plastic grocery bag to use as a barrier.

The CDC notes that the risk of infection transmission in the provision of home-based care is presumed to be minimal. This has been a challenge for home care providers, and practice has not always been based on evidence. Pathogens are invisible and impossible to test readily in the home. No one wants to take a chance of causing an infection, carrying a pathogen to another household, or picking up a visible insect, such as a bedbug, flea, or cockroach. There are no guarantees, but using a barrier technique is believed to reduce the risk.

One example is the use of "nursing bag technique," the practice in which barriers are placed between the nursing bag and environmental surfaces. Although the environment may not always look clean, the need for barriers has long been questioned. Research is needed to identify evidence-based practices.* At present, whether to use a barrier pad is a matter of personal preference and agency policy. When leaving the home, discard trash, including the barrier pad if used, into a plastic bag and tie the top closed. Some agencies require workers to bring trash with them for later disposal at the agency. Discard according to employer policy.

Before using items from your nursing bag:

1. Select a location to place your bag that is out of the reach of children and pets. Prepare a clean area for placement of supplies and equipment to use for the client, if necessary.

2. Wash your hands or use an alcohol-based hand cleaner.

3. Put on a plastic apron and remove necessary items from your bag. Close the bag.

4. When you are finished, wash and clean reusable equipment. The plastic apron may be left in the client's home or discarded.

5. Wash your hands and replace equipment in your bag. Store contaminated supplies in a plastic bag for later cleaning and disinfection.
   - If you used bandage scissors, wash them well with soap and water and dry well.

6. Discard contaminated disposable items. Seal these items in plastic bags and discard them in the outside trash cans when you leave, if possible. Never leave contaminated waste in an open wastebasket in the home.
   - Reusable containers in the home, such as plastic wastebaskets, may be used to hold medical waste temporarily, if lined with a plastic bag. Empty the wastebasket daily and replace the bag.
   - If the wastebasket is not lined completely with a plastic bag, it must be washed and thoroughly sanitized each time it is emptied.

PERSONAL SAFETY

Personal safety is always a concern for home care workers. Be alert to conditions and people around you. Inform your employer promptly if you believe unsafe conditions exist. Thousands of nursing personnel make daily home care visits, and incidents of violence are few. However, you must trust your own instincts. If something does not feel right, it probably is not.

Other ways of protecting your own safety include the following:
- Never give your personal phone number to your clients. If they ask for it, explain that the best way to contact you is through the agency office or by using the agency cell phone.
- Map out your travel route in advance so you know where you are going. If you have online access, print a map with written directions to each new client's residence.
- Your vehicle may be equipped with an online navigation system.
- Some smart phones have the ability to provide you a map of directions to your destination.
- Inform the client what time you will be arriving.
- If you have one, lock your purse in the trunk of your car at the beginning of your workday. Use pockets or a belt-type (fanny) pack for essentials such as driver's license and pens.
- Wear scrubs or clothing that identifies you as a nursing caregiver. Wear your name badge.
- In potentially dangerous areas, ask your agency if you can make joint visits with a co-worker or use an escort.

*Siegel, J. D., Rhinehart, E., Jackson, M., Chiarello, L, & The Healthcare Infection Control Practices Advisory Committee. (2007). 2007 guideline for isolation precautions: Preventing transmission of infectious agents in healthcare settings. This is from the CDC. (Centers for Disease Control and Prevention). It was last updated in 2019. The URL is https://www.cdc.gov/infectioncontrol/pdf/guidelines/isolation-guidelines-H.pdf

- If neighbors, relatives, or others become a safety problem, make visits when they are away from the home.
- If a client suggests that a family member escort you, never get into someone else's car.
- Keep your gas tank full.
- Avoid parking on deserted streets or in dark areas.
- Keep your car windows up and doors locked at all times.
- Attend classes on personal safety and self-defense.
- Carry a cellular telephone and keep it fully charged. Follow state and local laws on using a cell phone in the vehicle. Park the car before typing or sending text messages.
- Do not enter a client's home if:
  - Your safety may be at risk, such as with firearms or other weapons, drugs, alcohol, guard dogs.
  - People are intoxicated.
  - Someone's behavior is abusive.
  - Sexual comments/gestures are made.
  - Verbal, gestured, or other threats are made.
  - There is suspected illegal activity.
  - Someone is dressed inappropriately, such as not wearing clothing, wearing only underwear.

HOME HEALTH CARE DUTIES

The duties of the home health care assistant are planned around the family routine. These duties may include:

- Following the care plan
- Helping with activities of daily living
- Taking vital signs
- Doing special monitoring, such as measuring blood glucose and intake and output
- Monitoring the client and reporting to the nurse and/or case manager
- Giving special treatments, such as prescribed exercises
- Doing simple dressing changes
- Giving skin care
- Providing ostomy care
- Overseeing and assisting with the client's self-administration of medication
- Providing comfort measures, such as positioning and special mouth care
- Maintaining a safe environment
- Bathing the client

- Changing linens
- Interacting with family members
- Documenting care, observations, and other information, usually on an electronic device, such as a tablet PC

You will be expected to spend a certain amount of time with each client. The tablet may also serve as your time sheet. You will log in when you reach the client's bedside. The last thing to do before leaving is to ask the client to sign the tablet to acknowledge your services. Your agency will log this as your time out. In most cases, you must spend at least 30 minutes with the client, depending on the service.

Homemaker duties may include:

- Light housekeeping
- Shopping for meals
- Preparing meals

Your agency may instruct you to ask the client if they need anything else before you leave.

You may also have to transport the client to clinic or therapy visits (Figure 35-5). You must have specific permission from your agency to perform activities outside of the home. Homemaker duties *do not* include:

- Doing heavy housework such as washing windows, waxing floors, or moving heavy furniture
- Making decisions about food purchases, unless the client is unable to do so

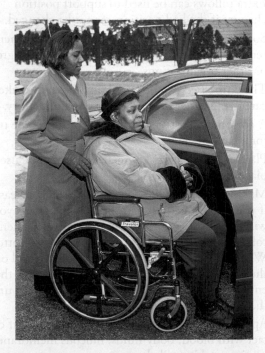

FIGURE 35-5 The home care nursing assistant may be responsible for transporting a client to a physician's appointment or clinic for care or therapy.

Difficult Situations

Sometimes an ice bag is ordered to treat a small area, or an area in which a full, large bag causes pain. Try uncooked rice. Measure a small quantity and place it in a sandwich bag. Tie the bag at the top, then freeze it. The bag can be custom-fitted to small areas, and can be reused when it warms up. Just return it to the freezer. Placing crushed ice in a glove and tying a knot in the end may also work, depending on the area you are treating and the length of the application. Tie the hand opening to the thumb, rather than knotting it closed or using a rubber band. Cover the glove with a washcloth or disposable cover. Gloves that are closed in this manner are less likely to leak than are plastic bags.

- Becoming involved in family disputes by offering opinions or taking sides

The skills you learned in the clinical setting can be adapted to the home environment. For example:

- Ice bags can be replaced by exam gloves or plastic bags sealed and wrapped in a towel.
- Reusable enema equipment can be substituted for disposable enema equipment.
- Extra pillows can be used to support position changes if the bed position cannot be changed.
- Some equipment may be rented from equipment rental companies or borrowed from religious groups or other organizations.
- The entire bed can be raised on blocks, to make caregiving easier if the client is not ambulatory.
- A cotton blanket or lightweight spread can be used for a bath blanket.
- Plastic covered with a twin-size sheet can be used in place of a draw sheet.
- Making an occupied bed by yourself may be easier if you make a bedroll first. Prepare the linens you will need by laying them out on the table. Then roll them up from side to side, then top to bottom. When the client is on their side, place the roll on the bed and unroll the linens halfway behind the client's back. Turn them on their other side and unroll the rest of the bedroll.
- Apply the principles of standard precautions if contact with blood, body fluids, mucous membranes, or nonintact skin is likely.
- A pillowcase hung on the back of a chair can serve as a laundry bag.

- If you are assigned to do dressing changes on minor skin wounds, use a plastic bag. Place your hand inside the bag and gently remove the dressing. Then turn the bag inside out, with the dressing on the inside. Tie or seal the bag and throw it away. Using this method prevents contamination. You can use a plastic bag in this manner any time you handle biohazardous or soiled material.
- Wind two rubber bands tightly around a slippery drinking glass to make it easier for a client to grasp the glass. Place the rubber bands about an inch apart.
- Some clients cannot suck forcefully enough to draw liquids up through a straw. Wash and dry your bandage scissors, and then cut the straw a few inches shorter. Place the cut end in the bottom of the glass and have the client suck from the smooth end. Removing a few inches is usually enough to enable the client to drink the liquid.
- Clients who use walkers and wheelchairs may become frustrated because of their inability to carry items with them. Attaching an inexpensive cloth tote bag, bicycle basket, or even a plastic grocery sack will work. Position the bag on the front of the walker or on one arm of the wheelchair. If the doorways are narrow, fasten the straps so the bag can be flipped up and held on the client's lap when going through the door. This is a good method for holding a cordless or cellular phone, or other important items. Although this may seem to be a small step, it is an excellent method of promoting client independence and helping them control the environment.
- A client who uses oxygen continuously is at risk for discomfort and skin breakdown behind the ears from the nasal cannula tubing. To solve this problem, cut a small foam hair curler lengthwise, and then wrap the foam around the tubing that rests on the ears. The cheekbones are also a tender area. Wrapping a corn or bunion pad (adhesive side in) around the tubing in the appropriate spot will also relieve pressure.
- If you care for a client who lives with a hard-of-hearing caregiver, suggest that they purchase a baby monitor. Place the receiver in the room near the client's head. Place the speaker in a room (or between two rooms) where the caregiver spends most of their time. Set the unit on "high" so the caregiver can hear it. Another option is to use a wireless or battery-operated doorbell. Give the client the bell button. Plug the bell into whichever outlet is closest to the caregiver.
- To weigh a client who has trouble balancing, ask the client to step onto the scale while holding onto a walker. The client will need to let go for about a second while you obtain the weight, but having the walker in front of the scale is usually adequate to maintain balance.

- Place a large piece of plastic on the car seat (you can cut a large trash bag, if necessary). The plastic enables the client to slide easily onto or off of the seat.
- Use a wire coat hanger to hang a catheter bag on the bed. Slide the hanger between the mattress and box spring, leaving only about an inch of the hook exposed. Hang the loop of the drainage bag on the hook. You can also pin a large safety pin horizontally to the fitted mattress pad or bottom sheet. Hang the hook for the drainage bag on the pin.
- Denture cleaner or dishwasher soap are both effective for removing sediment and stains on bedpans and urinals. Pour very hot water into the bedpan or urinal and then add one tablet of denture cleaner or 1/4 cup of dishwasher soap. Stir with a tongue blade and let sit for a few minutes. Empty the solution into the toilet and rinse. This eliminates odor and sediment.
- Use a turkey baster (that is reserved for this purpose) and warm water to rinse reusable ostomy pouches and other items.
- A bed tray can replace an overbed table for eating and activities.

Items that you or a family member can make are pictured in Figure 35-6.

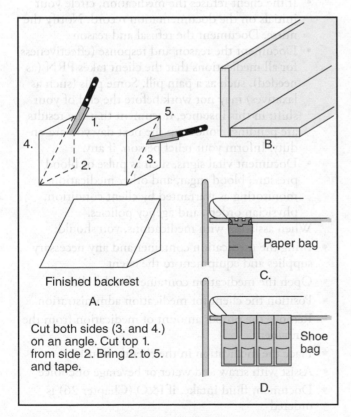

Cut both sides (3. and 4.) on an angle. Cut top 1. from side 2. Bring 2. to 5. and tape.

Finished backrest

Paper bag

Shoe bag

FIGURE 35-6 Items to facilitate client care in the home may be made with readily available materials.

- A cardboard box can be cut, taped, and padded for use as a backrest.
- Two lightweight pieces of wood nailed at right angles can be padded and used as a footrest to hold bedding off the toes.
- A paper bag can be taped to the bed frame, overbed table, or nightstand to discard soiled tissues. The entire bag can then be closed and properly handled for disposal.
- A shoe bag tucked under the mattress and hanging by the bedside can provide compartments for a remote control and other personal articles.

Difficult Situations

Dry, sore, burning, itchy eyes are a common problem in the elderly. If the person does not clean the eyes regularly, the eyelids fill with matter, which worsens the problem. Washing the eyelids with tearless baby shampoo several times a day and rinsing with warm water clears the condition quickly. A cotton pad is an excellent tool for washing and rinsing the eyes.

ASSISTING CLIENTS WITH MEDICATIONS

The physician may prescribe medications for clients who are receiving home health care. Nursing assistants are not legally responsible for giving medications. In many states, nursing assistants handing out medication is not permitted. However, you may have to supervise the client as they self-administer medications. The client may need assistance in opening a container. You may not read a label, remove a pill, or instruct a client to take it. However, you may remind and assist a client by bringing them a bottle, reading the label to them, informing them of the time, and opening the container. Many different containers are available to hold multiple drug doses in individual sections labeled for the days of the week (Figure 35-7). These containers simplify medication management, and it is easy to determine whether the medications have been taken. A nurse must fill the medication container.

Difficult Situations

If the client or a family member informs you of new problems with any of the following when no home care worker is on duty, notify your supervisor: eating, getting into or out of bed, maintaining continence or using the toilet, bathing, or dressing. Clients with new problems related to these activities require further nursing assessment.

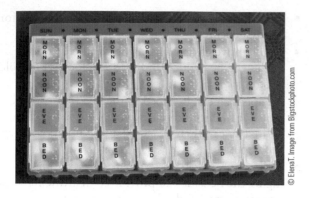

FIGURE 35-7 The nurse may fill containers that hold up to a week's supply of medication.

If you are instructed to assist a self-directed client with medications that are needed to maintain or improve health, the client must:

- Be able to make choices about activities of daily living
- Understand how these choices affect them
- Assume responsibility for the results of the choices
- Need assistance with the task or be physically unable to perform the activity

In addition, at least one of the following situations must be present:

- No informal caregiver is available at the time the medication must be given.
- The caregiver is unwilling or unable to perform the task.
- The caregiver's assistance is not acceptable to the client.

The "Six Rights" of Medication Administration

When assisting clients with medications, the home health assistant must remember the Six Rights of medication administration:

1. Right Medication
   - Compare the label to the order.
   - Check the medication three times:
     - Before pouring
     - After pouring
     - Before replacing the container
   - Make sure you have the correct preparation, such as tablet or liquid.
   - Always check the expiration date.
   - Always check for allergies before assisting with any medication.
2. Right Dose
   - Always double-check the dose.
   - Always review and question dosage changes.

Difficult Situations

If a client swallows a pill and complains it "didn't go down all the way," offer them a piece of a banana. Food works well if clients have problems swallowing pills, and bananas are thick, sticky, and usually effective for moving pills down the esophagus.

3. Right Route
   - Check to be sure you know the correct route of administration.
   - Check for special orders, such as giving with food, or before or after meals.
4. Right Time
   - Administer at the correct time.
5. Right Client
   - Be sure to give the correct medication to the correct client.
6. Right Documentation
   - Never chart medications in advance.
   - Initial each medication immediately after the client takes it.
   - Document fluid intake promptly, if client is on intake and output monitoring (I&O).
   - If the client refuses the medication, circle your initials on the documentation record. Notify the nurse. Document the refusal and reason.
   - Document the reason and response (effectiveness) for all medications that the client takes PRN (as needed), such as a pain pill. Some pills (such as laxatives) may not work before the end of your shift; in this instance, document that the results are pending. Follow up the next day you are on duty. Inform your relief person, if any.
   - Document vital signs, such as pulse or blood pressure, blood sugar, and other medication monitoring as warranted by client condition, physician orders, and agency policies.

When assisting with medications, you should:

- Bring the medication container and any necessary supplies and equipment to the client
- Open the medication container for the client
- Position the client for medication administration
- Remove the proper amount of medication from the container
- Place the medication in the client's mouth
- Assist with straw and water or beverage of choice
- Document fluid intake, if I&O (Chapter 26) is ordered
- Notify the case manager if you suspect a client or family member is abusing or diverting medication

GUIDELINES 35-1 Guidelines for Supervising Self-Administration of Medications

- Medicine must be taken at the correct time. Note whether it should be taken before meals, with food, or after meals.
- Check the expiration date to be sure the medicine is not outdated.
- Note whether the client is also taking over-the-counter medications (nonprescription) and check with your supervisor to find out whether these medications will interact with the prescription drugs.

- Perform any monitoring activities required, such as checking pulse, blood pressure, or blood sugar—*before* the drug is taken.
- Note how much medication is left in the container. Follow your instructions for getting the prescription refilled so that the client does not run out.

Clients with Diabetes

Approximately 25.8 million persons in the United States (8.3% of the population) have diabetes, so it is likely that you will be caring for clients with diabetes. The care plan will list your responsibilities. If you are responsible for providing meals or snacks, you must also understand:

- How to check blood glucose (Chapter 42)
- What normal and reportable blood glucose values are
- The nutritional needs of clients with diabetes
- The need for regular meals
- Special methods of meal preparation, if any
- How snacks are used in the daily regimen of persons with diabetes
- How exercise affects blood glucose levels
- That changes in schedules, activity, stress, and illness can affect blood sugar
- When to call the case manager and/or 9-1-1 for help

Technology has advanced to the point that many medications are delivered through programmable, battery-operated devices. One such commonly used device is the insulin pump (Figure 35-8). Home health care nursing assistants are not responsible for the pumps, but need to observe and report signs and symptoms of abnormal blood sugar (Chapter 42) or any other unusual changes.

THE HOME ENVIRONMENT

You are responsible for maintaining a safe and comfortable environment for the client. This means that you must:

- Be alert to unsafe situations
- Control the spread of infection
- Care for and maintain the client's furnishings, supplies, and appliances
- Learn the locations of items that may be needed in an emergency (such as a flashlight or fire extinguisher)

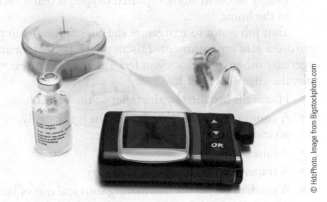

FIGURE 35-8 An insulin pump is an alternative to taking multiple daily injections of insulin. Some newer units do not require tubing.

Your first visit to a client's home gives you an opportunity to check for safety factors. Tell a family member or case manager about safety problems. For example, things to call to the attention of your supervisor include:

- Furniture or other items that obstruct the client's walkway
- Electrical cords that could cause the client to fall
- Stair railings and stair treads that need repair
- Unstable or lightweight chairs
- Highly polished floors that may be slippery
- The need to lock up specific items if the client is disoriented:
  - Chemicals such as household cleaning supplies, paints, insecticides, and cleaning fluids
  - Medications, both prescription and over-the-counter
  - Aerosol cans
  - Small appliances like toasters or irons that can be plugged in and used inappropriately
  - Power tools
  - Weapons or anything that could be used as a weapon

© HdcPhoto. Image from Bigstockphoto.com

- Fragile, breakable, or valuable items
- Smoking materials that should be used only with supervision
- Electrical outlets that require covering
- Thermostats that may need guards over them.
- Stove knobs
- Loose scatter rugs, which might cause a fall as the client ambulates
- Electrical cords that are under rugs, creating a fire hazard
- Lack of smoke detectors and fire extinguishers
- Overloaded electrical outlets or extension cords, which might cause a fire
- Ambulatory aids that require repair or replacement, such as broken straps on braces or worn rubber tips on walkers, canes, and crutches
- Family or client smoking when oxygen is being used in the home

Your job is not to reorganize the client's home but to ensure a safe environment. Discuss with the case manager any other conditions you feel are unsafe. For example, the client may need:

- Handrails installed by the toilet or the bathtub.
- A commode to use if the bathroom is not easily accessible.
- A raised toilet seat
- A trapeze to assist with bed mobility
- A mechanical lift for transferring into and out of bed

These items are readily available from durable equipment providers, and most insurance companies and Medicare will pay for equipment that is required for client care. However, the case manager must consult with the physician, who must write an order for the equipment.

 Safety **ALERT**

Pay close attention to safety risks in the following areas, which are the most common locations of injury in the home: stairs and steps, bathroom(s), kitchens, and basements. If you feel there are hazards or other safety or security risks, inform your supervisor promptly. If conditions in the home should be modified, an occupational therapist may be asked to make a home visit to make recommendations. Do not attempt to make mechanical or environmental modifications yourself.

The number 911 is used to contact emergency help everywhere in the United States and Canada. It is universal for any type of emergency.

Keep a list of other emergency numbers close to the telephone, or program them into the phone. The list should include:

- The agency
- The case manager and/or supervising nurse
- The physician
- A family member (emergency contact and/or primary caregiver)

You should find out if the client:

- Uses a medical alert bracelet or necklace.
- Has out-of-hospital code papers, advance directives, or a living will.
- Has state-specific documents or directives.
- Has a special storage place in the house for important medical information that would be needed in an emergency. Some people keep these in the refrigerator so they can be easily located.

Elder Abuse

As a home health assistant, you may care for clients who are suspected victims of abuse. Chapter 4 describes the various types of abuse that may be inflicted by staff members, family members, or others. These situations may also occur in the home:

- Some families provide loving, capable care for older dependent relatives for many years without assistance. They may be emotionally stressed and may have also depleted their financial resources.
- In some cases there has been a long family history of one spouse abusing the other.
- Self-abuse may occur when a person with a disability is unable to adequately carry out activities of daily living and is unwilling to accept help.

If you are a mandatory state reporter, follow your state rules for reporting abuse. If you are not required to report suspected abuse to your state, you must notify the case manager of your findings. You are not responsible for determining if an individual has been abused or what type of abuse has been inflicted. Report suspected signs or symptoms of abuse to your supervisor. These include:

- Statements of the client that reflect neglect or abuse
- Unexplained bruises or wounds
- Signs of neglect such as poor hygiene
- A change in personality

Remember, these indications do not necessarily mean that the person is being abused. However, they may signal a need for further investigation by your supervisor. The supervisor will assess the client and take the appropriate action.

GUIDELINES FOR FOOD MANAGEMENT

As a rule, most home health nursing assistants do not plan or shop for meals. For the most part you will be responsible for very simple meals, such as making soup and sandwich for lunch or cooking a prepared microwave meal.

Meal Preparation

You learned about therapeutic diets in Chapter 26. The physician may order a special diet to meet the needs of a home care client. You must know:

* What the diet order means
* How the diet affects the illness
* How to adjust planning, shopping, and preparation to comply with the diet
* How to assist the client to follow the diet
* How to prepare, weigh, and measure foods

Food Sanitation

Wash your hands well before preparing food. Wash them again if you touch an unclean item or surface, or touch your face or hair. All surfaces, dishes, and utensils that come into contact with food must be clean and sanitary.

Safe Minimum Cooking Temperatures

You cannot tell by appearance whether food is safely cooked (Figure 35-9). Always check the internal temperature of meat, poultry, seafood, and other cooked foods with a food thermometer to ensure that they have reached a safe minimum temperature. Suggested minimum internal temperature and rest time.

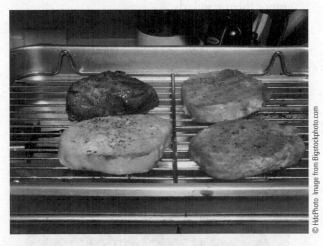

FIGURE 35-9 Preparing meals may be an expectation when caring for a client in the home.

Rest Time

Allow meat to rest after removing it from the heat source. The temperature remains constant or continues to rise during the rest period. This allows the food to finish cooking, and eliminates pathogens, if present.

INFECTION CONTROL

Some of the methods used in daily cleaning help to control the spread of infection. Other requirements are:

* Washing your hands (Figure 35-10) or using an alcohol-based hand cleaner
* Keeping the kitchen and bathroom clean
* Caring for food properly
* Disposing of tissues and other wastes properly
* Cleaning up dirty dishes
* Dusting daily
* Not allowing clutter to accumulate
* Wearing a plastic apron
* Wearing latex gloves for client care if contact with blood, body fluids, mucous membranes, or nonintact skin is likely
* Wearing utility gloves when cleaning environmental surfaces or doing laundry contaminated with blood, body fluids, secretions, or excretions

Discarding Medical Waste

Your agency will have policies and procedures for discarding disposable, contaminated items, and cleaning

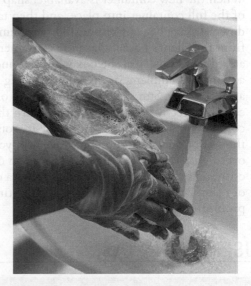

FIGURE 35-10 Handwashing is the most important infection control technique in health care. All handwashing rules and guidelines used in facilities also apply to home care.

permanent items for reuse. Apply the principles of standard precautions and apply personal protective equipment appropriate to the task. Follow your local regulations for disposal of all infectious medical waste. In general:

- Place contaminated supplies in a plastic bag and close tightly.
- Double-bag in a second plastic bag if the outside of the first bag is torn or contaminated.
- Seal the bag by using a twist tie, taping, or tying, or according to agency policy.
- Dispose of double-bagged waste in the household trash. Take it to the outside trash can, if possible, when you leave for the day.
- After discarding trash, wash your hands or use alcohol-based hand cleaner.
- Sanitize all contaminated equipment and surfaces appropriately.
- Blood, body fluids, secretions, and excretions may be discarded in the client's toilet. Pouring should be done slowly and carefully to minimize splashing, spattering, or aerosolizing. Wear eye protection, face mask, and gloves. Wear a gown or plastic apron if there is a potential for splashing, spattering, or aerosolizing the fluid.
- Place sharp items, such as needles, syringes, fingerstick lancets, and disposable razors in a sharps container, which is furnished by the home health care agency and left in the client's home.
  - Replace the container when it is three-quarters full. This is usually the nurse's responsibility. Inform the case manager when a new container will be needed.
  - When the new container is available, snap the lid of the full container into place, and then tape it down. It may be your responsibility to remove it from the client's home. Place the container inside a cardboard box. Seal the box with tape and affix a biohazard emblem, or mark it according to agency policy. Store the box in the trunk of your car. Go directly to your agency to return the container for disposal. Do not carry it around for the rest of the day and do not leave it in your car overnight. The United States is having an opioid crisis, and a full sharps container creates a degree of risk for you and your vehicle. Eliminating it promptly is the best action to take.

HOUSEKEEPING TASKS

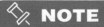 **NOTE**

Fabric-softener dryer sheets will eliminate static and soften clothes, but they have many other helpful uses as well:

- Wash dishes—loosen baked-on food from dishes by placing a dryer sheet on the dish, filling with cold water, and letting it soak, preferably overnight. Weight the dryer sheet with a spoon to keep it in place, if needed. The fabric softener will loosen the food, making it much easier to clean.
- Eliminate odors in sneakers, slippers, luggage, closets, basements, attics, and garages.
- Remove soap scum—clean glass shower doors by scrubbing them with damp dryer sheets.
- Dust—wipe static from your television and computer screens, as well as dust from blinds.

In some cases, the homemaker assistant (aide) will perform light housekeeping tasks. In other cases, the home health care nursing assistant may be assigned some or all of these duties.

Cleaning the Client's Room

Keeping the client's room clean is a way to prevent infection. It also helps raise the client's morale. Remember that you are not to rearrange the client's things without permission.

- Pick things up so clutter will not accumulate.
- Keep cleaning equipment in one place so you do not waste time gathering it for each job as you move from room to room (Figure 35-11).
- Clean and put equipment away as soon as you have finished with it.
- Dust the room daily.
- Damp-dust uncarpeted floors weekly and vacuum carpeted floors.
- Remove used dishes and glasses when finished and rinse right away.
- Put clean clothes away after laundering. Hang up robes when not in use.
- Line each wastepaper basket with a plastic bag and empty them regularly.

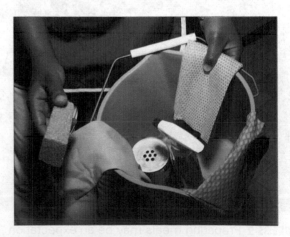

FIGURE 35-11 Keep cleaning supplies together for good organization and efficient time management.

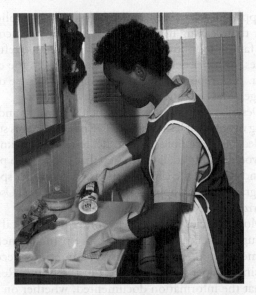

FIGURE 35-12 Clean the bathroom daily and whenever needed.

Cleaning the Bathroom

The bathroom can be a source of infection, so you must be careful and thorough in your daily cleaning (Figure 35-12). Use a disinfectant product (client/family's choice) to clean the:

- Inside and outside of the toilet
- Shower or tub after each use
- Sink and faucets
- Countertops
- Floor; if carpeted, vacuum daily

Put dirty towels and washcloths into the laundry. Replace them with clean towels and washcloths. Use a deodorant to keep the bathroom smelling fresh and clean.

Cleaning the Kitchen

The kitchen is another area that requires special attention. An unclean kitchen can be a source of infection.

- Clean up after each meal.
- Do not allow dirty dishes to accumulate in the sink. Clean up immediately after meals.
- Rinse dishes and wash by hand in detergent and hot water.
- Wash glasses first, then silverware, then dishes, utensils, and pots and pans.
- Rinse with hot water and allow to dry in drain rack.
- Put away when dry.
- You may wash items in the dishwasher by:
  - Rinsing well
  - Adding recommended detergent to the dishwasher
  - Loading the dishwasher—but do not run the dishwasher until it is full

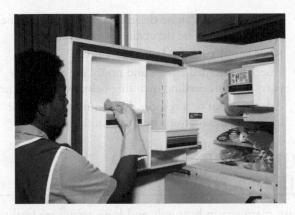

FIGURE 35-13 Wipe up spills immediately.

- Wash pots and pans as directed; some are not dishwasher-safe.
- Wash utensils with wooden handles by hand.
- Clean the sink, countertops, and stove.
- Dispose of garbage properly. It may be put in an in-sink disposal if one is available. Wrap bones tightly in newspaper and put them in the trash (or compactor if available).
- Sweep the floor after each meal.
- Place leftover foods in small covered containers and refrigerate. Use or discard within a few days.
- Keep the refrigerator clean and keep food covered. Clean up spills in the refrigerator and freezer immediately (Figure 35-13).
- Keep the microwave oven clean. Use a damp cloth to wipe up spills immediately and to clean after each use. Make sure you heat food in microwave-safe dishes only. Do not use metal of any kind (including dishes with any metallic trim) in a microwave oven.
- Wash the kitchen floor weekly, or more often if necessary.

Ask the client or a responsible family member for instructions on operating appliances before using.

Laundry

Laundry may also be your responsibility. Carefully launder the client's clothes. They represent a sizable investment. This may have to be done daily. Always:

- Read labels before laundering. Some clothes must be dry-cleaned, hand-washed, or washed at special temperatures.
- Use the client's choice of detergent and read the label for instructions on amount to use.
- Wear gloves when sorting clothing and loading the washing machine.
- Separate light and dark fabrics and wash them separately.
- Wash drip-dry fabrics separately so they can be hung and dried or folded.

- Be sure clothes can be dried in a dryer, and use the proper setting. Use dryer sheets as directed.
- After laundering, fold or hang clothes.
- Check for needed repairs and notify the responsible party of items needing mending before storing clothes.
- Ask the client or a responsible family member for operating instructions before using appliances.

COMMUNICATION VIA DOCUMENTATION

Team members in hospitals and long-term care facilities communicate face-to-face at the beginning and end of every shift. Handoff communication occurs whenever necessary throughout the shift. Home health care workers work independently, and workers are rarely in the same place at the same time. As a result, documentation becomes the primary means of communication. Because of this, documentation must be timely, complete, and concise. Follow the guidelines you learned in Chapter 8. Address the care plan goals and approaches. Document the client's response to the intervention, including unexpected responses. Include verbal and nonverbal responses and direct quotations, when appropriate.

If you are using paper documentation, make certain the client's name is on every page. If the documentation involves checking boxes, make sure they are accurate and complete. If information on a printed form does not apply to your client, write NA for "not applicable" rather than leaving it blank. Document any noncompliance, failure to follow health care instructions, refusal of services, or other behavior that poses a risk to the client's health. Also report this information to the nurse or case manager, and document that you have done so.

Describe all preventive care, such as turning and positioning or applying heel protectors. Avoid statements such as: "Applied fall precautions." The reader has no way of knowing what you did. Instead, list each step that you took to prevent falls and describe the client's response. Use proper spelling, good grammar, and appropriate medical phrases. Use only authorized abbreviations. Sign and date every entry.

Most agencies require each worker to take vital signs. Although tablets are now used as the primary means of documentation, the vital signs are sometimes recorded on a single paper form that is left in the home. Remember that the information documented, whether on paper or in electronic format, is confidential and protected under HIPAA. It should not be visible or accessible to unauthorized persons.

Agencies often ask the client to sign their name at the end of the visit to verify that the service was provided. If paper documentation is used, the client signs a form with a pen. Agencies that use electronic documentation ask the client to sign a touchscreen tablet. If the tablet is heat sensitive, the client signs the name with a fingertip on the tablet. Some sign their initials. If the tablet is not heat sensitive, a stylus may be used.

REVIEW

A. True/False

Mark the following true or false by circling T or F.

1. T F   The home health care nursing assistant may be responsible for both nursing care and limited household tasks.

2. T F   The home health care nursing assistant makes no contribution to the nursing process, because care is given at the client's home and not in a facility.

3. T F   Self-discipline is an important characteristic of the nursing assistant who works in a home.

4. T F   When washing dishes, wash the plates first, then the pots and pans, and then the glassware.

5. T F   As a home health assistant, your primary role is to do the housework and cooking.

6. T F   Your observations are important for monitoring the client's progress.

7. T F   Because the client is your responsibility, you need not be concerned with the client's family.

8. T F   The client who is disoriented does not require smoking supervision if they are in their own home.

9. T F   Adaptability is an important characteristic for home health nursing assistants.

10. T F   You should clean the bathroom daily.

11. T F   The rules for home health care nursing assistants are uniform throughout the United States.

12. T F   Home health care nursing assistants must have a minimum of 75 hours of education before working with clients.

13. T F   The home health care nursing assistant's certificate will expire if the assistant does not work for a period of 24 months.

14. T F   A voluntary certification program is available for home health care nursing and hospice assistants.

15. T F   There are eight levels of Medicare hospice care.

16. T F   Core values are deeply held principles and beliefs.

17. T F A hospice recipient may live in a nursing facility.

18. T F Clients who accept Medicare hospice care agree to give up their Part A hospital benefits.

19. T F The home health care nursing assistant is responsible for giving each client's medications.

20. T F Mrs. Tinker says she is hungry and asks you to make her a sandwich. As a home health nursing assistant, you are not permitted to prepare food for the client.

B. Multiple Choice

Select the best answer for each of the following.

21. A special characteristic needed by a home health care nursing assistant working in a home is:
- **a.** honesty.
- **b.** being a follower.
- **c.** being a fast worker.
- **d.** being able to take shortcuts.

22. Which household tasks would the home health care nursing assistant not be required to do?
- **a.** Shop for food
- **b.** Move heavy furniture
- **c.** Carry out nursing procedures
- **d.** Keep the kitchen clean

23. Home health assistant responsibilities include all but which of the following?
- **a.** Washing windows
- **b.** Cleaning the bathroom daily
- **c.** Documenting the care given
- **d.** Shopping for the client

24. The home health assistant should remember that:
- **a.** if you are running late clients can be skipped.
- **b.** infection control is as important in the home as it is in other settings.
- **c.** they must take directions from family members instead of the case manager.
- **d.** home health care workers are not required to follow agency policy and procedure manual.

25. Daily tasks may include:
- **a.** wiping the counter after preparing a meal.
- **b.** watering the lawn and shrubs.
- **c.** shampooing the carpets.
- **d.** washing windows.

26. The folder of home health information left in each client's home includes all of the following *except*:
- **a.** the client's rights and responsibilities.
- **b.** Medicare, HIPAA, and privacy information.
- **c.** the doctor's office chart.
- **d.** how to contact the agency.

27. A hospice recipient receiving continuous care is evaluated every:
- **a.** 8 hours.
- **b.** 24 hours.
- **c.** 72 hours.
- **d.** 5 to 7 days.

28. Respite care:
- **a.** is high-level care given to clients who are ill and unstable.
- **b.** involves transferring the client to a facility for 30 days.
- **c.** is short-term, time-limited, temporary care to relieve the family.
- **d.** is terminal care that is given when death is near.

29. Hospice:
- **a.** is a philosophy of care.
- **b.** is a location where one goes to die.
- **c.** focuses on curing the client.
- **d.** is based on religious principles.

C. Nursing Assistant Challenge

30. Protect your personal safety when working as a home care assistant by:
- **a.** informing the client of your estimated time of arrival.
- **b.** giving the client's family your personal phone number.
- **c.** using only public transportation to get to work.
- **d.** asking a client's family member to drive you home.

31. You are working for a home health agency, and Mrs. Fernandez is one of your clients. She has had a stroke and needs assistance with all activities of daily living. Your assignment includes a bath, personal care, dressing, making the bed, making her breakfast, making her lunch so she can have it after you have gone, cleaning the bathroom, and general "picking up" around her apartment. She asks if you will go to the drugstore before you leave to get her prescriptions refilled. Make a work plan that includes all of these tasks, as well as any other routine tasks you need to complete.

_____

_____

_____

_____

_____

_____

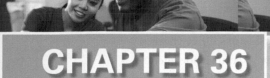

OBJECTIVES

After completing this chapter, you will be able to:

36.1 Spell and define terms.

36.2 Describe the purpose of subacute care.

36.3 Explain the differences between acute care, subacute care, and long-term care.

36.4 Describe special procedures provided in the subacute care unit.

36.5 Describe the responsibilities of the nursing assistant when caring for patients using subacute care.

36.6 Define sterile technique and explain why it is used.

36.7 List the guidelines for sterile procedures.

36.8 Describe the purpose of a sterile field.

36.9 Demonstrate how to establish a sterile field.

36.10 Explain when to use sterile gloves.

36.11 Describe how to use sterile gloves without contamination.

36.12 Describe the care of surgical drains.

36.13 Describe continuous sutures, interrupted sutures, and staples.

36.14 Demonstrate the following procedures:
- Procedure 83: Applying and Removing Sterile Gloves
- Procedure 84: Applying a Dry Sterile Dressing (Expand Your Skills)

VOCABULARY

Learn the meaning and the correct spelling of the following words and phrases:

central venous catheter (CVC)
continuous sutures
epidural catheter
exacerbation
infiltration

interrupted sutures
Kelly
multisensory stimulation
narcotic
oncology

patient-controlled analgesia (PCA)
peripheral intravenous central catheter (PICC)
piggyback
spasticity

subacute care
total parenteral nutrition (TPN)
transcutaneous electrical nerve stimulation (TENS)
transitional care unit (TCU)

DESCRIPTION OF SUBACUTE CARE

Subacute care is comprehensive, goal-oriented care for individuals with acute illness, injury, or **exacerbation** (worsening) of a chronic medical condition. It is provided instead of, or immediately after, hospitalization, at a lower cost than the acute care hospital. Subacute units can be located in freestanding facilities, or may be specialized units within a hospital or skilled nursing facility. The patients in the subacute unit do not need hospital services, but their needs are greater and more complex than the skilled nursing facility can provide. Thus, subacute care provides a transitional level of care from one setting to another. For this reason, subacute units may be called **transitional care units (TCUs)**. They help make the transition from one level of care to the next. When the patient reaches their goals, they are transferred to a lower level of care. The subacute unit bridges the gap between the acute care hospital and the chronic care setting or the patient's home. As a rule, the subacute unit is licensed as a skilled nursing facility. There is no separate or distinct license for a subacute care or transitional care unit in a licensed SNF. However, each unit will have eligibility criteria that patients must meet for admission.

Emphasis and Philosophy of Subacute Care

The emphasis and philosophy of subacute care are slightly different from those of long-term care. Subacute care focuses on managing new or acute problems, whereas long-term care manages chronic problems. (Subacute care also manages chronic conditions affecting patient recovery, such as an acute exacerbation of heart failure or chronic obstructive pulmonary disease (COPD).) The subacute unit is not a permanent place for patients to live. In contrast, long-term care facility placement may be permanent.

Patients in the subacute care unit require frequent nursing assessment, evaluation, and adjustment of the care plan. Assessment and adjustment continue until the patient's condition stabilizes and treatment goals are met.

On a subacute care unit, there are:

- More medications and treatments than on a regular skilled care unit
- More frequent physician's visits than in a skilled care unit
- More sophisticated types of equipment than in a skilled care unit

Types of Care Provided in a Subacute Care Unit

Most subacute care units provide specialized types of care in one or two areas of care. Each unit sets its own criteria for admission. Some examples are:

- Rehabilitation—all therapies are provided and the patient participates in rehabilitation for five hours a day, six or seven days a week.
- Peritoneal dialysis—a method of ridding the body of wastes for a person who has kidney failure (see Chapter 45).
- Ventilator weaning and tracheostomy care (see Chapter 39) for persons who have been unable to breathe without the help of a ventilator (Figure 36-1).

⚖ Legal ALERT

In some states and facilities, nursing assistants are not permitted to perform the procedures in this chapter. Your instructor will explain your responsibilities in your state and facility. Perform these procedures only if you are permitted to do so by state law and facility policies. Doing only tasks that you have been instructed to do, in the way that you were taught, protects patients from injury and protects you from injury, legal exposure, and liability.

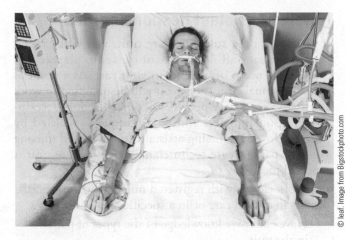

FIGURE 36-1 This patient is intubated and is on a ventilator for breathing.

© leaf. Image from Bigstockphoto.com

- Cardiac monitoring for persons who have a myocardial infarction (heart attack) or acute heart failure (see Chapter 40).
- Pain management and control for persons who have acute, unstable, or severe chronic pain (see Chapter 10).
- Oncology—for persons with cancer who are receiving treatments such as radiation or chemotherapy (see Chapter 47).
- Wound management for persons with stage 3 or stage 4 pressure injuries, other injuries (such as those related to peripheral vascular disease), or injuries such as burns (see Chapter 38).
- Specialized care for persons who have suffered brain damage resulting from trauma or stroke.
- AIDS care.
- Hospice care.
- Postoperative care for persons who have other complicating conditions such as chronic obstructive pulmonary disease (COPD) or diabetes.
- Infusion therapy for persons needing ongoing intravenous fluids, nutrition, medications, or antibiotic therapy.
- Pre- and posttransplant care for persons waiting for an organ transplant, and management and stabilization of patients after a major organ transplant.
- Coma care—weaning off drugs and tubes, **multisensory stimulation** (intense stimulation of sight, sound, touch, smell, pressure, and pain to help the patient awaken and use previously unused portions of the brain), and management of patients in a coma who have respiratory, nutritional, skin and eye care, contracture prevention, and elimination needs.

Nursing Assistant Responsibilities

If you work on a subacute care unit, you will participate in special staff development classes to prepare you to meet the needs of patients in your care. As a result of your additional education, you will be qualified to work as an advanced care provider. Your title, job description, responsibilities, and pay grade are specified by your employer. A nursing assistant (or advanced nursing assistant/patient care technician) on a subacute unit is expected to:

- Work closely with registered nurses who are specialists in critical care or in a specific area of nursing.
- Have extensive knowledge of the types of patients in the unit.
- Care for patients receiving complicated treatments.
- Have excellent observational and technical skills, because of the complex conditions of the patients.
- Be a member of an interdisciplinary team that includes professionals in physical therapy, occupational therapy, speech therapy, respiratory therapy, and social services.

Staff on a subacute care unit must be able to provide for patients' emotional well-being. Many patients will eventually be able to return to their own homes. They may still have concerns if they will have to rely on community services or family members to meet some of their needs. Other patients will have an uncertain future. For example:

- Will the patient receiving dialysis receive a kidney transplant?
- Will the oncology treatments cure the patient's cancer?
- Will ventilator weaning be successful, or will a ventilator be a lifelong need?
- Will the patient receiving rehabilitation regain the skills necessary to live independently at home?

SPECIAL PROCEDURES PROVIDED IN THE SUBACUTE CARE UNIT

You may be assigned to care for patients who are receiving special treatments that require use of equipment that is unfamiliar to you. As a nursing assistant, you will not be expected to provide highly technical procedures. However, you will be providing the same basic personal care and procedures that you would with any patients. The level of care or frequency may be slightly higher. For example, you may take vital signs once a day on a chronic care patient. However, patients in a subacute environment are less stable, and you may be asked to take vital signs four to six times daily. Some may require

continuous pulse oximetry monitoring or checking the pulse oximeter/oxygen saturation value more frequently (see Chapter 39).

Taking Vital Signs in the Subacute Unit

Patients in the subacute unit require close monitoring of their vital signs. When taking vital signs on patients:

- Avoid taking blood pressure on the side affected by a stroke.
- Avoid taking blood pressure in the arm with a dialysis graft or shunt.
- Avoid taking blood pressure in an arm with an IV.
- Avoid taking blood pressure in the arm on the side where a patient recently had surgery or breast removal.
- Avoid taking an oral temperature on patients with tubes in the nose or mouth.
- Report abnormal vital signs to the nurse immediately.

Caring for Patients Connected to Special Equipment

Patients in the subacute unit are frequently connected to electronic monitoring and caregiving devices. Many of these devices are used 24 hours a day and cannot be disconnected while personal care is provided. Be careful not to accidentally move, bump, or disconnect the equipment. Avoid bending, kinking, or placing traction on tubes entering surgical incisions or body cavities. In most cases, you will not be permitted to adjust or regulate the equipment. Respond immediately if an alarm sounds, and notify the nurse without delay.

Rehabilitation

Patients may require intense rehabilitation because they have had:

- A stroke that affected their mobility, their ability to carry out activities of daily living, or their speech
- Orthopedic surgery or an amputation (Figure 36-2)
- An accident that resulted in neurological or orthopedic problems

All caregivers working with these patients must have a knowledge of rehabilitation as well as a knowledge of the underlying condition (stroke, brain injury, etc.). You must become familiar with each patient's goals and approaches. Consistency is the key to successful rehabilitation.

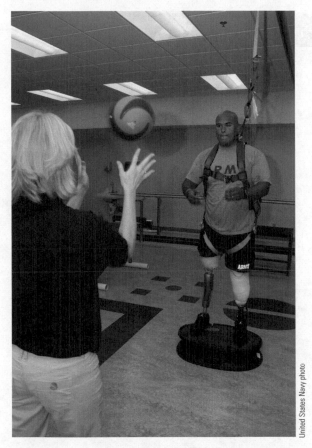

United States Navy photo

FIGURE 36-2 A patient may need extensive rehabilitation to recover from a traumatic injury.

STERILE TECHNIQUE

In many facilities, only licensed nursing personnel perform procedures using sterile technique. However, there are times when a nursing assistant may be asked to provide or assist with a sterile procedure. Common nursing procedures in which sterile technique is used are:

- All invasive procedures.
- Procedures in which the skin is broken, such as injections and insertion of intravenous needles or catheters.
- Procedures in which body cavities are entered, such as catheterization and tracheal suctioning.
- Changing surgical dressings.
- Changing dressings on central intravenous catheters.
- Procedures involving patients with severe destruction of the skin, such as burns and trauma.

Only sterile supplies contact the patient's body during sterile procedures. Sterile gloves are worn. Masks are worn during some sterile procedures. Follow Procedure 2 (see Chapter 13) for applying a mask. In some procedures, the patient also wears a mask. In others, a mask is not necessary. Check with the nurse if you are not sure whether to wear a mask.

Environmental Conditions

Check the environment before using a sterile item or creating a sterile field. The surface on which you open the sterile package must be clean, dry, flat, and stable. The area must be free from airborne contamination. Patients may accidentally contaminate sterile supplies and trays. Explain the procedure to the patient before beginning. Instruct them to avoid touching sterile supplies; crossing over the sterile field; or talking, coughing, or sneezing over sterile articles. Remind the patient during the procedure, as necessary.

A *sterile field* is a sterile surface that you create to use as a work area for sterile procedures. A one-inch border around the outside edge of the field is considered not sterile. Avoid placing sterile items in this border area. Only the top surface of the work area is considered sterile. A sterile drape often hangs over the edges of the table. The area below the tabletop is not sterile. Sterile supplies can touch only the sterile field. Avoid touching the field or items on it with your hands. Refer to Chapter 13 for additional information.

If a small surface is needed, the inside of a sterile package can be used as a sterile field. If a larger surface is needed, a sterile drape is used as the foundation for the sterile field.

Sterile Gloves

Using sterile gloves is essential when using aseptic (sterile) technique. Wearing sterile gloves permits you to touch sterile items without contaminating them.

Transfer Forceps

Some facilities use sterile transfer forceps to add supplies to the sterile field (Figure 36-4). When the sterile tray is packaged, the cup for liquids is turned on its side. The transfer forceps are also used to turn the cup upright without contaminating the sterile tray. The forceps are used for one procedure, then sterilized after use. Using transfer forceps eliminates the need to use sterile gloves to handle sterile supplies.

The handle of the sterile forceps is contaminated because you have touched it with your hands. Avoid touching the end of the forceps. The tips must remain sterile to contact sterile items. After using the forceps, rest the tips on a sterile surface to keep them sterile until the end of the procedure.

GUIDELINES 36-1 Guidelines for Sterile Procedures

- Always wash your hands before beginning a sterile procedure.
- Check the expiration date on the package. Avoid using items that are beyond the expiration date.
- If the sterility of an item is in doubt, consider it unsterile and avoid using it.
- If a sterile package is cracked, cut, or torn, it is contaminated and should not be used.
- If a sterile item or package becomes wet, it is contaminated.
- If a sterile item contacts an unsterile item, the sterile item is contaminated.
- Follow your facility's policy. You may be asked to sanitize and dry the table or other surface that sterile supplies will be placed on before establishing a sterile field.
- The outside of a sterile wrapper is not sterile, so you may handle it with your hands. Avoid touching the inside of the wrapper or items inside the package with your hands.

- The inside of a sterile package can be used as a sterile field.
- Never turn your back on a sterile field.
- Avoid reaching across or touching a sterile field. If you must add an item to the sterile field, drop it onto the field from the sterile package.
- Avoid touching unsterile articles when wearing sterile gloves. Avoid touching the outside of sterile packages when wearing sterile gloves. Keep your hands above your waist and make sure you can see them at all times. Avoid touching your clothing or body. If the gloves become torn or contaminated, change them immediately.
  - If sterile gloves touch an unsterile item, such as the outside of a package, they are contaminated. Change them before proceeding.
- Keep sterile items above waist level.
- Avoid talking, coughing, or sneezing over a sterile field.

PROCEDURE **83**   APPLYING AND REMOVING STERILE GLOVES

The following steps are written assuming the right hand is the dominant hand. All of the captions in the figures refer to dominant and non-dominant hands, not right/left.

1. Wash your hands.
2. Check the glove package for sterility.
3. Open the outer package by peeling the upper edges back with your thumbs.
4. Remove the inner package containing the gloves and place it on the inside of the outer package. Open the center fold and place it flat on the table (Figure 36-3A).
5. Open the inner package, handling it only by the corners on the outside (Figure 36-3B).
6. Pick up the cuff of the right-hand glove using your left hand. Avoid touching the area below the cuff.
7. Insert your right hand into the glove (Figure 36-3C). Spread your fingers slightly, sliding them into the glove fingers. If the glove does not go on correctly, do not attempt to straighten it at this time.

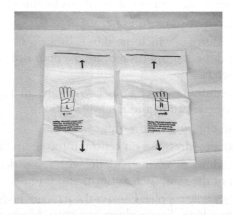

FIGURE 36-3A   Sterile gloves often are packaged with right and left clearly marked. Lay the package flat on the table.

(continues)

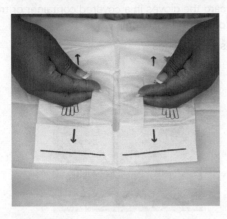

FIGURE 36-3B Using only the fingertips, reach in from each side and grasp the edges of the paper. Pull out and lay the paper flat without touching any area except the very edges.

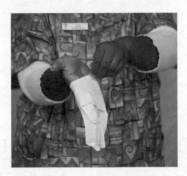

FIGURE 36-3C With the nondominant hand, grasp the inner cuffed edge of the opposite glove. Pick the glove up and step away from the sterile area, keeping the hands above the waist and away from the body. With palm up on the dominant hand, slide the hand into the glove.

8. Insert the gloved fingers of your right hand under the cuff of the left glove (Figure 36-3D).

9. Slide your fingers into the left glove, adjusting the fingers of the gloves for comfort and fit (Figure 36-3E). Because both gloves are sterile, they may touch each other. Avoid touching the cuffs of the gloves.

10. Insert your left hand under the cuff of the right glove and push the cuff up over your wrist (Figure 36-3F). Avoid touching your wrist or the outside of the cuff with your glove.

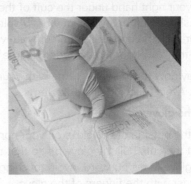

FIGURE 36-3D Step back to the sterile area. With the gloved hand, pick up the glove for the remaining hand by slipping four fingers under the outside of the cuff.

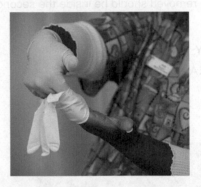

FIGURE 36-3E With palm up, slip the second hand into the glove. Keep the gloved thumb in a "hitch-hiking" position or extended away from the other fingers.

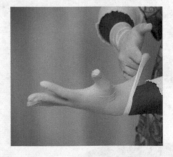

FIGURE 36-3F Keeping hands above the waist and away from the body, pull on the second glove. Pull the cuffs up. Avoid touching the skin with your glove.

(continues)

PROCEDURE **83** CONTINUED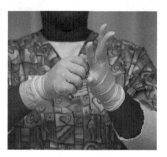

11. Insert your right hand under the cuff of the left glove and push the cuff up over your wrist. Avoid touching your wrist or the outside of the cuff with your glove. Adjust the gloves for fit as needed (Figure 36-3G).

12. You may now touch sterile items with your sterile gloves. Avoid touching unsterile items.

To remove the gloves:

13. Grasp the outside of the glove on your nondominant hand at the cuff. Pull the glove off so that the inside of the glove faces outward. Avoid touching the skin of your wrist with the fingers of the glove.

14. Place this glove into the palm of the gloved hand.

15. Put the fingers of the ungloved hand *inside* the cuff of the gloved hand. Pull the glove off inside out. The first glove removed should be inside the second glove.

ICON KEY:

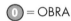 = OBRA

16. Discard the gloves in a covered container or trash, according to facility policy.

17. Wash your hands.

FIGURE 36-3G Adjust gloves if desired, staying away from the wrist area. Keep gloved hands above the waist and away from the body.

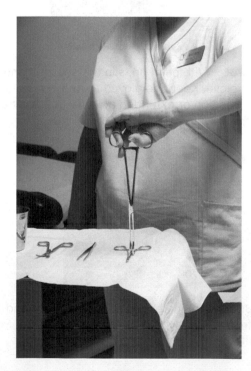

FIGURE 36-4 Use sterile forceps to add or move items on a sterile field. Do not allow the tips of the forceps to touch unsterile surfaces or objects. Wash the forceps after use and return them for sterilization according to facility policy. Do not use them for more than one procedure.

SKILLED NURSING PROCEDURES

Although nursing assistants are not allowed to perform skilled nursing procedures, they are frequently called upon to assist while the nurse is doing so, and must care for patients who have had such procedures.

Intravenous Therapy

Intravenous (IV) therapy refers to medication or solutions administered directly into a vein. Standard intravenous therapy is given into a peripheral vein (a large vein in the arm). The IV may consist of a single bag of solution connected to simple tubing with a needle or small catheter on the end. Sometimes an additional small bag of fluid is connected to the main (primary) tubing. This is called a **piggyback**. The small bag contains medication such as an antibiotic that is intermittently infused into the vein (Figure 36-5).

The IV tubing is usually threaded through an intravenous controller or pump that regulates the flow of solution (Figure 36-6). These electronic devices fasten to the IV standard and operate by electricity. Most automatically switch to battery mode in the event of a power failure. An alarm will sound for problems such as:

EXPAND YOUR SKILLS

PROCEDURE **84** APPLYING A DRY STERILE DRESSING

1. Carry out initial procedure actions.

2. Assemble supplies:
   - 1 pair disposable exam gloves
   - 1 pair sterile gloves
   - Normal saline or other cleansing solution
   - Sponges, applicators, or other supplies for cleaning wounds
   - Sterile gauze pads or other sterile dressing, as ordered, and according to facility policy
   - Bed protector(s), if needed
   - Bath blanket, if needed
   - Tape or bandage material
   - Plastic bag for used supplies

3. Holding gentle traction on the skin, loosen the tape that is holding the old dressing in place by pulling the ends toward the wound. Then remove the dressing. Discard in the plastic bag.

4. Cleanse and rinse the wound as ordered. If the wound appears abnormal or infected, notify the nurse.

5. Remove the gloves and discard in the plastic bag.

6. Wash your hands.

7. Set up your sterile field and prepare sterile dressing supplies. Arrange the field so that you do not have to cross over it when reaching for supplies.

8. Cut the tape, if used. Place on the edge of the overbed table, or as permitted by your facility's policy.

9. Apply sterile gloves.

10. Pick up sterile dressings by holding them only by the corners. Center them over the wound.

11. Tape the dressing securely in place, or cover it with a bandage (Procedure 85, Chapter 38).

12. Carry out ending procedure actions.

ICON KEY:

 = OBRA   = PPE

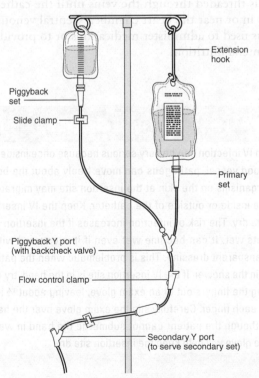

FIGURE 36-5 The large bag contains intravenous fluid that flows continuously into the vein. The small bag (piggyback) contains medication that is given for a short period of time.

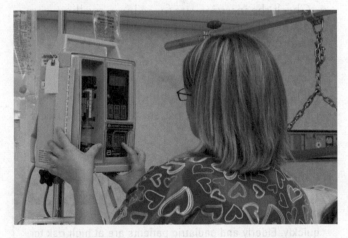

FIGURE 36-6 The nurse programming an intravenous infusion pump.

- Air in the line
- Line occlusion
- Interference with delivery of fluid at the designated rate
- Completion of the infusion
- Low battery

The alarm must always be in the on position when fluid is infusing. Sometimes an alarm is touchy and sounds repeatedly for no apparent reason. Although this can be annoying, never turn an alarm off. Some pumps will change to a "keep vein open" (KVO) rate if the alarm sounds. Some will shut off completely. Respond promptly to any alarm and take corrective action within the limits of your job description; notify the nurse promptly.

The nurse will immobilize the IV insertion site to prevent the catheter from moving. Movement is uncomfortable and increases the risk that the catheter will be dislodged. The nurse is responsible for the intravenous infusion. However, you must monitor the intravenous site and tubing each time you are in the room.

The most common problem of IV therapy is **infiltration**. This occurs when the catheter or needle comes out of the vein and fluid flows into the surrounding tissue. If an IV infiltrates, the drip rate usually slows or stops. Monitor the insertion site for swelling, cool skin temperature, and a white or pale skin color. The patient may complain of burning or pain. If the patient experiences these problems, or if you are unsure of the infiltration status of the IV, promptly notify the nurse. If infiltration occurs, the nurse will remove the IV and restart it in another area. The nurse may instruct you to remove the IV catheter and apply warm compresses to the area of infiltration.

On the subacute care unit, nursing assistants may be permitted to take limited nursing action if an IV infusion stops dripping. If you are permitted to troubleshoot an IV that has stopped dripping, you should:

- Confirm that fluid is present in the container.
- Check the insertion site for redness, swelling, complaints of pain or burning, or other signs of possible infiltration.
- Check the height of the IV solution; it should be at least 30 to 36 inches above the insertion site.
- Check for kinks in the tubing.
- Reposition the arm or patient to see if this affects the flow of solution.

- Straighten the arm with the IV to see if the fluid begins infusing again. Monitor the insertion site to see if it begins swelling, which indicates infiltration. If you observe other problems, such as blood backed up in the tubing, inform the nurse promptly. Do not attempt to correct the problem.

Move the patient carefully to avoid dislodging the IV. Avoid pulling on, kinking, or obstructing the tubing. Avoid positioning the patient with the tubing under the body. Position the arm with the IV at heart level when the patient is in bed. Instruct the patient to place the arm with the IV across the abdomen during ambulation. Advise the patient not to comb hair or brush teeth using the arm with the IV.

Discontinuing a Peripheral IV

An IV is discontinued if complications such as infiltration occur. In this situation, it is restarted in another location, preferably the opposite extremity. An IV is also discontinued upon the physician's order. In some facilities, nursing assistants are permitted to discontinue IVs. Follow your facility's policies and physician orders.

Central Venous Catheters

IV therapy can also be administered through a **central venous catheter (CVC)** (Figure 36-7A). A special catheter is inserted into a vein near the patient's collarbone and is threaded through the veins until the catheter tip ends in or near the heart chamber. Central venous therapy is used to administer medications or to provide total parenteral nutrition.

 Age-Appropriate Care ALERT

Occasionally, a pump error causes fluids to run in very quickly. Elderly and pediatric patients are at high risk for circulatory overload when IV fluids are given rapidly, and should be closely observed during IV therapy. Common signs of circulatory overload are elevated blood pressure, rapid pulse and respirations, coughing, shortness of breath, anxiety, and cyanosis. Inform the nurse immediately if you suspect a problem with a pump.

Infection Control ALERT

An IV infection can be very serious because once inside the blood vessel, pathogens can move freely about the body. Organisms on the skin at the insertion site may migrate to the inside or outside of the catheter. Keep the IV insertion site dry. The risk of infection increases if the insertion site gets wet. It can become wet even if it is covered with a transparent dressing. This is problematic when the patient is in the shower. If the IV insertion site is in the hand, try cutting the fingers out of an exam glove, leaving about ½ inch of each finger. Carefully slip the exam glove over the hand. Although the patient cannot submerge the hand in water, the glove will help keep the insertion site dry.

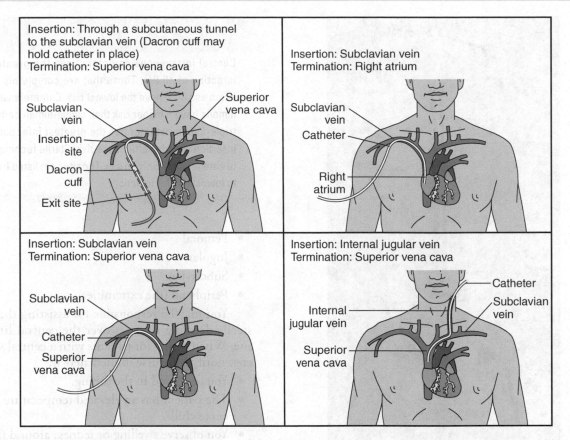

FIGURE 36-7A Locations for CVC insertion. The central intravenous catheter is threaded through the vein until the tip reaches the superior vena cava or right atrium.

Insertion: Basilic vein (peripheral)
Termination: Superior vena cava

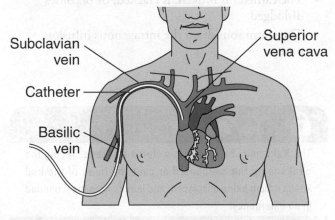

FIGURE 36-7B The PICC is usually inserted into the upper arm. The long catheter is threaded to the superior vena cava of the heart.

Peripheral Intravenous Central Catheter Line

A **peripheral intravenous central catheter** (**PICC**) line consists of a catheter that is inserted into a peripheral vein and threaded upward through the vein to the jugular or subclavian vein (Figure 36-7B). It is used to administer medications or to provide total parenteral nutrition.

Total Parenteral Nutrition

Total parenteral nutrition (**TPN**) is also called *hyperalimentation*. TPN is given to a patient whose digestive system needs complete rest. All required nutrients (carbohydrates, proteins, and fats) are given directly into the vein so the bowel does not have to work to digest food, allowing it to rest and heal. Patients receiving TPN may have to be weighed daily or every other day. Obtain the weight at the same time of day with the patient wearing the same type of clothing. The person may be gradually switched over to enteral feedings (Figure 36-8).

The nurse will care for the insertion site. Be sure the tubing is not obstructed or kinked. Be very careful to avoid dislodging the tubing when moving or caring for patients. Many health care facilities keep a special clamp, called a **Kelly** (Figure 36-9), at the bedside of patients with central intravenous lines. Serious complications occur if the tubing breaks or becomes dislodged. The Kelly is used to clamp the tubing close to the patient's body if the line breaks or is accidentally pulled loose. Air in the line can cause fatal complications. The Kelly should be readily available and visible at all times. Avoid storing it in a drawer or removing it from the room.

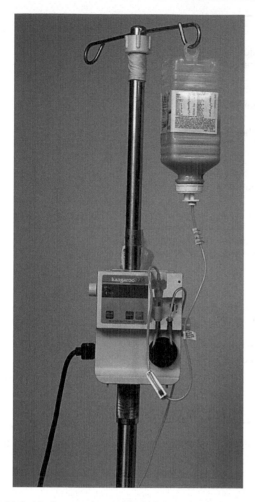

FIGURE 36-8 Unflavored nutritional supplements may be given through a nasogastric or gastrostomy tube. The flow of the supplement is controlled through a pump such as shown in this picture.

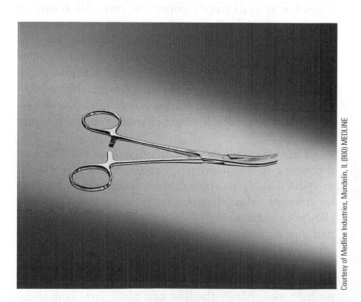

Courtesy of Medline Industries, Mundelein, IL (800) MEDLINE

FIGURE 36-9 A Kelly clamp is applied on a broken central line to prevent air from entering the circulation.

 Infection Control **ALERT**

Central intravenous catheters have the greatest risk of infection of all IVs. Those that are completely implanted (such as ports) have the lowest risk. Catheters with multiple lumens have a higher risk than single-lumen catheters. The triple-lumen catheter has the greatest infection risk. The insertion site also affects the risk. Sterile technique is used to care for any insertion site. The sites are listed from highest to lowest risk for infection:

- Femoral
- Jugular
- Subclavian
- Peripheral (the extremities)

You may be responsible for assisting the nurse with sterile dressing changes over the central line insertion site. When caring for patients with a central venous catheter, notify the nurse immediately if:

- You see blood in the tubing.
- The patient has an elevated temperature or experiences chills.
- You observe swelling or redness around the collarbone or near the infusion site.
- The patient complains of pain in the neck or chest.
- The patient becomes short of breath, or develops elevated blood pressure or edema.
- The catheter is broken, is cracked, or becomes dislodged.
- The alarm sounds on the intravenous infusion pump.

 Safety **ALERT**

The Kelly must be sealed in a sterile package. Taping the package on the headboard or over the head of the bed keeps it from being misplaced, and leaves it visible if needed in an emergency.

 Infection Control **ALERT**

Remember that all IV procedures are sterile. If you are assisting a nurse with any of these procedures, review sterile technique and avoid contaminating the sterile field or supplies.

PAIN MANAGEMENT PROCEDURES

Pain management may be the major reason some patients are admitted to the subacute unit. Other patients may be undergoing pain management related to conditions such as recent surgery or cancer. Both drug and nondrug treatments can be successful in helping to prevent and control pain. A 2006 study done at the Cleveland Clinic and Case Western Reserve University showed that listening to music for an hour a day will bring some relief to people suffering from chronic pain. Researchers noted that the kind of music patients listened to did not affect the pain relief experienced. Various types of relaxation techniques are also used for pain management.

Patient-Controlled Analgesia

Patient-controlled analgesia (PCA) is used for acute, chronic, or postoperative pain. *Analgesia* means pain relief. A device is inserted into the patient's vein and connected to a solution that contains a narcotic. A **narcotic** is a drug such as morphine that is used for pain relief. The dosage is controlled by equipment that has been preset by the nurse. The patient pushes the PCA button at times of discomfort. The controls on the pump are set to prevent accidental medication overdose. Report to the nurse if you note any change in the patient's:

- Level of consciousness
- Rate and pattern of respirations
- Pupil size
- Skin color

Other complications that you should report to the nurse are:

- Nausea and/or vomiting
- Inability to urinate or difficulty urinating
- Excessive drowsiness
- Confusion or change in mental status
- Itching
- Sounding of the preset pump alarm

Constipation is a common side effect of narcotic medications. Problems can become serious if not carefully monitored. Encourage patients to eat fiber foods on trays, drink liquids, and be as active as possible in keeping with the plan of care. Carefully monitor and document the patient's bowel activity. Report complaints or signs of constipation to the nurse.

GUIDELINES 36-2 Guidelines for Caring for Patients with Intravenous and Central Venous Lines

Use these guidelines in addition to the troubleshooting activities listed earlier.

- Make sure the solution is flowing. Know the drip rate in the drip chamber. Notify the nurse if the rate changes or the drip chamber is full.

- Avoid pulling or twisting tubing. Make sure the patient does not lie on the tubing.

- Note signs of moisture that may indicate the tubing is leaking.

- Make sure all junctions in the tubing are securely connected.

- Report immediately to the nurse:

  - Signs of dyspnea, cyanosis, chest pain, or back pain.

  - Wetness or moisture at the insertion site or where the tubing connects to the intravenous catheter.

  - If the solution in the intravenous bag or bottle is empty or low. The container should never run dry.

  - If the IV is not dripping, seems to be dripping too fast, or if the drip chamber is completely full.

  - If the needle becomes dislodged.

  - If the tubing pulls apart from the needle.

  - If the solution appears to be leaking.

- When caring for patients with any type of IV therapy, *never*:

  - Change the drip rate.

  - Disconnect any tubing.

  - Manipulate the catheter, needle, or tubing. If the tubing or needle accidentally separates, put firm pressure on the needle insertion site with a gloved hand and call for the nurse immediately.

  - Remove, change, or manipulate any dressing over the site.

  - Adjust the clamps on the tubing.

  - Take a blood pressure in the arm with an intravenous infusion.

  - Turn off an alarm on an IV pump or other infusion equipment.

Pain Management with an Epidural Catheter

Continuous medication infusion may be used to manage pain after major thoracic, abdominal, and orthopedic surgery. This therapy works by blocking transmission of pain at the spinal cord. Patients receiving continuous epidural analgesia receive stable, consistent doses of pain medication rather than experiencing the peaks and valleys associated with most other control methods. Patients are more willing to participate in their care plans when they are not having pain, and are usually satisfied with their care.

An **epidural catheter** is implanted beneath the skin and inserted into the epidural space near the spinal cord (Figure 36-10). Medication is administered either intermittently or continuously into the epidural space through the catheter. Narcotic pain-relieving medications and local anesthetics are usually given together, but either drug can be given individually. The patient may have leg numbness and weakness for the first 24 hours after the catheter is inserted. Limited mobility in areas not affected by the medication and decreased blood pressure when rising from bed are also common reactions. Instruct the patient to call for assistance when getting out of bed. Elevate the head of the bed 30° to 40°. Monitor the patient's blood pressure and pulse at least every hour for the first two hours after the catheter is inserted, then every two hours. Monitor the respirations every hour for the first day, and then every two hours.

Report the following to the nurse immediately:

- A catheter becomes dislodged from the insertion site.
- Changes in respiration rate and pattern.
- Patient complains of itching.
- Vomiting or complaints of nausea.
- Dressings covering the catheter become wet from leaking or an external cause.
- Respirations decrease to 12 or below.
- Oxygen saturation drops below 90 percent.
- The patient's level of consciousness decreases.
- Urinary retention (the patient complains of a need to urinate, but cannot).

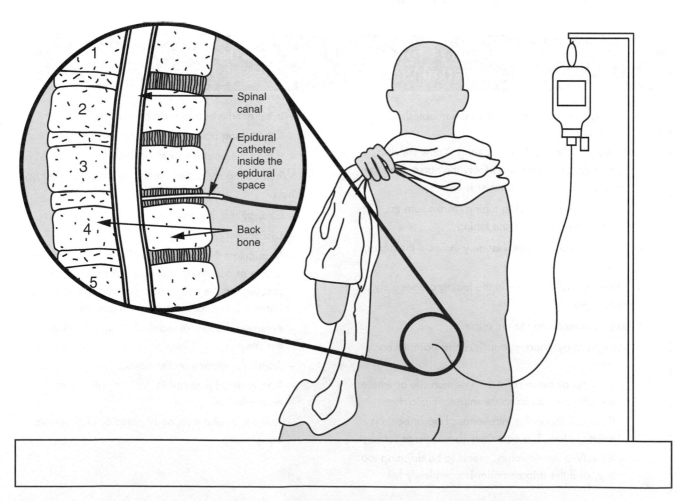

Spinal canal

Epidural catheter inside the epidural space

Back bone

FIGURE 36-10 The epidural catheter is used for intermittent or continuous pain medication.

- Low blood pressure (hypotension)
- Hives
- Rapid pulse (tachycardia)
- Redness, warmth, tenderness, swelling, itching, or drainage at the catheter insertion site
- Patient complains of inability to move the legs
- Patient complains of severe low back pain
- Patient complains of change in sensation or motor function

Implantable Medication Pumps

Implantable medication pumps are sometimes used for long-term medication delivery in both adults and children (Figure 36-11A). The pumps are surgically placed under the abdominal skin. A tiny catheter is threaded under the skin from the pump to the spine (Figure 36-11B). Medications are infused directly into the cerebrospinal fluid. This type of therapy has become common for patients with:

- Chronic, severe pain
- Severe **spasticity** (sudden, frequent, involuntary muscle contractions that impair function)
- Some types of cancer

The medication pump is implanted surgically. The patient will have two surgical sites, one on the abdomen and a smaller one near the spine. A physician or specially trained nurse will use a computer (Figure 36-11C) to adjust the medication dose over a period of time until the desired response is achieved.

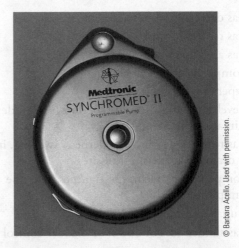

FIGURE 36-11B A medication pump can hold up to 40 mL of medication.

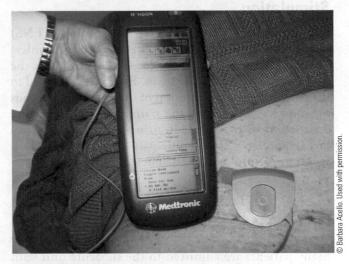

FIGURE 36-11C A handheld device is used to regulate the dose of medication.

Postoperative Care

The patient may remain on bed rest for 2 to 20 hours after surgery, depending on physician preference and patient response. An abdominal binder (see Chapter 29) may be used after surgery. The nurse may instruct you to apply a cool application or ice pack (see Chapter 27) to the site where the catheter tunnels under the skin. Some physicians permit patients to resume normal activity immediately, if they are able. If you are assisting the patient with transfers, avoid using a transfer belt until the surgical site is fully healed (usually several months after surgery, according to physician order and facility policy). In some facilities, a wide transfer belt is used for these patients, to prevent pressure on the pump or surgical site.

Patients with newly implanted medication pumps may have a complicated medication regimen in which they slowly withdraw from oral medications and depend increasingly on medications administered through the pump. Notify the nurse if the patient:

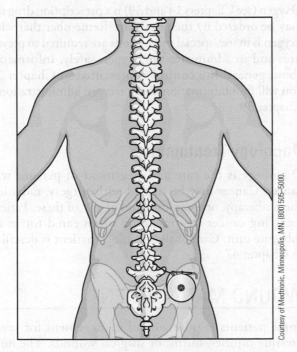

FIGURE 36-11A The implantable medication pump delivers medication directly into the cerebrospinal fluid.

- Has decreased responsiveness
- Has respirations of 12 or below
- Has a temperature over 100°F orally
- Complains of headache
- Experiences fluid leakage
- Develops a collection of blood or fluid under the skin at the insertion site
- Has redness, warmth, tenderness, swelling, itching, or drainage at the surgical sites
- Complains of a feeling of tightness over the pump site
- Is unable to move the legs
- Has sudden loss of bowel or bladder control

Transcutaneous Electrical Nerve Stimulation

Transcutaneous electrical nerve stimulation (TENS) is a nondrug method of pain relief. Mild, harmless electrical current stimulates nerve fibers to block the transmission of pain to the brain. Electrodes are taped to the patient's skin. The location of the electrodes depends on the areas related to the pain. The electrodes are attached to wires that are in turn attached to a control box (Figure 36-12). The intensity of the stimulation is set on the control box by the nurse.

CARING FOR SUBACUTE PATIENTS WITH SKILLED NURSING NEEDS

Many patients are admitted to the subacute unit with problems related to the respiratory system. Some conditions are caused by diseases within the lungs. Some patients experience respiratory problems as a result of complications of other conditions. Attention to the patient's oxygenation is a very important responsibility.

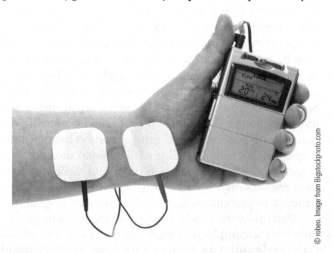

FIGURE 36-12 A TENS unit is used to block the transmission of pain impulses to the brain.

 Culture **ALERT**

Many individuals make a fashion statement by wearing tongue piercings (Figure 36-13). Countless risks accompany this practice. A tongue piercing can be especially problematic if the patient requires an oral airway or endotracheal tube. Notify the nurse promptly if a patient with a tongue piercing has pain, bleeding, increased flow of saliva, swelling, or signs of infection in the mouth. Swelling of the tongue can become severe, closing off the airway. To prevent patient injury, jewelry in tongue piercings will probably have to be removed when an airway is inserted.

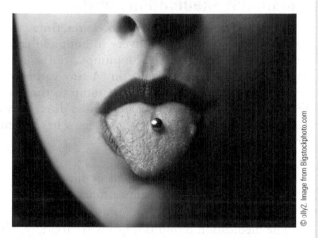

FIGURE 36-13 Tongue piercings create a high risk for complications.

Oxygen Therapy

Oxygen (see Chapters 14 and 39) is a prescription drug that may be ordered by the physician. Remember that when oxygen is in use, special precautions are required to prevent fires and to administer the oxygen safely. Information about general fire control is presented in Chapter 14. You will find information about oxygen administration in Chapter 39.

Oncology Treatments

Oncology is the care and treatment of persons with cancer. Cancer may be treated with surgery, radiation, chemotherapy, or a combination of any of these. Patients receiving cancer treatment are often cared for in the subacute unit. Care of the oncology patient is described in Chapter 47.

WOUND MANAGEMENT

Some patients require wound management for severe pressure injuries, burns, or surgical wounds. The nurse or physical therapist will perform frequent dressing changes on these areas using sterile technique. You may be required to assist with dressing changes, so a basic knowledge of sterile technique is necessary. The patient may have special positioning needs related to the injured area of the skin, or may be on a low air loss therapy bed or another type of specialty bed. Positioning with special devices and props may be ordered. Notify the nurse if any of the following occur:

- The wound appears red or swollen or has increased drainage.
- The dressing becomes saturated with drainage from the wound.
- Wound drainage has a foul odor.
- The patient complains of increased pain in the wound.
- The wound dressing becomes wet, is soiled, or falls off.
- The wound dressing accidentally becomes contaminated with urine or stool.

Managing Wounds with Drains

Drains (see Chapter 29) may be placed in wounds during surgical procedures to remove fluids that have collected below the skin. A drain may be sutured in place and exit the skin through a small incision. Some drains are hollow and empty directly to the outside of the body. Others have closed containers for collecting fluids, and must be emptied. Care of the device varies with the purpose of the drain, physician orders, and type of drain used. Use sterile technique when managing drains. A drain is a portal of entry (see Chapter 12) through which the patient can contract an infection. Apply the principles of standard precautions and use aseptic technique.

Caring for a Patient with a T-Tube

T-tubes are named for their shape. This T-shaped drain is used to drain bile and keep the common bile duct open after gallbladder removal surgery. One end exits the skin through an incision in the right upper quadrant. The tube fits tightly and is seldom sutured in place. It is usually attached to a sterile closed drainage system. Attaching the T-tube to a sterile urinary leg drainage bag provides the patient with more mobility. You may use the bag to collect the bile. Measure it in a

---

⚖ Legal ALERT

Some of the procedures related to tubes and drains in this chapter are considered advanced in some facilities. Perform the procedures only if you are qualified, approved, and permitted to do so according to your job description, facility policies, and state nurse practice act.

---

graduate pitcher. Applying dry sterile dressings around the insertion site will help protect the skin. Check the T-tube every few hours to make sure it is not kinked or obstructed.

Observe the patient closely for bile leakage, which will irritate the skin and may indicate obstruction. During the first 24 hours after surgery, the tube will drain approximately 300 to 500 mL of blood-tinged bile. Inform the nurse if drainage exceeds this amount. Daily drainage usually decreases to 200 mL or less after five days, although it may occasionally be more. Bile is normally thick, sticky, gummy or syrupy, and green-brown in color. To prevent excessive bile loss, secure the T-tube drainage system at abdominal level. If bile drainage exceeds 1,000 mL daily, the nurse or physician must return the bile to the patient's digestive system orally or through a nasogastric tube. Advanced nursing assistant responsibilities include:

- Checking the T-tube for patency and site condition every hour for the first eight hours
- After the first eight hours, checking the tube every four hours, or as instructed
- Providing good skin care, doing frequent dressing changes, and keeping the skin clean and well protected
- Using Montgomery straps to avoid irritating the skin with tape
- Monitoring the urine and stool carefully. Report color changes to the nurse
- Monitoring the patient for jaundice apparent in the skin and sclera, and notifying the nurse if noted
- Informing the nurse if the color or viscosity (thickness, stickiness) of the T-tube drainage changes, or if the drainage increases
- Monitoring and documenting strict intake and output

Clamping the T-Tube

The T-tube is usually clamped for one hour before and one hour after each meal. Clamping the tube alters the flow of bile so it moves back to the duodenum to aid digestion. Clamping the tube may be a licensed nurse procedure in your facility. However, you must understand the purpose of clamping the tube. You will monitor the patient's response to clamping and watch for signs of obstructed bile flow. Check the bile drainage level in the closed system drain bag regularly. Monitor for and report to the nurse:

- Fever
- Chills
- Rapid pulse
- Nausea and/or vomiting

- Complaints of pain or fullness in the right upper quadrant
- Jaundice
- Foamy, dark urine
- Clay-colored stools

Using a Closed Wound Drainage System

The Jackson-Pratt and Hemovac drains are commonly used closed drainage systems. These drains are placed directly in a wound, and drainage goes into an expandable container outside the body. The amount and character of drainage is recorded in the output record and the nursing notes. It is your responsibility to:

- Report both heavy and light drainage.
- Report a change in the appearance, amount, or character of drainage.
- Make sure the flow of drainage is not blocked.

If you observe any of the following, report it to the nurse:

- Drain is not intact or patent.
- Drain appears blocked, dislodged, or kinked.
- Surrounding skin appears abnormal (erosion, red, hot, swollen, macerated).
- Drainage is eroding surrounding healthy skin.
- Drainage is purulent, cloudy, foul-smelling, or abnormal smelling.
- Drainage color changes or appears abnormal.
- Amount of drainage decreases markedly or stops entirely.
- Amount of drainage increases markedly.
- Patient has fever, tachycardia, and/or hypotension.
- Urinary output decreases.

Closed wound drainage promotes healing and prevents swelling of the postoperative wound. Various systems apply gentle suction to the wound to remove fluid and reduce tension on the suture line. It also decreases the risk of skin breakdown, eliminates the need for many dressing changes, and helps reduce the risk of infection.

The Hemovac and Jackson-Pratt closed drainage systems use perforated tubing and a vacuum unit to remove wound drainage. The proximal end of the tube is in the wound bed. The tubing usually has its own exit site, and is commonly sutured to the skin to prevent displacement. It seldom extends through the suture line. Thus, the patient will have two surgical wounds. The length of time the drain is left in place is determined by the wound drainage. The collection container must be frequently emptied and measured to maintain suction and prevent pulling and stretching the suture line. When you empty a drainage container, select the proper PPE, and use good sterile technique.

REMOVING SUTURES AND STAPLES

Surgical wounds and large lacerations are closed with sutures and staples that are removed in 7 to 10 days, depending on the location of the wound and progress in healing (Figure 36-14). Sutures that close muscle and tissue below the skin surface are made of absorbable material and need not be removed.

Interrupted sutures are most commonly used. When this type of suture is used, each thread is tied off and knotted separately. A single thread is used to close an area when **continuous sutures** are used. Staples may be used to close abdominal and chest wounds. Patients may be apprehensive about suture and staple removal because of pain. Although there may be slight discomfort, the procedure is not painful.

DOCUMENTATION OF CARE IN THE SUBACUTE UNIT

Reimbursement for care in subacute units is frequently provided by insurance companies and managed care organizations. Reimbursement is often based on documentation. The main purpose of documentation is to provide a record of patient care. However, the medical record may also be used to evaluate the level and value of services the facility provides to each patient. The information on the record is used to determine payment to the facility.

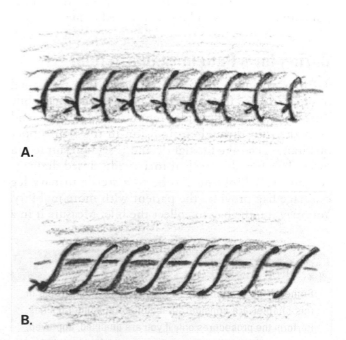

FIGURE 36-14 (A) Interrupted sutures; (B) Continuous sutures.

Payment may be denied if the documentation does not support the claims of the care given or what the patient required. The agencies that pay the bills will only pay for care that matches the patient's treatment plan and describes the patient's progress toward goals and response to treatment. If you are working with patients on special restorative nursing or therapy programs, you may be required to document additional information. Avoid subjective terms such as *good, fair,* or *poor.* Describe patient response to services or progress toward care plan goals in measurable terms, such as:

* "Ambulated 50 feet in hallway with walker"
* "Ate 90% of breakfast meal"
* "Consumed 975 mL of fluid orally this shift"

The survival of a facility and its staff depends on payment for services. This is what pays the bills and meets payroll. Therefore, documentation is important for many reasons. Documentation requirements change as reimbursement changes.

Complete, accurate documentation proves that workers have complied with physician orders, complied with the law, and met legal standards of care. It shows that the patients received good care. Properly completed records will show that the patients' risks and needs were identified, and that care was given to meet those needs. You will care for several patients each day, and remembering each small detail is difficult. Make notes if necessary, so you do not forget important information. Documentation is an important communication tool for all workers who care for the patient. Accurate, complete documentation protects both the facility and the individual workers. Missing, inaccurate, or absent information may cause problems with communication, reimbursement, facility inspections, or legal actions. Your facility will provide instruction on special documentation requirements related to subacute care and reimbursement in the subacute unit.

REVIEW

A. Multiple Choice

Select the best answer for each of the following.

1. Subacute care is given to persons who:
   a. have been acutely ill.
   b. have had a long, progressive illness.
   c. require only custodial care.
   d. require intensive care.

2. The purpose of subacute care is to:
   a. increase the use of long-term care facilities.
   b. discharge patients as quickly as possible.
   c. provide the care a person needs at a lower cost.
   d. provide care to unstable patients.

3. Patients treated in subacute care include persons:
   a. who are critically ill.
   b. requiring routine long-term care.
   c. who may require complex wound care.
   d. receiving obstetrical care.

4. A nursing assistant working in subacute care would need to:
   a. learn how to start intravenous fluids.
   b. have excellent observational skills.
   c. learn how to administer chemotherapy.
   d. instruct patients in pain management techniques.

5. If you accept a position in a subacute care unit, you may need to learn:
   a. how to administer medication.
   b. how to care for patients receiving dialysis.
   c. how to prepare special therapeutic diets.
   d. to manage unstable patients.

6. Documentation in the subacute unit:
   a. is for internal monitoring only.
   b. affects reimbursement for care.
   c. is the primary means of communication.
   d. is the responsibility of the unit secretary.

7. A central venous catheter is inserted into:
   a. a vein in the patient's foot.
   b. an artery in the patient's arm.
   c. the jugular or subclavian vein.
   d. the epidural space.

8. Total parenteral nutrition (TPN) is used for patients:
   a. who need to lose weight.
   b. who are unconscious.
   c. who refuse to eat.
   d. whose bowel needs rest.

9. The nursing assistant's responsibility in caring for patients with intravenous fluids is to:
   a. insert the needle into the vein.
   b. add medication to the bag of fluid.
   c. observe for complications.
   d. change the drip rate if it is too fast or too slow.

10. Patient-controlled analgesia is used:
   a. for acute, chronic, or postoperative pain.
   b. for oral pain and anxiety medications.
   c. to administer medication every four hours.
   d. for medication delivery on a fixed schedule.

11. An epidural catheter is used for:
   a. pain management.
   b. administering nutrition.
   c. emptying the bladder.
   d. intravenous fluids.

12. Sterile technique is used for:
   a. colostomy care.
   b. changing surgical dressings.
   c. routine stage I pressure injury care.
   d. administering enemas and suppositories.

13. Which of the following statements is true?
   a. A sterile package may be used more than once.
   b. Always wash your hands before applying sterile gloves.
   c. The sterile area of the sterile drape includes the top and area hanging over the edge.
   d. Regular exam gloves must be worn when assisting with a sterile dressing change.

14. When pouring liquid into a cup on a sterile field, a small amount splashes onto the sterile drape. The drape is:
   a. contaminated.
   b. clean.
   c. sterile.
   d. aseptic.

15. You are using transfer forceps to add supplies to a sterile field. You expect to add more supplies before the procedure is finished. Which of the following is true?
   a. The handle to the forceps is sterile.
   b. Store the forceps in liquid disinfectant so they remain sterile.
   c. Keep the tip of the forceps on a sterile area until the procedure is finished.
   d. The forceps may be used for 24 hours after the package is opened.

16. Oncology is the care and treatment of patients with:
   a. severe wounds.
   b. kidney failure.
   c. cancer.
   d. terminal illness.

17. The nursing assistant should avoid taking blood pressure:
   a. on the unaffected arm of a person who has had a stroke.
   b. with an electronic blood pressure unit.
   c. on an arm with an intravenous infusion.
   d. on the arm with the identification band.

18. Always keep the bag of intravenous solution:
   a. below the needle insertion site.
   b. exactly 6 feet off the floor.
   c. parallel to the needle insertion site.
   d. above the needle insertion site.

19. If the intravenous tubing accidentally becomes separated from the needle, the nursing assistant should:
   a. apply firm pressure to the needle insertion site with a gloved hand.
   b. quickly plug the tubing back into the needle or intravenous catheter.
   c. wrap the area with a pressure bandage and call the nurse.
   d. apply a dressing over the open intravenous catheter and call the nurse.

20. Constipation is a common side effect of:
   a. spasticity.
   b. narcotic medications.
   c. TPN.
   d. oncology treatments.

21. Do not use a transfer belt on a patient with a:
   a. ventilator.
   b. hip replacement.
   c. central intravenous catheter.
   d. newly implanted medication pump.

22. Transcutaneous electrical nerve stimulation is:
   a. implanted in the spine for medication delivery.
   b. a computer that controls implanted devices.
   c. a mild, harmless, nondrug method of pain relief.
   d. internally implanted in the epidural space.

23. Hospitals:
   a. care for persons with chronic illnesses.
   b. are not required to maintain accreditation.
   c. provide low-level services to elderly people.
   d. must keep patient information confidential.

24. Long-term care facilities:
    a. care for persons with chronic conditions.
    b. are not required to maintain confidentiality.
    c. admit only independent patients.
    d. provide acute care services.

25. When providing perineal care, you should use:
    a. clean gloves.
    b. no gloves.
    c. sterile gloves.
    d. shoe covers.

B. True/False

Mark the following true or false by circling T or F.

26. T F A sterile field is used whenever a body cavity is entered.

27. T F Clean technique is used when caring for surgical drains.

28. T F Surgical staples are removed three to four days after they are placed.

29. T F A single thread is used to place interrupted sutures.

30. T F Hospitals provide acute care.

31. T F Apply a sterile dressing surrounding a drain.

32. T F When applying a sterile dressing, use clean gloves.

33. T F Hold a sterile drape by the corners.

C. Word Choice

Choose the correct word from the following list to complete each statement in questions 34–44.

exacerbation	piggyback
hyperalimentation	spasticity
Kelly	transcutaneous electrical nerve stimulation
multisensory stimulation	transitional care
narcotic	
parenteral	

34. Subacute care is also called _____.

35. A _____ refers to a small bag of fluid containing intravenous medication that is connected with a tube to the primary tubing.

36. Total parenteral nutrition (TPN) is also called _____.

37. _____ nutrition is a feeding administered through a tube into the patient's vein.

38. A _____ is a potent drug used for pain relief.

39. The use of electrical current to treat pain is done with a procedure called _____.

40. Using various methods of sight, sound, touch, smell, pressure, and pain to help the patient awaken from a coma is called _____.

41. Worsening of the patient's condition is called _____.

42. A patient with severe _____ has sudden, frequent, involuntary muscle contractions that impair function.

43. A _____ is a curved clamp that is used to occlude central intravenous lines in an emergency.

44. Make sure a _____ clamp is available in the rooms of persons with central intravenous catheters.

D. Nursing Assistant Challenge

You have completed your nursing assistant course and have been working the night shift for three months in a skilled care facility. The director of nursing calls you into their office. They compliment you on your work and tell you they appreciate your dependability. They ask if you would like to work the day shift in the new subacute care unit of the facility. You tell them you would like to think about it for a day and then give your decision. Consider the types of care that are given in subacute care and then answer these questions.

45. What would your duties be in the new unit?

_____

_____

46. You feel confident of your nursing assistant skills. However, you know you will need to learn some new things to care successfully for subacute care patients. What new information or skills will you need to acquire?

_____

_____

47. How do you plan to obtain this education?

_____

_____

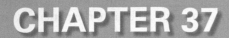

CHAPTER 37

Alternative, Complementary, and Integrative Approaches to Patient Care

OBJECTIVES

After completing this chapter, you will be able to:

37.1 Spell and define terms.

37.2 Define alternative medicine.

37.3 Differentiate alternative practices from complementary and integrative practices.

37.4 List five categories of alternative and complementary therapies.

37.5 Define holistic care.

37.6 List at least three ways in which the nursing assistant supports patients' spirituality.

VOCABULARY

Learn the meaning and the correct spelling of the following words and phrases:

acupuncture
alternative
alternative medical
  systems
Anthroposophically
  Extended Medicine
  (AEM)
aromatherapy
art therapy
Ayurveda
biofeedback
biological therapy
body-based therapy
chelation therapy

chiropractic care
color therapy
complementary/alternative
  medicine (CAM)
complementary medicine
cupping
dance therapy
doctor of osteopathy
  (DO)
electromagnetic therapy
energy therapy
guided imagery
herbal therapy
herbs

holistic care
homeopathy
hypnotherapy
integrative (integrated)
  health care
light therapy
massage therapy
meditation
mind–body therapy
modalities
movement therapy
moxibustion
naturopathic medicine
nutrition therapy

osteopathic manipulative
  treatment (OMT)
prayer
qigong
reflexology
Reiki
relaxation
supplements
therapeutic touch (TT)
traditional Chinese medicine
  (TCM)
visualization
yoga

ALTERNATIVES TO MAINSTREAM HEALTH CARE

When most people in Western society think of medical care, they think of medical, surgical, pharmaceutical, and technological treatment of patients. In the United States, these practices and techniques are the accepted, traditional, mainstream approaches to patient care and healing of illness. Throughout history, though, people have actively sought out other forms of healing the sick. Drawings in caves show early humans practicing healing. Medical practice in ancient Egyptian society was quite advanced. Native (North) American tribes have medicine men. The Bible describes healing of the sick. Some tribes of today have shamans (Figure 37-1), who practice divination and healing.

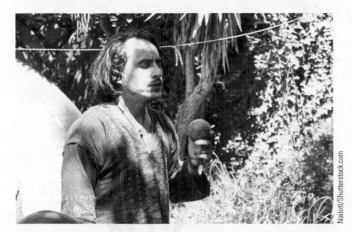

FIGURE 37-1 A shaman performing a healing ceremony.

Mainstream medicine involved many alternative practices before twentieth-century advances in technology, research, and medicine. In many ancient cultures, religion and medicine were closely connected. In the Middle Ages, medicine was the concern of either the church or the state. Because of this, many people used folk remedies that included herbs (Figure 37-2). People used various religious customs and charms for healing. These methods were more readily available and affordable than medical treatments.

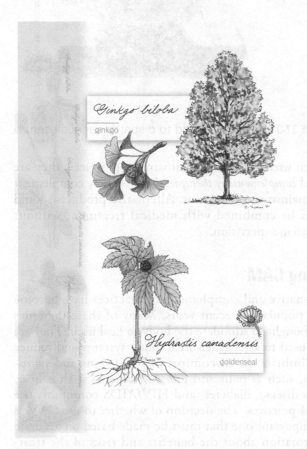

FIGURE 37-2 Herbs are potent natural substances with medicinal properties.

Today, some people prefer natural and spiritual treatments for illness. Others are afraid of the technology, drugs, and surgical procedures of today. Some patients believe that conventional medical treatments are worse than the discomfort of disease. They prefer using other methods of relieving symptoms and eliminating sickness. Because of this, many people use **alternative** health care practices and products to prevent and treat illness. Some people use alternatives instead of conventional health care. Most alternative strategies use natural products rather than those made from chemicals. Alternative therapies are used to treat every imaginable symptom and condition, from pain to menopause. Some people use natural products and practices to prevent illness. Most towns have at least one health food store that sells alternative products. Many books and magazines are available describing natural alternatives to mainstream health care. Some nontraditional practices have proven effective. Others have shown no real benefit, but this is a popular trend. The use of alternative therapy is not a passing fad; it is here to stay.

Many old remedies, practices, and traditions are being used today. The public and many medical professionals accept different forms of nontraditional healing. These nontraditional methods are called **complementary/alternative medicine (CAM)**. CAM is a group of diverse systems, practices, and products that are not presently considered part of conventional medicine. This is an area of much research and scientific study. Because of this, practices listed as CAM change continually. Safety is always a great concern in health care. Some CAM practices are unsafe or ineffective and are no longer used. Others have proven safe and effective and have moved into mainstream health care. For safety, a physician or other health care practitioner should always supervise a CAM program. New practices and techniques are always emerging.

Culture ALERT

Some patients may view an illness as having a supernatural cause. Others believe they need a traditional cure, diet, herb, or therapy for treatment.

Culture ALERT

Learn the patient's views about health. Accept the patient's practices whenever possible. Inform the nurse of practices that may affect the patient's overall care and those that pose special health risks, such as taking herbal remedies or eating items not permitted on the diet ordered.

Complementary and Alternative Practices

Hundreds of different alternative therapies are used instead of traditional medicine. For example, some patients use **herbs** (medicines made from plants), **supplements** (nutritional substances used to correct a deficiency or strengthen the whole), and diet to treat cancer instead of surgery, chemotherapy, and radiation therapy (Chapter 47). Supplements are also used in addition to mainstream methods. Nutritional products are usually slow to work and no immediate effect is seen when patients take them. The patient may have to take the preparation for a minimum of three to six months before seeing results.

A degree of caution is necessary when using nutritional preparations. Some are toxic or harmful when taken in large quantities. Some have negative interactions with other medications and foods. Some nutritional products contain combinations of vitamins and nutrients. Taking several combination products increases the risk that the patient will exceed the safe dosage range. An example is vitamin A, which is necessary for good eyesight and night vision. However, when taken in large amounts, vitamin A can cause blindness and liver failure. Water-soluble preparations are excreted from the body. Fat-soluble preparations are stored in the tissues for a period of time. Some preparations interfere with drugs and therapies given for other medical conditions. Several have caused serious liver and kidney damage.

Complementary medicine is a treatment regimen in which alternative practices are combined with conventional health care. For example, magnets may be used with medications to relieve pain. Various sound and music therapies are used to reduce complications, relieve stress, otherwise make patients feel better, and increase their sense of well-being. **Aromatherapy** (using natural scents and smells to promote health and well-being) (Figure 37-3) is used by chemotherapy patients to relieve nausea. Some people use **guided imagery** in combination with cancer treatment. People who use imagery believe that focusing on and visualizing positive changes causes these changes to occur. **Energy therapies** work with the energy field that allegedly surrounds and penetrates the body. (The existence of this energy has not been confirmed scientifically.) **Relaxation** (techniques and methods of reducing stress) and **meditation** (calming and quieting the mind by focusing attention) are used in combination with heat and medications to relieve pain.

Thousands of different treatments and therapies fall under the CAM umbrella. These **modalities** (forms of treatment or uses of therapeutic agents or regimens) can be placed into five broad categories, which are listed in Table 37-1. Most of these practices can be used alone or combined with treatment that is more conventional. When used alone, they are called *alternative treatments.*

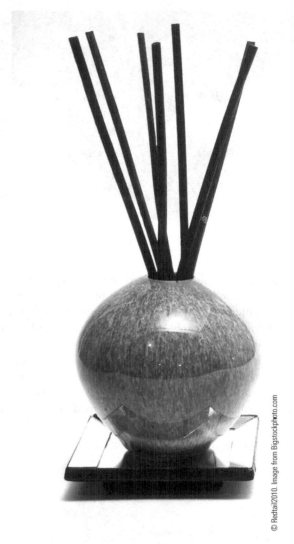

FIGURE 37-3 Reeds are used to disperse various scents.

When used with other mainstream practices, they are called *complementary therapies,* because they complement the mainstream treatment. Alternative products should never be combined with medical treatment without physician supervision.

Using CAM

Alternative and complementary practices have become very popular in recent years. Many of these therapies are thought to stimulate the body to heal itself. They are also used to strengthen weak body systems and reduce or eliminate the discomfort of some signs and symptoms, such as pain and nausea. Patients with cancer, heart disease, diabetes, and HIV/AIDS commonly use CAM practices. The decision of whether to use CAM is an important one that must be made based on accurate information about the benefits and risks of the treatment. The patient must look beyond advertisers' claims to find reliable, credible information about the method

TABLE 37-1 Common Complementary and Alternative Medicine Categories

Category	Description	Example
Alternative medical systems	Therapeutic or preventive health care practices that do not follow generally accepted methods and may not have a scientific explanation for their effectiveness. These treatments are usually based on complete systems of medical practice. Many were developed in other countries and have been used for centuries, predating conventional medical practices.	• Traditional Chinese medicine (TCM) • Ayurveda • Homeopathy • Naturopathy
Mind–body therapy	Practices that employ various techniques to enhance the mind's ability to affect bodily function and symptoms (mind-over-matter principle). Many have been accepted by the mainstream medical community and are part of integrative health care practices and treatments.	• Meditation • Art therapy • Music therapy • Dance therapy • Patient support groups • Cognitive therapy • Prayer • Guided imagery
Biological therapy	Biologically based practices using natural substances, such as vitamins, herbs, and foods. Other natural products, such as shark cartilage, are also used.	• Herbs • Nutritional products • Dietary supplements
Body-based therapy (may also be called manipulation, or manipulation therapy)	Practices that are based on direct body contact, including manipulation or movement of one or more parts of the body.	• Chiropractic adjustments • Osteopathic manipulation • Massage therapy
Energy therapy	The study of how living organisms interact with electromagnetic energy fields. Although some practitioners believe touch is necessary for healing, others believe they can effect healing by placing the hands within the field. Two types of energy therapy are commonly used. Biofield therapies work by laying hands on the body or through its energy field to transfer a healing force. The biofield may also be called an *aura*. The energy field is believed to permeate the body and extend outward for several inches. Biomagnetic-based therapy is a form of energy therapy in which the hands are placed in or through the energy field to apply pressure on the body.	• Reiki • Therapeutic touch • Magnet therapy and use of magnetic fields • Pulsed current fields • AC and DC current fields

being considered. Authoritative information is difficult to find for some treatments because little research has been done. When evaluating the negatives and positives, the patient should ask:

- What are the advantages, disadvantages, risks, side effects, expected results, and length of treatment?
- What is the safety record of the treatment? Are specific safety precautions necessary?
- Is the treatment effective in circumstances similar to mine? Is it harmful in circumstances similar to mine?
- What are the qualifications of the individual providing the treatment (if applicable)?
- Will the CAM therapy interfere with the conventional treatment or medication being used for my acute or chronic medical problem?
- Can I comfortably comply with the directions for using this treatment?

People use alternative therapies and programs for many different purposes. Many do this on their own, without medical supervision. Potential drawbacks of an

unsupervised alternative treatment program include the following:

- Some herbs and nutritional products are potentially toxic (especially in large amounts).
- Self-diagnosis may be inaccurate.
- The self-treatment regimen may not be appropriate, even if the diagnosis is correct.
- Self-treatment does not always work.
- The alternative regimen may delay necessary medical treatment.
- The program may interfere with prescription drugs and other medical care.
- Some herbs interfere with anesthesia and may cause complications during surgery, including unstable blood pressure and pulse, increased bleeding, and adverse reactions with other drugs.
- Self-treatment may cure the symptoms, but aggravate other health problems.

If you decide to pursue an alternative program, do so under medical supervision. Seek medical help if the condition you are treating does not respond within a week, if the original symptoms worsen, or if new symptoms develop.

INTEGRATIVE (INTEGRATED) HEALTH CARE PRACTICES

Some researchers estimate that at least 50 percent of the American public uses at least one form of alternative or complementary treatment. Because of this, many hospitals have opened specialized units and clinics in which **integrative (integrated) health care** is practiced. Integrative health care involves using both mainstream medical treatments and CAM therapies to treat patients. Approximately 25 percent of the hospitals in the United States offer some type of integrative medical services. Most integrative health care programs have two components. The wellness component helps participants stay well and prevent disease. The illness management component helps eliminate uncomfortable symptoms and strengthens the body to overcome the effects of illness and heal. Many patients in the illness track also use approaches from the wellness track to prevent worsening of their conditions. Thus, persons who are well can participate to prevent illness, and those who are ill can participate to aid in their recovery.

Usually, the CAM method is used to enhance mainstream treatment, or to relieve signs and symptoms. Some services combine drug therapy with nutrition, diet, exercise, or other nontraditional therapies. CAM practices that promote relaxation and relieve pain are some of the most commonly used in integrative care. This is based on the belief that when the mind and body are relaxed, pain and unpleasant symptoms decrease, and a healing environment is established within the body. Professionals who practice integrative care are very cautious, and CAM treatments are usually selected only when there is solid evidence that they are safe. If there is a substantive risk of harm to the patient, the treatment combination is not used.

Some patients practice integrative care on their own, without the knowledge of their health care provider. This can be dangerous, because some therapies increase the risk of complications when combined with some medical treatments and medications. For example, Mrs. Rosenberg has a strong family history of Alzheimer disease. She fears she will develop this condition. She has taken herbs regularly for several years, as a preventive measure. Mrs. Rosenberg is hospitalized for a routine surgical procedure. She does not tell the doctor about the herbs, because they are nonprescription, natural products. She did not deliberately withhold the information. The herbs were just part of her routine and she did not think about it. During surgery, she experienced a large, unexpected blood loss and required a blood transfusion. Mrs. Rosenberg did

> ### ⊕ Clinical Information **ALERT**
>
> A four-month study by researchers at Northwestern Memorial Hospital in Chicago showed that art therapy helped alleviate eight of nine symptoms in patients being treated for cancer, including pain, depression, poor appetite, and fatigue.

not know that some herbs have a blood-thinning effect. Because the physician did not know of the herb use, she did not take measures before surgery to reduce the increased risk of bleeding.

The use of herbs during pregnancy can also be risky. In fact, herbs are very powerful substances that should be treated with caution and respect. They interact with many different prescription and nonprescription medications. Patients should always inform the health care provider if they are using alternative products. If a patient advises you that they use alternatives, always inform the nurse, who will notify the physician.

Holistic Care

Standard medical care focuses on treating single body parts or systems. Most integrative medicine practitioners believe in using **holistic care** (practices that consider the whole person, including mind, body, and spirit). Holistic care (Figure 37-4) is designed to nourish, balance, and vitalize the whole individual. The patient's strengths are used to overcome weaknesses. Nursing care, in its purest form, has always been guided by principles of holistic care. In nursing, we look at the whole person. We know that one weakness can affect the patient's overall health

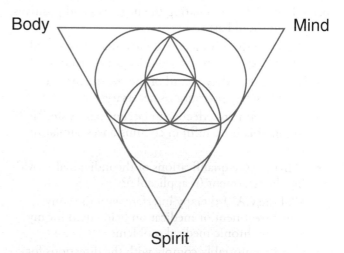

FIGURE 37-4 Holistic care looks at the body, mind, and spirit of the person. CAM therapists believe that these three aspects of the person must be balanced for health and wellness.

and well-being. By supporting and strengthening all body systems, holistic medical care provides additional tools with which to fight disease.

Practitioners of holistic care also consider the effect that disease has on the patient's family dynamics and relationships. This reaches beyond curing a disease. Holistic care considers the entire person as a complex being with many problems and needs. The patient is an active member of the health care team, not a passive participant. Besides standard medical care, consideration may be given to:

- Food and nutrition
- Fluid balance
- Elimination of body wastes
- Adequate rest and sleep
- Stress-relieving strategies
- Exercise
- Recreation
- Avoidance of unhealthy practices and substances
- Loving relationships and support systems
- Inner strength
- Creative expression
- Spiritual expression and well-being

CAM Practices and Holistic Care

When the patient and physician agree to consider an integrated approach to treatment, the assessment process begins. Integrative health care is based on certain principles:

- Each individual can be empowered to bring greater wellness and healing into their own life.
- Complementary therapies can be used to support and strengthen overall health. Some therapies promote healing. Others relieve symptoms, such as pain and nausea.

✚ Clinical Information **ALERT**

Nursing schools teaching holistic care have proven that each holistic theory embodies the art and science of nursing, while acknowledging the integrity and wholeness of the individual. They encourage students to enter each patient's room with healing intent and recommend stopping outside the door momentarily to clear the mind of one's own concerns, then entering the room with the ability to focus on the patient as a whole being.

- The mind affects the healing process.
- Every person is unique, and no single set of recommendations will be right for everyone. The integrative program must be individualized to meet the patient's needs and circumstances. More than one supportive therapy may be necessary.

The assessment for a holistic integrative care program will consist of:

- Evaluating the nature of the patient's medical and nursing problems.
- Determining if further diagnostic tests are needed (and obtaining tests, if necessary).
- Evaluating the patient's coping resources.
- Identifying the patient's goals and expectations.
- Evaluating the patient's knowledge about their disease.
- Evaluating the patient's knowledge about CAM.
- Identifying patient teaching needs and developing a patient teaching plan.
- Agreeing with the patient on treatments to use and goals of therapy.
- Developing an individualized integrative treatment plan.
- Making referrals, consultations, and appointments, if necessary.

Patient teaching is done so the patient can make informed decisions about their care. You may be asked to contribute information to the assessment. You may also reinforce patient teaching when you are caring for the patient. Always follow the plan of care. Teaching is an ongoing process during treatment. The patient's response to treatment will be evaluated frequently, and the treatment plan is adjusted as often as necessary to achieve a positive response.

COMMON CAM THERAPIES

Many CAM therapies are being used in health care facilities today. Modalities that are commonly used in integrative practice in hospital units and clinics include:

- **Acupuncture**, which is an ancient practice dating back thousands of years. Acupuncture is used to treat many acute and chronic conditions. Tiny, thin needles are placed in various parts of the body to correct imbalances in energy. It is safe and painless when done by a trained and qualified practitioner.
- **Anthroposophically Extended Medicine (AEM)**, a holistic Western system of natural medicine. AEM treats the whole person, not just the disease or symptoms. Practitioners consider

the human being as far more than a physical machine. Treatment is designed to harmonize the relationship of body, mind, and spirit. AEM practitioners may use herbal and homeopathic preparations to support and guide the natural healing processes in the body.

- *Aromatherapy*, which uses essential oils to stimulate the patient's sense of smell. Smelling the oils stimulates the olfactory nerve, sending messages to the brain. Although this treatment has many uses, it is commonly used to promote relaxation, relieve pain or nausea, and boost the immune system.

- **Art therapy**, **dance therapy**, and music therapy, all of which focus on use of the senses. Each helps the patient express themselves. They provide distraction and stress reduction. Art therapy helps the patient deal with emotional conflict, increase awareness, and express unspoken concerns. Dance therapy uses dance to decrease body tension, reduce pain, improve body image and self-esteem, decrease fear, and express anger. Music therapy has many therapeutic purposes and can be used alone or as part of other programs for relaxation, pain relief, and improved self-esteem.

- **Ayurveda**, a natural system of medicine that originated in India more than 3,000 years ago. Translated, *ayurveda* means "knowledge of life." This system is based on the belief that disease is due to an imbalance in the individual's consciousness. Practitioners encourage certain lifestyle interventions and use natural therapies to help the patient regain a balance between the body, mind, and environment. It begins with an internal purification process, followed by a special diet, herbal remedies, massage therapy, yoga, and meditation. It is commonly used to treat high blood pressure, reduce stress, and reduce blood cholesterol.

- **Biofeedback**, a method of retraining the mind to control various physical problems and stresses that one would normally not be aware of.

- **Chelation therapy**, which involves intravenous (IV) injection of an amino acid by a licensed professional. It is commonly used to treat serious circulatory problems and reduced blood flow in the legs because of a buildup on the walls of the blood vessels. The amino acid injection bonds with substances within the blood vessels and removes them into circulation, where they are excreted in the urine. Although chelation therapy is usually considered safe, side effects range from mild to serious. It is usually used in combination with diet and exercise.

- **Chiropractic care**, a common, accepted CAM treatment that many people consider part of the mainstream medical system (Figure 37-5). Health insurance and Medicare pay for chiropractic visits; they do not pay for treatments for which effectiveness has not been proven. Chiropractic treatment has proven effective in relieving some types of pain, headaches, and menstrual cramps. Chiropractic care is based on the premise that the nervous system must function properly for good health. Because the nerves run through the spinal cord, chiropractic adjustments are done to keep the vertebrae in good alignment. This relieves pressure on nerves, muscles, and joints. Most chiropractors also promote exercise, diet, and good nutrition for overall health.

- **Color therapy**. Many studies have been done on how color affects the human mind. Some of these have also shown that color affects the body. Color is believed to stimulate many different senses and

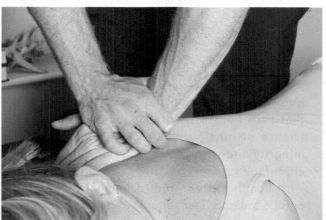

FIGURE 37-5 Chiropractic care is a common CAM treatment that many people find beneficial to treat specific health problems and support general wellness.

emotions. Marketing experts and advertisers use color to affect your moods and decisions. The color scheme on the packaging of most products is carefully designed to encourage you to buy. Past due bills are usually pink, which is associated with being very important. Red and orange color themes in restaurants are designed to increase your appetite. Many different alternative health care practices use color therapy, usually to affect mood, emotions, relationships, and sense of well-being. Color can be meditated upon, gazed at, worn, or beamed in with various lights. Spiritual light and color are used for healing the body and mind. Color is also used for deepening meditation and creating specific effects in and on the body's energy field.

- **Electromagnetic therapy**, which is based on the belief that electric and magnetic energies exist within the body. Treatment is given to correct imbalances in the electrical and magnetic fields, which are believed to cause illness and disease. Different forms of electrical energy are used to correct imbalances. Mainstream medicine has adopted many electromagnetic approaches, such as using a defibrillator (Chapter 51) to start the heart or a TENS unit (Chapter 36) to relieve pain.

- **Herbal therapy**, used throughout the world for its medicinal effect. Many food products we use today are herbs. *Herbs* are medicines made from plants that provide a different way of treating pain and illness. However, herbs are generally very strong, and some can be very toxic. The use of herbs as medicine should be supervised by a qualified practitioner.

- **Homeopathy**, a practice that uses a wide range of natural (plant and mineral) substances to stimulate the body's immune system to fight disease. Homeopathic medicines are given to stimulate the natural healing abilities of the body.

- **Hypnotherapy**, used to create an altered state of consciousness in which the patient is more open to the power of suggestion. It has many different applications, but in health care, it is commonly used to relieve pain, anxiety, depression, addiction, and insomnia.

- **Light therapy**, used to treat mood and sleep disorders, jet lag, and depression. Seasonal affective disorder (Chapter 30) is often treated with integrative medicine, and light therapy is an accepted approach. Treatment involves exposing patients to special lights covered with a plastic screen to block ultraviolet rays. The most common treatment involves sitting in front of a light box with the eyes open, but not looking directly into the

light. Treatment time is progressively increased up to 90 minutes a day. One treatment involves shining a light behind the patient's knees. Research is being done on using light in the treatment of many conditions, including obesity and premenstrual syndrome.

- **Massage therapy**, which is provided by licensed massage therapists. Massage stimulates and improves circulation, providing relaxation and pain relief. It is believed to stimulate the immune system to fight disease. Massage increases feelings of well-being and reduces stress and fatigue.

- *Meditation*, a form of body and mind relaxation. It has various applications, ranging from stress relief to pain relief. Meditation is an intensely personal and spiritual experience for most people. To meditate is to turn inward, to concentrate on the inner self. Meditation is a three-step process involving preparation, concentration, and merging with the object of concentration. It is commonly used for personal growth and developing tolerance. Meditation is said to channel awareness into a more positive direction by transforming one's state of mind.

- **Movement therapy**, a form of nonaerobic exercise and breath control that gives patients an awareness of how the body moves. Practitioners learn to alter posture and motion to reduce pain and stress. It is useful in chronic neurological disorders, such as Parkinson disease, multiple sclerosis, and stroke. It has been used for increasing self-esteem.

- **Naturopathic medicine**, whose doctors receive extensive education at one of five schools in North America. Naturopathic care focuses on whole-person wellness, emphasizing prevention and self-care. The doctor looks for the cause of illness, rather than strictly treating symptoms. Naturopathic practitioners cooperate with and refer patients for medical diagnosis and treatment when necessary. They use nontoxic, natural medications that are compounded and individualized to the patient's needs.

- **Nutrition therapy**, which evaluates the patient's diet to ensure that it contains optimal nutrition for health, wellness, and healing. This may mean eliminating some foods and adding others. Vitamins, minerals, and nutritional supplements (Table 37-2) may be added for wellness promotion or healing, such as calcium to prevent osteoporosis, or vitamin C to promote pressure-injury healing.

- **Prayer**, a CAM technique that is used alone and in combination with other treatments. Some people

TABLE 37-2 Vitamins

Vitamin	Purpose	Effects of Deficiency	Dietary Sources
Vitamin A	Helps maintain vision Promotes the growth of healthy skin, hair, bones, and teeth Assists with cell reproduction Strengthens the immune and reproductive systems The body converts beta-carotene to vitamin A	Reduced vision Night blindness Dry skin Poor bone and tooth health, growth, and development	Soy milk (and other dairy products) Carrots Spinach Green peas Tomato juice Watermelon Sweet potatoes Pumpkins Cantaloupe Sunflower seeds Fish liver oils Liver Lean ham Mango Broccoli Lean pork chops Egg yolks
Vitamin B1 (Thiamine)	Helps convert carbohydrates into energy Helps to maintain normal nervous system Helps maintain function of the muscles, heart, and digestion	Reduced concentration Loss of appetite Weakness, exhaustion, and fatigue	Lean pork Legumes Yeast Bananas Most fish Liver Nuts and seeds Potatoes Sweet potatoes Peas Watermelon Avocados Poultry Whole-grain and fortified cereals
Vitamin B2 (Riboflavin)	Body growth Growth of hair, nails, skin Helps prevent sores and swelling of mouth and lips Aids in reproduction and cell regeneration Aids in the release of energy from carbohydrates	Itching skin Irritation of lips, eyes, skin, and mucous membranes	Eggs Fish and shellfish Fortified cereals Meat Poultry Dairy products Kiwi fruit Avocados Broccoli Turnip greens Asparagus Spinach

(continues)

TABLE 37-2 (continued)

Vitamin	Purpose	Effects of Deficiency	Dietary Sources
Vitamin B3 (Niacin)	Helps release energy from carbohydrates Aids in the function of the digestive system and nerves	Depression, diarrhea, dizziness, fatigue, halitosis, headaches, indigestion, insomnia, limb pains, loss of appetite, low blood sugar, muscular weakness, skin eruptions, inflammation	Beef liver Peanuts Chicken (white meat) Tuna Salmon Almonds Mushrooms Corn Mango Lentils
Vitamin B9 (Folic acid, folate)	Helps produce and maintain red blood cells and the nervous system Essential for mental and emotional health; helps normalize brain functions	Anemia Reduction in growth rates Digestive disorders such as diarrhea, loss of appetite, and weight loss Weakness, sore tongue, headaches, heart palpitations Irritability, forgetfulness, behavior disorders	Dark green vegetables Dry beans Peas Lentils Enriched grain products Fortified cereals Liver Orange juice Wheat germ Yeast
Vitamin B12	Nerve and red blood cell functions Needed to make DNA	Demyelination Irreversible nerve cell death Numbness or tingling of the extremities Ataxic gait	Dairy products Eggs Cereals Soy-based products Liver Beef Clams
Vitamin C (Ascorbic acid)	Necessary for collagen production Helps the skin, connective tissues, and organs; promotes healing Can act as an anti-oxidant to help protect the body from free radicals	Scurvy, loose teeth, poor wound healing	Citrus fruit (oranges, grapefruit, lemons, limes) Berries Melons Tomatoes Potatoes Green peppers Green, leafy vegetables
Vitamin D	Promotes the absorption of calcium and phosphorus Helps form and maintain strong, healthy bones	Soft bones, deformities	Liver High-fat fish Fish oils Egg yolk Fortified cereals Fortified milk Sunlight
Vitamin E	Antioxidant that protects cells from the effects of free radicals, which are potentially damaging byproducts of energy metabolism	Intestinal disorders Cystic fibrosis Pancreatitis Impaired liver function Prevents absorption of dietary fats and fat-soluble nutrients	Margarine Nuts and seeds Peanuts and peanut butter Vegetable oils Wheat germ Whole-grain and fortified cereals

(continues)

TABLE 37-2 *(continued)*

Vitamin	Purpose	Effects of Deficiency	Dietary Sources
Vitamin K	Helps control blood clotting; necessary for making the liver protein that controls clotting	Bleeding, nosebleeds, internal and external hemorrhaging	Broccoli Brussels sprouts Cabbage Leafy green vegetables Mayonnaise Soybean, canola, and olive oils
Zinc	(Not a vitamin; an essential mineral) Essential for cellular metabolism, immune function, protein synthesis, wound healing, cell synthesis and division Supports normal growth and development during pregnancy, childhood, and adolescence Needed for proper sense of taste and smell	Malabsorption Chronic liver disease Chronic renal disease Sickle cell disease Diabetes Malignancy Depressed growth Diarrhea Impaired mental status Depressed immunity	Wheat (germ and bran) Sesame seeds Poppy seeds Alfalfa seeds Celery seeds Mustard seeds Beans Nuts Almonds Whole grains Pumpkin seeds Sunflower seeds Black currant

use it with meditation. Patients have many different religious rituals and activities. Prayer is a connection with a person's higher power. One large study showed that patients who received prayer recovered faster after surgery than patients who were not the recipients of prayer. Many of the study patients were not aware that others were praying for their recovery.

- **Qigong,** whose practitioners believe that everyone is born with a life-force energy called *qi* or *chi*. This treatment involves physical and mental activities to teach the patient to channel the chi, thereby improving health. It is used to treat a variety of problems, including arthritis, gastric ulcers, insomnia, headaches, allergies, and high blood pressure.

- **Reflexology** (Figure 37-6), an ancient form of healing used to reduce stress and treat illness. Certain reflex areas in the hands and feet are stimulated. The stimulation affects other parts of the body, reducing stress, stabilizing body functions, and correcting health problems.

- **Reiki,** which touches on various areas of the body to promote health and well-being. The practitioner's hands are placed in various positions, beginning with the head and working down. The hands are held in place on each area for three to five minutes. Practitioners believe that sickness

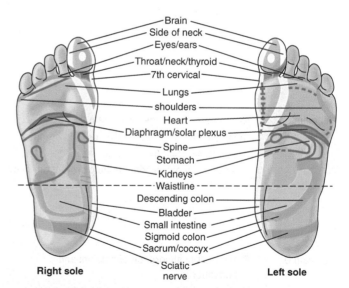

FIGURE 37-6 Practitioners of reflexology believe that body ailments can be healed by manipulating the feet. This is based on the principle that different areas of the foot are connected to specific areas of the body.

drains a person's physical and emotional energy. Reiki is used to promote spiritual and mental well-being, relieve stress, relieve pain, and promote relaxation.

- **Therapeutic touch (TT)**, a term commonly used to describe touching patients in a caring manner. However, in this context, it is a CAM treatment in which the hands are used to exchange energy and stimulate healing. Therapeutic touch practitioners believe that when energy is unbalanced, disease occurs. TT restores the energy field in the body to create a healing environment. The healer's hands do not touch the patient. The goal is to align the mind, body, and spirit for good health. TT is commonly used in the care of patients with AIDS, chronic pain, anxiety, and high blood pressure.

- **Traditional Chinese medicine (TCM)**, a complete health care system that is thousands of years old. It has changed little over the centuries. The basic idea is that a vital life force moves through the body. Any imbalance in the life force can cause illness. Disease is caused by an imbalance in the opposite and complementary energies that make up the life force, called *yin* and *yang*. The TCM doctor treats disease by restoring the balance between the internal body organs and the external elements of earth, fire, water, wood, and metal. Treatment may involve acupuncture, **moxibustion** (burning herbal leaves on or near the body), **cupping** (use of warmed glass jars to create suction on certain points of the body), massage, herbal remedies, movement, and concentration exercises.

- **Visualization**, one of the practices involved in guided imagery. This technique involves using the imagination to visualize something. Creating images in the mind helps reduce stress, pain, and symptoms associated with many medical conditions. The patient sets health goals and objectives. They are guided to visualize and work toward the goals. Two methods are commonly used. Visualization of colors is done to reduce stress. Another method involves visualizing the elimination of health care problems; for example, the patient may imagine a PacMan gobbling up cancer cells in the body.

- **Yoga**, which means the union between mind and body. Yoga involves a combination of breath control, postures, relaxation, and meditation. It is used to improve lung function and circulation, decrease pain, and reduce anxiety.

Osteopathic Medicine

Some individuals consider osteopathic medicine to be an alternative practice, but over the years this branch of medicine has been accepted as a form of mainstream medicine. The **doctor of osteopathy (DO)** has preparation similar to that of a medical doctor (MD). A DO receives a complete medical education. They receive additional training in **osteopathic manipulative treatment (OMT)**, a passive, thrusting motion similar to that used in chiropractic adjustment. OMT is used to restore normal body movement, in combination with regular medical treatment. For example, a DO treats a patient with an infection of the foot by prescribing antibiotic therapy. Additionally, they provide an OMT treatment to enhance blood and oxygen flow throughout the body. This is based on the belief that the antibiotic will be more effective in eliminating the infection if circulation to the foot is not impeded.

Osteopathic Medicine Versus Chiropractic Care

Some people believe that chiropractic and osteopathic treatments are identical, but they are not. Chiropractic care focuses mainly on the spine and involves many very fine maneuvers. The chiropractor focuses on preventing interruptions in nerve flow. The osteopathic physician

 Culture **ALERT**

Listen to how patients describe and otherwise talk about their conditions. For example, some cultures classify illnesses as "hot" or "cold" and treat each type differently. Ask questions if you need to understand better. However, you must be aware that occasionally a patient may expect you to have all the answers and will not ask questions. Inform the patient that learning their views helps you give better care. If direct questions make the patient uneasy, try indirect questions. For example, ask what the medicine man or other cultural healer would do in a given situation.

 Clinical Information **ALERT**

In 2002, the National Center for Complementary and Alternative Medicine (part of the National Institutes of Health) released a study showing that 36 percent of people over the age of 18 were using some form of complementary medicine. That number increased to 62 percent when the statistics included prayer specifically directed at health conditions.

focuses on how tight muscles and joints affect the function of all body systems. The emphasis is on ensuring proper movement of air (oxygen) and fluid within the body. This is based on the belief that the body works most effectively when:

- All tissues are nourished with oxygen.
- Wastes can be removed in body fluids.
- The body is in an optimum state of health; healing will occur when it is nourished with oxygen and wastes have been removed.

The osteopathic physician uses OMT along with regular medical treatment, whereas the chiropractor uses only spinal manipulation. Because of this, the DO can treat many conditions that do not respond to chiropractic care.

SPIRITUALITY

Spirituality and religion also have a place in nontraditional health care practices. Many people believe that spirituality and religion are the same thing, but they are not. Spirituality is more of an umbrella that defines:

- Our perceptions of our place in the universe.
- Higher power (if any).
- Our responsibilities to others.
- Our fears and beliefs about living and dying.

The need for spirituality may be fueled by experiences, relationships, opportunities that provide the motivation for deeper healing, and growth throughout life. Illness can be a powerful motivator for eliminating emotional, mental, and physical patterns that limit and restrict spiritual growth. A key to caring for patients' spiritual needs is respecting each patient as an individual, and appreciating that no two people are alike.

When patients use spirituality for healing, they allow the power of the spirit to work more fully in their lives, leading to greater harmony and balance. It is usually a quiet time for introspection and questioning. Healing may require making changes. It involves blending of the physical, mental, emotional, and spiritual aspects of self. When a person experiences deep physical or emotional healing, all parts of the self are changed. Physical problems often involve thoughts and emotions. Patients sometimes have surprises during periods of intense spirituality. They may release a great emotional burden instead of experiencing a physical recovery. The lifting of the emotional burden brings a great sense of inner peace.

Religion

Religion differs from spirituality in that it includes another element for the cause of disease. Religious beliefs vary widely, so making generalizations is difficult. However, members of various religions believe that other factors contribute to the development of disease, such as sin, assault from a demonic power or a lesser god, or the malevolence of others. Another common belief is that disease occurs to help a person learn an important life lesson or overcome a weakness. Most believe that although the higher power allows diseases to occur, that power is in no way responsible for them. Practitioners of some religions believe that the power of prayer, laying-on of hands, or another ritual is necessary to heal illness. Many believe that the power or intercession of a religious authority is necessary to effect a cure. The patient may practice certain religious rituals, such as fasting and prayer, to promote healing.

Nursing Assistant Actions

The nursing assistant must recognize that all humans are spiritual beings, although we all choose different paths. Be sensitive to each patient's paths and choices. Avoid making judgments about patients' religious, spiritual, ethnic, and cultural practices and choices in health care treatment. Although spiritual beliefs are usually considered a private concern, the need for spiritual caring is fundamental when serious health problems occur. The patient may question the meaning and purpose of life, their ability to hope, belief in themselves, belief in the caregiver's ability, belief in the physician's ability, and belief in a higher power.

Health care personnel are privileged to have a role in these very personal times of significant stress and turmoil in patients' lives. Pay attention to what the patient is saying. Your role is to listen, to reflect, and to clarify information. Never try to interpret or define spiritual meaning or truth to the patient. Avoid imposing your beliefs on the patient. Avoid pat, uncaring answers to questions. Never give patients false hope. Never use problem-solving techniques to analyze spiritual truths for patients. Admitting that you do not know an answer is acceptable.

Remember that caring for patients during very private moments is a privilege. Do not be so distracted with your workload or the environment that you fail to show sensitivity when patients express spiritual concerns. Provide privacy and support while they work through challenges to their health and well-being. Inform the nurse of the patient's concerns. They may be able to provide assistance, intervention, or referrals to other sources of help.

REVIEW

A. True/False

Mark the following true or false by circling T or F.

1. T F You should use problem-solving CAM techniques to teach patients to analyze spiritual truths.

2. T F Complementary therapies are used instead of traditional medical treatments.

3. T F Safety is a major concern when considering complementary and alternative health care and treatment methods.

4. T F Some CAM therapies involve manipulation of the body with the hands.

5. T F Herbs are medications made from plants.

6. T F Imagery involves focusing on and visualizing positive changes.

7. T F An osteopathic physician and a chiropractor have similar education and practice.

8. T F The nursing assistant should never admit that they do not know the correct answer to a question.

9. T F Complementary therapies have no place in health care.

10. T F Integrative health care involves a combination of mainstream medicine and alternative health care treatments.

11. T F Biofeedback involves training the mind to control physical problems.

12. T F Chiropractic adjustments are done to relieve pressure on nerves.

B. Matching

Choose the correct phrase from Column II to match the words or phrases in Column I.

Column I

13. _____ hypnotherapy
14. _____ homeopathy
15. _____ acupuncture
16. _____ Reiki
17. _____ movement therapy
18. _____ meditation
19. _____ aromatherapy
20. _____ therapeutic touch
21. _____ yoga
22. _____ Ayurveda
23. _____ qigong
24. _____ massage

Column II

a. stimulating sense of smell
b. concentrating on inner self
c. creates awareness of how body moves
d. rubbing the body to stimulate circulation, promote relaxation
e. views disease as an imbalance in a person's consciousness
f. activities to teach the patient to channel chi
g. alters the state of consciousness
h. uses natural substances to stimulate immune system
i. begins with hands on head, working down over body
j. restores energy field so healing can occur
k. uses thin needles
l. union between mind and body

C. Multiple Choice

Select the best answer for each of the following.

25. Holistic care includes:
    a. meditation and biofeedback.
    b. using strengths to overcome weaknesses.
    c. freeing nerves from entrapped vertebrae.
    d. focus on the disease process.

26. An integrative care program always begins with:
    a. patient teaching.
    b. goal-setting.
    c. assessment.
    d. assisting the patient to cope.

27. Cognitive therapy is a form of:
    a. mind–body therapy.
    b. energy therapy.
    c. manipulation.
    d. biological therapy.

28. Chelation therapy is used to:
    a. cleanse the mind.
    b. promote rest and relaxation.
    c. relieve stress.
    d. cleanse blood vessels.

29. Yin and yang are concepts used in:
    a. Ayurveda.
    b. traditional Chinese medicine.
    c. qigong.
    d. Reiki.

D. Nursing Assistant Challenge

Your patient, Mrs. Matassarin, has been diagnosed with colon cancer. She has chosen an integrative medicine program to treat her illness. She meditates and prays several times each day. The care plan states that you are to assist her in preparing to meditate at 3:15 p.m. each day. You are running a little late. You enter the room at 3:22 p.m. and find the patient deep in meditation.

30. What nursing assistant action should you take if the patient is meditating? Why?

_____

_____

31. What actions can you use in the future to assist the patient with the meditation care plan?

_____

_____

32. If you are unsure of what actions to take, how will you find out?

_____

_____

33. Based on your knowledge of integrative health practices, what effect will the meditation have on Mrs. Matassarin?

_____

_____

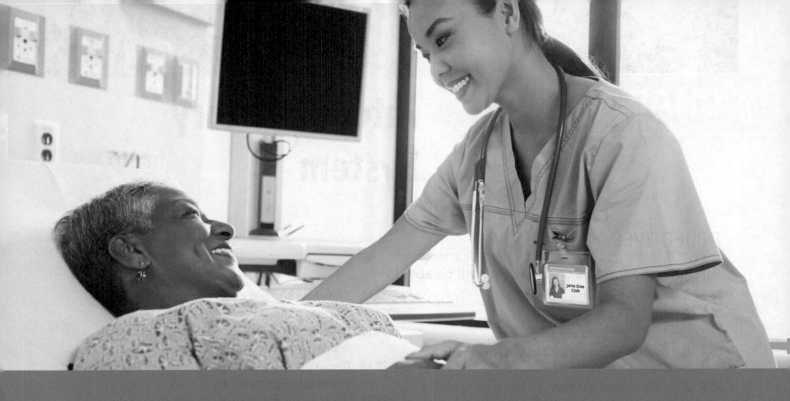

SECTION 11

Body Systems, Common Disorders, and Related Care Procedures

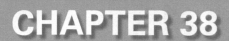

CHAPTER 38

Integumentary System

OBJECTIVES

After completing this chapter, you will be able to:

38.1 Spell and define terms.

38.2 Review the function of the skin.

38.3 Describe some common skin lesions.

38.4 List three diagnostic tests associated with skin conditions.

38.5 Describe nursing assistant actions relating to care of patients with specific skin conditions.

38.6 Identify persons at risk for the formation of pressure injuries.

38.7 Describe measures to prevent pressure injuries.

38.8 Describe the stages of pressure injury formation and identify appropriate nursing assistant actions.

38.9 List nursing assistant actions in caring for patients with burns.

38.10 State how skin tears occur and describe prevention measures.

38.11 Describe the guidelines for caring for patients with negative pressure wound therapy.

38.12 Discuss precautions to use when assisting with a pulsatile lavage treatment.

38.13 Describe the importance of nutrition in healing wounds and burns.

38.14 List the guidelines for cleansing and observing a wound.

38.15 Demonstrate the following procedure:
- Procedure 85: Changing a Clean Dressing and Applying a Bandage (Expand Your Skills)

VOCABULARY

Learn the meaning and the correct spelling of the following words and phrases:

abrasion	dermal ulcer	macule	rubra
allergen	dermis	malodorous	sebaceous gland
allergies	dressing	necrosis	senile purpura
anaphylactic shock	electrical burn	negative pressure wound	shearing
bandage	epidermis	therapy (NPWT)	skin tear
burns	eschar	nodule	slough
cartilage	excoriation	obese	subcutaneous tissue
chemical burn	friction	pallor	sudoriferous gland
contusion	hematoma	papule	tepid
crust	hydrocolloid dressing	pressure injury	thermal burn
cyanotic	integument	pulsatile lavage with	transparent film dressing
debride	Kaposi's sarcoma	suction (PLWS)	vesicle
decubitus ulcer	lesion	pustule	wheal

INTEGUMENTARY SYSTEM STRUCTURES

The integumentary system (Figure 38-1) includes:
- Skin
- Hair
- Nails

690

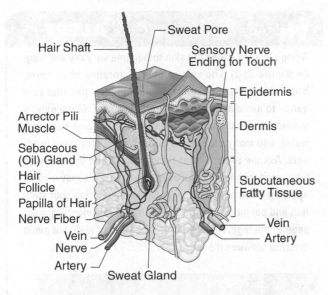

Hair Shaft
Sweat Pore
Sensory Nerve Ending for Touch
Epidermis
Arrector Pili Muscle
Sebaceous (Oil) Gland
Hair Follicle
Dermis
Papilla of Hair
Nerve Fiber
Subcutaneous Fatty Tissue
Vein
Nerve
Artery
Vein
Artery
Sweat Gland

FIGURE 38-1 Cross-section of the skin.

- Sweat glands
- Nerves
- Oil glands

The outermost layers of the skin make up the epidermis. The dermis lies under the epidermis. The **subcutaneous tissue** that attaches the skin to the muscles lies under the dermis.

The nails are horny cell structures found on the dorsal, distal surfaces of the fingers and toes. They protect the sensitive fingers and toes. The teeth are formed from the tissues of the **integument** (body shell).

Epidermis

The **epidermis** consists of dead outer cells that are constantly shed as new cells move upward from the dermis. No blood vessels are in the epidermis, so injury to this layer does not cause bleeding. Nerve endings reach into this outer layer. The nerves are sense organs that keep us in contact with changes in the environment. Nerve endings called *receptors* receive information about:

- Heat
- Cold
- Pain
- Pressure
- Temperature regulation (because the skin regulates body temperature)

Dermis

The **dermis** contains blood vessels, nerve fibers, and two kinds of glands:

- Sweat glands (**sudoriferous glands**)
- Oil glands (**sebaceous glands**)

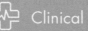 Clinical Information **ALERT**

The skin is the largest organ of the human body. In an average-size adult, the skin weighs approximately 4 kilograms (8.8 pounds). It covers an area of approximately 2 meters (78.4 inches). The average person's skin renews itself every 28 days. Each square inch of human skin consists of approximately 19 million cells; 60 hairs; 90 oil glands; 19 feet of blood vessels; 625 sweat glands; and 19,000 sensory cells. People of different races and skin color have about the same number of cells that produce skin color (melanocytes). A person's skin color depends on how much or how little melanin each melanocyte cell produces. Human skin has about 100,000 bacteria per square centimeter. Ten percent of human dry weight is attributed to bacteria. The normal flora that live on the skin help to protect you from harmful bacteria.

Sweat Glands

The sweat glands produce perspiration that reaches the skin surface through tubes or ducts that end in openings called *pores*. Blood vessels carry heat to the skin from deep inside the body. This heat is transferred to the perspiration. At the skin surface, the perspiration and the heat are lost through the pores to the air. The heat of the body is controlled by changes in the size of the blood vessels in the skin.

 Clinical Information **ALERT**

"Goose bumps" are caused by the contraction of an arrector pili muscle connected to each hair follicle. Although you may not notice it, the contraction also causes the hair to stand on end.

 Clinical Information **ALERT**

Sweat from the apocrine glands (those located mainly in the underarm and genital areas) is odorless. Body odor is caused by the action of the skin's normal bacteria on the sweat.

 Clinical Information **ALERT**

The average scalp has about 100,000 hairs. The hair on the head grows at a rate of approximately 1 cm per month (1 centimeter = 0.3937 inch). The average person sheds approximately 50–100 hairs from the head each day.

- When the central opening of a blood vessel becomes enlarged (dilated), more heat is brought to the body surface.
- When the central opening of a blood vessel becomes smaller (constricted), less heat is brought to the body surface.

Oil Glands and Hair

Oil glands lubricate and keep flexible the hairs found in the skin. Hair covers almost all body surfaces except for the palms of the hands and the soles of the feet.

SKIN FUNCTIONS

The skin has many functions that are critical to the well-being of the body:

- Protection—forms a continuous membranous covering for the body.
- Storage—stores fat and vitamins.
- Elimination—loses water, salts, and heat through perspiration.
- Sensory perception—contains nerve endings that keep us aware of environmental changes.
  The skin tells us much about the general health of the body:
- A fever may be indicated by hot, dry skin.
- Unusual redness—**rubra**, or flushing of the skin—often follows strenuous activity.
- **Pallor**, which is less color than normal, is a sign associated with many conditions.
- The oxygen content of the blood can be noted quickly by the color of the skin. When the oxygen content is very low, the blood is darker and the skin appears bluish or **cyanotic.**

AGING CHANGES

As a person ages, changes become evident in the skin and its elements. These changes include:

- Glands that are less active.
- Decreased circulation.
- Dryness, thinning, and scaling.
- Thickening of fingernails and toenails.
- Loss of fat and elasticity.
- Loss of hair color.
- Development of skin irregularities such as skin tabs or tags, moles, and warts.

Skin injury or disease can cause changes in skin structures. These changes are called **lesions**. The lesions may be caused by disease, injury, wear, or the aging process.

👪 Age-Appropriate Care **ALERT**

Aging changes cause the skin to become very dry and fragile (Figure 38-2). The skin of elderly persons often tears, breaks, and bruises readily. Handle elderly patients very gently to avoid accidental injury to the skin. Many elderly individuals avoid soap for routine bathing. Some use clear water, and many others use lotion-based cleansing products. Ask the patient what they prefer. Keep the skin well lubricated with lotion to prevent dryness. This may involve applying lotion to dry areas several times during your shift. Rub and pat lotion into the skin gently. Avoid vigorous massage of the legs. Apply lotion to the feet as well, but avoid the area between the toes.

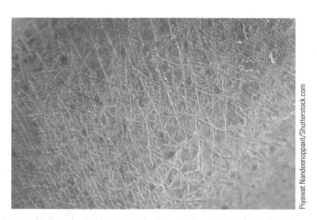

FIGURE 38-2 Dry skin is common in older people.

Piyawat Nandeenoppairt/Shutterstock.com

✚ Clinical Information **ALERT**

Babies with certain types of recurrent rashes appearing at 18 months old or younger may be more likely to develop common and chronic skin conditions.

Use standard precautions when caring for patients with skin lesions. Some of the most common skin lesions or eruptions are:

- **Macules**—flat, discolored spots, as in measles (Figure 38-3).
- **Nodules**—small, knotlike protrusions; small masses of tissue.
- **Papules**—small, solid, raised spots, as in chickenpox.
- **Pustules**—raised spots filled with pus, as in acne.

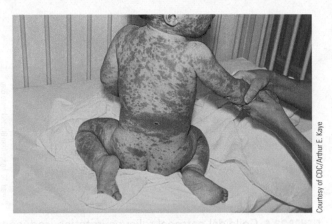

FIGURE 38-3 Macules on a baby that are caused by an allergy to a smallpox vaccination.

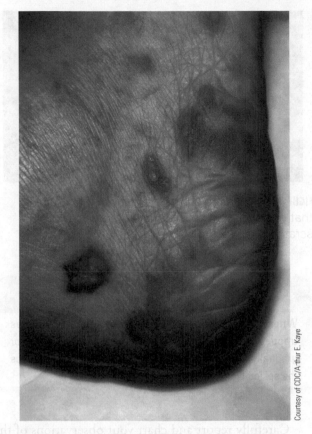

FIGURE 38-4 Kaposi's sarcoma is a malignant tumor caused by the human herpes virus 8 (HHV8) that commonly affects persons with weakened immune systems.

- **Vesicles**—raised spots filled with watery fluid, such as a blister.
- **Wheals**—large, raised, irregular areas frequently associated with itching, as in hives.
- **Excoriations**—portions of the skin that appear scraped or scratched away.
- **Crusts**—areas of dried body secretions, such as scabs.
  Skin lesions may be a result of systemic responses to:
- Communicable disease—diseases that are easily transmitted, directly or indirectly, from person to person. Measles and chickenpox are two such diseases. Each has characteristic skin lesions called *skin eruptions* or *rashes*.
- Immune system problems—Persons whose immune systems are depressed, such as those with HIV infection, may develop a type of cancer called **Kaposi's sarcoma** (Figure 38-4). It appears as lesions in the skin and eventually in other organs. The lesions are reddish-purple to dark blue in color and begin as macules, papules, or nodules that gradually become bigger and darker. In addition to persons with HIV infection, Kaposi's sarcoma is most common in men older than 60 years of age. Recent research suggests that it is caused by a herpes virus and may be spread by kissing an infected person. Kaposi's lesions can also appear in the mouth and internal organs. Progression of the disease may be slow or rapid.
- **Allergies**—also called *sensitivity reactions*, may have associated skin lesions. The vesicles of poison ivy are well known. The material causing the sensitivity is called an **allergen**. Individuals respond to allergens in different ways.
- **Anaphylactic shock**—a severe, sometimes fatal, sensitivity reaction.

SKIN INJURIES

Some lesions are seen when the skin is injured:

- **Abrasions** are injuries that result from scraping the skin.
- **Contusions** are mechanical injuries (usually caused by a blow) resulting in hemorrhage beneath the unbroken skin.
- An *ecchymosis* is a bruise.
- A **hematoma** is a localized mass of blood that is confined to one area.
- *Lacerations* are accidental breaks in the skin.
- **Senile purpura** (Figure 38-5) are dark purple bruises on the forearms and backs of hands; they are common in elderly individuals.
- *Skin tears* are shallow injuries in which the epidermis is torn. The shape is often irregular. These injuries are also common in elderly individuals.

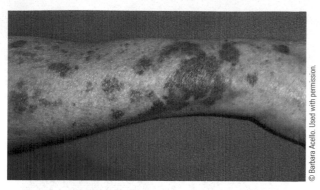
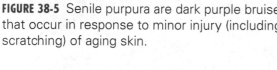

FIGURE 38-5 Senile purpura are dark purple bruises that occur in response to minor injury (including scratching) of aging skin.

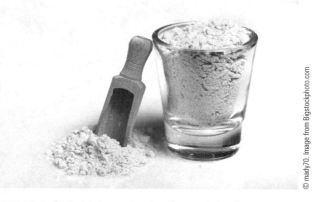

FIGURE 38-6 Colloidal oatmeal relieves irritation, reduces itching, and moisturizes, softens, and protects the skin.

⚕ Clinical Information **ALERT**

When a bruise (*ecchymosis*) occurs, blood becomes trapped under the skin, causing a reddish color. The color gradually changes as the area heals and the body absorbs the spilled blood.

Carefully report and chart your observations of the skin and accurate descriptions of what you see.

Diagnosing Skin Lesions

Your careful observations and accurate description of any skin lesions provide valuable information about the patient's condition. The physician may order diagnostic tests to help establish the cause of a lesion:

- Studying scrapings from the skin lesion under the microscope
- Culturing the skin lesion if an infection is suspected
- Performing skin testing if sensitivities are suspected, by introducing small quantities of substances (allergens) known to bring about an allergic (hypersensitivity) reaction in humans; allergens include pollens, foods, dust, animal dander, and medications, among other things

Care of Skin Lesions

Take the following precautions when skin lesions are present:

- Closely observe the patient's skin upon admission, but do not remove any dressings. Report abnormalities. Describe them accurately.
- Soap and water as well as rubbing lotions are often contraindicated (not permitted). Check the nursing care plan before bathing the patient or giving a backrub.
- Special products may be used for bathing or soaking the skin, such as *colloidal oatmeal* (Figure 38-6). This product is used for many different skin conditions to relieve irritation; reduce itching; and moisturize, soften, and protect the skin. You may be instructed to use **tepid** (lukewarm) water for bathing instead of hot water. Make sure that the patient does not get the treated bath water in the eyes. The product may make the tub slippery. Instruct the patient to use the handrail when rising from the tub and provide assistance as needed.
- Wear gloves when contact with blood, body fluids (including drainage from blisters or skin lesions), or nonintact skin is likely. Apply the principles of standard precautions and apply other PPE as needed, depending on the type and size of the skin lesion.
- Do not attempt to remove any crusts.
- Handle the patient gently. Avoid rubbing the skin.

⚕ Clinical Information **ALERT**

Therapeutic baths or soaks in tepid water are often used to treat skin conditions. Tepid water should be between 80°F and 93°F. The patient may need a therapeutic bath up to three times a day, depending on the severity of the underlying condition. Colloidal oatmeal is commonly added to the water. Add the product to the tub *as it is filling*. If the patient complains of feeling sticky after the bath, rinse with a few extra cups of tepid water from the faucet. Pat (do not rub) the skin dry.

Infection Control ALERT

Become familiar with the appearance of scabies and body lice on the skin. They may appear as numerous tiny scabs on the skin surface. The areas commonly itch, and the patient may scratch them. If the patient has multiple tiny scab-like areas, wear gloves when care requires skin contact. Report the presence of these lesions to the nurse for further assessment.

- Special bed linens may be used, such as sterile linens, linens that have been washed in special detergent, or disposable linens. Special bedding will be listed on the care plan.
- A bed cradle (Chapters 15 and 25) may be placed on the bed to prevent the sheet from contacting the open skin areas.
- Notify the nurse if the:
  - Skin lesions are draining.
  - Nature of the drainage changes.
  - Amount of drainage increases.
  - Drainage becomes **malodorous** (having a bad or foul odor).
  - Drainage changes in color.

SKIN TEARS

A **skin tear** is an injury that separates the epidermis from underlying structures as a result of friction alone or shearing and friction (Figure 38-7). It is common in aging skin. There is a close relationship between skin tears and pressure injuries. A thinning epidermis, water loss, thinning and fragile blood vessels, reduced elasticity, and loss of protective subcutaneous fat increase the risk of injury. These aging changes also interfere with the ability to heal.

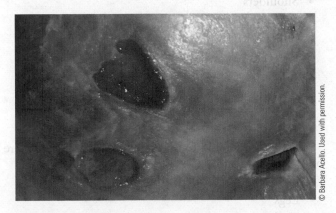

FIGURE 38-7 Friction injuries.

More than 1.5 million skin tears occur annually in health care facilities. They can be very serious and always increase the risk for infection. Patients who are dependent have the highest risk of injury, which usually occurs during ADL care. Independent, ambulatory persons sustain the second-highest number of skin tears, usually on the lower extremities. Persons with impaired vision are in the third-highest risk category. Approximately 50 percent of skin tears are of unknown origin. The other 50 percent are caused by accidental injuries. Approximately 80 percent of skin tears occur on the arms and hands.

Prevention

Patients with a known risk of skin tears will have preventive care listed on the care plan. Nursing assistant care includes:

- Protecting the skin with clothing or skin protectors.
- Using no-rinse skin care products or emollient soap.
- Applying a moisturizer twice a day. Cream works best. Applying the product immediately after bathing will help seal moisture in the skin.
- Keeping the environment safe.
- Providing good lighting.
- Handling the person with care during transfers. Be sure you have enough help. Use transfer techniques and mechanical aids that prevent friction or shear.
- Using a lift sheet and other aids for moving and turning whenever possible.
- Avoiding friction; shearing; sudden rough, harsh movement; or pulling on the skin.
- Applying a foam or sheepskin overlay to the bed. (This measure is for skin tear prevention. Other measures may be required for pressure injury prevention.)
- Padding bed rails, wheelchair arm and leg supports, and any other equipment that may be used; this will protect the person from accidentally bumping into a hard surface.
- Wrapping wheelchair arms and leg rests with sheepskin or a commercial padding.
- Using commercial side rail pads or sheepskin to cover side rails.
- Supporting dangling arms and legs with adjunctive devices, foam padding, pillows, or blankets.
- Making sure the person is wearing glasses and hearing aid(s), if used. Keep these items clean.
- Monitoring patients who wander. Provide a safe area for wandering.
- Providing good nutrition and hydration.
- Avoiding the use of tape on fragile skin. Use gauze bandage, stockinette, flexible net, stretch bandage (Kling, Kerlix), or other wraps to secure dressings instead of using tape, if possible.

PRESSURE INJURIES (DERMAL ULCERS)

Pressure injuries, formerly called pressure ulcers, decubitus ulcers, bedsores, or **dermal ulcers**, may occur in patients of any age who spend time mainly in bed or a chair. Although they commonly develop on the skin over a bony prominence as the result of pressure, they may occur in other areas and are common in patients whose fragile skin is already discolored, torn, or swollen and those who are:

- Elderly
- Very thin
- Overweight
- **Obese**
- Unable to move
- Incontinent
- Debilitated
- Poorly nourished (eat less than half of meals and snacks)
- Confined to bed or wheelchair
- Disoriented
- Dehydrated
- In prolonged contact with moisture
- Circulation-impaired
- Paralyzed
- Subjected to shearing

Shearing (Figure 38-8) occurs when the skin moves in one direction while the structures under the skin, such as the muscles and bones, remain fixed or move in the opposite direction. This can happen when patients are dragged rather than lifted up in bed, or when patients slide down in bed or in a wheelchair. Blood vessels become twisted and stretched, causing the tissues to lose essential oxygen and nutrients, leading to breakdown. In addition, shearing may tear fragile skin. Skin tears are painful, a portal of entry for infectious pathogens, and commonly lead to further breakdown. **Friction** (rubbing of the skin against another surface, such as bed

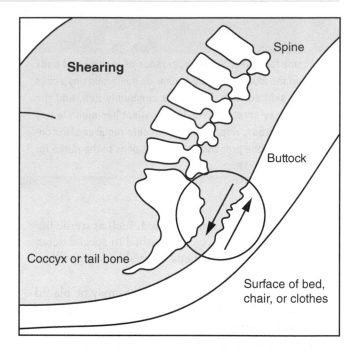

FIGURE 38-8 Shearing occurs when the skin is stretched in one direction while the underlying structures remain stationary or move in the opposite direction.

linens) also contributes to pressure injury formation. It usually occurs when the patient is being moved.

Pressure injuries are caused by prolonged pressure on an area of the body that interferes with circulation. The tissue first becomes reddened. As the cells die (undergo **necrosis**) from lack of nourishment, the skin breaks down and an ulcer forms. The resulting pressure injuries may become large and deep.

Pressure injuries occur most frequently over areas where bones come close to the surface. The most common sites (Figures 38-9A and 38-9B) are the:

- Elbows
- Heels
- Shoulders
- Sacrum, coccyx
- Hips
- Buttocks
- Ankles
- Ears
- Knees (inner and outer parts)
- Toes

Patients also tend to develop pressure injuries where body parts rub and cause friction. Common sites are:

- Between the folds of the buttocks
- Legs
- Under the breasts

⚕ Clinical Information **ALERT**

The five most common conditions in which pressure injuries develop are pneumonia, urinary tract infection, septicemia, aspiration pneumonitis, and congestive heart failure. Patients who are admitted to the hospital for pressure injury treatment often have diagnoses of spinal cord injury, paralysis, substance abuse, malnutrition, multiple sclerosis, stroke, and/or dementia.

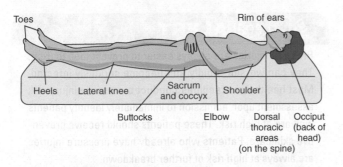

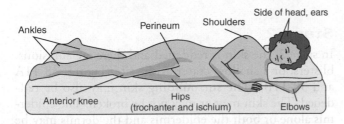

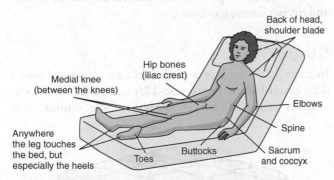

FIGURE 38-9A Potential areas of pressure when a patient is in bed.

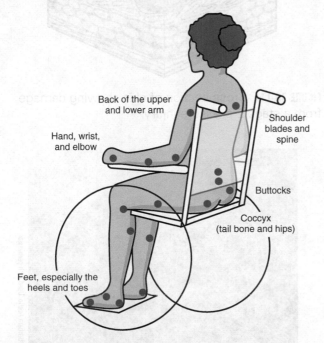

FIGURE 38-9B Potential areas of pressure when a patient is in a chair or wheelchair.

- Abdominal folds
- Ankles
- Knees

The rubbing of tubing and other patient care equipment can also cause pressure injuries.

Preventing Pressure Injuries

Pressure injuries are easier to prevent than to cure, and all caregivers are responsible for preventive care.

The nurse will assess the patient's risk for skin breakdown upon admission. This assessment gives a baseline against which all future assessments may be measured. The assessment may be documented in words, pictures, diagrams, and/or as a score. If a patient has a nursing diagnosis of actual or "risk for impaired skin or tissue integrity," the care plan will describe measures to prevent skin breakdown, limit any existing breakdown, and promote healing.

Clinical Information ALERT

Approximately 1.8 million people in the United States develop pressure injuries annually. Of these, approximately 70 percent occur in persons age 70 or older. Up to 23.9 percent of residents of skilled nursing facilities develop pressure injuries at some time. The numbers increase for residents with hip (femur) fractures. It is estimated that more than 60 percent of these individuals develop pressure injuries.* The annual cost of pressure injury care is approximately $1.3 billion. Other facts:

- Medicare and Medicare do not pay for the care of pressure injuries that develop during a hospitalization. The hospital is expected to absorb the cost of all care and treatment.
- 95 percent of pressure injuries occur on the lower part of the body.
- 36 percent of pressure injuries occur on the sacrum.
- 30 percent of pressure injuries occur on the heel.
- 8 percent of all deaths in nursing homes are the result of pressure injuries.
- Approximately 17,000 lawsuits concerning pressure injuries are filed each year.
- Annual treatment cost for pressure injuries is approximately $1.3 billion.

*Clinical trial shows 96% improvement in pressure injury healing among nursing home residents. (2006, March 11). *Medical News Today*. http://www.medicalnewstoday.com/articles/39327.php

Development of Pressure Injuries

Tissue breakdown occurs in four stages. Nursing intervention at each stage can stop the decline and prevent further damage.

Stage 1

In stage 1, the intact skin develops a redness (Figures 38-10A and 38-10B) or blue-gray discoloration over the pressure area that does not go away within 30 minutes after pressure has been relieved. In dark-skinned people, the area may appear drier, or it may appear dark blue or black. This stage is usually reversible if the area is identified promptly and pressure is relieved.

Stage 2

In stage 2, the skin is reddened and there are abrasions, blisters, or a shallow crater at the site (Figures 38-11A and 38-11B). The surrounding skin may also be reddened. The skin may or may not be broken. The epidermis alone or both the epidermis and the dermis may be involved. If this stage of involvement is neglected, further and deeper damage occurs.

Stage 3

In stage 3, all the layers of the skin are destroyed and a deep crater forms (Figures 38-12A and 38-12B). Subcutaneous tissue may be visible, but muscle, tendon, and

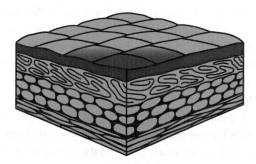

FIGURE 38-10A Cross-section of skin showing damage from a stage 1 pressure injury.

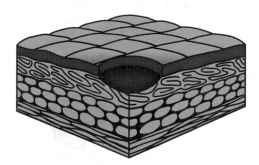

FIGURE 38-11A Cross-section of skin showing damage from a stage 2 pressure injury.

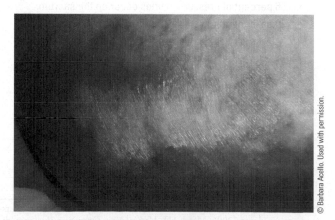

FIGURE 38-10B Stage 1 pressure injury.

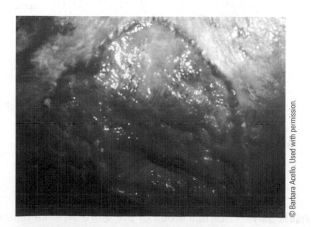

FIGURE 38-11B Stage 2 pressure injury.

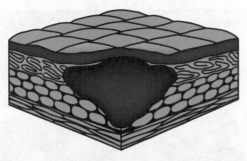

FIGURE 38-12A Cross-section of skin showing damage from a stage 3 pressure injury.

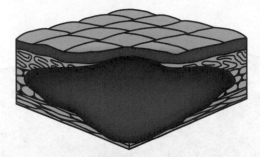

FIGURE 38-13A Cross-section of skin showing damage from a stage 4 pressure injury.

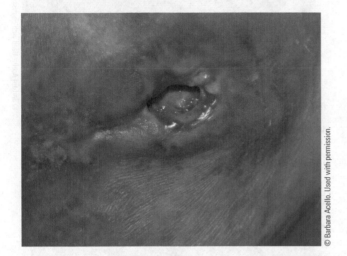

FIGURE 38-12B Stage 3 pressure injury.

© Barbara Acello. Used with permission.

bone are not exposed. The nurse documents the size of the lesion using a commercial scale.

Stage 4

In stage 4, the injury extends through the skin and sub-cutaneous tissues and may involve bone, muscle, and other structures (Figures 38-13A and 38-13B). At this stage, the patient will experience fluid loss and is at great risk for infection.

Cartilage is a connective tissue found in many areas of the body, such as the joints between bones, the rib cage, the ear, and the nose. Cartilage is somewhat flexible and serves the same purpose as bone. Pressure injuries that have exposed cartilage are also classified as stage 4.

Other Pressure-Related Skin Injuries

Two other skin injuries are often associated with pressure.

Suspected Deep Tissue Injury

A purple or maroon area of intact skin or a blood blis-ter may develop, caused by damage to underlying soft

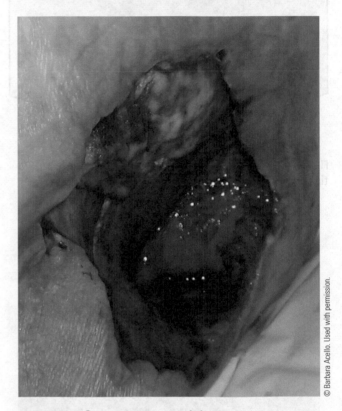

FIGURE 38-13B Stage 4 pressure injury.

© Barbara Acello. Used with permission.

tissue from pressure or shear (Figure 38-14). Before the problem becomes visible, the area may be painful, firm, mushy, boggy, or warmer or cooler than adjacent tissue. This area may be difficult to identify in persons with dark skin. A deep tissue injury may worsen rapidly.

Unstageable

A full-thickness area that is covered by **slough** (yellow, tan, gray, green, or brown; Figure 38-15A) and/or **eschar** (tan, brown, or black; Figure 38-15B) in the wound bed cannot be staged. The slough is typically yellow and hard to remove. Eschar is thick and leathery and can be removed only by debridement. Slough and eschar are necrotic (dead) tissue. The injury cannot be evaluated and the wound will not heal until the tough, fibrous tis-sues that cover the wound are removed.

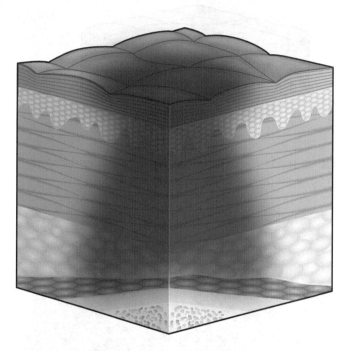

FIGURE 38-14A Cross-section of skin showing deep tissue injury.

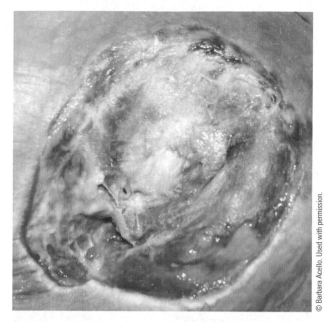

FIGURE 38-15A Yellow slough. This wound was much more serious than it appeared when the slough was finally removed.

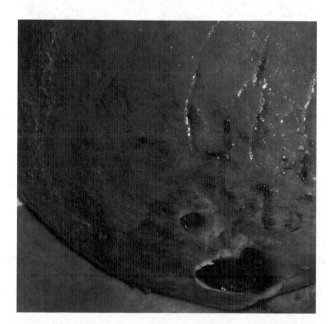

FIGURE 38-14B The bluish color of the skin indicates deep tissue injury.

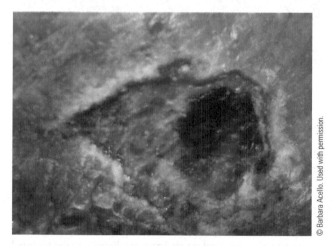

FIGURE 38-14B Brown eschar. The ulcer cannot be staged and the wound will not heal until the eschar is removed.

Actions to Take when Breakdown Occurs

Nursing assistant actions when skin breakdown occurs include:

- Performing the actions listed in Guidelines 38-1 to prevent further breakdown.
- Following the care plan exactly.

Clinical Information **ALERT**

Pressure injuries are very painful. Some health care workers believe that stage 4 injuries are not painful because they are below the nerve endings. This is not true. Although the base of the injury is stage 4, the nerve endings are exposed around the edges, which are usually the depth of a stage 2 or III lesion. The open area has passed through stages I, II, and III before becoming a stage 4 lesion. In each of these stages, nerve endings were exposed and painful. Even a minor stage 1 pressure injury can be very painful.

- Reporting signs of infection, such as fever, odor, drainage, bleeding, and changes in size.
- Keeping the patient clean and dry.

The nurse or physician may perform other procedures to care for areas of skin breakdown. For example:

- Patients may be placed on low air loss mattresses or pressure-reducing mattresses or beds.
- In some facilities, open lesions are packed loosely with gauze soaked in a wound gel. The gel keeps the lesions moist, breaks down dead cells, and promotes healing.
- The area may be protected and kept moist by using dressings that keep healing tissue moist and promote healing. A self-adhesive dressing must extend beyond the wound edge. The dressing is changed every three to five days unless there is leakage or it comes off.
- The wounds may be cleaned by the nurse or physician with saline solution and **debrided** (dead tissue removed) using instruments, treatment products, and specialty dressings. A necrotic lesion may look much larger and deeper after the dead tissue is removed.
- In severe cases, surgery may be needed to close the ulcerated area.

The Wound Care Team

It takes the expertise of an entire interdisciplinary team to care for each patient with a pressure injury. To be effective, communication between team members must be open and precise. Documentation must be objective and accurate. The pressure injury team members are determined by patient need. Members may include:

- Unit nurses
- Certified wound care nurse
- Infection control nurse, if needed
- Physician
- Surgeon, if needed
- Therapists as appropriate (physical and occupational therapy)
- Dietitian
- Social worker, if needed

The wound team will assess the wound, then plan care to meet the person's needs. A certified wound care nurse is consulted to coordinate care when the wound is first identified. As the plan of care is implemented, the team will regularly evaluate the progress of healing and document their findings. If the condition of the patient or wound declines, the team will reevaluate the treatment plan right away. Nurses will check the wound daily. A qualified wound care nurse will check the wound weekly, or more often, if needed. The physician will also assess the wound as often as needed.

Nutritional management is essential to the pressure injury treatment program. Wounds will not heal without good nutrition. The dietitian will assess the patient, write a nutritional plan of care, and continue to follow the patient's progress.

Pressure injuries *hurt*. Avoid assuming that pain does not exist in persons who cannot express pain or respond in a typical fashion. The person will also be assessed for pain. Unrelieved pain interferes with healing.

Therapists will be consulted if their services are needed for wound care, therapy, or adaptive equipment. A surgeon may be consulted if the wound requires surgical care. The social worker will make arrangements for equipment and ongoing care if the patient will be transferred to another setting.

GUIDELINES 38-1 Guidelines for Preventing Pressure Injuries

Nursing assistant actions are vital in identifying potential causes of breakdown and eliminating or minimizing them. The following care should be given:

- Change the patient's position at least every two hours. A major shift in position is required. Be careful to avoid friction, such as sliding the patient over bedclothes or against equipment. Use lifting devices to avoid dragging. Follow the turning schedule in the care plan. Figure 38-16 shows an example of the sequence of turns.
- Encourage patients sitting in chairs or wheelchairs to raise themselves every 15 minutes to relieve pressure, or assist patients to do so.

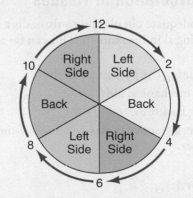

FIGURE 38-16 Example of a turning schedule.

(continues)

GUIDELINES 38-1 Guidelines for Preventing Pressure Injuries (continued)

- Encourage proper nutrition and adequate intake of fluids. Breakdown occurs more readily and healing is delayed when the patient is poorly nourished. Tube feedings or enriched high-protein and high-vitamin oral supplements may be needed to improve nutrition. Adequate fluids are essential.

- Immediately remove feces or urine from the skin. Wash and dry the area immediately.

- Inspect skin daily and report the condition.

- Keep the skin clean and dry at all times.

- Keep linens dry and free from wrinkles and hard objects such as crumbs and hairpins.

- Bathe patients frequently. Pay particular attention to potential pressure or friction areas. Avoid hot water and friction.

- Keep the skin supple and well lubricated with lotion. Do not massage directly on the injury site and do not use alcohol. Apply moisturizers on dry skin by patting. Do not rub vigorously.

- Do not use lotion on broken skin.

- Separate body areas that are likely to rub together, especially over bony prominences, by using pillows, foam wedges, or folded bath blankets, according to the care plan.

- Use mechanical aids, such as foam padding, sheepskin, or an alternating-pressure mattress, to relieve pressure, friction, and shearing.

- Protect areas at risk, such as heels and elbows.

- Use a turning sheet to move patients who are dependent in bed. Avoid friction and shearing on the heels when using the draw sheet to position the patient or move them up in bed.

- Elevate the head of the bed no higher than 30°, to prevent a shearing effect on the tissues. If the patient must have the head elevated, such as when a continuous tube feeding is infusing, relieve pressure on the buttocks, hips, and torso regularly. Turn the patient from side to side at least every two hours. You will not be able to turn the patient far enough to use the lateral position, but even a slight move and shift to the side will provide pressure relief.

- Carry out range-of-motion exercises at least twice daily to encourage circulation.

- Check nasogastric tubes and urinary catheters to be sure they are not causing pressure and irritation. Keep the nasal and urinary openings clean and free of drainage.

- Use foam, gel, or air cushions to reduce pressure on buttocks and sacrum for persons sitting in chairs or wheelchairs. Routinely monitor for skin problems.

- Use a pillow or pad between the legs when the patient is on their side.

- Report signs of infection, such as fever, odor, drainage, inflammation, or bleeding, to the nurse.

PREVENTING PRESSURE INJURIES

Blood Circulation to Tissues

Ensuring adequate circulation to tissues is a major factor in preventing skin breakdown. This can be accomplished by:

- Positioning the patient properly.
- Using mechanical aids.
- Giving backrubs.
- Performing active or passive range-of-motion exercises.

Positioning

Five basic in-bed positions are used to relieve pressure. Review the positioning procedure in Chapter 15. Remember that not all patients are able to assume the full range of positions, because of disabilities such as arthritis, contractures, and breathing limitations.

Patients with special problems require extra care when they are positioned in bed. For example:

- Be sure the patient can breathe properly.
- Remember that a fractured hip is never rotated over the unaffected leg.
- If the patient had a stroke, elevate the weak arm to reduce edema.
- Always maintain good body alignment.
- Turn the patient with a recent stroke on the unaffected side.

Protecting the Feet

Patients who are bedfast are at very high risk of developing pressure injuries on the feet and ankles (Figure 38-17). Patients with hip fractures have an especially

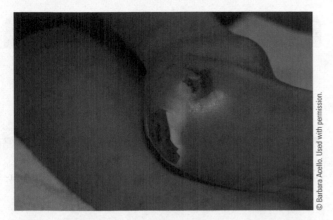

FIGURE 38-17 Heel ulcers develop rapidly and can become quite serious due to reduced blood flow in the feet.

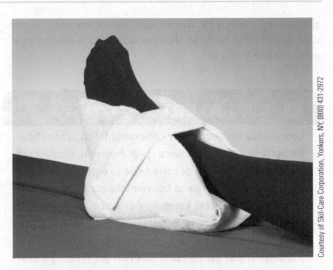

FIGURE 38-18A Heel protector.

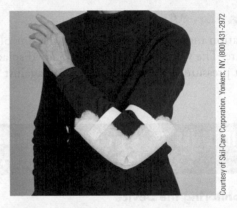

FIGURE 38-18B Elbow protector.

great risk. The skin in the feet and lower legs is thin, and there is little fatty padding. A shallow injury or pressure injury can become a stage 4 ulceration very quickly. Occasionally injuries develop on the toes and the sides of the foot. Foot and ankle injuries are easy to prevent by propping the calves on pillows positioned lengthwise to suspend the heels over the surface of the bed, relieving all pressure. Follow the patient care plan and use the pressure prevention measures listed in Guidelines 38-1. You can also use other measures to prevent pressure injuries on the feet and ankles:

* Keep the feet well lubricated with lotion (but avoid the area between the toes).
* Protect the feet from injury.
* Be sure shoes fit correctly and that the patient is wearing socks. Never allow a patient to ambulate barefoot or wearing only socks on the feet.
* Make sure bed linens are not too tight on the feet. Use a bed cradle to keep the bedding away from the skin.

Mechanical Aids

Mechanical aids are used to prevent pressure injuries. Examples are:

* Sheepskin pads (or artificial sheepskin).
* Foam pads, pillows, and overlays.
* Protectors for areas that are subject to friction as the patient moves in bed, such as heels (Figure 38-18A) and elbows (Figure 38-18B). Heel and elbow protectors reduce damage caused by friction and shearing, but they do not relieve pressure. Review Chapter 15 for other devices that reduce pressure.

Sheepskin Pads (or Artificial Sheepskin)

Sheepskin absorbs moisture and reduces friction and shearing when placed under the patient. It does not relieve pressure. Sheepskin also works well to prevent injuries when the patient is up in a wheelchair.

Foam Pads, Pillows, and Overlays

Foam pads and pillows are used to bridge areas to reduce pressure. *Foam overlays* are large foam pads that are placed on top of the mattress to provide a pressure-reducing surface. Some of these are cooler than other pads, which is important because trapped heat contributes to skin breakdown. Many foam overlays and pads lose their fire-retardant properties when washed and must be replaced if they become soiled. Protect the surface of the overlay with incontinent pads to prevent accidental soiling.

Alternating-Pressure Mattress

This type of mattress is used in some facilities. Air pressure is reduced in a different area of the mattress on an alternating basis. The air-pressure alteration reduces pressure against the body so that no skin area is continuously subjected to pressure.

 Safety **ALERT**

Low air loss beds are easily compressed. This is beneficial for persons needing pressure relief. However, incidents of injury and death have occurred due to entrapment of the neck and other body parts between the mattress and side rails. Monitor patients carefully. Remember that gaps can be created by movement, compression of the mattress, and other factors such as the patient's weight and position. If you suspect that a mattress or side rails are creating a dangerous situation for a patient, inform the nurse.

Flotation Mattress

A flotation mattress is a water bed with controlled temperature. The weight of the patient's body displaces water so that pressure is consistently equalized against the skin.

 OSHA **ALERT**

Water and gel flotation mattresses are very heavy when filled. Two or more workers are needed to lift, move, and position them correctly on the bed. To prevent injury to your back, never attempt to carry or move a full mattress by yourself.

Sheets should not be tucked tightly over a flotation mattress, because this will restrict its function.

Gel-Filled Mattress

The gel in this type of mattress has a consistency similar to body fat. It allows a more equal distribution of body weight because it conforms to the body contours. It is similar in appearance and design to the water-filled flotation mattress. Avoid using pins and other sharp objects when a patient is on one of these mattresses. They are punctured easily, and leaks can be difficult to patch. These mattresses are also quite heavy. Do not attempt to move or carry a full mattress by yourself.

GUIDELINES 2-1 Guidelines for Caring for a Patient with a Negative Pressure Wound Therapy System

Monitoring the Device

- Place the drainage collection device on a level surface, or hang it from the foot of the bed or an IV standard. If the unit tips over, an alarm will sound and the device will turn off.
- Keep the unit turned on at all times, if possible. The negative pressure may be off for no more than 2 hours per 24-hour period. Organize your time so you can shower or bathe the patient and provide other necessary care during this time.
- The care plan will list the control unit settings. Check to be sure that the unit is delivering the ordered amount of suction to the wound.
- The unit is usually quiet. If it suddenly becomes noisy or whistles, you have an air leak. Leaks usually occur around the tubing. Notify the nurse.

Patient Care

- Use the same measures that you would use when caring for a person with pressure injuries.
- Use pressure-relieving devices and other techniques to avoid pressure on the wound.
- The patient may be on a low air loss bed or other pressure-relieving surface.

- Bridge the area to relieve pressure on the wound, if necessary.
- Prevent friction and shearing.
- Ensure good nutrition and hydration. Inform the nurse if the patient's meal consumption or fluid intake are not adequate.
- Position the tubing on flat body surfaces and away from the perineal area, bony prominences, and pressure areas.
- Position the patient so they are not sitting on the tubing.
- Check the dressing every 2 hours. Be sure that the foam is firm and collapsed in the wound bed. If not:
  - Check the display screen; it should read "Therapy on."
  - If the screen is not on, inform the nurse.

Monitor for and Report

- Severe pain or an increase in pain.
- Signs of infection, such as fever, malaise, or lethargy.
- Increase in drainage.
- Heavy bleeding (this is a potential emergency that requires immediate nursing assessment).

Pillows

Pillows are used in a technique called *bridging*. In bridging, body parts are supported by pillows so that spaces are created to relieve pressure on specific areas.

NEGATIVE PRESSURE WOUND THERAPY SYSTEMS

Negative pressure wound therapy (NPWT) provides a closed, moist healing environment. This device is also called a wound VAC (vacuum-assisted closure). This treatment stimulates new tissue formation for many types of wounds. Therapy involves sealing a porous sponge on the wound under a transparent film dressing (Figure 38-19A) and then connecting it to a vacuum pump with tubing (Figure 38-19B). The pump removes drainage and potentially infectious materials, relieves edema, and improves circulation. You are responsible for monitoring the patient and the negative pressure unit.

PULSATILE LAVAGE

Pulsatile lavage with suction (PLWS) may also be called *pulse lavage, pulsed lavage, pulsatile jet lavage, negative pressure hydrotherapy*, or simply "the wound gun." Pulsed lavage is another form of negative pressure therapy in which the wound is irrigated and debrided with normal saline or another solution. A therapist or nurse uses a manual spray nozzle to deliver the solution under pressure, then suctions the wound to remove debris and the irrigation solution. The negative pressure pulsed action removes necrotic tissue and unwanted debris, cleanses the wound, helps eliminate infection, and stimulates growth of new tissue. Used as recommended, PLWS does not damage healthy tissue. Low-pressure irrigation is used. Higher pressure is avoided because it traumatizes the wound and forces pathogens deep into the tissue.

Treatment is usually once a day until the base is full of new tissue. Then the frequency is decreased to two or three times weekly. Each treatment takes about 15 to 30 minutes. Disadvantages of pulsatile lavage are:

- Increased pain for some patients.
- Chilling, hypothermia, and/or delayed healing due to cooling of the wound bed (this can be prevented if the irrigation solution is warm).
- High risk of infection if proper precautions are not used.
- Environmental contamination due to aerosolized fluids (splashes, spray, etc.).

These are precautions for assisting with a pulsatile lavage treatment:

- Use aseptic technique.

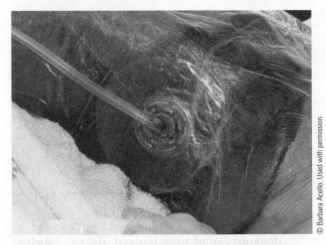

FIGURE 38-19A The Wound VAC foam is color-coded according to the therapeutic properties.

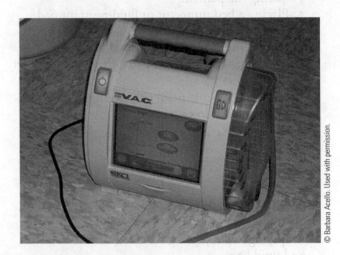

FIGURE 38-19B The Wound VAC unit.

- Apply the principles of standard precautions and use personal protective equipment.
  - Wear a fluid-resistant gown, gloves, mask/goggles or face shield, and hair cover. Consider shoe covers. This level of protection is needed because of the risk for aerosolization (spraying) of contaminated fluid.
  - You may be asked to assist with applying a surgical mask to the patient to serve as a droplet barrier.
  - Cover the patient's lines, ports, and wounds that are not being treated with a towel or drape.
  - Carefully follow manufacturer's directions for use of the device(s), including cleaning and disinfecting the equipment.
- Carry out the procedure in a private room enclosed with walls and doors (no privacy curtains or large open areas).

- The room should not have supplies stored on open shelves or cabinets (due to the risk of spraying).
- The room should be well ventilated.
- Bring only essential equipment into the treatment area.
- Cover exposed environmental surfaces during treatment to reduce the risk of aerosol contamination.

You will be responsible for:

- Preparing the treatment area.
  - A high–low stretcher, bed, or treatment table with adjustable height works best.
  - Be sure you have a strong light source so the therapist can identify internal structures such as blood vessels, if necessary.
- Gathering supplies.
- Preparing the patient.
  - Placing a bed protector or fluid-resistant pad under the area to be treated.
  - Positioning clean towels around the wound.
  - Covering adjacent body parts, IV sites, and other portals of entry.
- Establishing a sterile field with treatment and dressing supplies within easy reach.
- Assisting the patient with positioning during the procedure.
- Assisting the therapist with glove changes during treatment.
- Connecting the tubing to the suction source.
- Warming and spiking the bags of fluid.
- Emptying and replacing the filled suction canisters and fluid bags.
- Assisting the patient with drying and changing clothes (if needed) after the procedure.
- Discarding all single-use supplies immediately after use.
- Cleaning, sterilizing, or disinfecting any reusable items after each use (most of the supplies are disposable).
- Cleaning and disinfecting the treatment room and environmental surfaces after each treatment.

BURNS

Burns (Figure 38-20) are traumatic injuries to the skin and underlying tissues caused by heat, chemicals, or electricity. A **thermal burn** is caused by heat, fire, or flame. A **chemical burn** is caused by exposure to chemicals that damage the skin and mucous membranes. **Electrical burns** are caused by contact with electricity and lightning. These burns are the most severe. They create damage along a pathway in the body that extends from the

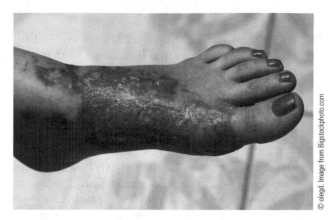

FIGURE 38-20 A painful second-degree burn.

point of entrance to a point of exit. Location of burns can also be an issue in treatment. For example, burns to the perineum often become infected. A catheter may have to be used to keep dressings dry. Burns to the face can cause disfigurement and emotional trauma. Scars and contractures are common complications. Burns are very painful injuries with a very high risk for infection and other serious complications. Extensive treatment is often required.

Whenever large sections of skin are destroyed, the body loses fluids and chemicals called *electrolytes* and is vulnerable to infection. Burns commonly cause the loss of large areas of skin.

Classification

The temperature and length of exposure determine the severity of a burn. Prognosis is based on the extent of the burns. Burns are commonly classified as first-, second-, and third-degree. Burns may also be classified according to the depth of tissue involvement:

- *First-degree burns* (partial thickness)
  - Epidermis. When only the epidermis is involved, the skin is pink to red. There may be some temporary swelling and pain. There is usually no permanent damage or scarring.

> ⊕ Clinical Information **ALERT**
>
> Approximately 2 million people in the United States are treated for burn injuries each year. Of these, approximately 100,000 require hospitalization. Approximately 4,500 people die from burn injuries each year. Burns are the sixth leading cause of death in older adults, with approximately 1,200 deaths a year. Patients' outcome is best when treatment is started immediately. Infection is the leading complication of burns.

- *Second-degree burns* (partial thickness)
  - Dermis. When both epidermis and dermis are involved in the burn, the color may vary from pink or red to white or tan. There is blistering and pain and some scarring.
- *Third-degree burns* (full thickness)
  - When the epidermis, dermis, and subcutaneous tissue are involved, the tissue is bright red to tan and brown. The area is covered with a tough, leathery coat (eschar). There is no pain initially because nerve endings have been destroyed. Later, pain and scarring will result from this injury.
  - When the epidermis, dermis, subcutaneous tissues, muscles, and bones are involved, the tissue appears blackened. Scarring will be extensive.

Management of Burns

Once a burn patient is in the medical facility, the care will involve:

- Assessment of the burn damage.
- Analgesia for pain.
- Management of fluids and electrolytes.
- Prevention of infection.
- Clean technique using cap, gown, mask, and gloves.
- Complete reverse isolation technique in some cases.
- Monitoring the patient for respiratory distress, shock, and anemia.
- Cleaning of the burned areas and removal of all debris.
- Application of topical antibiotics.
- Emotional support.

Some hospitals have established burn centers where specially trained personnel care for patients with burns. One of two approaches is in common use:

- Open method—the burns are left uncovered. Sterile technique is used to care for the patient.
- Closed method—the burns are covered by special ointments and wrapped in layers of gauze. The body part is checked for circulation distal to the dressing and maintained in proper alignment.

New techniques, such as keeping the patient submerged in a silicone solution, are also being used. There are four goals of treatment, whatever method is selected:

1 Replacement of lost fluids and electrolytes to combat shock.
2 Relief of pain and anxiety.
3 Prevention of contractures, deformities, and infections; a *contracture* is a shortening of a muscle, which limits motion and causes deformities; plastic surgery may also be required.
4 Provision of emotional support and motivation.

Nursing Assistant Care

Special care emphasizes:

- Monitoring for and reporting pain.
- Maintaining proper alignment.
- Gentle positioning to prevent contractures.

⚖ NOTE

A wide variety of burn recovery beds are available to permit frequent rotation to relieve pressure.

- Encouraging a high-protein diet.
- Carefully measuring intake and output.
- Giving emotional support and encouragement.
- Carrying out procedures that prevent infection.
- Applying the principles of standard precautions and wearing the correct protective apparel if contact with burned skin areas is likely.

IMPORTANCE OF NUTRITION IN HEALING WOUNDS AND BURNS

Good nutrition is essential for healing. You learned in Chapter 26 that protein is the only nutrient that can make new cells and rebuild tissue. Protein is nature's building block that supplies the material needed for tissue growth. Correcting protein deficiencies is essential to wound healing and preventing infection. Vitamins A and C, along with zinc, are also important to healing.

The dietitian may recommend that the patient increase protein foods such as meat, poultry, fish, eggs, cheese, milk and other dairy products, and beans. For example:

- Powdered milk added to whole milk, pudding, yogurt, or baked goods
- Protein powders added to drinks or moist foods
- Cheese added to sandwiches, vegetables, potatoes, omelets, burritos, or beans
- Nuts and peanut butter added to cookies
- Extra cheese or eggs added to casseroles
- Extra meat added to lasagna or spaghetti
- Yogurt and milk added to fruit smoothies
- Beans, cheese, and nuts added to salads

In addition, the doctor may order vitamins and/or liquid amino acid and protein nutritional supplements, such as ProStat, Resource, or Juven (Figure 38-21). These products speed healing and growth of new tissue by

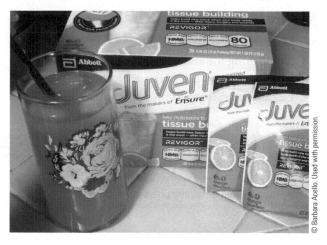

© Barbara Acello. Used with permission.

FIGURE 38-21 Juven® enhances healing of skin problems.

TABLE 38-1 Integumentary System Problems to Observe and Report

- Rash
- Redness in the skin that does not go away within 30 minutes after pressure is relieved from a bony prominence or pressure area
- In dark- or yellow-skinned residents, spots or areas that are darker in appearance than normal skin tone
- Abrasions, skin tears, lacerations
- Irritation
- Bruises
- Skin discoloration
- Swelling
- Lumps
- Abnormal skin growths
- Change in color of a wart or mole
- Abnormal sweating
- Excessive heat or coolness to touch
- Open areas/skin breakdown (pressure ulcers) at bony prominences
- Red or weeping tissue in skin folds
- Drainage
- Foul odor
- Complaints such as numbness, burning, tingling, itching
- Signs of infection
- Unusual skin color, such as blue or gray color of the skin, lips, nail beds, roof of mouth, or mucous membranes
- Skin growths
- Poor skin turgor; tenting of skin on forehead or over sternum
- Sunken, dark eyes
- Any other signs of tissue injury

promoting collagen production. Collagen is an essential building block that helps repair the skin.

Monitor for and report the problems listed in Table 38-1.

 Infection Control **ALERT**

Your bandage scissors, stethoscope, and other personal items may transfer pathogens from one patient to the next, as well as to your own hands and pockets. Wash personal equipment items with an alcohol product or soap and water before and after each use.

DRESSINGS AND BANDAGES

You may be responsible for caring for skin tears, stage 1 and 2 pressure injuries, and other uninfected wounds.

Dressings are gauze or composite products that are used to directly cover a wound. Some dressings are adhesive; others are held in place with tape. **Bandages** may also be used to hold dressings in place. Bandages are wrapped around the dressing and are made of flexible fabric, gauze, net, or elastic material (such as an Ace bandage). Gauze bandages are the most common. Elastic bandages reduce edema and support injured areas. Wrap bandages from the bottom upward. Be sure the bandage is not so tight that it restricts circulation.

Clean dressings keep minor, uninfected wounds clean. Handle dressings by the corners. Avoid touching the center that contacts the wound. Be sure to wash your bandage scissors and dry them well before and after using them for a dressing change.

Applying a Clean Dressing

Prepare a clean work surface. The overbed table is a good surface for clean supplies. Covering the table with a disposable bed protector or other clean barrier further reduces the risk of contamination. Open packages and prepare your supplies before beginning. Avoid bringing large facility stock bottles (such as normal saline) into a room. Pour what you need into a paper cup or plastic medicine cup. Some facilities permit nursing assistants to apply nonprescription products to minor wounds. All clean supplies that you bring into the room must be used or discarded. They cannot be used for another person. If you are using a treatment cart, lock it and leave it in the hallway.

Transparent Film and Hydrocolloid Dressings

Transparent film dressings are adhesive membranes of various sizes and thicknesses (Figure 38-22A). These dressings are easily molded over various parts of the body. Transparent film dressings are waterproof and protect

GUIDELINES 38-3 Guidelines for Removing a Dressing

- Position a trash bag at the end of the bed, away from clean supplies. Position it so you do not have to cross over clean items to discard soiled items. Make a cuff on the end of the bag so it stays open.
- Apply clean gloves.
- Apply traction to the skin while gently loosening the edges of the tape. Lift the dressing off.
- Pour a little saline on the dressing if it sticks to the wound. Let it sit for a minute to loosen, and then

hold gentle traction on the skin and carefully lift the dressing off. Check it for color, odor, and amount of drainage. Discard the soiled dressing in a plastic bag placed at the foot of the bed.
- Use tape remover or baby oil to remove the adhesive if the skin feels sticky.
- Discard your trash in a plastic bag in the biohazardous waste.

GUIDELINES 38-4 Guidelines for Cleansing and Observing the Wound

- The texture of some gauze is very rough and irritating to the skin. Select gauze sponges with a soft cotton surface.
- Apply cleansing solution to a gauze sponge, and then squeeze it so it is not dripping.
- Gently clean the wound with normal saline or the ordered cleanser. (Use normal saline unless a specific cleansing solution is ordered.)
- Work from clean areas to less clean areas. When cleansing an injury, minor wound, or pressure injury, work in half circles or full circles, beginning in the center of the wound and working outward. Use a new sponge for each circle. Cleanse the skin at least one inch beyond the anticipated edge of the dressing.
- Avoid rubbing back and forth. Rinse using the same technique.
- Avoid contaminating an entire bottle of cleansing solution with used swabs or gauze. Pour solution into a smaller container or directly onto the dressing.

- If a cotton swab is used, swab the wound once, then discard the swab. If more solution is necessary, use a clean swab. Never dip a used swab into a bottle of cleansing solution.
- Some wound cleansers must be rinsed off. Others are no-rinse. Follow the product directions. If in doubt, rinse with a sponge moistened with normal saline, and gently pat dry with a clean sponge.
- After cleansing the wound, remove and discard your gloves.
- Wash your hands (and scissors, if used) for at least 20 seconds, or use an alcohol-based hand cleaner.
- If the wound has changed since the last dressing change, or if signs or symptoms of infection are present, ask the nurse to assess it before applying a new dressing.

GUIDELINES 38-5 Guidelines for Estimating Amount of Drainage

- *None*—wound tissue dry
- *Scant*—no measurable drainage, but wound tissue is moist
- *Small*—wound tissue is very moist, with drainage on less than 25 percent of the dressing
- *Moderate*—wound tissue is wet; drainage covers 25 to 75 percent of the dressing

- *Large*—wound tissue is filled with fluid and drainage covers more than 75 percent of the dressing
- *Copious*—wound tissue is saturated and dressing is saturated; may be leaking

the wound from bacteria. They maintain a moist environment, which is recommended for healing. Transparent film is used for minor pressure injuries, skin tears, and wounds with necrotic tissue. The moist environment under the dressing debrides the necrosis. They are not recommended for deep, infected, or draining wounds or for patients with very fragile skin, as they increase the risk of skin tears. Dressings are usually changed every three to five days but may remain in place for up to seven days. Because they are transparent, the nurse can evaluate progress in wound healing. No cover dressing or bandage is used. Patients can bathe or shower with a dressing in place. Some types are difficult to handle and stick together after the paper backing is removed. Select a dressing size that allows at least 1¼ inch of dressing surrounding the entire wound. To remove the dressing, push down on the skin and stretch (Figure 38-22B). Do not pull on the dressing.

Hydrocolloid dressings are made of materials such as gelatin and pectin. They are self-adhesive and come in various sizes and thicknesses. Hydrocolloids provide a moist environment for wound healing. They are used for pressure injuries and some other wounds. They can be used for wounds with light to moderate drainage. These dressings will debride necrotic tissue. Hydrocolloids should not be used on persons with fragile skin, deep or infected wounds, or wounds in which tendon or bone is exposed. The dressing is left in place for up to seven days, or according to physician's order. The dressing expands to absorb exudate. It protects the wound from contamination and requires no cover dressing or bandage. You cannot see through this type of dressing, so the nurse cannot assess the wound with a dressing in place. Select a dressing size that allows at least 1¼ inch of dressing surrounding the entire wound. Some hydrocolloids curl at the edges and must be taped.

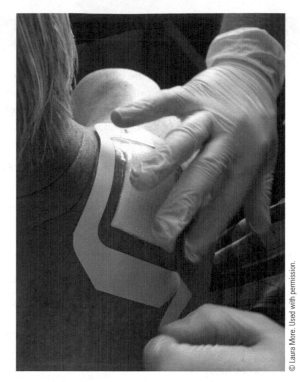

FIGURE 38-22A A transparent film dressing may be left in place for up to 7 days.

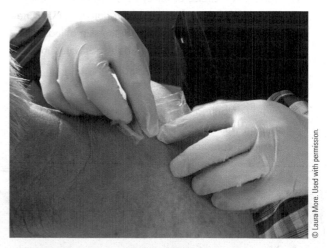

FIGURE 38-22B To remove the dressing, push the skin down and stretch the dressing.

🔓 Safety **ALERT**

Check to see if the patient is allergic to adhesive tape before applying a transparent film or hydrocolloid dressing. Some patients with tape allergies can use these dressings successfully. Others have allergic reactions. A rash, hives, redness, and heat in the area are signs of an allergic reaction to the dressing. Overall, the incidence of allergies to these dressings is low.

EXPAND YOUR SKILLS

PROCEDURE **85** CHANGING A CLEAN DRESSING AND APPLYING A BANDAGE

1. Carry out initial procedure actions.

2. Assemble equipment:
   - 2 pairs of clean, disposable exam gloves
   - Normal saline or other cleansing solution
   - Sponges, applicators, or other supplies for cleaning wound
   - Clean or sterile gauze pads or other dressing, as ordered, and according to facility policy
   - Bed protector(s), if needed
   - Bath blanket, if needed
   - Treatment product, if ordered
   - Tape or bandage material
   - Plastic bag for used supplies

3. Holding gentle traction on the skin, loosen the tape by pulling the ends toward the wound, and remove the old dressing. Discard in the plastic bag.

4. Cleanse and rinse the wound with normal saline or ordered solution. If the wound appears abnormal or infected, notify the nurse.

5. Remove your gloves and discard them in the plastic bag.

6. Wash your hands.

7. Set up your dressing supplies and open packages.

8. Apply clean exam gloves.

9. Apply the treatment product to the patient's skin according to directions. Use an applicator, tongue blade, or gauze sponge to spread the product on the wound. Do not contaminate the product package. Discard applicator or gauze in the plastic bag.

10. Pick up the clean dressing, holding it only by the corners.

11. Center the dressing over the wound.

12. Tape the dressing securely in place, or cover it with a bandage.

13. Carry out ending procedure actions, or wrap with a bandage (following).

Applying a Bandage

14. After applying the dressing, apply the bandage. Most bandaging materials are conforming, self-adhering gauze. Brand-name products, such as Kling® and Kerlix®, or generic products, such as conforming gauze, are commonly used.

15. The bandage must cover the dressing completely. Begin by holding the bandage in your dominant hand. Hold the bandage against the skin with your nondominant thumb, approximately 1 inch below the dressing.

16. Wrap the bandage around the extremity two or three times to hold it securely in place.

17. Wrap the bandage from distal to proximal, in overlapping spiral turns (refer to procedure 80 in Chapter 29). Each turn should overlap half to three-quarters of the previous turn. The bandage should be snug so it does not fall off. However, it must not be so tight that it restricts blood flow.

18. Wrap the bandage at least one inch above the top of the dressing. Wrap it completely around the extremity twice, and then cut the end. Tape the end to the bandage itself, not the skin.

19. Check the circulation distal to the bandage to ensure that the circulation is adequate.

20. Carry out ending procedure actions.

ICON KEY:
 = OBRA   P = PPE

REVIEW

A. True/False

Mark the following true or false by circling T or F.

1. T F Obesity predisposes a patient to pressure injury formation.

2. T F The sacrum is a common site for the development of pressure injuries.

3. T F To avoid pressure injuries, change the patient's position at least every two hours.

4. T F Massage directly over reddened areas.

5. T F The nails and hair are part of the integumentary system.

6. T F Burns to the epidermis are not painful.

7. T F Collagen is an essential building block that helps repair the skin.

8. T F The skin will blister if both the dermis and epidermis are damaged by burns.

9. T F Prevention of infection is an important consideration when caring for a patient with burns.

10. T F The patient with burns needs great emotional support.

11. T F Friction and shearing are not related to pressure injury development.

12. T F A sheepskin is an excellent pressure-relieving device.

13. T F A stage 1 pressure injury will fade when pressure is relieved for more than 30 minutes.

14. T F Cover the low air loss bed tightly with a sheet to reduce pressure.

15. T F Nodules are small tissue protrusions.

16. T F When assisting with a colloidal oatmeal bath, keep the solution out of the patient's eyes.

17. T F Ninety-five percent of pressure injuries occur on the upper part of the body.

18. T F Medicare and Medicaid do not pay for the care of pressure injuries that develop while the patient is in the hospital.

19. T F Suspected deep tissue injury may look like a bruise.

20. T F If a wound VAC suddenly becomes noisy or whistles, it has an air leak.

21. T F Wounds with slough and eschar are always stage 4.

22. T F Slough and eschar are dead tissue.

23. T F There is a low incidence of allergies to transparent film dressings.

24. T F Wash personal equipment items with an alcohol product or soap and water before and after each use.

B. Matching

Choose the correct item from Column II to match each word or phrase in Column I.

Column I

25. _____ no measurable drainage, but wound tissue is moist

26. _____ wound tissue filled with fluid and covers more than 75 percent of the dressing

27. _____ wound tissue and dressing are both saturated; may be leaking

28. _____ wound tissue wet; drainage involves 25 to 75 percent of the dressing

29. _____ wound tissue is very moist, with drainage on less than 25 percent of the dressing

Column II

a. no drainage
b. copious drainage
c. scant drainage
d. moderate drainage
e. large drainage
f. small drainage

C. Multiple Choice

Select the best answer for each of the following.

30. Flat, discolored spots such as those seen in measles are called:

a. pustules.
b. macules.
c. papules.
d. vesicles.

31. Raised spots filled with fluid, such as blisters, are called:

a. pustules.
b. macules.
c. papules.
d. vesicles.

32. Anaphylactic shock is:
- **a.** a severe sensitivity reaction.
- **b.** never fatal.
- **c.** a communicable disease.
- **d.** associated with partial-thickness burns.

33. When caring for patients with skin lesions:
- **a.** rub the skin vigorously.
- **b.** use soap and water when bathing.
- **c.** do not attempt to remove any crusts.
- **d.** use rubbing lotion.

34. To help ensure adequate circulation to prevent skin breakdown, you could:
- **a.** change the patient's position frequently.
- **b.** position the patient on bony prominences.
- **c.** rub red areas well.
- **d.** apply rubbing alcohol to the skin after bathing.

35. A skin tear:
- **a.** separates the epidermis from subcutaneous fat.
- **b.** results from shearing and friction.
- **c.** is a normal aging change.
- **d.** is most common in ambulatory patients.

36. When assisting a patient with a colloidal oatmeal bath, the nursing assistant should:
- **a.** use tepid water.
- **b.** give a bed bath.
- **c.** use very hot water.
- **d.** scrub the skin well.

37. Safety precautions to follow when assisting a patient with an oatmeal bath include:
- **a.** using sterile water to prevent infection.
- **b.** scrubbing the lesions well with a sponge.
- **c.** adding plenty of hot water so the oatmeal will dissolve.
- **d.** advising the patient to use the hand rail to prevent slipping.

38. In a dark-skinned patient, a stage 1 pressure injury may appear:
- **a.** red or pink.
- **b.** gray or green.
- **c.** blue or black.
- **d.** shiny and oily.

39. Patients using low air loss beds:
- **a.** do not require repositioning, as the bed relieves pressure.
- **b.** are at risk for entrapment between the mattress and rails.
- **c.** must have multiple stage 1 injuries to qualify for a bed.
- **d.** should be turned and positioned every 30 to 45 minutes.

40. Special precautions are needed for pulsatile lavage treatment because:
- **a.** there may be aerosolization of contaminated fluid.
- **b.** the device must be specially wrapped and discarded after use.
- **c.** the patient's body will be exposed during the treatment.
- **d.** the patient may get cold and need a warm blanket.

41. To promote healing in a pressure injury, the doctor may order:
- **a.** six large, high-protein meals a day.
- **b.** vitamins A and C, zinc, and Juven.
- **c.** vitamins B6, B12 and D, and SAM-E.
- **d.** multivitamin, vitamin E, and milk.

42. Dressings:
- **a.** hold bandages in place.
- **b.** must be applied tightly.
- **c.** should be sterile.
- **d.** directly cover a wound.

43. Bandages:
- **a.** should be sterile.
- **b.** must be applied tightly.
- **c.** directly cover a wound.
- **d.** hold dressings in place.

D. Completion

Complete the statements by filling in the correct word(s).

44. Three nursing assistant actions related to the care of patients with skin lesions are:
- **a.** _____
- **b.** _____
- **c.** _____

45. Three diagnostic tests used to identify skin-related lesions are:

a. _____

b. _____

c. _____

46. Five types of patients at risk for the development of pressure injuries are:

a. _____

b. _____

c. _____

d. _____

e. _____

47. Name five common sites of pressure injury formation.

a. _____

b. _____

c. _____

d. _____

e. _____

48. It is especially important to encourage proper nutrition and fluids in patients who have pressure injuries because _____

_____

E. Nursing Assistant Challenge

Agnes Finlay has been transferred to your facility from a long-term care facility. She uses a wheelchair but fell and fractured her arm. You notice a reddened area around the base of her spine. Answer the following by selecting the correct word.

49. People sitting in wheelchairs should raise themselves every _____ minutes. (60) (15)

50. The head of the patient's bed should not be elevated more than _____. (30°) (40°)

51. While she is in bed, Ms. Finlay's position should be changed at least every _____ hours. (three) (two)

52. Range-of-motion exercises should be carried out at least _____ a day. (once) (twice)

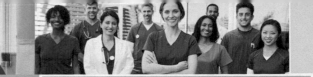

Respiratory System

OBJECTIVES

After completing this chapter, you will be able to:

39.1 Spell and define terms.

39.2 Review the location of the respiratory organs.

39.3 Explain the function of the respiratory organs.

39.4 Describe some common diseases of the respiratory system.

39.5 List five diagnostic tests used to identify respiratory conditions.

39.6 Describe nursing assistant actions related to the care of patients with respiratory conditions.

39.7 Identify patients who are at high risk of poor oxygenation.

39.8 Describe the care of patients with a tracheostomy, laryngectomy, or chest tubes.

39.9 List five safety measures for the use of oxygen therapy.

39.10 Describe the care of patients who have an endotracheal tube and are mechanically ventilated.

39.11 State the purpose of the oral airway and nasal airway.

39.12 Discuss the care of patients who have airways in place.

39.13 Discuss the use of the incentive spirometer.

39.14 Discuss the use of the nebulizer.

39.15 Explain (or discuss) the use of BiPAP and CPAP masks.

39.16 Demonstrate the following procedure:

- Procedure 86: Collecting a Sputum Specimen (Expand Your Skills)

VOCABULARY

Learn the meaning and the correct spelling of the following words and phrases:

adjunctive device	chronic obstructive	nasopharyngeal airway	stoma
alveoli	pulmonary disease (COPD)	nebulizer	trachea
asthma	continuous positive airway	oropharyngeal airway	tracheostomy
bag-valve-mask (BVM)	pressure (CPAP)	orthopneic position	tripod position
bilevel positive airway	dyspnea	oxygen	upper respiratory
pressure (BiPAP)	emphysema	oxygenation	infection (URI)
biopsy	endotracheal intubation	oxygen concentrator	ventilation
bronchi	endotracheal tube (ET tube)	oxygen mask	ventilator
bronchioles	expectorate	pharynx	vocal cords
bronchitis	high Fowler's position	pleura	Yankauer catheter
cannula	humidifier	pleural effusion	
capillary refill	incentive spirometer	pneumonia	
carbon dioxide	laryngectomee	pulse oximetry	
chest tubes	laryngectomy	respiratory care	
chronic obstructive lung	larynx	practitioner (RCP)	
disease (COLD)	nasal cannula	sputum	

INTRODUCTION

Oxygen is essential to life and good health. Carbon dioxide, a cellular waste product, must be eliminated from the body. Diseases of the respiratory tract that interfere with this vital exchange of oxygen and carbon dioxide cause acute distress. Nursing care is directed toward making breathing easier and preventing infection.

STRUCTURE AND FUNCTION

The respiratory system (Figure 39-1) is the lifeline of the body. It extends from the nose to the tiny air sacs (**alveoli**) that make up the bulk of the lungs. The organs of the respiratory system include the:

- Nose
- Pharynx (throat)
- Larynx (voice box)
- **Trachea** (windpipe)
- Bronchi
- Lungs

The sinuses, diaphragm, and intercostal muscles between the ribs are auxiliary structures.

Air is warmed, moistened, and filtered as it passes through the nasal cavities, which are separated by the nasal septum. The air passes through the **pharynx**, a passageway for both air and food, into the larynx and trachea. It then passes into the **bronchi** to go through the upper respiratory tract to the lungs. Within the lungs, the bronchi branch into smaller and smaller divisions called **bronchioles** (Figure 39-2A). The *alveoli* are tiny air sacs that extend from the bronchioles. The exchange of gases takes place in the alveoli (Figure 39-2B). The alveoli, bronchioles, and the important pulmonary blood vessels form the lungs.

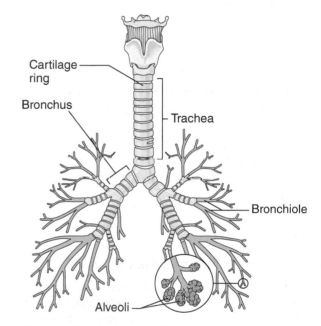

FIGURE 39-2A The lower respiratory tract.

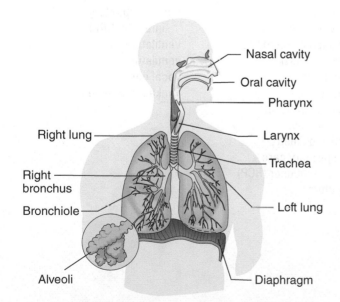

FIGURE 39-1 The respiratory system.

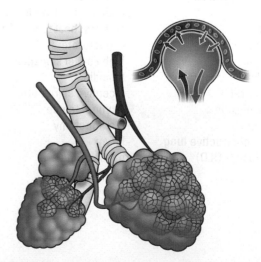

FIGURE 39-2B Illustration of the exchange of oxygen and carbon dioxide that occurs inside pulmonary alveoli.

The purpose of the respiratory system is to bring **oxygen** (O_2) into the body to meet cellular needs and to expel carbon dioxide (CO_2). **Carbon dioxide** is a gaseous metabolic waste produced by the cells.

Each cell in the body must have a constant supply of oxygen. The oxygen is used to produce the energy for cellular activity:

Nutrients + oxygen yields energy + water + CO_2

There is a close connection between the respiratory and circulatory systems. Oxygen is delivered throughout the body by means of the bloodstream. Every cell in the body produces carbon dioxide. It is transported in venous blood. When it reaches the lungs, it is exhaled into the atmosphere. When the body does not eliminate carbon dioxide, it creates chemical reactions, causing an acid buildup. Death will result if levels of acid and carbon dioxide become too high. Signs and symptoms indicating problems with oxygen use that should be reported to the nurse promptly are listed in Table 39-1.

Aging Changes to the Respiratory System

The respiratory system is vital to health and survival because it provides oxygen to the body. Lung function

TABLE 39-1 Respiratory Signs and Symptoms to Observe and Report

- Respiratory rate below 12 or above 20
- Unusual skin color, such as dusky, pale, blue, or gray
- Unusual color of the lips, mucous membranes, nail beds, tongue, lining or roof of mouth
- Cool, clammy skin
- Slow, rapid, noisy, or irregular breathing
- Shortness of breath, gasping, or labored breathing
- Respirations are irregular, very deep, or shallow
- Nasal flaring is present during inspiration
- Changes in mental status, including decreased responsiveness, drowsiness, sleepiness for no apparent reason, restlessness, increased confusion
- Tachycardia
- Cheyne-Stokes respirations
- Coughing (dry or moist/productive), wheezing
- Retractions (the muscles and skin pull inward under and between the ribs)
- Movement in the chest is absent, minimal, or irregular
- Breathing movement appears to be in the abdomen, not the lungs
- Air movement cannot be detected by listening and feeling for breath sounds on your cheek and ear
- Patient is unable to speak at all, or cannot speak in sentences because of shortness of breath
- Capillary refill takes more than 3 seconds
- Pulse oximeter value below 90%

The respiratory system is *very* powerful. The air released from an explosive cough moves at speeds up to 60 miles per hour (mph). A sneeze creates a force of air moving nearly 99 mph (Figure 39-3). It is impossible to sneeze with your eyes open.

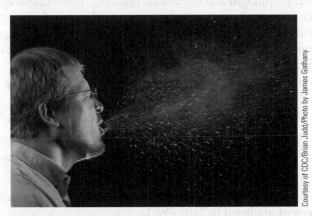

Courtesy of CDC/Brian Judd/Photo by James Gathany

FIGURE 39-3 A photograph of a sneeze that shows droplets being expelled from an open mouth. Because of this, the mouth should be covered when sneezing or coughing. Hands should be washed if they come in contact with droplets.

and efficiency change with the normal aging process. Aging changes to the respiratory system include:

- Loss of elasticity, reducing the lungs' ability to inflate and deflate
- Increased risk of hypoxia, because lungs cannot expand fully
- Reduced movement of the rib cage, which does not move or expand as freely because of muscular and arthritic changes
- Reduced respiratory volume
- Decreased size of the inner lumen of the trachea
- Increased mucus production
- Decreased number of cilia
- Less effective cough, so there is increased difficulty clearing secretions
- Loss of tone in the throat and upper airway, which reduces oxygen intake and increases risk of snoring and sleep apnea

Emphysema is common in people aged 50 to 70. Aging changes are usually worse in long-time smokers.

The Act of Respiration

The two lungs are located in the thorax. A double-walled membrane called the **pleura** surrounds each lung. Between the layers of the pleura is a small amount of fluid that reduces friction as the lungs alternately expand and contract, filling with and then expelling air.

The size of the thorax depends on the contraction of the diaphragm and intercostal muscles. As the diaphragm contracts, the thorax enlarges, expanding the lungs. Air carrying oxygen enters the lungs. When the diaphragm relaxes, the thorax becomes smaller, pushing the air carrying carbon dioxide out.

- *Inspiration* (or inhalation) is the act of drawing air into the lungs.
- *Expiration* (or exhalation) is the act of expelling air.
- **Ventilation** is the combination of these two actions.
- **Oxygenation** is the movement of oxygen from the lungs into the blood to be carried to the cells.

Respiratory signs and symptoms to observe and report are listed in Table 39-1.

Voice Production

The **larynx**, or voice box, is part of the respiratory tract. It is important in voice production. Two membranes called the **vocal cords** stretch across the inside of the larynx. As air moves upward through the larynx, it passes through an opening between the vocal cords. Changes in the shape of the vocal cords and the size of the opening permit controlled amounts of air to reach the mouth, nasal cavities, and sinuses, where specific speech sounds are made when formed by the teeth, lips, and tongue.

PATIENTS AT RISK OF POOR OXYGENATION

The human body eliminates three main waste products. You have learned about problems with urinary and bowel elimination. The third important waste product is carbon dioxide (CO_2). Every cell in the body produces carbon dioxide. It is transported in venous blood to the lungs, where it is exhaled into the atmosphere. When the body does not sufficiently eliminate carbon dioxide, chemical reactions cause an acid buildup. Death will result if levels of acid and carbon dioxide become too high. Patients who are immobile and those on bedrest have an increased risk of hypoxemia. When hypoxemia develops, immobility makes a positive outcome less likely. High-risk conditions are:

- Cardiac disease
- Pulmonary disease
- Being postoperative (for up to a week after surgery)
- Sleep apnea

👪 Age-Appropriate Care ALERT

Researchers have concluded that a mild decrease of oxygen in the blood, once thought to be of limited harm, contributes to long-term impairment of mental function and behavioral disorders. This is an area of ongoing research and study.

- Decreased level of consciousness
- Neuromuscular diseases
- Morbid obesity
- Kyphoscoliosis (curvature of the spine)
- Trauma

Capillary Refill

Checking **capillary refill** is a quick, easy, painless test to evaluate how well oxygen is getting to the body tissues. It is an indication of the patient's peripheral circulation and shows how well the tissues are being nourished with oxygen. A light-skinned person should have pink skin, indicating an adequate supply of oxygen. The nail beds, mucous membranes in the mouth, and lips are also an indication of how well the patient's body is using oxygen. The color of these areas should also be pink. Look at the nail beds, oral mucous membranes, and lips of a dark-skinned person to determine how well they are using oxygen, because you cannot evaluate the skin. Cyanosis in any of these areas indicates a problem due to lack of oxygen in the blood or poor circulation.

The capillary refill test will help you identify problems with oxygen delivery. Check all four extremities. Although capillary refill varies with age, skin color should return to normal within two to three seconds in all patients. This is approximately the length of time it takes to say the words *capillary refill*.

You can check capillary refill at any time when you are taking vital signs or caring for the patient. If the capillary refill time is more than three seconds, inform the nurse.

Nail Polish

Several procedures involve using and evaluating the patient's fingernail beds. The color of the fingernails is a good indication of how much oxygen is in the blood. Nail polish will interfere with the ability to evaluate the patient. Follow your facility's policy for removing polish. Some facilities remove polish from one finger only. Other facilities remove all nail polish. If a patient has acrylic or sculpted nails, remove the polish with a nonacetone polish remover. Some facilities completely remove the acrylic material from one nail. Know and follow your facility's policy. Check with the nurse if necessary.

The Pulse Oximeter

Pulse oximetry (Figure 39-4) is another simple, painless test to determine how well the body is using oxygen. The pulse oximeter measures the level of saturation of the patient's hemoglobin with oxygen. *Hemoglobin* is the part of the blood that carries oxygen to the cells. The measurement is usually continuous, but can be intermittent. Having these data readily available enables the nurse to treat the patient quickly. Pulse oximetry will detect critical changes in the patient's oxygen levels as soon as they occur. The outcome is better when early treatment is provided.

If oxygen is in use, document the liter flow before applying the pulse oximeter. Attach the pulse oximeter to the patient's skin with a sensor. Several different types are available. They can be placed on the finger, toe, earlobe, foot, forehead, or bridge of the nose. The tip of the finger and the earlobe are most commonly used. In these areas, a clothespin-like sensor is attached to both sides. The finger and toe sensors work best with dark-skinned patients. Poor circulation, cold extremities, and nail polish interfere with pulse oximeter values.

🔓 Safety ALERT

Always monitor the patient, not the equipment. For example, the pulse oximeter alarm sounds and the oxygen saturation value reads 63 percent, suggesting that the patient is in severe distress. However, the patient is visiting with their family, smiling, and talking. Their color is good, nail beds and mucous membranes are pink, and capillary refill is less than three seconds. You are having an equipment problem, not a patient problem. If you cannot identify and correct the problem, ask the nurse or respiratory professional to help. Although your findings indicate an equipment problem, inform the nurse of the problem and your evaluation of the patient and situation.

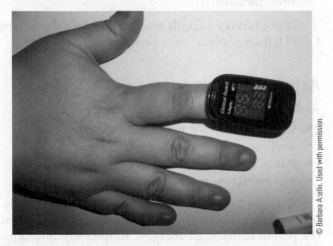

© Barbara Acello. Used with permission.

FIGURE 39-4 The fingertip sensor is the most common type of pulse oximeter.

The pulse oximeter measures light as it passes through the tissue, and shows a numeric value for the amount of oxygen in the arterial blood (Figure 39-5). The percent of oxygen saturation can be viewed on the digital display. Pulse oximeter values are listed in Table 39-2.

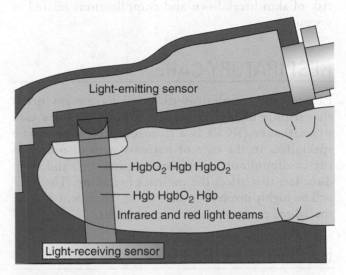

FIGURE 39-5 The pulse oximeter uses light to measure the amount of oxygen in the arterial blood.

TABLE 39-2 Pulse Oximeter Values

Pulse Oximeter Reading	Interpretation
95% to 100%	Normal
Below 90%	Suggests complications, impending hypoxemia
85%	Inadequate oxygen for body function; condition worsening, potential impending crisis
Below 70%	Life-threatening

Never turn the pulse oximeter alarm off.

Monitoring the Patient

Monitor the patient regularly when a pulse oximeter is being used. Reporting to the nurse is part of your ending procedure actions. In this case, make sure to report the patient's initial pulse oximeter reading and vital signs. This is important information on which the nurse will act. They will further assess the patient and provide care for abnormal values. The nurse must know the initial values as a basis for comparison.

If the patient's vital signs or appearance change significantly from baseline values, notify the nurse promptly. Also inform the nurse immediately if the patient's pulse oximetry value declines markedly. Each time you are in the room, monitor the liter flow for the oxygen to verify it is set at the ordered rate.

Rotate the position of the tape finger sensor at least every four hours. Move the spring-clip sensor every two hours. Rotating the location of the sensor reduces the risk of skin breakdown and complications related to pressure.

RESPIRATORY CARE

Patients with respiratory disorders have many needs that require highly skilled care. The **respiratory care practitioner (RCP)** is a licensed professional who specializes in the care of patients with disorders of the cardiopulmonary system, respirations, and sleep disorders that affect the patient's breathing. The RCP will be highly involved in the care of the patient and the specialized equipment used for treatment.

UPPER RESPIRATORY INFECTIONS

An **upper respiratory infection (URI)** follows invasion of the upper respiratory organs by pathogens. The upper respiratory organs include the nose, sinuses, and throat. A common cold, which is caused by a virus, is an example of a URI. It is one of the most ordinary illnesses found in people. Symptoms include:

- Elevated temperature (fever)
- Runny nose
- Watery eyes

This usually self-limiting disease is best treated by:

- Use of a drug to reduce fever, such as acetaminophen
- Rest
- Increased fluid intake

Patients with respiratory infections should be taught to:

- Cover the nose and mouth with a tissue when coughing or sneezing.
- Dispose of soiled tissues by placing them in a plastic or paper bag to be burned.
- Turn the face away from others when coughing or sneezing.
- Wash hands (or use alcohol-based hand cleaner) after handling soiled tissues.

You have learned that respiratory infections are spread by the airborne and droplet methods of transmission. Secretions containing pathogens make their way to the environment, where you pick them up. Good handwashing is the best method of preventing infection, including respiratory infection.

You must take special note of and report the following:

- **Dyspnea** (difficult breathing)
- Changes in the rate and rhythm of respiration
- Presence and character, color, and amount of respiratory secretions
- Cough
- Changes in skin color, such as pallor or cyanosis

URIs sometimes move down into the chest and develop into bronchitis or even pneumonia.

Pneumonia

Pneumonia is a serious inflammation of the lungs. It can be caused by a variety of infectious organisms. Three common causes of pneumonia are:

- Viruses.
- Bacteria.
- Protozoa.

Pneumocystis carinii pneumonia (PCP) is most often seen in patients who have poorly functioning immune systems. Today, most pneumonias, though serious and potentially life-threatening, respond favorably to antibiotic therapy.

CHRONIC OBSTRUCTIVE PULMONARY DISEASE

Chronic obstructive pulmonary disease (COPD) is also called **chronic obstructive lung disease (COLD)**. These terms refer to conditions that result in chronic blockage or obstruction of the respiratory system that is not reversible. Several conditions constitute COPD, including:

- Emphysema
- Chronic bronchitis
- Bronchiectasis

It can be very difficult to differentiate asthma from COPD, particularly in older patients.

Asthma

Asthma is a breathing disorder resulting from:

- Constriction of the muscles of the bronchioles
- Swelling of the respiratory membranes
- Production of large amounts of mucus that fill the narrowed passageways

A person having an asthma attack has labored breathing and frequent coughing. An attack may result when the person contacts an allergen. Respiratory infections can also cause an asthma attack. Common allergens are:

Asthma is caused by narrowing and clogging of the bronchi, the small tubes that carry air into and out of the lungs (Figure 39-6). The bronchi normally narrow during the night, in everyone. This increases resistance to air flow. People who do not have asthma probably will not notice the change. However, in people with asthma, the change may be enough to bring on an asthma attack, whether the patient is awake or asleep.

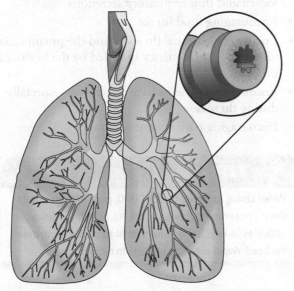

FIGURE 39-6 In asthma, the size of the airways is decreased due to inflammation, making breathing very difficult.

- Pollen
- Medications
- Dust
- Feathers
- Foods such as peanuts, eggs, or chocolate
- Cigarette and cigar smoke
- Cockroaches
- Dust mites
- Furry pets
- Mold
- Certain chemicals

Known allergies (hypersensitivity to specific items) should be listed in the patient's health record. Long-term treatment consists of identifying the allergen and eliminating it or exposure to it. To relieve an attack, the patient is given medication to decrease the swelling and

dilate the bronchioles. Low levels of supplemental oxygen may also be necessary.

The incidence of asthma in children is increasing. Children from low-income households, minorities, and children living in the inner city experience higher morbidity and mortality due to asthma. Asthma accounts for at least 14 million lost school days annually. It is the third leading cause of hospitalization among children ages 15 and under. Currently, there are no preventive measures or cures for asthma; however, children and adolescents can control their asthma by taking medication and controlling environmental triggers.

Chronic Bronchitis

Chronic **bronchitis** is prolonged inflammation in the bronchi due to infection or irritants (Figure 39-7). Signs and symptoms include:

- Swollen and red bronchial tissues, resulting in narrowed bronchial passageways
- Persistent cough
- Sputum production
- Respiratory distress
  Treatment includes:
- Antibiotics to fight the infection

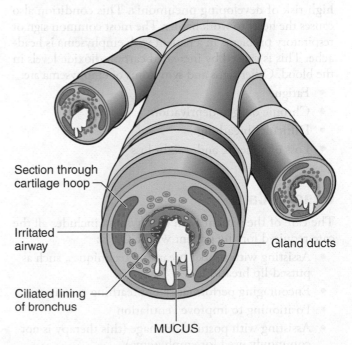

Section through
cartilage hoop

Irritated
airway

Gland ducts

Ciliated lining
of bronchus

MUCUS

FIGURE 39-7 In chronic bronchitis, the air passages are swollen and mucus production is excessive.

- Drugs to loosen secretions deep in the respiratory tract
- Techniques to improve ventilation and drainage
- Adequate fluid intake to keep secretions thin so they can be coughed up

Emphysema

Emphysema develops after chronic obstruction of the air flow to the alveoli. The air sacs:

- Become distended
- Lose their elasticity and recoil ability
- Finally become nonfunctional
- Lose the ability to exchange gases

The patient can bring air into the lungs, but it becomes more difficult to expel air from the lungs because of the loss of elasticity. As a result, there is less and less room for air to reenter.

Risk factors for emphysema are:

- Genetics
- Airways that are very responsive to irritants
- Exposure to tobacco smoke
- Exposure to dust and chemicals in the workplace
- Exposure to indoor and outdoor air pollution
- Repeated lung infections

Emphysema alone (without chronic bronchitis, which often accompanies it) is a dry disease. There is no sputum production. However, patients with emphysema are at high risk of developing pneumonia. This condition also causes the heart to work harder. The most common sign of respiratory problems in a patient with emphysema is headache. This is caused by increased carbon dioxide levels in the blood. Other signs and symptoms of emphysema are:

- Fatigue
- Chronic oxygen deprivation
- Difficulty breathing
- Loss of appetite and weight loss

General Care

The care of the patient with emphysema includes all the care required for any patient with COPD:

- Assisting with proper breathing techniques, such as pursed-lip breathing
- Encouraging performance of breathing exercises
- Positioning to improve ventilation
- Assisting with postural drainage (this therapy is not commonly used for emphysema)
- Providing care during low-flow oxygen therapy

 Infection Control ALERT

Patients with asthma, bronchitis, COPD, or weakened immune systems readily contract fungal infections from pillows. The typical pillow contains many fungi. Use disposable pillows, if possible, or make sure the pillow is encased in a plastic pillow cover.

- Assisting with and encouraging good nutrition
- Treating infections with antibiotics and drugs to loosen and thin respiratory secretions
- Encouraging fluid intake
- Encouraging annual flu shots and the pneumonia vaccine at the frequency specified by the health care provider
- Encouraging patients to avoid crowds, especially during flu season
- Encouraging patients not to smoke

 TIPS

When caring for patients with COPD, pace activities. Help them conserve energy as much as possible. Minimize activities in which the patient must raise the arms over the head. Avoid exposing patients to aerosol sprays.

Wear gloves if your hands may contact the patient's respiratory secretions. Wear a gown, goggles or face shield, and a surgical mask if the patient is coughing and spraying respiratory secretions into the air.

 Clinical Information ALERT

Pursed-lip breathing is one of the most effective methods of controlling shortness of breath. Have the patient breathe in slowly through the nose for two breaths, with the mouth closed. Next, take a normal breath. Pucker (purse) the lips as if preparing to whistle and exhale. **Pursed-lip breathing** slows the respirations and enables the patient to take more air in. Over time, it will strengthen the lungs and improve their efficiency.

SURGICAL CONDITIONS

Most respiratory problems are not treated with surgery. However, several problems require surgical correction to ensure uninterrupted air flow.

Tracheostomy

A **tracheostomy** (Figure 39-8) is inserted into a surgical opening in the patient's trachea (windpipe). It is used when the person cannot breathe in air through the nose. The tube directs air into the trachea and then into the lungs. A person who uses a ventilator for a long time will have a tracheostomy. The patient may have secretions coming from the chest and through the tube. The nurse will use suction to remove these secretions.

A tracheostomy may be temporary or permanent. The external opening on the skin surface is the **stoma**. Eventually, the stoma will heal and remain permanently open. A plastic or metal tube is inserted through the stoma to maintain patency until the stoma has healed open. This tube is the **cannula**. An outer and inner cannula are used. Several types of outer cannulae are available. The most common has an inflatable cuff (Figure 39-9). It seals or reduces the air flow to the nose and throat, so virtually all breathing is done through the tracheostomy. The cuff also

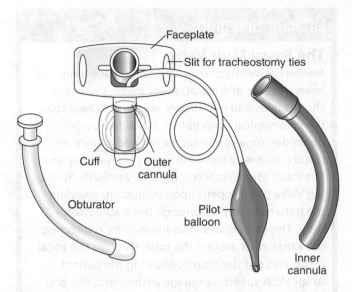

FIGURE 39-10 Parts of a tracheostomy.

helps reduce the risk of aspiration of feedings. Care of the cuff is not a nursing assistant responsibility. The nurse or RCP will inflate and deflate the cuff periodically. The cuff must be inflated before feeding the patient or providing mouth care. A cuffless tube may also be used, but this is less common. Patients with a cuffless tube are able to breathe through the nose, mouth, and tracheostomy. The outer cannula has a flat plate, with a flange on each side that is fastened to twill tape or a Velcro fastener that encircles the patient's neck. The tape helps hold the device securely in place. The inner cannula has an adapter on the distal end that can be attached to the manual resuscitation bag. The parts of the tracheostomy apparatus are shown in Figure 39-10.

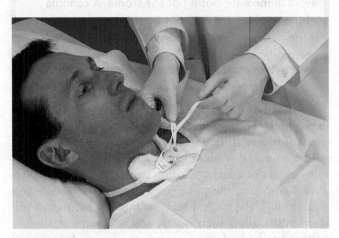

FIGURE 39-8 A tracheostomy stoma is a surgical opening in the trachea. The cannula keeps the stoma open.

Nursing Assistant Care of a Person with a Tracheostomy

Persons with tracheostomies can usually take a bath or shower, but must keep the water from entering the opening. Avoid using powders, sprays, or shaving cream around the tube. When caring for a patient with a tracheostomy, observe for:

- Changes in respiratory rate, depth, and quality
- Changes in mental status, such as confusion, restlessness, or irritability that indicate the patient's brain is not getting adequate oxygen

Report to the nurse immediately if the:

- Tube becomes dislodged.
- Patient is having trouble breathing.
- Patient needs suctioning.
- Alarm sounds on the respirator.

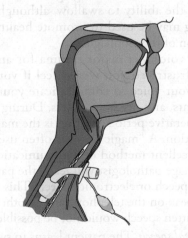

FIGURE 39-9 A tracheostomy with the cuff inflated.

Difficult Situations

The Passy Muir Valve

Nonverbal means of communication have long been a source of frustration for persons with tracheostomies and health care workers. To help solve the communication problem, David Muir, who depended on a ventilator, developed a positive-closure, one-way speaking valve that is widely used. The Passy Muir Tracheostomy and Ventilator Speaking Valve (PMV) opens upon inhalation, enabling the patient to inspire through the tracheostomy tube. The valve closes after inspiration, redirecting the exhaled air around the tube, through the vocal cords, and out the mouth, allowing the patient to speak. A speech-language pathologist, RN, and RCP will all be involved in fitting, monitoring, and teaching the patient to use the device. Some patients will only be able to wear the PMV for a few minutes at a time, building up time gradually. Monitor blood pressure, pulse, and respirations closely when a patient starts using the valve. Inform the nurse at once if the patient shows signs and symptoms of distress, such as:

- A significant change in blood pressure or pulse
- Increased respiratory rate
- Dyspnea
- Diaphoresis
- Anxiety
- Uncontrollable coughing
- Pulse oximeter value of less than 90 percent

Be sure you know how the patient communicates. The opening in the trachea interferes with the patient's ability to talk.

Caring for the tracheostomy is the nurse's responsibility. Notify the nurse immediately if the ties are loose or the device comes apart. You should be able to slide a finger underneath the tie on either side of the neck. If you cannot, it is too tight, and you should notify the nurse immediately.

Malignancies

Malignant tumors can develop in any part of the respiratory tract. Although the exact causes of malignancy are not fully understood, cigarette smoking and exposure to cancer-producing agents in the environment are known to be contributing factors. Lung cancers are treated by surgery, radiation, chemotherapy, or a combination of all three therapies.

Cancer of the Larynx

Cancer of the larynx may require removal of the larynx, resulting in loss of the voice. A **laryngectomy** is the surgical removal of the larynx. During this procedure, the airway is separated from the mouth, nose, and esophagus. The patient breathes through an artificial opening in the neck and trachea. A person who has had this surgery may be called a **laryngectomee**. When the larynx is removed, there is no longer a connection between the upper and lower airways (Figure 39-11).

Difficult Situations

If a cannula becomes dislodged, stay with the patient and call for the nurse or RCP immediately. The stoma may close quickly, so this has the potential to become a serious emergency. A second, smaller cannula set is kept at the bedside at all times. The smaller set is used for rapid insertion, to avoid immediate closing of the stoma. A cannula of the original size may not fit. Inform the nurse if the neck ties become moist with secretions or perspiration.

A laryngectomy stoma is a special kind of opening in the neck. Though it may look like a regular tracheostomy, it is very different. If you are caring for a patient with a stoma, you must know whether it is a tracheostomy stoma or a laryngectomy stoma. If the patient has a tracheostomy, the passageway from the mouth and nose through the trachea remains intact. Patients can still smell odors, blow their noses, and suck on a straw. If a patient has had a laryngectomy, the larynx (voice box) has been removed. The upper airway is no longer connected to the trachea. The patient will not be able to talk, smell, blow their nose, whistle, gargle, or suck on a straw. They retain the ability to swallow, although initially a tube feeding may be used to promote healing and prevent irritation of the esophagus.

Loss of voice is a major trauma for anyone. Just think how frustrated you would feel if you could no longer use your voice to communicate your thoughts, feelings, wants, and needs to others. During the immediate postoperative period, writing is the major form of communication. A "magic slate" is often used. A tablet is also an excellent method of communication. Later, a speech-language pathologist will teach the patient to use esophageal speech or electronic speech. This enables the patient to speak on the telephone and in other situations in which written speech would not be possible.

- *Esophageal speech*. The patient learns to swallow air and then bring it back up through the esophagus into the mouth. Here the air is formed by the teeth

Before

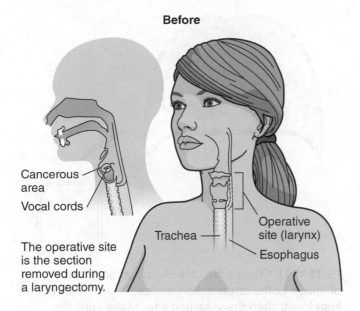

Cancerous area

Vocal cords

The operative site is the section removed during a laryngectomy.

Trachea

Operative site (larynx)

Esophagus

After

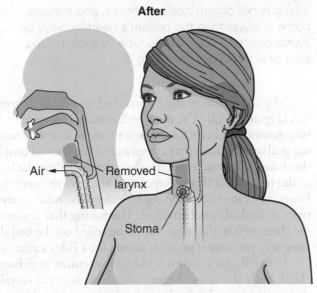

Air

Removed larynx

Stoma

FIGURE 39-11 The anatomy of the face and neck before and after laryngectomy surgery.

and tongue into words, as it would be if it were being exhaled from the lungs. Esophageal speech is difficult to learn, but motivated patients can succeed.

- *Electronic speech.* Patients who cannot use esophageal speech may be able to use an electronic artificial larynx to create speech. Some patients may use a combination of both techniques.

Patients with laryngectomies need patience and understanding from all health care providers. Communication is possible, but the voice does not sound normal. The patient needs extra time to formulate the sounds. The loss of one's voice requires a difficult psychological adjustment, similar to that undergone when losing

a loved one. Expect periods of depression, anger, and hostility.

Caring for a Patient with a Tracheostomy or Laryngectomy Stoma

When people breathe normally, the structures in the nose and mouth capture microbes and other foreign particles, preventing them from entering the airway. In addition, the body moistens and warms air before it enters the lungs. Inhaling cold, dry air is very uncomfortable, and it irritates the lungs. Because the stoma bypasses the normal breathing structures, the patient's body cannot use its normal protective mechanisms to warm, moisten, and filter the air. Thus, care is designed to replace these body functions. Warm, humidified oxygen may be administered to patients with a stoma.

The stoma now provides a direct passageway into the lungs. Because of this, some patients wear a mask similar to a surgical mask over the opening. The risk of inhaling a foreign particle is greatly increased. Inhaling small particles or water (such as during a shower) can cause serious complications. Check with the nurse or care plan for precautions to take when showering the patient. Avoid getting powder, lint, dust, water, shaving cream, or other objects near or in the stoma.

Infection Control **ALERT**

The nasal hairs and tonsils filter pathogens and other substances from the air, preventing them from reaching the lungs. Patients with stomas do not have this advantage. The stoma provides a direct, unfiltered passageway to the lungs for irritating foreign substances and pathogens. Practice good infection control techniques when caring for patients with a stoma.

Likewise, the opening in the neck provides an open pathway for pathogens to enter, causing infection. Use standard precautions and frequent handwashing when caring for a patient with a stoma. Secretions may be expelled from the stoma when the patient coughs. The patient has no control over this. If they are expelling secretions, you will also need to wear a gown, mask, and eye protection when caring for the patient.

The stoma in the patient's neck is the primary airway. If the tube becomes blocked, dislodged, disconnected, or otherwise damaged, the patient's airway will be seriously compromised. Be especially careful when turning and bathing the patient. Monitor the skin color closely. Watch for cyanosis, changes in color of the nail beds or mucous membranes, and respiratory distress. Important, early signs of ineffective airway clearance and poor gas exchange to observe for and report are:

- Restlessness
- Dyspnea
- Anxiety
- Increased heart rate
- Lethargy
- Disorientation

Chest Tubes

Chest tubes (Figure 39-12) are sterile, plastic tubes that are inserted through the skin of the chest, between the ribs, and into the space between the pleural membrane that covers the lung and the pleural membrane that lines the chest wall. They are used after surgery to drain any bloody fluid drainage from the chest. These tubes also allow air to escape if there is a leak of air at the suture line after lung surgery.

Common reasons for using chest tubes are:

- To address an air leak after lung surgery that is slow to heal
- To drain fluid that collects around the lungs (often seen in patients who have cancer). This fluid is called a **pleural effusion**
- To treat a collapsed lung. Although this condition occurs spontaneously in some people, it is commonly the result of trauma, such as an auto accident

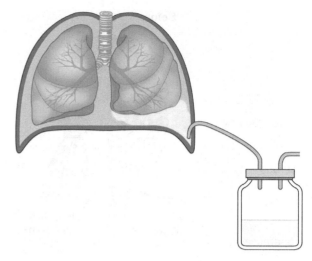

FIGURE 39-13 Chest tubes are always attached to a drainage bottle or collection device, which must be kept lower than the insertion site. Make sure the tubing is not obstructed or pinched, and that the bottle is lower than the patient's heart. Always be aware of the location of the tube to avoid pulling on it or accidentally removing it.

The chest tube is always attached to a drain of some sort (Figure 39-13). The nurse will manage this system. To help monitor and care for the patient, make sure that nothing pulls on the tube that comes out of the chest. Position the drainage system in an upright position, below the level of the heart at all times. Reposition the patient every two hours, or as instructed. Make sure the chest tube is never twisted, kinked, or obstructed. The tubing that connects the chest tube to the drain should be coiled on the bed the same way you would position tubing for a Foley catheter.

If the drain is connected to a vacuum regulator, check with the nurse before you disconnect it to take the patient to the bathroom, for example. Do not hesitate to get the patient up in a chair and to keep them mobile if their condition allows, even though they have a chest tube. The patient with a chest tube should always have oxygen and suction set up at the bedside. A tray of emergency equipment will also be kept in the room. Never remove these items.

Notify the nurse promptly if the:

- Vital signs change.
- Pulse oximeter alarm sounds.
- Dressing on the chest wall is loose.
- Color or amount of drainage from the chest tube changes.
- Patient coughs up blood.
- Patient becomes short of breath or cyanotic.
- Patient develops new swelling on the torso, neck, or face that "crackles" when you touch it.
- The tube comes out of the chest wall.

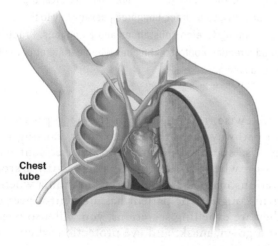

Chest tube

FIGURE 39-12 Chest tubes are sterile plastic tubes that are inserted through the skin of the chest, between the ribs, and into the space between the pleural membrane that covers the lung and the pleural membrane that lines the chest wall. The chest tube is securely covered with dressings.

DIAGNOSTIC TECHNIQUES

Some techniques used to diagnose problems of the respiratory system include:

- Tissue **biopsy** (microscopic examination of a specimen of tissue removed from the patient)
- Cultures of secretions
- Volume studies that measure the amount of air entering or leaving the lungs during various respiratory movements
- Radiographic techniques such as X-rays, CT scans, and MRIs
- Direct visualization procedures such as bronchoscopy

SPECIAL THERAPIES RELATED TO RESPIRATORY ILLNESS

Nursing assistants aid patient breathing by proper positioning and by helping provide moisture and oxygen. They also are assigned to collect sputum specimens for examinations.

Oxygen Therapy

Oxygen is necessary for life. Humans take in oxygen from the air during breathing. Some diseases and conditions prevent the body tissues from getting enough oxygen. Some patients have normal oxygen levels, but are at increased risk of hypoxemia. Oxygen is a prescription item, and a physician's order is needed to furnish it to a patient through an oxygen delivery system. The doctor will specify how much oxygen to use and the method of oxygen delivery. Check the flow rate each shift to ensure that it is set at the ordered amount. You should not start, stop, or change the flow rate of oxygen.

Culture **ALERT**

Oxygen is a basic need at the lowest level of Maslow's hierarchy of needs. Needs at the lower levels must be fulfilled before needs at the higher levels become important. The patient who is having trouble breathing cannot focus on much else. Keep conversation short and succinct. Give the patient verbal and nonverbal reassurance. Find alternate means of communicating, such as writing, if necessary.

Most facilities have a respiratory care practitioner on staff to oversee the use of oxygen therapy. Nursing personnel monitor patients who use oxygen, and notify the RCP as needed. Although an RCP may be responsible for the patients' oxygen needs, you still must have a working knowledge of oxygen administration. You must know where portable oxygen cylinders are stored, how to assemble them, and how to transport them safely.

Humidifiers

Some facilities attach a **humidifier** (Figure 39-14) to the oxygen administration equipment if the patient's flow exceeds five liters. Use of oxygen humidifiers is a controversial subject. Humidification is not necessary with liter flows below five. Some facilities do not use humidifiers at all.

The humidifier is a water bottle that moistens the oxygen for comfort and prevents drying of the mucous membranes in the nose, mouth, and lungs. The bottle fastens to a male adapter on the flow meter. Oxygen passes through the water in the humidifier, picking up moisture before it reaches the patient. When the system is functioning correctly, the water in the humidifier will bubble. Oxygen will not exit the tubing if it is obstructed. If this occurs, pressure builds up in the unit and discharges through a pressure relief valve. When setting up a humidifier, check this valve by turning the oxygen on and pinching the connecting tubing. If the oxygen does not flow through the tubing, the valve will be obstructed and pop open.

Two types of humidifiers are used. Acute care hospitals commonly use the *prefilled* type of humidifier. Change the unit when it is empty, or according to the manufacturer's directions or facility policies. Discard the

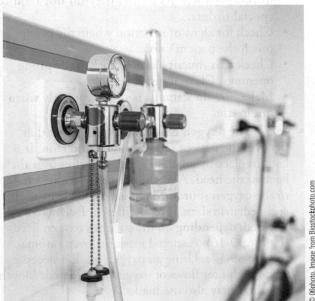

FIGURE 39-14 A humidifier for oxygen.

bottle after replacing it with a new one. Attach a sticker to the bottle showing the date and time it was changed and your initials.

Wash *refillable* humidifiers with soap and water or 2 percent alkaline glutaraldehyde solution every 24 hours. Rinse well, and then sterilize. Refill the sterile bottle with sterile distilled water. Never add water to a partially filled humidifier. Avoid tap water, which is associated with an increased incidence of Legionnaire's disease. The water level in the humidifier should always be at or above the "minimum fill" line on the bottle.

Methods of Oxygen Delivery

Several different methods are used for oxygen delivery. The same basic care is required for each method, with modifications.

- *Nasal cannula.* Delivery of oxygen by **nasal cannula** is the most common method. The oxygen flows through a tube that has two small plastic prongs (Figure 39-15). Position the prongs at the entrance to the patient's nose. Tubing that can be hooked over the patient's ears helps to hold the cannula in place.
  - Make sure the strap is secure but not too tight. Soft tubing is available for persons who complain of discomfort from the regular, rigid tubing. Protective covers are available for the earpieces to prevent them from cutting nto tender skin above and behind the ears. These are things that the respiratory therapy department should normally stock. As a rule, they do not require special orders.
  - Check for signs of irritation where the prongs touch the patient's nose.
  - Check that mucus has not blocked the prong openings. Clean if necessary.
  - Make sure the cannula is stored correctly when not in use.
- *Mask.* The **oxygen mask** is a cuplike mask that fits over the patient's nose, mouth, and chin. It is held in place by an elastic strap that slips over the back of the head. A small tube connects the mask to the oxygen source. Masks are available in adult and pediatric sizes. Several different face masks are used, depending on the patient's oxygen needs (Figure 39-16). A special mask fits over a stoma (Figure 39-17). Using an oxygen mask is necessary when high liter flows of oxygen are ordered. Mouth breathers may also use masks.

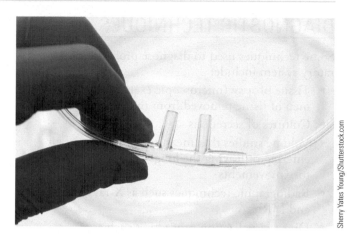

FIGURE 39-15 Nasal cannula for oxygen delivery.

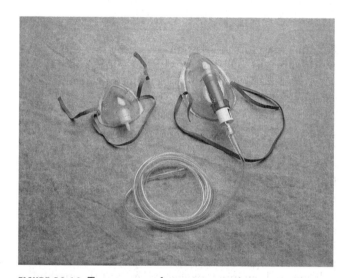

FIGURE 39-16 Two types of oxygen masks.

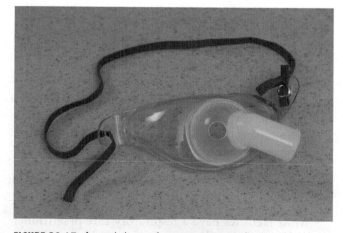

FIGURE 39-17 An adult tracheostomy mask.

Some masks have inflatable bags at the bottom. The bag should be inflated at all times. Notify the nurse if the bag collapses more than halfway during inspiration. This type of mask provides very high amounts of oxygen.

Caring for a Patient Who Is Receiving Oxygen Therapy

Elevating the head of the bed will make it easier to breathe. A patient using an oxygen mask cannot eat while wearing the mask. The physician may order a nasal cannula for mealtimes. Follow the instructions on the care plan or critical pathway for patient care measures.

> 🔓 Safety **ALERT**
>
> Oxygen is a prescription medication. Using oxygen is safe if you follow facility policies and safety guidelines. Never change the fittings from one type of oxygen bottle to another. Make sure you use the correct adaptor and plug for the unit. Avoid sparks; static electricity can start a fire. Do not use electric appliances, such as razors or hair dryers, when oxygen is in use.

> 🔓 Safety **ALERT**
>
> When using cylinder oxygen, identify the contents of the cylinder. Oxygen cylinders are always colored green in the United States. Transport oxygen cylinders carefully. Chain the cylinder to a carrier during transport. Secure it in a base or chain it to a carrier or wall when in use. Avoid dropping the tank. Cylinders can explode if the tank is dropped and the cylinder valve is damaged.

Being unable to breathe is very frightening. Patients who are receiving oxygen often need reassurance and emotional support. Check on the patient frequently and spend as much time in the room as possible. Difficulty breathing also makes it hard to talk. The patient may be unable to hold a normal conversation. Just being with the patient without talking is very reassuring.

You will care for patients using different devices for the administration of oxygen. Carefully check the skin under the device to be sure it does not become red or irritated. Pad the straps with cotton, if necessary. Oxygen is drying, and patients receiving oxygen will need extra liquids to drink. However, patients who are short of breath may be unable to suck on a straw. Assist the patient by holding the cup, if necessary. Patients who use oxygen will also need frequent care of the mouth and nose. They may feel warm and perspire heavily. Assist with bathing and linen changes as needed. Adjust the temperature in the room and help the patient change into a hospital gown. The care plan or critical pathway will provide information on patient preferences and needs.

Use of Oxygen in an Emergency

There are several differences between routine oxygen use and use of oxygen in an emergency. High concentrations of oxygen are necessary in emergencies. Cylinders, liquid oxygen, or piped-in oxygen are used. An oxygen concentrator cannot supply the high liter flows necessary for emergency care. Oxygen may be delivered dry. Do not take the time to search for a humidifier.

Oxygen Concentrator

An **oxygen concentrator** (Figure 39-18) takes in room air and removes impurities and gases other than oxygen, allowing the oxygen to become concentrated in the unit. The air delivered to the patient from the concentrator is more than 90 percent oxygen. It is delivered by tubing attached to a nasal cannula. The flow rate is usually two liters per minute (L/min or LPM).

General Oxygen Concentrator Precautions

Follow these precautions when a concentrator is used:

- Place the concentrator at least five feet away from any heat source and at least four inches away from the wall.
- Smoking is not permitted in the same room.

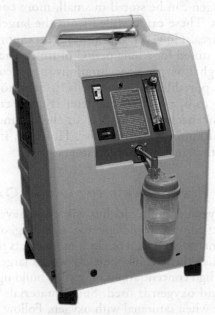

FIGURE 39-18 An oxygen concentrator delivers low liter flows of oxygen. It may have an attachment for a humidifier; however, humidification is not required for low liter flows.

- Be sure the unit is plugged in and grounded.
- Do not use an extension cord with the concentrator.
- Never change the flow meter setting.
- Notify the nurse if the alarm sounds.
- Do not use a mask on the patient.
- Wipe the cannula daily with a damp cloth (do not use alcohol- or oil-based products).
- Clean concentrator surfaces using a damp cloth only.
- Remove the filter weekly. Wash in warm soapy water, rinse, squeeze dry, and replace.
- Store the nasal cannula according to facility policy when not in use. Keep it covered and off the floor.
- Some patients may use long oxygen extension tubing so they can move about the room. The tubing presents a trip hazard for both patient and staff. Position it out of the flow of traffic as much as possible.
- Change the cannula every 24 to 48 hours, or according to facility policy, if this is your responsibility. Fold a piece of bandage tape or a label in half over the distal end of the tubing, affixing it to itself. Use a permanent marker to write the date and time the tubing was changed and your initials.
- When changing the cannula, replace the packaging used to store the cannula when not in use.

Liquid Oxygen

Oxygen also comes in a liquid canister. Liquid oxygen is made by cooling the oxygen gas. As it cools, it changes to a liquid form. One advantage is that large amounts of liquid oxygen can be stored in small, more convenient containers. These can be filled from the larger unit in a special area. However, liquid oxygen evaporates and cannot be stored for a long period of time. The canister delivers higher oxygen concentrations than a concentrator, and is portable and convenient. It does not require electricity to operate. The canister is quiet compared with a concentrator, which has an electric motor and makes a humming/puffing noise. However, it is more expensive than using a concentrator.

Safety Precautions for Liquid Oxygen

Liquid oxygen is nontoxic, but will cause severe burns upon direct contact. Avoid opening, touching, or spilling the container. If your skin or clothing contacts the liquid oxygen, flush the area immediately with a large amount of water. High concentrations of oxygen build up quickly when liquid oxygen is used. Some materials are very flammable when saturated with oxygen. Follow all safety precautions for preventing sparks and fires (Chapter 14). Never seal the cap or vent port on the liquid oxygen.

Doing so will increase pressure within the system, creating a potentially dangerous situation. Never try to fill the small, portable liquid oxygen cylinder. This must be done by a qualified person in a specially ventilated area.

 Safety ALERT

Oxygen concentrators are used only for patients who use low liter flows of oxygen. The concentrator cannot convert room air when high liter flows are necessary. For this reason, an oxygen concentrator should not be used in an emergency. If you are sent for an external oxygen source in an emergency, a small tank is best.

INTRODUCTION TO ADVANCED AIRWAY MANAGEMENT

If you work in subacute or critical care units, you will work with various patients who have advanced airways and those who need airway support to prevent or treat hypoxemia. Advanced health care providers, nurses, and RCPs will be responsible for managing patients' airways and ventilation devices. You must be able to identify the airways and ventilation devices and understand basic patient care. You must also be able to identify a patient who is in distress and needs immediate attention.

Oropharyngeal Airway

An **oropharyngeal airway** (Figure 39-19), or oral airway, is a curved plastic device that is inserted into the mouth to the posterior pharynx. It is used to keep the airway open in an unconscious patient.

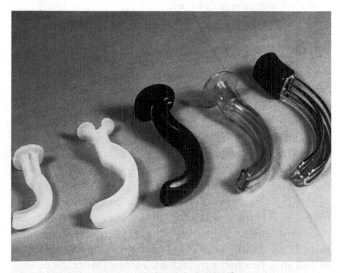

FIGURE 39-19 Various types and sizes of oral airways.

The most common cause of airway obstruction is the tongue. The oral airway prevents the tongue from falling to the back of the throat and obstructing the airway. The airway has a flange at the end, which fits between the patient's lips. The curve of the airway holds the tongue forward. It is not the airway of choice for patients who have had recent oral surgery or those with loose teeth.

When caring for a patient with an oral airway, use gloves and other personal protective equipment as needed to apply the principles of standard precautions. The patient may move the hand to the face to remove the airway. Do not attempt to stop them. If they can pull it out, they do not need the airway, even if they are not fully awake.

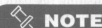

> **NOTE**
>
> This applies only to an oral airway, not an endotracheal tube.

> **Difficult Situations**
>
> Inserting an oral airway into a conscious or semiconscious patient will induce vomiting. *If the patient is awake enough to spit the airway out, they do not need it.*
>
>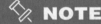
>
> **NOTE**
>
> This applies only to an oral airway, not an endotracheal tube.

Check the patient's respirations immediately after the airway is removed to ensure that they are adequate. If you have concerns about the patient's ability to maintain the airway, discuss them with the nurse. Make sure the airway is in the correct position and that the patient's tongue and lips are not positioned between the airway and the teeth.

Nasopharyngeal Airway

A **nasopharyngeal airway** (Figure 39-20) is a curved, soft rubber device that extends from one nostril to the posterior pharynx area, keeping the tongue off the back of the throat. You may hear this airway called a nasal trumpet. It is used in persons who are responsive. It is not used for patients receiving

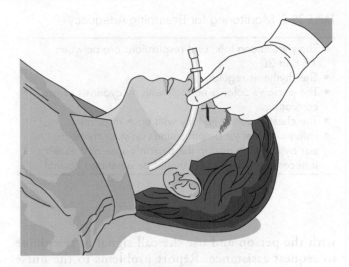

FIGURE 39-20 The nasopharyngeal airway (nasal trumpet) may be used with responsive patients. A length of airway is used to measure from the tip of the nose to the earlobe. It should be approximately one inch longer than this distance.

anticoagulant (blood-thinning) medications or for those who have a nasal deformity, bleeding disorders, or sepsis. The nasal trumpet is the airway of choice for patients who:

- Are awake and responsive
- Have had recent oral surgery, loose teeth, or trauma of the mouth
- Need frequent nasal suctioning

The care plan may instruct you to keep the patient's head turned to the side to prevent aspiration. The airway is removed once every shift to provide nasal care and check for irritation in the nose.

If the patient gags or coughs, the airway may be too long. Notify the nurse or RCP promptly. Wear a mask and eye protection in addition to gloves until the problem subsides. A gown is also needed if the patient cannot contain the secretions.

MAINTAINING THE PATIENT'S BREATHING

The normal respiratory rate is determined by age. *Respiratory failure* occurs when breathing cannot sustain life. *Respiratory arrest* occurs when breathing stops. It is caused by many conditions, including heart attack and stroke. Follow the criteria in Table 39-3 to determine if the person's breathing is adequate. Stay

TABLE 39-3 Monitoring for Breathing Adequacy

- The person can talk, and respirations are between 12 and 20.
- The rhythm is regular.
- The person's color is normal, with no cyanosis or gray coloration.
- The chest expands equally with each inspiration.
- Listen and feel for breath sounds on your cheek and ear by kneeling next to the person's nose and mouth, if necessary. The sounds should be quiet and normal.

with the person and use the call signal or telephone to request assistance. Report problems to the nurse immediately.

Opening the Airway

If you discover a person is in respiratory failure or respiratory arrest, remain in the room and call for help. Open the patient's airway. The most common cause of airway obstruction is the tongue falling back into the throat. Opening the airway lifts the tongue from the back of the throat, making breathing easier. This procedure is most effective when the patient is lying in the supine position. Always remove the pillow. Position the patient on the back before beginning.

The *head-tilt, chin-lift maneuver* is the most common method of opening the airway. If the person has a neck injury, do not perform this procedure. Instead, use the jaw-thrust maneuver. The jaw-thrust maneuver is used to open the airway of persons with known or suspected neck injuries, and in those whose airways cannot be opened using the head-tilt, chin-lift method.

Mask-to-Mouth Resuscitation

When a person stops breathing, their respirations must be sustained by artificial means to prevent brain damage and other complications. If you have taken a CPR class, you may have learned mouth-to-mouth ventilation. This is a technique of breathing for the person. Avoid this method on patients because of the risk of disease transmission. Various **adjunctive devices** are used instead. An airway adjunct is a secondary device used to maintain respirations. This is done by a trained and qualified health care professional.

Mask-to-mouth ventilation is performed using a *pocket mask*. This is a temporary measure until more

advanced airway support becomes available. The mask has a special valve that prevents the patient's exhaled air and secretions from entering the caregiver's mouth.

Endotracheal Intubation

Endotracheal intubation provides complete control over the airway. It is commonly called *intubation*. An **endotracheal tube (ET tube)** is passed through the mouth, or less commonly the nose, into the patient's lungs (Figure 39-21). The patient is ventilated and suctioned through the tube. Patients are routinely intubated for surgical procedures; in some emergencies, including code (CPR) situations; or when complete airway control is needed. Intubating the patient has many advantages over other methods of controlling the airway.

The endotracheal tube is inserted by a qualified health care professional who is certified in advanced cardiac life support (ACLS). Although you will provide many aspects of patient care, only a licensed nurse, RCP, or physician should care for the endotracheal tube.

Caring for the Patient Who Has an Endotracheal Tube

Patients who are intubated need a great deal of care, comfort measures, and reassurance. The patient will be unable to speak because the tube is between the vocal cords. This causes anxiety and fear. Patients who are intubated are ventilated mechanically. This involves using a ventilator, a positive-pressure mechanical device that forces air into the lungs. The RCP and nurse will

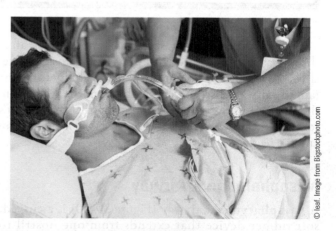

FIGURE 39-21 An endotracheal tube is placed into the trachea and is used to oxygenate seriously ill patients.

© leaf. Image from Bigstockphoto.com

care for the ventilator. The patient may be restrained to prevent them from removing the endotracheal tube. They will need total nursing care, including turning and repositioning, and restraint care and observation. The care plan or critical pathway will provide instructions.

Difficult Situations

Some bariatric surgery patients (Chapter 31) require prolonged intubation, and continued mechanical ventilation is sometimes necessary after surgery. The airway can be difficult to manage in these patients because of the configuration of the head and neck. An emergency tracheostomy tube and tray must be visible at the bedside and readily available at all times. Patients who are morbidly obese often cough more forcefully than smaller persons. The forceful cough can cause the tube to move out of position. To prevent exposure to oral, nasal, or airway secretions, select and wear the correct PPE if the patient is coughing. To prevent accidental removal of the tube, work with a partner when:

- Transporting a patient who is morbidly obese and who has an endotracheal tube
- Turning the patient and providing routine personal care
- Assisting with portable chest X-rays

Caring for a Patient Who Is Mechanically Ventilated

A **ventilator** is a mechanical device that assists breathing in patients with impaired respiratory or diaphragm function. It is connected to an endotracheal tube or tracheostomy. Ventilators are used primarily in critical care and subacute care units. Patients who are using ventilators usually have serious medical problems, and may be very unstable. Most of the skilled services will be provided by the nurse or RCP. You will assist with ADLs and routine nursing care.

The risk of infection is a great concern. Use good handwashing (or alcohol-based hand cleaner), standard precautions, and aseptic technique. Your job description and facility's policy and procedure manuals will list your responsibilities.

Assisted Ventilation for a Patient with an Endotracheal Tube

There will be times when the patient with an endotracheal tube or tracheostomy is not connected to the ventilator, such as during transportation or when tracheostomy care is being done. When a mechanical ventilator cannot be used, the **bag-valve-mask (BVM)** device is used to manually ventilate a patient. You may have seen the BVM used to support ventilation when CPR was being given. It consists of a face mask and a ventilation bag. When the patient is intubated or has a tracheostomy, the mask is removed and a sterile bag is connected directly to the endotracheal tube or tracheostomy cannula. The nurse or RCP will ventilate the patient. You may be responsible for cleaning the bag and ensuring that it is sterilized according to facility policy. If a BVM is in a patient's room, keep it visible and readily available. Do not put it away or remove it from the room.

Suction

Suction is used to remove fluid, food, and secretions from a patient's nose, mouth, and airway, reducing the risk of aspiration. This keeps the airway clear in patients who are unable to cough effectively to maintain the airway on their own. Suctioning is done as often as necessary to remove secretions.

GUIDELINES 39-1 Guidelines for Caring for Mechanically Ventilated Patients

- Monitor the patient frequently and anticipate their needs.
- Never turn the alarm off. Respond to alarms immediately. Remember, if an alarm sounds, check the patient first, not the machine.

- If an oral or nasal airway is used, keep the patient's head turned to the side to prevent aspiration.
- Monitor the patient's tolerance to the ventilator by checking pulse oximetry, vital signs, cardiac monitor, anxiety, ability to sleep, and mental status.

(continues)

GUIDELINES 39-1 Guidelines for Caring for Mechanically Ventilated Patients (continued)

- If the person is breathing independently, observe for changes in respiratory rate and depth, shortness of breath, and use of accessory muscles in breathing.

- When monitoring the vital signs of patients using mechanical ventilation, count spontaneous respirations as well as ventilator-delivered breaths.

- Visually inspect the chest when monitoring respirations. If both sides do not expand equally upon breathing, inform the nurse.

- Check for tube displacement each time you are in the room. The endotracheal tube is usually marked at the lips, teeth, or nares, so you can see if the tube has moved.

- Make sure the endotracheal tube is taped securely. Inform the nurse if the tape is loose or comes off.

- Inform the nurse or RCP if the person requires suctioning (is unable to manage oral or nasal secretions, is coughing or choking, or has loose or rattling respirations).

- Provide frequent oral and nasal care. Monitor the mucous membranes for signs of pressure, irritation, dryness, cracking, and breakdown from the breathing apparatus.

- Keep the lips and mucous membranes moist.

- Monitor the patient regularly for pain, and report to the nurse.

- Elevate the head of the bed 60° to 90°, or as directed in the care plan.

- Remember that elevation of the head of the bed increases the risk of skin breakdown. Reposition the patient every two hours or more often. Provide preventive skin care with lotion. Apply a therapeutic mattress, if ordered.

- Elevate the heels off the surface of the bed to prevent pressure injuries. Heel protectors relieve friction and shearing. They do not relieve pressure.

- Condensation in the ventilator tubing causes resistance to air flow and increases the risk of aspiration. Inform the nurse or RCP if condensation forms. Do not attempt to empty condensation in the ventilation tubing backward into the humidifier or in a way that causes you to get sprayed in the face with contaminated fluid.

- Make sure that adequate sterile supplies are available in the room in case they are needed quickly. Get a list of supplies from the care plan or nurse and restock the room every shift and as needed. If supplies are used, replace them immediately.

- Items needed for emergency care, such as a Kelly clamp, clean airway, or tracheostomy tray, may be stored in plain view, close to the patient. Small items may be taped to the headboard or over the head of the bed. Leave them in packages so they do not collect dust or become contaminated. Do not store these items in a drawer or cupboard. Make sure everyone can see them.

- Monitor the patient for constipation; inform the nurse if the patient has not had a bowel movement in three days.

- Provide active and passive range of motion, according to the plan of care. Use positioning aids to support the patient, promote comfort, and reduce the risk of contractures.

- Monitor restraints, if used; release restraints according to facility policy.

- Monitor bony prominences for signs of redness, irritation, or breakdown.

- Be compassionate and empathetic to the patient's circumstances; reassure the patient and family.

- Use nursing comfort measures (Chapter 10), such as a backrub or supporting the patient's position, to promote comfort.

- Ask the patient yes and no questions. They can respond by blinking or holding fingers up; for example, one blink (or finger) for yes and two blinks (or fingers) for no.

- Always explain what you are doing, even if the person seems unable to respond.

- Develop a means for communicating with the patient, such as using a magic slate or writing.

- Answer the call signal immediately.

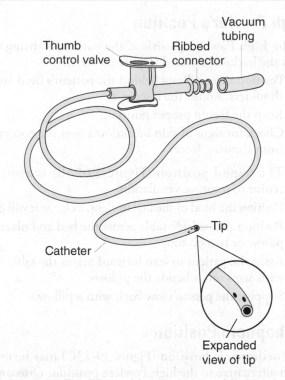

Clinical Information ALERT

In some facilities, personnel bring extra supplies to the room in anticipation of needing them during a procedure. For example, sterile gloves and sterile suction and urinary catheters may have to be replaced. Once supplies have been brought to a patient's room, they cannot be returned to stock and used in the care of another patient. Thus, if the "extra" sterile supplies are not used, they must be discarded. This is costly, in terms of replacement supplies and waste disposal. Some of the patient conditions discussed in this chapter are unstable, making it necessary to keep some stock items in the room. Know and follow your facility's policies for bringing extra supplies into patients' rooms in anticipation of needing them during sterile procedures. Bring only what is needed. Avoid overstocking. Do so only if permitted, and obtain directions on how to manage unused sterile items.

FIGURE 39-22A Flexible suction catheter with thumb control valve. Some do not have a valve and are controlled by pinching and releasing the tubing.

A flexible, plastic suction catheter (Figure 39-22A) or rigid plastic suction, called a **Yankauer catheter** (tonsil tip) (Figure 39-22B), are used for oral suctioning. This is a clean procedure. The flexible catheter is inserted into the mouth or nose to remove secretions. The Yankauer is used only for oral suctioning. Apply the principles of standard precautions when caring for the patient and handling suction equipment. Wear a mask and face protection if this is your facility's policy, or if there is a risk that the patient will cough in your face. Tracheal suctioning is always a sterile procedure, as is suctioning through a tracheostomy, laryngectomy, or endotracheal tube. Although an advanced care provider, nurse, or RCP will do the suctioning, you must understand the purpose of the procedure, keep sterile suction supplies stocked, clean and maintain the equipment, recognize when the patient needs suctioning, and use standard precautions when assisting.

RESPIRATORY POSITIONS

Positioning to permit expansion of the lungs and a straightened airway is helpful to patients with respiratory distress. These positions work best when used in combination with pursed-lip breathing and diaphragmatic breathing. The RCP will work with the patient on these activities.

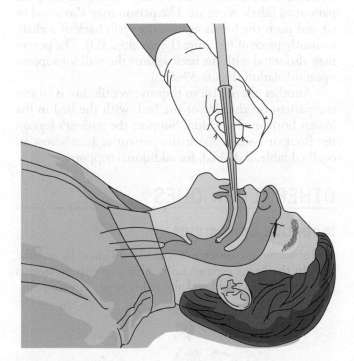

FIGURE 39-22B A Yankauer catheter should never be placed farther back than the base of the tongue.

High Fowler's Position

In the **high Fowler's position**, the patient is sitting up with the backrest elevated (Figure 39-23A).

- Position three pillows behind the patient's head and shoulders. Adjust the knee rest.
- Keep the feet in proper position.
- Check for signs of skin breakdown over the coccyx from shearing forces.

The **tripod position** (Figure 39-23B) is another alternative to improve ventilation.

- Position the head of the bed upright, as far as it will go.
- Position the bedside table across the bed and place a pillow or two on top.
- Assist the patient to lean forward across the table with arms on or beside the pillows.
- Support the person's low back with a pillow.

Orthopneic Position

The **orthopneic position** (Figure 39-23C) may be used as an alternative to the high Fowler's position. *Orthopnea* means "needing to sit up to breathe comfortably." The patient sits as upright as possible with the forearms and feet supported. They may lean slightly forward, supporting themselves with the forearms, if desired. This position makes the thorax larger on inspiration, enabling the patient to inhale more air. The person may also stand or sit and push the hands against the wall, back of a chair, or sturdy piece of furniture (Figure 39-23D). The person may also stand with the back against the wall for support upon inhalation (Figure 39-23E).

Another alternative to improve ventilation is to seat the patient on the side of the bed, with the bed in the lowest horizontal position. Support the patient's legs on the floor or a stool. Assist the patient to lean across an overbed table, if desired, for additional support.

OTHER TECHNIQUES

Incentive Spirometer

An **incentive spirometer** (Figure 39-24) may be ordered to help the lungs expand fully. This prevents atelectasis (collapse of the alveoli) and also helps prevent pneumonia.

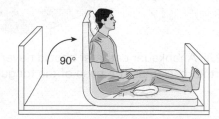

FIGURE 39-23A A patient in the high Fowler's position.

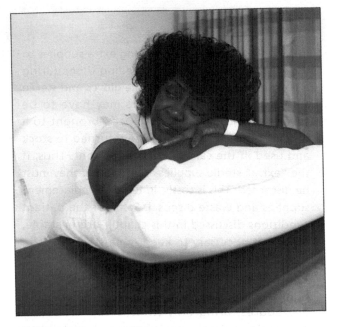

FIGURE 39-23B A patient in the tripod position.

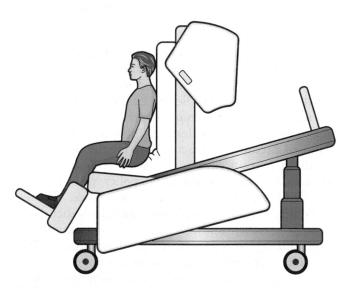

FIGURE 39-23C A patient in the orthopneic position is fully upright with arms and feet supported. Providing arm and foot support helps relax the abdominal muscles, enabling the person to breathe more deeply. Special orthopneic beds are available for optimal positioning.

The patient may use the incentive spirometer in bed, with head and shoulders well supported. Monitor the patient the first few times to ensure that they do it correctly.

- The RCP or nurse will instruct the patient on how to use the incentive spirometer.
- The patient exhales normally and then, with the lips placed tightly around the mouthpiece, inhales

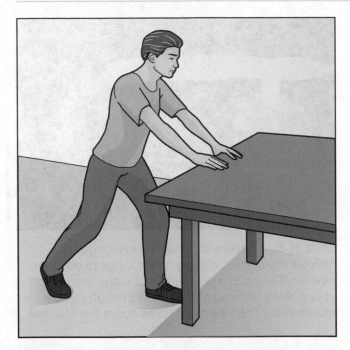

FIGURE 39-23D Push against the wall or heavy furniture.

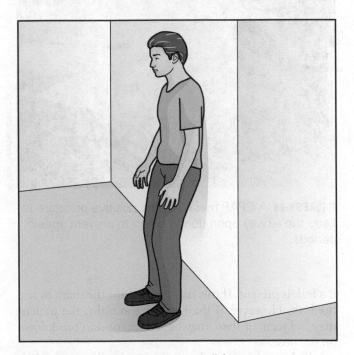

FIGURE 39-23E Lean against the wall for support.

through the mouth strongly, enough to raise the balls in the chambers.

- Encourage the patient to keep the balls suspended by holding the deep breath as long as possible.

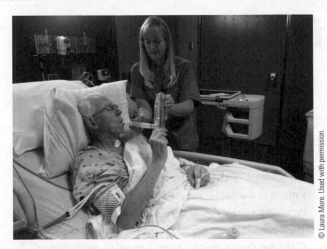

FIGURE 39-24 An incentive spirometer is a device used to improve oxygenation. Inhaling through the attached tube causes the ball inside the plastic chamber to rise.

- The patient then removes the mouthpiece and exhales normally.
- The exercise is repeated as many times as is ordered. The following are nursing assistant responsibilities:
- Remind the patient to use the device according to care plan instructions. For example, a postoperative patient may be instructed to use the spirometer 10 times every hour. The RCP will develop this plan of care and set the slide bar to a level on the side of the instrument. The slide bar represents the patient's inhalation goal.
- Observe the patient for correctness of procedure.
- Advise the patient not to take in too many deep breaths in a row, as this will cause dizziness.
- Be sure the patient does not become overly fatigued.
- Encourage the patient to cough and clear the respiratory passages.
- Report to the nurse if the patient seems overly fatigued during the procedure.
- Carefully observe and report any unusual responses, such as pain, dizziness, or throat and airway irritation.
- When the patient has completed the pulmonary exercise, wash the spirometer mouthpiece in warm water, dry it, replace it in the plastic bag, and leave it at the bedside.
- Provide mouth care as needed or desired.
- Praise patients for their efforts. Many times this encourages greater effort the next time the incentive spirometer is used.

The incentive spirometer is usually left at the bedside. The patient will be prompted to use it throughout the day. They are instructed to take slow, deep breaths using the spirometer, as ordered. If the patient becomes dizzy or complains of tingling in the fingers, they may be breathing too fast. Have the patient relax and breathe normally until the sensation passes. Monitor the patient's breathing before and after the treatment. Report your observations to the nurse. Please note that the bottom of the incentive spirometer is very slippery on the tabletop. The device is top-heavy and falls over and cracks easily. Place the device on its side on a towel or washcloth to reduce the risk of falls.

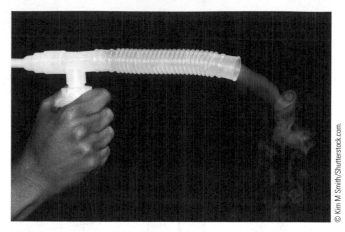

FIGURE 39-25 A handheld, small-volume nebulizer delivers medication directly to the lungs to open the airways. The liquid medication in the cup produces steam that is inhaled and exhaled through the mouthpiece. The treatment takes about five minutes.

Aerosol Therapy

Nebulizers deliver moisture or medication deep into the lungs. Small-volume nebulizers (Figure 39-25) turn liquid medicine into a mist that can be inhaled. Drugs are ordered to dilate the bronchi and open up obstructed airways for patients with COPD and asthma. The nebulizer may be powered by oxygen or compressed air. Encourage the patient to cough after the treatment is given.

Continuous Positive Airway Pressure (CPAP)

Some patients stop breathing periodically while they sleep. This condition is called *sleep apnea*. It is commonly caused by a blockage or obstruction in the patient's airway that occurs when the muscles relax. Patients with sleep apnea may stop breathing hundreds of times a night, and they snore loudly when they start to breathe again. This interrupts their sleep, and they are often very tired during the day. Treatment uses a device that delivers pressure to the airway while the patient sleeps; this pressure holds the airway open.

The device is called **CPAP** (pronounced SEE-pap) which stands for **continuous positive airway pressure** (Figure 39-26). A mask is placed on the patient's face and held in place with a head strap. Large-diameter corrugated tubing connects the mask to a device (sometimes called a blower) that creates low levels of pressure. The mask must fit tightly against the face.

Many patients will put on their own masks at bedtime. Remind them to wash and dry the face so that less skin oil will get on the mask. Monitor the patient while they are connected to a CPAP machine. Make sure the mask is comfortable. Air will blow into the patient's eyes

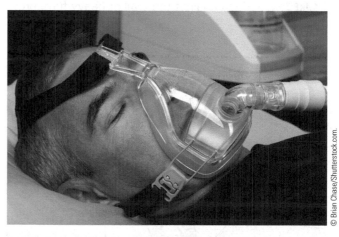

FIGURE 39-26 A CPAP mask applies positive pressure to keep the airway open during sleep to prevent apneic periods.

if a leak is present. If this happens, adjust the mask to seal the leak. However, if the mask is too tight, the patient may feel pain, or there may be redness or skin breakdown on the nose.

If the patient complains of excessive dryness in their nasal passages, a humidifier can be added to the CPAP system. The nurse may also get an order for saline spray or nose drops to reduce the irritation. If a patient swallows a lot of air from the mask, belches frequently, and feels pressure in the abdomen, elevate the head of the bed.

Wash the mask with soap and water each morning, after the patient takes it off. Store the dry mask in a clean plastic bag until use at bedtime.

Bilevel Positive Airway Pressure (BIPAP)

Bilevel positive airway pressure (BiPAP) is another treatment for sleep apnea that is similar to CPAP. The BiPAP has two airway settings, whereas the CPAP only has one. Exhalation pressure is lower with a BiPAP than it is with the CPAP, making it easier for the person to exhale air and breathe more comfortably. It is used for people with congestive heart failure and those who need some form of breathing assistance.

COLLECTING A SPUTUM SPECIMEN

Sputum is matter that is brought up (**expectorated**) from the lungs. A culture of the specimen identifies the cause of an infection. Make sure that the specimen comes from the lungs and is not saliva from the mouth.

If the patient cannot expectorate sputum, suctioning may be needed to obtain the specimen. (The nurse performs this procedure.) It is easier to collect the specimen when the patient wakes up in the morning and after they take two or three deep breaths.

EXPAND YOUR SKILLS

PROCEDURE 86   COLLECTING A SPUTUM SPECIMEN

1. Carry out initial procedure actions.

2. Assemble equipment:
   - Disposable gloves
   - Mask, eye protection, gown if spraying of sputum is likely
   - Sterile container and cover for specimen
   - Glass of water
   - Label, including:
     – Patient's full name
     – Room number
     – Patient number
     – Date and time of collection
     – Physician's name
     – Examination to be done
     – Other information as requested
   - Tissues
   - Emesis basin
   - Biohazard specimen transport bag
   - Laboratory requisition

3. Wash your hands and put on disposable gloves.

4. Ask the patient to rinse their mouth with water and spit into the emesis basin.

5. Ask the patient to breathe deeply and then cough deeply to bring up sputum. The patient spits the sputum into the container.

   a. While coughing, have the patient cover their mouth with a tissue to prevent the spread of infection.

   b. Collect one to two tablespoons of sputum unless otherwise ordered.

   c. Do not contaminate the outside of the container.

   d. Avoid touching the inside of the container or lid. Instruct the patient not to touch the inside of the container or lid.

6. Remove your gloves and discard them according to facility policy.

7. Wash your hands.

8. Cover the specimen container tightly and attach a completed label.

9. Place the specimen container in a biohazard transport bag and attach a laboratory requisition.

10. Carry out ending procedure actions.

11. Follow facility policy for transporting specimens to the laboratory.

ICON KEY:

 = OBRA   **P** = PPE

REVIEW

A. True/False

Mark the following true or false by circling T or F.

1. T F In asthma, there is increased production of mucus, which blocks the respiratory tract.
2. T F Drugs to reduce fever also fight infection.
3. T F An allergen causes a sensitivity reaction.
4. T F URI stands for underrated respiratory incentive.
5. T F Use of the incentive spirometer can help prevent pneumonia.
6. T F Always post a sign when oxygen is in use.
7. T F The oxygen flow rate is ordered by the physician.
8. T F Immobility is a risk factor for hypoxemia.
9. T F When oxygen is administered by mask, make sure the straps are very tight.
10. T F In the high Fowler's position, the patient leans forward across the overbed table.

B. Matching

Choose the correct word from Column II to match each phrase or statement in Column I.

Column I

11. _____ inflammation of the lungs
12. _____ an example of COLD
13. _____ difficult breathing
14. _____ cough up
15. _____ material brought up from lungs

Column II

a. emphyscma
b. sputum
c. pneumonia
d. dyspnea
e. spirometer
f. expectorate

C. Multiple Choice

Select the best answer for each of the following.

16. Patients with respiratory disease should:
    a. cover the nose and mouth when coughing.
    b. turn the face toward others when sneezing.
    c. wash their hands only after toileting.
    d. carry a plastic bag to dispose of soiled tissues.

17. When an oxygen tank is in use:
    a. store empty tanks in the patient's room.
    b. attach the tank to the patient's bed.
    c. inform the nurse when the tank is empty.
    d. chain the tank to a carrier or secure it in a base.

18. Nursing care for a male patient who is using oxygen includes:
    a. keeping the head of the bed elevated 10°.
    b. shaving the patient with an electric razor.
    c. covering the patient with a wool blanket.
    d. providing frequent mouth care.

19. When your patient is receiving oxygen, you should:
    a. monitor intake and output.
    b. know the ordered rate.
    c. check the flow rate once each shift.
    d. check the flow rate every three hours.

20. When administering oxygen by mask, in addition to routine care and precautions, you should:
    a. pull the straps until they are very tight.
    b. provide emotional support and reassurance.
    c. make sure the mask covers only the mouth.
    d. remove the mask for bathing and meals.

21. Aging changes to the respiratory system include all of the following *except*:
    a. loss of elasticity in the lungs.
    b. decreased ability to inflate lungs.
    c. increased risk of hypoxia.
    d. increased size of the trachea.

22. Capillary refill is used to evaluate:
    a. how much oxygen is in the venous blood.
    b. how well oxygen is getting to body tissues.
    c. cyanosis and changes in color.
    d. the strength of the pulse.

23. Normal capillary refill is:
    a. 2 to 3 seconds.
    b. 3 to 6 seconds.
    c. 5 to 10 seconds.
    d. 15 to 20 seconds.

24. The pulse oximeter measures:
    a. how much oxygen is in the venous blood.
    b. saturation of hemoglobin with oxygen.
    c. the amount of blood in the fingertip.
    d. the pulse and level of oxygen in the lungs.

25. Which of the following pulse oximeter values suggests that the patient is becoming hypoxemic?
    a. 96 percent
    b. 98 percent
    c. 90 percent
    d. 89 percent

26. An asthma attack is usually triggered by:
    a. the patient's pillow.
    b. an allergen.
    c. cold.
    d. heat.

27. Chronic obstructive pulmonary disease (COPD) is caused by:
    a. prolonged inflammation in the bronchi.
    b. narrowing and clogging of the bronchi.
    c. loss of elasticity of the alveoli.
    d. normal aging changes in the trachea.

28. The most common sign of hypoxemia in a patient with emphysema is:
    a. pain.
    b. nausea.
    c. moist cough.
    d. headache.

29. The external skin opening for the tracheostomy is the:
    a. ventilator.
    b. stoma.
    c. cannula.
    d. flange.

30. The primary purpose of the Passy Muir valve is to:
    a. enable the person to speak.
    b. reduce the risk of dyspnea.
    c. keep foreign bodies out of the trachea.
    d. prevent uncontrolled coughing.

31. A change in mental status in a person with a tracheostomy suggests that:
    a. something is wrong with the tube.
    b. the patient needs suctioning.
    c. the patient is not getting enough oxygen.
    d. the patient is having shortness of breath.

32. A patient with a laryngectomy can:
    a. smell.
    b. swallow.
    c. suck on a straw.
    d. blow their nose.

33. Pleural effusion is:
    a. a treatment for cancer.
    b. a complication of a laryngectomy.
    c. a collection of fluid around the lungs.
    d. part of the chest tube water suction.

34. Which of the following is true about oxygen humidifiers?
    a. Oxygen from a concentrator should pass through a humidifier.
    b. Fill the humidifier bottle with normal saline.
    c. Persons with COPD need humidified oxygen.
    d. Oxygen may be given without humidification.

35. Your patient has removed their oral airway and handed it to you with a smile. After this, they went back to sleep. Your first action should be to:
    a. run and find the nurse.
    b. check the patient's blood pressure.
    c. put the airway back in.
    d. check the pulse oximeter.

36. The nasal airway:
    a. may be used for conscious patients.
    b. is needed when a ventilator is used.
    c. is molded from hard plastic.
    d. is used during anticoagulant therapy.

37. A mechanical ventilator is used with a:
    a. CPAP device.
    b. endotracheal tube.
    c. nasopharyngeal airway.
    d. refillable humidifier.

38. Make sure your patient who is mechanically ventilated:
    a. is restrained if they may try to pull the tube out.
    b. has condensation in the tubing at all times.
    c. has a means of communicating their needs.
    d. wears heel protectors at all times to relieve pressure.

39. Which of these positions will enable the patient to inhale the most air?
    a. Fowler's position
    b. orthopneic position
    c. supine position
    d. semiprone position

40. The Yankauer catheter is a(n):
    a. nasal airway.
    b. three-way urinary catheter.
    c. sterile endotracheal catheter.
    d. oral suction device.

41. Diagnostic techniques used for identifying respiratory problems include all of the following except:

    a. culture of secretions.

    b. X-rays.

    c. checking for edema.

    d. volume studies.

42. Mr. Lyons's pulse oximeter reading is 88 percent. The nursing assistant knows that:

    a. this value is normal.

    b. it should be documented at the end of the shift.

    c. the nurse should be notified right away.

    d. the patient's blood pressure is too low.

D. Nursing Assistant Challenge

Mrs. Harvey has had asthma all her life. She is sensitive to many allergens. She is admitted to your facility for emphysema. She is receiving respiratory assistance with an oxygen concentrator. Complete the following questions related to her care.

43. The flow rate of the concentrator is usually _____.

(10 L/min) (2 L/min)

44. Smoking in the same room as oxygen _____ permitted.

(is) (is not)

45. The flow of oxygen on a concentrator _____ be changed by the nursing assistant.

(may) (may not)

46. The concentrator should be placed at least _____ from a heat source.

(two feet) (five feet)

47. The concentrator filter should be cleaned _____.

(monthly) (weekly)

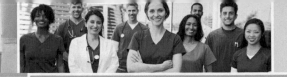

Circulatory (Cardiovascular) System

OBJECTIVES

After completing this chapter, you will be able to:

40.1 Spell and define terms.

40.2 Review the location of the organs of the circulatory system.

40.3 Describe the functions of the organs of the circulatory system.

40.4 Describe some common disorders of the circulatory system.

40.5 Describe nursing assistant actions related to care of patients with disorders of the circulatory system.

40.6 List five specific diagnostic tests for disorders of the circulatory system.

40.7 State the purpose of the pacemaker and implantable cardioverter defibrillator.

VOCABULARY

Learn the meaning and the correct spelling of the following words and phrases:

anemia
angina pectoris
arteries
ascites
atheroma
atherosclerosis
atrium
capillaries
cardiac cycle
cardiac decompensation
compensate
congestive heart failure
    (CHF)

coronary embolism
coronary occlusion
coronary thrombosis
diuresis
dyscrasia
embolus
endocardium
erythrocyte
heart block
hypertrophy
implantable cardioverter
    defibrillator (ICD)
infarction

ischemic
leukemia
leukocyte
lymph
lymphatic vessel
myocardial infarction (MI)
myocardium
orthopnea
pacemaker
pericardium
peripheral
phlebitis

plasma
stent
thrombocyte
thrombus
transient ischemic attack
    (TIA)
varicose vein
vein
ventricle

INTRODUCTION

The circulatory system is a transportation system that carries nourishment and oxygen to the cells and removes waste products. The force of the heartbeat keeps this closed system in motion. Diseases that attack any part of the system interfere with overall body function. Long-standing diseases of the cardiovascular system eventually affect the pulmonary system as well.

STRUCTURE AND FUNCTION

The organs of the cardiovascular system include:

1. Heart—a central pumping station.
2. Blood vessels
   a. **Arteries**—tubes that carry blood away from the heart. They:
      - Have muscular, elastic walls with smooth linings.
      - Branch to form arterioles with thinner walls. Arterioles then become capillaries.
      - Carry blood with a high concentration of nutrients and oxygen to the body cells.
   b. **Veins**—tubes that carry blood toward the heart. They:
      - Have thinner muscular walls.
      - Carry blood back to the heart.
      - Carry blood with a lower concentration of oxygen, more carbon dioxide, and more waste products.
      - Have cuplike valves that help move the blood.
   c. **Capillaries**—tubes that connect arteries and veins. They:
      - Have walls only one cell thick.
      - Are the site of exchange of nutrients and oxygen from the blood to the cells, and carbon dioxide and waste products from the cells to the blood.
3. **Lymphatic vessels**—tubes that carry lymph or tissue fluid to the bloodstream. Fluid from the bloodstream passes into the tissue spaces, where it is called *tissue fluid*. Some of the tissue fluid returns to the bloodstream by way of the capillaries. Some of it is first drawn off into the lymphatic vessels, where it is called **lymph**. Eventually the lymph returns to general circulation and becomes part of the blood.
4. Lymph nodes—masses of lymphatic tissue along the pathway of the lymph. They filter the lymph.
5. Spleen—a lymphatic organ. The spleen produces some of the blood cells and helps destroy worn-out blood cells. It acts as a blood reservoir or blood bank.
6. Blood—a connective tissue made up of a liquid (plasma) and cellular elements.

The Blood

Blood is a red body fluid composed of plasma and cellular elements. The body contains four to six quarts (liters) of blood. Fifty-five percent of the blood is formed of the liquid plasma. **Plasma** is a watery solution containing:

- Antibodies (gamma globulin)—chemicals to fight infection
- Nutrients—such as glucose, amino acids, fats, salts
- Gases—such as oxygen and carbon dioxide
- Waste products—such as urea and creatinine

The blood cells are produced in the bone marrow and lymphatic tissues of the body. The bone marrow, liver, and spleen destroy worn-out blood cells. The blood cells include red blood cells, white blood cells, and thrombocytes.

- Red blood cells (RBCs)—**erythrocytes**—carry most of the oxygen and small amounts of carbon dioxide. There are 4.5 to 5 million RBC per cubic millimeter (mm^3).
- White blood cells (WBCs)—**leukocytes**—fight infection. There are 7,000 to 8,000 WBCs/mm^3.

Thrombocytes (or platelets)—are not whole cells but only parts of cells. They seal small leaks in the walls of blood vessels and initiate blood clotting. There are 200,000 to 400,000 thrombocytes/mm^3.

The Heart

The heart is a hollow, muscular organ about the size of a fist (Figure 40-1). It is divided into a right and left side by a muscular wall called the *septum* and into four chambers. There are three layers in the heart wall. The **endocardium** lines the heart chambers. The **myocardium** is the muscle layer. The **pericardium** is a membranous outer covering.

The four chambers are:

- The right **atrium** (RA) (right upper heart chamber) receives blood from all over the body. This blood has a low oxygen content and a relatively high carbon dioxide level. It is called *deoxygenated blood*.

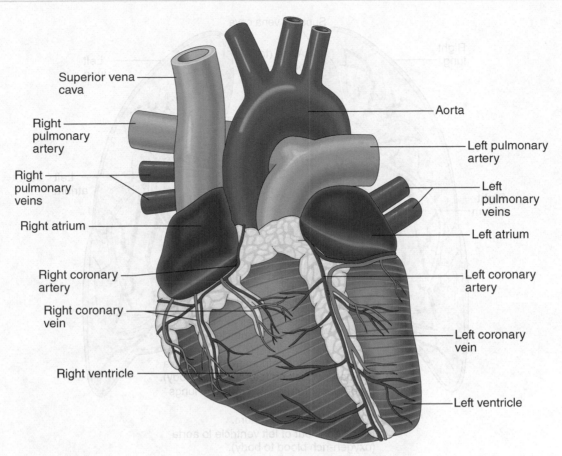

Superior vena cava

Right pulmonary artery

Right pulmonary veins

Right atrium

Right coronary artery

Right coronary vein

Right ventricle

Aorta

Left pulmonary artery

Left pulmonary veins

Left atrium

Left coronary artery

Left coronary vein

Left ventricle

FIGURE 40-1 The heart.

- The right **ventricle** (RV) (right lower heart chamber) receives blood from the right atrium and sends it out to the lungs through the pulmonary artery to pick up oxygen and deliver carbon dioxide for excretion.
- The left atrium (LA) (left upper heart chamber) receives oxygenated blood from the lungs and sends it to the left ventricle.
- The left ventricle (LV) (left lower heart chamber) receives blood from the left atrium and sends it out through the aorta to the entire body.

Valves separate the chambers. They also guard the exit of the pulmonary artery and aorta to prevent backflow and maintain a constant forward motion. The pulmonary artery carries blood to the lungs. The aorta is the largest blood vessel in the body. The valves are located as follows:

- Tricuspid valve—between right atrium and right ventricle
- Bicuspid (mitral) valve—between left atrium and left ventricle
- Pulmonary semilunar valves—between right ventricle and pulmonary artery
- Aortic semilunar valve—between left ventricle and aorta

Nerve impulses make the heart contract regularly according to body needs. For example, when you run, your body cells need more oxygen. The cells signal the brain that they need more oxygen. The brain sends a signal to the heart through the nerves, telling it to supply more blood. These nerve impulses cause the heart to beat faster. Thus, more oxygenated blood is pumped to the body cells to supply the oxygen required. These impulses cause the heart to beat faster.

The Cardiac Cycle

The heart pumps blood through the body by a series of movements known as the **cardiac cycle**. First, the upper chambers of the heart, the *atria*, relax and fill with blood as the lower chambers contract, forcing blood out of the heart through the aorta and pulmonary arteries. Next, the lower chambers relax, allowing blood to flow into them from the contracting upper chambers. Then the cycle is repeated (Figure 40-2). Each cycle lasts about 0.8 second. This happens about 70 to 80 times per minute.

The pulse you feel at the radial artery corresponds to ventricular contraction. The sounds you hear when listening to the heart and taking a blood pressure are the sounds made by valves closing during the cardiac cycle.

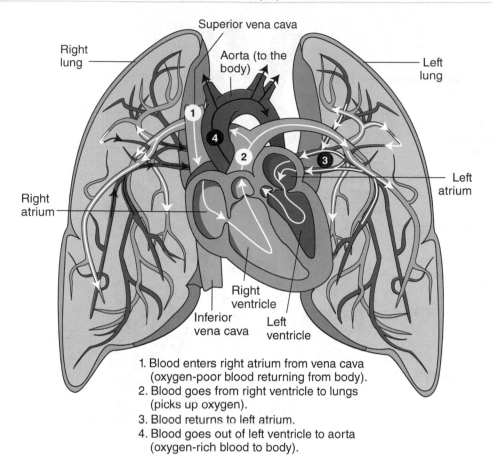

1. Blood enters right atrium from vena cava (oxygen-poor blood returning from body).
2. Blood goes from right ventricle to lungs (picks up oxygen).
3. Blood returns to left atrium.
4. Blood goes out of left ventricle to aorta (oxygen-rich blood to body).

FIGURE 40-2 Blood flows from the heart to the lungs, to the body, and back to the heart to begin the cycle again.

The rate and rhythm of the cardiac cycle are regulated by the conduction system. The conduction system is made up of special neuromuscular tissue that sends out impulses. The impulses eventually reach the myocardial cells, which respond by contracting.

- The impulses begin at the sinoatrial (SA) node in the right atrium and spread across the two atria. All heart tissue can act as a pacemaker. However, the SA node is the natural pacemaker of the heart. The patient experiences problems if other areas are pacing. The atria contract.
- Impulses from the SA node reach the atrioventricular (AV) node in the right atrium.
- Messages from the AV node then spread through the bundle of His in the septum. From there they go through the Purkinje fibers to the walls of the ventricles.
- The ventricles contract, forcing the blood forward.

An *electrocardiogram*, called an ECG or an EKG, is a test that traces the electrical impulses of the heart. Heart disease may be detected with this test.

Blood Vessels

Many large arteries and veins take their names from the bones they are near or from the part of the body they serve. For example, the femoral artery and vein run close to the femur (thigh bone). The subclavian arteries and veins are found under the clavicle. The axillary arteries and veins are found in the axillary (armpit) area. Figure 40-3 shows the arterial system that distributes blood from the heart. Figure 40-4 shows the venous system that returns blood to the heart.

Aging Changes to the Cardiovascular System

Aging changes to the cardiovascular system can be very serious and often affect other vital organs and systems. Common aging changes are:

- The heart rate slows, causing a slower pulse and less efficient circulation.
- Blood vessels lose elasticity and develop calcium deposits, resulting in stiffening and narrowing.
- Blood pressure increases because of stiffening and other changes to the walls of the blood vessels. This change alone increases the risk of heart attack, stroke, and other serious conditions.

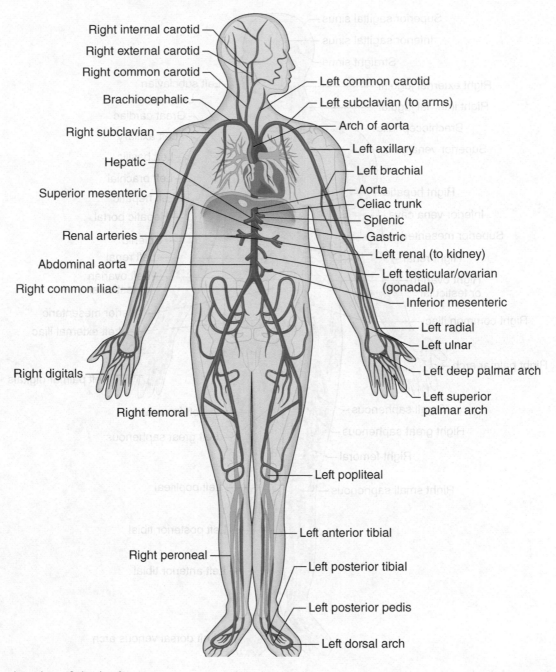

Right internal carotid
Right external carotid
Right common carotid
Brachiocephalic
Right subclavian
Hepatic
Superior mesenteric
Renal arteries
Abdominal aorta
Right common iliac

Right digitals

Right femoral

Right peroneal

Left common carotid
Left subclavian (to arms)
Arch of aorta
Left axillary
Left brachial
Aorta
Celiac trunk
Splenic
Gastric
Left renal (to kidney)
Left testicular/ovarian (gonadal)
Inferior mesenteric
Left radial
Left ulnar
Left deep palmar arch
Left superior palmar arch

Left popliteal

Left anterior tibial

Left posterior tibial

Left posterior pedis

Left dorsal arch

FIGURE 40-3 Arteries of the body.

- It takes longer for the heart rate to return to normal after exercise.
- Veins become enlarged, causing the blood vessels near the surface of the skin to become more prominent.
- Heart muscle becomes stiffer and heart walls become thicker. The amount of blood the chambers can hold is decreased and pumping is less efficient.
- Changes in the heart cause blood pressure and pulse to take longer to return to normal after stress.

- Heart rate slows slightly due to a loss of pacemaker cells.
- Fat deposits and fibrous tissue may interfere with the electrical pathways, causing abnormal (and potentially serious) heart rhythms.
- Changes in blood vessels may reduce blood flow to vital organs such as the kidneys by as much as 50 percent, and to the brain by 15 to 20 percent.
- The incidence of heart murmurs increases because heart valves become less flexible and calcium deposits build up in them.

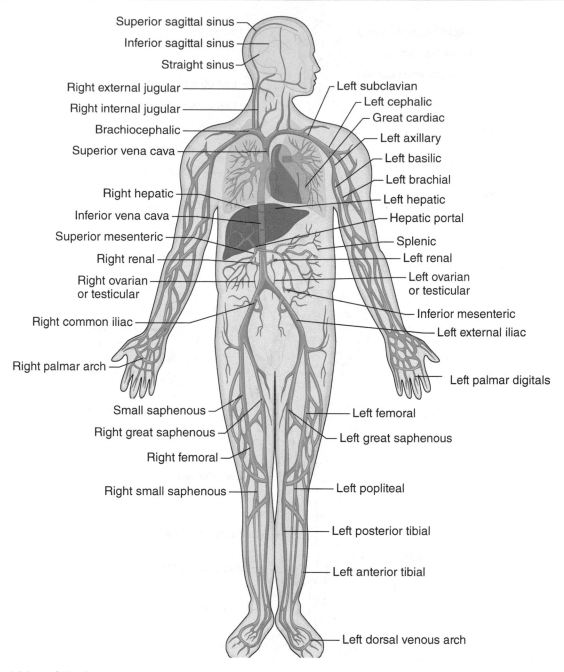

FIGURE 40-4 Veins of the body.

COMMON CIRCULATORY SYSTEM DISORDERS

Common disorders of the circulatory system include:
- Diseases relating to the blood vessels.
- Diseases of the heart.
- Blood **dyscrasias** (abnormalities); these conditions may involve the bone, bone marrow, liver, or spleen.

Observations to make and report for patients with disorders of the circulatory system are listed in Table 40-1.

PERIPHERAL VASCULAR DISEASES

The blood vessels that serve the outer parts of the body, particularly those of the hands and feet, are referred to as **peripheral** (toward the outer part) blood vessels. Diseases of these vessels affect the parts of the body through which they pass. The health of these vessels also influences heart function.

Peripheral vascular diseases that affect the arteries diminish the flow of blood to the extremities. Tissues through which the narrowed arteries pass may not get the oxygen and nutrients that provide the nourishment

TABLE 40-1 Signs and Symptoms of Cardiopulmonary Disorders That Should Be Reported to the Nurse Immediately

- Abnormal pulse below 60 or above 100
- Pulse irregular, weak, bounding, or other marked change in pulse rate or rhythm
- Blood pressure below 100/60 or above 140/90 or marked change from previous value
- Unable to hear blood pressure or palpate pulse
- Pain over center, left, or right chest
- Chest pain that radiates to shoulder, neck, jaw, or arm
- Shortness of breath (dyspnea) or other unusual respiratory problem
- Headache, dizziness, weakness, paralysis, vomiting
- Cold, blue, or gray appearance
- Cold, blue, numb, painful feet or hands
- Coughing (dry or moist/productive)
- Retractions (the muscles and skin pull inward under and between the ribs)
- Edema
- Disorientation or other change in mental status
- Blue color of lips, nail beds, or mucous membranes
- Feeling faint or lightheaded, losing consciousness
- Capillary refill greater than three seconds
- Pulse oximeter value less than 95 (or less than 90, depending on facility policy; a progressive decrease in pulse oximeter value suggests a deterioration in condition)

Also review respiratory signs and symptoms. These systems are closely related and may be symptomatic at the same time.

⊕ Clinical Information **ALERT**

Patients with some types of heart disease will have a fever. This is usually an inflammatory response to heart cell damage after conditions such as a heart attack or acute infection of the heart. Monitor the temperature closely and inform the nurse of abnormalities.

---

they need. Areas affected are the extremities: the arms, legs, and brain. The signs and symptoms associated with decreased peripheral circulation are:

- Burning pain during exercise
- Hair loss over feet and toes
- Thick and rigid toenails
- Dusky red skin or cyanotic brownish skin
- Dry and scaly or shiny skin
- Chronic edema of the feet and legs
- Cool skin temperature of feet and legs
- Difficulty with ambulation

When the arteries are affected, the blood flow may be seriously interrupted. This condition requires immediate medical treatment. These sores are caused by poor blood circulation in the legs. These ulcers are difficult to treat and may take months or even years to heal.

Treatment is aimed at increasing local circulation and preventing injuries that may heal poorly.

- Positioning and specific prescribed exercises are done to promote arterial flow and venous return.
- Sometimes an oscillating (rocking) bed is employed to improve the circulatory flow. The oscillating bed rocks up and down in cycles, raising the patient's feet 6 inches above the head and then lowering them 12 to 15 inches. The steady rhythm provides both passive exercise for the patient and some circulatory stimulation.
- Nothing that would further hamper the patient's circulation is permitted.

Protecting the Feet

Patients with impaired circulation are at great risk of ulceration, gangrene, and eventual amputation due to pressure or injuries to the feet and ankles. A small injury or ulcer can lead to major complications. Nursing assistant care for patients with peripheral vascular disease includes:

- Checking the feet and legs daily and reporting abnormalities to the nurse.
- Protecting the feet from injury.
- Making sure the patient is wearing footwear that fits properly when out of bed. The patient should always wear socks with shoes. They should never ambulate barefoot or when wearing only socks on the feet.
- Not cutting toenails; this is a licensed health care provider responsibility in most facilities. Some facilities will not let nursing assistants cut fingernails. Many restrict nail cutting on patients with diabetes only. There are so many variables that it is important to learn and follow your facility's policy. Do not take someone's word for it. Look it up in your policy and procedure manual. In any event, avoid using sharp objects such as a nail file. An orange (orangewood) stick is the usual substitute for a nail file for cleaning nails. Make sure bed linens are not too tight on the feet. Use a bed cradle, if ordered.
- Checking the skin under support hose regularly. Remove the hose for bathing and according to the care plan.

- Making sure footwear is not too tight; if footwear fits tightly, notify the nurse.
- For patients who are bedfast, propping their calves on pillows that are positioned lengthwise so that the heels are elevated from the surface of the bed. You may also position the patient so that the heels hang over the end of the mattress, with the soles of the feet against a footboard. Do not position the pillow widthwise under the calves. Heel protectors are helpful, but remember that they do not prevent pressure on the heels. Other devices are available to keep the heels off the surface of the bed to relieve pressure. Follow the care plan and the nurse's instructions.
- Making sure the feet are supported on footrests when the patient is using a wheelchair; avoid dragging them across the floor.

- The feet should not dangle when a patient is in a wheelchair. Positioning begins with the feet, and the feet should always be supported.

Atherosclerosis

Atherosclerosis is a common form of vascular disease. Roughened areas known as **atheromas**, which are growths developed over deposits of fatty materials, form on the inner walls of the arteries and narrow the vessels. The vessels of the heart and brain, and those leading to the legs from the body, are often affected. The atheromas gradually grow larger until they eventually block blood flow to the parts and organs served by the affected vessels (Figure 40-5). Sometimes clots that have formed over the

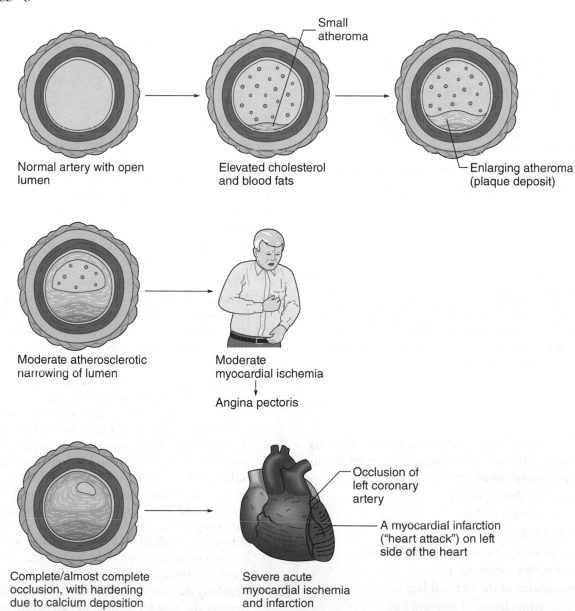

Normal artery with open lumen

Elevated cholesterol and blood fats

Small atheroma

Enlarging atheroma (plaque deposit)

Moderate atherosclerotic narrowing of lumen

Moderate myocardial ischemia

Angina pectoris

Complete/almost complete occlusion, with hardening due to calcium deposition

Severe acute myocardial ischemia and infarction

Occlusion of left coronary artery

A myocardial infarction ("heart attack") on left side of the heart

FIGURE 40-5 Cross-sections of a coronary artery showing atherosclerotic changes.

AFFECTED SITE   **COMPLICATION**

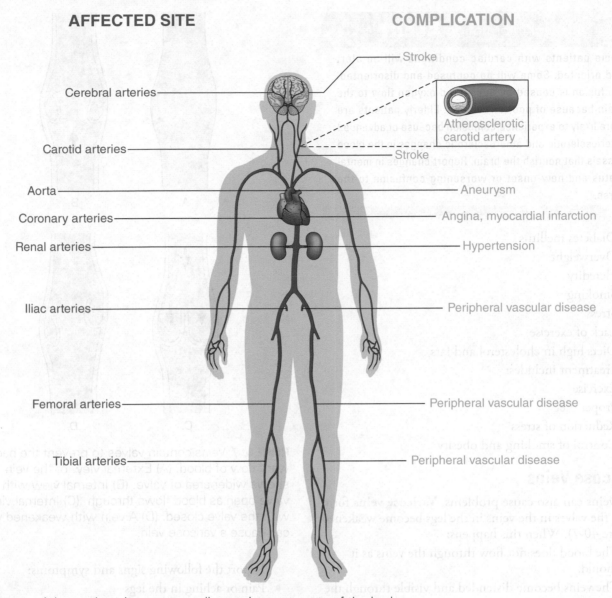

FIGURE 40-6 Atherosclerosis can cause disease in many parts of the body.

Clinical Information **ALERT**

Edema develops when the heart cannot pump blood efficiently. In right-sided heart failure, blood backs up into the peripheral veins. Extra fluid has nowhere to go, so it enters the tissues in lower parts of the body, such as the feet and ankles. It may also enter the hands, fingers, and area over the sacrum. To check for edema, gently press two fingers into the skin and release immediately. If the marks from the fingers remain, the patient has pitting edema. This is a potentially serious problem. Notify the nurse promptly.

---

irregular areas in the vessel walls break off and travel as emboli to block distant vessels.

The narrowing of vessels can lead to serious complications (Figure 40-6), such as:

- Formation of blood clots
- Angina pectoris
- Myocardial infarction (MI)
- Stroke (cerebrovascular accident [CVA]) (also known as brain attack)
- Gangrene

The exact cause of atherosclerosis is unknown, but several factors seem to increase the risk that a person will develop it. These factors include:

- Hypertension

- Diabetes mellitus
- Overweight
- Heredity
- Smoking
- Stress
- Lack of exercise
- Diets high in cholesterol and fats
  Treatment includes:
- Exercise
- Proper diet
- Reduction of stress
- Control of smoking and obesity

Varicose Veins

The veins can also cause problems. **Varicose veins** form when the valves in the veins in the legs become weakened (Figure 40-7). When this happens:

- The blood does not flow through the veins as it should.
- The veins become distended and visible through the skin.
- The veins may become inflamed (**phlebitis**).
- A blood clot may form in the vein.

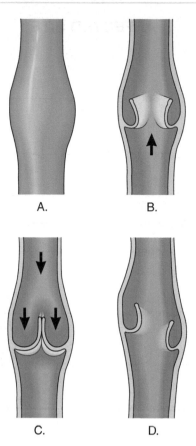

FIGURE 40-7 Veins contain valves to prevent the backward flow of blood. (A) External view of the vein shows wider area of valve. (B) Internal view with the valve open as blood flows through. (C) Internal view with the valve closed. (D) A vein with weakened valve can cause a varicose vein.

Report the following signs and symptoms:
- Pain or aching in the legs
- Signs of inflammation (warmth and redness)
  Remember that you *never* rub or massage the area of a varicose vein.

GUIDELINES 40-1 Guidelines for Caring for Patients with Peripheral Vascular Disease

- Elevate the feet when the patient will be sitting in a chair for a long time. When the feet are not elevated, make sure that the patient's feet are flat on the floor. If they are not, support the feet with a footstool. Discourage the patient from crossing the legs when sitting. Discourage the patient from using circular garters or socks with tight elastic tops.
- Discourage smoking—it interferes with circulation.

- Avoid pressure caused by elevating the knee rest of the bed.
- Avoid using heating pads or hot water bottles. The patient may not feel the heat and could be burned.
- Maintain body warmth. Make sure the patient has warm clothes, including socks that fit well. Provide blankets for the bed.

(continues)

GUIDELINES 40-1 Guidelines for Caring for Patients with Peripheral Vascular Disease (continued)

- Prevent injury to the feet:
    - Instruct the patient to wear shoes when out of bed.
    - Check to see that the shoes are in good repair and that they fit well.
    - Avoid pressure on the legs and feet from any source.
- Inspect the feet carefully when you bathe the patient or if the patient complains of any discomfort in the feet. Promptly report any signs of inflammation, injury, or circulatory problems:
    - Broken skin
    - Color change (redness, whiteness, or cyanosis)
    - Heat or coldness

- - Cracking between toes
    - Corns or calluses
    - Swelling
    - Pain
    - Loss of function
    - Drainage
- Bathe the feet regularly.
    - Dry thoroughly and gently between the toes.
    - Use a moisturizing lotion on the feet and legs if the skin is dry.
- Do not cut the toenails of patients who have peripheral vascular disease. In many facilities, nursing assistants are not permitted to clip toenails. Know and follow your facility's policies.

CARDIOVASCULAR DISORDERS

Two common cardiovascular disorders are transient ischemic attacks and hypertension.

Transient Ischemic Attack

Transient ischemic attack (TIA) is a temporary interruption of the blood flow to part of the brain (Chapter 43). The patient may experience:

- Weakness or paralysis of any extremity or the face
- Vision problems
- Difficulty with speech
- Difficulty with swallowing

These symptoms come on quickly and may last from just a few minutes to 24 hours. There are no permanent effects. However, a TIA is usually a warning that a stroke will occur at some time. If a patient has any of the symptoms listed, report them to the nurse immediately.

Hypertension

Hypertension is another name for high blood pressure. It may have no known origin, or it may follow illnesses that affect such organs as the:

- Heart
- Blood vessels
- Kidneys
- Liver

High blood pressure:

- Promotes the development of atherosclerosis, which further narrows the vessels. This increases the blood pressure even more.

- Increases stress on the heart.
- Increases the damage to blood vessel walls, so they are more apt to rupture.
- Further limits blood flow to the organs of the body.

Treatment may consist of:

- Drugs that lower the blood pressure
- A low-sodium diet
- A diet that promotes weight loss
- A regular exercise program
- Quitting smoking
- Moderation in lifestyle
- Biofeedback techniques to lower the blood pressure

Report immediately any of the signs and symptoms of hypertension:

- Flushed face
- Dizziness
- Nosebleeds
- Headaches
- Changes in speech patterns
- Blurred vision

HEART CONDITIONS

Heart disease may sometimes be due to an infection, but most heart disease develops because of changes in the blood vessels. As the openings of the blood vessels become smaller, the heart must work harder and harder to do its job of pumping blood to the body.

Clinical Information ALERT

Poor circulation is common in patients with disorders of the cardiovascular system. The poor circulation reduces blood flow to body organs and systems. Pain is a common sign of reduced blood flow, which in this case is called *ischemia*. Chest pain is caused by ischemia of the heart muscle. Pain in the legs is also common. This is caused by lack of oxygen in the leg muscles. Observe cardiovascular patients for pain. If noted, inform the nurse promptly.

TIPS

Always take complaints of chest pain seriously. If a patient complains of chest pain, assist them to stop all activity and assume a comfortable position. Notify the nurse promptly.

Angina Pectoris

Angina pectoris is known as cardiac "pain of effort." You will recall that the blood vessels nourishing the heart are the coronary arteries. These vessels are often the site of atherosclerotic changes. In an angina attack, the vessels are unable to carry enough blood to meet the heart's demand for oxygen. This may develop:

- Gradually over a period of time, as atheromas develop
- Suddenly, as the vessels constrict
  Factors that precipitate (bring on) an attack include:
- Exertion
- Heavy eating
- Emotional stress
  The signs and symptoms of angina pectoris that you should immediately report include:

- Pain when exercising or under stress. Stress causes a need for an immediate increase in coronary circulation. The pain is described as dull, with increasing intensity. It is usually centered under the breast bone (sternum), spreading to the left arm and up into the neck.
- Pale or flushed face.
- Heavy perspiration.
  Signs and symptoms may differ with individuals, but the symptoms are usually the same each time a person experiences an attack.
  Treatment of angina pectoris consists of:
- Diagnosing hidden causes. A treadmill stress test is one method of doing this.
- Teaching the patient to avoid stress and sudden exertion.
- Drugs that relax the coronary arteries.

Clinical Information ALERT

Patients with cardiac conditions may have skin color or temperature changes. Make sure you have good light when checking the skin. You will see cyanosis on the lips and mucous membranes of the mouth, as well as on the earlobes, skin, and nail beds. Caucasian patients with pallor may appear as if they have no blood. In African American, Asian, and Hispanic patients, pallor may appear as a gray color. If the patient has a circulation problem, check the arms and legs. Make sure the skin color and temperature are equal on both sides of the body. Thick toenails and little to no hair growth on the legs indicates a circulatory problem. Varicosities may also be present.

- Coronary artery bypass surgery.
- Angioplasty, a surgical procedure to open the vessels. You may assist the patient who has angina pectoris by:
- Helping the person avoid unnecessary emotional or physical stress.
- Encouraging the patient not to smoke.
- Reporting any signs or symptoms of an attack to the nurse at once.

Myocardial Infarction (Coronary Heart Attack)

The term **myocardial infarction (MI)**, or *heart attack*, refers to a period in which the heart suddenly cannot function properly. There are different kinds of heart attacks. They differ in severity and prognosis (expected outcome). Remember that the heart is muscle tissue and may become tired just as any muscle may tire. The cells of the heart require nourishment and oxygen like all other cells.

An acute myocardial infarction occurs when the coronary arteries, which nourish the heart, are blocked. Part of the heart muscle supplied by these vessels becomes **ischemic** (loses its blood supply). Unless circulation is restored quickly, the cells die (**infarction**). If too much tissue dies, the person cannot survive. Coronary heart attack is also called:

- **Coronary occlusion**—blockage of coronary arteries
- **Coronary thrombosis**—when a **thrombus** (stationary blood clot) forms at the site, blocking the blood flow
- **Coronary embolism**—when a moving clot or insoluble particle (**embolus**) moves to the heart from another part of the body and becomes lodged in the artery

Signs and Symptoms

The signs and symptoms of a heart attack include:

- Pain—may resemble severe indigestion. It is often described as "crushing" chest pain that radiates to the jaw and left arm.
- Nausea/vomiting.
- Irregular pulse and respiration.
- Perspiration (diaphoresis).
- Feelings of anxiety and weakness.
- Indications of shock, which include drop in blood pressure and pallor.
- Shortness of breath.
- Syncope (fainting).
- Restlessness.
- Cyanosis or gray skin color.

The signs and symptoms of a heart attack vary with the individual. The pain may be in the chest in some patients, and radiate to the jaw or either arm. If a patient has chest pain combined with any other signs or symptoms, they should be evaluated by a health care professional. Instruct the patient to stop all activity immediately and assume a comfortable position. Stay with the patient and call for assistance.

Immediate treatment has saved many people. The treatment is directed toward:

- Relieving the pain
- Reducing heart activity
- Altering the clotting ability of the blood
- Administering drugs to dissolve the clot

Nursing Care

During the acute stage, heart attack patients require professional care. Many hospitals provide intensive and/or cardiac care units for these patients. Nursing care supports the therapy ordered. Special attention must be given to:

- Noting signs of a recurrence and reporting immediately to the nurse
- Watching for bleeding and reporting immediately.
- Assisting with activities of daily living
- Monitoring vital signs
- Patient teaching to eliminate risk factors

Implantable Cardioverter Defibrillator (ICD)

Ventricular dysrhythmias occur in the lower chambers of the heart. The ability to pump blood is impaired when abnormal ventricular rhythms occur.

Some heart problems are very serious and cause rapid loss of consciousness and sudden death if not reversed quickly. Reversal is done by delivering an electric shock.

The **implantable cardioverter defibrillator (ICD)** is inserted under the skin on the chest. Wires extend to the heart to monitor and sense heart activity. The ICD is programmed to deliver an impulse similar to a shock when a life-threatening abnormal rhythm occurs.

Persons with ICDs know when the device delivers a shock. Sometimes they are aware of the onset of symptoms that will result in the delivery of a shock. If this occurs, have the patient stop all activity and assume a comfortable position. Remain with the patient and use the call signal to summon help. Inform the nurse of what the patient was doing before the shock was delivered, any signs and symptoms, and the patient's response to the shock.

If you are touching the patient when a shock is delivered, you will notice tension and muscular rigidity in the upper arms and chest. The shock will not harm you.

Congestive Heart Failure (CHF)

The heart, like any other muscle, will enlarge and tire if it has to work against increasing pressure. The heart must pump harder to maintain the internal flow of blood (circulation) when blood vessels narrowed by atherosclerosis increase the resistance to blood flow, and when there is severe damage to major organs like the liver and spleen. Under these conditions, the heart does not pump well enough to meet the body's demands for oxygen. The heart muscle may also have been damaged and weakened by myocardial infarction. Other common causes of heart failure are heredity, long-term high blood pressure, alcohol abuse, and viral infection.

At first, the heart enlarges (**hypertrophy**) to make up (**compensates**) for the additional workload. Eventually, however, it reaches a point when it can no longer compensate. Heart failure follows.

This form of heart disease is known as **congestive heart failure (CHF)** or **cardiac decompensation**. The condition got its name because of *failure* of the *heart* to pump efficiently, which results in *congestion* of the lungs. The heart tries to compensate for the problem, but this worsens the condition.

Signs and Symptoms

The signs and symptoms are the result of the heart being unable to pump the blood with sufficient force:

- Hemoptysis (spitting up blood)
- Cough
- Dyspnea (difficulty breathing)
- **Orthopnea** (difficulty in breathing unless sitting upright)
- **Ascites** (fluid collecting in the abdomen)
- Neck vein swelling
- Fatiguing easily

- Hypoxia (hypoxemia; inadequate oxygen levels)
- Confusion
- Edema (swelling), which develops in dependent tissues and slows blood flow, congesting the vessels and allowing more fluid to enter the body spaces and tissues; is most common in the abdomen, ankles, and fingers
- Waking up at night with breathlessness
- Being unable to lie flat at night
- Fluid accumulation in the lungs
- Cyanosis, which occurs because fluid in the lungs makes gas exchange less efficient
- Irregular and rapid pulse
- High blood pressure
- Palpitations (galloping heartbeat)
- Kidney malfunction in later stages
- Liver malfunction

Treatment

Treatment involves:

- Drugs to help the heart beat more strongly and regularly and to increase the output of fluids (**diuresis**) by the kidneys.
- Minimally invasive procedures that may be done to open the arteries. These involve inserting a long tube into an artery in the groin. The tube is threaded through the system to the heart. A balloon on the tube is inflated to open blocked arteries (Figure 40-8A). The balloon-tipped catheter is removed and replaced with a **stent** (Figure 40-8B), a device that keeps the arteries open. This procedure pushes the fatty deposits back against the artery walls, making more room for blood to flow through and preventing heart attack.
- A low-sodium diet.
- Restriction of fluids, if ordered.
- Weighing the patient daily to monitor level of fluid retention.
- Monitoring the apical pulse and observing for pulse deficit (Chapter 20).
- Positioning the patient in orthopneic position or high Fowler's position supported by pillows, or supported in a chair. The position must be changed frequently, but move the patient slowly. Keep the weight of the bedding off the toes.
- Applying elasticized stockings or *TED hose* (Chapter 29). TED hose are elastic anti-embolism stockings. TED hose and Ace bandages help channel blood to the deeper vessels. Remove and reapply the hose as specified on the care plan. Check the extremities carefully for adequate circulation. The skin should be normal color and warm.
- Assisting with activities of daily living as needed.

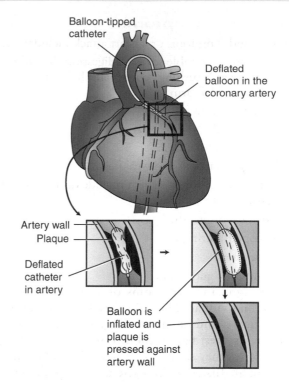

FIGURE 40-8A A balloon presses the plaque against the walls of the artery, making the vessel larger.

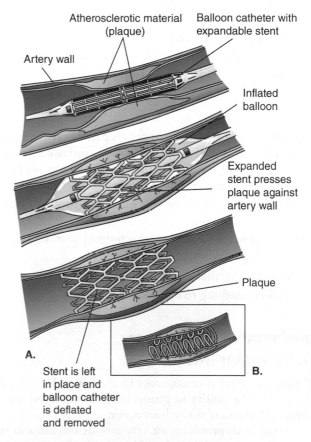

FIGURE 40-8B A stent is left in place to keep the artery open, and the balloon is removed.

- Attending to general hygiene. Complete bathing is tiring, but partial baths can stimulate circulation and provide comfort. Special attention must be given to the skin because the combination of position, edema, and poor circulation contributes to tissue breakdown. Allow the patient to be as independent with bathing as possible, unless you are instructed otherwise. Bathing is not normally a strenuous activity, but the patient with CHF may tire easily. Check the patient frequently while they are is bathing. Be prepared to take over and complete the bath if the patient becomes short of breath or too tired.

- Assisting with oxygen therapy. Oxygen therapy may be provided either by face mask or by nasal cannula. Because cardiac patients often breathe through the mouth, the mouth tends to be very dry. Special mouth care may be needed.

- Providing for elimination. A bedside commode is convenient. The use of a commode is less tiring for the patient than using a bedpan for elimination.

- Encouraging adequate nutrition. Small, easily digested meals should be provided. You may need to assist in feeding the patient to prevent fatigue.

- Monitoring and recording fluid intake. Patients with acute heart failure may be given drugs that increase the output of urine and alter the heart rate. Measuring the intake and output and taking daily weights are ways of determining if fluid is being retained. The patient may be on fluid restrictions (Chapter 26) in the acute phase of the illness.

- Regularly checking vital signs. Sometimes the heart contraction, which propels the blood forward into the blood vessels, is not forceful enough to make the vessels expand.

- Keeping the feet elevated when the patient is up in a chair or wheelchair.

- Encouraging regular rest periods throughout the day.

- Assisting with exercise, as specified on the care plan.

🔒 Safety **ALERT**

Keep magnets and devices containing magnets at least 12 inches away from a pacemaker or ICD. Telephones contain magnets. Advise the patient to hold the telephone in the hand opposite where the device is implanted.

Keep it away from the implant. Defibrillators are safe with some magnets, but pacemakers are not. If the patient complains of dizziness in the presence of a magnetic (or potentially magnetic) device, remove it or the patient from the area.

Heart Block

Heart block is a condition that develops due to interference in the electrical current through the heart. (The flow of electrical current through the heart muscle makes the normal cardiac cycle possible.)

An electronic device called a **pacemaker** (Figure 40-9) is implanted under the chest muscles or in the abdomen. An electrode carries electrical current from the pacemaker directly into the heart muscle to replace the lost natural control. The electrical current signals the heart to contract. Some pacemakers send messages only if normal messages carried by the conduction system are delayed. This type of pacemaker is called a *demand pacemaker*. Other pacemakers send regular signals to keep the heart contracting at a preset rate.

When caring for a patient who has a pacemaker:

- Count and record the pulse rate.
- Report any irregularities or changes below the preset rate.
- Report discoloration over the implant site.
- Report hiccupping, because this may indicate problems.
- Teach the patient to hold a cell phone or cordless phone on the opposite side of the body from the ICD or pacemaker. Phones with an antenna must be 12 inches or more away from the implant.

A pacemaker weighs an ounce or less and must be replaced every six years to prevent battery failure. Newer pacemakers can monitor blood temperature, respiratory rate, and other factors. The device adjusts the heart rate to changes in the internal body environment and patient activity. Newer ICDs can function as pacemakers as well.

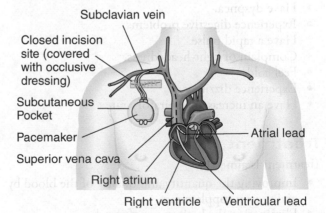

Subclavian vein

Closed incision site (covered with occlusive dressing)

Subcutaneous Pocket

Pacemaker

Superior vena cava

Right atrium

Atrial lead

Right ventricle   Ventricular lead

FIGURE 40-9 A pacemaker sends electrical impulses to the heart muscle, causing it to contract. It is inserted under the skin with the electrode placed inside the heart, resting on the heart muscle.

Older-type pacemakers must be kept away from microwave ovens. Very few of these are still in use because of the need for device replacement every six years. Newer pacemakers are safe in the presence of a microwave.

Patients usually function very well with pacemakers as long as they are adequately monitored.

BLOOD ABNORMALITIES

Blood abnormalities are often called *blood dyscrasias*.

Anemia

Anemia is a condition that results from a decrease in the quantity or quality of red blood cells that carry oxygen to nourish the body. There are several causes, including:

- Poor diet
- Low production of new red blood cells
- Blood loss, as in hemorrhage
  Types of anemia include:
- Pernicious—inability to absorb vitamin B12 (most often seen in the elderly). The body needs vitamin B12 to produce red blood cells.
- Sickle cell—inability to form normal hemoglobin. Sickle cell anemia is transmitted genetically. It is seen most often in African Americans.
- Iron deficiency—inadequate intake of iron, inability to absorb iron, or excessive loss of iron.
- Dietary—inadequate intake of iron or vitamins in diet.

Signs and Symptoms

The person with anemia may:
- Have little energy.
- Be pale or jaundiced.
- Have dyspnea.
- Experience digestive problems.
- Have a rapid pulse.
- Complain of light-headedness.
- Feel cold.
- Experience dizziness.
- Have an increased respiratory rate.

Treatment

Treatment is aimed at:
- Improving the quantity and quality of the blood by giving iron supplements.
- Eliminating the basic cause of the disease.
- Giving blood transfusions as needed.
- Providing nutrients and nutritious meals.

Leukemia

Leukemia is sometimes called *cancer of the blood*. The causes of the many forms of leukemia are not known. This disease may strike young or old. The number of white blood cells increases, but the white blood cells may be of poor quality. The number of erythrocytes and platelets decreases. Patients with leukemia are highly susceptible to infection. During the course of the disease, even minor trauma causes bleeding.

Treatment

Treatment is determined by the type of leukemia and the person's age. The overall goals are to:
- Ease symptoms and keep the person comfortable.
- Maintain normal blood levels. Transfusions may be needed to combat the anemia that accompanies this condition.
- Prevent infection.
- Combat infection, if present, by using antibiotics.
- Slow the production of abnormal white cells through chemotherapy and/or radiation therapy.

Special Care

Patients who have cancer or anemia require special care. You must:
- Check vital signs.
- Encourage rest.
- Handle the patient very gently.
- Encourage good nutrition and fluid intake.
- Give special mouth care, because the mouth and tongue become sensitive.
- Be sure to report any signs of bleeding, such as bruises or discolorations, because further blood loss makes the condition worse.
- Keep the patient warm.
- Protect the patient from falls that may result from dizziness or weakness.
- Change the patient's position often, at least every two hours.
- Provide emotional support.

✿ Infection Control **ALERT**

Patients with leukemia are at high risk of infection because the immature white blood cells do not protect the body effectively. Conscientiously apply the principles of standard precautions in all patient care. Notify the nurse promptly of signs or symptoms of infection.

DIAGNOSTIC TESTS

Some techniques used to diagnose problems of the cardiovascular system include:

- Blood chemistry tests, such as electrolyte panels.
- Complete blood cell count (CBC).
- Electrocardiogram (ECG or EKG).
- Cardiac catheterization and angiogram—introduction of catheter and dyes into the vascular system under fluoroscopy.
- Ultrasound—sound waves are bounced against tissues to reflect variations in tissue density.

PERFORMING AN ECG

The heart is a three-dimensional muscle. The ECG gives us the ability to look at the heart from different dimensions. The ECG uses of 12 leads (wires), which record the same cardiac activity simultaneously. Each provides a picture of the heart's activity from a different angle. The waves from each lead look slightly different because they are viewing the electrical activity from different positions. Each lead has a positive pole and a negative pole. The unit measures the electrical difference between the poles.

REVIEW

A. True/False

Mark the following true or false by circling T or F.

1. T F Smoking is not harmful to a person with atherosclerosis.
2. T F The treadmill test is done to detect hidden cardiac stress.
3. T F When someone with peripheral vascular disease needs warmth, a heating pad should not be used.
4. T F Another name for a heart attack is atrial infarction.
5. T F In leukemia, there is an increase in the number of white blood cells.
6. T F The heart muscle shrinks as it undergoes hypertrophy.
7. T F An embolus is a moving blood clot.
8. T F Anemia is an example of a blood dyscrasia.
9. T F Hypertension is best treated with a high-sodium diet.
10. T F A person with CHF should be monitored for pulse deficit.

B. Matching

Choose the correct term from Column II to match each phrase in Column I.

Column I

11. _____ inflammation of a vein
12. _____ death of the heart muscle
13. _____ another term for stroke
14. _____ high blood pressure
15. _____ blocking of the blood supply to the heart

Column II

a. hypertension
b. edema
c. myocardial infarction
d. plasma
e. phlebitis
f. CVA
g. hypotension
h. coronary occlusion

C. Multiple Choice

Select the best answer for each of the following.

16. Which of the following is not a predisposing cause of atherosclerosis?
    a. Emboli
    b. Diabetes mellitus
    c. Heredity
    d. Stress

17. You suspect that a patient needs immediate attention for a possible heart attack because the person:
    a. has chest pain.
    b. complains of not feeling well.
    c. has ankle edema.
    d. has pink nail beds.

18. Nursing care of a patient with anemia might include:
    a. bloodletting.
    b. good nutrition.
    c. a pacemaker.
    d. chemotherapy.

19. A patient with anemia has:

    a. a high energy level.

    b. pink, rosy skin.

    c. a low energy level.

    d. a slower-than-normal respiratory rate.

20. An attack of angina pectoris could be brought about by:

    a. bathing in the evening.

    b. resting in bed.

    c. emotional stress.

    d. walking in the hallway.

21. The purpose of the implantable cardioverter defibrillator (ICD) is to:

    a. strengthen the heart in persons with congestive heart failure.

    b. deliver a shock when a life-threatening heart rhythm occurs.

    c. keep arteries open by pushing fatty deposits against artery walls.

    d. regulate the heart rate through an electrical current in the ventricles.

22. All of the following are aging changes to the cardiovascular system *except*:

    a. the heart rate slows, causing a slower pulse and less efficient circulation.

    b. blood vessels lose elasticity and develop calcium deposits, resulting in narrowing.

    c. blood pressure increases because of stiffening and changes to the blood vessels.

    d. veins get smaller, causing blood vessels near the skin to become less prominent.

23. When fluid has nowhere to go in right-sided heart failure, it will:

    a. collect in the tissues in the feet and ankles.

    b. cause overflow of urine from the bladder.

    c. gather in the abdomen, causing enlargement.

    d. increase the person's risk for stroke.

24. When a patient has peripheral vascular disease, it is important to protect the:

    a. arms.

    b. hands.

    c. thighs.

    d. feet.

25. Conditions that increase the risk of vascular disease include:

    a. allergies.

    b. smoking.

    c. thyroid disease.

    d. hepatitis.

26. Inflammation of the veins is:

    a. dema.

    b. vascular disease.

    c. phlebitis.

    d. atheroma.

27. A temporary interruption of blood flow to the brain with no lasting effects is:

    a. heart attack.

    b. brain attack.

    c. angina pectoris.

    d. transient ischemic attack.

28. Cardiac pain of effort is:

    a. angina pectoris.

    b. hypertension.

    c. peripheral vascular disease.

    d. ischemia.

29. Signs and symptoms of heart attack may include all of the following *except*:

    a. high blood pressure.

    b. shortness of breath.

    c. irregular pulse.

    d. cyanosis.

30. Signs and symptoms of heart failure may include all of the following *except*:

    a. cough.

    b. neck vein swelling.

    c. low blood pressure.

    d. ascites.

D. Completion

Complete the statements in the spaces provided.

31. Five specific tests used to diagnose cardiac, vascular, or blood abnormalities are:

    a. _____

    b. _____

    c. _____

    d. _____

    e. _____

32. Six predisposing factors for atherosclerosis are:

    a. _____

    b. _____

    c. _____

    d. _____

    e. _____

    f. _____

E. Nursing Assistant Challenge

Mrs. O'Brien is only 38 years old but has been diagnosed with hypertension. Recently she experienced dizziness and weakness and had difficulty speaking for a short period. The doctor suspects that she had a TIA. Complete the statements in questions 33–40 by choosing the correct word from the following list.

blurred vision	low
brain	permanent
discouraged	potassium
encouraged	sodium
exercise	stroke
high	temporary
hypertension	

33. Hypertension means this patient has _____ blood pressure.

34. The TIA means there was a(n) _____ interruption of the blood flow to the _____.

35. The diet for this patient should be low in _____.

36. Smoking should be _____.

37. The TIA indicates that a _____ will probably occur in the future.

38. Treatment for hypertension includes regular _____.

39. _____ is a sign that should be reported immediately.

40. Nosebleeds are a danger sign for people with _____.

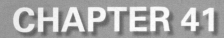

CHAPTER 41

Musculoskeletal System

OBJECTIVES

After completing this chapter, you will be able to:

41.1 Spell and define terms.

41.2 Describe the location of the musculoskeletal system.

41.3 Explain the functions of the musculoskeletal system.

41.4 Describe some common conditions of the musculoskeletal system.

41.5 Describe nursing assistant actions related to the care of patients with conditions and diseases of the musculoskeletal system.

41.6 List at least seven specific diagnostic tests for musculoskeletal conditions.

41.7 Demonstrate the following procedure:
- Procedure 87: Performing Range-of-Motion Exercises (Passive)

VOCABULARY

Learn the meaning and the correct spelling of the following words and phrases:

abduction
abduction pillow
adduction
amputation
arthritis
atrophy
avulsion fracture
bursa
bursitis
cardiac muscle
cartilage
cervical traction
closed (simple) fracture
comminuted fracture
compartment syndrome
complete fracture
compound (open) fracture
compression fracture
continuous passive motion (CPM)

countertraction
degenerative joint disease (DJD)
depressed fracture
diarthrotic joint
discectomy
dorsiflexion
ecchymosis
eversion
exacerbation
extension
fibromyalgia
flexion
fracture
fusion
gout
greenstick fracture
impacted fracture
incomplete fracture
insertion

inversion
involuntary muscle
laminectomy
ligament
oblique fracture
open (compound) fracture
open reduction/internal fixation (ORIF)
origin
osteoarthritic joint disease (OJD)
osteoporosis
passive range-of-motion (PROM) exercises
pathologic fracture
pelvic belt traction
phantom pain
plantar flexion
pronation
radial deviation

range-of-motion (ROM) exercises
remission
rheumatoid arthritis (RA)
rotation
spica cast
spiral fracture
stimulus
supination
tendon
total hip arthroplasty (THA)
transverse fracture
ulnar deviation
vascular
vertebrae
visceral muscle
voluntary muscle

THE MUSCULOSKELETAL SYSTEM

The bony frame of the body is called the *skeleton*. Tissue that is made up of contractile fibers (fibers that contract and relax) or cells that produce movement are called *muscles*. Together, the skeleton and muscles are termed the *musculoskeletal system*. The musculoskeletal system includes:

- Skeletal muscles
- Bones
- Joints
- Tendons
- Ligaments

The system functions to:

- Give shape and form to the body.
- Protect and support organs and body parts.
- Permit movement.
- Produce some blood cells.
- Store calcium and phosphorus.

When muscles, bones, or joints are injured, a long period of rest and inactivity may be required for the parts to heal. During this period, it is important that all other moving parts get sufficient exercise. Bones that are not stressed lose calcium and become less functional.

Structure and Function

Bones

It will be helpful for you to learn the names and general location of the bones of the body. To learn the names, study the skeleton in Figure 41-1A and the skull in Figure 41-1B. Note that the same number and kinds of bones are found on one side of the midline as on the other.

The bones:

- Number 206.
- May share the same name. For example, there are:
  - 24 ribs helping to form the chest.
  - 56 phalanges, the finger bones.
  - 2 femurs, the thigh bones.
  - 31 bones (**vertebrae**) in the spinal column. Small discs or pads of **cartilage** with soft, gel-like centers between the vertebrae help to cushion these bones. The anterior (front) of the vertebrae support the head and body. The posterior (rear) portions form a tunnel that surrounds and protects the delicate spinal cord and nerves.

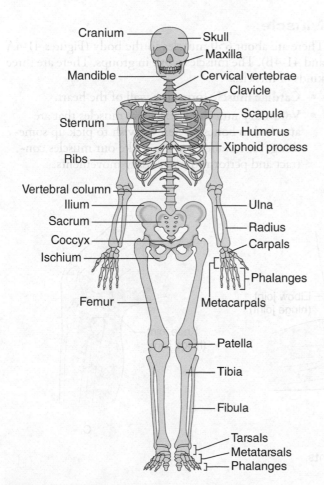

FIGURE 41-1A The human skeleton anterior.

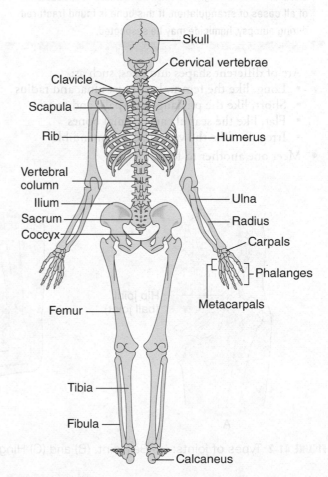

FIGURE 41-1B The human skeleton posterior.

- Are of different shapes and sizes, such as:
  - Long, like the femur, humerus, ulna, and radius
  - Short, like the phalanges, carpals, and tarsals
  - Flat, like the scapula and cranial bones
  - Irregular, like the vertebrae and mandible
- Meet one another to form joints.

Joints

Joints are points where bones come together and there is the possibility of movement. Without movable joints, walking, bending, lifting, and sitting would be impossible. Joints are capable of different movements depending the type of joint (Figure 41-2). **Ligaments** are strong bands of fibrous tissues that hold the bones together and support the joints. **Bursae** are small sacs of synovial fluid that are located around joints to help reduce friction.

Special terms are used to describe the different movements in a **diarthrotic joint**, which is a joint that permits free movement.

- **Flexion:** Decreasing the angle between two bones (Figure 41-3A). For example, bending the elbow.
- **Extension:** Increasing the angle between two bones (Figure 41-3B). For example, straightening the elbow.
- **Rotation:** Circular motion in a ball-and-socket joint (Figure 41-3C). For example, the shoulder and hip joints, which can move in all directions.
- **Abduction:** Moving away from the midline (Figure 41-3D).
- **Adduction:** Moving toward the midline (Figure 41-3E).

Muscles

There are about 650 muscles in the body (Figures 41-4A and 41-4B). The muscles work in groups. There are three kinds of muscles:

- **Cardiac muscle** forms the wall of the heart.
- **Voluntary muscles** are skeletal muscles that are attached to bones. When we wish to pick up something, for instance, we can make our muscles contract and perform the necessary movements.

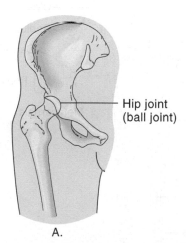

A.

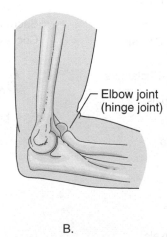

B.

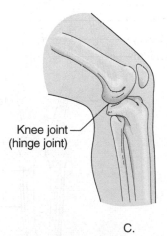

C.

FIGURE 41-2 Types of joints: (A) Ball joint. (B) and (C) Hinge joints.

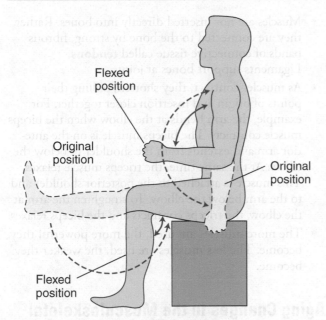

FIGURE 41-3A Flexion—bending a joint.

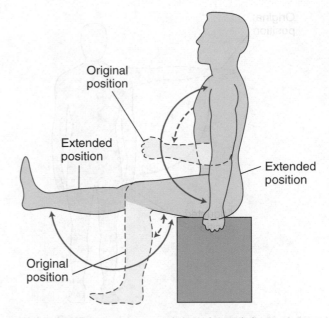

FIGURE 41-3B Extension—straightening a joint.

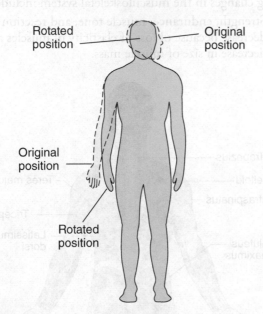

FIGURE 41-3C Rotation—moving a joint in a circular motion.

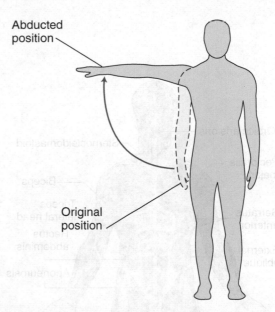

FIGURE 41-3D Abduction—moving an extremity away from the body.

- **Involuntary** or **visceral muscles** form the walls of organs. These muscles operate without our conscious control.
Muscles receive their names in three ways:
- Their location; for example, the rectus femoris near the femur
- Their shape; for example, the trapezius—trapezoidal shape
- Their action; for example, flexors—bring about flexion

You can easily locate the major muscle groups responsible for an activity if you remember that:
- Muscles can only shorten (contract) and lengthen (relax). Contraction occurs when nerves bring a message (**stimulus**) to do so to the muscle cells. Muscles relax when there is no stimulus.
- Muscles have two points of attachment to the bone. As they stretch from one point (**origin**) to the other (**insertion**), they cross over one or more joints.

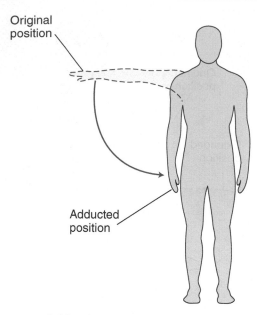

FIGURE 41-3E Adduction—moving an extremity back toward the body.

- Muscles are not inserted directly into bones. Rather, they are connected to the bone by strong, fibrous bands of connective tissue called **tendons**. Ligaments support bones at joints.
- As muscles contract, they shorten, pulling their points of origin and insertion closer together. For example, the arm bends at the elbow when the biceps muscle contracts. The biceps muscle is on the anterior arm and extends from the shoulder to below the elbow. At the same time, the triceps muscle relaxes. This muscle is attached to the posterior shoulder and to the arm below the elbow. To straighten the arm at the elbow, the triceps contracts and the biceps relaxes.
- The more muscles are used, the more powerful they become. The less muscles are used, the weaker they become.

Aging Changes to the Musculoskeletal System

Aging changes in the musculoskeletal system include:
- Strength, endurance, muscle tone, and reaction time decrease because of loss of elasticity of muscles and decrease in size of muscle mass.

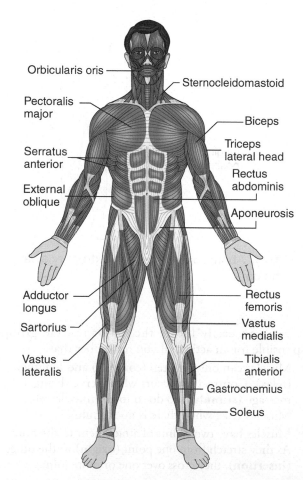

FIGURE 41-4A Major muscles of the body, anterior view.

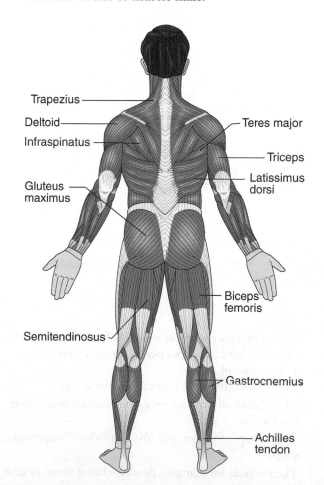

FIGURE 41-4B Major muscles of the body, posterior view.

- The spine becomes less stable, less flexible, and more easily injured.
- Posture may become slumped or hunched over because of weakness in back muscles.
- Deterioration in the joints results in limited movement, stiffness, and pain.
- Most people lose two inches of height by age 80.
- Bones lose calcium, bone density (mass) decreases; osteoporosis may develop; bones lose strength, become brittle, and break more easily.
- Lean muscle mass is lost.
- Muscle strength and endurance decrease.
- Ability to perform activities of daily living (ADLs) decreases.
- Changes in balance and gait increase both fall risk and fracture risk.

COMMON CONDITIONS

Many conditions can affect the bones, muscles, tendons, ligaments, and joints. Often, when one of these structures is diseased or injured, the surrounding tissues are also involved.

Bursitis

Bursae are small sacs of fluid found around joints. They help to reduce friction when muscles move. At times, the bursae can become inflamed and the tissues around a joint may become painful. This condition is known as **bursitis**. Treatment of bursitis includes:

- Applications of heat to promote healing
- Immobilization so that the joint cannot move, to relieve pain around the joint
- Removal of excess fluid from the joint by aspiration with a needle
- Administration of steroids

Arthritis

The term **arthritis** (Figure 41-5A) refers to inflammation of the joints. It may develop following an acute injury, or it may be chronic and progressive.

Three forms of chronic arthritis are the most common.

- **Rheumatoid arthritis (RA)** affects the joint tissues and the joint lining, and can affect any other body system. It is a serious form of arthritis that can occur in persons of any age. The cause is not specifically known, but it is believed to be an autoimmune response. It usually follows an intermittent course. RA has **exacerbations**, which are times when the condition seems to worsen. and **remissions**, times when the disease appears stable. The involved joints may feel hot to the touch. The condition causes reduced joint function and deformities. These can be severe and disabling. (Also refer to Chapter 6.)

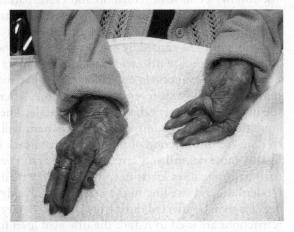

FIGURE 41-5A Deformities caused by rheumatoid arthritis make hand movement difficult.

- **Osteoarthritic joint disease (OJD)** or **degenerative joint disease (DJD)** affects the cartilage covering the ends of the bones that form a joint. Cartilage breaks down and the ends of the bones rub together, causing pain and deformity. The joints most often affected are the weight-bearing joints. Several factors seem to contribute to the disease process:

  - Aging
  - Trauma
  - Obesity

  The most common symptom of osteoarthritis is pain. This is usually described as a deep, aching pain that occurs after exercise, weight bearing, or exertion. It is often relieved by rest. Changes in the weather may also cause pain. Other symptoms include limited ability to move and stiffness, particularly upon arising in the morning. This also may occur after strenuous exercise or physical overactivity. In some individuals, an audible grating sound can be heard in the joints during movement. Osteoarthritis may cause redness and swelling in the joints. Conditions such as obesity and stress aggravate the symptoms.

- **Gout** (gouty arthritis) is a metabolic disease that can be severely disabling. It is caused by increased uric acid in the bloodstream, which deposits in the joints and forms crystals that cause pain. It can occur in any joint, but is most common in the feet and legs. The great toe is often the first joint affected. Gout also follows a course of remission and exacerbation. It can lead to complete disability, hypertension, and chronic renal disease. The cause is unknown, but it is thought to be caused by a genetic defect in the ability to metabolize uric acid. The affected joints may be red or cyanotic in appearance. The patient may have a low-grade fever during this time. After the initial, painful period, symptoms subside. The condition goes into remission and the patient will be pain-free for a period of time. The next attack is usually more painful and severe than the first. Eventually, chronic disease sets in. It is marked by pain, tenderness, and swelling in the joints. Other body systems may be affected during this stage. Dietary restrictions are used to reduce the uric acid level in the blood. The dietitian will plan a diet that restricts the amount of red meat and foods rich in purines.

Arthritis can cause mild discomfort to severe deformities and disability. Patients with arthritis are at high risk of contractures (Figure 41-5B). If permitted by your facility, place patients with this condition in the prone position periodically. This reduces the risk of contractures of the hips and knees. Avoid placing pillows under the knees or elevating the knee area of the bed. Using a small, flat pillow under the head and neck is best. A large pillow pushes the neck into a position of flexion. You may be assigned to perform range-of-motion exercises

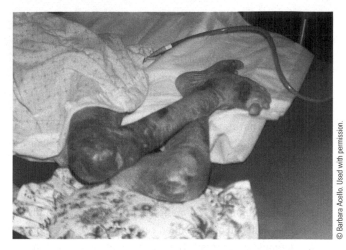

FIGURE 41-5B Arthritic deformities can affect the legs.

© Barbara Acello. Used with permission.

on patients with arthritis. Be very gentle. Avoid moving joints past the point of pain or resistance. Avoid the neck area unless you have a specific physician's order.

Treatment of arthritis includes:

- Relief of pain
- Balance of rest and exercise
- Joint immobilization where there is pain
- Weight control to relieve pressure on the joints
- Medication to relieve pain and reduce inflammation
- Physical therapy when inflammation subsides, to maintain joint mobility
- Surgical replacement of badly damaged joints
- Use of splints, braces, and adaptive equipment to enable the patient to get the most range of motion from injured joints
- Exercise of arthritic joints in warm water (with or without whirlpool action) to maintain function and relieve pain
- Prevention of deformities and contractures

Osteoporosis

Osteoporosis is a metabolic disorder of the bones. It is most common in elderly females, but can occur in males. Bone mass is lost, causing bones to become porous and spongy (Figure 41-6). Because of this, affected bones are at very high risk for fracture. Fractures can occur spontaneously, such as when the patient is walking. They can also occur when the patient is moved or turned in bed or during transfers.

The cause of osteoporosis is unknown. It is thought to result from years of inadequate calcium intake. Other potential causes are declining adrenal function, faulty protein metabolism, estrogen deficiency, and lack of exercise or activity.

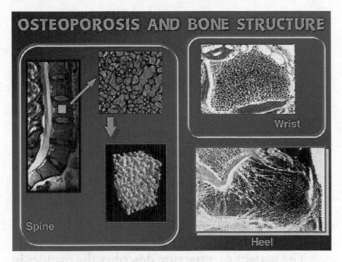

FIGURE 41-6 Bone loss from osteoporosis causes painful, disabling fractures in both sexes. One half (50%) of women over age 50 and one fourth (25%) of men will experience an osteoporosis-related fracture in their lifetime.

Signs and Symptoms

The first sign of osteoporosis may be a fracture. Commonly, the patient moves or lifts something and hears a "pop" or snapping sound in a bone, usually in the lower back or hip. The patient who is walking may suddenly fall. In this case, the fall is the *result* of the fracture; in most other falls, the opposite is true. After the initial incident, the area is very painful, particularly upon movement. Sometimes the onset of osteoporosis begins with a curvature of the spine and loss of height. The back progressively weakens, straining the neck, hips, and low back. Spontaneous fractures may occur during movement or as a result of a minor injury.

Treatment

The goals of treatment are to prevent further fractures and control pain. Gentle range-of-motion and other exercises may be ordered. Splints, braces, and other devices may be ordered to support weakened bones. Female patients may be given estrogen replacement and other drugs to replace calcium and bone mass. For bone to withstand mechanical stresses, old bone mass is constantly being broken down and new bone is being formed. This is called *bone remodeling*. Disruption of bone remodeling can lead to osteoporosis and other disorders. *Bisphosphonates* are a class of medications that inhibit the breakdown of bones. These drugs are a newer method of preventing and treating osteoporosis. Patients taking drugs in this category have specific requirements for eating, drinking, and maintaining an upright position. The nurse and the care plan will provide information about special monitoring.

You must handle the patient with osteoporosis very gently. If you are assigned to perform range-of-motion exercises, do so slowly and carefully. Avoid stretching the joint past the point of resistance. Use a mechanical lift for transfers whenever possible. This is less traumatic than pulling on the patient. Make sure you have extra help for all procedures in which you will be moving or positioning the patient. Follow the care plan exactly.

Fibromyalgia

Fibromyalgia is a common chronic pain syndrome for which there is no known cause or cure. It affects more women than men. The area between the shoulder blades and the bottom of the neck is often painful. The pain is described as either a general soreness or a gnawing ache, and stiffness is usually worst in the morning. Although this is a common problem, it is very controversial. Some physicians believe that there is no physical cause, and that psychiatric problems or sleep disorders are responsible for the patient's symptoms. The condition can be very painful and interfere with the patient's quality of life and daily activities. To be diagnosed with this condition, the patient must meet certain criteria, such as:

- Having pain on both sides of the body
- Having pain both above and below the waist
- Having pain upon palpation in at least 11 of 18 specified body sites (Figure 41-7)

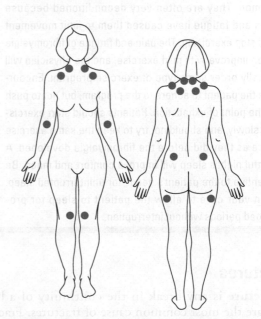

FIGURE 41-7 Pain must be present in 11 of 18 specific body areas for fibromyalgia to be diagnosed.

Signs and Symptoms

Signs and symptoms of fibromyalgia are:

- Pain and stiffness
- Feeling abnormally tired
- Waking up tired
- Pain upon touch in certain areas of the body

Treatment

Treatment involves pain medications and exercise. Muscle-relaxant medications and antidepressants are sometimes used. Some patients use alternative and complementary therapies to relieve pain and stiffness. The most common complementary therapies used to treat this condition are:

- Massage
- Biofeedback
- Acupuncture
- Hypnosis
- Relaxation, meditation, and other forms of stress management

Because the cause of fibromyalgia is not known, there is no prevention or cure for this condition. Fibromyalgia complicates treatment for many other medical problems because of the underlying pain and difficulty in assuming some positions necessary for examination and treatment.

⚖ TIPS

Most patients with fibromyalgia are middle-aged women. They are often very deconditioned because pain and fatigue have caused them to limit movement and stop exercising. The pain and fatigue of fibromyalgia often improve with mild exercise, and the physician will usually order some type of exercise program. Encourage the patient to adhere to the program, but not to push to the point of exhaustion. Patients should start exercising slowly, and should not try to keep the same exercise pace as they did before the fibromyalgia developed. A restful night's sleep will improve comfort and mood. Be attentive to the patient's needs for uninterrupted sleep. Plan your care to allow the patient to sleep for prolonged periods without interruption.

Fractures

A **fracture** is any break in the continuity of a bone. Falls are the most common cause of fractures. Fractures (Figure 41-8) are classified by the type of break in the bone and whether the skin is broken:

- A **complete fracture** involves a break across the entire cross-section of the bone. It is often displaced, or improperly aligned, and must be reduced and straightened.
- An **incomplete fracture** involves only part of the cross-section of bone.
- A **closed (simple) fracture** (Figure 41-8A) occurs when the skin is intact, not broken.
- An **open (compound) fracture** (Figure 41-8B) occurs when the skin over the fracture is broken. The bone may or may not protrude.
- A **pathologic fracture** is a fracture in a diseased bone. It occurs as a result of osteoporosis, a tumor, or cancer.

The pattern of a fracture describes the manner in which the bone is broken:

- A **greenstick fracture** (Figure 41-8C) occurs when only one side of the bone is broken and the other side is bent. This fracture is common in children, whose bone growth is incomplete. The bones tend to bend like young trees; hence the name "greenstick" fracture.
- A **transverse fracture** (Figure 41-8D) breaks completely across the bone.
- An **oblique fracture** (Figure 41-8E) runs at an angle across the bone.
- A **spiral fracture** (Figure 41-8F) twists around the bone.
- A **comminuted fracture** (Figure 41-8G) involves shattering and splintering of the bone into more than three fragments.
- A **depressed fracture** (Figure 41-8H) is seen only in fractures of the skull and face. This type of fracture depresses the bone and drives fragments inward.
- A **compression fracture** (Figure 41-8I) is seen only in the vertebrae of the spine. This type of fracture collapses the bone inward.
- An **avulsion fracture** (Figure 41-8J) occurs when a bone fragment is pulled off at the point of ligament or tendon attachment.
- An **impacted fracture** (Figure 41-8K) occurs when a fragment from one bone is wedged into another bone.

Signs and Symptoms

Signs and symptoms of fractures will vary with the type of fracture and location. Fractures are painful conditions. Movement is limited, or the patient may be unable to move the injured area. The skin surrounding the fracture may appear deformed. Edema is common. **Ecchymosis**, or bruising, may occur. Some parts of the body, such as the area over the femur, are very **vascular**. Areas that are

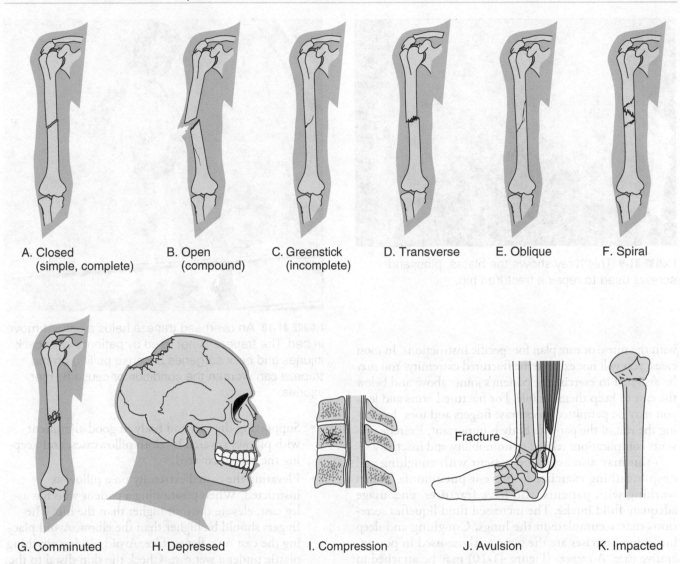

A. Closed
(simple, complete)
B. Open
(compound)
C. Greenstick
(incomplete)
D. Transverse
E. Oblique
F. Spiral

G. Comminuted
H. Depressed
I. Compression
J. Avulsion
K. Impacted

FIGURE 41-8 Types and patterns of fractures.

vascular contain many blood vessels. They bleed readily under the skin. An ecchymosis the size of an adult's fist over the femur indicates loss of approximately one pint of blood.

Treatment

A new fracture is usually treated in the hospital emergency department. Admission for surgical correction of the fracture may be necessary. The immediate goals of care are to:

- Control pain.
- Prevent complications of immobility.
- Prevent or reduce edema.
- Keep the fracture in good alignment.
- Keep the fractured extremity immobile.

Fractures of any kind are treated by keeping the part that is injured immobilized in proper position until healing takes place. Injured bones take from several weeks to several months to heal. Immobilization is achieved through the use of:

- Pins (Figure 41-9)
- Screws
- Splints
- Bone plates
- Casting
- Traction

Special beds and attachments are used to make nursing care easier. The patient may be placed on a Stryker frame or a CircOlectric bed. Be sure you know how to operate each bed and attachment before attempting to give care. In many facilities, a nurse must be present when the bed is turned. Know and follow the policy of your facility.

You will assist patients who have fractures with range-of-motion exercises several times each day. Check

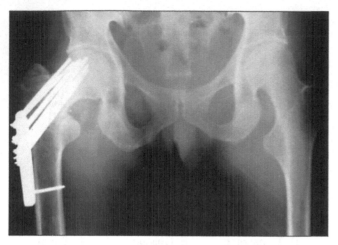

FIGURE 41-9 This X-ray shows the plates, pins, and screws used to repair a fractured hip.

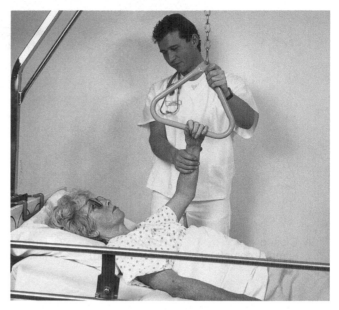

FIGURE 41-10 An overhead trapeze helps a patient move in bed. The trapeze is not used by patients with back injuries and back surgeries because pulling on the trapeze can worsen the condition or cause further injuries.

with the nurse or care plan for specific instructions. In most cases, you will not exercise the fractured extremity. You may be assigned to exercise the patient's joints above and below the cast to keep them mobile. For fractured arms and legs, you may be permitted to exercise fingers and toes. Exercising the rest of the patient's body is important. Exercise prevents complications related to immobility and inactivity.

You may also assist the patient with coughing and deep breathing exercises to prevent pneumonia. When working with patients who have fractures, encourage adequate fluid intake. The increased fluid liquefies secretions that accumulate in the lungs. Coughing and deep breathing exercises are the same as those used in postoperative care. A *trapeze* (Figure 41-10) may be attached to the bed to assist the patient with movement. The nurse will teach you how to move and reposition the patient without interfering with the traction. The casted extremity is elevated on pillows if traction is not used.

Treatment for patients with fractures begins soon after admission. The type of treatment is determined by the location and type of fracture, and method of fracture reduction. Patients with fractures will be evaluated by physical and occupational therapists. Therapists will design rehabilitation programs to meet patients' needs and help them to regain as much mobility as possible.

Care of Patients with Casts

Two types of cast materials are commonly used:

- Plaster of Paris, which can take up to 48 hours to dry completely
- Fiberglass, which dries very rapidly

Cast material is wet when it is applied. During the drying period, the cast gives off heat. Special care for the newly casted patient includes:

- Supporting the cast and body in good alignment with pillows covered by cloth pillowcases, and keeping the cast uncovered.
- Elevating the casted extremity on a pillow as instructed. When positioning a patient who has a leg cast, elevate the foot higher than the hip. The fingers should be higher than the elbow. Avoid placing the cast on a flat surface. Avoid placing anything plastic under a wet cast. Check the skin distal to the cast frequently for signs of poor circulation.
- Turning the patient frequently to permit air circulation to all parts of the cast. Maintain support. Use the palm of your hand, not your fingers, to support the wet cast.
- Not positioning the cast against the footboard or side rail. It is best to leave the cast open to air until it dries. If the patient is cold, cover the cast loosely with a sheet. Avoid tucking the sheet under the mattress. A bed cradle may be helpful. The greatest area of heat loss is the head. Covering the upper body and back and top of the head with a blanket may help keep the patient warm.
- Closely observing the uncasted areas of the extremities, such as the fingers and toes, for signs of decreased circulation. Immediately report coldness, capillary refill of more than three seconds, cyanosis, swelling, increased pain, numbness, or tingling.
- Closely observing skin areas around the cast edges for signs of irritation (Figure 41-11). Cover rough edges with adhesive strips to prevent skin irritation.

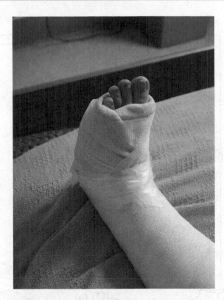

FIGURE 41-11 The skin around the edges of a cast should be checked for signs of irritation. Circulation in the toes is assessed regularly.

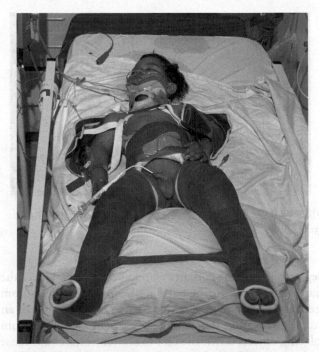

FIGURE 41-12 A spica cast is commonly used to treat hip fractures and after hip surgery in children.

Clinical Information **ALERT**

To warm a patient quickly, fashion a hat using six-inch stockinette. This is the sock-like material that is used to protect a leg before a cast is applied. Cut a length of stockinette, then fasten it closed with a rubber band. Warm the hat in the blanket warmer or microwave, if available. Applying a warm hat helps to warm and comfort a cool patient quickly, and they will appreciate your concern.

Recall the following key of reportables when checking the patient:

C = color

M = motion

E = edema

T = temperature

Special Care After the Cast Is Dry

After the cast has dried completely:

- Turn the patient to the noncasted side. This is particularly important in moving a patient with a body cast (**spica cast**) (Figure 41-12), because turning to the casted side may crack the cast.
- Always support the cast when turning or moving a patient.
- Encourage use of a trapeze to assist the patient in helping themselves.

Safety **ALERT**

A fiberglass cast dries immediately. A plaster arm or leg cast will take 24 to 48 hours to dry completely. A plaster body or spica cast will take 48 to 72 hours to dry. Proper positioning of the cast is essential during the drying period to prevent depressions that can cause pressure and edema. Never use a table or hard object to support the cast during the drying period. Avoid rubber or plastic pillows, which increase heat under the cast. When the cast is dry, it will look white and shiny. It will not appear to be soft or damp.

- Tape the edges of casts to prevent pressure and abrasive areas, if edges were not covered when the cast was applied.
- Use plastic to protect cast edges that are near the genitals and buttocks, to help prevent soiling during toileting.

After the cast dries, you may observe changes that indicate infection or ulceration under the cast:

- Odor from the cast
- Drainage through the cast

The care plan may instruct you to keep the casted extremity elevated to prevent edema. A sling (Figure 41-13) may be used to elevate an arm cast when the patient is out of bed. A wheelchair with an elevated

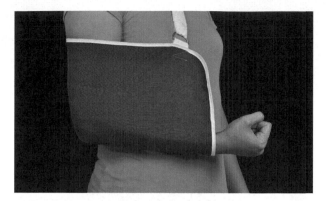

FIGURE 41-13 A sling may be used to elevate the hand and wrist.

leg rest is used for patients who have leg casts. Cover the cast with plastic during bathing. Keep small objects from getting inside the cast. The patient may complain of an itching sensation under the cast. Discourage them from placing objects down the cast to scratch. This could cause a skin injury and infection. Report complaints of itching to the nurse.

Care of Patients in Traction

Traction is designed to pull two body areas slightly apart to:

- Relieve pressure.
- Help tightly contracted (spasmodic) muscles relax.
- Keep them in proper position as healing takes place.

    There are two types of traction:
- Skin traction, in which traction is applied to the skin or outside of the body (Figure 41-14A)
- Skeletal traction, in which traction is applied through the skin to the bone (Figure 41-14B)

    Traction is applied by attaching weights to a part of the body above or below the area to be treated. The patient's body weight serves as **countertraction** by pulling in the direction opposite to the traction. Belts, head halters, or tapes may be applied to the patient's skin to hold the traction. Traction may be applied continuously or intermittently.

    Skeletal traction uses tongs or pins placed into bones with weights applied to the tongs or pins. Caring for the pins is an advanced procedure. Skeletal traction is always continuous once applied. The weights for skeletal traction must not be lifted or removed until the traction is to be discontinued.

    When patients are in traction:
- Review the correct placement of straps and weights with the therapist or nurse. Get instructions for moving the patient up in bed and turning from side to side, as ordered.

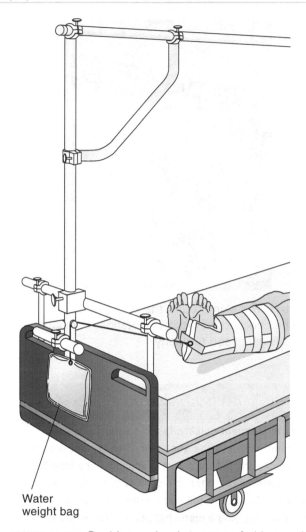

Water weight bag

FIGURE 41-14A Buck's traction is a type of skin traction that is used to stabilize the bone before surgery or until the fracture heals in patients who are not candidates for surgery.

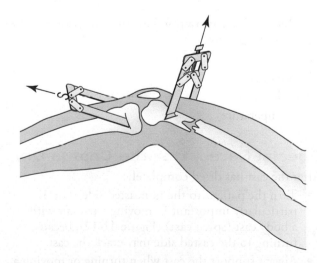

FIGURE 41-14B Skeletal traction immobilizes a body part by attaching weights directly to the bones with pins, screws, wires, or tongs.

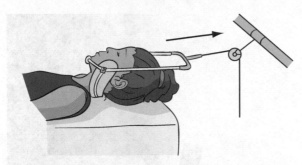

FIGURE 41-14C Cervical traction is not frequently used; however, it relieves pain and muscle spasms associated with neck fractures.

- Do not disturb the weights or permit them to swing, drop, or rest on any surface. Avoid moving, dropping, or releasing the weights. They should not touch the bed, swing back and forth freely, or rest upon any object or surface. The water bag or weight hangs motionless at the end of the bed.
- Keep the patient in good alignment in the center of the bed. Make sure that the body is acting properly as countertraction by keeping the head of the bed low. The feet should not rest against the end of the bed.
- Check under straps and belts for areas of pressure or irritation.
- Make sure straps and belts are smooth, straight, and properly secured.
- Keep bed covers off ropes and pulleys.

Not all patients remain in traction continuously. Although not common, belt and halter traction is used occasionally. If **pelvic belt traction** or **cervical traction** with a head halter (Figure 41-14C) is to be discontinued, take the following steps:

1. Slowly raise the weights to the bed. Avoid abrupt or jerking movements, as this may cause the patient pain. If two sets of weights are being used, raise them at the same time and rate.
2. Remove the weight holder and weights from the connection with the halter or belt and place them on the floor. Remove the head halter or pelvic belt.
3. To reapply traction, reverse the procedure.
4. Remember never to jerk or drop the weights quickly or lower them unevenly. Always apply weights smoothly to avoid causing the patient pain.

Bedmaking

Bedmaking for orthopedic patients varies according to the type of traction.

- Two half-sheets are often used in place of a large sheet for the bottom.
- Bottom linens may be changed from top to bottom rather than side to side.

- The top linen is arranged according to the patient's special needs. Half-sheets and folded bath blankets can be worked around the traction to keep the patient covered and comfortable.

Clinical Information **ALERT**

Some problems, such as hip fractures and amputations, are very hard on the bodies of older persons. There is a high risk of morbidity and mortality. Amputations can become life-threatening in persons over age 60 who have peripheral vascular disease.

Fractured Hip

Hip fractures are the most common type of fracture in the elderly. It is not unusual for a patient to be admitted to the hospital or long-term care facility for treatment of another problem, then fall and break a hip. The most common cause of hip fractures is falls, but fractures may also occur because of ostcoporosis. The term *hip fracture* really is not accurate. This term refers to a fracture anywhere in the upper third or head of the femur.

Signs and Symptoms of Hip Fracture

A patient with a fractured hip is usually found on the floor. They will be unable to get up or move the injured leg. The leg on the affected side may be shortened and in a position of external rotation. In this position, the toes point outward. The shortening and rotation occur because the strong muscles in the upper leg contract. This causes the bone ends to override each other.

The patient will complain of severe pain in the hip. The pain of a hip fracture is usually localized in the hip. Some patients complain of pain in the knee. This may be confusing or misleading. Edema and ecchymosis may be present in the hip, thigh, groin, or lower pelvic area.

Emergency Care

Avoid moving the patient until you are instructed to do so by a nurse. You will use a sheet, backboard, or other device to move the patient. Avoid excessive movement, which can worsen the injury. Moving a patient with a hip fracture requires four or five individuals. The patient is logrolled onto the lifting device. The device is lifted to the bed or stretcher. You may be assigned to monitor the patient's vital signs and check for signs of shock. Patients who are poor surgical risks may be treated with Buck's traction.

Open Reduction/Internal Fixation

The most common treatment for a fractured hip is a surgical procedure called **open reduction/internal fixation (ORIF)**. In this procedure, the surgeon makes an incision, manipulates the fractured bone into alignment, and then inserts a device such as a nail, pin, or rod to hold the ends of the fractured bone in place (Figure 41-15). If you are assigned to a patient who has had this surgery, you must:

> ### ⚕ Clinical Information **ALERT**
>
> Hip fractures account for 350,000 hospital admissions each year, and 60,000 nursing home admissions. Hip fractures are more common in women. More than 4 percent of hip fracture patients die during their initial hospitalization. Only 25 percent of persons who have sustained a hip fracture will make a full recovery; 50 percent will lose the ability to walk and require nursing home care; 50 percent will need a cane or walker; and 24 percent of those over age 50 will die within 12 months because of complications related to the injury. Several studies have shown that the incidence of death doubles after a hip fracture in an elderly person.[1] The cost of hip fracture care averages $26,912 per patient.

- Know how to position the patient in bed. It is important to avoid adduction and internal and external rotation of the affected hip.
- Know the correct procedure if the patient is allowed to ambulate. The patient is usually not allowed to bear weight on the affected side for a few weeks after surgery. The activity order is determined by the location of the fracture and the type of corrective surgical procedure performed.

Total Hip Arthroplasty

Total hip arthroplasty (THA), or insertion of a hip prosthesis (artificial body part), is a common procedure (Figure 41-16A). This surgery is done because the patient:

- Has fractured a hip and the bone cannot be set by traditional methods
- Has degenerative arthritis that has caused the hip joint to deteriorate

In THA, the patient's hip joint is surgically removed and a metal or synthetic ball and socket are inserted (Figure 41-16B). There are specific body positions that the patient must avoid to prevent damage to the new joint.

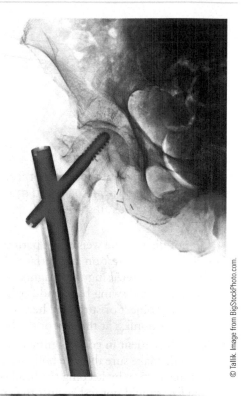

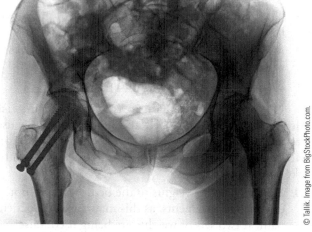

© Tallik. Image from BigStockPhoto.com.

FIGURE 41-15 When an ORIF is done, a nail, pin, or rod is inserted to hold the ends of the fractured bone in place.

> ### Difficult Situations
>
> A patient who has had hip surgery will probably have physician orders for anti-embolism hosiery and an incentive spirometer. Following hip surgery, the patient will be at high risk for pressure injury development, particularly on the heels. Take active measures to prevent pressure. Follow the care plan. Check the skin regularly for redness, irritation, and breakdown.

[1]Basaraba, S. (2019). *Hip Fracture Dangers and Mortality Rates.* Retrieved October 18, 2019, from https://www.verywellhealth.com/how-dangerous-is-a-broken-hip-when-youre-older-2223520

*American Academy of Orthopaedic Surgeons Online. Accessed September 15, 2012, at https://orthoinfo.aaos.org/en/diseases

Caring for the Patient Who Has Had Hip Surgery

After hip surgery, the following general procedures are commonly ordered:

- A trapeze is attached to the bed to assist with movement. Instruct the patient not to press down on the foot of the affected leg when using the trapeze.
- Apply anti-embolism stockings (Chapter 29). Follow the care plan for circulation checks.
- A fracture bedpan is used initially for elimination. When the patient is able to use the toilet, an elevated toilet seat is used.
- Do not elevate the head of the bed more than 45° without a specific order.
- Avoid acute flexion of the hip and legs. The physician will give directions for positioning and the degree of flexion permitted.
- These patients will usually use a special pillow, called an **abduction pillow**, to keep the legs apart (Figure 41-17). This is particularly important when the patient is turned on the side. The patient will be instructed to avoid crossing the legs, which can cause a dislocation. Keep the pillow in place when the patient is turned to the side. Support the lower leg on pillows, if necessary.

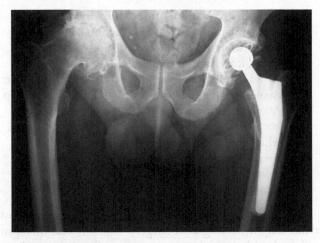

FIGURE 41-16B A THA is the replacement of the ball of the femur and socket.

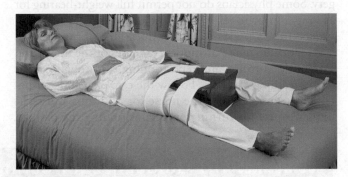

FIGURE 41-17 An abduction pillow is commonly used after hip surgery to keep the legs from crossing over at the ankles or adducting.

- Maintain the affected leg in good alignment without internal or external rotation.
- Avoid rolling the affected leg toward the other leg when turning the patient. Make sure the abduction pillow is in place during turning to prevent the legs from crossing.
- Support the affected leg when moving the patient to the side of the bed.
- Instruct the patient to:
  - Avoid sleeping on the stomach or operative side.
  - Avoid crossing the legs, as this may cause hip dislocation.
  - Avoid sitting on low chairs or couches. Position the patient only in chairs with arms where the knees remain lower than the hips.
  - Avoid leaning forward while sitting, and avoid picking up items from the floor or bending to put on shoes and socks.
  - Avoid flexing the hips more than 80° or rotating the foot and leg inward.
  - Avoid raising the knee higher than the hip on the operative side.

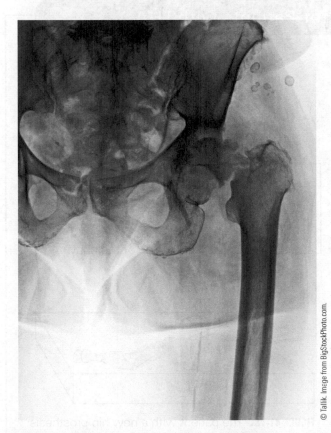

© Tallik. Image from BigStockPhoto.com.

FIGURE 41-16A A THA is done to treat a hip fracture or replace a hip with degenerative changes.

- Keep the legs at least three to six inches apart when sitting, or use the abduction pillow.
- Avoid stretching the affected hip backward.
- Avoid kneeling on one knee.
- Avoid turning the foot outward on the affected side.
- Avoid twisting the body away from the affected hip.
- Avoid standing with the toes pointed outward; keep the toes of the affected leg pointed forward when standing, sitting, or walking.
- Avoid swinging the affected leg outward away from the body.
- Avoid assuming a straddling position.

The physician will specify how long the patient must avoid weight-bearing after surgery. The physical therapist will work with the patient to restore mobility. Some patients are able to ambulate soon after surgery. A walker, crutches, or cane are commonly used for a period of time after surgery. Some physicians do not permit full weight-bearing for as long as four to six weeks. Initially, you will assist with procedures to prevent the complications of immobility. These include range-of-motion exercises of the unaffected extremities, turning and repositioning, and coughing and deep breathing exercises. Follow the care plan and get specific instructions from the nurse for positions and techniques to use for turning and repositioning the patient.

Relieve pressure from the heels and check the patient's skin carefully each day for signs of red or open areas.

Total Joint Replacement

Sometimes joints are completely replaced because of arthritis or severe damage to the joint. The goal of joint replacement surgery is to relieve pain, which is often so severe that the patient avoids using the joint as much as possible. This weakens the muscles and worsens the problem. Hip and knee replacements are the most common, but joint replacement surgery can be done on the ankle, foot, shoulder, elbow, and fingers. Postoperative care will vary with the surgical procedure. General care for joint replacement surgery includes:

- Preventing infection
- Preventing blood clots
- Administering anticoagulant medication to thin the blood
- Applying anti-embolism hosiery (Chapter 29)
- Doing exercises to increase blood flow in the leg muscles, if not contraindicated
- Using sequential compression therapy (Chapter 29)
- Using continuous passive motion (CPM)

GUIDELINES 41-1 Guidelines for Caring for Patients with THA

The patient should *not*:

- Flex the hip more than 90° (Figure 41-18A).
- Cross the affected leg over the midline of the body, whether in bed or sitting in a chair (Figure 41-18B).
- Internally rotate the hip on the affected side (Figure 41-18C).

Never do passive range-of-motion exercises on a joint that has had surgery, unless you are specifically instructed to do so—and then only if you have been given instructions as to which actions can safely be performed.

The patient will have limited weight-bearing on the affected leg for several days or weeks after surgery.

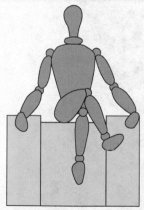

FIGURE 41-18B The patient with a new hip prosthesis should never cross the affected leg over the midline of the body.

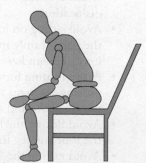

FIGURE 41-18A The patient with a new hip prosthesis should never flex the affected hip more than 90°.

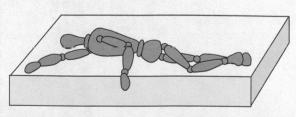

FIGURE 41-18C The patient with a new hip prosthesis should never internally rotate the hip on the affected side.

Difficult Situations

As a rule, patients who have had hip replacement surgery may have the head of the bed elevated up to 45° for comfort. Some physicians write more permissive orders, but check with the nurse before elevating the head more than this. Try to limit head elevation to 30-minute periods of time, if possible. Never allow the person to remain in a position of hip flexion for more than 90 minutes, because longer periods increase the risk of prosthesis dislocation. Positioning the person in the supine position, with the affected leg in extension, for 1 hour three times a day will help prevent contractures of the hip joint.

Continuous Passive Motion

Continuous passive motion (CPM) therapy (Figure 41-19) may be ordered following joint replacement and other orthopedic procedures. Moving a surgically repaired joint is painful. If the patient fails to move the joint, stiffness will develop and the range of motion will be limited. Months of physical therapy will be necessary for the patient to fully recover. CPM therapy prevents stiffness by delivering a form of passive range-of-motion exercise so the joint is moved without the patient's muscles being used. CPM therapy is effortless for the patient. A machine moves the affected joint through a prescribed range of motion for an extended period of time. CPM therapy:

- Enhances circulation, which lowers the risk of blood clots
- Reduces edema
- Promotes collagen formation within the joint, which enhances healing

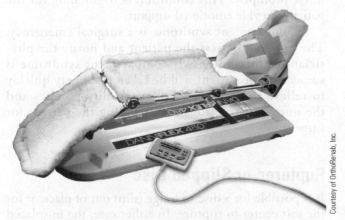

FIGURE 41-19 The continuous passive motion (CPM) machine performs passive range-of-motion exercises on the affected joint without straining the patient's muscles.

Courtesy of OrthoRehab, Inc.

- Reduces scarring
- Decreases stiffness
- Improves range of motion (which decreases postoperatively without movement)
- Reduces the risk of complications in the joint, such as contractures and adhesions
- Helps reduce pain

Many orthopedic surgeons prescribe CPM therapy following knee replacement and other surgical procedures. CPM devices are available for the knee, ankle, toes, jaw, shoulder, elbow, wrist, and hand. Indications for using CPM therapy are:

- Crush injuries of the hand without fractures or dislocations
- Burn injuries
- Stable fractures
- Joint and tendon repair
- Surgical release of contractures
- Knee or hip replacement
- Reconstructive surgery on bone, cartilage, tendons, and ligaments
- Prolonged joint immobilization

The physician prescribes how the CPM unit should be used. They order the settings on the CPM unit that control the speed, duration of use, range of motion, pause settings, hours of use per day, and rate of increase of motion. The directions for use will vary slightly depending on the body area being treated, the type of CPM machine being used, and the physician's orders. In some facilities, this procedure is done only by licensed nurses. In others, the nursing assistant can set up the unit, but the nurse must check the settings for accuracy. This is a key step. Improper settings can damage reconstructive work in the joint. Follow your facility policies and procedures.

Contraindications for CPM therapy include:

- Untreated infections
- Unstable fractures
- Known or suspected blood clots (deep vein thrombosis)
- Hemorrhage

If the patient develops any of the following signs or symptoms upon using the device, stop the unit and inform the nurse promptly:

- Fever
- Increasing redness or irritation
- Increasing warmth
- Edema
- Bleeding
- Increased or persistent pain

Safety **ALERT**

Make sure the side rail is up on the side where the CPM unit is placed. Position the edge of the tibia sling slightly above the support bar.

Do not proceed with treatment until the nurse informs you that the physician has approved continued use of the device.

Check the patient periodically when using the CPM machine. Each time the settings are changed, stay with the patient for several cycles to be sure they tolerate the change. Check the skin every two hours for signs of redness, irritation, or breakdown. Report problems and abnormalities to the nurse.

Compartment Syndrome

Compartment syndrome is a very painful condition that occurs when pressure within the muscles builds up, preventing blood and oxygen from reaching muscles and nerves. This serious complication may develop following an injury or surgical procedure. It may also occur following athletic injuries, burns, snake bites, IV infiltration, frostbite, and musculoskeletal conditions in which there is no fracture. Patients of all ages can be affected.

Compartment syndrome is usually seen after a traumatic injury, such as a long-bone fracture. It may develop if an injury or surgical site swells after a cast has been applied. A tough membrane, called *fascia*, surrounds the muscles in the arms and legs. Fascia does not expand readily. Compartment syndrome develops gradually over several hours. Bleeding or swelling occurs in the muscle tissue, under the fascia. In some cases, pressure from a cast or compression device also increases the pressure from the outside. If the swelling is not relieved, pressure on the muscles and nerves builds. Eventually, the pressure inside the fascia compartment will exceed the blood pressure, causing the capillaries to collapse. Blood flow to the muscles and nerves stops. If it is not restored promptly, tissue death begins.

Difficult Situations

The most common location of compartment syndrome in adults is near a fractured tibia. The most common location of compartment syndrome in children is the humerus.

Signs and Symptoms

The most common symptom of acute compartment syndrome is severe pain, especially when the muscle is moved. The pain may seem out of proportion to the injury. The patient may also complain of:

- Severe pain when the muscle is gently stretched
- Tenderness when the area is touched gently
- Pain during deep breathing
- Tingling
- Burning
- Numbness
- Feeling tight or full in the affected muscle
- Abnormal sensations in the affected area
- Weakness or inability to use the muscle

You may observe that:

- The color of the extremity appears pale, cyanotic, or red.
- The skin of an extremity with no cast may feel warm to the touch.
- The fingers or toes of a casted extremity may feel cool to the touch.
- Edema (swelling) develops.

Loss of the pulse in the extremity is a late sign. Rapid identification and treatment of this condition is necessary.

Nursing Assistant Responsibilities

Follow the care plan and monitor patients who have musculoskeletal injuries and casts frequently. Monitor for changes in the extremity. Check the color and temperature of the extremity distal to a cast. Ask the patient if they are able to move the fingers or toes. If the patient complains of severe pain, or if the pain is not relieved after the patient receives pain medication, notify the nurse promptly. This condition is frightening for the patient. Provide emotional support.

Compartment syndrome is a surgical emergency. The nurse will assess the patient and notify the physician of the findings. If compartment syndrome is suspected, the patient will be taken to surgery quickly to relieve the pressure. Follow facility policies and the nurse's instructions for preparing the patient for surgery.

Ruptured or Slipped Disc

It is possible for a disc to bulge (slip) out of place or for the soft center to rupture. In either case, the misplaced

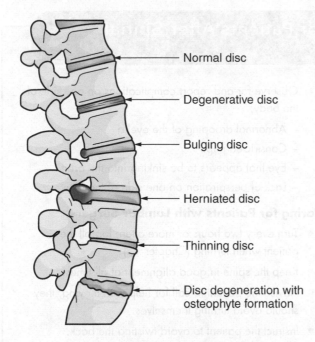

- Normal disc
- Degenerative disc
- Bulging disc
- Herniated disc
- Thinning disc
- Disc degeneration with osteophyte formation

FIGURE 41-20 When a person has a slipped disc, uneven pressure on the nerve root causes the disc to bulge. The disc is herniated (ruptured) when the pressure on the nerve root causes the gel-like center to ooze out.

disc applies pressure on the spinal nerves (Figure 41-20). Depending on which disc is injured, the patient may experience, in different parts of the body:

- Pain
- Numbness
- Tingling
- Weakness of one or more muscles

Treatment

The goal of treatment is to relieve pressure on the nerve roots. Early treatment is very conservative and includes rest, medication, ice, compresses, physical therapy, and exercise. Some people use complementary and alternative therapies, most commonly:

- Acupuncture
- Chiropractic care
- Massage
- Yoga
- Biofeedback

Other methods that may be ordered to relieve pressure on the spinal cord are:

- Traction. This is an older treatment that is seldom used.
- The physician may order a firm mattress or bed boards.
- Surgery to remove the protruding portion of the disc (**laminectomy**). The surgery sometimes includes a fixation (**fusion**) of the vertebral bones.
- A surgical procedure called **discectomy**. This is a minimally invasive procedure with rapid recovery. In this procedure, a tiny wand is inserted through the back into the disc. Tissue is removed through the wand, and the channel is thermally sealed. This may be done as an outpatient surgery in some facilities.

Lower Extremity Amputation

You may care for patients who have had one or both legs surgically removed (amputated). A leg may have to undergo **amputation** because of circulatory problems, a malignancy, or an accident in which the leg was severely damaged.

It is common for people to experience **phantom pain** after the removal of a limb. Patients with phantom pain may feel pain or tingling where the limb used to be. These feelings may persist for months or even years. The pain is real, although it is difficult to explain.

When you are positioning a patient who has had an amputation of the lower extremities, remember:

- Avoid abduction and flexion of the patient's hip. Because the weight of the lower leg is not there, the hip on the affected side will quickly become contracted if flexion is allowed.
- If the patient has a below-the-knee amputation (BKA), avoid flexion of the knee, so that a contracture does not form.
- Avoid placing pillows under the amputated extremity. Position the leg flat on the bed.
- Avoid elevating the head of the bed for prolonged periods.
- Keep the legs in a position of adduction. A trochanter roll is helpful. Avoid positioning the patient with pillows between the legs.
- Assist the patient to lie in the prone position twice a day, if permitted.
- Encourage and assist the patient to move in bed frequently.

GUIDELINES 41-2 Guidelines for Caring for Patients After Spinal Surgeries

- Monitor vital signs as ordered.
- Assist with coughing, deep breathing, and incentive spirometer treatments, as ordered.
- Monitor the dressing for bleeding and clear fluid leakage. If noted, inform the nurse promptly.
- Use the fracture bedpan for elimination.
- Inform the nurse if the patient is unable to void or voids less than 240 mL in eight hours.
- Assist with log rolling and positioning in good alignment.

Caring for Patients with Cervical Surgery

- Do not remove the cervical collar.
- Encourage the patient to keep the head straight in midline position; avoid turning to sides.
- Support the patient's head, neck, and upper shoulders when repositioning or moving from lying to sitting to standing position, and when getting into and out of a chair.

- Observe for and report complications on one side of the body:
  - Abnormal drooping of the eyelid
  - Constricted pupil
  - Eye that appears to be sinking into the orbit
  - Lack of perspiration on one side of the face

Caring for Patients with Lumbar Surgery

- Turn every two hours or more often; logroll the patient when turning (Chapter 15).
- Keep the spine in good alignment at all times.
- Advise the patient to call for help with moving; they should avoid turning themselves.
- Instruct the patient to avoid twisting the back.
- During the first postoperative week, the patient should sit in a straight-backed chair.
- Teach the patient to avoid prolonged sitting and avoid slumping.
- Remind the patient to use good body mechanics and bend from the knees and hips, not the waist.

After the surgery, the patient will either have the stump wrapped with elastic bandage or will wear a stump shrinker to make sure that the stump heals in the appropriate shape. This must be in place at all times except during the bath. It is the nurse's responsibility to apply either of these items. If you bathe a patient with an amputation:

- Gently wash the stump with soap and warm water, rinse well, and pat dry.
- Observe the stump for:
  - Redness
  - Swelling
  - Drainage from the incision
  - Open areas in the incision or anywhere else on the stump
- Do not apply lotion to the stump. Lotion softens the skin, making safe prosthesis use difficult.
- Never apply a prosthesis over unprotected skin.

🔒 Safety ALERT

Make sure that the stump shrinker, sock, or wrap is smooth, with no wrinkles or exposed skin. Inform the nurse promptly if the patient complains of throbbing under the stump shrinker. Throbbing is an indication of impaired circulation, a potentially serious complication.

After an amputation, most patients are fitted with an artificial leg (prosthesis). They must learn to walk and sit while wearing the prosthesis. A prosthesis is custom-made for the person who will be wearing it. A special health care professional measures the patient and makes the prosthesis. The physical therapist teaches the patient how to apply the prosthesis and how to use it. If you are responsible for helping a patient put on a prosthesis, be sure you know how to attach and secure it, because each device is different.

Difficult Situations

When the stump is healed and the patient prepares to use the prosthesis, the physician may order special care. This involves not shaving the stump, as shaving increases the risk of rash and irritation. Bathing of the stump may be ordered for bedtime, because warm water may increase swelling and make application of the prosthesis difficult. The physician may also order alcohol rubs to the stump several times a day to toughen the skin. Avoid powders and lotions, which soften the skin. Monitor the stump for irritation and report to the nurse, if present. The stump sock may require frequent changing to avoid wetness. The socks must be hand-washed. Muscle-strengthening exercises will be ordered to prepare the patient to lift the weight of the prosthesis.

Various types of materials are used to make prostheses. They must be cleaned regularly, and the method of cleaning depends on what materials were used to make the prosthesis.

Wipe the inside of the prosthesis daily with a damp, soapy cloth to remove sweat and body oils. Rinse with a second damp cloth. Dry the inside of the socket well. Avoid placing a damp prosthesis on a patient. Never attempt to adjust the prosthesis. Consult the nurse if you believe an adjustment is necessary.

RANGE OF MOTION

Patients who have been ill or confined to bed are not as active, so joints may not move through the normal range of motion daily. Weakness and muscle wasting from lack of use is called **atrophy**. Over time, muscles become rigid. The joints do not move as freely as they once did. Joint movement may be painful because the muscles have shortened from lack of use. When the joint moves, the muscle stretches. This causes discomfort or pain, and the patient may move even less because of it.

Contractures and deformities develop when the patient is immobile. *Contractures* are disfigurements caused by muscle shortening. They are serious, painful complications of inactivity. Contractures make caring for the patient more difficult. There is a direct relationship between contractures and pressure injuries. Patients with contractures of the knees, feet, and

ankles cannot walk. A footboard is used to prevent contractures. If permitted, placing patients in the prone position for 15 to 30 minutes daily helps stretch the muscles, which prevents contractures. Avoiding the sitting position for prolonged periods also helps prevent flexion contractures.

If patients cannot move independently, you will be responsible for exercising their joints. All patients should be exercised regularly to prevent deformities. This includes patients with no potential for rehabilitation. Like pressure injuries, contractures are much easier to prevent than to reverse. However, they can be reversed, particularly in the early stages. Reversing contractures requires a diligent effort by staff and takes a long time—much longer than it took for the contracture to develop.

Other complications of inadequate exercise are:

- Mineral loss from bones.
- Slowing of general body circulation.
- Blood clots.

Active **range-of-motion (ROM) exercises** are done by the patient during activities of daily living. **Passive range-of-motion (PROM) exercises** are performed for patients when independent movement is impossible. Passive range-of-motion exercises maintain movement and prevent deformities. They do *not* strengthen the muscles. You will perform PROM for patients with conditions such as:

- Paralysis
- Contractures
- Orthopedic conditions
- Neurologic disorders
- Severe cognitive impairment

Passive range-of-motion exercises are also ordered when active movement:

- Increases spasticity
- Causes pain
- Creates excessive stress on the heart
- Makes patients unable to move joints safely

The patient must be comfortable and relaxed during the exercises. Take each joint through the normal range of movement.

The nurse will instruct you as to the type or limitation of range-of-motion exercises to be done. Exercises are usually done during or after the bath and before the bed is made. They may be carried out at other times as well.

Precautions and Special Situations

Patients with certain conditions require special care and handling. Avoid exercising extremities with fractures or dislocations. When assisting patients with healed hip or other joint replacements, avoid internal rotation. Also avoid adduction beyond the midline. Patients with osteoporosis can sustain fractures with little or no trauma. Check with the nurse and the care plan when your patient has a special situation or osteoporosis.

If the patient has a wound or pressure injury, check to see if exercise will harm the healing tissue. If a patient is combative or resists exercise, avoid forcing them. Gently explain and demonstrate the procedure. Try to coax the patient into participating. Sometimes singing an old song will distract the patient. Encourage the patient to sing along with you. If distracted, they may allow you to perform the exercises. The patient may even have fun! Performing range-of-motion exercises in the bathtub or whirlpool may also be an option, if permitted. Notify the nurse if the patient continues to refuse.

Some patients have muscle spasms and rigidity. When exercising patients with these conditions, move the joint slowly and smoothly. Stop at the point of pain or resistance. Apply gentle, steady pressure until the muscle relaxes. Avoid rapid, jerking movements. Do not stretch the joint too far. These activities cause pain and worsen the condition. Suspect muscle spasms if resistance progressively increases during exercise. Rigidity presents as resistance to movement in any direction. Slow, continuous, sustained movements help prevent spasticity and rigidity. If rigidity and muscle spasms develop, hold steady, gentle pressure on the muscle. Avoid forcing the muscle past the point of resistance. This should enable you to complete the exercise. Report the problems to the nurse. The nurse or therapist will provide specific instructions.

⚖ Legal **ALERT**

Passive range of motion that involves the neck is usually carried out by a physical therapist or a nurse. Patients who can exercise this area themselves are encouraged to do so. Check your facility policy regarding ROM neck exercises.

GUIDELINES 41-3 Guidelines for Assisting Patients with Range-of-Motion Exercises

- Check the care plan or ask the nurse for specific guidelines and limitations.
- Explain the procedure to the patient.
- Before beginning, make sure the patient is comfortable.
- Position the patient in good body alignment, in the supine position, before beginning.
- Elevate the bed to a comfortable working height.
- Use good posture and apply the principles of good body mechanics.
- Encourage the patient to assist, if able, but keep your hands in position to provide support.
- Make sure you have enough space for full movement of the extremities.
- Expose only the part of the body you are exercising.
- Support each joint by placing one hand above and one hand below the joint.
- Move each joint slowly and consistently. Stop briefly at the end of each motion.
- Work systematically from the top of the body to the bottom.

- Never push the patient past the point of joint resistance. Move each joint only as far as it will comfortably go.
- In many facilities, the neck is not exercised without a physician's order. Know and follow your facility policy.
- Perform each joint motion 5 to 10 times, or according to the therapist's evaluation, physician's order, care plan, and facility policy.
- Stop the exercise and report to the nurse if the patient complains of pain. Watch the patient's body language and facial expression for signs of pain.
- Be alert for changes in the patient's condition during the activity. If you feel that the activity is harming the patient, stop. Notify the nurse. Changes that suggest a potential problem are pain, shortness of breath, sweating, and change in color.
- Help the patient relax during exercise.
- Use the session as quality time to communicate with the patient.
- For patients who are stiff or combative, consider doing the exercise in the bathtub or whirlpool. Check with the nurse.

PROCEDURE **87** **PERFORMING RANGE-OF-MOTION EXERCISES (PASSIVE)**

NOTE

This procedure may be carried out as an independent procedure or as part of the bath. Repeat each action 5 to 10 times, or as noted above.

1. Carry out initial procedure actions.

2. Assemble equipment:
   - Bath blanket

3. Position the patient on their back close to you.

4. Adjust the bath blanket to keep the patient covered as much as possible.

5. Supporting the elbow and wrist, exercise the shoulder joint nearest you as follows:

   a. Bring the entire arm out at a right angle to the body (horizontal abduction) (Figure 41-21).

   b. Return the arm to a position parallel to the body (horizontal adduction).

6. a. With the arm parallel to the body, roll the entire arm toward the body (internal rotation of shoulder).

   b. Maintaining the parallel position, roll the entire arm away from the body (external rotation of shoulder).

7. With the shoulder in abduction, flex the elbow and raise the entire arm over the head (shoulder flexion) (Figure 41-22).

8. With the arm parallel to the body (palm up— **supination**), flex and extend the elbow (Figures 41-23A and 41-23B).

9. Flex and extend the wrist (Figure 41-24). Flex and extend each finger joint (Figure 41-25).

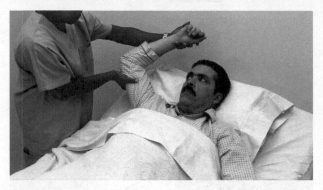

FIGURE 41-22 Shoulder flexion. With the shoulder in abduction, flex the elbow and raise the entire arm over the head.

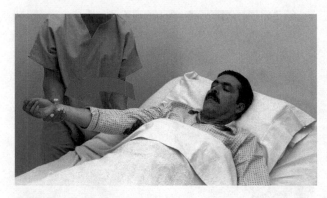

FIGURE 41-23A Elbow extension and flexion. Support the upper arm and wrist, and then straighten the elbow.

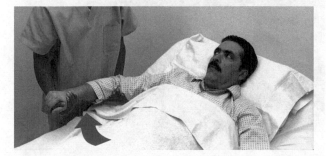

FIGURE 41-21 Shoulder abduction and adduction. Support the arm at the elbow and wrist, and then bring the entire arm out at a right angle from the body.

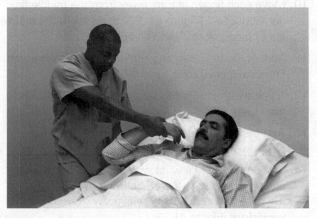

FIGURE 41-23B Flex the lower arm toward the upper arm.

(continues)

PROCEDURE **87** CONTINUED   **0**

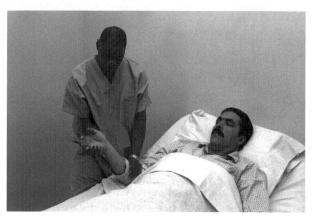

FIGURE 41-24 Wrist extension and flexion. Supporting the arm above the wrist and hand, straighten the wrist.

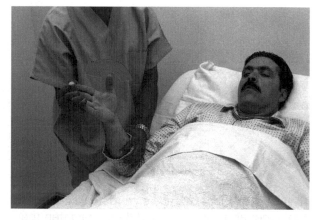

FIGURE 41-25 Finger extension. Slip the figures over the patient's flexed fingers and then straighten the fingers.

10. Move each finger, in turn, away from the middle finger (abduction) (Figure 41-26A) and toward the middle finger (adduction) (Figure 41-26B).

11. Abduct the thumb by moving it toward the extended fingers (Figure 41-27).

12. Touch the thumb to the base of the little finger, and then to each fingertip (opposition) (Figure 41-28).

13. Turn the hand palm down (**pronation**), and then palm up (supination).

14. Grasp the patient's wrist with one hand and the patient's hand with the other. Bring the wrist toward the body (**inversion**) and then away from the body (**eversion**) (Figure 41-29).

15. Point the hand in supination toward the thumb side (**radial deviation**), and then toward the little-finger side (**ulnar deviation**).

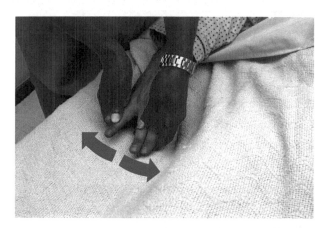

FIGURE 41-26A Abduction of the fingers.

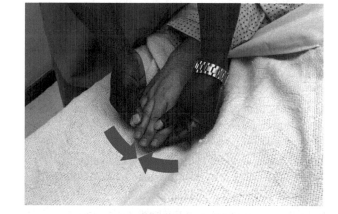

FIGURE 41-26B Adduction of the fingers.

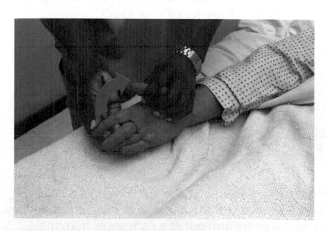

FIGURE 41-27 Abduction and adduction of the thumb and fingers. Supporting the hand, draw the thumb toward and away from the extended fingers.

(continues)

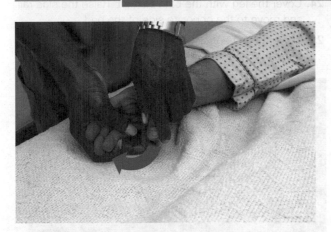

FIGURE 41-28 Thumb opposition. Supporting the hand, touch each finger with the thumb.

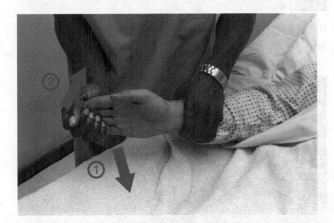

FIGURE 41-29 Wrist inversion (supination) and eversion (pronation). Grasp the patient's wrist with one hand. Grasp the patient's hand with the other hand. Bring the wrist toward the body and then away from the body.

16. Cover the patient's upper extremities and body. Expose only the leg being exercised. Face the foot of the bed.

17. Supporting the knee and ankle, move the entire leg away from the body center (abduction) (Figure 41-30) and toward the body (adduction).

18. Turn to face the bed. Supporting the knee in bent position (flexion), raise the knee toward the pelvis (hip flexion) (Figure 41-31A). Straighten the knee (extension) (Figure 41-31B), as you lower the leg to the bed.

19. a. Supporting the leg at the knee and ankle, roll the leg in a circular fashion away from the body (lateral hip rotation).

    b. Continuing to support the leg, roll the leg in the same fashion toward the body (medial hip rotation).

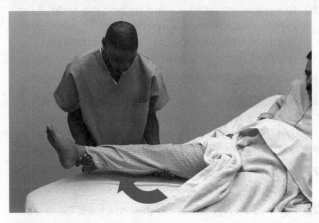

FIGURE 41-30 Abduction of the hip. Supporting the patient's knee and ankle, move the entire leg away from the center of the body.

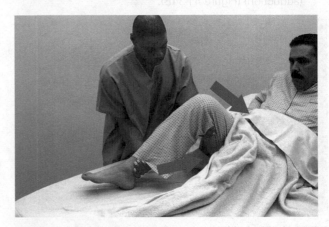

FIGURE 41-31A Hip and knee flexion. Supporting the leg, return toward the center of the body.

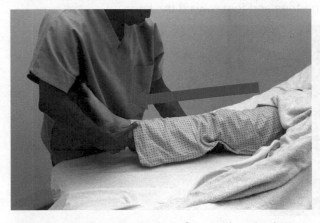

FIGURE 41-31B Knee extension. Supporting the knee and ankle, straighten the leg.

(continues)

PROCEDURE **87** **CONTINUED**   **0**

20. Grasp the patient's toes and support the ankle. Bring toes toward the knee (**dorsiflexion**) (Figure 41-32A). Then point the toes toward the foot of the bed (**plantar flexion**) (Figure 41-32B).

> ### ✎ NOTE
>
> The patient may be more comfortable if the knee is slightly flexed during this motion.

21. Gently turn the patient's foot inward (inversion) (Figure 41-33) and outward (eversion).

22. Place your fingers over the patient's toes. Bend the toes (flexion) and straighten them (extension).

23. Move each toe away from the second toe (abduction) (Figure 41-34A) and then toward the second toe (adduction) (Figure 41-34B).

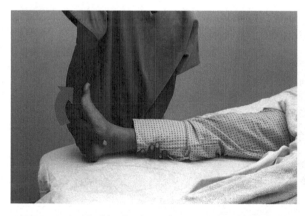

FIGURE 41-32A Ankle flexion. Grasp the patient's heel with one hand, using the upper arm to support the foot. Dorsiflex the ankle by bringing the toes and foot toward the knee.

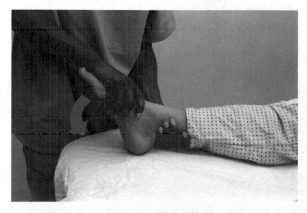

FIGURE 41-32B Plantar flex the ankle by drawing the foot into a downward position.

ICON KEY:
 = OBRA

24. Cover the leg with the bath blanket. Raise the side rail and move to the opposite side of the bed.

25. Move the patient close to you and repeat steps 5 through 23 on the other side.

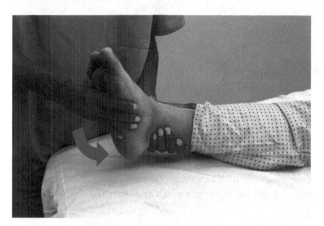

FIGURE 41-33 Foot inversion. Grasp the patient's foot and gently turn it inward.

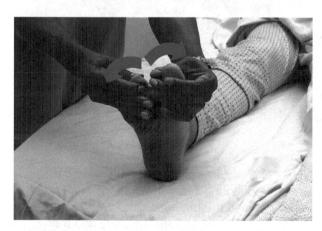

FIGURE 41-34A Toe abduction. Move each toe away from the second toe one at a time.

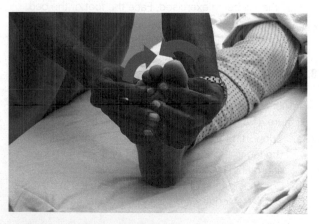

FIGURE 41-34B Toe adduction. Move each toe toward the second toe one at a time.

Observation and Reporting

Signs and symptoms of musculoskeletal system problems to make and report to the nurse are listed in Table 41-1.

DIAGNOSTIC TECHNIQUES

Some techniques used to diagnose problems of the musculoskeletal system include:

- Radiographic techniques such as X-ray.
- Electromyography (EMG) test to measure the effectiveness of muscle/nerve interaction.
- Measurements of alkaline and acid phosphatases.
- Bone marrow examination, in which a sample of the bone marrow is removed and evaluated.
- Computed tomography (CT or CAT) scan to check for bone, muscle, and joint conditions.
- Radioisotope scanning, a technique that often can detect early bone and joint changes.
- Arthroscopy for direct visualization of a joint.

TABLE 41-1 Observations to Make and Report Related to the Musculoskeletal System

- Pain when at rest
- Deformity
- Edema
- Immobility
- Inability to move arms and legs
- Inability to move one or more joints
- Limited/abnormal range of motion
- Shortening and external rotation of one leg in patient with a history of fall
- Sudden onset of falls, difficulty balancing
- Jerking, tremors, shaky movements, muscle spasms
- Weakness
- Sensory changes
- Changes in the ability to sit, stand, move, or walk
- Pain upon movement

- Magnetic resonance imaging (MRI) to show conditions of tissues around bones. This helps to diagnose tumors, a ruptured disc between two vertebrae, and other conditions.

REVIEW

A. True/False

Mark the following true or false by circling T or F.

1. T F Men have the highest risk of osteoporosis, a type of arthritis caused by abnormalities of the reproductive hormones.

2. T F If ROM exercises are not carried out faithfully, the patient's future mobility may be threatened.

3. T F When carrying out ROM exercises, always support the parts being exercised at the joint.

4. T F The nursing assistant will carry out special corrective exercises on the neck.

5. T F Aging is a contributing factor in osteoarthritis.

6. T F When the patient has a painful arthritic joint, it should be exercised vigorously.

7. T F An overbed bar (trapeze) will assist orthopedic patients to move more easily and enable them to help themselves.

8. T F A fracture is any break in a bone.

9. T F Before operating beds or attachments used with orthopedic patients, the nursing assistant must be sure of their competency to operate this equipment.

10. T F It only takes a few moments for a plaster cast to dry completely.

11. T F Patients recovering from fractured hips must be encouraged to get up and ambulate the evening after the surgery.

12. T F If a patient has an open reduction/internal fixation for a fractured hip, a cast will have been applied.

13. T F Phantom pain after an amputation is imaginary and of no concern to caregivers.

14. T F The nursing assistant is responsible for assisting patients with amputations to use the new prosthesis.

15. T F It is important to prevent contractures after an amputation.

B. Matching

Choose the correct word from Column II to match each word or phrase in Column I.

Column I

16. _____ abduction
17. _____ adduction
18. _____ alignment

19. _____ dorsiflexion
20. _____ eversion
21. _____ extension
22. _____ external rotation
23. _____ flexion
24. _____ internal rotation
25. _____ inversion
26. _____ plantar flexion
27. _____ pronation
28. _____ radial deviation
29. _____ rotation
30. _____ supination
31. _____ ulnar deviation

Column II

a. moving away from the body

b. toes pointed up

c. turning outward

d. with hand in supination, lateral movement toward the little-finger side

e. extending the foot in a downward movement

f. moving toward the body

g. extremity rolled inward

h. turning on the axis; rotating of a joint

i. decreasing the angle between two bones

j. increasing the angle between two bones

k. facing downward

l. wrists are turned toward the thumb side

m. turning inward

n. extremity rolled outward

o. position in which the body can function properly

p. facing upward

C. Multiple Choice

Select the best answer for each of the following.

32. When assigned to perform ROM, you should:
    a. exercise every joint.
    b. exercise joints to the point of pain.
    c. check for any limitations before starting.
    d. perform each exercise four times.

33. A greenstick fracture:
    a. occurs mainly in children.
    b. fragments the bone.
    c. occurs mainly in the elderly.
    d. twists around the bone.

34. While a leg cast is drying:
    a. cover it tightly so moisture will not be lost.
    b. maintaining general alignment is not important.
    c. carefully observe the extremities for circulation.
    d. use only fingertips to handle the cast.

35. When caring for a patient in traction:
    a. maintain proper alignment.
    b. lift the weights rapidly.
    c. allow weights to rest on the floor.
    d. position the patient's feet against the footboard.

36. Your patient has a ruptured disc. You should note and report:
    a. crossing of the legs.
    b. ambulation in the room.
    c. numbness and tingling.
    d. complaints of feeling tired.

37. The most common symptom of osteoarthritis is:
    a. swollen joints.
    b. pain.
    c. redness.
    d. limited mobility.

38. Gout is caused by:
    a. renal disease.
    b. hypertension.
    c. arthritic changes in aging.
    d. elevated uric acid levels in the blood.

39. When positioning a patient who has had hip replacement surgery, you should:
    a. elevate the head of the bed at least 60°.
    b. cross the legs at the ankles.
    c. avoid elevating the head more than 45°.
    d. position the hips and knees in complete flexion.

40. Compartment syndrome is a:
    a. serious surgical emergency.
    b. normal side effect of a fracture.
    c. chronic condition related to arthritis.
    d. side effect of medications.

41. Position the patient who has had a leg amputation:
    a. with both legs in abduction.
    b. with pillows between the legs.
    c. with the head elevated at least 90°.
    d. with the legs in adduction.

42. The adult human body contains:
  a. 156 bones.
  b. 206 bones.
  c. 300 bones.
  d. 406 bones.

43. The longest, strongest bone in the human body is the:
  a. humerus.
  b. fibula.
  c. femur.
  d. radius.

44. Bursae:
  a. hold bones together.
  b. support joints.
  c. help rotate joints.
  d. help reduce friction.

D. Nursing Assistant Challenge

You are assigned to care for 62-year-old Mrs. Nellie Goldstein, who had a total hip arthroplasty two days ago. She will be starting rehabilitation today and will continue her therapy as an outpatient after she is discharged to her daughter's home in three more days. Mrs. Goldstein is a very active person and is eager to be "up and moving."

45. What restrictions do you need to be aware of when taking care of Mrs. Goldstein?

  _____

  _____

  _____

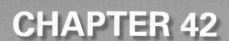

CHAPTER 42

Endocrine System

OBJECTIVES

After completing this chapter, you will be able to:

42.1 Spell and define terms.

42.2 Review the location of the endocrine system.

42.3 Explain (or Describe) the functions of the endocrine system.

42.4 List five specific diagnostic tests associated with conditions of the endocrine system.

42.5 Describe some common diseases of the endocrine system.

42.6 Recognize the signs and symptoms of hypoglycemia and hyperglycemia.

42.7 Describe nursing assistant actions related to the care of patients with disorders of the endocrine system.

42.8 Perform blood tests for glucose levels if facility policy permits.

42.9 Perform the following procedure:

- Procedure 88: Obtaining a Fingerstick Blood Sugar (Expand Your Skills)

VOCABULARY

Learn the meaning and the correct spelling of the following words and phrases:

acetone
Addison disease
adrenal glands
assimilate
Cushing syndrome
diabetes mellitus
endocrine glands
estrogen
fingerstick blood sugar
  (FSBS)
glucagon
glucose
glycated hemoglobin (A1C)
glycogen

glycosuria
gonads
hormones
hypercalcemia
hyperglycemia
hypersecretion
hyperthyroidism
hypertrophy
hypoglycemia
hyposecretion
hypothyroidism
insulin
insulin-dependent diabetes
  mellitus (IDDM)

iodine
islets of Langerhans
lancet
metabolism rate
non-insulin-dependent
  diabetes mellitus
  (NIDDM)
ovaries
ovum
parathormone
parathyroid gland
pineal body
pituitary gland
polydipsia

polyphagia
polyuria
progesterone
scrotum
simple goiter
sperm
testes
testosterone
tetany
thyrocalcitonin
thyroid gland
thyroxine

STRUCTURE AND FUNCTION

The **endocrine glands** (Figure 42-1):

- Secrete **hormones,** chemicals that regulate the body's activities.
- Control body activities and growth.
- Are found as distinct glands or clusters of cells.
- Are subject to disease that can result in **hyposecretion** (underproduction) or **hypersecretion** (overproduction) of hormones.

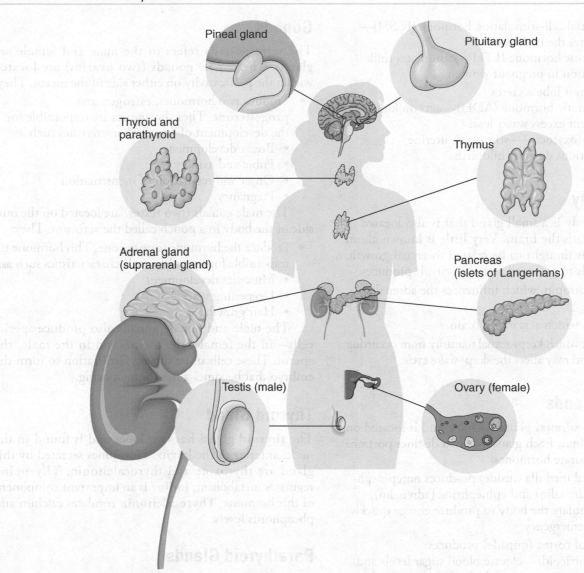

FIGURE 42-1 Endocrine system.

Labels: Pineal gland; Pituitary gland; Thyroid and parathyroid; Thymus; Adrenal gland (suprarenal gland); Pancreas (islets of Langerhans); Testis (male); Ovary (female)

Pituitary Gland

Because it controls most of the other glands, the **pituitary gland** is called the *master gland*. The pituitary gland has two portions called *lobes*. Each of the lobes secretes more than one hormone.

1. The anterior lobe secretes:
   - Somatotropic hormone (STH)—a growth hormone that stimulates the growth of long bones.
   - Thyroid-stimulating hormone (TSH)—stimulates the thyroid gland.
   - Follicle-stimulating hormone (FSH)—promotes growth of the ovarian follicle in which the egg develops during the menstrual cycle.
   - Adrenocorticotropic hormone (ACTH)—stimulates production by the adrenal glands.
   - Luteinizing hormone (LH)—in females, helps stimulate ovulation during the menstrual cycle.

Clinical Information **ALERT**

Hormones from the endocrine system travel through the bloodstream to various body sites. The human body produces more than 30 hormones to regulate such things as hunger, body temperature, stress reactions, and growth. The purpose of some hormones is to stimulate other glands to secrete their own hormones. Regardless of external factors, hormones are responsible for regulating organ function and normalizing the body, keeping it in a balanced, normal state. Of the glands in the endocrine system, the adrenal glands produce the greatest number of hormones. The parathyroids are the smallest endocrine glands (there are four of these), and the largest pure endocrine gland is the thyroid. The thymus is the largest at birth.

- Interstitial cell-stimulating hormone (ICSH)—stimulates the male testes.
- Lactogenic hormone (LTH)—stimulates milk production in pregnant women.
2. The posterior lobe secretes:
   - Antidiuretic hormone (ADH)—acts on kidneys to prevent excess water loss.
   - Pitocin (oxytocin)—stimulates uterine contractions during childbirth.

Pineal Body

The **pineal body** is a small gland that is also located in the skull beneath the brain. Very little is known about this gland. It is thought to be related to sexual growth, because it tends to get smaller at maturity. It produces:

- Glomerulotropin, which influences the adrenal gland.
- Serotonin, which acts in the brain.
- Melatonin, which keeps sexual maturity from occurring too early and may affect the sleep–wake cycle.

Adrenal Glands

There are two **adrenal glands**. One gland is located on top of each kidney. Each gland has two distinct portions that secrete separate hormones.

1. The adrenal medulla (inside) produces norepinephrine (noradrenalin) and epinephrine (adrenalin), which stimulate the body to produce energy quickly during an emergency.
2. The adrenal cortex (outside) produces:
   - Glucocorticoids—elevate blood sugar levels and control the response of the body to stress and inflammation. They also depress inflammation.
   - Mineral corticoids—manage sodium and potassium levels.
   - Gonadocorticoids—influence both male and female sex hormones.

Clinical Information **ALERT**

The adrenal glands are responsible for the "fight-or-flight" stress reaction when we perceive a threat. In this reaction, adrenalin flows throughout the body, causing changes that the body needs to react quickly for possible defense. The senses sharpen, so you feel more alert. The pupils dilate, enabling you to see more clearly. Hairs stand on end; heart rate and respirations increase. Blood supply to the muscles increases and blood flow to nonessential organs is reduced.

Gonads

The term **gonads** refers to the male and female sex glands. The female gonads (two **ovaries**) are located within the pelvic cavity on either side of the uterus. They:

- Produce two hormones, **estrogen** and **progesterone**. These hormones are responsible for the development of female characteristics such as:
  - Breast development
  - Pubic and axillary hair
  - Onset and regulation of menstruation
  - Pregnancy

The male gonads (two **testes**) are located on the outside of the body in a pouch called the **scrotum**. They:

- Produce the hormone **testosterone**. This hormone is responsible for secondary male characteristics such as:
  - Muscular development
  - Deepening voice
  - Hair growth

The male and female gonads also produce special cells—in the female, the **ovum**, and in the male, the **sperm**. These cells unite during fertilization to form the embryo that becomes a new human being.

Thyroid Gland

The **thyroid gland** has two lobes and is found in the neck, anterior to the larynx. Hormones secreted by this gland are thyroxine and thyrocalcitonin. **Thyroxine** regulates metabolism. **Iodine** is an important component of this hormone. **Thyrocalcitonin** regulates calcium and phosphorus levels.

Parathyroid Glands

The tiny **parathyroid glands** are embedded in the posterior thyroid gland. The hormone they manufacture is called parathormone. **Parathormone** helps control the body's use of two minerals, calcium and phosphorus. Insufficient amounts of calcium result in severe muscle spasms or **tetany**. Untreated tetany can lead to death.

Islets of Langerhans

The **islets of Langerhans** are small groups of cells found within the pancreas. These cells produce two hormones: insulin and glucagon. **Insulin** lowers blood sugar. **Glucagon** elevates blood sugar.

AGING CHANGES TO THE ENDOCRINE SYSTEM

Aging changes to the endocrine system include:

- Increased blood sugar level caused by delayed release of insulin, a hormone that regulates sugar use in the body.

- Lower **metabolism rate**, or slower body function, which reduces the amount of calories needed for the body to function normally.
- Changes in the way that hormones control body systems. Some tissues become less sensitive to their controlling hormone. The total amount of hormone production may change, but this is highly variable. Blood levels of some hormones increase, some decrease, and some will be unchanged. Hormones are also broken down more slowly.

COMMON CONDITIONS OF THE THYROID GLAND

The thyroid gland may secrete too much or not enough hormones. Either situation is treatable. If not treated, severe illness or death will occur.

Hyperthyroidism

Hyperthyroidism, or overactivity of the thyroid gland, results in production of too much thyroxine (hypersecretion). The person shows:

- Irritability and restlessness
- Nervousness
- Rapid pulse
- Increased appetite
- Weight loss
- Sensitivity

Nursing Assistant Actions

When caring for these patients, the nursing assistant must be understanding and have patience. Keep the room quiet and cool. Meet the patient's increased nutritional needs by serving foods that they like.

Treatment

Treatment of hyperthyroidism is designed to reduce the level of thyroxine through:

- Surgical thyroidectomy.
- Radiation to reduce the number of functional cells.

Thyroidectomy

It may be necessary to treat hyperthyroidism with surgery. If you will be assisting with postoperative care, you will:

- Position the patient in a semi-Fowler's position, with neck and shoulders well supported. Support the back of the neck at all times. Avoid hyperextension of the neck, which may damage the operative site.
- Assist with oxygen, if ordered, using all oxygen precautions.

- Give routine postoperative care.
- Check for and report:
  - Any signs of bleeding (this may drain toward the back of the neck). Check the pillows behind the patient, as well as the dressings.
  - Signs of respiratory distress.
  - Inability of the patient to speak. Initial hoarseness is common, but report any increase in speech problems.
  - Greatly elevated temperature and pulse, pronounced apprehension, or irritability.
  - Numbness, tingling, or muscular spasm (tetany) of the extremities.

Hypothyroidism

Hypothyroidism results in an undersecretion of thyroxine. Recall that iodine is an essential component of thyroxine. A lack of iodine in the diet can result in low thyroxine production.

- The condition is called **simple goiter**.
- The thyroid gland enlarges (**hypertrophies**).
- Secretions produced have low thyroxine content.

Hypothyroidism can usually be successfully managed with thyroxine replacement.

Observation and Reporting

Signs and symptoms of thyroid problems to observe and report are listed in Table 42-1.

TABLE 42-1 Observations of Thyroid Problems to Make and Report

Hyperthyroidism	Hypothyroidism
Increased appetite	Decreased appetite, loss of appetite
Intolerance to heat	Intolerance to cold
Elevated body temperature	Low body temperature
Weight loss despite increased appetite	Weight gain despite loss of appetite
Tachycardia	Bradycardia
Moderate hypertension	Hypotension
Irritability	Lethargy, sleepiness
Restlessness	Pale, cool, dry skin
Nervousness	Face appears puffy
Anxiety	Hair coarse
Insomnia	Nails thick and hard
Tremors	Heavy menses
Flushed, warm, moist skin	May be unable to conceive
Irregular or scant menses	If pregnant, loss of fetus possible

COMMON CONDITIONS OF THE PARATHYROID GLANDS

Parathormone, secreted by the parathyroid glands, regulates the levels of electrolytes, calcium, and phosphates. Hypersecretion of this hormone results in:

- Excessively high levels of blood calcium (**hypercalcemia**)
- Development of renal calculi (kidney stones)
- Loss of bone calcium

Hypersecretion is usually caused by tumors. Tumors can be treated by surgical removal.

Hyposecretion can lead to:

- Abnormal muscle-nerve interaction
- Severe muscle spasm (tetany)

Tetany can be an emergency situation, requiring management of the muscle spasms and administration of calcium. In the chronic state, calcium replacements and increased dietary calcium are prescribed.

COMMON CONDITIONS OF THE ADRENAL GLANDS

Adrenal gland secretions regulate:

- Development and maintenance of sexual characteristics
- Carbohydrate, fat, and protein metabolism
- Fluid balance
- Electrolyte levels of sodium and potassium

Hypersecretion results in **Cushing syndrome**, which is characterized by:

- Weakness due to loss of body protein
- Increased blood sugar levels (hyperglycemia)
- Edema
- Hypertension
- Loss of potassium and retention of sodium
- Masculinization of a female

Therapy is primarily surgical and supportive.
Hyposecretion results in **Addison disease**, which is characterized by:

- Loss of sodium and retention of potassium
- Abnormally low blood sugar (hypoglycemia)
- Dehydration
- Low stress tolerance

Addison disease is treated by hormone replacement therapy and techniques to combat dehydration.

DIABETES MELLITUS

Most cases of diabetes (about 95 percent) are type 2. Approximately 9.4 percent of the U.S. population (30.3 million) had diabetes in 2015. Of these, 23.8 percent (7.2 million) did not have or did not report having been diagnosed with diabetes. Diabetes occurs in people of all ages and races but is most common in African Americans/Blacks, Native Americans, Latinx, Asian Americans, Alaska Natives, and Pacific Islanders. The incidence of diabetes increases with age.

Diabetes mellitus is a chronic disease that results from a deficiency of insulin or a resistance to the effects of insulin. The problems with insulin cause the body to be unable to properly process food into energy. The glucose from the food breakdown remains in the blood, resulting in elevated blood sugar. Persistent, elevated glucose levels affect the blood vessels and nerves, making the person with diabetes more likely to develop heart attack, stroke, blindness, renal disease, and other serious complications and conditions.

The reason diabetes develops is not fully understood. Factors that seem to play a role in the incidence of diabetes are:

- Heredity
- Obesity
- Age
- Diet
- Lack of exercise

All people with diabetes should wear or carry a medical alert identification so that proper and immediate care can be provided in an emergency. People with diabetes are also advised to carry food that provides a quick source of carbohydrates.

Disease Mechanism

In diabetes, the normal metabolism of fats, carbohydrates, and proteins is unbalanced. Normally, when carbohydrates are absorbed into the bloodstream, the blood sugar (glucose) level rises. The pancreas responds to an increase in **glucose** by secreting more insulin. Insulin is the hormone primarily responsible for:

- Lowering the blood sugar level by allowing glucose to cross the cell membrane.

Clinical Information ALERT

Almost 1 in 20 people worldwide have diabetes. Approximately 2,000 cases are diagnosed every day. Before developing type 2 diabetes, most people develop a condition called *prediabetes*. In this condition, the blood glucose is higher than normal, but not high enough to be called diabetes. Damage to the body associated with diabetes may be caused in this stage. People with prediabetes may be able to delay or prevent development of type 2 diabetes through diet and exercise.

- Increasing the oxidation of glucose by the tissues.
- Stimulating the conversion of glucose to glycogen by the liver. **Glycogen** is a storage form of energy.
- Decreasing glucose production from amino acids.
- Stimulating the transformation of glucose into fat for storage.

In diabetes, there is insufficient insulin for these metabolic functions.

- Glucose cannot be properly utilized for energy.
- Fats and proteins are incompletely broken down. This leads to an accumulation of ketone bodies and nitrogenous waste products.
- The excess glucose is eliminated, along with water and salts, through the kidneys. This causes dehydration and electrolyte imbalance.
- The characteristic symptoms of excessive thirst, hunger, and increased urination are directly related to the loss of fluids, electrolytes, and sugar.

Types of Diabetes Mellitus

Diabetes mellitus is typed and named according to the need for insulin. The two main types are insulin-dependent diabetes mellitus (IDDM) and non-insulin-dependent diabetes mellitus (NIDDM). IDDM appears more commonly in the young, and NIDDM is more common in older people.

Insulin-dependent diabetes mellitus (IDDM) (type 1) accounts for approximately 5 to 10 percent of diabetes cases. This type tends to run in families. It is most commonly diagnosed in children and young adults. Initial symptoms may mimic the flu in young children. People with type 1 diabetes must take daily insulin injections to stay alive. Typical signs and symptoms are:

- **Polyuria**—excessive urination
- **Polydipsia**—excessive thirst
- **Polyphagia**—excessive hunger
- **Glycosuria**—sugar in the urine

Non-insulin-dependent diabetes mellitus (NIDDM) (type 2) is a metabolic disorder that occurs when the body does not make enough insulin, or does not properly use insulin. This is the most common form of diabetes and accounts for 90 to 95 percent of all diabetes cases. It is said to be nearing epidemic proportions due to the high incidence of obesity and sedentary lifestyles. Type 2 diabetes was once seen only in adults. Over the past few decades, the incidence has risen dramatically in young people. More than 26.9 percent of the population aged 65 and older now has diabetes.

People may not be aware they have the condition until symptoms become severe or complications develop. The risk for type 2 diabetes increases with age. Common signs and symptoms of type 2 diabetes are:

- Easy fatigue
- Skin infections
- Slow healing
- Itching
- Pruritus vulvae (itching of the vulva)
- Burning on urination
- Vision changes
- Obesity
- Weight loss

Often only one or two symptoms are apparent in elderly persons. An older person may:

- Complain of constant fatigue.
- Have a skin lesion that takes an unusually long time to heal.
- Experience vision changes that may be mistakenly attributed to aging.

Care of the person with diabetes is directed toward maintaining a normal blood glucose level so that complications may be prevented. To regulate blood glucose, the person with diabetes must:

- Eat a healthful, well-balanced diet as prescribed by the physician.
- Exercise regularly in a manner appropriate for the person's age and ability.
- Check the blood sugar regularly.
- Use insulin or oral antidiabetic agents correctly if ordered by the physician.

For some persons, this may require lifestyle changes. Nurses and dietitians are responsible for teaching patients who are newly diagnosed with diabetes how to care for themselves. People with diabetes who are knowledgeable about the disease and who are willing to manage their lives accordingly can live happily and productively (Figure 42-2).

Illness

High blood sugar increases the risk of infection, slows healing, and can lead to complications. Blood sugar levels often increase during illness and after injury due to stress. Some people are admitted to the hospital with high blood sugar, or their glucose increases during hospitalization. Some medications and decreased physical activity also contribute to elevated blood sugar.

Diet

Blood sugar control forms the basis of treatment for diabetes. Diet is an important part of this treatment. Physicians do not fully agree as to how strictly a diet must be followed by all patients. The American Diabetes Association (ADA) recommends that a consistent-carbohydrate

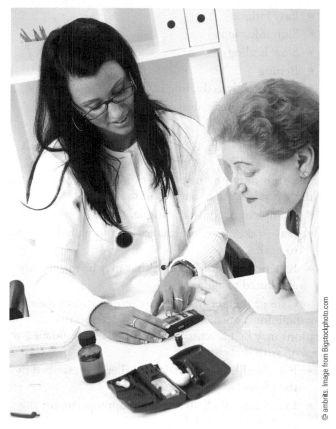

FIGURE 42-2 A patient is instructed by a nurse on ways to manage diabetes.

diet (Chapter 26) be served to persons with diabetes who are hospitalized. It does not endorse any special diets, calorie counts, or meal plan.

- Weight reduction is favored.
- Weight reduction alone may be sufficient to bring the condition under control in NIDDM.

Meal Planning

The dietitian is a key member of the health care team for patients with diabetes. The dietitian helps the person plan meals in keeping with the person's goals, lifestyle, laboratory values, caloric and nutritional needs, and food preferences. Refer to Chapters 26 and 35 for information about diabetic diets.

The American Diabetes Association and U.S. Department of Agriculture (USDA) promote balancing food intake with physical activity. Such a balance is essential in promoting health, including the prevention of diabetes and its complications. The Diabetes Prevention Program (DPP) proved that type 2 diabetes can be prevented or delayed by keeping weight under control and by increasing physical activity.

The goals of the diet include maintaining near-normal blood sugar, optimal fat levels, and adequate calories based on individual needs. Meal plans are flexible. The diet should be well balanced, with sufficient fiber.

Exercise

Exercise (Figure 42-3) is an important part of the overall treatment. The amount and type of exercise the patient routinely engages in are balanced by the food intake and insulin or hypoglycemic drug requirements.

Hypoglycemic Drugs

Diabetes mellitus is treated by one of two main drug groups. One is insulin(s) administered by injection. The other is given orally.

At present, there are several types of insulin. They vary in:

- Speed of action
- Duration of action
- Potency or strength
  Insulin is:
- Administered by the nurse. The nurse rotates the administration sites.
- Given by injection.
- Increasingly given through use of an insulin pump. The insulin pump delivers a prescribed amount of insulin on a regular basis into the patient's body.
- Used to treat IDDM and some patients with NIDDM.

Persons living at home are taught to administer their own insulin.

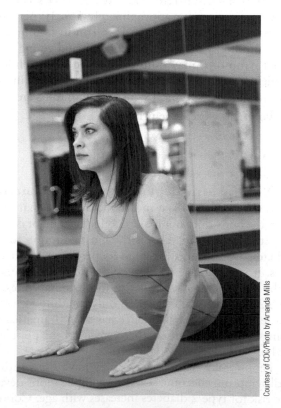

FIGURE 42-3 Exercise helps balance food intake and diabetic medication requirements.

NOTE

When insulin is self-administered, it is important to report any missed injections or signs of infection around the administration site.

Oral hypoglycemic drugs are:

- Administered by the nurse
- Given by mouth
- Used to treat NIDDM

Some people use CAM therapy to treat diabetes. Products such as chromium, magnesium, brewer's yeast, and vanadium are common alternatives. Several herbs are also used, but little is known about their long-term safety. Currently, there are no formal recommendations for the use of alternatives.

Complications

Because persistently high glucose levels cause damage to the nerves and blood vessels, the following complications can occur:

- Renal disease
- Circulatory impairments that often result in gangrene (Figure 42-4) and amputation
- Poor healing
- Hypertension
- Cardiovascular problems
- Diabetic coma
- Vision problems and blindness

Hypoglycemia (Low Blood Sugar)

Hypoglycemia occurs when the blood glucose level is below normal. It:

- May occur rapidly.
- Is referred to as *insulin reaction* or *insulin shock* when due to an overdose of insulin.
  Hypoglycemia can be brought on by:
- Skipping meals, not eating enough food, Omission of planned snacks or meals
- Unusual activity
- Stress

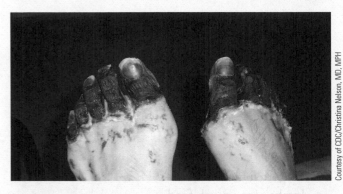

FIGURE 42-4 A small injury can cause gangrene, resulting in the loss of body parts.

- Vomiting
- Diarrhea
- Interaction of drugs
- Too much insulin or antidiabetic medication

Signs and Symptoms

The signs and symptoms of hypoglycemia include:

- Complaints of hunger, weakness, dizziness, shakiness
- Skin cold, moist, clammy, pale
- Rapid, shallow respirations
- Nervousness and excitement
- Rapid pulse
- Unconsciousness
- No sugar in the urine
- Low blood sugar test results

If the patient is awake and alert, treatment includes intake of orange juice, milk, or another easily absorbed carbohydrate such as hard candy. If the patient is unconscious, the physician or nurse may give an injection of glucagon, which causes a rapid elevation of blood sugar. A glucose paste can be rubbed on the mucous membranes of the mouth; from there it is quickly absorbed into the bloodstream.

Hyperglycemia (High Blood Sugar)

Hyperglycemia (diabetic coma):

- Occurs when there is insufficient insulin for metabolic needs.

Difficult Situations

Persons with diabetes are at very high risk for skin breakdown and pressure injuries. Pressure injuries on the feet can be very serious, eventually leading to amputation. Pay close attention to risk factors. Relieve pressure from the feet and check the feet each day for abnormalities.

- Usually develops slowly, sometimes over a 24-hour period.
- May be seen as confusion, drowsiness, or a slow slippage into coma in a patient who is confined to bed. Hyperglycemia may be brought on by:
- Stress.
- Illness such as infection.
- Dehydration.
- Injury.
- Forgotten medication.
- Intake of too much food.

Signs and Symptoms

The signs and symptoms of diabetic coma include:
- Early headache, drowsiness, or confusion
- Sweet, fruity odor to the breath
- Deep breathing, labored respirations
- Full, bounding pulse
- Low blood pressure
- Nausea or vomiting
- Flushed, dry, hot skin
- Weakness
- Unconsciousness
- Sugar in the urine
- High blood sugar test results

Treatment includes administration of insulin, fluids, and electrolytes.

Other Complications

Persons with diabetes should have regular health monitoring so that complications may be detected early and treated promptly. Health monitoring should include:
- Eye examinations by an ophthalmologist for early detection of diabetic retinopathy, which can lead to impaired vision and eventually blindness
- Urinalysis and other urological examinations to evaluate the condition of the kidneys
- Cardiac evaluation; monitoring of heart action and blood pressure
- Circulatory evaluation
- Care and treatment of any wounds
- Blood sugar monitoring
- Regular tooth cleaning and evaluation by a dental professional

Nursing Assistant Responsibilities

When caring for patients with diabetes, you should:
- Know the signs of insulin shock and diabetic coma.
- Be alert for the signs of diabetic coma or insulin shock and report them immediately to the nurse.
- Know the storage location of orange juice or other easily **assimilated** (absorbed) sources of carbohydrates.
- Keep easily assimilated carbohydrates, such as orange juice, crackers, hard candy, or Karo syrup, available if caring for a patient with diabetes at home.
- Make sure you serve the patient proper trays of food.
- Do not give extra nourishments without permission.
- Document food consumption on the patient's chart, and report uneaten meals to the nurse (Figure 42-5).
- Give special attention to care of the feet of a patient with diabetes.
  - Wash daily, carefully drying between toes.
  - Inspect feet closely for any breaks or signs of irritation. Check every two to four hours if the person wears anti-embolism hosiery.
  - Report any abnormalities to the nurse.

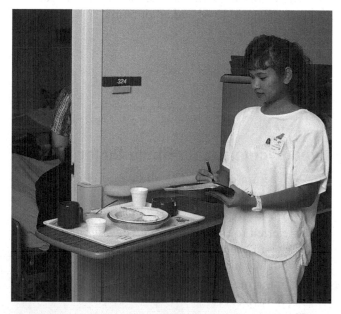

FIGURE 42-5 The amount and type of food consumed by a patient with diabetes is closely monitored and documented.

Difficult Situations

People with diabetes need to pay special attention to care of the teeth. A 2005 study showed that periodontal disease was a strong predictor of mortality from heart disease and kidney disease.

Difficult Situations

Attention to personal hygiene, oral care, and cleanliness is particularly important in individuals with diabetes. They must bathe regularly to prevent localized skin infections. However, they should avoid prolonged soaking in a tub, which can soften the tissues and lead to breakdown. If you observe unusual areas, such as yellowish pimples or boils on the skin of a patient with diabetes, or red areas in skin folds (such as under the breasts, underarms, or groin), inform the nurse. Assist the patient with toothbrushing and flossing. The teeth have five surfaces, and toothbrushing only reaches three. Flossing effectively cleans the areas that are not accessible with the brush. Good foot care and drying well between the toes are essential. Report signs and symptoms of infection, even if they seem minor.

- Do not allow moisture to collect between toes.
- The toenails should be cut only by a nurse or a podiatrist.
- Shoes and stockings should be clean, be free of holes, and fit well. Anything that might injure the feet or interfere with the circulation must be avoided.
- Do not allow the patient to go barefoot or to wear shoes without socks.

Inform the nurse of:
- Inadequate food intake
- Eating food not allowed on diet
- Refusal of meals, supplements, or snacks
- Nausea, vomiting, or diarrhea
- Inadequate fluid intake
- Excessive activity
- Complaints of dizziness, shakiness, racing heart
- Blood sugar values outside of normal range

DIAGNOSTIC TECHNIQUES

Techniques used to diagnose problems of the endocrine system include:
- Blood analysis for hormone levels
- Urine analysis for hormone levels
- Radioisotope scanning for thyroid disease
- Radioactive iodine uptake testing for thyroid function
- Basal metabolic rate (BMR) testing to measure the speed of oxygen uptake

BLOOD GLUCOSE MONITORING

Blood glucose levels are monitored both over a period of time and for immediate current values.

Glycated Hemoglobin

Glycated hemoglobin (A1C) is a term used to describe a series of stable minor hemoglobin components formed from hemoglobin and glucose. It is commonly called A1C. The A1C test is a measurement of glucose levels in the blood over a prolonged period of time. It differs from the fingerstick blood sugar test because it provides a snapshot of the patient's diabetic control over the past two to three months. The percentage of A1C in whole blood is approximately:

- 50 percent from the most recent 30 days
- 25 percent from the previous 30 to 60 days
- 25 percent from the previous 60 to 90 days

The A1C test is not a screening test. It is used only for testing ongoing glucose control in persons who have been diagnosed with diabetes. Regular testing helps predict the risk for development of many serious, chronic complications. The ADA recommends A1C testing twice a year for patients who are meeting treatment goals, and four times a year for persons who are not meeting goals or those who need more intensive monitoring. Home testing kits are now available. Single-use, disposable kits are also being used in physicians' offices, and as a point-of-care bedside test in the hospital and long-term care facility.

Having the A1C profile information enables the physician to evaluate the patient's control; order additional diagnostic tests, if necessary; regulate medications; and establish a monitoring routine. Patient teaching is a very important part of care. Knowing the degree of diabetic control enables the nurse and certified diabetes educator to plan and provide specific patient teaching targeted toward good control. The information helps the dietitian assist the patient with diet management, food preparation, and methods of meeting individual dietary wants and needs.

Bedside glucose testing has become very common in the management of patients with diabetes. Many individuals perform this testing at home several times each day. The antidiabetic medication may be adjusted according to the patient's blood sugar. A blood sample is taken from a capillary and inserted into a meter. The test meter will display the blood sugar value in one minute or less. This is a convenient, accurate method of monitoring. Nursing assistants perform this procedure in some facilities. Know and follow your facility's policy.

Safety **ALERT**

In 2005, the U.S. Food and Drug Administration issued a warning that in some cases, mistaken blood glucose readings have resulted in the blood sugar of people with diabetes becoming dangerously high. This occurred because the meters were accidentally set to report the blood sugar level in the foreign standard of units, millimoles per liter, instead of milligrams per deciliter, which is the measurement value used in the United States. The switch can occur:

- When the time and date on the meter are set.
- If the meter is dropped.
- During battery replacement.

Make sure the meter you are using is set for the correct value.

Infection Control **ALERT**

The CDC has had reports of multiple incidents of hepatitis B infection as a result of shared blood glucose meters in health care facilities. Other diseases may also be spread in this manner, such as hepatitis C and human immunodeficiency virus, the virus that causes AIDS. These viruses are stable on environmental surfaces at room temperature, and infected patients often have no symptoms. Because of this, viruses may easily be passed to workers and other patients if improper techniques are used. This emphasizes the need for education, use of standard precautions, and careful monitoring of diabetes care procedures in all health care settings.

Some hospitals issue a new, individual glucose meter to each patient who requires periodic blood glucose monitoring. Blood glucose is regularly checked on patients with diabetes and those receiving high-dose steroids. The glucose meter is discarded or the person takes it home upon hospital discharge. All facilities have policies and procedures for disinfecting meters that are to be reused after each use. Learn your facility's policies and take your responsibility for cleaning the equipment very seriously.

The physician will order specific times for blood sugar testing. The specimen may be collected at a fixed time, such as before meals. The nurse may administer insulin based on the blood sugar value. Collect the capillary sample exactly as ordered. Specimens must be collected at the right time for accurate results. Always report the value to the nurse, and document according to facility policy.

Fingerstick Blood Sugar

A **lancet** is a tiny needle used for collecting a capillary blood sample for **fingerstick blood sugar (FSBS)** testing. The blood is transferred to a test strip. For most reagent strips, you must place a hanging drop of blood onto the reagent pad. Avoid smearing the strip against the finger. The Multistix (Figure 42-6) and Chemstrip BG can be read visually, by comparing the color on the reagent strip with the key on the bottle.

Many new meters do not use a reagent strip. A test strip is inserted into the meter before beginning. The finger is pierced with the lancet and the blood is drawn into the tip of the test strip on contact. An audible beep sounds when the tube has collected enough blood.

Many different blood glucose meters are available. All are accurate and simple to use. Each meter has its own reagent or test strip. For accuracy, make sure the strip is compatible with the meter you are using. Also, check the expiration date on the bottle or package. Do not use strips that are beyond the expiration date. Follow the directions for the meter and reagent strips you are using. All are slightly different.

Many different lancets are also available for performing blood glucose checks. Retractable lancets, which are spring-loaded, have the lowest incidence of injury. The needle withdraws after the finger has been punctured, reducing the chance of needlestick injuries. Discard lancets into a puncture-resistant sharps container. Many health care workers have been injured by lancets that were inadvertently dropped in the bed or on the floor.

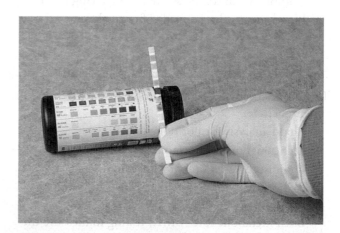

FIGURE 42-6 Multistix are used for many different blood tests.

The blood sugar values that the health care facility considers normal vary by facility. The normal fasting range in most facilities is somewhere between 65 and 120, with the normal value commonly being 70 to 110. Values below 70 suggest hypoglycemia. Fasting values above 110 suggest hyperglycemia. Learn the normal values for your facility. Values that are well above or below

Infection Control **ALERT**

When doing a fingerstick test, ask the patient to wash their hands under warm, running water and then dry them. This reduces the risk of infection and increases blood flow to the hand. After piercing the skin with the lancet, squeeze lightly. Avoid prolonged pressure, as this may cause incorrect results by introducing tissue fluids. The fingerstick should be deep enough so that hard pressure is not required. If gentle pressure is not effective in starting blood flow, repeat the puncture in a different location.

Difficult Situations

Ketone bodies are created when body fat, instead of sugar, is burned for fuel. The ketone bodies cause a chemical imbalance, resulting in accumulation of acids and upset of the patient's buffer system. If a patient's blood sugar is over 250 mg/dL, the nurse may instruct you to check the patient's urine for ketones. If the patient is very ill, the nurse may request a ketone test even if the blood sugar is not high.

the normal range suggest diabetic complications. Notify the nurse immediately of blood sugar values outside of the normal range or of other potential problems, such as:

- Inadequate food intake
- Eating food not permitted on the patient's diet
- Refusal of meals, supplements, or snacks
- Nausea, vomiting, or diarrhea
- Inadequate fluid intake
- Excessive activity
- Complaints of dizziness, shakiness, racing heart
- Abnormal vital signs

Some blood glucose meters have a narrow range. Typically, handheld blood glucose meters will read a blood sugar value as low as 40. A few measure blood sugars as low as 20. For values below the lowest meter reading, the screen will display the word *low*. On the high end, most meters do not read values above 400 or 500. If the FSBS exceeds the meter capacity, the display will read *high*. If the screen displays the word *low* or *high*, the patient's condition may deteriorate quickly. Inform the nurse immediately.

Acetone Monitoring

You may be expected to test the patient's urine for acetone. **Acetone** is a substance that accumulates in the body when the blood glucose is out of balance. A simple urine test detects the presence of acetone. Some blood glucose meters also check for ketones in the blood. However, urine monitoring is usually done by using a reagent strip when the ketone level must be measured.

EXPAND YOUR SKILLS

PROCEDURE **88** OBTAINING A FINGERSTICK BLOOD SUGAR

 Legal **ALERT**

Be sure this is a nursing assistant procedure in your facility.

 NOTE

This procedure is generic and applies the principles used for most blood glucose meters. Follow the directions for the meter and strip you are using. The operating directions are slightly different for each.

1. Carry out initial procedure actions.

2. Assemble equipment:
- Disposable exam gloves
- Alcohol sponge
- Lancet
- Blood glucose meter
- Reagent strip or test strip for the blood glucose meter being used
- Sharps container
- Plastic bandage strip
- Plastic bag for used supplies
- Disinfectant wipes or other supplies to clean the meter according to facility protocol

(continues)

PROCEDURE **88** CONTINUED

3. Wipe the patient's finger with the alcohol sponge. Allow the alcohol to dry.

4. Pierce either side of the middle or ring finger using the lancet (Figure 42-7A).

5. Discard the lancet in the sharps container.

6. Squeeze the sides of the finger gently to obtain a drop of blood.

7. Hold the puncture site directly over the reagent strip, and place a hanging drop of blood onto the reagent pad. If using capillary tube (straw-like) strips, peel the package back to open it. Hold the package firmly with your thumb and forefinger over the test end (patient end) of the strip. Insert the strip into the meter (Figure 42-7B). Remove and discard the package. Hold the strip next to the puncture site to draw blood into the straw (Figure 42-7C).

8. Insert the strip into the meter, if this was not done previously.

9. Wipe the patient's finger with the alcohol sponge. Apply pressure until bleeding stops. Then allow the finger to dry. Apply a bandage strip, if necessary.

10. Wait the designated period of time for the meter you are using. An audible beep will indicate when the blood sugar value is displayed on the screen (Figure 42-7D). Read and document this result.

11. Carry out ending procedure actions.

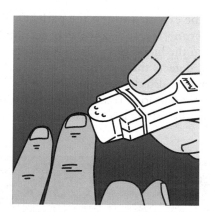

FIGURE 42-7A Pierce the side of a finger with the lancet.

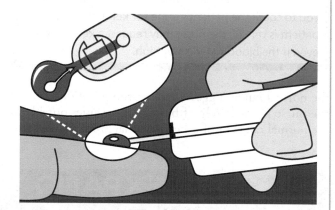

FIGURE 42-7C This strip is like a straw that will draw blood into the base.

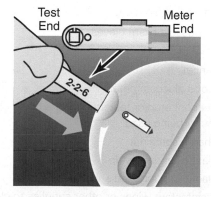

FIGURE 42-7B Insert the strip in the meter.

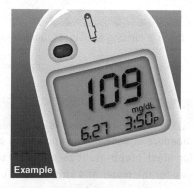

FIGURE 42-7D Read the meter after the designated period of time.

ICON KEY:
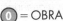 = OBRA

REVIEW

A. True/False

Mark the following true or false by circling T or F.

1. T F   A person with polyphagia has a high urine output.

2. T F   In type 2 diabetes, the body does not make enough insulin, or does not properly use insulin.

3. T F   Glucose is another name for blood sugar.

4. T F   A person with hyperthyroidism is slow-moving and lethargic.

5. T F   Hyperthyroidism causes people to lose weight.

6. T F   You should keep the room of a patient with hyperthyroidism quite warm.

7. T F   Obesity may play a role in the incidence of diabetes mellitus.

8. T F   If a patient with IDDM appears drowsy and confused, you should suspect the possibility of hyperglycemia.

9. T F   Foot care is especially important for a patient with diabetes.

10. T F   Disposable gloves should be worn when testing urine for ketones.

B. Matching

Choose the correct item from Column II to match each word or phrase in Column I.

Column I

11. _____   chemical messenger
12. _____   diabetic coma
13. _____   excessive thirst
14. _____   sugar in urine
15. _____   produces hormones
16. _____   excessive hunger
17. _____   blood sugar
18. _____   overweight
19. _____   master gland
20. _____   located above kidneys

Column II

a. polydipsia
b. polyphagia
c. glycosuria
d. endocrine gland
e. hormone
f. obesity
g. hyperglycemia
h. glucose
i. adrenal glands
j. pituitary gland

C. Multiple Choice

Select the best answer for each of the following.

21. Your patient has had a thyroidectomy. You should:
    a. keep the patient flat in bed.
    b. watch for and report signs of respiratory distress.
    c. carry out ROM exercises immediately.
    d. position the patient in a left Sims' position.

22. Lack of iodine in the diet can result in:
    a. hypothyroidism.
    b. hyperthyroidism.
    c. diabetes mellitus.
    d. ketosis.

23. The pituitary gland is responsible for secreting hormones that:
    a. stimulate ovulation during the menstrual cycle.
    b. manage sodium and potassium levels.
    c. control calcium and phosphorus.
    d. regulate blood sugar.

24. Your patient has insulin-dependent diabetes. You know that this:
    a. is a stable form of the disease.
    b. affects only older persons.
    c. requires oral hypoglycemic drugs.
    d. is a less stable form of the disease.

25. Insulin is an important hormone because it:
    a. lowers blood sugar.
    b. raises blood sugar.
    c. converts glycogen to glucose.
    d. breaks fat down to form glucose.

26. The most common type of diabetes is:
    a. type 1.
    b. type 2.
    c. juvenile late onset.
    d. adult early onset.

27. The human body produces:
    a. 7 hormones.
    b. 11 hormones.
    c. more than 30 hormones.
    d. more than 50 hormones.
28. Which gland(s) produce the greatest number of hormones?
    a. Endocrine
    b. Ovaries
    c. Pineal
    d. Adrenal
29. Aging changes to the endocrine system include:
    a. slower body function.
    b. reduced release of insulin.
    c. increased fluid retention.
    d. need for additional calories.

D. Nursing Assistant Challenge

You are assigned to two patients who both have diabetes. Sally Sakowski is 29 years old and has had diabetes for 10 years. She is considered to be IDDM. Ruth Young is 72 years old and has just been diagnosed with NIDDM. Although these patients both have diabetes, there may be many differences in their signs, symptoms, and problems. Consider these questions:

30. Hypoglycemia and hyperglycemia may be a complication for either patient. List the differences in the signs and symptoms of both complications.

_____

_____

_____

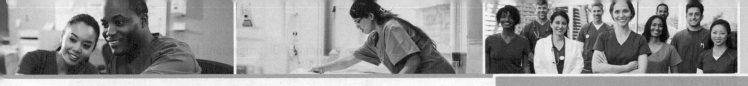

Nervous System

CHAPTER 43

OBJECTIVES

After completing this chapter, you will be able to:

43.1 Spell and define terms.

43.2 State the location of the organs of the nervous system.

43.3 Describe the functions of the organs of the nervous system.

43.4 List five diagnostic tests used to determine conditions of the nervous system.

43.5 Describe 15 common conditions of the nervous system.

43.6 Describe nursing assistant actions related to the care of patients with conditions of the nervous system.

43.7 Explain the proper care and handling when caring for an artificial eye and mucous membranes in the eye socket.

43.8 Explain the proper care, handling, and insertion of a hearing aid.

VOCABULARY

Learn the meaning and the correct spelling of the following words and phrases:

absence seizure	conjunctiva	intention tremor	Parkinson disease
akinesia	convulsion	intracranial pressure	petit mal seizure
amyotrophic lateral	cornea	iris	position sense
sclerosis (ALS)	dendrite	lacrimal gland	post-polio syndrome (PPS)
aphasia	diplegia	Lhermitte's sign	pupil
aura	emotional lability	macular degeneration	quadriplegia
autonomic dysreflexia	epilepsy	meninges	receptive aphasia
axon	eustachian tube	meningitis	retinal degeneration
brain attack	expressive aphasia	monoplegia	semicircular canal
brainstem	flaccid paralysis	multiple sclerosis (MS)	spastic paralysis
cataract	generalized tonic-clonic	nerve	spatial-perceptual deficit
cerebellum	seizure	neuron	status epilepticus
cerebrospinal fluid (CSF)	Glasgow Coma Scale	neurotransmitter	stroke
cerebrovascular accident	glaucoma	nystagmus	synapse
(CVA)	global aphasia	ossicle	tetraplegia
cerebrum	grand mal seizure	otitis media	tremor
chorea	hemianopsia	otosclerosis	tympanic membrane
cochlea	hemiparesis	paralysis	unilateral neglect
cochlear implant	hemiplegia	paraplegia	vertigo
cognitive impairment	Huntington disease (HD)		

STRUCTURE AND FUNCTION

The nervous system controls and coordinates all body activities, including the production of hormones. Special parts of the nervous system are concerned with maintaining normal day-to-day functions. Other parts act during emergency situations. Still others control voluntary activities. Neurological conditions require highly specialized nursing care. You will assist with the less technical aspects of that care.

Neurons

Cells of the nervous system are called **neurons** (Figure 43-1A). They are specialized to conduct electric-like impulses. The neuron has extensions called **axons** and **dendrites**. Impulses enter the neuron only through the dendrites and leave only through the axons.

Although neurons do not actually touch each other, the axon of one neuron lies close to the dendrites of many other neurons. In this way, impulses may follow many different routes. The space between the axon of one cell and the dendrites of others is called a **synapse**. Axons and dendrites in the periphery are covered with *myelin*, which acts as insulation.

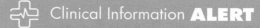

Clinical Information **ALERT**

There are 31 pairs of spinal nerves and 12 pairs of cranial nerves. One nerve can send up to 1,000 impulses per second. A nerve impulse travels at approximately 224 miles per hour. One square inch of skin on the back of your hand has 12,000 nerve endings. There are 45 miles of nerves in the skin of a human being. If all the nerves in the body were laid out end to end, they would measure 167 miles. There are 30 times more pain receptors than cold sensors. The body is more sensitive to pain late in the afternoon.

Neurotransmitters

Neurotransmitters are chemicals that enable messages (nerve impulses) to pass from one cell to another (Figure 43-1B). If the chemicals are not produced in the right amounts, the message pathway becomes confused or blocked.

Nerves

Some axons and dendrites are long. Others are short. Axons and dendrites of many neurons are found in bundles that are held together by connective tissue. These bundles resemble telephone cables and are called **nerves** (Figure 43-1C). The cell bodies of the axons and dendrites in these nerves may be found far from the ends of the nerves in clusters called *ganglia*.

Sensory nerves are made up of dendrites. They carry sensations to the brain and spinal cord from the various body parts. Feeling is lost when these nerve impulses are interrupted. Motor nerves carry impulses from the brain and spinal cord to muscles that cause body activity. Paralysis or loss of function occurs when these nerves are damaged.

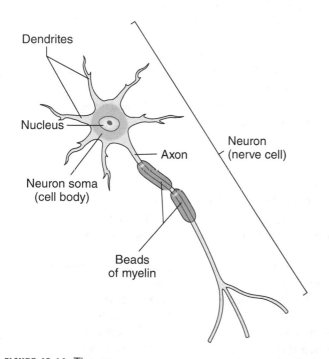

FIGURE 43-1A The neuron.

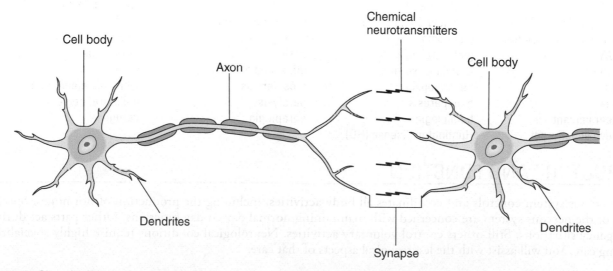

FIGURE 43-1B Chemicals called neurotransmitters help pass the message across the synapse from one neuron to another.

Anatomy of a Nerve

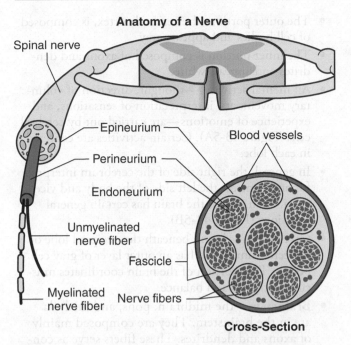

FIGURE 43-1C Anatomy of a nerve. The nerve fibers appear like bundles of cables in the cross-section.

For easier study, the nervous system can be divided into two parts: the central nervous system (CNS) and the peripheral nervous system (PNS). The CNS is composed of the brain and spinal cord (Figure 43-2). The PNS is composed of the 12 pairs of cranial nerves and

31 pairs of spinal nerves that reach throughout the body (Figure 43-3). Remember, though, that the nervous system is one interwoven system, a complex of millions of neurons.

The Central Nervous System

The brain and spinal cord are:

- Surrounded by bone.
- Protected by membranes called *meninges*.
- Cushioned by cerebrospinal fluid.

The brain and spinal cord are a continuous structure found within the skull and spinal canal. Nerves extend from the brain and the spinal cord.

The Brain

The brain (encephalon) is a large, soft mass of nerve tissue contained within the cranium. It is composed of gray matter and white matter. Gray matter consists principally of nerve-cell bodies. White matter consists of nerve cells that form connections between various parts of the brain.

The brain can be further subdivided into the:

- **Cerebrum**—the largest portion of the brain. The outer portion is formed in folds known as *convolutions* and separated into lobes. The lobes take their names from the skull bones that surround them (Figure 43-4).

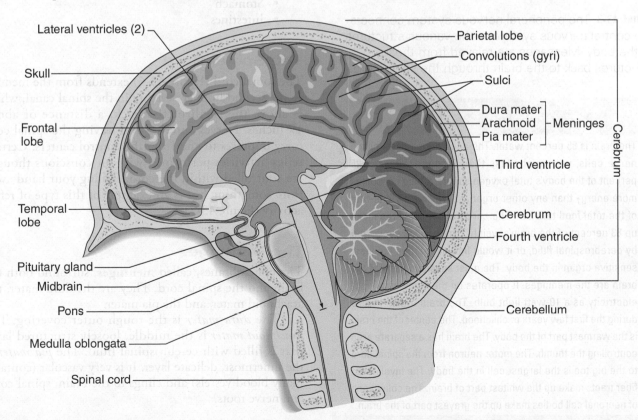

FIGURE 43-2 The central nervous system is composed of the brain and the spinal cord.

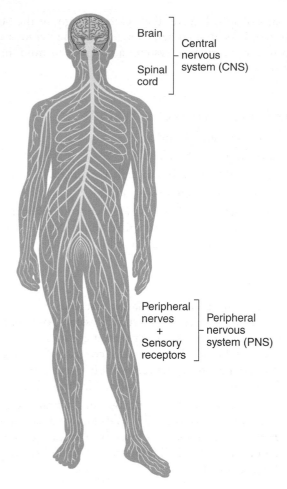

FIGURE 43-3 The peripheral nervous system connects the central nervous system to the various structures of the body. Messages are relayed from these structures back to the brain through the spinal cord.

Clinical Information **ALERT**

The brain is 85 percent water. The adult brain has 14 billion nerve cells, yet weighs less than 3 pounds. It uses 25 percent of the body's total oxygen supply. It also consumes more energy than any other organ, approximately one-fifth of the total food taken in. The cerebral hemispheres make up 83 percent of the brain's weight. The brain is supported by cerebrospinal fluid, or it would flatten out. It is the least sensitive organ in the body. The most sensitive parts of the brain are the meninges. It operates on the same amount of electricity as a 10-watt light bulb. The brain triples in size during the first few years of childhood. The center of the brain is the warmest part of the body. The brain has a separate area controlling the thumb. The motor neuron from the spinal cord to the big toe is the largest cell in the body. The myelinated fiber tracts make up the whitest part of brain. The collections of neuronal cell bodies make up the grayest part of the brain.

- The outer portion, the cerebral cortex, is composed of cell bodies and appears gray.
- The inner portion is composed of axons and dendrites and appears white.
- All mental activities—thought, direction of voluntary movements, interpretation of sensations, and experience of emotions—are carried out by cerebral cells (Figure 43-5A). Certain activities are centered in each lobe.
- In general, the right side of the cerebrum interprets for and controls the left side of the body and vice versa. Each side of the brain has certain general functions (Figure 43-5B).
- **Cerebellum**—found beneath the occipital lobe of the cerebrum. It too has an outer layer of gray cell bodies. This portion of the brain coordinates muscular activities and balance.
- **Brainstem**—the midbrain, pons, and medulla are in the brainstem. They are composed mainly of axons and dendrites. These fibers serve as connecting pathways between the control centers in the cerebrum and cerebellum and the spinal cord. Control centers in the brainstem regulate important involuntary movements of vital organs, such as the:
  - Heart
  - Blood vessels
  - Lungs
  - Stomach
  - Intestines

The Spinal Cord

The spinal cord (Figure 43-6) extends from the medulla to the second lumbar vertebra in the spinal canal, which is above the small of the back, a distance of about 17 inches. Nerves entering and leaving the spinal cord carry impulses to and from the control centers. Certain reflex activities performed without conscious thought are controlled within the cord. Pulling your hand away from something hot is an example of this type of reflex activity (Figure 43-7).

The Meninges

Three membranes, called **meninges**, surround both the brain and the spinal cord. They are the dura mater, the arachnoid mater, and the pia mater.

The *dura mater* is the tough outer covering. The *arachnoid mater* is the middle, loosely structured layer that is filled with cerebrospinal fluid. The *pia mater* is the innermost, delicate layer. It is very vascular (contains many blood vessels) and clings to the brain, spinal cord, and nerve roots.

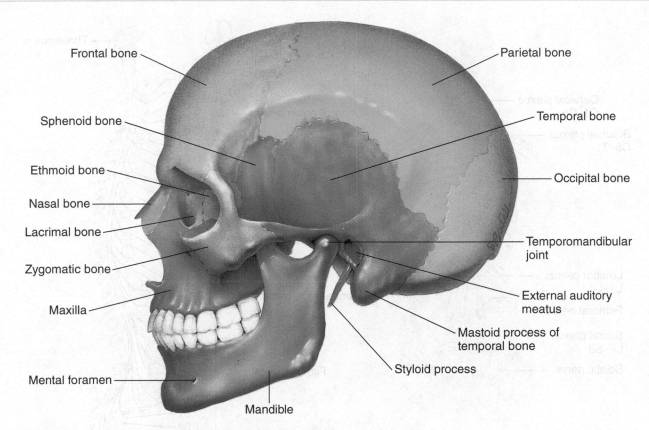

Frontal bone

Sphenoid bone

Ethmoid bone

Nasal bone

Lacrimal bone

Zygomatic bone

Maxilla

Mental foramen

Mandible

Parietal bone

Temporal bone

Occipital bone

Temporomandibular joint

External auditory meatus

Mastoid process of temporal bone

Styloid process

FIGURE 43-4 The lobes of the brain are named according to the nearest skull bones.

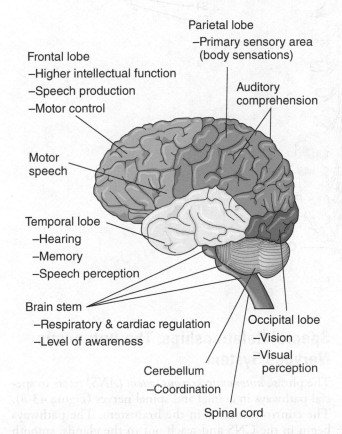

Parietal lobe
  –Primary sensory area (body sensations)

Frontal lobe
  –Higher intellectual function
  –Speech production
  –Motor control

Auditory comprehension

Motor speech

Temporal lobe
  –Hearing
  –Memory
  –Speech perception

Brain stem
  –Respiratory & cardiac regulation
  –Level of awareness

Occipital lobe
  –Vision
  –Visual perception

Cerebellum
  –Coordination

Spinal cord

FIGURE 43-5A Each area of the brain is responsible for a different function.

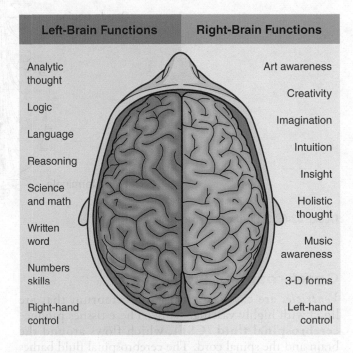

Left-Brain Functions	Right-Brain Functions
Analytic thought	Art awareness
Logic	Creativity
Language	Imagination
Reasoning	Intuition
Science and math	Insight
Written word	Holistic thought
Numbers skills	Music awareness
Right-hand control	3-D forms
	Left-hand control

FIGURE 43-5B Activities controlled by the left and right brain. This information is important when caring for a patient recovering from a stroke.

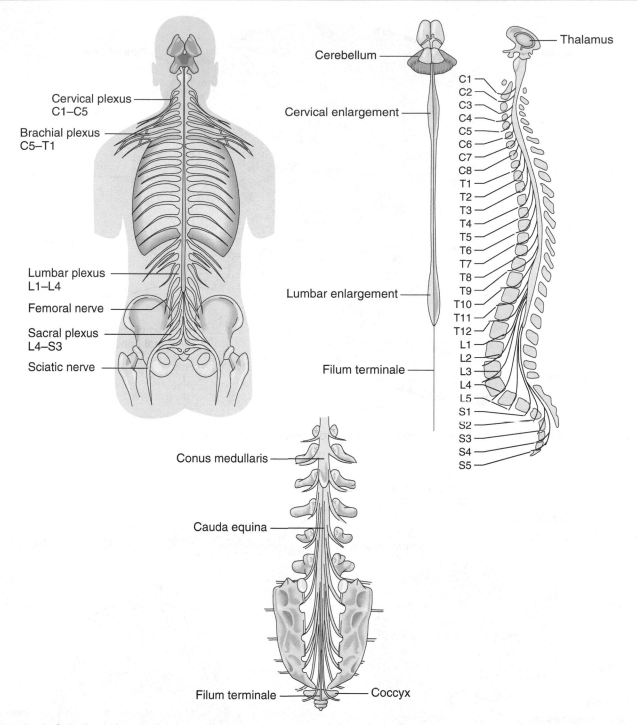

FIGURE 43-6 Spinal cord and nerves.

Cerebrospinal Fluid

Ventricles are cavities within the cerebrum that are lined with highly vascular tissue. These tissues produce **cerebrospinal fluid (CSF)**, which flows around the brain and the spinal cord. The cerebrospinal fluid bathes the central nervous system and cushions it against shock and possible injury.

Special Relationships: The Autonomic Nervous System

The phrase *autonomic nervous system (ANS)* refers to special pathways in cranial and spinal nerves (Figure 43-8). The control center is in the brainstem. The pathways begin in the CNS and reach out to the glands, smooth muscle walls of organs, and heart.

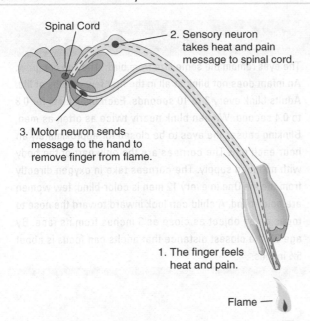

Spinal Cord

2. Sensory neuron
takes heat and pain
message to spinal cord.

3. Motor neuron sends
message to the hand to
remove finger from flame.

1. The finger feels
heat and pain.

Flame

FIGURE 43-7 Reflex arc.

The autonomic nervous system consists of two parts: sympathetic fibers and parasympathetic fibers. Sympathetic fibers stimulate activities that prepare the body to deal with emergency situations. This is the mechanism of "fight or flight." Parasympathetic fibers control the usual functions of moderating heartbeat, digestion, elimination, respiration, and glandular activity.

AGING CHANGES TO THE NERVOUS SYSTEM

Aging changes to the nervous system include:

- Increased length of time for tasks involving speed, balance, coordination, and fine motor activities, such as those involving the fingers.
- Problems with balance and coordination as a result of deterioration to the nerve terminals that provide information to the brain on the movement and position of the body.

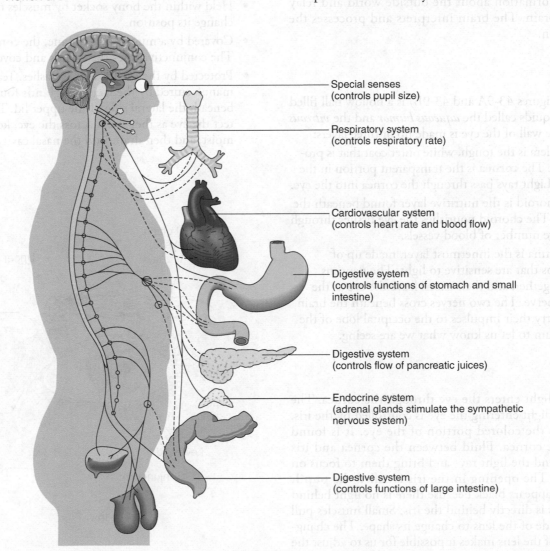

Special senses
(controls pupil size)

Respiratory system
(controls respiratory rate)

Cardiovascular system
(controls heart rate and blood flow)

Digestive system
(controls functions of stomach and small
intestine)

Digestive system
(controls flow of pancreatic juices)

Endocrine system
(adrenal glands stimulate the sympathetic
nervous system)

Digestive system
(controls functions of large intestine)

FIGURE 43-8 Autonomic nervous system.

- Loss of ability to feel pressure and temperature decreases, resulting in higher potential for injury.
- Decreased blood flow to the brain. This may result in mental confusion and memory loss.

SENSORY RECEPTORS

The ends of the dendrites carrying sensations to the central nervous system are found throughout the body.

- Some begin in joints and bring information about body positions to the brain.
- Others in the skin carry sensations of pain, heat, pressure, and cold.
- Those in the nose carry the sense of smell.
- The dendrites in the tongue carry the sense of taste.

Sensory dendrites also receive stimulation through two very special end organs, the eye and the ear. All of these structures are called *sensory receptors* because they receive information about the outside world and relay it to the brain. The brain interprets and processes the information.

The Eye

The eye (Figures 43-9A and 43-9B) is a hollow ball filled with two liquids called the *aqueous humor* and the *vitreous humor*. The wall of the eye is made up of three layers:

- The sclera is the tough, white outer coat that is protective. The **cornea** is the transparent portion in the front. Light rays pass through the cornea into the eye.
- The choroid is the nutritive layer found beneath the sclera. The choroid nourishes the eye tissues through its large number of blood vessels.
- The retina is the innermost layer, made up of neurons that are sensitive to light. The neurons join together, and their axons leave the eye as the optic nerve. The two nerves cross beneath the brain and carry their impulses to the occipital lobe of the cerebrum to let us know what we are seeing.

Seeing

We see as light enters the eye through the cornea. The amount of light entering the eye is controlled by the iris. The **iris** is the colored portion of the eye. It is found behind the cornea. Fluid between the cornea and iris helps to bend the light rays and bring them to focus on the retina. The opening in the iris is called the **pupil**. The pupil appears black because there is no light behind it. The lens is directly behind the iris. Small muscles pull on either side of the lens to change its shape. The changing shape of the lens makes it possible for us to adjust the range of our vision from far to near or from near to far.

The eye is:

- Held within the bony socket by muscles that can change its position.
- Covered by a mucous membrane, the **conjunctiva**. The conjunctiva lines the eyelids and covers the eye.
- Protected by the eyelids and eyelashes. Tears are manufactured by the **lacrimal glands** found beneath the lateral side of the upper lid. Tears protect the eye as they wash across the eye, keeping it moist, and then drain into the nasal cavity.

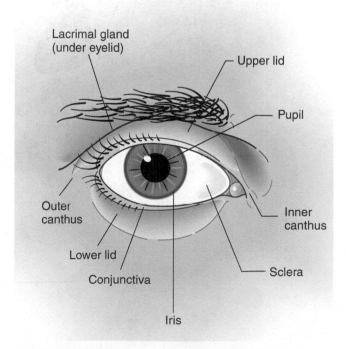

FIGURE 43-9A External view of the eye.

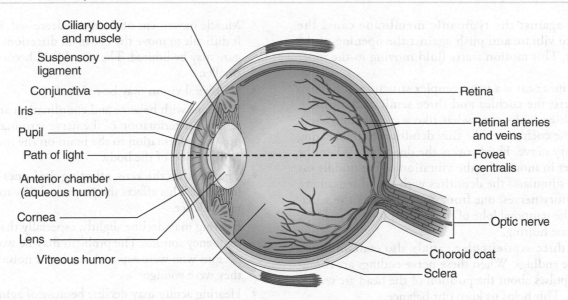

Ciliary body
and muscle

Suspensory
ligament

Conjunctiva

Iris

Pupil

Path of light

Anterior chamber
(aqueous humor)

Cornea

Lens

Vitreous humor

Retina

Retinal arteries
and veins

Fovea
centralis

Optic nerve

Choroid coat

Sclera

FIGURE 43-9B Internal view of the eye.

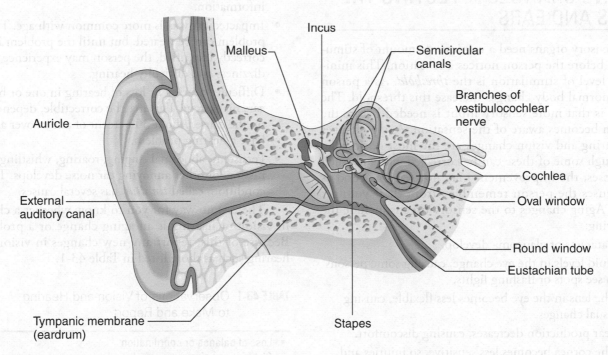

Incus

Malleus

Auricle

External
auditory canal

Tympanic membrane
(eardrum)

Semicircular
canals

Branches of
vestibulocochlear
nerve

Cochlea

Oval window

Round window

Eustachian tube

Stapes

FIGURE 43-10 Internal view of the ear.

The Ear

Just as the eye is sensitive to light, the ear is sensitive to sound (Figure 43-10). The ear is responsible for hearing and equilibrium (balance). The ear has three parts: the outer ear, the middle ear, and the inner ear. The outer ear consists of the visible external structure known as the *pinna* and a canal, which directs sound waves toward the middle ear. At the end of the canal is the eardrum, or **tympanic membrane**. Sound waves cause the eardrum to vibrate.

The middle ear is made up of three tiny bones called **ossicles**. The ossicles form a chain across the middle ear from the tympanic membrane to an opening in the inner ear. These bones are known as the:

- Incus or anvil
- Malleus or hammer
- Stapes or stirrup

Small tubes, called the **eustachian tubes**, lead from the nasopharynx into the middle ear to equalize pressure on either side of the eardrum. Sound waves pushing against the tympanic membrane cause the ossicles to vibrate and push against the opening of the inner ear. This motion starts fluid moving in the inner ear.

The inner ear is a very complex structure. It has two main parts: the cochlea and three semicircular canals. The **cochlea** looks somewhat like a coiled snail shell. Within the cochlea are the tiny dendrites of the hearing or auditory nerve. Fluid covers the dendrites. When the fluid is set in motion by the vibration of the middle ear bones, it stimulates the dendrites with sound sensations. The auditory nerves, one from each ear, carry the sensations to the temporal lobe of the cerebrum to let us know what we are hearing.

The three **semicircular canals** also contain liquid and nerve endings. When these nerve endings are stimulated, impulses about the position of the head are sent to the brain. This helps us keep our balance.

AGING CHANGES AFFECTING THE EYES AND EARS

The sensory organs need a minimum amount of stimulation before the person notices a sensation. This minimum level of stimulation is the *threshold*. As a person ages, normal body changes increase this threshold. The result is that more sensory input is needed before the person becomes aware of the sensation. Aging changes in hearing and vision changes are the most noticeable. Although some of these can be corrected with aids such as glasses, the improvement may not seem as good as the senses the person remembers from their younger years. Aging changes to the sensory organs include the following:

- Cataracts or glaucoma develop.
- Fluid levels in the eye change, causing some persons to see spots or flashing lights.
- The lens in the eye becomes less flexible, causing visual changes.
- Tear production decreases, causing discomfort.
- The cornea becomes less sensitive, so injuries and foreign bodies may not be noticed.
- By age 60, the size of the pupils decreases to about one-third of the size they were at age 20.
- The pupils react more slowly in response to darkness or bright light. The person may have difficulty adapting to glare and bright light.
- Visual acuity may gradually decline. Almost everyone older than age 55 needs glasses at least part of the time. Most also need bifocals.
- All people have more difficulty distinguishing blues and greens compared with reds and yellows. This problem worsens with age.

- Muscle movement of the eye is decreased, making it difficult to move the eye in all directions. Upward gaze may be limited. The visual field becomes smaller.
- Peripheral vision may be reduced.
- Problems with balance and coordination arise as a result of deterioration of the nerve terminals that provide information to the brain on the movement and position of the body.
- The eardrum thickens, affecting the bones of the inner ear. This affects the person's ability to maintain balance.
- Hearing may decline slightly, especially that of high-frequency sounds. The problem may be worse in persons who were exposed to a lot of noise when they were younger.
- Hearing acuity may decline because of aging changes in the auditory nerve. This problem worsens if aging or disease has reduced the brain's ability to process or translate sounds into useful information.
- Impacted ear wax is more common with age. This problem can be treated, but until the problem is correctly identified, the person may experience dizziness and difficulty hearing.
- Difficulty hearing or loss of hearing in one or both ears may occur. This may be correctible, depending on the cause. About 30 percent of adults over age 65 have a hearing problem.
- Persistent, abnormal ringing, roaring, whistling, hissing, or other annoying ear noise develops. This condition, called *tinnitus*, has several causes.

There is no way for you to know whether a change in vision or hearing is an aging change or a problem. Because of this, report any new changes in vision and hearing such as those listed in Table 43-1.

TABLE 43-1 Observations of Vision and Hearing to Make and Report

- Loss of balance or coordination
- Change in pupil size; unequal pupils
- Abnormal color of sclera (yellow, red)
- Complaints of pain or pressure in eyes or ears
- Drainage from eyes or ears
- Ability to hear on one side, but not the other
- Impaired vision, change in ability to see
- Eating food on one side of meal tray, but not the other
- Frequently rubbing the eyes
- Presence of foreign body in eyes or ears
- Dizziness on sudden movement of head
- Complaining of ringing in ears
- Complaining of spots or "lightning" in front of eyes
- Eyes appear swollen or inflamed
- Excessive tear production

COMMON CONDITIONS INVOLVING THE NERVOUS SYSTEM

The nervous system usually remains healthy. However, injury or disease to the brain, spinal cord, or nerves requires appropriate treatment.

Increased Intracranial Pressure

The structures within the skull normally exert a certain amount of pressure, called **intracranial pressure**. The pressure is due to:

- Nervous tissue
- Cerebrospinal fluid
- Blood flowing through cerebral vessels

Any change in the size or amount of these components changes the pressure. Increased intracranial pressure can result from:

- Head injury. Bleeding from damaged blood vessels and edema puts pressure on the delicate nervous tissue.
- Inflammation or infection plus edema.
- Intracranial bleeding due to ruptured blood vessels. This is called a *cerebrovascular accident (CVA)*.
- Toxins.
- High temperature.
- Blockage of the normal flow of cerebrospinal fluid.
- Tumors.

Signs and Symptoms

Indications of increased intracranial pressure include:

- Alteration in pupil size and response to light. In the normal eye, the pupil becomes smaller when a flashlight is directed at each eye. The equality of the pupils and their ability to react to light is an important observation when a head injury occurs.
- Headache.
- Vomiting.
- Change in mental status.
- Loss of consciousness and sensation.
- **Paralysis**—loss of voluntary motor control.
- **Convulsions** (seizures)—uncontrolled muscular contractions that may seem violent.

How long all or part of the symptoms remain depends on the extent and cause of damage to the brain cells. Remember also that paralysis is not always accompanied by sensory loss.

Specific Nursing Care

Patients who are acutely ill with head injuries or increased intracranial pressure require skilled nursing care. The nurse is responsible for monitoring the patient's:

- Level of consciousness
- Degree of orientation to time and place
- Reaction to pain and stimuli
- Vital signs

If you note any change in the patient's response or behavior as you are assisting in care, bring it to the nurse's attention immediately. Changes that might be very significant include:

- Incontinence (new onset)
- Uncontrolled body movements
- Disorientation
- Deepening or lessening in the level of consciousness
- Dizziness
- Vomiting
- Alterations in speech
- Change in ability to follow directions

Once improved, the patient may be moved from a critical unit to an intermediate unit. From there, the patient may go to a long-term care facility for a possibly long period of convalescence. The patient may require extensive rehabilitation to regain functional skills. The nursing measures first established in the critical care unit must be maintained throughout this extended period.

Loss of sensation and decreased mobility make these patients more prone to pressure injuries, infection, and contractures. You must continue to:

- Give special skin care.
- Carry out range-of-motion exercises.
- Check skin over pressure points frequently.
- Change the patient's position regularly.
- Report early signs of infection.
- Monitor elimination. Loss of muscle tone and inactivity may lead to constipation and impaction.
- Check drainage tubes such as indwelling catheters.
- Provide reality orientation as needed.
- Be alert to any signs of mood change and plan extra time to provide essential support. Patients recovering from these illnesses often experience anxiety and depression.
- Keep a careful check on vital signs of any patient with a head injury. A special record (neurological monitoring record) may be kept for recording all observations.

Observations to make and report related to the nervous system are listed in Table 43-2.

Glasgow Coma Scale

The **Glasgow Coma Scale** is used to monitor neurologic problems after trauma, stroke, and other illnesses and injuries. The examiner determines the best response the patient can make to stimuli. The score is determined

TABLE 43-2 Observations to Make and Report Related to Neurological Problems

- Headache
- Dizziness
- Double vision
- Paralysis on one side
- Inability to move a body part
- Hypertension
- Slow, full, bounding pulse
- Impaired coordination
- Temporary unilateral paralysis
- Droopy eyelid
- Double vision
- Distortion of visual field
- Visual disturbances such as flashing lights or wavy lines
- One pupil larger than the other
- Weakness
- Tingling
- Numbness; loss of sensation
- Spasticity; abnormal involuntary movement
- Confusion, disorientation to day, date, time
- Difficulty speaking or loss of ability to speak
- Changes in ability to respond verbally or nonverbally
- Difficulty understanding or inability to understand
- Difficulty swallowing; changes in ability to swallow
- Change in mood, behavior, or emotional status
- Change in ability to follow directions
- Difficulty concentrating
- Fatigue
- Nausea and vomiting
- Loss of coordination
- Sensitivity to light
- Irritability
- Lethargy, excessive sleepiness
- Change in level of consciousness

by adding the total of all three categories. Higher point values are assigned to responses that indicate increased awareness and arousal. A score of less than 8 indicates a neurological crisis. A score of 9–13 indicates moderate dysfunction, and a score of 13–15 indicates moderate to minor dysfunction.

Transient Ischemic Attack

A *transient ischemic attack (TIA)* is a temporary period of diminished blood flow to the brain. It may be called a mini stroke, but it is really a major warning.

Culture ALERT

Men, African Americans/Blacks, and Mexican Americans have higher rates of TIA than women and non-Hispanic Whites.

- Approximately 15 percent of all strokes are preceded by a TIA.
- The short-term risk of stroke after TIA has been shown to be as high as 10 percent at 2 days and as high as 17 percent at 90 days.
- Individuals who have a TIA have a 10-year stroke risk of approximately 19 percent.
- Within 1 year of TIA, 25 percent of patients will die.
- In 2016, stroke accounted for about 1 of every 19 deaths in the United States.
- On average in 2016, someone died of stroke every 3 minutes, 42 seconds.

The attack comes on rapidly and may last from 2 to 15 minutes or for as long as 24 hours. Symptoms are similar to those of a stroke but are sometimes temporary and reversible. Transient ischemic attacks may occur once or several times in a lifetime. Persons experiencing TIAs are at risk for eventually experiencing a stroke. Several scales and a simple drawing test are available to help predict stroke risk.

Stroke

A **stroke** is also called a **cerebrovascular accident (CVA)** or **brain attack**. It affects the vascular system and the nervous system. The complete or partial loss of blood flow to the brain tissue is frequently a complication of atherosclerosis or brain hemorrhage. Causes of CVA include:

- Vascular occlusion due to a thrombus, atherosclerotic plaques, or emboli that obstruct the flow of blood.
- Intracranial bleeding as blood vessels rupture, releasing blood into the brain tissue.
  Stroke types are summarized in Table 43-3.
  Remember, most nerve pathways cross from one side to the other in the brain. Because of this, damage on one side of the brain results in signs and symptoms on the opposite side of the body. Symptoms vary depending on the extent of interference with the circulation and on the area and amount of tissue damaged. Patients with damage to the right side of the brain will exhibit:

- **Spatial-perceptual deficits.** This means it is difficult to distinguish right from left and up from down. The world may appear "tilted" to the person with right-brain damage. The patient will have problems propelling a wheelchair, setting down items, and carrying out activities of daily living.
- Change in personality. The individual with right-brain damage becomes very quick and impulsive.

If the left side of the brain is damaged, you will note:

The average stroke takes 10 hours to evolve and involves about 3 cubic inches of brain tissue. Oxygen deprivation causes the brain to age about 3.6 years each hour; 1.9 million nerve cells in the brain die each minute after a stroke. Getting rapid treatment is essential to preventing further damage to the brain. A popular saying is "Time is brain," a reminder that outcomes decline when treatment is delayed. Stroke is the leading cause of long-term disability in the United States. Each year, 795,000 people experience a new or recurrent stroke. Approximately 610,000 of these are first attacks, and 185,000 are recurrent attacks.

- More women than men have a stroke.
- Someone in the United States has a stroke approximately every 40 seconds.
- Stroke ranks fifth among all causes of death.

When the patient with a suspected stroke arrives at the hospital, doctors will determine what type of stroke they are having (Figure 43-11). Ischemic strokes can be treated with newer clot-busting drugs if the patient arrives at the hospital quickly.

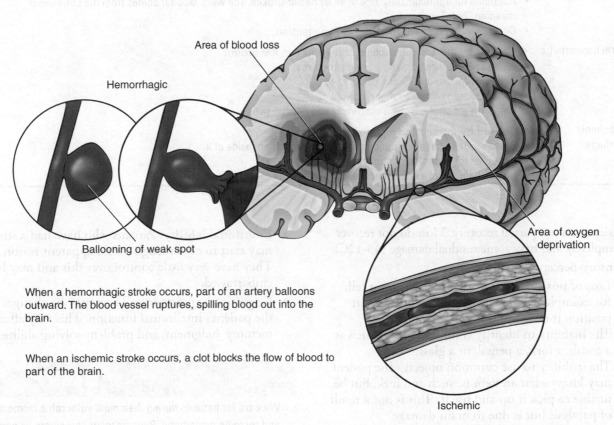

Area of blood loss

Hemorrhagic

Ballooning of weak spot

Area of oxygen deprivation

When a hemorrhagic stroke occurs, part of an artery balloons outward. The blood vessel ruptures, spilling blood out into the brain.

When an ischemic stroke occurs, a clot blocks the flow of blood to part of the brain.

Ischemic

FIGURE 43-11 Thrombotic strokes are more common in older adults, and hemorrhagic strokes are more common in younger persons. Drugs may be given to break a clot causing a thrombotic stroke if the condition is identified and treated within three hours of the onset of symptoms. No comparable drugs are available to treat hemorrhagic stroke, and the prognosis for this type of stroke is not as good.

- **Aphasia**—an inability to express or understand speech.
- Change in personality. The individual becomes very cautious, anxious, and slow to complete tasks.

   Other symptoms are often present with either right- or left-brain damage. These include:

- **Hemiparesis** (weakness) or **hemiplegia** (paralysis) on one side of the body, on the opposite side from the area of the brain in which the stroke occurred. You will notice a difference when comparing the sides of the body, from head to foot (Figures 43-12A and 43-12B). With early, aggressive treatment, some

TABLE 43-3 Types and Causes of Stroke

Type of Stroke	Cause and Information
Ischemic stroke	• Most common type of stroke; about 87% of all strokes. • Caused by a clot or other blockage within an artery leading to the brain. • Can be treated with clotbuster drugs if treatment is started early.
Embolic stroke	• A clot develops in a part of the body other than the brain (commonly the heart). • The clot travels to the brain, where it lodges in a small artery. • Stroke occurs suddenly and without warning. • Approximately 15% percent of embolic strokes occur in persons with atrial fibrillation.
Thrombotic stroke	• Clot forms in the brain, usually in one of the cerebral arteries. • Clot remains attached to the artery wall until it grows large enough to block the artery. • May be preceded by one or more TIAs.
Lacunar infarct	• Small, deep infarcts occur, usually in the basal ganglia and thalamus. • Results from small vessel disease; most likely caused by atherosclerotic occlusion of perforating branches. • May also affect the brainstem and other vital structures. • Accounts for approximately 25% of all *ischemic* strokes. The word *lacunar* comes from the Latin word meaning "hole" or "cavity." • Common in persons with diabetes or hypertension.
Cerebral hemorrhage	• Caused by the sudden rupture of an artery in the brain. • Blood spills out, compressing brain structures. • Accounts for about 10% of strokes. • Most common type in younger individuals. • Hemorrhagic stroke is the most deadly and difficult to treat.
Subarachnoid hemorrhage	• Caused by the sudden rupture of an artery. • Blood fills the space surrounding the brain rather than inside of it. • Accounts for about 3% of strokes. • Hemorrhagic stroke is the most deadly and difficult to treat.

patients make a partial recovery. Most do not recover completely and have some residual damage (43-12C).

- Sensory-perceptual deficits:
  - Loss of **position sense**. The person cannot tell, for example, where an affected foot is or what position it is in without looking at it.
  - The inability to identify common objects such as a comb, a fork, a pencil, or a glass.
  - The inability to use common objects. The patient may know what an item is, such as a fork, but be unable to pick it up and use it. This is not a result of paralysis but is due to brain damage.
- **Unilateral neglect.** The patient ignores the paralyzed side of the body. For example, the affected arm may hang over the side of the wheelchair without the patient realizing where the arm is.
- **Hemianopsia.** This is impaired vision. Both eyes have only half vision. For example, if the patient has left hemiplegia, the left half of both eyes is blind (Figure 43-13). Remember this if a patient who has had a stroke eats the food on one side of the tray and leaves the food on the other side. The patient probably cannot see it. Turn the tray around.

- **Emotional lability.** Patients who have had a stroke may start to cry or laugh for no apparent reason. They have very little control over this and may be embarrassed.
- **Cognitive impairments.** There may be changes in the patient's intellectual function. This may affect memory, judgment, and problem-solving abilities.

⛑ Clinical Information **ALERT**

We care for patients during their most vulnerable moments and try to be empathetic. Patients view caregivers as compassionate, talented, professional healers who accept patients' loss of independence with grace and dignity. Unfortunately, patients often do not accept their losses well. Each time we touch them, they want us to make it all right and ease their pain, which is often emotional. Understanding how tangible independence is, along with the dynamics, grief, and pain associated with a loss of this magnitude, will enhance your insight into patients' needs. It will give you insight into why some patients take risks. Their physical, mental, emotional, and psychosocial challenges are often enormous.

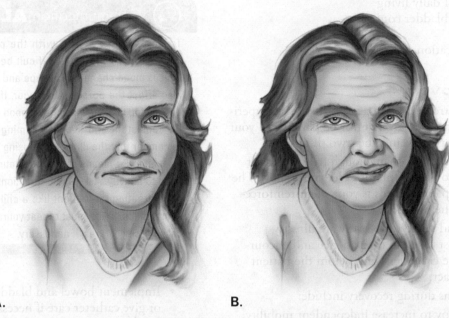

FIGURE 43-12A Weakness or paralysis occurs in the face, arm, and leg on the opposite side of the area of the brain in which the stroke occurred. (A) Normal. (B) Stroke on left side of brain (right side of picture).

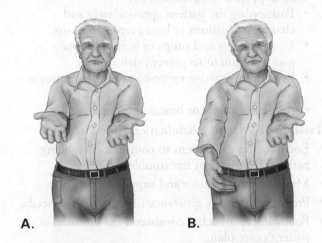

FIGURE 43-12B Picture (A) shows a person with no deficits. Picture (B) shows a person that has had a stroke. The right side of the body (left side of picture) is weaker than it was previously.

Nursing Care

The goals of poststroke care include:

- Maintaining the skills and abilities that the patient has left.
- Preventing complications caused by immobility:
  - Contractures
  - Pressure injuries
  - Pneumonia
  - Blood clots
- Helping the patient regain functional abilities:

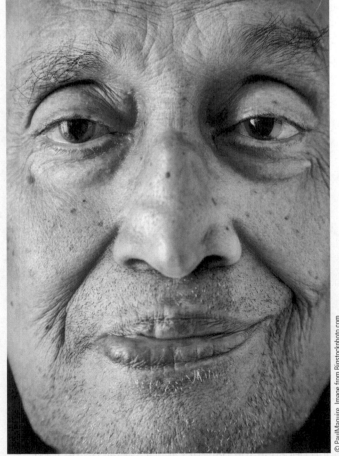

FIGURE 43-12C This patient who had a stroke is smiling. Note that only one side of the mouth curves up. The other side is paralyzed.

- Activities of daily living
- Bowel and bladder control
- Mobility
- Communication skills

During Recovery

Recovery from a stroke is often a very frustrating experience for the patient. Caregivers must be patient. In your approach to the patient, remember two things:

- The patient has more than enough frustration for both of you, so be careful not to let yours show. The last thing the patient needs is your silent reinforcement of their helplessness.
- The degree and speed of recovery are directly related, in most cases, to the patience and encouragement of the caregivers with whom the patient has close contact.

Other interventions during recovery include:

- Physical therapy to increase independent mobility: bed movement, getting to the side of the bed, standing by the side of the bed, transferring out of bed and into a chair, and ambulation.
- Occupational therapy to regain the ability to perform the activities of daily living, such as bathing, grooming, dressing, and eating, with little or no assistance.
- Speech therapy to regain or to learn different methods of communication. The speech therapist also works with swallowing problems caused by the stroke.
- Nursing care to:

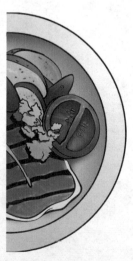

FIGURE 43-13 Hemianopsia is blindness in one-half of the visual field. This can cause a problem with eating because the patient cannot see all of the food. The problem is solved by turning the plate around. Because of changes in the brain after the stroke, do not expect the patient to turn the plate.

 Communication ALERT

Try to develop rapport with the patient on your first contact. At times, this is difficult because a stroke often causes mood changes. The type and location of the stroke also affect the person's behavior. If the patient is newly dependent, they may also have mood or behavior problems. Be consistent and avoid becoming discouraged. Try to remember that the illness is causing the problem. Find the most effective means of communicating the information you need to convey. Ask yes/no questions whenever possible. Avoid treating the patient like a child and do not correct their speech. If you must repeat yourself, do so quietly and calmly. Use gestures, if necessary.

- Implement bowel and bladder training programs, or give catheter care if necessary.
- Implement pressure injury prevention programs.
- Reinforce the therapy programs.
- Care to prevent contractures by:
  - Positioning the patient appropriately and changing positions at least every two hours.
  - Using pillows and props to keep the person in good alignment to prevent deformities.
  - Performing passive range-of-motion exercises as directed.
  - Applying splints or braces as ordered.

All staff can help with rehabilitation efforts by:

- Encouraging the patient to communicate; being patient if the patient has trouble.
- Maintaining a positive and supportive attitude.
- Providing only the assistance that the patient needs.
- Following approaches consistently as outlined in the patient's care plan.

Convalescence is often long. The nursing care is demanding, requiring much patience and understanding.

Aphasia

Stroke victims often suffer from aphasia or language impairment. They have difficulty forming thoughts or expressing them in coherent ways. This is extremely frustrating and frightening for the patient and family.

- **Receptive aphasia** means that the person cannot comprehend communication.
- **Expressive aphasia** means that the person cannot properly form thoughts or express them coherently.
- **Global aphasia** means that the person has lost all language abilities.

Review the Chapter 7 guidelines for communicating with patients who have aphasia.

Parkinson Disease

Parkinson disease is believed to be caused by not having enough neurotransmitters (dopamine) in the brainstem and cerebellum. The symptoms are progressive over many years. Some people will show minor changes. Others will have much more obvious symptoms (Figure 43-14).

Signs and Symptoms

Signs and symptoms of Parkinson disease include:

- **Tremors** (uncontrolled trembling). Tremors of the hands commonly affect the fingers and thumb in such a way that an affected person will appear to be rolling a small object (such as a pill) between them. These tremors occur frequently. They usually begin in the fingers, then involve the entire hand and arm, and finally affect an entire side of the body. Starting on one side, the tremors eventually involve both sides of the body. Tremors are more evident when the person is inactive. A typical posture of a patient suffering from Parkinson disease is shown in Figure 43-15.

- Muscular rigidity (loss of flexibility). The muscular rigidity is more evident when the patient is inactive. It seems to be lessened when the person sleeps or engages in activities such as walking or other exercises that require large-muscle involvement. The rigidity makes the person with Parkinson disease more prone to falls and injury.

- **Akinesia** (difficulty and slowness in carrying out voluntary muscular activities). Persons with advanced Parkinson's typically have:
  - A shuffling manner of walking.
  - Difficulty starting the process of walking.
  - Difficulty stopping smoothly once walking has started.
  - Affected speech, causing words to be slurred and poorly spoken (enunciated).
  - Facial muscles that lose expressiveness and emotional response.
  - Difficulty chewing and swallowing.

- Loss of autonomic nervous control. Because of loss of autonomic nervous control, persons with Parkinson's may:
  - Drool.
  - Become incontinent.
  - Become constipated.
  - Retain urine.

- Mood swings and gradual behavioral changes. A patient may appear happy and positive one moment, and then be depressed the next. The depression tends to be progressive. Personality and behavioral changes may occur, with psychotic breakdowns and dementia in later stages.

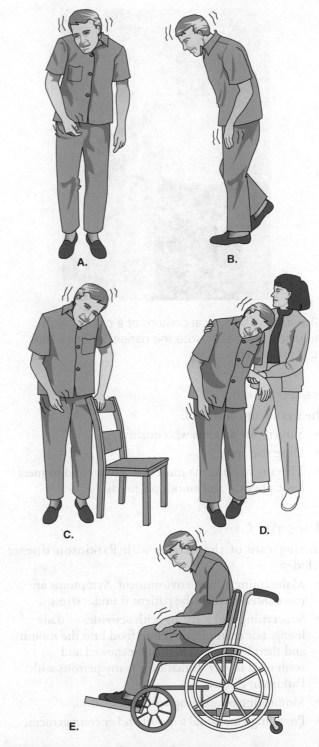

FIGURE 43-14 Progression of Parkinson's disease. (A) The patient leans slightly forward and develops flexion of the affected arm. (B) The patient stoops forward slightly and walks with a shuffling gait. (C) As the disease progresses, the patient needs support to prevent falling. The patient tends to shuffle faster and faster, leaning farther forward and may fall on the face. (D) The disease progresses to the point of needing assistance for ambulation. (E) The patient has profound weakness and severe tremors. Ambulation becomes impossible.

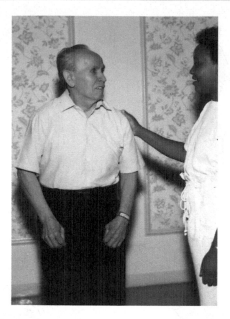

FIGURE 43-15 The typical posture of a patient with Parkinson's disease. Note the patient's hands and facial expression.

Treatment

The treatment consists of:

- Surgery for patients who qualify
- Drug therapy
- Therapy to limit the muscular rigidity and to meet basic physical and emotional needs

Nursing Care

Nursing care of the person with Parkinson disease includes:

- Maintaining a calm environment. Symptoms are more intense when the patient is under stress.
- Supervising and assisting with activities of daily living. For example, directing food into the mouth and then keeping it there to be chewed and swallowed is very difficult for many persons with Parkinson disease.
- Monitoring or assisting with ambulation.
- Providing emotional support and encouragement.

Difficult Situations

Patients with Parkinson disease may have inconsistent needs for physical support and assistance. If the patient is tired, they may need more support than when they are rested. When the patient is stressed, the tremors may worsen, increasing the need for hands-on assistance.

- Carrying out a program of general and specific exercises.
- Providing protection for patients with dementia.

Huntington Disease

Huntington disease (HD) is also called *Huntington's chorea*. This is a hereditary disease. In recent years, a genetic test has become available to identify the presence of the Huntington's gene. If the gene is present, development of the disease is inevitable. Some people with a family history are not tested because they do not want to know if they will develop the condition. They have seen family members with the disease and fear the diagnosis.

Signs and Symptoms

Clinical signs of HD usually begin when individuals are in their forties or fifties, but symptoms first appear in childhood or young adulthood. Signs and symptoms include hallucinations, delusions, and poor judgment. The disease is progressive and there is no cure. Disability and death occur within 15 to 20 years. Abnormal movements, called **chorea**, are the primary sign of HD. The movements are subtle early in the course of the illness. The individual will appear anxious or restless and will move frequently. The person may try to disguise the activity with voluntary movements, such as scratching the head or crossing the legs. As the disease progresses, rapid, jerking choreiform movements develop. These movements involve the entire body. The patient will eventually lose voluntary control of all movement. They also lose control of the bowel and bladder. They will have difficulty speaking, chewing, and swallowing. The involuntary movement increases with stress and attempts to control the choreiform motions.

Nursing Care

There is no known treatment or cure for HD. Persons with Huntington disease are commonly admitted to a long-term care facility because they cannot function safely at home. They may be hospitalized for complications, such as aspiration and pneumonia, which are common with this condition. Urinary tract infection and pressure injuries are also problematic. As the disease progresses, the patient's response to pain as well as heat and cold sensitivity may be delayed. Anticipate these sensation abnormalities and monitor food and bath water temperature closely. Nursing care is designed to:

- Maintain a consistent routine, avoiding change as much as possible.
- Keep the patient as independent as possible for as long as possible.
- Maintain the person's current abilities.

- Prevent weight loss by replacing calories used by the spastic movements.
- Promote safe swallowing and prevent choking.
- Prevent falls and other injuries.
- Maintain the patient's ability to communicate.
- Prevent complications such as pressure injuries and contractures.

Poor muscular control makes communication difficult. The speech therapist will assess the patient and establish a communication program. The patient will be taught to use hand signals, cards, or a communication board. Give the patient feedback when they speak. Repeating what the patient says is a good way to show that the communication was successful.

Ambulation and Mobility

As the disease progresses, the patient will develop a strange gait in which they sway back and forth and extends the hips in an attempt to balance. If the patient is ambulatory, they are at very high risk of falls. Allow them to walk, but provide support and assistance as necessary. Sitting in a chair may be difficult for some patients. The involuntary movements may cause the patient to fall out of the chair and onto the floor. Approaches to assist with mobility include supervising ambulation for safety and ambulating the patient with a gait belt.

A recliner with adaptations and padding may be necessary to enable the person to be out of bed. A seat belt may also be necessary when the patient is in the chair. When the patient is in bed, the side rails should be well padded to prevent injury caused by banging arms and legs into the rails because of spasticity.

Cognitive Changes

Individuals with HD develop mental changes. Early in the condition, the individual becomes nervous, suspicious of others, and irritable. Mood swings are common, as is depression. As the condition progresses, the individual develops dementia. They become totally dependent on others.

Loss of control, power, and autonomy are major issues in HD. The patient loses impulse control with disease progression and may become angry at caregivers' efforts to protect them. Some patients view cigarette smoking as a bridge between independence and dependence. They insist on smoking because it is "the last remaining pleasure" they have. Unfortunately, they may exhibit unsafe smoking behavior. They lose sensitivity to heat and cold and may burn themselves when lighting a cigarette, or when smoking down to the filter. Give patients as much control over daily routines as possible, and empower them by offering choices. Other approaches are to:

- Treat the patient with dignity and respect.
- Monitor smoking closely.
- Inform the nurse if you find smoking materials in the room of a patient with HD.
- Despite cognitive changes, the patients usually know what is going on around them. Avoid treating them like children or making insensitive remarks.

Nutrition

The rapid choreiform movements burn many calories. The patient is at very high risk for weight loss. Provide extra nutrition and hydration. The patient may have difficulty with the texture of some foods. Saliva may run from the mouth, and the tongue may be difficult to control. The patient will develop difficulty swallowing and is at very high risk for choking. They may need to be spoon-fed. Increased movements of the tongue may tend to push the food out of the mouth, making chewing and swallowing difficult. Assist the patient at mealtime by:

- Keeping mealtime as stress-free as possible.
- Applying a clothing protector; avoid calling this garment a bib.
- Allowing extra time for the patient to eat. You may have to reheat the food.
- Serving a mechanical soft or pureed diet, or other foods that are easy to swallow.
- Feeding slowly.
- Encouraging use of adaptive utensils listed on the care plan to help maintain independence.
- Seating the patient completely upright at meals to prevent choking.
- Following the care plan for approaches to use at mealtime.
- Avoiding conversation at mealtime. Limit conversation to cues and instructions for eating.
- Checking the mouth for retained food after each meal.
- Providing oral hygiene after meals. This is important because of the risk of aspiration of food particles and saliva.

Multiple Sclerosis

Multiple sclerosis (MS) generally occurs in young adults. The exact cause is unknown, but it is considered an autoimmune disorder. It results from loss of insulation (myelin) around central nervous system nerve fibers. This interferes with the ability of the nerve fibers to function.

Many individuals live the usual life span even though they have this chronic condition. The symptoms are variable and may not be the same for all individuals. Symptoms may include:

- Loss of sensation with regard to temperature, pain, and touch.
- Feelings of numbness and tingling.
- **Vertigo** (a spinning or dizzy sensation).
- **Lhermitte's sign** (a tingling, shocklike sensation that passes down the arms or spine when the neck is flexed).

Problems with vision occur in almost half of the people who have MS. The problem may be temporary or permanent. Vision symptoms may include:

- Blurriness, color blindness, or difficulty seeing objects in bright light.
- Double vision.
- **Nystagmus** (jerky eye movements).

Mobility is usually affected:

- Pain in the legs that disappears with rest.
- **Paraplegia** (paralysis of both legs) and **quadriplegia** (paralysis of all four extremities) in advanced cases. The preferred term for paralysis of the arms and legs is **tetraplegia**. When a person is paralyzed, voluntary movement, strength, and sensation are limited or absent. This condition involves much more than the loss of ability to move a body part.
- Spasticity of muscles.
- **Intention tremor** (shaking of the hands that gets worse as the individual tries to touch or pick up an object).

In severe MS, speech is affected because of muscle weakness in the chest, face, and lips. The speech may be slow, with poor articulation. The mind usually remains alert. Incontinence of bowel and bladder is common in advanced cases. One of the most disabling features of MS is fatigue. The fatigue is very real and is not psychological.

MS may follow one of four courses:

- *Benign course*—mild attacks with long periods of no symptoms.
- *Exacerbating-remitting*—severe attacks (exacerbations) followed by periods of partial or complete recovery (remissions). Often the periods of exacerbation get longer and more severe with shorter periods of remission.
- *Slowly progressive*—slow, steady deterioration.
- *Rapidly progressive*—deterioration is rapid and progressive and may be life-threatening.

Nursing Care

Nursing care of the patient with multiple sclerosis includes:

- Implementing a pressure injury prevention program.
- Implementing contracture prevention programs through consistent changes of position and passive range-of-motion exercises. Apply splints correctly, if ordered.

- If the patient has an indwelling catheter, providing regular catheter care to prevent bladder infections.
- Encouraging independence. Follow instructions from the nurse or the therapists for specific techniques to use.
- Helping the patient maintain a balanced schedule of rest and activity.
- Providing emotional support and encouragement.

Treatment

There is no known way to stop the progression of the disease. Treatment consists of maintaining functional ability as long as possible through general health practices and physical therapy.

Post-polio Syndrome (PPS)

Polio is a very serious neurological disease that has been with us since at least 1350 BCE This disease is caused by a virus that attacks the motor neurons in the spinal cord. There were large annual outbreaks of polio in the United States every summer until 1955, when the first vaccine became available.

Post-polio syndrome (PPS) is marked by increased weakness and abnormal muscle fatigue in persons who had polio many years earlier. It is believed to be related to the loss of motor neurons. Most polio survivors have about 10 to 50 percent as many motor neurons as other people. These neurons have served the person by adapting so that they innervate areas that are five to seven times larger than normal. The neurons are wearing out from years of overuse. As the neurons die, the muscles stop responding.

Signs and Symptoms

Signs and symptoms of PPS range from annoying to debilitating. Any new injury strains the remaining neurons, reducing function and increasing pain and fatigue. Signs and symptoms include:

- Fatigue that may be debilitating.
- New joint and muscle pain. Most experience pain daily.

Difficult Situations

A warm bath or shower is often very relaxing to a patient with multiple sclerosis. However, you must make sure that the water is not too hot, which temporarily intensifies some symptoms of MS. Keeping bath water at about 100°F to 105°F is best. Provide ROM to maintain joint mobility and muscle tone, reduce spasticity, improve coordination, and boost self-esteem.

- New weakness in muscles affected by polio; formerly unaffected muscles are also now affected.
- New dyspnea and other respiratory problems.
- Severe cold intolerance, which causes muscle weakness to worsen, the arms or legs to become pale or cyanotic, and the extremities to feel cold to the touch.
- Muscle spasms and cramps that are sometimes severe and painful.
- Difficulty swallowing.
- Difficulty falling asleep and waking frequently during the night.

Surgical Procedures

Patients with PPS are much more sensitive to anesthesia than persons who have not had polio. They require less medication and half the anesthesia, yet take twice as long as others to recover from the anesthesia. Because of this, the patient with PPS must be monitored closely in the postoperative period.

Nursing Assistant Care

Patients with post-polio syndrome are usually in the hospital for treatment of another condition. The problems caused by PPS itself are seldom severe enough to require hospitalization. However, they complicate the care of other conditions and procedures. Remember that these patients have lived with their condition for years and have found ways to adapt to it. Overall, they are experts in their own care. Respect their expertise. Coping with the new problems from PPS is often much more difficult than recovery from the original illness. Be prepared to help with activities of daily living, bed mobility, transfers, and ambulation. Patients with PPS may have many special needs.

Most patients with PPS have their homes arranged so they can function independently. Temporarily staying in a different environment, such as a hospital, can be very troublesome for the patient. They may need help with tasks that they could do independently at home. Most patients with PPS fear becoming dependent on others. The patient may have great difficulty asking for help. Anticipate their needs, and ask if assistance is needed. Do not be surprised if the patient refuses your offer of help. Respect the refusal, but advise the patient that accepting assistance is different from being dependent. In fact, assistance may help the patient remain independent. Even if the patient refuses your help, stand by to see if they can perform the task or procedure safely. Adapt the environment, whenever possible, for optimal independent function. You may do this by moving furniture or bringing a bedside commode, for example. Most polio survivors are attuned to what their bodies are telling them. If the patient says they cannot do something, pay attention.

Amyotrophic Lateral Sclerosis (ALS)

Amyotrophic lateral sclerosis (ALS) is a progressive neuromuscular disease that causes muscle weakness and paralysis. ALS is also called *Lou Gehrig's disease*, after a famous baseball player who had the condition. It is a disease of the motor nerves that control voluntary movement. The cause is unknown, and there is no cure. There seems to be a familial link in about 10 percent of cases. ALS occurs in all races and both genders, although it is more common in men. The most common age of onset is 55, but it can occur in persons of any age. ALS is almost always fatal. About half of patients diagnosed with ALS die within 18 months, although some may live for many years. One drug has been successful in slowing progression of the disease, but there is no known cure. Some medications are used to relieve the symptoms.

Signs and Symptoms

ALS takes months to be diagnosed definitively because the signs and symptoms are similar to those of other neurologic conditions. Common signs and symptoms of ALS are:

- Stumbling, tripping, and falling
- Loss of strength and muscle control in the hands, arms, and legs
- Difficulty speaking
- Difficulty swallowing
- Drooling
- Breathing that becomes progressively more difficult
- Muscle cramping, shaking, and twitching, progressing to spasticity
- Muscle weakness and atrophy
- Abnormal reflexes

ALS is not a painful disease, but the effects of ALS often cause pain. These are:

Difficult Situations

Many patients with post-polio syndrome are fiercely independent, sometimes to their detriment. They may not complain because most were taught that part of their recovery includes being "normal." They were supposed to be like everyone else. They were bullied if they did things differently. They continue to strive for normalcy to this day. Asking for help may be very difficult for these patients.

- Muscle cramps
- Contractures
- Constipation
- Burning eyes
- Swelling feet
- Muscle aches
- Pressure injuries

ALS does not affect the entire body. The patient's mental acuity is intact. Depression is common. The heart, bowel and bladder control, and sexual function are not affected. The muscles controlling eye and eyelid movement are the last muscles affected. Sometimes they are not affected at all.

Progression of ALS

Progression of ALS varies with the patient. Worsening occurs over several months to several years. A common pattern is:

- Difficulty walking, causing the patient to use a cane, then a walker, then a wheelchair.
- As the legs weaken, the hands and arms also become weaker.
- The person loses the ability to write and feed themselves.
- The patient experiences difficulty speaking, chewing, swallowing, and talking.
- Eventually a feeding tube becomes necessary.
- The patient needs an alternative communication system. Some people use computers to speak for them. If they have financial resources available, the patient or family will often purchase a computer to manage other aspects of daily life.
- Chest and diaphragm muscles weaken, causing lung problems.
- The patient needs a ventilator to stay alive.

Nursing Assistant Care

Most patients with ALS are cared for at home, with brief hospitalizations to manage complications. Because of this, ALS often involves the whole family. Patients are taught to manage their own illness. Allow the patient to be in control of daily routines, and respect their intelligence. Adaptive equipment is used to maintain independence for as long as possible.

Many patients with ALS are not bedridden, despite being completely paralyzed. Special wheelchairs and portable ventilators are often used so patients can get out of bed. Follow the patient's care plan for mobility. If the patient does not get out of bed, reposition and turn them at least every two hours, or more often, as instructed.

Nursing care is designed to prevent complications of immobility. The most common problems are constipation, contractures, and pressure injuries. You will also take measures to prevent choking and infection. Care of the patient is largely determined by the stage of the patient's disease at admission to the health care facility. Follow the care plan and the nurse's instructions. Care of the typical patient with ALS involves:

- Attention to positioning. An upright position (such as high Fowler's) may be ordered to ease respiration.
- Range-of-motion and light exercises to prevent deformities and maintain the strength of muscles that are not yet affected.
- Assisting the patient to use the incentive spirometer (Chapter 39).
- Having the patient rest before meals to conserve muscle strength and reduce the risk of choking.
- Providing small, frequent feedings.
- Taking swallowing precautions when feeding the patient. The speech therapist may have taught the patient positions and techniques to use to prevent choking. Commonly, the patient is as upright as possible, with the neck flexed slightly forward.
- Not washing solid foods down with liquids. This increases the risk of choking and aspiration in ALS patients.
- Checking the mouth after meals to make sure that no food particles remain. Provide mouth care promptly after each meal.
- Scheduling rest and activities to preserve the patient's strength and energy.
- Using good infection control measures, handwashing, and standard precautions to reduce the risk of infection.

Seizure Disorder (Epilepsy)

Seizure disorder (convulsions, **epilepsy**) involves recurrent, transient attacks of disturbed brain function. It is characterized by various forms of convulsions called *seizures*. Not all seizures are alike. A seizure occurs when one or more of the following is present:

Difficult Situations

ALS is a particularly cruel disease that causes rapid degeneration of the nervous system, making the patient dependent. The mind remains intact and alert, so the patient is aware of each small change and its implications. Strive to develop a good rapport with the patient and provide generous emotional support and compassion.

- An altered state of consciousness, which may be momentary or prolonged
- Convulsive uncontrolled movements
- Disturbances of feeling or behavior
  Seizures may develop:
- Congenitally, associated with a difficult birth.
- Following a head injury.
- As a result of increased intracranial pressure.
- As a result of lesions of the brain such as tumors.
- As a result of cerebrovascular accidents.
- As a result of high fever or infection, especially in infants and children.
- From taking certain medications or street drugs.

Some persons experience an aura just before the seizure occurs. An **aura** involves one of the senses. The person may smell an unusual odor or hear a sound. The aura is usually consistent and remains the same each time it is experienced. For some people the aura serves as a warning so the person can get to a safe place. Other people may not remember the aura.

Some people have service dogs that warn them of an impending seizure so they can take safety precautions before the seizure begins. A dog's sense of smell is much more sensitive than a human's. It is believed that the dog smells a chemical reaction that signals the onset of a seizure. Your facility will have policies regarding the use of service animals.

There are many different types and categories of seizure activity. The most common are classified as follows.

1. Partial seizures:
   - There may or may not be loss of consciousness.
   - Seizures generally begin in one part of the body and involve only one side of the body.
2. Generalized seizures (Figure 43-16):
   - These include **grand mal seizures**. A newer name is **generalized tonic-clonic seizures**. There is bilateral generalized motor movement and muscular rigidity. Consciousness is lost. An aura in the form of lights, sounds, or aromas may occur before the seizure. When this seizure begins, the patient cries out, then falls to the floor. The muscles stiffen (tonic phase), then the extremities begin to jerk and twitch (clonic phase). The patient may lose bladder control. Consciousness returns slowly. After the seizure, the patient may feel tired or be confused and disoriented for anywhere from a few minutes to several hours or days. The patient may fall asleep, or gradually become less confused, until full consciousness returns.
   - **Petit mal seizures** are characterized by momentary loss of muscle tone. A more recent name is **absence seizures**. The seizure begins

without warning, and consists of a period of unconsciousness, in which the patient blinks rapidly, stares blankly, breathes rapidly, or makes chewing movements. The seizure lasts 2 to 10 seconds, then ends abruptly. The patient usually resumes normal activity immediately. Because these seizures are mild, they may go unnoticed. Children with absence seizures may have learning problems if the seizures are not identified and treated.
   - **Status epilepticus** is a seizure that lasts for a long time or repeats without recovery. It is a serious medical emergency. Death may result if the patient is not treated immediately. Status epilepticus can be convulsive (tonic-clonic) or nonconvulsive (absence). A person in nonconvulsive status epilepticus may become confused or appear dazed. The highest incidence of status epilepticus occurs during the first year of life and after age 60. In elderly adults, most cases are related to cerebrovascular accidents.

Nursing Care During Seizures

The main nursing focus during a seizure is to:

- Prevent injury by:
  - Staying with the person.
  - Assisting the person to lie down, if there is time.
  - Making no attempt to restrain the person's movements or to put anything in their mouth.
  - Moving away any object the person might hit, to prevent injury.
- Maintain an airway by:
  - Loosening clothing, particularly around the neck.
  - Turning the person's head or body to one side so that saliva or vomitus drains out.
  - Opening the airway, if necessary, by using the head-tilt, chin-lift method (Chapter 51), or lifting the person's shoulders and allowing the head to tilt back.

> ## Difficult Situations
>
> Patients with epilepsy commonly take a drug called *phenytoin* to prevent seizures. This drug causes a condition of the gums in which the normal cells increase, causing excess bulk and thickness. Careful, regular oral hygiene and mouth care can relieve the problem slightly. Do not overlook this important activity of daily living in patients with epilepsy or seizure disorder.

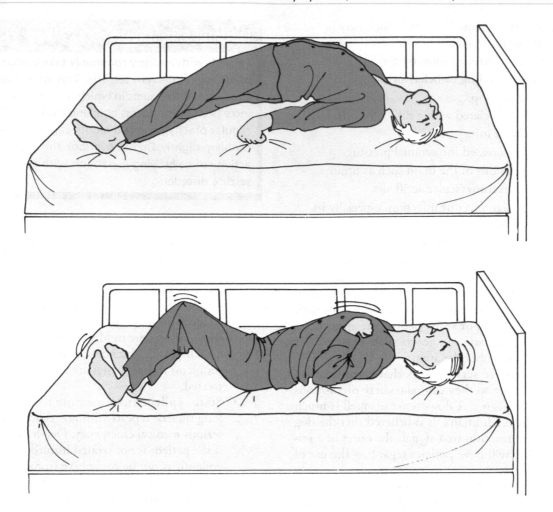

FIGURE 43-16 Generalized tonic-clonic seizures involve the entire body. Side rails should be padded for patients with seizure disorder. (Side rails in this picture are down for clarity only.)

If you find a person who is having a seizure, ring for assistance, if possible, but do not leave the patient alone. As much as possible, protect the patient from injuring themselves during the seizure.

- Do not move the person.
- Do not put anything in the person's mouth.
- Maintain an airway.
- Ring or call for assistance.
- Protect the person from self-inflicted injury.
- Watch the person carefully.
- Apply standard precautions when caring for a patient with seizure activity. There is a high probability of contact with blood, bodily fluids, secretions, and excretions during the care of this patient.
- Observe the patient during and after the seizure. Breathing should be carefully monitored.

Nursing Care after a Seizure

When the seizure stops, tell the patient where they are and what happened. Assist them to bed. The patient will be very tired. Allow them to sleep. They may be confused and require periodic reorientation. Leave the patient in a position of comfort and safety with the call signal and needed personal items within reach. Other care includes:

- Providing incontinence care, if necessary.
- Checking the vital signs as instructed; you may take vital signs frequently until the patient is stable.
- Monitoring the patient closely for return of seizure activity.
- Assisting the nurse to administer oxygen or suctioning, if needed.
  Report to the nurse:
- Any change in the patient before the seizure, such as an aura, confusion, or change in behavior.

- A description of the way the seizure looked, including the body parts involved.
- Loss of bowel or bladder control, eyes rolling upward, rapid blinking, or biting tongue.
- The time the seizure started and stopped, if known.
- The condition of the patient after the seizure.
- Vital signs.

Spinal Cord Injuries

Injuries to the spinal cord result in loss of function and sensation below the level of the injury. These patients are particularly prone to contractures and pressure injuries.

Paralysis is seen in many medical conditions but is most commonly associated with spinal cord injury. Paralysis may involve a single muscle, but usually involves an entire region of the body. A spinal cord injury causes loss or impaired function resulting in reduced mobility and feeling (sensation) below the level of the injury to the cord. The word *lesion* is a general term used to describe an alteration or change in tissue, which may be due to many causes. The most common of these are wounds and injuries. The damage to the spinal cord is also called a *lesion*. Terms used to describe paralysis are:

- **Diplegia**—paralysis affecting the same region on both sides of the body (such as both arms).
- *Hemiplegia*—paralysis on one entire side of the body (such as the arm and leg).
- **Monoplegia**—paralysis affecting one limb only.
- *Paraplegia*—paralysis of the trunk (usually below the waist) and both legs.
- *Tetraplegia* (*quadriplegia*)—paralysis of the trunk (usually below the neck), both arms, and both legs.

Flaccid paralysis involves loss of muscle tone and absence of tendon reflexes. Some patients have **spastic paralysis**. These patients have no voluntary movement. The extremities move in an involuntary pattern, similar

---

Clinical Information **ALERT**

In the United States, the term *quadriplegia* was used for many years to describe paralysis. It is derived from a combination of Greek and Latin words. In Europe, the term used to describe this condition has always been *tetraplegia*. In 1991, the American Spinal Cord Injury Classification system was revised and the terminology thoroughly researched. Since then, the American Spinal Cord Association has recommended that the term *tetraplegia* be used so that there are not two different words in English referring to the same thing.

---

to muscle spasms. The patient is aware of the movements, but cannot stop them. The type of paralysis is determined by the level of injury. Patients with upper motor injuries are more likely to exhibit spastic paralysis.

Signs and Symptoms

Signs and symptoms of paralysis vary with the level of the injury. The patient will be paralyzed below the level where the spinal cord was damaged. For example, an injury to the upper vertebrae in the neck will cause respiratory depression. The patient will be unable to move the arms and legs. They will lose bowel and bladder control. An injury near the waist will also cause loss of bowel and bladder control. The patient will be unable to move the legs but can use the arms and hands.

Treatment

Treatment depends on the level of injury. Overall, treatment is directed at:

- Keeping the lungs clear.
- Preventing complications of immobility.
- Preventing deformities.
- Restoring the patient to the highest degree of independence possible.

Responsibilities of the Nursing Assistant

Patients with spinal cord injury need long-term nursing care, which includes:

- Encouraging and allowing patients to direct their own care. Give the person as much control as possible.
- Encouraging the patient to make choices about things that affect them.
- Listening. Many persons with spinal cord injury are taught to give directions to caregivers who are doing for the person what the individual cannot do for themselves.
- A consistently calm and patient approach, because the loss of sensory and motor functions makes self-care difficult or impossible.
- Acceptance of the patient's expressions of anger, fear, and depression, as well as clumsy attempts at self-care. Remember that the patient's ability to think is not necessarily impaired. Frustration is even greater because these patients can no longer act according to their will or intention.
- Careful skin care, because:
  - Incontinence not only causes the patient embarrassment and discomfort but also makes the skin prone to breakdown.

- The lack of nervous stimulation decreases circulation to the skin.
- Pain and pressure cannot be felt.
- Attention to elimination needs. For example, suppositories may be given daily. A catheter may be inserted into the bladder, so catheter and drainage care will be needed. Special pads within plastic incontinence pants may also be used.
- Avoidance of contractures and deformities, which occur rapidly after the onset of paralysis. When moving and positioning patients with paralysis, move the extremities slowly and gently. Rapid, rough movements will cause spasticity. If a patient's extremities move into a position of flexion, position them in extension. If the extremities move into a position of extension, position them in flexion. Positioning devices may be necessary to maintain position. Attention to proper positioning is a major key to preventing contractures and deformities in these high-risk patients.
- Provision of ROM exercises. These will be needed for the rest of the patient's life.
- Proper attention and care to prevent:
  - Respiratory infections.
  - Urinary tract infections.
  - Pressure injuries.

Autonomic Dysreflexia

Autonomic dysreflexia (Figure 43-17) is a potentially life-threatening complication of spinal cord injury. It usually occurs in patients with injuries above the mid-thoracic area. It indicates uncontrolled sympathetic nervous system activity. Problems that seem minor can trigger this condition. As a rule, injuries that would normally cause pain below the level of spinal injury can set this life-threatening chain of events in motion. For example:

- Overfull bladder (this is the most common cause)
- Urinary retention
- Urinary tract infection

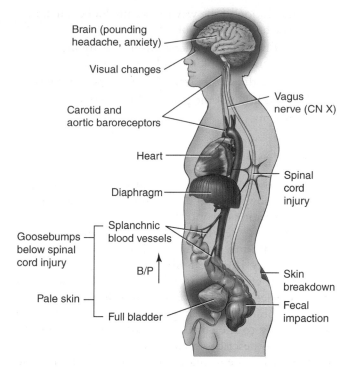

FIGURE 43-17 In autonomic dysreflexia, lower motor neurons sense a painful stimulus and send a signal to the brain. However, the signal cannot penetrate the area of spinal cord injury, so it cannot reach the brain. This triggers hypertension, pounding headache, gooseflesh (goosebumps) below the level of the spinal cord injury, and generalized pallor, visual changes, and anxiety. The body tries to notify the brain of the hypertension, but again the message cannot penetrate because of the spinal cord injury. This triggers the vagus nerve to slow the heart rate, and the patient develops bradycardia as a result of the body's attempt to normalize internal conditions.

- Blocked catheter
- Overfilled urinary drainage bag
- Constipation or fecal impaction
- Hemorrhoids
- Infection or irritation in the abdomen, such as appendicitis or acute abdominal conditions
- Pressure injuries
- Prolonged pressure by an object in the chair, shoe, wrinkled clothing, and the like
- Minor injury, such as a cut, bruise, or abrasion
- Ingrown toenails
- Burns, including sunburn
- Pressure on skin from tight or constrictive clothing
- Menstrual cramps
- Labor and delivery
- Overstimulation during sexual activity
- Fractured bones

Signs and symptoms of autonomic dysreflexia are:

- Extremely high blood pressure, greater than 200/100 mm Hg
- Severe headache
- Red, flushed face
- Red blotches on the skin above the level of spinal injury
- Sweating above the level of spinal injury
- Stuffy nose
- Nausea
- Bradycardia (pulse below 60 beats per minute)
- Goosebumps below the level of injury
- Cold, clammy skin below the level of injury

If you observe any of these signs and symptoms, notify the nurse immediately. Treatment for this condition involves identifying the offending stimulus and removing it. If you believe something has triggered the condition, inform the nurse. Remove tight and constricting clothing and shoes. Check the catheter and drainage bag. Follow the nurse's instructions.

Meningitis

Meningitis is an inflammation of the meninges. It is usually caused by viruses or bacteria. The signs and symptoms of meningitis are:

- Headache
- Nausea
- Stiffness of the neck
- Seizures
- Chills
- Elevated temperature

If the cause is bacterial, meningitis is treated with antibiotics. If it is communicable, droplet precautions are used.

Cataracts

Cataracts (Figure 43-18A) are the leading cause of vision loss in adults over the age of 55. Because of this, cataract surgery is one of the most common surgeries in the United States today.

Cataracts cause the normally clear lens of the eye to become cloudy. The cloudy (opaque) lens will not allow light rays to pass through, so the person is no longer able to see.

Treatment

Removal or replacement of the lens permits light rays to enter the eye, restoring sight. The latest innovations in cataract surgery increase comfort and convenience for the patient. Until recently, most surgeries for cataracts involved removing the center (nucleus) of the

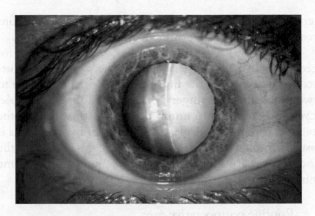

FIGURE 43-18A A cataract turns the lens of the eye cloudy.

Lens Implant Surgery for Cataracts

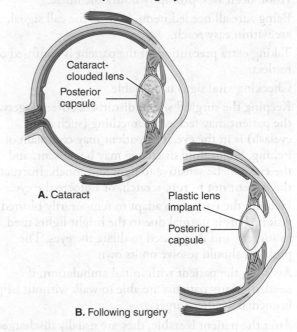

Cataract-clouded lens
Posterior capsule

A. Cataract

Plastic lens implant
Posterior capsule

B. Following surgery

FIGURE 43-18B The lens is removed and the plastic intraocular lens is permanently placed in the eye.

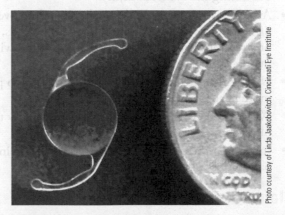

Photo courtesy of Linda Jaakobovitch, Cincinnati Eye Institute

FIGURE 43-18C The lens implant is similar to a contact lens and smaller than a dime. It is left in place but cannot be felt after the eye heals.

lens through a large incision. Currently, most surgeons remove cataracts with a small incision and ultrasound.

The surgery is performed either as an outpatient procedure or in a day surgery center. The patient is admitted to the center in the morning and remains for one to two hours after the surgery, or until vital signs are stable. Eye drops are used to numb the eye. In this surgery, the cataract is removed. A plastic, silicone, or hydrogel lens is usually implanted (Figures 43-18B and 43-18C), and the incision is naturally sealed. Stitches are not used. Some surgeons apply a patch to the eye, but most do not.

Nursing care of the cataract patient includes:

- Routine postoperative care.
- Relief of pain. Discomfort is usually mild. If pain worsens, the patient complains of sharp pain, or vision decreases, promptly notify the nurse.
- Being sure all needed items, such as the call signal, are within easy reach.
- Taking extra precautions if the patient is confused or restless.
- Checking vital signs until stable.
- Keeping the surgical site undisturbed. After surgery, the patient may feel as if something (such as an eyelash) is in the eye. The patient may complain of itching. Slight fluid discharge may be present, and the eye may be sensitive to light and touch. Instruct the patient not to rub, scratch, or squeeze the eye.
- Helping the patient to adapt to temporarily blurred vision. This is normal due to the bright lights used in surgery and drops used to dilate the eyes. The problem should resolve on its own.
- Assisting the patient with initial ambulation, if needed. Many patients are able to walk without help immediately after surgery.

After the patient is stable, they are usually discharged home. Orders regarding postoperative activity usually include:

- Protecting the eye from injury.
- Avoiding straining activities such as bending over, lifting objects that weigh more than 20 pounds, or strenuous coughing. The surgeon or nurse will instruct the patient on the level of activity.
- Using medicated eye drops for several weeks to promote healing and control pressure.
- Wearing an eye shield at night, if instructed by the physician.
- Informing the physician if there is an increase in pain or loss of vision.

Glaucoma

Glaucoma is a condition of increased pressure within the eye. The most common type of glaucoma is *open-angle*

glaucoma, a slowly progressive, chronic condition. There are no early signs and symptoms. As the problem progresses, the patient begins to experience vision loss. The problem causes gradual loss of peripheral vision. The patient:

- Develops eye pain.
- Has difficulty adjusting to darkness.
- May be unable to detect color.
- Sees halos around lights.

Untreated, this condition progresses to loss of central vision and blindness. The problem is usually detected during a routine eye examination. Untreated, the condition compresses the lens into the vitreous humor. This places pressure on the neurons in the retina, leading to blindness. Open-angle glaucoma commonly occurs in both eyes at the same time.

An acute glaucoma, called *closed-angle glaucoma*, is less common. This type usually occurs in only one eye. When the pressure within the eye increases, the iris will bulge out. The patient usually has severe pain and vision loss in the eye. Other signs and symptoms are:

- Nausea and vomiting
- Headache
- Feeling very tired
- Blurred vision
- Rainbow-like halos around lights

This is an emergency situation that must be promptly treated.

Care of the Patient with Glaucoma

Glaucoma is treated with medications and special eye drops that reduce pressure within the eye. Surgery may be done to drain fluid and relieve pressure. The patient must have regular eye examinations to measure the pressure within the eye. Care of the patient with glaucoma includes:

- Monitoring accurate intake and output if the patient is on intravenous medication to reduce eye pressure.
- Checking vital signs every two to four hours.
- Reporting complaints of eye pain promptly to the nurse.
- Arranging needed items so the patient can see them; avoid moving things unless the patient gives permission.
- Avoiding strain and exertion that will increase intraocular pressure.
- Keeping the patient from stooping or lifting.
- Avoiding tight and constrictive clothing, which also increases pressure.
- Keeping the patient safe, if vision is limited.

Retinal Degeneration

Breakdown of the retina, known as **retinal degeneration** or **macular degeneration**, occurs over a period of months or years. The incidence increases with age. Central vision is progressively lost as the macula (area of acute central vision) is damaged. Subretinal hemorrhages lead to scarring of this important area.

Early treatment with laser therapy can seal the tiny capillaries to prevent further damage to the macula.

Vision Impairment

Cataracts, glaucoma, retinal degeneration, eye infections, and other eye conditions such as ocular tumors can cause blindness. Persons who are legally blind may still have partial vision. When giving care, consider the degree of visual limitation and the patient's attitude to the limitations. Adjustment to blindness is both a physical and an emotional process.

Allow the person who is blind or nearly blind the opportunity to do as much as possible in personal care and other activities. Many blind people are capable and independent. In fact, most blind people do well with minimal help and support once they are fully oriented to their surroundings. Review the guidelines in Chapter 7 for working with persons who have visual impairments.

Artificial Eye

Situations such as severe injury to the eye or untreatable cancer may require surgical removal of an eye. An eye prosthesis (artificial eye) is usually inserted after the surgery. The care plan should provide information if the patient has an artificial eye.

Some patients remove the artificial eye at night. Others prefer not to remove the eye at all. You may be responsible for removing the eye. If the eye is to remain out of the socket, store it in a marked cup in contact lens disinfectant solution or sterile saline. The socket is usually cleansed and irrigated when the eye is removed. Irrigation of the socket may be a licensed nursing procedure in your facility. Know and follow your facility's policy. Apply the principles of standard precautions when caring for the artificial eye and mucous membranes in the eye socket.

Warm and Cool Eye Compresses

Many elderly patients have dry, itchy eyes. This may be caused by allergies, irritants, squinting, rubbing, or blinking the eyes. The eyes may appear red, with swollen eyelids. If a patient rubs or scratches the eyes, they may become infected. Patients with dry, itchy eyes may complain of:

- Burning
- Scratchy feeling
- Itching
- Light sensitivity
- Difficulty moving eyes
- Excess mucus production
- Severe pain
- Blurred vision
- Seeing halos

Observe the patient for:

- Drainage from the eyes
- Redness of eyelid rims
- Scaly, flaky skin around the eyes
- Edema of the eyelids

Report your observations to the nurse. You may be instructed to apply warm or cool soaks to the eyelids. Apply the principles of standard precautions when performing this procedure. If an infection is suspected, use separate gloves and equipment for each eye. This will prevent the infection from spreading.

Otitis Media

Otitis media is an infection of the middle ear. Infections of the nose and throat can move along the eustachian tube to the middle ear, causing inflammation. Fluid and pus form within the middle ear. This may result in fusion (locking) of the middle ear bones. Increased pressure may cause the eardrum to rupture. Both conditions decrease the ability to transmit sound waves. This condition, which is rare in adults, is common in children.

Antibiotics are usually given. A surgical opening (myringotomy) is sometimes made in the eardrum to drain the pus. Small tubes may be inserted for drainage.

Otosclerosis

Otosclerosis is a progressive form of deafness of unknown cause. The process involves the growth of new, abnormal bone in the bony labyrinth. This growth prevents the stapes from vibrating properly.

Hearing is improved by the use of a hearing aid. Surgery (stapedectomy) removes the excess bone and replaces it with a prosthesis.

Hearing Impairment

Some of your patients will be hard of hearing or completely deaf. A hearing aid (Figures 43-19A and 43-19B) will sometimes improve the patient's level of hearing and comprehension. Lip reading or sign language may be needed to communicate. Review the Chapter 7 guidelines for working with persons who have hearing impairments.

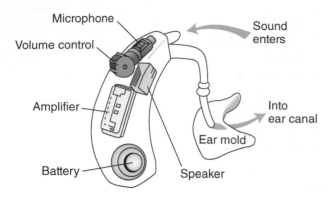

FIGURE 43-19A Parts of a behind-the-ear hearing aid. The ear mold is placed in the ear canal. The rest of the hearing aid is worn outside and over the top of the ear.

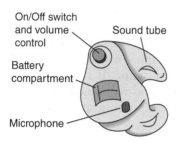

FIGURE 43-19B This is a diagram of a hearing aid that is worn inside the outer ear canal.

Caring for Hearing Aids

A hearing aid is a delicate and expensive prosthesis. It requires safe handling and regular care.

Cochlear Implant

A **cochlear implant** is a complex device that can be used to help persons with certain types of hearing loss. An external portion sits behind the ear. A second part is surgically implanted under the skin (Figure 43-20). An implant does not restore hearing, but it can help a deaf person understand speech and provides a useful representation of sounds in the environment. A cochlear implant is different from a hearing aid. The implant bypasses damaged portions of the ear and stimulates the auditory nerve. The person must learn how to use it over time, but it improves quality of life and makes it possible to hear sirens and other safety warnings.

DIAGNOSTIC TECHNIQUES

Numerous tests and techniques help physicians diagnose problems of the nervous system. Diagnostic tests include:

- Magnetic resonance imaging (MRI).
- Computerized axial tomography (CAT or CT) scan.

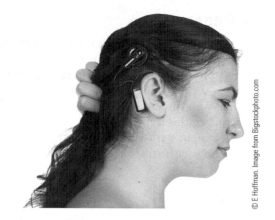

FIGURE 43-20 Part of the cochlear implant is internal and part is external.

- Electroencephalogram (EEG) to measure electrical activity of the brain.
- Myelogram, which introduces dye or contrast material into the spinal canal so an X-ray can be done.
- Tonometry, to measure intraocular pressure.
- Audiometry, to evaluate hearing.
- Spinal puncture, to collect cerebrospinal fluid.

Spinal Puncture

Spinal or lumbar punctures are done to withdraw cerebrospinal fluid (CSF) for examination or to introduce medication or anesthetic into the spinal column. The physician inserts a long, sterile needle between the lumbar vertebrae into the fluid-filled space between the arachnoid mater and pia mater. The pressure of the CSF is measured. A sample is withdrawn and placed in a sterile test tube. This test may be performed in the patient's room with nurses or nursing assistants helping with the procedure. The patient is positioned to make it easier for the needle to enter the spinal column. The patient must be very still and not move during the procedure. If the physician wants the patient positioned in a lateral position:

- Position the patient on the side facing away from the physician.
- Draw the patient's knees up to the abdomen, with the chin bent down on the chest.
- Flex the arms in a comfortable position (Figure 43-21A).

If the physician wants the person positioned in a sitting position (Figure 43-21B):

- Assist the patient to sit on the edge of the bed facing away from the physician.
- Provide an overbed table to lean on for support.

GUIDELINES 43-1 Guidelines for Caring for a Hearing Aid

- Store hearing aids at room temperature when they are not being worn. Temperature extremes can damage hearing aids. They should not be worn for more than a few minutes in very cold weather.

- Keep hearing aids dry. If an aid is accidentally worn in the shower, ask the nurse how to dry it. Avoid exposing them to hair dryers. The heat will damage the aid, and the noise is very annoying to the patient.

- Store extra batteries in a cool, dry place. Remove the batteries from the hearing aid at night or open the battery compartment. This allows trapped moisture to evaporate.

- Keep hearing aids safe. They break easily if dropped on a hard surface.

- Remove the hearing aid if hair spray is being used, as the spray may cause damage.

- Turn the hearing aid off when it is not in use. Turn the aid off before removing it.

- Wipe in-the-ear aids daily with a dry tissue.

- Check regularly to make sure the opening of the aid or ear mold is free of wax. In-the-ear types come with a cleaning tool. This should be used only by someone who has been instructed on how to use it. Never use a toothpick, paper clip, or other sharp object to clean the hearing aid.

- Insert the hearing aid properly. Sometimes the shape of the ear changes with aging and the hearing aid may have to be refitted. This may be the problem if the patient complains of pain or the aid is difficult to insert. Advise the nurse if this occurs.

- When communicating with the patient, follow the same guidelines that you use when communicating with a patient who has hearing impairment.

- Check bed linens carefully before placing them in the soiled linen hamper. A hearing aid is small, expensive, and easily lost. It will not survive a trip through the washer and dryer!

- Always shave the male patient with an electric razor *before* the hearing aid is put in the ear, or remove the hearing aid before using the electric razor. The hearing aid will amplify the noise from the razor, making it quite loud and annoying.

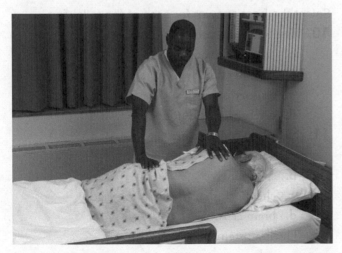

FIGURE 43-21A Position the patient on the side with the upper body and legs flexed for a lumbar puncture.

- Instruct the patient to hunch the shoulders forward.
- Position the feet firmly on the floor.
- Steady the table to prevent the patient from sliding or falling.

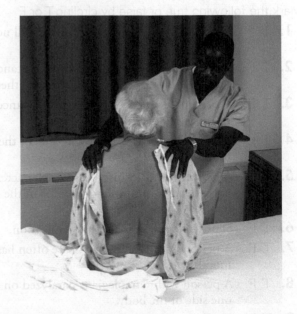

FIGURE 43-21B An alternate position for a lumbar puncture. The patient may be more comfortable leaning on a pillow on an overbed table. Be careful that the table does not slip.

GUIDELINES 43-2 Guidelines for Troubleshooting Hearing Aids

If the aid is not producing sound, before inserting it in the patient's ear:

- Check to make sure the "+" (positive) side of the battery is next to the "+" marking inside the hearing aid battery case or compartment.

- Try a new battery—the old one may be dead. Hold the hearing aid in the palm of your hand. Turn the volume all the way up. Cup the aid between your hands. You should hear a loud whistle. A weak or absent sound indicates that the battery is low.

- Before changing the battery, check the position of the old battery so you can put the new one in the same way. When inserting a new battery, place it in the unit gently. If you meet resistance, do not force it. Consult the nurse.

- Check the ear mold to see if it is plugged with wax.

- Make sure the hearing aid is set on "M" (microphone), not "T" (telephone switch).

- If the hearing aid works intermittently or makes a scratchy sound, check for dirt under and around the battery. Also check the volume control and connections. If the hearing aid has a connecting wire, make sure it is plugged in tightly and is not cracked or bent.

If the hearing aid is making squealing sounds:

- If the hearing aid is in the patient's ear and makes a loud, whistling sound, check the position. The aid should be securely in the ear. Make sure that hair, ear wax, or clothing are not interfering with the position. Check the tubing (if any) for cracks. Whistling usually indicates an air leak.

- Determine if the ear mold fits properly. It should be completely in the ear. If it does not fit well, report it to the nurse.

- Check the volume on the aid. If it is too high, turn it down until the squealing stops.

- Check the plastic tubing on a behind-the-ear aid. If it is cracked or split, it must be replaced.

REVIEW

A. True/False

Mark the following true or false by circling T or F.

1. T F   A patient with right-brain damage will not be able to speak.

2. T F   A patient with aphasia cannot understand you, so it is not necessary to speak to them.

3. T F   A patient with a CVA will need assistance in carrying out ROM exercises.

4. T F   Hemiplegia is paralysis on one side of the body.

5. T F   A person with Parkinson disease characteristically has a "pill-rolling" tremor in the hands.

6. T F   Status epilepticus is a serious condition.

7. T F   A person with Parkinson disease often has mood swings.

8. T F   A person with tetraplegia is paralyzed on one side of the body.

9. T F   Fluid may be withdrawn from the spinal canal for examination.

B. Multiple Choice

Select the best answer for each of the following.

10. The brain and spinal cord make up the:
    a. central nervous system.
    b. peripheral nervous system.
    c. sensory organs.
    d. cerebrospinal fluid space.

11. Neurotransmitters are:
    a. neurons.
    b. special nerves.
    c. chemicals that help pass messages.
    d. brain cells.

12. The brainstem controls:
    a. voluntary movement.
    b. thinking.
    c. vital functions.
    d. emotions.

13. A condition that causes the lens of the eye to become cloudy and impair vision is called:
    a. glaucoma.
    b. macular degeneration.
    c. diabetic retinopathy.
    d. cataract.

14. Hearing aids should be kept:
    a. wrapped in tissue.
    b. dry.
    c. disassembled.
    d. in a cold area.

15. Persons with Parkinson disease generally have:
    a. pain.
    b. rigidity.
    c. spasticity.
    d. hearing impairment.

16. A person who has had a stroke on the left side of the brain will:
    a. have left hemiplegia.
    b. become quick and impulsive.
    c. have aphasia.
    d. have no personality changes.

17. A person who has had a stroke on the right side of the brain will:
    a. have left hemiplegia.
    b. have aphasia.
    c. become slow, anxious, and cautious.
    d. have hearing loss in the right ear.

18. Patients with stroke:
    a. need proper positioning to prevent contractures.
    b. must be repositioned every four hours.
    c. will be unable to speak during the acute phase.
    d. will always be NPO during the acute phase.

19. Multiple sclerosis occurs because:
    a. the myelin sheath of the neuron is damaged.
    b. of a hemorrhage in the brain.
    c. of a lack of a certain neurotransmitter.
    d. of muscle damage.

20. Patients with multiple sclerosis may experience:
    a. hemiplegia.
    b. no obvious signs or symptoms.
    c. loss of sensation to temperature, pain, and touch.
    d. inability to swallow.

21. Increased intracranial pressure can develop from:
    a. Parkinson disease.
    b. head injuries.
    c. ruptured disc.
    d. post-polio syndrome.

22. If you are assisting in the care of a patient with a head injury, you should note and report:
    a. blood pressure of 112/74.
    b. pulse rate of 96.
    c. changes in levels of consciousness.
    d. skin warm and dry.

23. You come into a room and find a patient having a seizure. You should:
    a. leave and find help.
    b. restrain the patient's movements.
    c. raise the foot of the bed.
    d. remove any object the patient might hit.

24. A patient with post-polio syndrome experiences:
    a. nausea and vomiting.
    b. visual disturbances and facial droop.
    c. cold intolerance and weakness.
    d. hemiplegia.

25. After surgery, patients with post-polio syndrome:
    a. take longer to recover from the anesthesia than other patients.
    b. experience bowel and bladder incontinence.
    c. do not feel pain as acutely as other patients.
    d. commonly experience tachycardia for 24 hours.

26. Patients with ALS commonly experience:
    a. hemiplegia.
    b. muscle weakness and atrophy.
    c. difficulty hearing.
    d. mental confusion.

27. When caring for a patient who has ALS, the nursing assistant should:
    a. encourage the patient to feed themselves so they do not lose this ability.
    b. allow the patient to set the routines, because their mental clarity is unaffected.
    c. keep the patient in bed and as still as possible.
    d. limit fluids to prevent choking and aspiration.

28. Autonomic dysreflexia can be caused by:
    a. hunger.
    b. thirst.
    c. overfull bladder.
    d. drowsiness.

29. Autonomic dysreflexia is:

   a. a life-threatening condition.

   b. a minor complication of surgery.

   c. very painful.

   d. common in patients with multiple sclerosis.

30. Glaucoma is:

   a. a clouding of the lens of the eye.

   b. caused by chemical exposure.

   c. related to retinal degeneration.

   d. caused by very high pressure in the eye.

31. When caring for a patient who has glaucoma, the nursing assistant should:

   a. apply patches to the patient's eyes at bedtime.

   b. perform tasks that would strain or exert the patient.

   c. apply eye drops to the affected eye every hour.

   d. apply cool eye compresses every two hours.

C. Matching

Choose the correct item from Column II to match each word or phrase in Column I.

Column I

32. _____ uncontrolled trembling

33. _____ CVA

34. _____ difficulty and slowness in carrying out voluntary muscular activities

35. _____ language impairment

36. _____ convulsion

37. _____ aura

38. _____ nystagmus

Column II

  a. akinesia

  b. aphasia

  c. tremors

  d. seizure

  e. sclera

  f. stroke

  g. involuntary movement of the eye seen in multiple sclerosis

  h. sensation experienced by some persons just before having a seizure

D. Nursing Assistant Challenge

You are assigned to care for Mr. Johnson, who has had a stroke. You learn from his care plan that he has right hemiplegia and aphasia. Answer these questions about this patient and his condition.

39. From this information, you know that which part of Mr. Johnson's brain was affected by the stroke?

   a. _____

40. What does right hemiplegia mean?

   a. _____

41. What will you expect from Mr. Johnson's attempts to communicate verbally?

   a. _____

42. What complications is he at risk for? What can you do to prevent these complications?

   a. _____

   b. _____

43. What observations would indicate that Mr. Johnson has cognitive impairment?

   a. _____

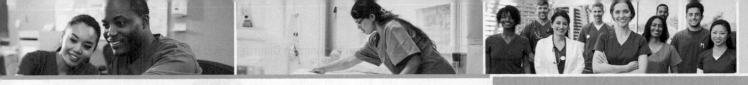

Gastrointestinal System

CHAPTER 44

OBJECTIVES

After completing this chapter, you will be able to:

44.1 Spell and define terms.

44.2 Review the location of the organs of the gastrointestinal system.

44.3 Explain the functions of the organs of the gastrointestinal system.

44.4 List specific diagnostic tests associated with disorders of the gastrointestinal system.

44.5 Describe some common disorders of the gastrointestinal system.

44.6 Describe nursing assistant actions related to the care of patients with disorders of the gastrointestinal system.

44.7 Explain the purpose of the different types of enemas.

44.8 List the guidelines for caring for an ostomy.

44.9 Demonstrate the following procedure:
- Procedure 89: Collecting a Stool Specimen (Expand Your Skills)
- Procedure 90: Testing for Occult Blood Using Hemoccult and Developer (Expand Your Skills)
- Procedure 91: Inserting a Rectal Suppository (Expand Your Skills)
- Procedure 92: Giving a Soap-Solution Enema (Expand Your Skills)
- Procedure 93: Giving a Commercially Prepared Enema (Expand Your Skills)
- Procedure 94: Giving Routine Stoma Care (Colostomy) (Expand Your Skills)
- Procedure 95: Giving Routine Care of an Ileostomy (with Patient in Bed) (Expand Your Skills)

VOCABULARY

Learn the meaning and the correct spelling of the following words and phrases:

abdominal distention	diarrhea	hernia	proctoscopy
bile	duodenal resection	herniorrhaphy	pyloric sphincter
bolus	duodenal ulcer	hydrochloric acid (HCl)	sigmoidoscopy
cholecystectomy	enema	ileostomy	stool
cholecystitis	fecal impaction	incarcerated (strangulated)	suppository
cholelithiasis	fecal material	hernia	ulcer
chyme	flatus	jejunostomy tube (J-tube)	ulcerative colitis
colon	gastrectomy	nasogastric tube (NG tube)	urgency
colostomy	gastric resection	occult blood	
constipation	gastric ulcer	pepsin	
defecation	gastroscopy	peristalsis	

INTRODUCTION

The digestive tract extends from the mouth to the anus. The teeth, tongue, salivary glands, liver, gallbladder, and pancreas break food into simpler substances that supply nutrition and eliminate wastes.

STRUCTURE AND FUNCTION

The gastrointestinal system is also called the *GI* or *digestive tract*. It extends from the mouth to the anus and is lined with mucous membrane (Figure 44-1). The organs along the length of this system change food into simple forms that can pass through the walls of the small intestine and into the circulatory system, which carries the nutrients to the body cells. The gastrointestinal system includes the:

- Mouth, teeth, tongue, and salivary glands
- Pharynx
- Esophagus (gullet)
- Stomach
- Small intestine
- Liver, gallbladder, and pancreas
- Large intestine

In the digestive system:

- Proteins are changed to amino acids.
- Carbohydrates are changed to simple sugars like glucose.
- Fats are changed to fatty acids and glycerol.

Mechanical actions and chemicals called *enzymes* cause these changes. The nondigestible portions of what we eat pass through the intestines and are excreted from the body as feces. Several organs contribute to the digestive process, and many disease conditions affect them.

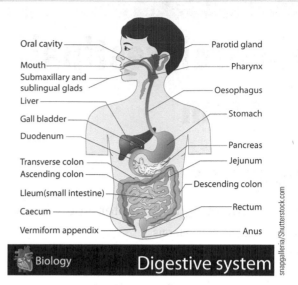

FIGURE 44-1 Digestive tract.

Labels (left): Oral cavity, Mouth, Submaxillary and sublingual glads, Liver, Gall bladder, Duodenum, Transverse colon, Ascending colon, Lleum(small intestine), Caecum, Vermiform appendix

Labels (right): Parotid gland, Pharynx, Oesophagus, Stomach, Pancreas, Jejunum, Descending colon, Rectum, Anus

Biology — Digestive system

snapgalleria/Shutterstock.com

Mouth

Food is chewed so it can be swallowed easily (Figure 44-2). The digestive process begins with the help of the:

- Tongue—a skeletal muscle that is covered by taste buds. The tongue pushes the food between the teeth to be broken up. It assists in mastication (chewing). It propels the food backward toward the pharynx to assist in swallowing and aids in speech formation.
- *Papillae*—tiny bumps on the tongue that are commonly called taste buds. Salt and some other substances amplify the response of the taste buds, probably by acting as electrical conductors. Humans can detect five known tastes, although further study is ongoing in this area. The tastes that have been identified are:
  - Sweet
  - Salt
  - Bitter
  - Sour
  - *Umami* (This was first established as a taste in 2000. It was formerly considered a "flavor enhancer." Umami is a Japanese word for a savory, meaty, or protein taste. Examples of umami tastes are steak and sautéed mushrooms.)
- Salivary glands—secrete saliva containing a digestive enzyme called salivary amylase.
  - Salivary amylase initiates carbohydrate digestion.
  - 1½ quarts of saliva are secreted daily.
  - Saliva moistens food to help in swallowing.

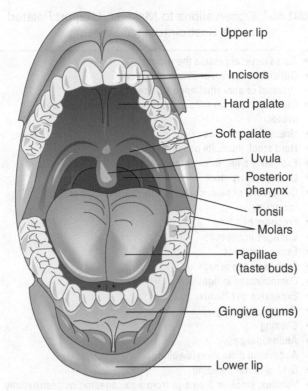

- Upper lip
- Incisors
- Hard palate
- Soft palate
- Uvula
- Posterior pharynx
- Tonsil
- Molars
- Papillae (taste buds)
- Gingiva (gums)
- Lower lip

FIGURE 44-2 Mouth.

- Teeth—mechanically break up food into smaller particles, forming a **bolus** of food that is swallowed. There are two natural sets of teeth. The first set (deciduous or temporary) numbers 20. The second set (permanent) numbers 32 and gradually replaces the deciduous set.
- Pharynx—allows the passage of both food and air. It leads to the esophagus.
- Esophagus—a tube 10 to 12 inches long that carries the food to the stomach. Strong muscular contractions called *peristaltic waves* move the food along the tract. These waves begin in the esophagus and continue throughout the intestinal tract.

The Stomach

The stomach:
- Is a hollow, muscular, J-shaped organ.
- Is found in the peritoneal cavity.
- Is two-thirds to the left of the midline.
- Is just below the diaphragm.
- Has circular muscles at either end that hold food while it is thoroughly mixed with digestive enzymes.
- Begins the chemical process of digestion.

Clinical Information **ALERT**

The digestive system is open at both ends and is about 25 to 30 feet long. The narrowest part of the digestive system is the esophagus, and the widest part is the stomach. The stomach can stretch to 50 times its empty size and can hold about a gallon (4 liters). Hydrochloric acid in the stomach is the most acidic substance in the body. The stomach must produce a new layer of mucus every two weeks; otherwise, it would digest itself.

- Holds food between 3 to 4 hours.

The stomach has three parts:
- Fundus—the area above the entrance of the esophagus.
- Body—holds food.
- Pylorus—the long, narrowly tapered distal end that connects with the small intestines. The muscle guarding this exit point is called the **pyloric sphincter**.

The stomach cells produce gastric juice, which contains:
- Proteolytic enzyme (**pepsin**) to begin protein breakdown.
- Hydrochloric acid (HCl).
- Intrinsic factor, which is needed for the absorption of vitamin B12.

The Intestines

When food leaves the stomach, it is in a semiliquid form called **chyme**. Chyme enters the small intestine, where any undigested nutrients are broken down by intestinal and pancreatic enzymes and bile from the liver.

Clinical Information **ALERT**

The liver is the largest gland in the body. The pancreas is the source of the most diverse mixture of digestive enzymes. The jejunum has the richest blood supply in the digestive system. The cells in the digestive system with the shortest life span are those found on the epithelium of the duodenum. These cells live for approximately three days. The small intestine is the largest internal organ in the body.

Materials move through the intestines by waves of **peristalsis**. Food digestion is completed in the small intestine, where most of the nutrients are absorbed into the bloodstream.

The small intestine is about 23 feet long and coils within the peritoneum. There are three main portions:

- The duodenum—about 12 inches long. Has an opening in the back to receive the bile and pancreatic secretions.
- The jejunum—about 8 feet long.
- The ileum—the last 12 to 13 feet. Terminates in the ileocecal valve (prevents food from traveling backward) and is connected to the large intestine.

The large intestine (colon) is about 4½ feet long. It is divided into several sections:

- Cecum
- Ascending colon
- Transverse colon
- Descending colon
- Sigmoid colon
- Rectum
- Anus

No digestive enzymes are secreted in the colon. The colon is the place where:

- Some vitamins are absorbed into the circulatory system.
- More complex carbohydrates are acted upon by bacteria.

Much of the remaining water is absorbed through the walls of the large intestine, changing wastes to a more solid form. In this way, the large intestine helps to maintain the water balance of the body.

Peristalsis continues to move waste through the large intestine until it reaches the rectum. When a certain amount has been collected in the rectum, it is eliminated as feces through the anus. This process is called **defecation**.

The Appendix

The appendix is located in the lower-right quadrant, attached to the cecum. Its function is not known. Inflammation of the appendix is called *appendicitis*.

The Liver and Gallbladder

The *liver* is a large gland with four lobes that is located just beneath the right side of the diaphragm. It performs numerous metabolic functions. For example, the liver helps control the amount of protein and sugar in the blood by changing and storing excess amounts. It produces blood proteins such as prothrombin and

TABLE 44-1 Observations to Make and Report Related to the Gastrointestinal System

- Sores or ulcers inside the mouth
- Difficulty chewing or swallowing food
- Unusual or abnormal appearance of feces
- Blood, mucus, parasites, or other unusual substances in stool
- Unusual color of feces
- Hard stool; difficulty passing stool
- Extremely small or extremely large stool
- Loose, watery stool
- Complaints of pain, constipation, diarrhea, bleeding, impaction
- Frequent belching
- Changes in appetite
- Excessive thirst
- Fruity smell to breath
- Complaints of indigestion
- Excessive gas (flatus)
- Nausea, vomiting
- Choking
- Abdominal pain
- Abdominal distention (swelling)
- Oral or rectal bleeding
- Vomitus, stool, or drainage from a nasogastric or gastrostomy tube that looks like coffee grounds

fibrinogen, which are important factors in the blood clotting process. The liver also produces bile, which is carried directly to the small intestine for use in digestion or to the gallbladder for storage. Bile prepares (emulsifies) fats for digestion.

The *gallbladder* is a small hollow sac that is attached to the underside of the liver. It holds about two ounces of bile that it receives from the liver. It releases bile into the small intestine to help digest a fatty meal. The presence of bile in the digestive tract gives solid wastes their usual brown color.

The Pancreas

The *pancreas* is a glandular organ that produces both exocrine secretions (digestive enzymes) and endocrine secretions (insulin and glucagon). It extends from behind the stomach into the curve of the duodenum. It manufactures pancreatic juice, which is sent into the duodenum to aid in the digestion of foods. The pancreas also produces insulin and glucagon, sending them directly into the bloodstream.

Observations to make and report related to the gastrointestinal system are listed in Table 44-1.

COMMON CONDITIONS

The tubelike mucous membrane structure of the alimentary canal lends itself to the possibility of malignancies, ulcerations, obstructions, and herniations.

Malignancy

Malignancies (cancers) of the gastrointestinal tract are very common. The symptoms they cause depend on their location. Among the symptoms are:

- Obstruction. Blockage of the passageway is sometimes the first major indication of a long-growing tumor.
- Indigestion.
- Vomiting.
- Constipation.
- Changes in the shape of the **stool** (feces or bowel movement).
- **Flatus** (gas).
- Blood in the stool.

Treatment

Malignancies of the intestinal tract are usually treated surgically by removing the affected part. For example:

- Esophagectomy—removal of the esophagus.
- Subtotal gastrectomy—removal of part of the stomach.
- Colectomy (bowel resection)—removal of a part of the **colon** (large intestine).
- **Colostomy**—creation of an artificial opening in the abdominal wall and bringing a section of the colon to it for the elimination of feces.
- **Ileostomy**—creation of an artificial opening in the abdominal wall and bringing a section of ileum through it for the elimination of waste.
- **Jejunostomy tube (J-tube)**—a long, small-bore tube that is threaded through the GI tract until the tip reaches the small intestine. These tubes may be placed through the nose (nasojejunostomy), or surgically through an incision in the abdominal skin. Used for providing enteral nutrition for patients who do not have a stomach and those in whom recurrent formula aspiration is a problem.

Ulcerations

An **ulcer** (sore or tissue breakdown) can occur anywhere along the digestive tract. Common places are the:

- Colon—**ulcerative colitis**. In colitis, malnutrition and dehydration are brought about by loss of fluids in frequent, watery, foul-smelling stools containing mucus and pus.
- Stomach—**gastric ulcer**.
- Duodenum—**duodenal ulcer**.

Treatment

Treatment of ulcerative colitis includes:

- Medication to slow peristalsis (the wavelike contractions of the intestines) and reduce patient anxiety.
- Modification of diet to include high protein, high calories, and low residue. The low-residue diet is one in which the foods are almost completely digested. There is little waste with this type of diet.
- Medication (steroids) to reduce inflammation.
- Antibiotics to control infection by the microorganism *Helicobacter pylori* (*H. pylori*).

Patients with gastric or duodenal ulcers have periodic burning pain about two hours after eating. Most patients improve when foods that cause distress are not eaten. Medications are given to neutralize the **hydrochloric acid (HCl)** in the stomach, to coat the stomach, and to decrease anxiety. Removing part of the stomach (**gastrectomy** or **gastric resection**) or duodenum (**duodenal resection**) may be necessary. Following such surgery, the patient is:

- NPO. Special mouth care is needed.
- Placed on gastrointestinal drainage. A **nasogastric tube (NG tube)** (Figure 44-3) is inserted through the patient's nose and into the stomach. The tube is attached to a drainage bottle. Additional tubes are inserted into the intestinal tract. Be careful not to disturb the tubes. Check frequently to ensure that the drainage is not blocked. If drainage becomes blocked, notify the nurse at once. Note and record the type and amount of drainage on the intake and output worksheet.

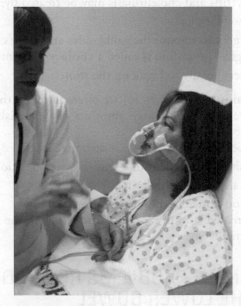

FIGURE 44-3 A nasogastric tube should be taped securely to the patient. Care should be taken when turning or moving a patient with a nasogastric tube to avoid dislodging or pulling on the tube.

Hernias

A **hernia** results when a structure such as the intestine pushes through a weakened area in the muscle that normally restrains it. The danger is that some of the protruding tissue can become trapped in the weakened area, reducing circulation so that the tissue is in danger of dying. This is called an **incarcerated (strangulated) hernia**.

Frequent sites of herniation are:

- Groin area (inguinal hernia).
- Near the umbilicus (umbilical hernia).
- Through a poorly healed incision (incisional hernia).
- Through the diaphragm (hiatal hernia).

Hernias are usually repaired surgically with a **herniorrhaphy**.

Gallbladder Conditions

Two common conditions affecting the gallbladder are:

- **Cholecystitis**—an inflammation of the gallbladder.
- **Cholelithiasis**—the formation of stones in the gallbladder. The stones may obstruct the flow of **bile** (fluid that aids digestion), giving rise to signs and symptoms such as:
  - Indigestion
  - Pain
  - Jaundice (yellow discoloration of the skin and whites of the eyes)

Treatment

Cholecystitis and cholelithiasis may be treated by:

- A low-fat diet.
- Surgery to remove the gallbladder and stones. This surgical procedure is called a **cholecystectomy**.
- Laser therapy to break up the stones.

Drains (see Chapter 36) are often placed in the operative areas. Initially, large amounts of yellowish-green drainage may be expected.

In addition to routine postoperative care:

- Position the patient in a semi-Fowler's position.
- Do not disturb drains.
- If you notice fresh blood on the dressing, increased jaundice, or dark urine, inform the nurse immediately.

COMMON PROBLEMS RELATED TO THE LOWER BOWEL

The frequency of bowel elimination varies with the individual. Some people have more than one bowel movement (BM) a day, but others have a BM every two or three days. **Fecal material** (solid body waste, feces, stool, bowel movement, BM) is normally brown, but the color can be affected by certain foods, medications, and diseases. The bowel movement is normally soft and formed. If it passes through the colon too quickly, it is loose and watery. When a patient has multiple watery stools, it is called **diarrhea**. If stool passes through the colon too slowly, the fecal material becomes hard, dry, or sticky and pasty in consistency and is difficult to pass. This is called **constipation**.

Certain foods, medications, infections, and diseases can cause constipation and diarrhea. Gas forms as foods move through the gastrointestinal tract by peristalsis. When the gas is expelled from the body, it is called flatulence or passing flatus. A healthy person expels about 3.5 ounces of intestinal gas in a single flatulent emission, or a little more than a pint each day. Most is caused by swallowed air. Some is due to breakdown of undigested food.

Gas that is not passed accumulates in the intestine. The abdomen will enlarge and appear bloated. This is called **abdominal distention** and is an important observation to report to the nurse. Abdominal distention may also be caused by constipation and urinary retention.

Changes in Function of the Gastrointestinal System Associated with Aging and Disease

Aging, disease, surgery, diet, and medications will cause a change in bowel function. Lack of privacy may also affect the patient's ability to have a bowel movement. Movement in the colon slows down, reducing the speed of food absorption and elimination. Other aging changes in the digestive system are:

- Taste buds are lost, beginning with sweet and salt. This helps explain why some elderly persons put a great deal of sugar and salt on their food. To a younger person with intact taste buds, the amount used may seem excessive.
- Saliva production in the mouth decreases, interfering with digestion of starch, making swallowing difficult, and increasing the potential for tooth decay.
- The gag reflex in the throat is less effective, increasing the risk of choking and aspiration.
- Movement of food into the stomach through the esophagus is slower.
- The stomach takes longer to empty into the small intestine, so food remains there longer.
- Fewer digestive enzymes are present in the stomach, causing indigestion and slower absorption of fat.
- Movement of the food mass through the large intestine is slower, resulting in constipation.

Other factors that affect bowel function are:

- Bedrest
- Inactivity
- Inadequate exercise
- Inability to chew foods properly
- Loose or missing teeth
- Inadequate fluid intake
- Stress
- Change in environment
- Change in diet
- Diet that does not contain enough fiber, fruits, or vegetables
- Some medications

Observations to Make when Assisting Patients with Bowel Elimination

Observe the patient's bowel movement before discarding it (Figure 44-4). If you note something unusual, save the stool for the nurse to assess. Observations of bowel elimination to make and report are listed in Table 44-2.

Constipation and Fecal Impaction

The patient is probably constipated if they have not had a bowel movement in more than three days; strains; or passes hard, marblelike stools. **Fecal impaction** (Figure 44-5) is the most serious form of

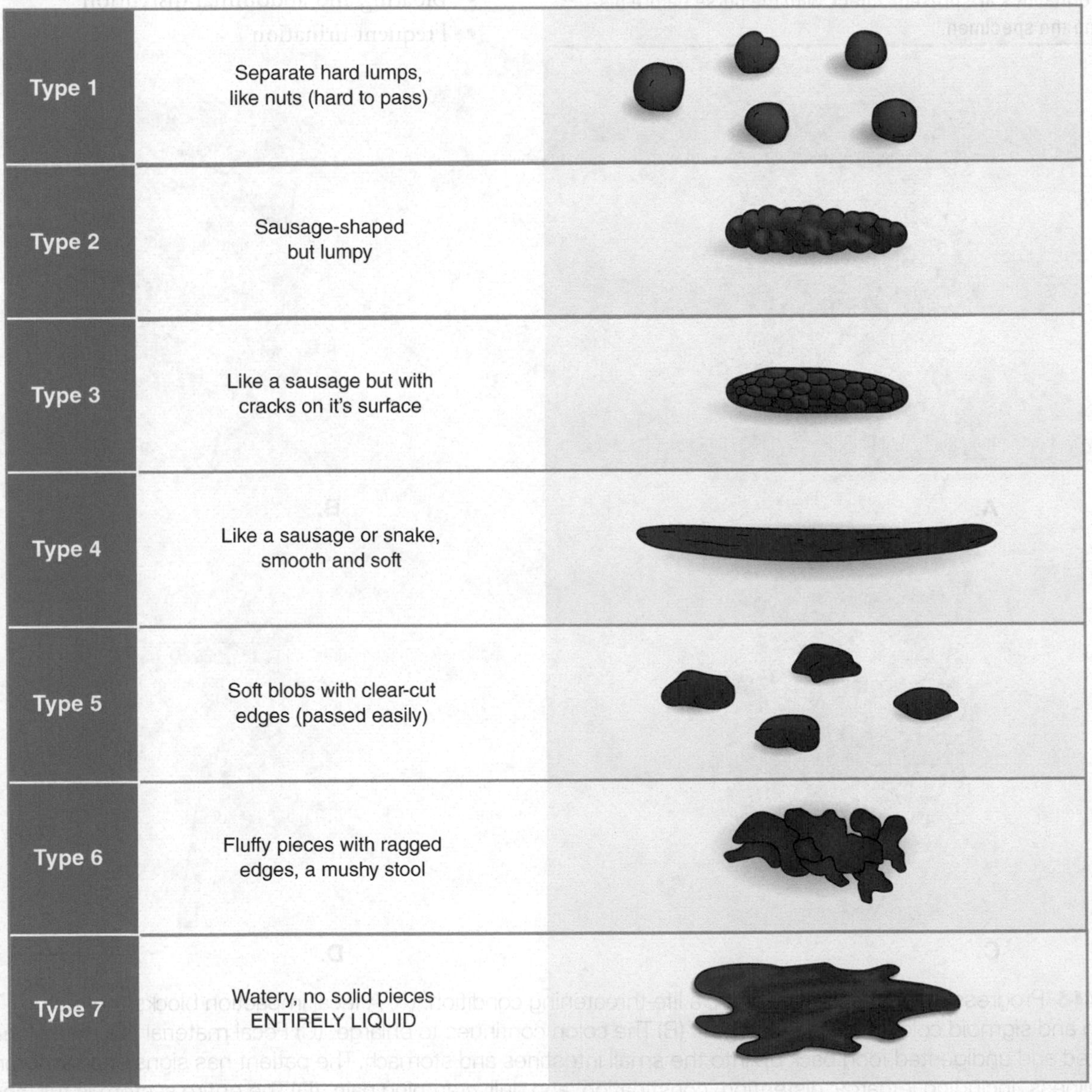

Type 1	Separate hard lumps, like nuts (hard to pass)	
Type 2	Sausage-shaped but lumpy	
Type 3	Like a sausage but with cracks on it's surface	
Type 4	Like a sausage or snake, smooth and soft	
Type 5	Soft blobs with clear-cut edges (passed easily)	
Type 6	Fluffy pieces with ragged edges, a mushy stool	
Type 7	Watery, no solid pieces ENTIRELY LIQUID	

Based on Bristol Stool Chart developed by Dr. K.W. Heaton, Reader in Medicine at the University of Bristol.

FIGURE 44-4 Types 1 and 2 indicate constipation. Stools 3 and 4 are more normal and easiest to pass. Types 5, 6, and 7 are looser.

TABLE 44-2 Observations of Bowel Elimination

Observe for potential abnormalities:
- Color
- Odor
- Consistency (loose, watery, dry, etc.)
- Character (hard, soft, pasty, etc.)
- Amount (unusual amount for person; extremely small or large)
- Frequency of stools
- Absence of stools; no BM in 3 days
- Cramping
- Pain
- Blood, pus, mucus, etc.
- Undigested food (except corn and raisins)
- Presence of parasites
- Distention
- Excessive flatulence
- Involuntary stools when previously had bowel control

If abnormalities are present, check with the nurse before discarding the specimen.

constipation. It is caused by retention of stool in the rectum, where water is absorbed. Over time, the stool becomes hard and dry. The patient may be unable to pass it. The dried waste irritates the bowel. Mucus dissolves the hard, outer part of the mass. The rectum becomes so full that fluid escapes around the impaction and is eliminated from the rectum as diarrhea. The patient may complain of:

- Abdominal or rectal pain
- Nausea
- Loss of appetite
- Feeling the need to have a bowel movement, but being unable

Other signs and symptoms of impaction are:
- Passing excessive flatus
- Bloating and abdominal distention
- Frequent urination

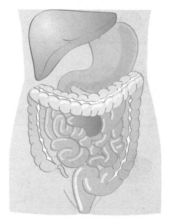

A.

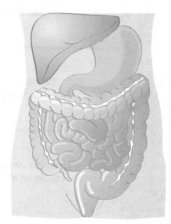

B.

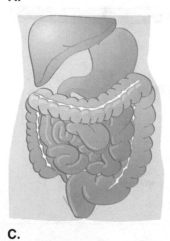

C.

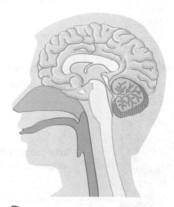

D.

FIGURE 44-5 Progression of a fecal impaction, a life-threatening condition: (A) A fecal impaction blocks the rectum. The rectum and sigmoid colon become enlarged. (B) The colon continues to enlarge. (C) Fecal material fills the colon. Digested and undigested food back up into the small intestines and stomach. The patient has signs and symptoms of acute illness, including lethargy, distention, constipation, and dull, cramping pain. (D) The entire system is full, and the patient vomits fecal material. The feces may be aspirated into the lungs.

- Inability to empty the bladder
- Leaking around the catheter
- Mental confusion
- Fever
- Liquid stool or mucus seeping from the rectum

Fecal impaction is usually treated by manual removal of the mass by the nurse or advanced care provider. Laxatives and enemas are also used. Prevention is the best approach. Carefully observe and document bowel elimination. Alert the nurse if a patient has not had a BM for three days.

Diarrhea

Diarrhea occurs when peristalsis in the intestines is very rapid. The need to defecate is usually very urgent if the patient has diarrhea. The force with which the fecal material moves through the intestines may cause the person to become incontinent. They may also complain of abdominal pain and cramping.

Diarrhea can cause dehydration and other serious medical problems if undetected or untreated. Most health care facilities have a definition of diarrhea, such as three or more loose stools within a defined period of time. One loose stool is not diarrhea. Remember to be objective in reporting your observations.

Bowel Incontinence

Bowel incontinence is involuntary passage of fecal material from the anus. It has many causes, including trauma, neurological diseases, inability to reach the toilet on time, and mental confusion. It is not as common as urinary incontinence. Fecal material is very irritating to the skin, so the patient must be cleansed well after each episode of incontinence. Skin exposed to fecal material will break down quickly. Bowel incontinence may lower the patient's self-esteem. Be professional, compassionate, and understanding when assisting patients with bowel elimination and incontinence.

Patients with bowel incontinence may be placed on a bowel retraining or incontinence management program. If this is ineffective, a fecal incontinence collector may be used.

Role of the Nursing Assistant in Assisting Patients with Bowel Elimination

Assisting with bowel elimination is a very important responsibility. Always apply the principles of standard precautions when assisting with elimination. Avoid

Infection Control **ALERT**

Clostridium difficile (C. difficile) (Chapter 12) is usually transmitted on workers' hands after they touch feces or contaminated surfaces. *C. difficile* spores can exist for five months on hard surfaces. One study showed that the level of worker hand contamination increases as levels of environmental contamination increase. The pathogen and spores can survive under fingernails, in skin folds, and on jewelry. Workers' hands may also contaminate bathrooms, faucets, clean linens, side rails, call signals, and toilets. Remember not to use alcohol-based hand cleaner if the patient is suspected of having infectious diarrhea that is spread by spores.

Clinical Information **ALERT**

Moisture from urinary and fecal incontinence increases the risk of skin damage from friction and shearing. Continued exposure to moisture weakens the skin and reduces its protective function, setting the stage for more irritation and continued weakening of the skin. Enzymes pass through the digestive system in feces. These enzymes break down food during digestion. They also break down the skin during prolonged exposure to stool, such as in diarrhea, an ostomy, or incontinence. Studies have shown that fecal incontinence is a contributing factor in more than half of all pressure injuries in the torso and buttock area.

contaminating environmental surfaces with your gloves. Wear a gown, eye protection, and face mask if splashing is likely. If an adult must wear a protective garment to contain incontinence, avoid calling the garment a diaper, which is demeaning. Use another term, such as *brief*, *adult brief*, or *clothing protector*, or call the garment by the product name, such as Depends.

Stool Specimens

A specimen of stool is a sample of fecal material (solid body waste or bowel movement) collected in a special container. The specimen is sent to the laboratory, where it may be examined for:

Communication **ALERT**

Remember that bowel activity is a normal body function. Avoid showing disgust in your facial expressions or body language when assisting patients with elimination. Documenting bowel activity is a very important responsibility. Unrelieved constipation is a serious, uncomfortable condition. The nurse depends on the accuracy of your documentation in the elimination record. They will use this record to contact the physician and administer medications and other treatments related to bowel elimination.

Clinical Information **ALERT**

Sometimes the doctor will order stool specimens ×3 for ova and parasites (O&P), various toxins, or occult blood. These specimens should be obtained 24 hours apart, unless otherwise ordered. A 12-hour minimum may be acceptable, depending on the circumstances. Always check with the nurse:

- Before discarding a specimen.
- If the patient just had a lower GI series (barium enema).
- After the administration of a prep for lower colon X-rays.
- After the nurse has given a laxative or suppository.

Normal saline enema specimens are acceptable, but must be labeled "saline enema specimen." If in doubt about the preparation for the specimen, check with the nurse.

- Pathogenic microorganisms (germs)
- Parasites
- **Occult blood** (hidden blood or blood that cannot be seen with the eye)
- Chemical analysis

GUIDELINES 44-1 Guidelines for Assisting Patients with Bowel Elimination

- Apply the principles of standard precautions when assisting with bowel elimination. Avoid environmental contamination from your gloves.
- Encourage patients to consume an adequate amount of fluid. Maintaining fluid intake is as important for bowel elimination as it is for urinary elimination.
- Encourage patients to eat a well-balanced diet.
- Allow adequate time for patients to eat meals.
- Encourage patients to chew food well. Cut it into small pieces if necessary. Report chewing problems to the nurse for further assessment.
- Offer a substitute if a patient does not eat fiber foods, fruits, or vegetables. The dietitian may visit the patient to discuss likes and dislikes, and ensure that the patient will eat the foods served.
- Encourage exercise and activity, as allowed and tolerated.
- Assist patients with toileting at regular intervals and provide privacy.
- Position patients in a sitting position, if allowed, for bowel elimination.
- Use a bath blanket to cover a patient who is using the bedpan or commode, for privacy and warmth.

- Leave the call signal and toilet tissue within reach and respond to the call signal immediately.
- Allow adequate time for defecation.
- Provide perineal care as needed, or according to facility policy. Feces are very irritating to the skin, and prolonged contact promotes skin breakdown and infection.
- Assist patients with cleaning the anal area (this may be called the rectal area by some health care providers).
- Apply a barrier product if the skin becomes irritated.
- Assist patients with handwashing and other personal hygiene after bowel elimination.
- Monitor bowel elimination and report irregularities as listed in Table 44-2.
- Record bowel movements on the flow sheet or designated area on the electronic documentation. Ask independent patients each day if they have had a bowel movement.
- Note that people who take narcotic analgesics (opioid drugs) absorb food by a slightly different route than other people. The rectum may be empty, yet the person is very constipated because water is absorbed from the stool higher up in the large intestine. Reduced peristalsis and slow transit time may also contribute to the problem.

SPECIAL DIAGNOSTIC TESTS

Some techniques used to diagnose problems of the gastrointestinal system include:

- Gastrointestinal (GI) series—a liquid containing *barium* is either swallowed (upper GI series) or given as an enema (lower GI series) before X-rays are taken.
- Direct visualization procedures:
  - **Proctoscopy**—visualization of the rectum
  - **Sigmoidoscopy**—visualization of the sigmoid colon
  - **Gastroscopy**—visualization of the stomach

The entire GI tract must be emptied before the X-rays are taken.

- No food is permitted for 8 hours or longer.
- Enemas are given repeatedly until only the clear liquid returns.
- Laxatives are given the night before the test.

Cholecystogram (Gallbladder Series)

A gallbladder (GB) series is an X-ray examination similar to the GI series except that the dye tablets are swallowed. Orders for preparing patients for this test vary.

Cleansing enemas may be ordered. A special diet may also be required beforehand.

Ultrasonography

Ultrasound is very high-frequency sound that cannot be heard. A concentrated beam can be directed at body organs and tissues to make a picture of the tissues being examined. *Ultrasonography* is the use of sound to produce an image of an organ or tissue.

Rectal Suppositories

Rectal **suppositories** may be given to stimulate bowel elimination. Medications are sometimes given in suppository form. Medicinal suppositories must be given by a nurse. In many states, nursing assistants can administer suppositories that soften the stool and promote elimination. Your instructor will inform you if this is a nursing assistant responsibility in your state. To be effective, the rectal suppository must be positioned above the rectal sphincter and against the bowel wall. Body heat will melt the suppository, stimulate bowel elimination, and lubricate the rectum. Apply the principles of standard precautions for this procedure.

EXPAND YOUR SKILLS

PROCEDURE 89 COLLECTING A STOOL SPECIMEN

1. Carry out initial procedure actions.
2. Assemble equipment:
   - Disposable gloves
   - Bedpan and cover or collection container
   - Specimen container and cover
   - Biohazard specimen transport bag
   - Label, including the following:
     - Patient's full name
     - Room number
     - Date and time of collection
     - Physician's name
     - Examination to be performed
     - Other information required
   - Toilet tissue
   - Tongue depressors
   - Basin
3. Wash your hands and put on disposable gloves.
4. Uncover the specimen collection container and use tongue depressors to obtain a specimen (Figure 44-6A).

Do not contaminate the outside of the specimen container or the cover. If possible, take a sample (about 1 teaspoon) from each part of the specimen. Transfer the sample to a specimen cup (Figure 44-6B).

5. Assist the patient with handwashing, if needed. If the patient is incontinent, carefully clean and dry the area around the anus.

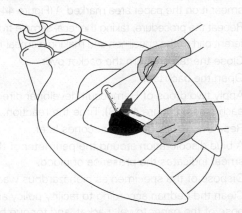

FIGURE 44-6A Use tongue blades to collect a sample from each part of the specimen.

(continues)

PROCEDURE **89** CONTINUED

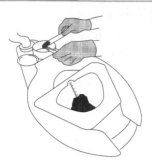

FIGURE 44-6B Use tongue blades to transfer the specimen from the collection device to the specimen cup.

6. Empty the collection container into the toilet. Clean or discard the container according to facility policy. If the patient was incontinent, dispose of the soiled brief or padding as biohazardous waste.
7. Remove and dispose of your gloves according to facility policy.
8. Wash your hands.
9. Cover the container and attach the completed label. Place the container in a biohazard transport bag.
10. Take or send the specimen to the laboratory promptly. (Stool specimens are never refrigerated.)
11. Carry out ending procedure actions.

ICON KEY:
 = OBRA   = PPE

EXPAND YOUR SKILLS

PROCEDURE **90** TESTING FOR OCCULT BLOOD USING HEMOCCULT AND DEVELOPER

1. Wash your hands.
2. Assemble equipment:
   - Disposable gloves
   - Bedpan with fresh specimen
   - Hemoccult slide packet
   - Hemoccult developer
   - Tongue blade
   - Paper towel
3. Place the paper towel on a flat surface and open the flap of the Hemoccult packet, exposing the guaiac paper.
4. Put on gloves.
5. Using a tongue blade, take a small sample of feces and smear it on the paper area marked *A* (Figure 44-7A).
6. Repeat the procedure, taking the fecal sample from a different part of the specimen and making a smear in area *B*.
7. Close the tab and turn the packet over.
8. Open the back tab.
9. Apply two drops of Hemoccult developer directly over each smear (Figure 44-7B). Time the reaction.
10. Read the results 30 to 60 seconds later.
11. A blue discoloration around the perimeter of the smear indicates the presence of blood.
12. Dispose of the specimen as biohazardous waste.
13. Clean the bedpan according to facility policy and dispose of the paper towel, packet, and tongue blade.

14. Remove and dispose of gloves according to facility policy. Wash your hands.

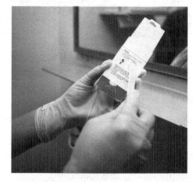

FIGURE 44-7A Place a small amount of stool on the identified area on the card when performing an occult blood test.

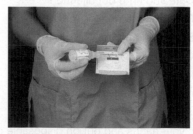

FIGURE 44-7B Apply the Hemoccult developer to the exposed guaiac paper.

ICON KEY:
 = OBRA   = PPE

EXPAND YOUR SKILLS

PROCEDURE **91** **INSERTING A RECTAL SUPPOSITORY**

1. Carry out initial procedure actions.
2. Assemble supplies:
   - 2 pairs disposable exam gloves
   - Bed protector
   - Suppository
   - Clean paper towel
   - Water-soluble lubricant
   - Toilet tissue
   - Bedpan and cover, if needed
   - Plastic bag
   - Bath blanket, if needed
   - Supplies for peri care, if needed
3. Wash your hands or use alcohol-based hand cleaner.
4. Apply gloves.
5. Place the bed protector under the patient's hips.
6. Adjust the bed linens to expose only the buttocks, or cover the patient with a bath blanket, exposing only the rectal area.
7. Place a clean paper towel on the table.
8. Unwrap the suppository. Place it on the paper towel.
9. Open the package of water-soluble lubricant and squeeze a small amount onto the tip of the suppository on the paper towel.
10. Apply a small amount of lubricant to the anus.
11. Separate the buttocks. Ask the patient to bear down gently and take slow, deep breaths through the mouth.
12. Carefully insert the lubricated tip of the suppository approximately two to three inches (Figure 44-8).
13. Assist the patient to the bathroom, or place them on a bedpan or commode.

14. Instruct the patient to relax, and take slow, deep breaths if uncomfortable, until the urge to defecate occurs. (This should take 5 to 20 minutes.)
15. Remove gloves and discard them in the plastic bag.
16. Wash your hands or use alcohol-based hand cleaner.
17. Adjust the bedding and make the patient comfortable. Make sure the call signal is in reach.
18. Return to the unit to check on the patient in five minutes and whenever they signal.
19. Wash your hands or use alcohol-based hand cleaner.
20. Apply gloves.
21. When the patient has finished, assist with the bedpan, commode, or toilet, as needed. Observe results of elimination and characteristics of the stool. If abnormal, save for the RN. Discard stool and soiled items, and clean equipment, as needed.
22. Assist the patient with hygiene, if needed. Cleanse hands and reapply gloves as needed.
23. Carry out ending procedure actions.

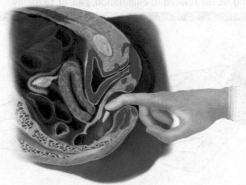

FIGURE 44-8 Carefully insert the lubricated suppository 2 to 3 inches into the rectum.

ICON KEY:
 = OBRA   = PPE

ENEMAS

A cleansing **enema** uses the technique of introducing fluid into the rectum to remove feces and flatus (gas) from the colon and rectum. (Refer to Procedures 92 and 93.) Enemas are given:

- To aid illumination during X-rays.
- Before surgery.
- Before testing.
- During bowel retraining programs.
- To relieve constipation and impaction.
- To instill drugs.

The fluids often used for enemas are:
- Soap solution (SSE)
- Salt solution (saline)
- Tap water (TWE)
- Phosphosoda

These solutions create a feeling of urgency in the patient's bowel. **Urgency** is the term used to describe the need to empty the bowel. Solutions are expelled a short time after they are given. Instruct the patient to retain the fluid as long as possible.

General Considerations

Here are some general considerations to keep in mind regarding enemas:

- Apply the principles of standard precautions. Avoid environmental contamination from your gloves.
- Administer an enema only upon the direction of a licensed nurse.
- Make sure the bathroom is available and not in use if the patient will be using the bathroom to expel the enema.

Culture **ALERT**

Patients from some cultures may be resistant to using a bedpan or urinal or may refuse to use it at all. A bedside commode may be much more acceptable, particularly when a treatment such as an enema or suppository is necessary. Some of these individuals may try to avoid having BMs while hospitalized and will be very constipated when they return home. Monitor elimination carefully and report no BM in three days to the nurse. Members of these cultures (Central American, Chinese American, Cuban, Filipino, Gypsy, Haitian, Iranian, Mexican American, Puerto Rican, and Samoan) are often very modest. They may avoid discussing issues related to elimination, sex, or sexuality.

- Give the enema before the patient's bath or before breakfast, if possible.
- Do not give an enema within an hour following a meal.
- Consult the care plan or the nurse for the amount and type of solution to use, and any special instructions.

NOTE

Avoid giving an enema within an hour after meals, because the increased peristalsis makes it difficult for the patient to retain the solution. Avoid administering an enema to a patient in a sitting position, such as on the toilet. The solution will not flow high into the colon when administered to a patient who is seated. It will cause the rectum to enlarge, causing rapid expulsion of the fluid.

Position

The best position for the patient to receive an enema is the left Sims' position. Figure 44-9 shows several alternative positions. The supine position can be used if the patient is unable to hold the fluid or to assume Sims' position.

At times, the enema may have to be administered with the patient on the bedpan in the supine position.

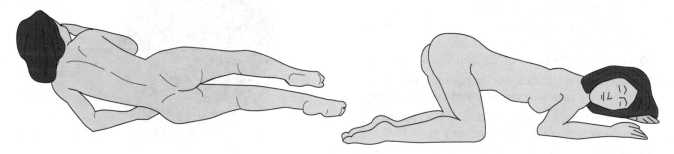

Sims' (left-lateral) position

Knee-chest position

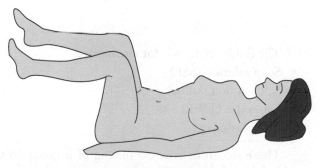

Position for self-administration

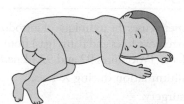

Child's position

FIGURE 44-9 Alternative positions for enema administration and rectal treatments.

- Flex and separate the patient's knees.
- A bariatric bedpan or an orthopedic (fracture) bedpan is more comfortable than a regular bedpan.

Disposable Enema Units

Disposable enema units are available to give:

- Soap-solution enemas
- Commercially prepared enemas

- Phosphosoda enemas
- Oil-retention enemas

Disposable enemas are simple to administer and save time in preparing and cleaning the equipment. The techniques for using reusable equipment for oil-retention or soap-solution enemas are the same.

EXPAND YOUR SKILLS

PROCEDURE 92 GIVING A SOAP-SOLUTION ENEMA

 NOTE

Be sure this is a nursing assistant procedure in your facility.

1. Carry out initial procedure actions.
2. Assemble equipment:
   - Disposable gloves
   - Disposable enema equipment (consists of a plastic container, tubing with rectal tube, clamp, and lubricant; this equipment is commercially available as a kit)
   - Bedpan and cover
   - Bed protector
   - Toilet tissue
   - Bath blanket
   - Castile soap packet
   - Towel, soap, basin
3. In the utility room:
   a. Connect the tubing to the solution container.
   b. Adjust the clamp on the tubing and snap it shut (Figure 44-10A).
   c. Fill the container with warm water (105°F) to the 1,000-mL line (500 mL for children) (Figure 44-10B).
   d. Open the packet of liquid soap and put the soap in the water (Figure 44-10C).
   e. Using the tip of the tubing, mix the solution (mix gently so that no suds form) or rotate the bag to mix. Do not shake.
   f. Run a small amount of solution through the tube to eliminate air and warm the tube (Figure 44-10D). Clamp the tubing.
4. Place a chair at the foot of the bed and cover it with a bed protector. Place the bedpan on it.
5. Elevate the bed to a comfortable working height. Be sure the opposite side rail is up and secure for safety.

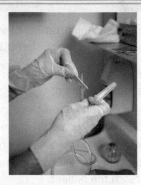

FIGURE 44-10A Slip the clamp over the tubing.

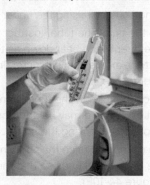

FIGURE 44-10B Fill the container with warm water. Use a bath thermometer to make sure the temperature is about 105°F.

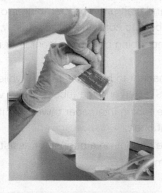

FIGURE 44-10C Add soap from the packet.

(continues)

PROCEDURE 92 CONTINUED   O   P

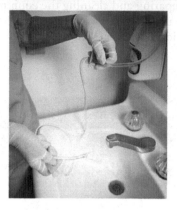

FIGURE 44-10D Run a small amount of water through the tubing to expel air, then reclamp the tubing.

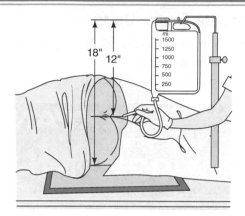

FIGURE 44-10E Raise the container above the anus so the flow of fluid is unobstructed.

6. Cover the patient with a bath blanket and fanfold linen to the foot of the bed.

7. Wash your hands and put on gloves.

8. Place a bed protector under the patient's buttocks.

9. Help the patient turn on the left side and flex the knees.

10. Place the container of solution on the chair so the tubing will reach the patient.

11. Adjust the bath blanket to expose the anal area.

12. Expose the anus by raising the upper buttock.

13. Lubricate the tip of the tube. Instruct the patient to breathe deeply and bear down as the tube is inserted, to relax the anal sphincter. Insert the tube two to four inches into the anus.

14. Never force the tube. If the tube cannot be inserted easily, get help. There may be a tumor or a mass of feces (impaction) blocking the bowel.

15. Open the clamp and raise the container 12 inches above the level of the anus so that the fluid flows in slowly (Figure 44-10E).
   – Ask the patient to take deep breaths to relax the abdomen.
   – If the patient complains of cramping, clamp the tube and wait until the cramping stops. Then open the tubing to continue the fluid flow.

16. Clamp the tubing before the container is completely empty.

17. Tell the patient to hold their breath while the upper buttock is raised and the tube is gently withdrawn.

18. Wrap the tubing in a paper towel. Put it in the disposable container.

19. Place the patient on a bedpan or assist them to the bathroom.

20. Using a paper towel, so your glove does not contaminate the control or crank, raise the head of the bed to a comfortable height if the patient is on the bedpan. Raise the side rail for safety if needed.

21. Place toilet tissue and the call signal within reach of the patient. If the patient is in the bathroom, stay nearby. Caution the patient not to flush the toilet.

22. Discard disposable materials as biohazardous waste, according to facility policy.

23. Remove your gloves and discard them according to facility policy. Wash your hands.

24. Return to the bedside. Put on fresh gloves.

25. Remove the bedpan. Place it on a bed protector on the chair and cover it.

26. Cleanse the patient's anal area.

27. Remove the bed protector and discard it according to facility policy.

28. Remove your gloves and discard them according to facility policy. Wash your hands.

29. Give the patient soap, water, and a towel to wash and dry their hands.

30. Replace the top bedding and remove the bath blanket.

31. Put on gloves. Take the bedpan to the bathroom. Dispose of the contents according to facility policy. If the patient used the toilet, flush the toilet using a paper towel over the handle.

32. Remove your gloves and dispose of them according to facility policy.

33. Wash your hands.

34. Leave the room in order.

35. Unscreen the unit.

36. Clean and replace all equipment.

37. Carry out ending procedure actions.

ICON KEY:
O = OBRA   P = PPE

Giving an Enema with a Commercially Prepared Chemical Enema Solution

Commercially prepared enemas are convenient to administer and more comfortable for the patient. The enema may be either an oil-retention enema or a phosphosoda enema. It may be followed by a cleansing (soap-solution) enema.

- The solution is already measured and ready to use.
- A small amount of fluid will remain in the container after administration.
- The phosphosoda enema stimulates peristalsis and draws fluid from the body.

- The oil-retention enema softens the feces, making them easier to expel.
- The amount of solution administered is about four ounces.
- The tip of the container is prelubricated.
- The enema solution is in an easy-to-handle plastic container.
- The solution is sometimes used at room temperature.
- You may be asked to warm the solution by placing the container in warm water before administration. Check with the nurse regarding your facility's policy.

EXPAND YOUR SKILLS

PROCEDURE 93 GIVING A COMMERCIALLY PREPARED ENEMA

 NOTE

Be sure this is a nursing assistant procedure in your facility.

 NOTE

Use this procedure when giving an oil-retention or a phosphosoda enema.

1. Carry out initial procedure actions.

2. Assemble equipment:
   - Disposable gloves
   - Disposable prepackaged enema
   - Bedpan and cover
   - Bed protector
   - Pan of warm water (if enema solution is to be warmed)

3. Open the package and remove the plastic container of enema solution. Place the solution container in warm water (if it is to be warmed).

4. Lower the head of the bed to a horizontal position and elevate the bed to a comfortable working height. Raise the side rail on the opposite side of the bed for safety.

5. Put on gloves.

6. Place a bedpan and cover on the chair close at hand.

7. Assist the patient to turn to the left side and flex the right leg.

8. Place a bed protector under the patient.

9. Expose only the patient's buttocks by drawing the bedding upward in one hand.

10. Remove the cover from the enema tip. Gently squeeze to make sure the tip is undamaged (patent).

11. Separate the buttocks, exposing the anus, and ask the patient to breathe deeply and bear down slightly.

12. Insert the lubricated enema tip two inches into the rectum.

13. Gently squeeze and roll the container until the desired quantity of solution is administered. A small amount of solution will remain in the container. Avoid releasing pressure on the container, or the solution will return.

14. Remove the tip from the patient and place the container in the box. Encourage the patient to hold the solution as long as possible.

15. Remove gloves and dispose of them properly. Wash your hands.

16. Discard the used enema as biohazardous waste.

17. Provide privacy. This enema should be retained for 20 minutes. Give the patient the call signal and leave.

18. When the patient feels the urge to defecate, lower the bed and assist the patient to the bathroom or commode, or position the patient on the bedpan.

19. Raise the head of the bed to a comfortable height if the patient is using a bedpan.

20. Place toilet tissue and the call signal within reach of the patient. Raise the side rail for safety if the bed is left in high position. If the patient is in the bathroom, stay nearby. Caution the patient not to flush the toilet.

21. Return to the patient when signaled. Wash your hands. Lower the nearest side rail, if it is up. Put on gloves.

22. Remove the bedpan and place it on the bed protector covering the chair. Observe the contents of the bedpan. Cover the bedpan.

23. Clean the patient's anal area, if required.

(continues)

PROCEDURE **93** CONTINUED

24. If the patient has used a commode or toilet:
- Clean the anal area, if required.
- Observe the contents of the commode or toilet.
- Flush the toilet using a paper towel, or cover the commode.
- Remove your gloves and discard them according to facility policy. Assist the patient into bed.

25. Put on gloves. Take the bedpan or commode container and equipment to the bathroom. Dispose of contents according to facility policy.

26. Remove and dispose of gloves properly. Wash your hands.

27. Give the patient soap, water, and a towel to wash their hands. Return equipment. Leave the side rails down unless needed for safety and leave the bed in low position.

28. Carry out ending procedure actions.

ICON KEY:

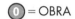 = OBRA   = PPE

Rectal Tube and Flatus Bag

The rectal tube reduces flatus (gas) in the bowel. Flatus distends the intestines, causing pain and stress on incisions. Placing a rectal tube into the anus provides a passageway for the gas to escape. You can assist the patient as follows:

- Encourage activity.
- Promote regularity.
- Accept the expulsion of gas as a natural body function. Do not contribute to the patient's embarrassment.
- Use flatus-reducing procedures when ordered.
- Insert a rectal tube with flatus bag if ordered. (Remember that your facility's policies must state that nursing assistants can perform this procedure.)

The disposable tube is used once in a 24-hour period for no more than 20 minutes.

- Relief may occur as soon as the tube is inserted.
- Check the amount of abdominal distention (stretching).
- Question the patient about the amount of relief.

OSTOMIES

The surgical removal of a section of diseased bowel requires the creation of an artificial opening (ostomy) in the abdominal wall for elimination of solid waste and flatus.

Care of the Patient with a Colostomy

When the colon is brought through the abdominal wall, the opening is called a *colostomy*. The mouth of the opening is called a *stoma* (Figure 44-11). The ostomy may be temporary or permanent. The location of the ostomy

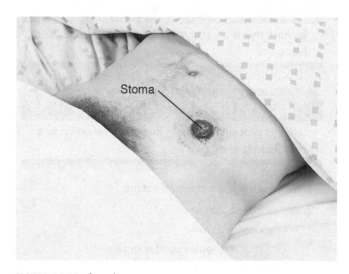

FIGURE 44-11 A colostomy stoma.

(Figure 44-12) determines if the feces are formed, soft and mushy, semiliquid, or liquid.

The patient with a colostomy does not have normal sphincter control and cannot voluntarily control emptying of the bowel. If the colostomy is located in the bowel where stool is formed, regularity of elimination may be established. As elimination is controlled, the stoma may be covered with a simple dressing between evacuations. Liquid to mushy fecal drainage from a stoma is collected in a disposable drainage pouch, called an *appliance*, that is attached over the stoma. (Refer to Procedure 94.) Proper stoma care is required to maintain healthy tissue, because the area around the opening comes into contact with liquid or semiliquid stool. At the stoma, there may be problems of:

- Leakage
- Odor control
- Irritation of the surrounding area

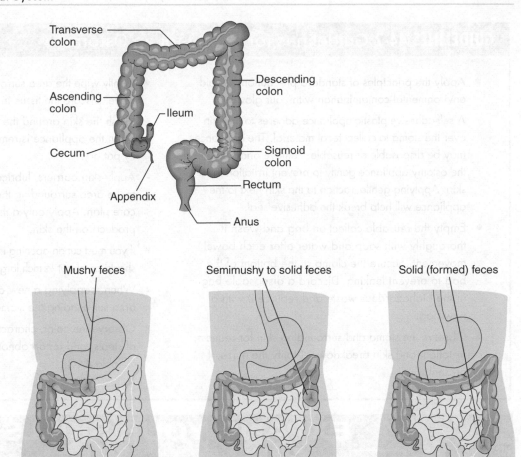

FIGURE 44-12 The location of the ostomy determines the character of the feces.

You can assist the patient who has a colostomy by keeping the area clean and dry, and by performing routine stoma care, including removing drainage and/or replacing the appliance.

Remember:

- Initial irrigations will be performed by the nurse.
- If the colostomy is to be permanent, patients are taught to carry out the irrigation procedure for themselves.
- In some facilities, qualified nursing assistants are permitted to irrigate well-established ostomies.

The two-piece system has an outer ring that snaps onto the pouch. The size of the ring in the pouch is very important. It must seal the appliance around the stoma, but not fit so tightly that it squeezes the stoma. An improper fit can injure the stoma. An improperly applied belt may also injure the stoma. Read the directions and make sure you understand how to use the type of device you have.

Difficult Situations

Having an ostomy alters the way in which solid waste (fecal material) is eliminated. This change in body image can be very traumatic for the patient. Covering the pouch with an attractive cover (check with the enterostomal therapy nurse) may help the patient's self-esteem. The ostomy may also have a profound effect on the patient's sex life. Be supportive and empathetic. Occasionally, a patient may become aroused or feel sexual pleasure when the ostomy is touched. Remain calm and professional and do not overreact. Avoid sending the patient mixed sexual messages, even in a joking manner. If the patient persists, inform them that sexual advances are not appropriate. The patient will most likely be very embarrassed about becoming involuntarily sexually aroused.

GUIDELINES 44-2 Guidelines for Caring for an Ostomy

- Apply the principles of standard precautions. Avoid environmental contamination with your gloves.

- A self-adhesive plastic appliance adheres to the skin over the stoma to collect fecal material. The appliance may be disposable or reusable. Remove and apply the ostomy appliance gently to prevent irritation to the skin. Applying gentle traction to the skin next to the appliance will help break the adhesive seal.

- Empty the reusable collection bag and wash it thoroughly with soap and water after each bowel movement. Secure the clamp at the bottom of the bag to prevent leaking. Discard a disposable bag in the biohazardous waste and replace it with a new bag.

- Observe the stoma and surrounding skin for redness, irritation, and skin breakdown. Notify the nurse, if present.

- Gently wipe the area surrounding the stoma with toilet tissue. Discard the tissue in the toilet or a plastic bag.

- Wash the skin around the stoma with mild soap when the appliance is removed. Rinse well and gently pat dry.

- Apply skin barriers, lubricants, or medicated creams to the area surrounding the stoma as stated on the care plan. Apply only a thin layer. Avoid caking any products on the skin.

- If you must cut an opening into the appliance, the area should be about ⅛ inch larger than the size of the stoma.

- When reapplying a new appliance, seal the entire area surrounding the stoma, to prevent leaking.

- Observe the color, character, amount, and frequency of stools, and report abnormalities to the nurse. Refer to Table 44-2.

EXPAND YOUR SKILLS

PROCEDURE 94 GIVING ROUTINE STOMA CARE (COLOSTOMY)

1. Carry out initial procedure actions.

2. Assemble equipment:
   - Disposable gloves
   - Washcloth and towel
   - Basin of warm water
   - Bed protectors
   - Bath blanket
   - Disposable colostomy bag and belt
   - Bedpan
   - Skin lotion as directed
   - Prescribed solvent and dropper
   - Cleansing agent
   - Adhesive wafer
   - 4 × 4 gauze square
   - Toilet tissue
   - Plastic bag

3. Cover the patient with a bath blanket. Fanfold the top bedding to the foot of the bed.

4. Wash your hands and put on gloves.

5. Place a bed protector under the patient's hips.

6. Place a bedpan and cover on a bed protector on the chair.

7. Remove the soiled disposable stoma bag (appliance) and place it in the bedpan or plastic bag—note the amount and type of drainage.

8. Remove the belt that holds the stoma bag and save it, if clean.

9. Gently clean the area around the stoma with toilet tissue to remove feces and drainage (Figure 44-13A). Dispose of used tissue in the bedpan or plastic bag.

10. Wash the area around the stoma with soap and water. Rinse thoroughly and dry.

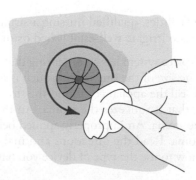

FIGURE 44-13A Clean the area carefully.

(continues)

PROCEDURE **94** CONTINUED

11. If ordered, apply barrier cream lightly around the stoma. Too much lotion may interfere with proper sealing of the fresh ostomy bag.

12. Position a clean belt around the patient. Inspect the skin under the belt for irritation or breakdown.

13. Use a commercial guide to size the stoma if you must replace the adhesive wafer (Figure 44-13B).

14. Replace the adhesive wafer (Figure 44-13C). Place a clean ostomy bag over the stoma and secure the belt.

15. Remove the bed protector. Check to be sure the bottom bedding is not wet. Change it if necessary.

16. Remove your gloves and discard them according to facility policy. Wash your hands.

17. Replace the bath blanket with the top bedding, and make the patient comfortable.

18. Using a paper towel to protect your hands, gather and cover the soiled materials and bedpan or plastic bag. Take them to the utility room. Dispose of materials according to facility policy.

19. Empty, wash, and dry the bedpan. Store it according to facility policy.

20. Carry out ending procedure actions.

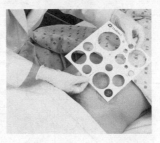

FIGURE 44-13B Check the stoma size to make sure the correct size wafer is used.

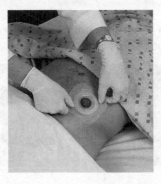

FIGURE 44-13C Apply a new barrier adhesive wafer around the stoma.

ICON KEY:
 = OBRA = PPE

Difficult Situations

Most ostomy appliances are odor-free. If odor control is a problem, consult the nurse. Commercial products are available to eliminate odors in the bag. Leave a small amount of air in the bag when changing it, to allow stool to fall to the bottom.

Care of the Patient with an Ileostomy

An *ileostomy* is a permanent artificial opening in the ileum (Figure 44-14) that drains through a stoma on the surface of the abdomen. The drainage from the ileum is in liquid form and contains digestive enzymes that are irritating to the skin. (Refer to Procedure 95.)

Considerations for caring for a patient with an ileostomy include:

- The licensed nurse cares for the patient with a new ileostomy.
- Routine care for a patient with a well-established ileostomy may be given by nursing assistants.
- The drainage from an ileostomy is very irritating to the skin, so care of the skin surrounding the stoma is crucial.
- The fit of the ileostomy ring is important so that leakage does not occur. This is true for both the disposable and reusable types of appliances (Figure 44-15).

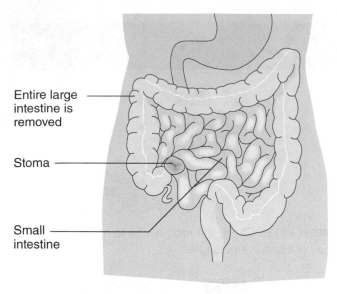

Entire large
intestine is
removed

Stoma

Small
intestine

FIGURE 44-14 An ileostomy brings a section of the ileum
through the abdominal wall.

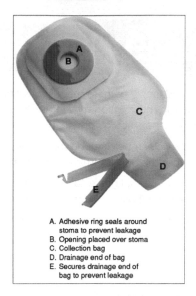

A. Adhesive ring seals around
   stoma to prevent leakage
B. Opening placed over stoma
C. Collection bag
D. Drainage end of bag
E. Secures drainage end of
   bag to prevent leakage

FIGURE 44-15 Stoma protector and collection bag.
(Courtesy of Hollister, Inc, Libertyville, Illinois)

EXPAND YOUR SKILLS

PROCEDURE **95** **GIVING ROUTINE CARE OF AN
ILEOSTOMY (WITH PATIENT IN BED)**

1. Carry out initial procedure actions.

2. Assemble equipment:
   - Disposable gloves
   - Basin of warm water
   - Bed protector
   - Bath blanket
   - Bedpan and cover
   - Fresh appliance and belt
   - Clamp for appliance
   - Prescribed solvent and dropper
   - Cotton balls
   - Deodorant (if permitted)
   - Cleansing agent
   - Karaya ring
   - 4 × 4 gauze squares
   - Toilet tissue
   - Paper towels
   - Plastic bag

3. Raise the opposite side rail for safety. Elevate the
head of the bed and assist the patient to turn on the
side toward you.

4. Replace bedding with a bath blanket.

5. Wash your hands. Put on gloves.

6. Place a bed protector under the patient.

7. Place a bedpan on the bed protector next to the
patient.

8. Place the end of the ileostomy bag in the bedpan
or plastic bag. Open the clamp and allow the bag to
drain. Note the amount and character of drainage.

9. Wipe the end of the drainage sheath with toilet paper
and move it out of drainage. Place the used tissue in
the bedpan. Cover the bedpan.

10. Disconnect the belt from the appliance and remove
the belt from the patient. Place it on paper towels.

11. With a dropper, apply a small amount of solvent
around the ring of the appliance. This will loosen it so
it can be removed. Wait a few seconds. Do not force
the appliance free.

12. Cover the stoma with gauze.
   - Carefully inspect the skin area around the stoma.
   - If the area is irritated or the skin is broken, cover
     the patient with a bath blanket, raise the side rail,
     and lower the bed.
   - Remove your gloves and dispose of them properly.
   - Wash your hands.
   - Report to the nurse for instructions.
   - Put on fresh gloves before continuing the
     procedure.

13. Remove the gauze from the stoma and place it on
paper towels.

(continues)

PROCEDURE 95 CONTINUED

14. If the appliance has a Karaya ring, moisten the ring, allow it to become sticky, and apply it to the stoma. If the appliance uses a paper-covered adhesive strip around the stoma opening, remove the paper and apply the strip around the stoma.

15. Clamp the appliance bag and apply it to the ring.

16. Remove your gloves and dispose of them properly. Wash your hands.

17. Adjust a clean belt in position around the patient and connect it to the appliance.

18. Remove the bath blanket and assist the patient to wash hands.

19. Wash your hands. Put on gloves.

20. Clean the patient's bathroom. Wash the belt and appliance, if reusable, and allow them to dry.

21. Carry out ending procedure actions.

ICON KEY:

O = OBRA   **P** = PPE

 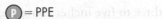

REVIEW

A. True/False

Mark the following true or false by circling T or F.

1. T F A herniorrhaphy is the surgery performed for bowel malignancy.

2. T F The drainage from a new cholecystectomy incision is normally yellowish-green.

3. T F A patient is positioned on the left side, if possible, for enema administration.

4. T F When a prepackaged enema is administered, approximately four ounces are given.

5. T F Be sure the bathroom is free before giving an enema.

6. T F A flatus tube is used to reduce abdominal distention from gas.

7. T F An enema may be given only upon direction from the nurse.

8. T F When giving a soap-solution enema, approximately 2,000 mL are used.

9. T F Gastric ulcers are located in the esophagus.

10. T F A stool with occult blood will appear bloody.

11. T F The Hemoccult test is used to determine the presence of bile in the feces.

12. T F Gloves must be worn when doing tests on feces or urine.

13. T F The proper amount of time to observe a Hemoccult packet after placing a fecal smear and adding the developer is five minutes.

14. T F Odor control can be a problem when a patient has an ostomy.

15. T F Drainage from a colostomy is always watery.

16. T F Apply the principles of standard precautions when caring for an ostomy.

17. T F Waste products from ostomy care are discarded in the biohazardous trash.

B. Matching

Choose the correct word from Column II to match each word or phrase in Column I.

Column I

18. _____ large bowel

19. _____ feces

20. _____ gallstones

21. _____ opening

22. _____ artificial opening in large intestine

23. _____ artificial opening in small intestine

24. _____ hidden

25. _____ drainage pouch

Column II

a. appliance

b. cholelithiasis

c. colon

d. colostomy

e. ileostomy

f. occult

g. stoma

h. stool

C. Multiple Choice

Select the best answer for each of the following.

26. A sign of possible gastrointestinal malignancy is:
   a. good appetite.
   b. change in stool color.
   c. weight gain.
   d. nausea.

27. Your patient has just returned from surgery for gallstones. They will be most comfortable in the:
   a. dorsal recumbent position.
   b. lithotomy position.
   c. semi-Fowler's position.
   d. left Sims' position.

28. Enemas are given:
   a. after the patient showers.
   b. at bedtime.
   c. before diagnostic testing.
   d. after surgery.

29. The oil-retention enema is usually:
   a. preceded by a soap-solution enema.
   b. retained for one hour.
   c. done to soften the feces so they are easier to expel.
   d. given in the semi-Fowler's position.

30. *Urgency* is a term that means:
   a. inability to have a BM.
   b. need to eliminate.
   c. pain from flatus.
   d. need to vomit.

31. Persons who are elderly often put extra sugar on their food because:
   a. a craving for sweets is normal.
   b. they need extra calories.
   c. taste buds have been lost.
   d. they need to prevent weight loss.

32. Jaundice is:
   a. abnormal appearance of stools.
   b. strangulation of the intestine.
   c. yellow skin and whites of the eyes.
   d. a malignancy of the lower bowel.

33. Removal of the gallbladder and stones is:
   a. gastrectomy.
   b. cholecystitis.
   c. cholelithiasis.
   d. cholecystectomy.

34. Inform the nurse if the patient does not have a bowel movement:
   a. daily.
   b. in two days.
   c. in three days.
   d. in five days.

35. *C. difficile* spores can exist on hard surfaces for:
   a. 24 hours.
   b. 30 days.
   c. 5 months.
   d. 1 year.

36. Insert the rectal suppository:
   a. six inches above the rectal sphincter.
   b. one to two inches above the rectal sphincter.
   c. three to five inches above the rectal sphincter.
   d. two to three inches above the rectal sphincter.

37. The fluids used for enemas include all of the following *except*:
   a. milk of magnesia.
   b. salt solution.
   c. tap water.
   d. phosphosoda.

38. An artificial opening in the colon is known as a(n):
   a. tracheostomy.
   b. colostomy.
   c. ileostomy.
   d. proctostomy.

39. The reaction time for a Hemoccult test is:
   a. 2 to 4 seconds.
   b. 30 to 60 seconds.
   c. 2 to 3 minutes.
   d. 90 to 120 seconds.

40. Before urine withdrawal, the port of a closed urinary drainage system should be cleaned with:
   a. soap and water.
   b. a paper towel.
   c. alcohol.
   d. a sterile 4 × 4 gauze pad.

41. During routine care, the area around a colostomy should:
   a. be cleaned with an alcohol sponge.
   b. be covered with petroleum jelly.
   c. be washed with soap and water.
   d. be cleaned with an antiseptic.

42. As compared to a colostomy, an ileostomy:

    a. has more formed stool.

    b. tends to be more irritating.

    c. has drainage containing blood clots.

    d. has a larger stoma.

43. You are giving routine stoma care to a patient with a colostomy and find the area surrounding the stoma red and irritated. You should:

    a. complete the procedure.

    b. clean the area with alcohol.

    c. apply powder and attach the ostomy bag.

    d. cover the area and notify the nurse.

44. If the skin around an ileostomy stoma is broken, you should:

    a. wipe it with alcohol.

    b. wash it with soap and water.

    c. seal it with appliance adhesive.

    d. inform the nurse.

D. Completion

Complete the statements in the spaces provided.

45. The tip of the commercially prepared enema is _____.

46. The purpose of a soap-solution enema is to _____.

47. A _____ occurs when the intestine pushes through a weakened area in the abdominal muscle.

48. Gallstones may obstruct the flow of _____.

49. Flatus is intestinal _____.

50. _____ is the most serious form of constipation.

E. Nursing Assistant Challenge

Mr. Rayburn has been admitted with a provisional diagnosis of gastric ulcers. He had been complaining of a burning sensation in his stomach halfway between meals. He is scheduled for an upper GI series at 8:00 a.m. tomorrow. Answer the following questions regarding Mr. Rayburn and his care.

51. What acid is naturally found in Mr. Rayburn's stomach?

_____

_____

52. Before the GI series, will it be all right to serve Mr. Rayburn breakfast in the morning?

_____

_____

53. What procedure will you be asked to carry out before the test?

_____

_____

54. Will Mr. Rayburn swallow the barium, or will he be given a barium enema?

_____

_____

55. Will X-rays be taken?

_____

_____

Mrs. Knight, who is 60 years old, was in an accident and received a broken right leg and two broken wrists. She has a long-standing colostomy, but because of her injuries cannot provide her own colostomy care. Answer the following questions about her care.

56. Will you need to wear gloves to give her colostomy care?

_____

_____

57. What will you use to remove feces from around the stoma?

_____

_____

58. What will happen if you apply lotion around the stoma?

_____

_____

59. How will the ostomy bag be held in place?

_____

_____

60. What are the three major problems associated with having a stoma?

_____

_____

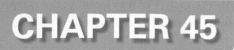

CHAPTER 45

Urinary System

OBJECTIVES

After completing this chapter, you will be able to:

45.1 Spell and define terms.

45.2 Review the location of the urinary system.

45.3 Review the function of the urinary system.

45.4 List five diagnostic tests associated with conditions of the urinary system.

45.5 Describe some common diseases of the urinary system.

45.6 Describe nursing assistant actions related to the care of patients with urinary system diseases and conditions.

45.7 State the purpose of the renal dialysis.

45.8 Give an overview of the two types of dialysis.

45.9 Describe the care of a person with an indwelling catheter.

45.10 State the reasons for removing an indwelling catheter as soon as possible.

45.11 Demonstrate the following procedures:

- Procedure 96: Collecting a Routine Urine Specimen (Expand Your Skills)
- Procedure 97: Collecting a Clean-Catch Urine Specimen (Expand Your Skills)
- Procedure 98: Collecting a 24-Hour Urine Specimen (Expand Your Skills)
- Procedure 99: Collecting a Urine Specimen Through a Drainage Port (Expand Your Skills)
- Procedure 100: Routine Drainage Check (Expand Your Skills)
- Procedure 101: Giving Indwelling Catheter Care
- Procedure 102: Emptying a Urinary Drainage Unit
- Procedure 103: Disconnecting the Catheter
- Procedure 104: Connecting a Catheter to a Leg Bag
- Procedure 105: Emptying a Leg Bag
- Procedure 106: Removing an Indwelling Catheter
- Procedure 107: Ultrasound Bladder Scan

VOCABULARY

Learn the meaning and the correct spelling of the following words and phrases:

Bowman's capsule
catheter
condom catheter
continuous ambulatory peritoneal dialysis (CAPD)
cortex
cystitis
cystoscopy
dialysis
dysuria
fistula
Foley catheter
glomerulus

graft
hematuria
hemodialysis
hydronephrosis
indwelling (retention) catheter
intermittent catheter
intravenous pyelogram (IVP)
kidney
lithotripsy
medulla
nephritis

nephron
oliguria
pelvis
peritoneal dialysis
port
pyelogram
pyuria
renal calculi
renal colic
renal failure
retention
retention (indwelling) catheter

retrograde pyelogram
suppression
suprapubic catheter (S/P cath)
ureter
urethra
urinalysis
urinary bladder
urinary incontinence
urinary meatus
void

INTRODUCTION

The urinary system consists of the kidneys, ureters, bladder, and urethra. The functions that this system performs are vital. It:

- Excretes liquid wastes.
- Manages blood chemistry.
- Manages fluid balance.

A **urinalysis** is a test performed on a urine specimen. The chemistry of the blood and urine reflect the chemistry of the cells and provides information about how well the body is functioning. Urine samples must be obtained and preserved properly.

STRUCTURE AND FUNCTION

The urinary system is shown in Figure 45-1. As the name implies, the organs of this system produce *urine*—liquid waste—that is excreted from the body. The urinary system also helps to control the vital water and salt balance of the body. Inability to secrete urine by the kidneys is known as **suppression**. Inability to excrete urine that has been produced by the kidneys is called **retention**. The organs of this system include:

- **Kidneys**—organs that produce the urine.
- **Ureters**—tubes that carry the urine from the kidneys to the urinary bladder. These tubes are 10 to 12 inches long and about ¼ inch wide.
- **Urinary bladder**—holds the urine until expelled. The urge to urinate (micturate or void) occurs when 150 to 300 mL of urine are in the bladder, although the bladder can hold much more urine than this.
- **Urethra**—the tube that carries the urine to the outside. The female urethra is about $1\frac{1}{2}$ inches long. The male urethra is about 6 to 8 inches long. The opening to the outside is called the external **urinary meatus**. The meatus is guarded by a round sphincter muscle that relaxes to release the urine.

The Kidneys

The two bean-shaped kidneys are located behind the peritoneum. They are held in place by capsules of fat. Each kidney weighs about 5 ounces. The outer portion of the kidney is called the **cortex**. This area produces the urine. The middle area is known as the **medulla**. It is a series of tubes that drain the urine from the cortex. The **pelvis** of the kidney receives the urine and directs it to the ureter.

Urine Production

The renal arteries carry blood to each kidney. Their many branches pass through the medulla to the cortex. In the cortex, urine is produced in filtering units called **nephrons** (Figure 45-2). It is estimated that each kidney contains 1 million nephrons.

Blood arriving at the kidneys carries waste products such as acids and salts that must be eliminated from the body. Urine is a liquid waste solution containing water and dissolved substances. In the kidneys:

- Waste products, helpful products, and large quantities of water pass through the capillary walls of the **glomerulus** (capillary bed) into **Bowman's capsule**, *forming a liquid called filtrate.*
- The filtrate moves slowly along the convoluted tubules, where some water and helpful substances like sugar are reabsorbed into the blood.
- The liquid remaining in the convoluted tubules is urine, which contains wastes.
- The urine passes into the collecting tubules of the medulla, and then out of the kidney to the ureter and into the urinary bladder.
- Normal urine is acidic and pale to deep yellow in color.
- Dilute urine has more water and fewer dissolved substances, so it is colorless to pale yellow.
- Concentrated urine has less water and more dissolved substances, so it is darker in color and has a stronger odor.
- The amount of urine produced depends on the amount of intake and various physical conditions. Inadequate water intake leading to dehydration results in a small amount of concentrated urine.

✚ Clinical Informatiom **ALERT**

An average human drinks about **16,000** gallons of water in a lifetime. The human body is about **66** percent water. Death will result if you lose **12** percent of your body fluids. An average person urinates **6** times per day. The yellow color of urine is caused by pigment derived from bile. The left kidney is slightly higher than the right. About **440** gallons of blood flow through the kidneys each day. If all the renal tubules were laid end to end, they would measure about **66** yards. The kidneys have about a million structures that filter out liquids and wastes in the blood.

Culture **ALERT**

Females from some cultures may prefer to do their own peri care with soap and water (or water only) after toileting. Some use toilet tissue; others cleanse with water instead of using tissue.

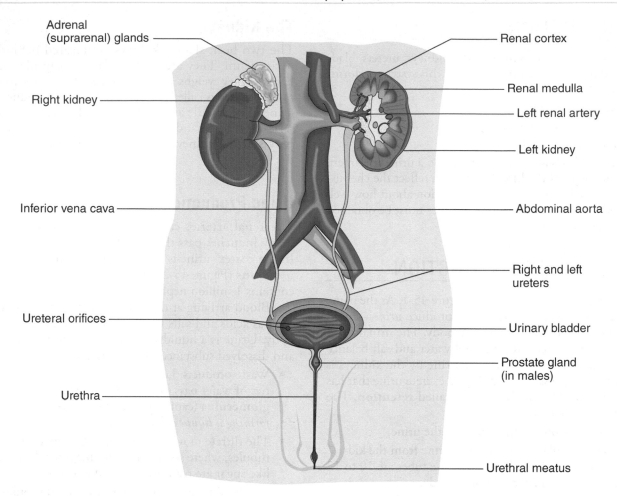

FIGURE 45-1 Structures of the urinary system.

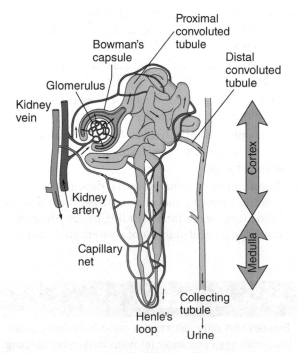

FIGURE 45-2 Nephron and related structures. Arrows indicate the flow of blood through the nephron. The urine produced by the nephron flows through the collecting tubule.

AGING CHANGES OF THE URINARY SYSTEM

The urinary system plays a major role in maintaining fluid balance in the body. Aging changes in the urinary system include:

- Bladder capacity decreases, increasing the frequency of urination.
- Kidney function increases at rest, causing the aging person to get up during the night to urinate.
- Bladder muscles weaken, causing leaking of urine or inadequate emptying of the bladder.
- The prostate gland (a tubular gland that encircles the urethra just below the bladder, in the male) frequently enlarges, causing frequency of urination, dribbling, urinary obstruction, and urinary retention.

COMMON CONDITIONS

Infection and inflammation are the most common conditions of the urinary system. These problems can result in permanent damage to the kidneys. Complications can lead to acute or chronic renal failure. An overview of common problems affecting the urinary system is given in Table 45-1.

Signs and symptoms of genitourinary disorders that should be reported to the nurse are listed in Table 45-2.

RENAL FAILURE

Renal failure is the inability of the kidneys to maintain fluid and electrolyte balance, excrete waste products, and regulate essential body functions. Dehydration and inadequate fluid intake are a major contributing cause of renal failure in elderly persons. The average adult requires at least 1.35 liters (1,350 mL) of fluid each day to maintain kidney function. The kidneys filter the blood. When the amount of circulating fluid decreases, the kidneys do not function correctly. Filtration of wastes decreases. Waste products accumulate in the bloodstream. The kidneys continue to filter wastes, but without adequate fluid, the rate of filtration is slow, so waste products are reabsorbed into the blood instead of being excreted in the urine.

Renal failure can occur in patients of any age. Two types of renal failure are acute and chronic. Patients with *acute renal failure* (ARF) have a sudden, rapid decrease in renal function. This condition can sometimes be reversed if it is identified promptly and the cause is corrected. *Chronic renal failure* (CRF) is characterized by progressive and irreversible damage. It usually develops over a long period of time. Signs and symptoms of renal failure to monitor for and report are listed in Table 45-3.

TABLE 45-1 Common Conditions of the Urinary System

Cystitis	Inflammation of the Urinary Bladder
Hematuria	Blood in the urine
Dysuria	Pain or burning on urination
Nephritis	Inflammation of the kidney
Oliguria	Decreased urine production
Dialysis	The process of removing wastes from the blood with a hemodialysis machine, commonly called an artificial kidney
Renal calculi	Kidney stones
Renal colic	Severe renal pain
Lithotripsy	Using sound waves to crush kidney stones
Hydronephrosis	A condition resulting from too much fluid on the kidney
Urinary incontinence	Loss of control over urination

TABLE 45-2 Signs and Symptoms of Genitourinary Disorders That Should Be Reported to the Nurse

Urinary output too low
Oral intake too low
Urinary output greatly exceeds fluid intake
Fluid intake and output not balanced
Fluid intake exceeds fluid restriction
Signs of dehydration, including low fluid intake; low output of dark urine with strong odor; weight loss; dry skin; dry mucous membranes of the lips, mouth, tongue, eyes; drowsiness; confusion
Edema; obvious fluid in tissues, particularly face, fingers, legs, ankles, feet
Abnormal appearance of urine: dark, concentrated, red, cloudy
Unusual substances in urine: blood, pus, particles, sediment
Complaints of difficulty urinating
Foul-smelling urine
Complaints of pain, burning, urgency, frequency, pain in lower back
Urinating frequently in small amounts
Sudden-onset incontinence
Sudden weight loss or gain
Respiratory distress
Changes in mental status
Complaints of inability to empty bladder, or cannot empty bladder completely

RENAL DIALYSIS

When end-stage renal disease develops, the person is in renal failure. In this condition, the kidneys perform at less than 10 percent of the necessary function. Many complications develop throughout the body. High blood pressure and weight gain occur. **Dialysis** is a process by which the blood is artificially cleansed of liquid wastes when the kidneys are unable to remove the wastes.

TABLE 45-3 Signs and Symptoms of Renal Failure to Monitor for and Report

Early signs and symptoms:
- Reduced urine production; little or no urine produced
- Confusion, decreased alertness, progressively worsening
- Pallor
- Rapid pulse
- Dry mouth
- Thirst
- Edema
- Abdominal pain
- Increased urination at night
- Signs or symptoms of infection elsewhere in the body

Late signs and symptoms:
- Low blood pressure
- Signs of shock
- Decreased pulse pressure

This procedure is needed when a person has kidney failure. If the waste products continue to accumulate in the bloodstream, the person will die without dialysis.

Dialysis is usually considered a temporary treatment to be used until a suitable organ is found for a kidney transplant. People who are not transplant candidates remain on dialysis for life. The two types of dialysis are hemodialysis and peritoneal dialysis.

Hemodialysis

During **hemodialysis** treatment, the patient's blood is circulated outside of the body into an artificial kidney machine. Dialysis is usually done three to four times a week and each treatment takes several hours. Treatment is usually given in an outpatient dialysis center. You may care for patients who are outpatients at the dialysis center. They spend several days a week receiving treatments (Figure 45-3A).

Hemodialysis treatments are done through a connection between the patient's circulatory system and the artificial kidney machine. A fistula or a graft is created during a minor surgical procedure. The **fistula** (Figure 45-3B) is created by attaching a vein to an artery, either in an arm or a leg. When a **graft** is used (Figure 45-3C), synthetic material is inserted to form a connection between an artery and a vein. Two needles are inserted for treatment with either a fistula or a graft. The needles are connected to tubes that go to and from the artificial kidney machine (Figure 45-3D). The dialysis machine cleans the blood with a liquid substance called *dialysate*, and then returns the blood to the patient's body (Figure 45-3E).

As a nursing assistant, you are not expected to care for the fistula or the graft. You need to be aware that the patient on dialysis will:

- Have fluid restrictions.
- Have dietary restrictions for calories, sodium, protein, potassium, calcium, and phosphorus.

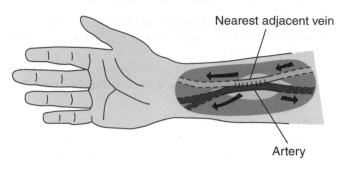

Edges of incision in artery and vein are sutured together to form a common opening.

FIGURE 45-3B The arteriovenous fistula.

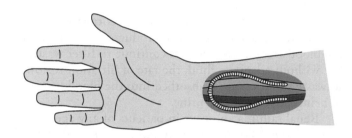

Ends of natural or synthetic graft sutured into an artery and a vein.

FIGURE 45-3C The arteriovenous vein graft.

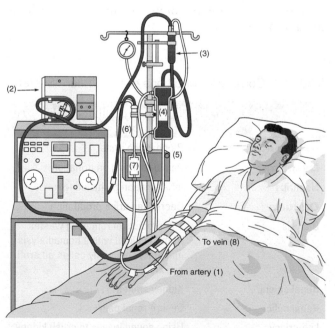

FIGURE 45-3D Hemodialysis is done through a graft or fistula. As an outpatient the person remains fully dressed and sits in a reclining chair during the procedure. It may also be done at the bedside of an unstable patient.

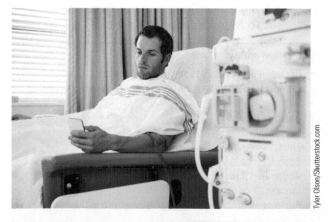

FIGURE 45-3A Patients receiving outpatient dialysis must remain in the recliner for three to five hours, three or more times per week. This patient is passing time by using a smartphones.

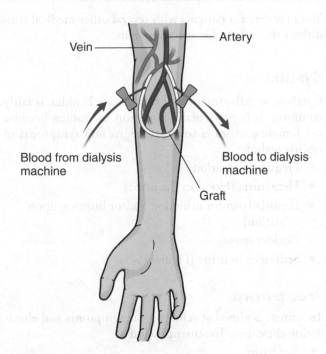

Vein

Artery

Blood from dialysis machine

Blood to dialysis machine

Graft

FIGURE 45-3E Dialysate solution removes impurities from the blood, and then returns the clean blood to the person's body.

- Need all fluid intake and output measured accurately and recorded (this is called *strict* I&O).
- Need to be weighed regularly at the same time of day, using the same scale, and with the same type of clothing.
- Need to be monitored and have vital signs taken frequently after dialysis. Remember not to take blood pressure in the arm used for dialysis. Patients may be weak when they return from dialysis. Monitor them closely when they ambulate. Watch for dizziness and loss of balance.

Dialysis is a time-consuming process, and many patients get very bored waiting for procedure completion. Look for sources of entertainment, which will vary with the setting. Providing a book or magazine, music via headset, television, video, electronic game, laptop computer, or tablet is a nice touch that will help pass the time faster.

Report to the nurse if the patient has:
- Swelling (edema) of the hands, feet, or face

 Infection Control **ALERT**

Caring for the dialysis catheter is a sterile procedure. All personnel in the room should wear masks when the system is open or entered.

- Changes in vital signs
- Changes in weight
- A change in intake or output measurements
- Shortness of breath
- Complaints of pain at the site of the fistula or graft

Peritoneal Dialysis

Peritoneal dialysis is also a process of cleansing the blood. The dialysate is introduced into the abdominal cavity, allowed to stay in for some time, and then drained out. As blood flows through the vessels in the peritoneum, waste products are filtered and excess fluids are removed. The nurse uses sterile technique to instill the dialysate through a catheter that has been surgically placed into the abdominal cavity. You may be asked to assist with sterile dressing changes. The type of dialysis used in the patient's room, subacute care unit, long-term care facility, or home care setting is called **continuous ambulatory peritoneal dialysis (CAPD)** (Figure 45-4A). A cycler unit may also be used at the bedside (Figure 45-4B).

Nursing assistants are not expected to administer peritoneal dialysis. You may be responsible for monitoring the patient's vital signs every 10 to 15 minutes for the first 1 to 2 hours after a treatment and then every 2 to 4 hours. Notify the nurse if there are any changes in vital signs.

Other signs and symptoms to report to the nurse are:
- Dialysate that appears bloody or has blood clots in the solution.
- Patient complaints of abdominal pain.
- Wet or soiled dressing.
- Fluid leaks around the insertion site.
- Tubing or catheter that becomes disconnected.
- Solution that does not appear to be running, or is running very slowly.
- Drainage container that is almost full.
- Patient who is weak or unsteady.
- Patient who has low blood pressure or complains of dizziness.
- Patient who is short of breath, in respiratory distress, or complains of difficulty breathing.

 Safety **ALERT**

Assist the patient with positioning for maximum lung expansion during dialysis. Make sure the dialysis tubing is not kinked or obstructed. You may be instructed to assist the patient with deep breathing exercises to promote lung expansion.

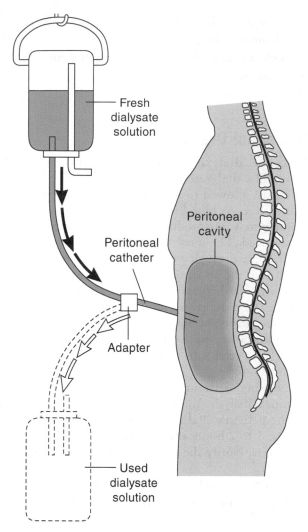

FIGURE 45-4A The peritoneal cavity is filled with fresh dialysis solution from the hanging bag. Waste products and excess fluid are removed as the dialysate flows out of the peritoneal cavity. These fluids are collected in a drain bag.

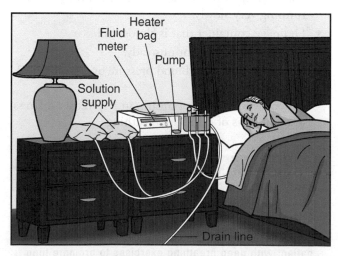

FIGURE 45-4B A cycler may also be used to perform four or five exchanges overnight while the person sleeps.
Source: National Kidney and Urologic Diseases Information Clearinghouse.

OTHER MEDICAL CONDITIONS

You may care for patients with several other medical conditions that affect the urinary system.

Cystitis

Cystitis, or inflammation of the urinary bladder, is fairly common. It is particularly common in women because the female urethra is so short. Signs and symptoms of cystitis include:

- Frequent urination
- Hematuria (blood in the urine)
- Dysuria (painful urination and/or burning upon urination)
- Bladder spasm
- Sediment in urine (Figure 45-5)

Treatment

Treatment is aimed at relieving the symptoms and eliminating the cause. Treatment includes:

- Sitz baths
- Rest
- Bacteriostatic agents
- Increased fluid intake
- Antibiotics

Nephritis

Nephritis is inflammation of the kidney. Nephritis:

- May follow an attack of infectious disease or may result from general arteriosclerosis. In either case, kidney cells are destroyed. This results in decreased urine production.
- May follow a disease course that is acute (rapid) or chronic (slow).
- Causes hypertension and edema.

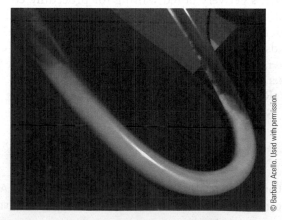

FIGURE 45-5 A urinary tract infection can cause white sandlike material or sediment in the tubing.

Signs and symptoms of nephritis are:

- Edema
- Hematuria
- Cloudy urine
- **Pyuria**—pus in urine
- Proteinuria—protein in the urine
- Hypertension
- Pain in kidney, abdomen, or pelvis
- Frequent urination
- Burning on urination
- Oliguria—decreased urination; occasionally

Treatment

Treatment includes:

- Absolute bedrest
- Low-sodium diet
- Restricted fluid intake, at times
- Frequent checks on vital signs
- Accurate intake and output (I&O) measurement
- Steroid medication, in some cases

If both kidneys are involved, the patient will require regular dialysis. The kidneys may recover with rest and increased fluid intake. If not, a kidney transplant will be necessary. *Dialysis* is the process of removing the waste products from the blood with a hemodialysis machine, commonly called an artificial kidney.

Many patients on dialysis receive treatment in a hospital dialysis unit or in special outpatient dialysis centers. Portable equipment is brought to the patient's bedside, if necessary. Other patients receive dialysis at home, using portable dialysis machines. The patient's overall physical condition is an important factor in determining whether home dialysis is an option.

Renal Calculi

Renal calculi are kidney stones. They can cause obstructions when they become lodged in the urinary passageways. There may be no signs or symptoms until an obstruction develops. Then:

- The pain is sudden and intense. It is called **renal colic**.
- Calculi may be passed in the urine.
- As stones pass along the tract, tissue damage may occur, resulting in hematuria (blood in the urine).

Treatment

The goal of treatment is to relieve the blockage and eliminate the stones. Encouraging fluids increases urine output, which helps move the stones along the tract.

All urine must be strained through gauze or filter paper, which is inspected for stones before it is discarded (Figure 45-6A). Some facilities pour urine through filters similar to coffee filters, or through gauze sponges, to catch small particles. Others use disposable paper funnels with a straining screen in a flat bottom. The urine passes through the filter, leaving stones behind. Save every particle, even if they are very tiny. Transfer the stones and all solid material to a

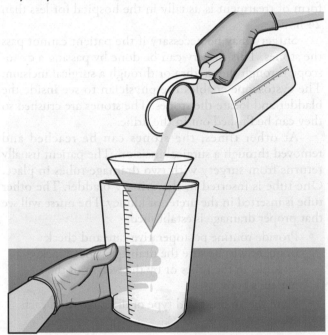

FIGURE 45-6A For a patient who needs to have urine strained, urine from every voiding is poured through filter paper to retrieve kidney stones.

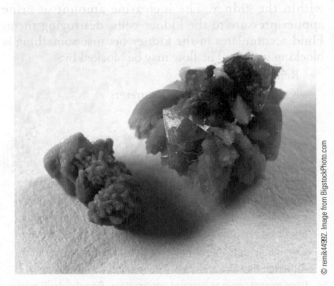

FIGURE 45-6B Renal calculi (kidney stones) are very painful. They are analyzed in the laboratory and based upon the findings, medication or diet changes may be prescribed.

specimen cup and send the specimen to the laboratory for analysis (Figure 45-6B). With information from the stones, the diet can sometimes be changed to make the formation of stones less likely. You will also use this procedure to check for brachytherapy seeds (Chapter 47).

Lithotripsy is a technique that uses carefully directed sound waves to crush the stones without the need for any surgical incision. The patient receiving this form of treatment is usually in the hospital for less than 24 hours.

Surgery may be necessary if the patient cannot pass the stones. This surgery can be done by passing a cystoscope through the urethra or through a surgical incision. The cystoscope enables the physician to see inside the bladder and locate the stones. The stones are crushed so they can be flushed out in the urine.

At other times, the stones can be reached and removed through a surgical incision. The patient usually returns from surgery with two drainage tubes in place. One tube is inserted in the urinary bladder. The other tube is inserted in the ureter or kidney. The nurse will see that proper drainage is established.

- Provide routine postoperative care and check frequently to be sure the drainage is not blocked by kinks in the tubes or by the weight of the patient's body.
- Note the amount and type of drainage from each area.

Hydronephrosis

Hydronephrosis results from accumulation of fluid within the kidney. The increasing amount of urine applies pressure to the kidney cells, destroying them. Fluid accumulates in the kidney because something is blocking its flow. The flow may be blocked by:

- Renal calculi
- Kinking or twisting of the ureters

- Tumors, especially benign prostatic hypertrophy
- A distended bladder

Symptoms may be acute and similar to those of renal calculi, or they may occur so gradually that they go unnoticed until much damage has been done.

Treatment

The condition is treated by draining the urine above the blockage to relieve pressure and then correcting the cause.

RESPONSIBILITIES OF THE NURSING ASSISTANT

Be sure you understand each patient's orders for positioning, drainage, and activity.

There are some important measures that will apply to most urinary patients in your care:

- Accurately measure intake and output (Figure 45-7).
- Promptly report signs and symptoms of:
  - Bleeding
  - Chilling
  - Elevated temperature
  - Reduced output
  - Increased edema
  - Pain
- Properly care for urinary drainage.
- Know the proper steps to take for encouraging fluid intake (forcing fluids) and for limiting fluids.
- When assisting with urination, collecting a urine specimen, or observing and recording I&O, note and report the following:
  - Amount of urine
  - Color of urine
  - Odor of urine
  - Presence and type of sediment

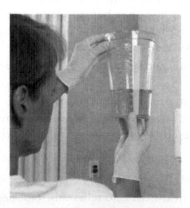

FIGURE 45-7 Accurately measure and record intake and output.

URINARY INCONTINENCE

Urinary incontinence (loss of control of urination) may be due to one or a combination of factors. Several factors may be present at the same time.

- Any interruption of cerebral control can lead to incontinence, including stroke, brain damage that destroys the control centers or pathways, confusion and decreased awareness due to general cerebral degeneration, or aphasia leading to the patient's inability to communicate the need for help.
- Incontinence may occur simply because the patient is unable to reach the proper facilities in time. The condition may be related to fecal impaction. Fecal impaction acts as a mechanical obstruction, causing the urine to be retained. The incontinence in this case is actually overflow.
- Infection, which is probably the most common reason for incontinence. Inflammation irritates sensory nerve endings in the bladder. Mucosal and bladder contractions are increased, causing the incontinence.
- Incontinence may be temporary, lasting only a few days. For example, after a period of illness, continence may improve as the patient becomes more able to respond to the environment. Attention to the underlying causes and the temporary use of incontinence pads may be all that is needed. Make every effort to help the patient regain control as soon as possible, with little reference to the temporary incontinence. Provide emotional support and reassurance.
- Incontinence of an established nature continues even though the patient is ambulatory. This is a more difficult, but still not impossible, form of incontinence to treat. Some drugs help improve bladder control. Retraining may also be needed.

Estimating Amount of Incontinence

Some facilities estimate the amount of each incontinent voiding. There is little difference between a small amount and a large amount:

- Small incontinence is 30 mL or less. This is the amount that will soak through the underwear.
- Moderate incontinence is 31 to 60 mL. This is the amount that will run down the legs if no underwear is worn.

- Large incontinence is 61 mL or greater. This is the entire bladder and includes soaking clothing, floor, and furniture.

Some facilities estimate the amount by weighing the incontinent pad or brief. A baby scale with metric measurements is used for this procedure.

DIAGNOSTIC TESTS

Techniques used to diagnose problems of the urinary tract include:

- Magnetic resonance imaging (MRI).
- Computed tomography (CT or CAT) scan.

👪 Age-Appropriate Care ALERT

Incontinence is up to five times more common in persons over age 50 than in younger adults. However, incontinence is not a normal aging change. It is always associated with another medical or psychological problem. Approximately one-third of all hospitalized adults are incontinent of stool. About half of all long-term care facility residents are incontinent of urine.

- Urinalysis—one common method of learning about the condition of the kidneys is to examine and test the urine.
- **Cystoscopy**—a test usually performed during surgery that enables the physician to look inside the bladder. An instrument called a *cystoscope* is inserted through the urethra. Following this examination, frequency of urination is to be expected, but heavy bleeding or a complaint of sharp, intense pain should be reported at once.
- **Pyelogram**—an X-ray examination of the urinary tract, similar to the GB and GI series. The dye may be given intravenously (**intravenous pyelogram** or IVP) or inserted during cystoscopy (**retrograde pyelogram**) through the urethra. Preparation of the patient usually includes cleansing enemas. Satisfactory results of the X-ray examination depend largely on proper patient preparation.
- Blood chemistry tests.
- Blood urea nitrogen (BUN).
- Creatinine.

GUIDELINES 45-1 Guidelines for Caring for the Patient with Incontinence

Nursing assistant responsibilities include:

- Assisting patients who need help to toilet regularly.
- Answering call lights promptly.
- Always being courteous and patient when assisting patients with toileting.
- Maintaining a positive attitude when changing soiled garments and bed linens, and never being critical.
- Performing good perineal care and being sure skin is clean and dry.
- Checking the skin for signs of irritation whenever toileting or bathing a patient or performing perineal care.

- Giving special attention to patients who are confused, are forgetful, or have communication problems because they may be unable to clearly state their need for assistance.
- Changing wet linens immediately to reduce the patient's discomfort and embarrassment. Prolonged skin exposure to urine is a major cause of skin breakdown. In addition, pathogens grow rapidly on the warmth and moisture and can quickly move upward through the urinary tract, causing life-threatening infection.
- Helping the patient become continent. Provide emotional support and reassurance.

GUIDELINES 45-2 Guidelines for Weighing an Incontinent Pad or Brief

The facility will post the weight of a dry pad or brief on or near the scale. You will:

1. Remove the wet brief. Weigh the wet pad or brief on an empty scale.

2. According to this formula, 1 g of weight = 1 mL of urine. For example, the wet brief weighs 500 g. The dry weight is 150 g. The difference is 350 g. 1 mL of urine × 350 mL = 350 mL.

Consider this hypothetical situation with a patient:

1. Remove the wet brief. Give perineal care, put a dry brief on the patient.

2. Weigh the wet brief. You find that it weighs 434 g.

3. The size large brief that the patient is wearing weighs 120 g in your facility.

4. Subtract: 434 g − 120 g = 314 g/mL.

5. Multiply: 314 mL × 1 mL = 314 mL total amount of incontinence.

EXPAND YOUR SKILLS

PROCEDURE **96** COLLECTING A ROUTINE URINE SPECIMEN

1. Carry out initial procedure actions.
2. Assemble equipment:
   - Disposable gloves
   - Bedpan/Urinal with cover
   - Bed protector
   - Toilet tissue
   - Small plastic bag
   - Specimen container and cover
   - Label, including:
     - Patient's full name
     - Room number
     - Facility identification

   - Date and time of collection
   - Physician's name
   - Examination to be done
   - Other information requested or required
   - Graduated pitcher
   - Laboratory requisition slip, properly filled out
   - Biohazardous specimen transport bag

3. Completely fill out the label for the specimen container.

4. Wash your hands and put on gloves.

5. If the patient cannot ambulate, offer the bedpan or urinal.

(continues)

PROCEDURE 96 CONTINUED

O P

- Instruct the patient not to discard toilet tissue in the pan with the urine. Provide a small plastic bag in which to place the soiled tissue.

- After the patient has voided, cover the pan and place it on the bed protector on the chair.

- Remove your gloves and dispose of them properly. Offer wash water to the patient. (Leave gloves on and use standard precautions if you will be assisting with perineal care.)

6. If the patient can ambulate to the bathroom, place a specimen collector in the toilet.

- Assist the patient to the bathroom. Ask the patient to void into the specimen collector. Remind the patient to discard soiled toilet tissue in the plastic bag provided. Do not place tissue in the collector.

7. Remove your gloves and dispose of them properly.

8. Provide privacy.

9. Wash your hands and put on fresh gloves. Remove the specimen collector from the toilet. If the patient is on I&O, note the amount of urine (Figure 45-8A). If the patient used a bedpan, pour the urine into a graduated container to measure it. Note the amount.

Remove your gloves and discard them according to facility policy. Wash your hands.

10. Remove the cap from the specimen container, and place it (inside up) on a shelf or other flat surface in the bathroom or utility room. Place the specimen container on a clean paper towel on the counter. Do not touch the inside of the cap or container.

11. Put on gloves. Hold the specimen container in one hand or leave it on the paper towel, and steady it with your other hand so it does not tip. Carefully pour about 120 mL of urine into the specimen container from the collector.

12. Remove and discard your gloves according to facility policy.

13. Wash your hands.

14. Place the cap on the specimen container. Do not contaminate the outside of the container. Attach the completed label to the container. Place the specimen container in a biohazardous specimen transport bag and attach a laboratory requisition slip (Figure 45-8B).

15. Carry out ending procedure actions.

16. Follow facility policy for transporting the specimen to the laboratory.

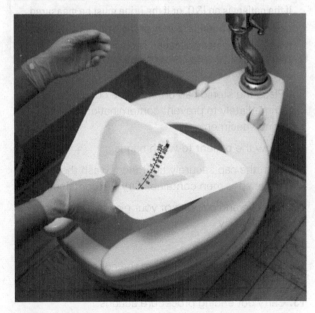

FIGURE 45-8A Remove the collection device. Note the total amount if the patient is on I&O.

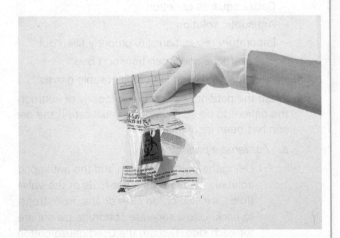

FIGURE 45-8B The properly labeled specimen container is placed in a transport bag with the laboratory requisition attached.

ICON KEY:
 = OBRA   = PPE

EXPAND YOUR SKILLS

PROCEDURE **97** COLLECTING A CLEAN-CATCH URINE SPECIMEN

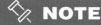 **NOTE**

The guidelines for this procedure vary slightly from state to state, and from one facility to the next. Your instructor will inform you if the sequence in your state or facility differs from the procedure listed here. Know and follow the required sequence for your facility and state.

1. Carry out initial procedure actions.
2. Assemble equipment:
   - Disposable gloves
   - Small plastic bag
   - Sterile specimen container and cover
   - Label for container, with:
     - Patient's full name
     - Room number
     - Facility identification
     - Date and time of collection
     - Physician's name
     - Type of specimen test to be performed
     - Any other information requested
   - Gauze squares or cotton
   - Antiseptic solution
   - Laboratory requisition slip, properly filled out
   - Biohazardous specimen transport bag
3. Wash your hands and put on disposable gloves.
4. Wash the patient's genital area properly or instruct the patient to do so. Provide perineal care if the person has been incontinent.
   a. *For female patients:*
      i. Using the gauze or cotton and the antiseptic solution, cleanse the outer folds of the vulva (folds are also called *labia* or *lips*) from front to back. Use a separate cotton/gauze square for each side. Discard the used gauze/cotton in the plastic bag.
      ii. Cleanse the inner folds of the vulva with two pieces of gauze and antiseptic solution, again from front to back. Discard the used gauze/cotton in the plastic bag.
      iii. Cleanse the middle, innermost area (meatus or urinary opening) in the same manner. Discard the used gauze/cotton in the plastic bag.

      iv. Keep the labia separated so that the folds do not fall back and cover the meatus.
   b. *For male patients:*
      i. Using the gauze or cotton and the antiseptic solution, cleanse the tip of the penis. Work downward in a circular motion. Wash the remainder of the penis using downward strokes.
      ii. Discard the used gauze/cotton in the plastic bag.
5. Open the container. Place the cap on the counter with the clean inside facing up. Do not touch the inside of the cup or lid with your hands.
6. Instruct the patient to void, allowing the first part of the urine to escape. Then:
   a. Catch the urine stream that follows in the sterile specimen container.
   b. Allow the last portion of the urine stream to escape.

 NOTE

If the patient is on I&O, or if the urine must be measured, catch the first and last part of the urine in a bedpan, urinal, or specimen collection container.

7. Place the sterile cap on the urine container immediately to prevent contamination of the urine specimen.
8. Allow the patient to wash hands.
9. With the cap securely tightened, wash the outside of the specimen container. Dry the container.
10. Remove and dispose of your gloves according to facility policy.
11. Wash your hands.
12. Attach a completed label to the container and place the specimen in the transport bag.
13. Carry out ending procedure actions.
14. Follow facility policy for transporting the specimen to the laboratory.

ICON KEY:
 = OBRA   = PPE

Urine Specimens

Routine Urine Specimen

Urinalysis is the most common laboratory test. The specimen is usually taken when the patient first **voids** (urinates) in the morning. The properties of fresh urine begin to change after 15 minutes. Take the sample to the laboratory or refrigerate it until it can be delivered.

Catheterized Urine Specimen

The nurse will insert a sterile tube called a **catheter** to collect a urine specimen that is free from external contamination.

Twenty-Four-Hour Specimen

If a 24-hour urine specimen is ordered, all urine excreted in a 24-hour period is collected and saved. The patient must start the 24-hour time period with an empty bladder, so the first specimen is discarded.

- Save all urine in a large, carefully labeled container that is supplied by the laboratory and may contain a preservative.
- The container is usually surrounded by ice. If the patient has an indwelling catheter, place the catheter bag in a container surrounded by ice. Empty the bag into the container supplied by the laboratory.
- Ask the patient to void. Discard the urine to ensure that the bladder is empty when the test begins.
- Save all other urine, including that voided as the test time finishes.
- Do not place toilet tissue in the container.
- Inform the nurse if you or the patient forget to save a specimen. If this occurs, the test will be discontinued and started again for another 24 hours.
- Apply disposable gloves and remove and dispose of them properly each time you collect a specimen.

EXPAND YOUR SKILLS

PROCEDURE 98 COLLECTING A 24-HOUR URINE SPECIMEN

1. Carry out initial procedure actions.

2. Assemble equipment:
   - Disposable gloves
   - 24-hour specimen container (supplied by health care facility)
   - Label
   - Bedpan, urinal, or commode; or specimen collector for toilet
   - Plastic bag
   - Sign for patient's bed
   - Biohazard bag

3. Label the container with:
   - Patient's name
   - Room number
   - Test ordered
   - Type of specimen
   - Time started
   - Time ended
   - Date
   - Physician's name

4. Instruct the patient to save all urine.

5. Place the specimen collection container in the bathroom in a pan of ice (Figure 45-9A). Refresh the ice as needed to keep the specimen cool for 24 hours.

6. Put on gloves.

7. Allow the patient to void.
   a. Assist with the bedpan or urinal as needed.
   b. Measure the amount of urine passed if the patient is on I&O.
   c. Discard the urine specimen.
   d. Note the date and time of voiding. This time marks the start of the 24-hour collection.

8. Place a sign on the patient's bed to alert other health care team members that a 24-hour urine specimen is being collected. (The sign may read: *Save all urine—24-hour specimen*.)

9. From this time on, for a period of 24 hours, all urine is added to the specimen container (Figure 45-9B). Check facility policy regarding handling of the specimen container.

(continues)

PROCEDURE **98** CONTINUED

10. Instruct the patient not to discard toilet tissue into the specimen collection container. Provide small plastic bags for this purpose.

11. At the end of the 24-hour period:
    a. Put on disposable gloves.
    b. Ask the patient to void one last time.
    c. Add this urine to the specimen container.

12. Remove the sign from the patient's bed. Check the container label for accuracy and completeness. Attach the appropriate requisition slip.

13. Remove and dispose of your gloves according to facility policy.

14. Place the specimen in a protective biohazard bag for transport.

15. Carry out ending procedure actions.

16. Clean and replace all equipment used, according to facility policy.

17. Follow facility policy for transporting the specimen to the laboratory.

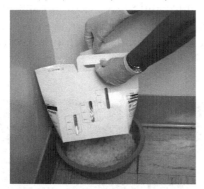

FIGURE 45-9A Close the container with the plastic fastener. Place the 24-hour specimen container in the patient's bathroom in a pan of ice. Refresh the ice as often as needed.

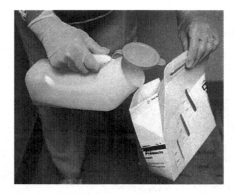

FIGURE 45-9B Open the mouth of the container wide to avoid spilling the specimen.

ICON KEY:
 = OBRA   = PPE

⚠ OSHA **ALERT**

Most facilities do not permit personnel to wear gloves or other PPE in the hallway because the OSHA Bloodborne Pathogen Standard states that PPE must be removed prior to leaving the work area. In this situation, the patient's room is the work area. Some facilities allow staff to use the one-glove technique (Chapter 13) to carry wet or soiled linen and other items into the hallway in close proximity to a patient's room. Know and follow your facility policies.

Urine Testing

The HemaCombistix is used to test for the presence of protein, blood, and glucose, and for pH (acidity) of urine.

URINARY DRAINAGE

Many patients with urinary problems will have urine drained from the bladder through a tube called a *catheter*.

- An **intermittent catheter** is inserted to empty the bladder, and then immediately removed. Many people have medical conditions that cause them to be unable to void. They catheterize themselves using this method five to eight times a day. The risk of infection is lower than using an indwelling catheter. French catheters or straight catheters (Figure 45-10A) are used for this purpose. These hollow tubes made of soft rubber or plastic. They are used to obtain a specimen or drain the bladder. An intermittent catheter does not remain in the bladder.

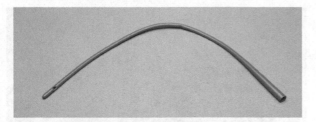

FIGURE 45-10A A straight catheter is inserted to collect a specimen or empty the bladder, and then removed.

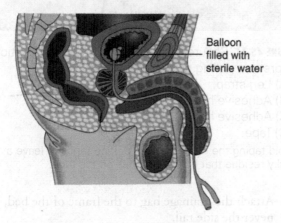

Balloon filled with sterile water

FIGURE 45-10B An indwelling urinary catheter is left in place to empty the bladder. The balloon is inflated with sterile water to hold the catheter in place. A catheter should only be used when medically necessary.

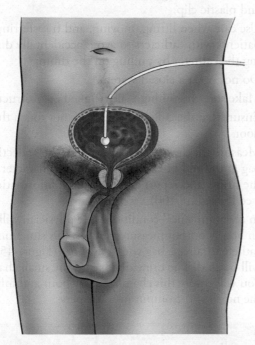

FIGURE 45-10C A suprapubic catheter is surgically inserted into the bladder through the abdominal wall. The urethra is not used to expel urine.

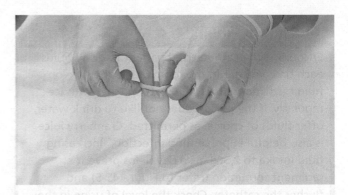

FIGURE 45-10D Keep the skin clean and dry under a condom catheter.

- **Foley catheters** (Figure 45-10B) have a balloon surrounding the neck. The balloon is inflated to hold the catheter in the bladder. This is known as an **indwelling catheter** or **retention catheter**. The insertion of a catheter is a sterile procedure. Closed urinary drainage systems protect the patient from infection. The patient may complain of feeling the urge to urinate due to the pressure of the balloon on the internal sphincter of the urethra. The pressure feels the same as the sensation of urine pressing on the sphincter. If the patient with a catheter complains of feeling the urge to void, notify the nurse.
- A **suprapubic catheter** (Figure 45-10C) is inserted surgically through the abdominal wall directly into the bladder.
- A **condom catheter** (Figure 45-10D) is an external catheter used in the care of incontinent males. It is applied over the penis and attached to drainage tubing. Remove the catheter daily and wash and dry the penis well. The risk for complications is very high, and keeping the patient clean helps reduce the risk.

> ### ❋ Infection Control **ALERT**
>
> As many as 13,000 patients die each year in the United States because of catheter-related infections. Careful handling and attention to technique when caring for and emptying the catheter will reduce the risk of infection. Catheters should be used only as a treatment of last resort because of the risk of complications. Possible complications are urinary tract or kidney infections, blood infections (septicemia), urethral injury, skin breakdown, bladder stones, and blood in the urine (hematuria). After many years of catheter use, bladder cancer may also develop.

Difficult Situations

Encourage the catheterized patient to drink fluids each time you are in the room unless they are on fluid restrictions. Refill the water pitcher with ice regularly. If the person does not like to drink water, offer fluids of choice, as permitted. Cranberry juice is also helpful in preventing infection.* Increasing fluid intake to 2,500 mL a day helps prevent sediment formation (refer to Figure 45-5) and flushes the catheter. Check the level of urine in the drainage bag each time you are in the room. Empty the bag if it is full.

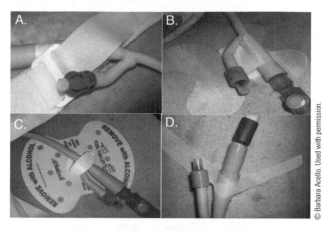

© Barbara Acello. Used with permission.

FIGURE 45-11 Secure the long part of the Y-connection to prevent pulling on the internal balloon.
(A) Leg strap.
(B) Adhesive holder.
(C) Adhesive holder.
(D) Tape.

Avoid taping the tube, if possible. Tape tends to leave a sticky residue that holds microbes on the tube.

You have definite responsibilities when patients are using urinary drainage systems:

- Apply the principles of standard precautions.
- Use aseptic technique when caring for the catheter or the drainage system.
- Keep the urinary meatus clean.
- Wash the area around the meatus daily with a solution approved by your facility.
- Check regularly for signs of irritation or urinary discomfort and report them to the nurse.
- Secure the tubing so that there is no strain on the catheter or tubing. Apply a catheter strap or adhesive holder (Figure 45-11) to secure the tubing.
  - Secure the catheter to the inner thigh of a female patient.
  - Although there is no single correct spot for fastening the catheter strap or adhesive holder, fastening it just after the junction of the tubing works well because this is the most rigid spot on the catheter. Anchoring one side of the tubing prevents accidental slipping and pulling.
  - Secure the catheter to the abdomen of the male patient with an adhesive catheter holder or tape (Figure 45-12). Fastening it to the leg may cause a fistula, or abnormal passageway between the penis and outside of the body.
  - Avoid placing the catheter under the leg, which may pinch and obstruct the flow of urine.
- Maintain the drainage bag below the level of the bladder. Never elevate the bag, as this allows urine to flow back into the bladder. Instruct the patient to carry the bag below the level of the bladder when ambulating.

- Attach the drainage bag to the frame of the bed, never the side rail.
- Attach the closed drainage bag to the frame of the chair or wheelchair.
- Many facilities place the drainage bag in a cloth catheter bag for privacy.
- Attach the tubing to the bed with a rubber band and plastic clip.
- Use care when lifting, moving, and transferring patients with catheters to avoid accidentally dislodging the catheter by pulling on the tubing.
- Do not open a closed system.
- Make sure the tubing is not kinked or obstructed.
- Ensure that the collection bag does not touch the floor.
- Measure the amount of drainage in the collection bag at the end of each shift, note the character of the urine, and report and record the information (see Procedure 100).
- In certain medical conditions, the physician will order an hourly output measurement. In this situation, a catheter drainage bag with a *urimeter* (Figure 45-13) will be used. The urine drains into the small chamber. You will empty this chamber every hour and inform the nurse of the output measurement.

  Infection Control **ALERT**

The presence of sediment in a catheter suggests infection. Inform the nurse.

---

*Stapleton, A. E., Dziura, J., Hooton, T. M., Cox, M. E., Yarova-Yarovaya, Y., Chen, S., & Gupta, K. (2012, February). Recurrent urinary tract infection and urinary *Escherichia coli* in women ingesting cranberry juice daily: A randomized controlled trial. *Mayo Clinic Proceedings, 87*(2), 143–150.

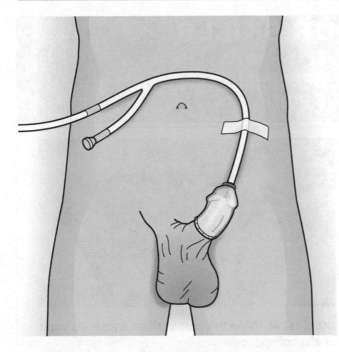

FIGURE 45-12 Securing the catheter to the abdomen reduces the risk of complications such as the development of a fistula or abnormal passageway between the penis and the outside of the body.

- Check the entire drainage setup each time care is given and at the beginning and end of your shift (see Procedure 100).
- Monitor the level of urine in the drainage bag. Most people excrete about 50 to 80 mL of urine each hour. Inform the nurse if the level of urine in the bag does not change; if the catheter is leaking; if no urine is present in the bag; or if the urine has an abnormal color, odor, or appearance.
- Notify the nurse if redness, irritation, drainage, crusting, or open areas are present at the catheter insertion site.
- Inform the nurse if the patient complains of pain, burning, or tenderness, or has other signs or symptoms of urinary tract infection.
- Do not disconnect the closed drainage system unless you have the nurse's permission.

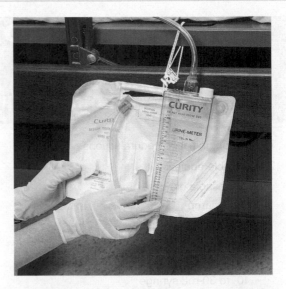

FIGURE 45-13 A drainage bag with a urimeter is used when hourly output measurements are required.

>  Infection Control **ALERT**
>
> The presence of sediment in a catheter suggests infection. Inform the nurse.

Collecting a Specimen from a Closed Urinary Drainage System

At some time, it may be necessary to collect a fresh specimen of urine when the patient has a closed urinary drainage system. Keep in mind that the:

- Urine sample must be fresh.
- Urine in the bag has accumulated over a period of time.
- The specimen may not be taken from the drainage bag.
- Fresh specimen must be taken directly from the catheter.

The procedure to be followed is determined by the type of Foley catheter that is in place. If the catheter has a **port** (opening) for fluid withdrawal, follow Procedure 99. Proper technique must be used to avoid introducing infectious organisms into the system.

EXPAND YOUR SKILLS

PROCEDURE **99** **COLLECTING A URINE SPECIMEN THROUGH A DRAINAGE PORT**

1. Carry out initial procedure actions.

2. Assemble equipment:
   - Disposable gloves
   - Tube clamp
   - Laboratory requisition
   - Completed label
   - Emesis basin
   - 10- to 30-mL syringe
   - 21- or 22-gauge needle
   - Specimen cup and lid
   - Sharps container
   - Alcohol wipe
   - Bed protector
   - Biohazardous specimen transport bag
   - Plastic trash bag

3. Go to the bedside 30 minutes before the sample is to be collected.

4. Clamp the drainage tube below the specimen port.

5. Wash your hands. Return to the bedside after 30 minutes.

6. Put on gloves.

7. Place a bed protector on the bed and place an emesis basin on the bed protector under the catheter drainage port.

8. Wipe the drainage port with an alcohol wipe (Figure 45-14A).

9. Carefully remove the cap on the syringe. Do not contaminate the tip.

10. Attach the sterile, capped needle carefully.

11. Open the package with the specimen container. Remove the lid and lay it, inside up, on the table. Do not touch the inside of the cup or the lid with your hands.

12. Clean the port with the alcohol sponge and allow to dry.

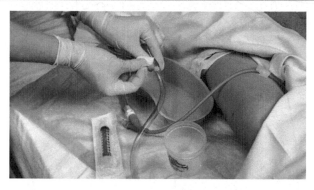

FIGURE 45-14A Wipe the port with an antiseptic wipe or alcohol sponge.

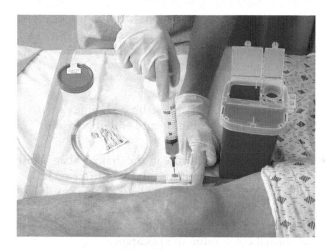

FIGURE 45-14B Draw the specimen into the syringe.

13. Remove the cap from the needle. Do not contaminate the needle tip.

14. Insert the needle into the port and withdraw the specimen (Figure 45-14B).

15. Carefully withdraw the needle.

16. Wipe the port with the alcohol wipe.

17. Transfer the urine sample to the specimen container (Figure 45-14C).

(continues)

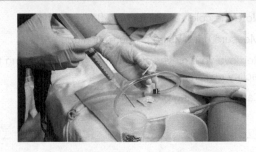

FIGURE 45-14C Transfer the specimen to the sterile container.

18. Do not recap the needle. Do not detach the needle from the syringe. Discard the assembled needle and syringe into the sharps container at the bedside.

19. Handling the lid by the top only, cover the container.

20. Remove the catheter clamp.

21. Remove your gloves and dispose of them according to facility policy. Wash your hands.

22. Complete the information on the label and put the label on the container. Compare the label to the requisition to be sure that the information is complete and accurate.

23. Place the specimen container in a biohazard transport bag, seal the bag, and attach the completed laboratory requisition (Figure 45-14D).

24. Carry out ending procedure actions.

25. Follow instructions for care and transport of the specimen.

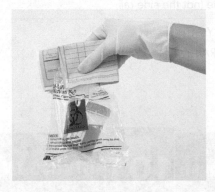

FIGURE 45-14D Place the specimen in the biohazard transport bag, seal the bag, and attach the laboratory requisition.

ICON KEY:

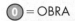 = OBRA  = PPE

Catheter Care

The urinary meatus must be kept clean and free of secretions. Wash the area around the meatus daily with a solution approved by your facility or with soap and water. In some facilities, this procedure is done each shift. This care is called *indwelling catheter care*.

Indwelling catheter care may be performed during routine morning care, as part of perineal care, or as a separate procedure (see Procedure 101). Report signs of irritation or complaints of discomfort, and changes in the character or quantity of drainage.

EXPAND YOUR SKILLS

PROCEDURE **100** ROUTINE DRAINAGE CHECK

1. Carry out initial procedure actions.

2. Wash your hands. Put on gloves.

3. Raise the bedding to observe the tubing.

4. Check the condition of the catheter and the meatus.

5. Keep the drainage tubing coiled on the bed so there is a direct drop to the collection bag.

(continues)

PROCEDURE 100 CONTINUED

6. Position the collection bag so it is lower than the patient's hips.

7. Keep the end of the drainage tube above the urine level in the bag. Check to be sure that neither the tubing nor the drainage bag is touching the floor.

8. Be sure the drainage bag is attached to the bed frame (not the side rail).

9. Note the color, character, and flow of urine.

10. Measure urine using proper technique.

11. Remove your gloves and discard them according to facility policy.

12. Carry out ending procedure actions.

ICON KEY:

O = OBRA   **P** = PPE

PROCEDURE 101 GIVING INDWELLING CATHETER CARE

1. Carry out initial procedure actions.

2. Assemble equipment:
   - Disposable gloves
   - Bed protector
   - Bath blanket
   - Plastic bag for disposables
   - Daily catheter care kit (if available)
   - Washcloth, towel, basin, and soap if kit is unavailable
   - Antiseptic solution
   - Sterile applicators
   - Adhesive or Velcro catheter holder

3. Raise the bed to a comfortable working height. Be sure the opposite side rail is up and secure. Position the patient on the back, with legs separated and knees bent, if permitted.

4. Cover the patient with a bath blanket and fanfold bedding to the foot of the bed.

5. Ask the patient to raise the hips. Place a bed protector underneath the patient.

6. Position a bath blanket so that only the genitals will be exposed.

7. Arrange a catheter care kit on the overbed table. Open the kit. Position the open bag at the foot of the bed. You may use a basin of warm water, soap, and several washcloths instead of a catheter care kit. Turn the washcloth with each stroke so that no surface is reused.

8. Wash your hands. Put on gloves and draw the drape or bath blanket back.

9A. *For the male patient:*

   a. Gently grasp the penis and draw the foreskin back, if not circumcised (Figure 45-15).

   b. Using a new applicator dipped in antiseptic solution for each stroke, cleanse the glans from the meatus toward the shaft for approximately four inches.

   c. After each stroke, dispose of the used applicator in a plastic bag.

Alternate action: Clean around the catheter first and then around the meatus and glans. Wash with soap and water, using a circular motion. Dry in the same manner. Make sure to return the foreskin (if not circumcised) to its proper position.

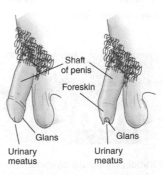

FIGURE 45-15 Comparison of circumcised and uncircumcised penis.

(continues)

9B. *For the female patient:*

   a. Separate the labia.

   b. Using a new applicator dipped in antiseptic for each stroke, cleanse from front to back. Begin at the center, and then cleanse each side.

   c. After each stroke, dispose of the used applicator in a plastic bag.

   d. Clean the catheter down about four inches.

   e. Dry carefully.

10. Remove your gloves and discard them in the plastic bag. Wash your hands.

11. Secure the catheter to the leg (female) or abdomen (male).

ICON KEY:

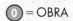 = OBRA   = PPE

12. Check to be sure the tubing is coiled on the bed and that it hangs straight down into the drainage container. Empty the bag and measure the contents, if necessary. Do not raise the bag above the level of the patient's hips. Check to be sure that neither the tubing nor the drainage bag is touching the floor.

13. Replace bedding and remove the bath blanket.

14. Fold the bath blanket and store, or put it in the linen hamper.

15. Lower the bed. Adjust side rails for safety.

16. Carry out ending procedure actions.

Ambulating with a Catheter

Carefully position the drainage bag for persons who are ambulatory or using a geriatric chair or wheelchair. Remember that the drainage bag must always be lower than the bladder so the urine cannot flow back into the bladder. The bag may be secured to the patient's leg or clothing when the patient ambulates.

When the patient is seated in a wheelchair, the tubing should run below and under the wheelchair so the drainage bag can be secured to the wheelchair frame. The drainage bag and tubing must never touch the floor.

There are times when you may have to disconnect the catheter. Follow your facility's policies for performing this procedure. In some facilities, a licensed nurse must give permission to disconnect a closed drainage system.

SUPRAPUBIC CATHETERS

A suprapubic catheter (S/P cath; see Figure 45-10C) is inserted surgically through the abdominal wall directly into the bladder. This type of catheter may also be called a *cystostomy tube.* It is believed to have a lower incidence of infection than a urethral catheter and is sometimes used for persons who need permanent or long-term urinary catheters. It may be inserted after prostate or bladder repair surgery. It is attached to a regular drainage bag and may be used with a leg bag or belly bag when the patient is ambulatory.

Caring for a Patient with a Suprapubic Catheter

GUIDELINES 45-3 Guidelines for Caring for a Patient with a Suprapubic Catheter

General care of the patient with a suprapubic catheter is very similar to care for a patient with an indwelling urethral catheter.

- Use aseptic technique when caring for the catheter or opening the closed drainage system.
- Perform catheter care as ordered, including careful cleansing of the insertion site and proximal catheter

- Maintain a sterile closed drainage system. Avoid opening the system, if possible.
- Anchor the tube with an adhesive tube holder to avoid tension and promote drainage.

(continues)

GUIDELINES 45-3 Guidelines for Caring for a Patient with a Suprapubic Catheter (continued)

There are a few variations from regular indwelling catheter care:

- Hairs should be trimmed (clipped, not shaved) surrounding the stoma (insertion site) to reduce the risk of bacterial contamination.

- Monitor the skin around the catheter daily. A small amount of redness and clear drainage is normal. Report any large area of redness, along with colored or foul-smelling, drainage to the nurse.

📖 NOTE

In some states, nursing assistants may not be permitted to care for the suprapubic catheter. Your instructor will inform you if this is a nursing assistant skill in your state. Care for the suprapubic catheter only as permitted by state law and facility policies.

- Place a split sterile 4 × 4 pad around the stoma (Figure 45-16). Change daily or as ordered. After the area has healed, no dressing is necessary.

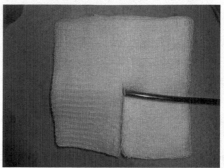

FIGURE 45-16 Fenestrated gauze is split so it can be used around tubes and drains. Make sure that the area is well-healed. If there are threads hanging on the gauze, keep them away from an open wound.

PROCEDURE 102 EMPTYING A URINARY DRAINAGE UNIT Ⓞ Ⓟ

1. Carry out initial procedure actions.

2. Assemble equipment:
   - Disposable gloves
   - Graduated container
   - Paper towel or disposable bed protector for floor
   - Antiseptic wipes
   - Plastic bag

3. Wash your hands and put on gloves.

4. Place a paper towel on the floor under the drainage bag. Place a graduated container on the paper towel under the drain of the collection bag.

5. Remove the drain from the holder. Disinfect the outlet with an antiseptic wipe and open the drain. Allow the urine to drain into the graduated container, using aseptic technique. Do not allow the tip of the tubing to touch the sides of the graduated container (Figure 45-17).

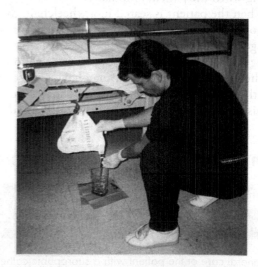

FIGURE 45-17 Center the graduated container under the drainage spout. If the spout accidentally contacts the fingers or the edge of the graduate, cleanse it with an alcohol sponge.

(continues)

6. Close the drain and wipe the tip with an antiseptic wipe before returning it to the holder. Dispose of used antiseptic wipes in a plastic bag.

7. Check the position of the drainage tube.

8. Pick up the paper towel, touching the top surface only, and discard it.

9. Take the graduated container to the bathroom and empty it.

10. Wash and dry the graduated container and store it according to facility policy.

11. Record the amount of urine and note its character.

12. Remove your gloves and discard them according to facility policy.

13. Carry out ending procedure actions.

ICON KEY:

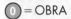 = OBRA   = PPE

Infection Risk

Disconnect the urinary catheter carefully because the catheter increases the risk for infection. There are several sites where infection can enter the drainage system (Figure 45-18):

- Urinary meatus, where the catheter is inserted
- Connection between the catheter and the drainage tube
- Opening used to empty the drainage bag

Disconnecting the Catheter

Avoid disconnecting the drainage setup, if this is possible. Use aseptic technique if you must disconnect the closed system. Use a sterile cap and plug, if available (Figure 45-19). If not, protect the disconnected ends with sterile gauze sponges.

External Drainage Systems (Male)

External urinary drainage systems are preferred for male patients who require long periods of urinary drainage because there is less danger of infection. A condom (sheath) catheter is applied to the penis and connected to the drainage system. Some patients find it easier to manage.

Complications, ranging from minor irritation to circulatory impairment, can occur. The external catheter is applied over the penis and attached with an adhesive strip. Always wrap the strip in a spiral. Severe injury can occur if it completely encircles the penis. Some external catheters have a self-adhesive film on the inside, making the adhesive strip on the outside unnecessary. About

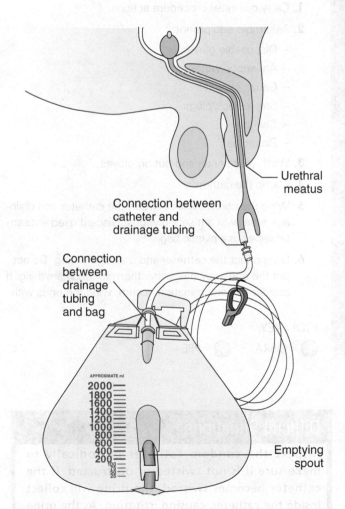

FIGURE 45-18 Handle the closed drainage system carefully to avoid accidental contamination of the closed system.

one inch of the catheter should extend beyond the tip of the penis and attach to the drainage tubing. Always apply the principles of standard precautions when caring for an external catheter.

The condom is attached to drainage tubing and a collection bag. The catheter can be attached to a regular closed drainage system or to a leg bag. Remove the condom every 24 hours to wash and dry the penis. Apply a new catheter and reconnect the drainage system.

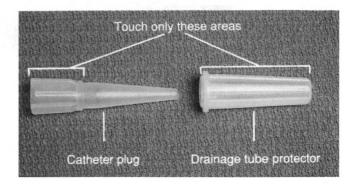

FIGURE 45-19 Sterile catheter plug and protective cap.

PROCEDURE 103 DISCONNECTING THE CATHETER (O) (P)

1. Carry out initial procedure actions.

2. Assemble equipment:
   - Disposable gloves
   - Antiseptic wipes
   - Gauze sponges
   - Sterile caps/plugs
   - Clamps
   - Plastic bag

3. Wash your hands and put on gloves.

4. Clamp the catheter.

5. Wipe the connection between the catheter and drainage tube with antiseptic wipes. Discard used antiseptic wipes in a plastic bag.

6. Disconnect the catheter and drainage tubing. Do not put the ends down or allow them to touch anything. If accidental contamination occurs, wipe the ends with antiseptic wipes before inserting the plug or placing the cap.

7. Insert a sterile plug in the end of the catheter. Place a sterile cap over the exposed end of the drainage tube. Empty the bag, if necessary.

8. Secure the drainage tube to the bed frame so that the tube will not touch the floor.

9. Remove and dispose of gloves according to facility policy. Wash your hands.

10. Carry out ending procedure actions.

🔨 NOTE

Reverse the procedure to reconnect the catheter. If you find an unprotected, disconnected tube in the bed or on the floor, *do not reconnect it. Report it at once.*

ICON KEY:
(O) = OBRA   (P) = PPE

Difficult Situations

Inspect the condom catheter periodically to make sure it is not twisted or obstructed. If the catheter becomes twisted, the urine will collect inside the catheter, causing irritation. As the urine accumulates, the catheter will expand until it eventually comes off.

Leg Bag Drainage

Some patients find it easier to ambulate when urine drainage is collected in a leg bag instead of the larger urinary drainage bag. The leg bag is held to the patient's leg by Velcro or vinyl straps, around either the thigh or the lower leg (Figure 45-20). Points to keep in mind when patients use a leg bag are:

- The leg bag is smaller than a regular drainage bag and must be emptied more often.
- Position the bag so there is a straight drop down from the catheter.

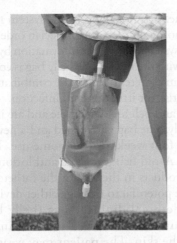

FIGURE 45-20 A leg bag is held in place by adjustable straps. The bag is smaller than a bed collection bag and must be emptied more often.

- Avoid tension on the catheter tubing.
- Apply the principles of standard precautions when connecting and disconnecting the catheter and emptying the drainage bag.

PROCEDURE 104 CONNECTING A CATHETER TO A LEG BAG

⚒ NOTE

Always check with the nurse before using a leg bag.

1. Carry out initial procedure actions.

2. Assemble equipment:
   - Disposable gloves
   - Antiseptic wipes
   - Leg bag and tubing
   - Emesis basin
   - Bed protector
   - Sterile cap/plug
   - Plastic bag

3. Wash your hands and put on gloves.

4. Place a bed protector under the connection between the catheter and the drainage tube.

5. Wipe the connection between the catheter and drainage tube with antiseptic wipes. Discard used antiseptic wipes in a plastic bag.

6. Disconnect the catheter and drainage tubing. Do not put them down or allow them to touch anything.

7. Insert a sterile plug in the end of the catheter. Place a sterile cap over the exposed end of the drainage tube.

8. Secure the drainage tube to the bed frame. The drainage tube must not touch the floor.

⚒ NOTE

If accidental contamination occurs, wipe the area with antiseptic wipes before inserting a sterile plug or replacing a sterile cap over the exposed end of the drainage tubing. Dispose of used antiseptic wipes in a plastic bag.

9. Remove the catheter plug.

10. Insert the end of the leg bag tubing into the catheter.

11. Secure the leg bag to the patient's leg so there is no tension on the tubing. Be sure there is a straight drop down from the catheter to the bag for urine flow. Check for leakage.

12. Remove the bed protector and discard it.

13. Remove your gloves and discard them according to facility policy. Wash your hands.

14. Assist the patient to get out of bed. A used single-use leg bag should be discarded in a biohazardous waste container.

15. Carry out ending procedure actions.

⚒ NOTE

To reconnect the regular drainage bag, reverse this procedure.

ICON KEY:

 = OBRA   = PPE

Infection Control ALERT

Avoid putting the patient to bed while they are wearing a leg bag. The urine may flow back into the bladder from the bag when the patient is in bed. Disconnect the leg bag and connect the catheter to the regular drainage bag when the patient is in bed.

Abdominal Drainage

People with some medical conditions use a catheter all the time. Patients with permanent suprapubic or indwelling urethral catheters may wear a device called an *abdominal urine bag* (belly bag; Figure 45-21) at home. (Belly bag is a

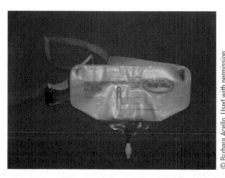

© Barbara Acello. Used with permission.

FIGURE 45-21 A disposable abdominal drainage bag is worn 24 hours a day and changed after 2 to 4 weeks of home use.

product name. It is not slang.) This system may be left in place in the hospital unless the physician orders a change in the drainage system. Verify this information by checking the care plan or with the nurse. The belly bag is contraindicated with a condom catheter because the combination of devices increases the risk for irritation and infection.

The bag and belt are disposable and are intended for a single use only. The bag is removed and a new bag applied every two to four weeks during home use. The used bag is discarded. Avoid using creams and lotions containing petroleum products in the area of the catheter and bag, as they have the potential to damage either device.

The abdominal drainage bag (belly bag) may be worn 24 hours a day. It has a soft backing, so it does not irritate the skin. The patient may wear a T-shirt or padding under the webbed belt if it is irritating. The belly bag is worn at the waist, under the clothing, and has many advantages over traditional drainage systems. The bag holds more than a leg bag and is less likely to leak. An antireflux valve behind the catheter port prevents backflow of urine from the bag into the bladder. The bag is emptied through a drainage tube that twists open and closed. The drain spout is in the approximate position of the urethra. Most patients sleep with the bag in place. Patients who use this type of bag find it superior to bed and leg drainage bags and may refuse to use anything else while hospitalized. Consult the nurse before using any substitute bag that you are not familiar with. Become familiar with the use instructions for the bags stocked by your facility or provided by the patient.

PROCEDURE 105 EMPTYING A LEG BAG

1. Carry out initial procedure actions.

2. Assemble equipment:
   - Disposable gloves
   - Antiseptic wipes
   - Emesis basin
   - Graduated pitcher
   - Paper towels

3. Position the patient safely.

4. Wash your hands and put on gloves.

5. Release the straps holding the leg bag so the bag can be moved away from the patient's leg.

6. Place a paper towel on the floor under the drainage outlet of the leg bag.

7. Place a graduated pitcher on the paper towel under the drainage outlet.

8. Remove the cap, being careful not to touch the tip. Drain the collected urine into the graduated pitcher. Do not put the cap down and do not touch the inside of the cap. If accidental contamination occurs, wipe the area with antiseptic wipes before replacing the cap. Dispose of used antiseptic wipes in a plastic bag.

9. Wipe the drainage outlet with an antiseptic wipe and replace the cap.

10. Refasten the straps to secure the drainage bag to the leg.

11. Make sure the patient is comfortable and safe.

12. Discard the paper towel.

13. Measure the urine and note the amount, if required.

14. Discard the urine. Clean the graduated pitcher and store it.

15. Remove your gloves and discard them according to facility policy.

16. Carry out ending procedure actions.

ICON KEY:

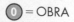 = OBRA   = PPE

Removing an Indwelling Catheter

An indwelling catheter is removed as soon as possible to reduce the risk of infection. A catheter must also be removed if it is obstructed, or for a routine change ordered by the physician. If a new catheter is not reinserted, monitor the patient's voiding after catheter removal. Follow your facility's policy for reporting to the nurse. If the patient has not voided within four to six hours, or if they complain of abdominal pain, notify the nurse.

PROCEDURE **106** REMOVING AN INDWELLING CATHETER

1. Carry out initial procedure actions.

2. Assemble equipment:
   - 2 pairs of disposable exam gloves
   - 10-mL syringe
   - Bed protector
   - Plastic bag for used supplies
   - Washcloth
   - Towel
   - Washbasin
   - Soap

3. Position the bed protector under the patient's buttocks.

4. Remove the device that secures the catheter to the leg.

5. Manipulate the tubing so that any urine in the tubing flows into the drainage bag.

6. Open the syringe. Attach the syringe to the inflation port (Figure 45-22).

7. Allow the inflation balloon to deflate into the syringe on its own. Follow facility policy for pulling on the plunger to withdraw fluid. If this method is used, pull very gently to avoid collapsing the inflation tube. (When the inflation tubing is collapsed, deflation of the balloon cannot occur.) The amount of fluid in the balloon may be marked on the catheter. Make sure you remove this amount. Depending on the catheter used, the port may flatten when the fluid is withdrawn. Empty the fluid from the syringe, reattach the syringe, and attempt to remove fluid again. When you are satisfied that the balloon is empty, proceed to the next step.

8. Grasp the catheter close to the perineum. Gently pull the catheter. If you feel resistance, stop. The balloon may not be completely deflated. Repeat steps 6 and 7.

9. If no resistance is met, withdraw the catheter. Observe the tip for the presence of sediment, blood, or mucus. If present, inform the nurse, who may request a culture.

10. Disconnect the catheter from the drainage tubing. Discard the catheter in the plastic bag, or according to facility policy.

11. Remove your gloves and discard them in the plastic bag.

12. Wash your hands.

13. Apply clean gloves.

14. Perform perineal care according to facility policy.

15. Empty the catheter drainage bag and measure output. Discard the empty bag in the plastic bag, or according to facility policy.

16. After the catheter is removed, instruct the patient to drink fluids, if permitted. Offer to take the patient to the bathroom, or offer the bedpan or urinal in two to four hours. Inform the nurse if the patient cannot void, or has complaints of urgency, pain, or burning.

17. Carry out ending procedure actions.

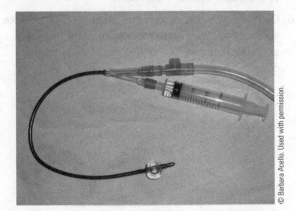

© Barbara Acello. Used with permission.

FIGURE 45-22 The syringe will begin removing fluid and deflating the balloon as soon as it is connected.

NOTE

Some facilities routinely culture the tip of the catheter after it is removed. As a rule, this is a dated practice that is not done. A physician's order is required. If the physician orders a culture, you will need a sterile specimen cup and sterile scissors. After removing the catheter, hold the end over the open specimen cup, and clip it three inches from the tip. Cover the cup and discard the remainder of the catheter.

ICON KEY:
 = OBRA   = PPE

BLADDER ULTRASOUND

It may be necessary to learn how much urine remains in the bladder after voiding or after a catheter has been removed. Doing an ultrasound scan is a noninvasive, painless method of learning the answer. The procedure will vary with the equipment and facility policy.

PROCEDURE 107 ULTRASOUND BLADDER SCAN

1. Carry out initial procedure actions.

2. Assemble equipment:
   - 2 pairs disposable exam gloves
   - Hospital gown
   - Bed protector
   - Plastic bag for used supplies
   - Washcloth
   - Towel
   - Washbasin
   - Soap
   - Dry tissue wipes to remove gel
   - Wet wipes to cleanse skin
   - Drinking water, cup, straw
   - Ultrasound gel
   - Ultrasound machine
   - Disinfectant wipes to cleanse handheld transducer

3. Assist the person to put on a hospital gown, if needed.

4. Encourage the person to drink at least 900 mL of water (or amount ordered) in the hour preceding the exam. Instruct them to avoid using the bathroom.

5. Assist the person into the supine position, with a pillow under the head.

6. Position the bed protector under the patient's buttocks.

7. Expose the abdomen, keeping the rest of the body covered.

8. Apply a generous amount of the ultrasound gel to the abdomen or scan head, according to facility policy.

9. Place the scan head on the abdomen and move in a circular motion (or according to the manufacturer's directions) in the gel. The ultrasound will automatically calculate and display the volume, recording it in the handheld unit. Wipe the gel off the skin with a dry wipe or paper towel. Discard in a plastic bag. Use a wet wipe to remove residue remaining on the skin.

10. Assist the patient with voiding in the bathroom, or the bedpan/urinal as needed.

11. Measure and document the amount of urine voided.

12. Return the patient to bed and assist back into the supine position.

13. Repeat the scan after the bladder is empty.

14. Assist the patient with cleansing the skin and dressing, as needed.

15. Cleanse the scan head with disinfectant, according to the manufacturer's directions.

16. Carry out your procedure completion actions. Make sure to document the amounts of urine from the ultrasound display, if this has not already been done.

REVIEW

A. True/False

Mark the following true or false by circling T or F.

1. T F Insertion of a sterile catheter into the urinary bladder is a routine nursing assistant task.

2. T F Gloves should be worn when emptying a urine collection bag.

3. T F Avoid disconnecting a closed urinary drainage system, if possible.

4. T F The pain associated with kidney stones is referred to as renal colic.

5. T F If you find an unprotected, disconnected catheter or tubing on the floor, you should reconnect it immediately.

6. T F The hemodialysis machine takes the place of nonfunctioning kidneys.

7. T F Ample fluid intake encourages increased output, which is important in treating kidney stones.

8. T F A catheter with an inflatable balloon is called a Foley catheter.

9. T F Foley catheters are indwelling catheters.

10. T F Cystitis is a fairly common problem for women.

11. T F Clamp the urinary drainage tube for 30 minutes before collecting a sample from a drainage port.

12. T F Reinsert the indwelling catheter if the patient does not void within four hours of catheter removal.

13. T F It is impossible to safely collect a sample of urine from a closed urinary drainage system.

B. Matching

Choose the correct term from Column II to match each word or phrase in Column I.

Column I

14. _____ indwelling catheter
15. _____ inability to expel formed urine
16. _____ urinate
17. _____ inflammation of the bladder
18. _____ blood in the urine

Column II

a. void
b. hematuria

c. cystitis
d. retention
e. dysuria
f. Foley catheter
g. suppression

C. Multiple Choice

Select the best answer for each of the following.

19. Your patient has a diagnosis of nephritis. Your care will include:
    a. keeping the patient very active.
    b. serving a high-sodium diet.
    c. measuring I&O accurately.
    d. eliminating vital sign measurements so the patient can rest more.

20. Your patient has renal calculi. One of your responsibilities will be:
    a. saving all urine.
    b. straining urine.
    c. limiting fluids.
    d. inserting a catheter.

21. A common cause of hydronephrosis is:
    a. renal calculi.
    b. pain in the bladder.
    c. bladder infection.
    d. drinking too much fluid.

22. Important signs and symptoms to report when there is a diagnosis involving the urinary system include:
    a. hunger.
    b. thirst.
    c. temperature elevation.
    d. voiding every three to four hours.

23. Indwelling catheter care is:
    a. a licensed nurse responsibility.
    b. performed during a.m. care.
    c. safely omitted as long as the patient is in bed.
    d. performed twice a week.

24. Dialysis is a procedure for:
    a. cleansing the blood of liquid wastes.
    b. relieving postoperative pain.
    c. administering oxygen.
    d. giving total parenteral nutrition.

25. A patient on dialysis will have:
  a. a regular diet.
  b. vital signs taken every hour.
  c. weight taken frequently.
  d. physical therapy.

26. When caring for patients who are on dialysis, you should observe for:
  a. edema of the face, hands, and feet.
  b. diarrhea.
  c. constipation.
  d. thirst.

27. When removing an indwelling catheter:
  a. cut the inflation port close to the catheter to remove fluid from the balloon.
  b. tell the patient to take a deep breath, and then quickly remove the catheter with the balloon inflated.
  c. withdraw fluid from the inflation port with a syringe.
  d. remove half the fluid from the balloon before removing the catheter.

28. Before collecting a specimen, clean the port of a closed urinary drainage system with:
  a. soap and water.
  b. a paper towel.
  c. alcohol.
  d. a sterile 4 × 4 gauze pad.

D. Completion
Complete the following statements.

29. The nursing assistant should apply the principles of _____ when caring for a catheter.

30. A routine check of a patient who uses urinary drainage should include _____.

E. Nursing Assistant Challenge
Mr. Starkman is 68 years of age. An external urinary condom is to be applied. Answer the following regarding his care while the condom is being applied.

31. You should wear gloves to apply the condom. _____
(yes)　(no)

32. The condom should be applied by _____ of the penis.
(pulling it up toward the tip)　(rolling it down toward the base)

33. When applying the condom, you should _____ space between the drainage tip and the glans of the penis.
(leave)　(not leave)

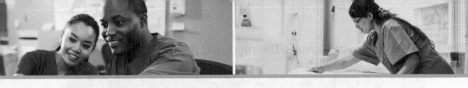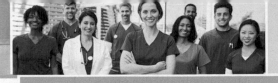

Reproductive System

OBJECTIVES

After completing this chapter, you will be able to:

46.1 Spell and define terms.

46.2 Review the location of the organs of the female reproductive system.

46.3 Review the location of the organs of the male reproductive system.

46.4 Explain the functions of the organs of the female reproductive system.

46.5 Explain the functions of the organs of the male reproductive system.

46.6 Describe some common disorders and conditions of the male reproductive system.

46.7 Describe some common disorders and conditions of the female reproductive system.

46.8 List six diagnostic tests associated with conditions of the male and female reproductive systems.

46.9 Describe nursing assistant actions related to the care of patients with conditions and diseases of the reproductive system.

46.10 State the nursing precautions required for patients who have sexually transmitted infections.

VOCABULARY

Learn the meaning and the correct spelling of the following words and phrases:

amenorrhea
benign prostatic
   hypertrophy
biopsy
brachytherapy
chancre
chlamydia
circumcision
climacteric
clitoris
colporrhaphy
Cowper's glands
cystocele
dilatation and curettage
   (D & C)
douche
dysmenorrhea
ejaculatory duct

endometrium
epididymis
fallopian tubes
genitalia
gonorrhea
hemorrhoid
herpes simplex II
hysterectomy
labia majora
labia minora
leukorrhea
lumpectomy
mammogram
mastectomy
menopause
menorrhagia
menstruation
metrorrhagia

Mycoplasma genitalium
oophorectomy
orchiectomy
ovary
oviduct
ovulation
ovum
panhysterectomy
Pap smear
pelvic inflammatory
   disease (PID)
penis
prolapsed uterus
prostatectomy
prostate gland
puberty
radical mastectomy
rectocele

salpingectomy
seminal vesicles
sexually transmitted
   infection (STI)
simple mastectomy
sperm
sterility
syphilis
testes
trichomonas vaginitis
uterus
vagina
vas deferens
venereal warts
vulva
vulvovaginitis

STRUCTURE AND FUNCTION

Both the male and female reproductive organs have dual functions. They:

- Produce reproductive cells. The male produces the **sperm**. The female produces the **ovum** (egg).
- Produce hormones that are responsible for sex characteristics.
  - Males produce testosterone.
  - Females produce estrogen and progesterone.

In the reproductive process, the:

- Male and female engage in sexual intercourse.
- Male ejaculates (propels) the sperm and the seminal fluid in which they swim into the female vagina.
- Sperm and egg meet in the female fallopian tube. One sperm penetrates the egg and conception takes place.
- Baby (fetus) develops in the uterus until birth.
- Female breasts (mammary glands) produce milk to nourish the newborn.

The Male Reproductive Organs: Structure and Function

The male organs (Figure 46-1) include the:

- **Testes**—two glandular organs located in the scrotum. The testes produce sperm and the hormone testosterone.
- **Epididymis**—a 20-foot-long coiled tube located on the top and back of each testis. The epididymis stores the sperm and allows them to mature.
- **Vas deferens**—a tube that leads from the epididymis. It carries the sperm upward into the pelvic cavity to the seminal vesicles during ejaculation. The vas deferens is accompanied by nerves and blood vessels. Together, they form the spermatic cord.

> ### ✚ Clinical Information **ALERT**
>
> Every human spent about half an hour as a single cell. All the seminiferous tubules in a male's body, laid end to end, would measure about 0.5 mile. Sperm travel about 3.5 millimeters per minute, for a total distance of about 4 inches to the site of fertilization. At the moment of ejaculation, some 350 million spermatozoa are deposited around the cervix. Of these, only about 100 get near the female egg. At birth, a female child has between 40,000 and 300,000 ova. Of these, only about 500 will ripen.

- **Seminal vesicles**—located behind the bladder. They receive and store the sperm from the vas deferens. They contribute nutrients to the seminal fluid. The small ejaculatory duct leads from the seminal vesicles to the urethra just below the prostate gland.
- **Ejaculatory duct**—carries the fluid produced in the seminal vesicles. Fluids are added as the sperm are propelled forward. The sperm and fluid form

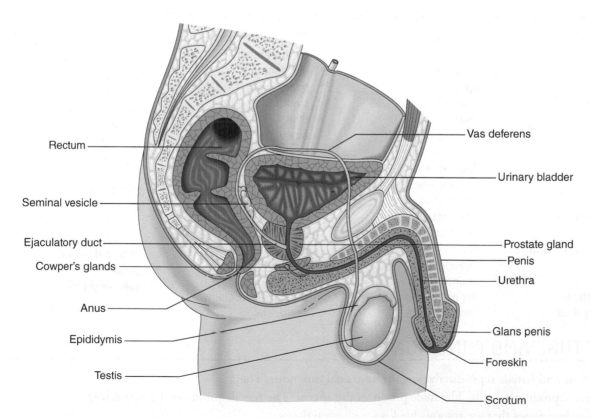

FIGURE 46-1 Cross-section of the male reproductive organs.

the seminal fluid or ejaculate. The fluid contains nutrients and other substances needed by the sperm.

- **Prostate gland**—found just below the urinary bladder surrounding the urethra. It secretes a fluid that increases the ability of the sperm to move in the seminal fluid. Enlargement of the prostate gland may impede or prevent urine from passing through the urethra. This is a fairly common occurrence in older men.

- **Cowper's glands**—two small glands located beside the urethra. They produce mucus for lubrication.

- **Penis**—composed of special tissue that can become filled with blood, making the organ enlarge and become stiffened so that it may enter the vagina to deposit seminal fluid. Loose-fitting skin (the prepuce or foreskin) covers the penis. The surgical removal of the foreskin is called **circumcision**.

The male urethra passes through the penis and serves two purposes. It carries:

- Reproductive fluid during intercourse.
- Urine during voiding.

The two activities cannot occur at the same time because they are under the control of different parts of the nervous system.

The Female Reproductive Organs: Structure and Function

The external female structures (**genitalia**) (Figure 46-2) include the:

- **Vulva**—made up of two liplike structures, the **labia majora** and **labia minora**. When the labia are separated, other external structures may be seen.

- **Clitoris**—a very sensitive structure found just behind the juncture of the labia minora. It functions during sexual stimulation to begin the rhythmic series of contractions associated with female climax (orgasm).

- **Urinary meatus**—the opening of the urethra to the outside.

- **Vaginal meatus**—the opening to the vagina or birth canal.

The Internal Female Structures

The internal female reproductive organs (Figure 46-3 and 46-4) include the following structures:

- **Ovaries**—two small glands, found on either side of the uterus, at the ends of the oviducts (fallopian tubes) in the pelvis. They produce two hormones, estrogen and progesterone, and the egg (ovum). The eggs are contained in many little sacs called follicles. About once each month, a follicle matures and releases an ovum. The ovum makes its way into one of the four-inch-long oviducts. This process is called **ovulation**. The cells of the follicles that are left produce progesterone. The progesterone causes changes within the uterus, readying it for the possibility of receiving a fertilized ovum.

- **Fallopian tubes** (**oviducts**)—two tubes, approximately four inches long, that serve as a pathway between the ovary and uterus. The sperm and egg meet in the tubes. Fertilization takes place here.

- **Uterus**—a hollow, pear-shaped organ. Its walls are made up of involuntary muscles. It is lined with special tissue called **endometrium**. The uterus has three main parts: the fundus, body, and cervix. The body and the fundus can stretch enough to hold a fetus, the amniotic sac, and the afterbirth (placenta). The cervix extends into the vagina.

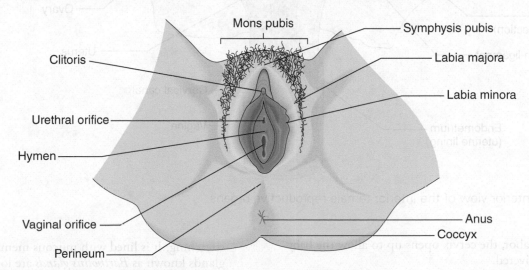

FIGURE 46-2 External female reproductive organs.

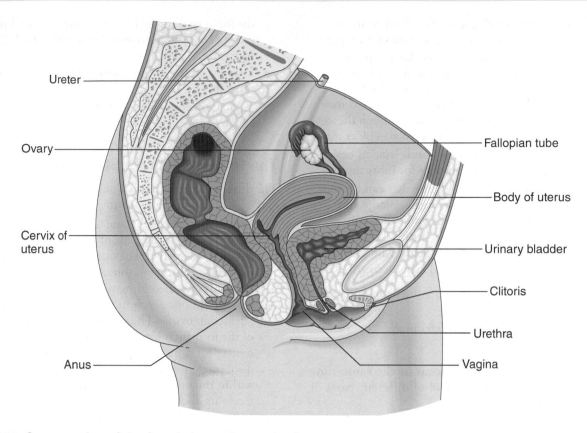

Ureter

Ovary

Cervix of uterus

Anus

Fallopian tube

Body of uterus

Urinary bladder

Clitoris

Urethra

Vagina

FIGURE 46-3 Cross-section of the female internal reproductive organs.

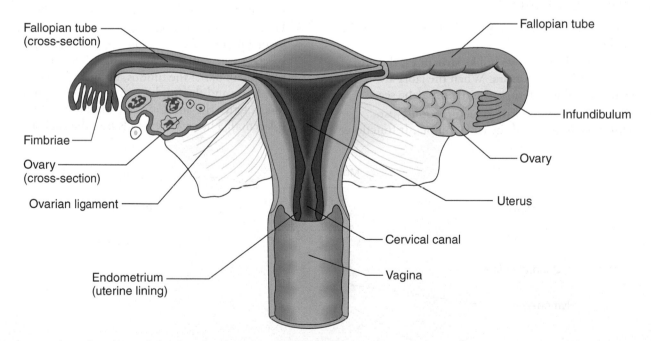

Fallopian tube (cross-section)

Fimbriae

Ovary (cross-section)

Ovarian ligament

Endometrium (uterine lining)

Fallopian tube

Infundibulum

Ovary

Uterus

Cervical canal

Vagina

FIGURE 46-4 Anterior view of the interior female reproductive organs.

During labor, the cervix opens up to allow the baby to be delivered.

• **Vagina**—found between the urinary bladder and the rectum. Its muscular walls are capable of much stretching. It is lined with mucous membrane. Two glands known as *Bartholin's glands* are located on either side of the external vaginal opening. They provide lubrication.

Menstruation and Ovulation

The menstrual cycle (female sexual cycle) begins at **puberty**. Puberty occurs in girls between the ages of 9 and 17. The cycle varies in length, usually between 25 and 30 days. The average is 28 days, which is why it is considered a monthly cycle.

During the menstrual cycle, a mature egg, or ovum (plural, *ova*):

- Is released from one of the ovaries.
- Travels from the ovary to one of the fallopian tubes.
- May be fertilized by a male sperm.

At the same time that the ovum is being matured and expelled from the ovary (ovulation), the lining of the uterus (endometrium) is being built up and made ready to receive the fertilized ovum. If fertilization does not occur, the endometrium is no longer needed, so it is carried out of the body as the menstrual flow. This process is known as **menstruation**.

Unlike the sperm cells, all the special cells that will become the ova exist when a female is born. When the last ova are released, the menstrual cycle ceases and **menopause** begins.

Menopause

As women age, the menstrual cycle becomes irregular and gradually ceases altogether. This is called the menopause, **climacteric**, or change of life.

Menopause usually occurs around the age of 55 and involves a natural series of changes that stop the menstrual cycle. These changes are not abrupt but usually take place over a period of years. Because eggs are no longer being matured and released, pregnancy cannot occur.

Some women may undergo menopause earlier in life after surgical removal of the ovaries.

AGING CHANGES TO THE REPRODUCTIVE SYSTEM

Aging changes in the male reproductive system are:

- Hormone production decreases, causing decreased size of testes and a lower sperm count.
- More time is needed for an erection to occur.
- The prostate gland may enlarge, causing urinary problems.
- The risk of prostate cancer increases.

Aging changes in the female reproductive system include:

- Cessation of menstrual periods.
- Fewer female hormones are produced, resulting in uncomfortable symptoms and loss of ability to conceive a child.

- The vagina becomes shorter and narrower.
- Vaginal secretions decrease.
- Breast tissue decreases and the muscles supporting the breasts weaken.
- The risk of breast cancer increases.

CONDITIONS OF THE MALE REPRODUCTIVE ORGANS

The male organs are subject to the same kinds of disease processes that affect other body parts. Examples of these conditions are tumors and infections. A very common problem experienced by many men involves the prostate gland.

Prostate Conditions

Benign prostatic (of the prostate gland) **hypertrophy** or *hyperplasia* (Figure 46-5) is an enlargement of the prostate gland without tumor development. It:

- Causes narrowing of the urethra, which passes through the center of the prostate gland.
- Can cause sufficient enlargement to cause urinary retention.
- Is noncancerous.

Signs and symptoms of prostate conditions include difficulty in starting the stream of urine or in emptying the bladder completely.

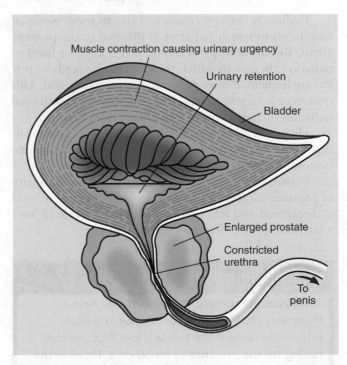

FIGURE 46-5 Cell growth causes the prostate to enlarge, constricting the urethra. The bladder may not empty completely, causing discomfort and increasing the risk of infection.

Prostate cancer is the second leading cause of cancer deaths in males. A blood test, the prostate-specific antigen (PSA), is used to screen for abnormalities. Because of the widespread use of the blood test, many prostate cancers are identified early, and the outcome is usually favorable. Prostate cancer usually grows very slowly. In the early stages, there may be no symptoms. As the condition progresses, signs and symptoms develop. The most common are:

- Difficulty with urination
- Decreased force of the urine stream
- Frequency of urination
- Urgency (an intense need to urinate)
- Urinary retention
- Repeated urinary tract infections
- Blood in the urine or semen

Treatment

Various surgical approaches are used to remove all or part of the prostate gland (**prostatectomy**) to relieve urinary retention.

- Transurethral prostatectomy (TURP)—only enough of the gland is removed, working from inside the urethra, to permit urine to pass.
- Perineal prostatectomy—the entire gland is removed through surgical incisions in the perineum.
- Suprapubic prostatectomy—an incision is made just above the pubis, and part of the gland is removed.

Radiation therapy consists of five to seven weeks of treatments in which radiation is directed to the prostate gland. **Brachytherapy** (Chapter 47) is another form of radiation therapy in which tiny radioactive seeds or pellets are implanted directly inside the prostate gland. This treatment is very successful and preferred over traditional radiation therapy because it has fewer side effects.

Hormone therapy is used to treat some prostate cancers. This treatment suppresses the male sex hormone (testosterone) that stimulates the cancer to grow.

Patients are likely to be disturbed by the necessity of prostate surgery. Men often feel that their manhood is threatened and fear that they will not be able to have sexual intercourse after a prostatectomy.

Difficult Situations

After prostate surgery, the patient may have a three-way catheter with continuous irrigation. Inform the nurse if the bottle is low. Monitor the tubing for the presence of blood clots. Monitor the patient for signs of excess bleeding, cold or clammy skin, pallor, restlessness, falling blood pressure, or rapid pulse. If noted, report them promptly.

Urinary incontinence is also a common problem and a great concern. In most cases, the rate of leakage decreases over time. Nevertheless, incontinence has a substantial impact on quality of life.

POSTSURGICAL CARE

In addition to routine postoperative care, the person who has had a prostatectomy:

- Will have a Foley catheter in place following the surgery. A 30 French with a 30-mL balloon is used for this purpose. A person who has had prostate surgery generally has heavy bleeding. The catheter and balloon are used to apply pressure to stop the bleeding. This is the only time that a catheter and balloon this large are recommended.
- May have a drain extending from a suprapubic incision.
- May have a perineal drain extending from a perineal incision.

The nursing assistant should:

- Wear personal protective equipment and apply the principles of standard precautions.
- Be careful that the tubes do not become twisted, stressed, or dislodged when the patient is being positioned.
- Carefully note the amount and color of drainage from all areas.
- Report at once any sudden increase in bright redness or the appearance of clots that seem to block the tube.
- Inform the nurse if dressings become wet.
- Be patient and understanding of the patient's emotional stress.
- Refer questions about possible sexual limitations and urinary incontinence to the nurse so that the patient can get information and support.

At times, it will be necessary to irrigate (wash out) the drainage tubes. This is a sterile procedure that will be carried out by the nurse or physician.

Cancer of the Testes

Cancer of the testes is fairly common. Treatment may require removal of the testicles (**orchiectomy**). This procedure is performed when there is testicular malignancy. Orchiectomy can be avoided if the condition is diagnosed and treated early.

CONDITIONS OF THE FEMALE REPRODUCTIVE ORGANS

Female reproductive organs are also subject to disease processes, including tumors and infections.

Rectocele and Cystocele

Rectoceles and cystoceles are hernias. They may occur simultaneously.

- **Rectoceles** (Figure 46-6A) are a weakening of the wall shared between the vagina and the rectum. They frequently cause constipation and **hemorrhoids** (varicose veins of the rectum).
- **Cystoceles** (Figure 46-6B) are a weakening of the muscles between the bladder and the vagina that cause urinary incontinence.

Treatment and Nursing Care

A surgical procedure called **colporrhaphy** tightens the vaginal walls.

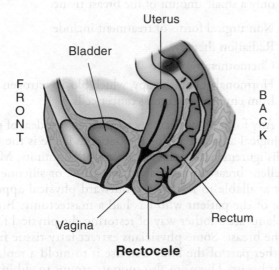

Rectocele

FIGURE 46-6A A rectocele causes the rectum to bulge into the vagina.

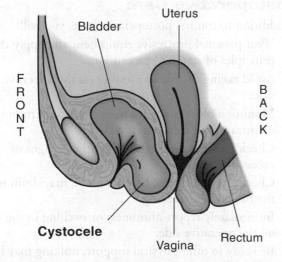

Cystocele

FIGURE 46-6B A cystocele causes the bladder to bulge into the vagina.

In addition to routine postsurgical care, you may assist in:

- Applying ice packs.
- Giving sitz baths.
- Giving vaginal douches (irrigations).
- Checking carefully for signs of excessive bleeding or foul-smelling discharge.

Vulvovaginitis

Vulvovaginitis is most often caused by a fungal infection of *Candida albicans*. Signs and symptoms are:

- Thick, white, cheesy vaginal discharge.
- Intense inflammation and itching.

Special drugs and creams are prescribed to fight the infection. Douches are not given for this condition.

Tumors of the Uterus and Ovaries

Both benign and malignant tumors of the uterus and ovaries are frequent. Malignancies of the cervix are very common. The cure rate is very high if treated in time.

The most common indications of tumors of the uterus and ovaries are changes in the menstrual flow, such as:

- **Menorrhagia**—excessive flow
- **Amenorrhea**—lack of menstrual flow
- **Dysmenorrhea**—difficult or painful menstrual flow
- **Metrorrhagia**—bleeding at completely irregular intervals

Ovarian cancer is very dangerous because usually there are no symptoms until it is well advanced and has spread beyond the ovaries. Even then, the symptoms are often mild, such as bloating, and may be attributed to other problems. It cannot usually be detected by a pelvic examination. This cancer accounts for more deaths than any other cancer of the female reproductive system. The disease has a strong familial link, and is most common in women over age 50. Women who have never had children and those who have taken fertility drugs are also at high risk. Women who take birth control pills have a lower risk.

Signs and Symptoms of Ovarian Cancer

Signs and symptoms of ovarian cancer are:

- Abdominal discomfort and pain
- Bloating
- Nausea
- Diarrhea
- Frequent urination
- Sudden weight gain or loss
- Abnormal vaginal bleeding

Treatment

Several different types of procedures may be performed to treat tumors of the female reproductive tract, including chemotherapy, radiation, and surgery. Some surgical procedures are:

- Total **hysterectomy**—removal of the entire uterus, including the cervix.
- **Oophorectomy**—removal of an ovary. In younger women, a portion of the ovary may be left to continue hormone production whenever possible.
- **Salpingectomy**—removal of a fallopian tube.
- **Panhysterectomy**—removal of the uterus as well as both ovaries and fallopian tubes.

The surgical approach may be abdominal or vaginal. If a panhysterectomy is performed, the patient experiences surgically induced menopause. The more uncomfortable symptoms of menopause are usually relieved with hormone supplements.

If cancer is present, nonsurgical forms of treatment may be used, including radiation therapy and chemotherapy.

Postoperative Care

In addition to the usual postoperative care, the care following a hysterectomy will include:

- Caring for catheter drainage.
- Caring for a nasogastric tube, which may be in place to relieve abdominal distention and nausea.
- Giving special attention to maintaining good circulation, because slowing of the blood supply to the pelvis may result in clot formation.
- Introducing fluids and foods gradually after the initial nausea subsides.
- Carefully observing the patient for low back pain.
- Monitoring urine output and bleeding.
- Checking both the abdominal incisional area and the vagina for presence and type of drainage.
- Providing emotional support.

Tumors of the Breast

Tumors, both benign and malignant, are commonly found in the breasts. Breast cancer is the second most common cancer in women. However, men can also develop breast cancer. Signs and symptoms include:

- Painless lump or mass
- Nipple discharge
- Retraction of nipple
- Scaly skin around nipple
- Dimpling of the skin
- Enlarged lymph nodes

Treatment

The stage of breast cancer is one of the most important factors in determining treatment options. Cancer doctors use a variety of tests to evaluate breast cancer and develop a personalized treatment plan. In 2019, a press release revealed that there is a relationship between treatment for breast cancer and heart disease.

Mastectomy is removal of the breast. All or part of the breast tissue may be removed in a mastectomy.

- A **simple mastectomy** removes the breast tissue only.
- A **radical mastectomy** removes the breast tissue, underlying muscles, and the glands in the axillary area. This procedure is not performed as often as it was previously.
- A **lumpectomy** removes the abnormal tissue and only a small amount of the breast tissue.

Nonsurgical forms of treatment include:
- Radiation therapy.
- Chemotherapy.
- Hormonal chemotherapy, which blocks estrogen from entering the breast cancer cells.

Any form of mastectomy requires a great deal of psychological adjustment for the patient. There is the fear of disfigurement and the fear of loss of femininity. Many excellent breast forms made from saline or silicone are now available to restore the outward physical appearance of the patient who has had a mastectomy. Breast implants are another way of restoring the physical form of the breast. Some physicians extract fatty tissue from another part of the body and use it to mold a replacement breast. There are also support groups to aid in the psychological adjustment.

Postoperative Care

In addition to routine postoperative care, you will:
- Wear personal protective equipment and apply the principles of standard precautions.
- Avoid taking the blood pressure on the operative side.
- Monitor a blood transfusion as you would monitor an intravenous infusion, if ordered.
- Check pressure dressings frequently for signs of excess bleeding.
- Check the bed linens, because blood may drain to the back of the dressing.
- Immediately report numbness or swelling in the arm on the operative side.
- Be ready to offer physical support; walking may be difficult for the patient, who may feel unbalanced.
- Offer your fullest emotional support.

- Assist the patient in rehabilitative exercises.
- Refer questions about disfigurement and loss of femininity to the nurse, who will see that the patient is provided with accurate information and support.

Prolapsed Uterus

A **prolapsed uterus** may also be called a *pelvic floor hernia*. It occurs when the uterus slips downward into the vaginal canal. The uterus is held in place by ligaments, which are weakened during childbirth, especially with large infants and difficult labor and delivery. Loss of muscle tone and muscle relaxation, combined with normal aging changes and a reduction of estrogen, is the most common cause of uterine prolapse. Signs and symptoms are pain during sexual activity, low backache, a feeling of heaviness or fullness, feeling as if sitting on a tennis ball, and protrusion of the uterus from the vaginal opening.

Kegel exercises involve contracting the pelvic floor to strengthen the muscles surrounding the urethra and vagina that support the pelvic structures. Surgery may be necessary in some cases.

SEXUALLY TRANSMITTED INFECTIONS (STIs)

Sexually transmitted infections (STIs) affect both men and women. Although most sexually transmitted infections can be treated and cured, patients do not develop immunity to repeated infections. It is possible to transmit the organisms causing STIs from:

- Mucous membrane to mucous membrane (Figure 46-7A)—genitals to mouth or mouth to genitals.
- Mucous membrane to skin, such as genitals to hands (Figure 46-7B).
- Skin to mucous membrane, such as hands to genitals.

Using standard precautions correctly will protect the nursing assistant from contracting these diseases when caring for patients.

There are many sexually transmitted infections. Some are seen more commonly than others. Patients may:

- Not always be aware that they have been infected.
- Be too embarrassed to tell you about the problem.
- Not realize the serious damage these infectious diseases can do to the body.

The most common sexually transmitted infections are gonorrhea, chlamydia, herpes simplex II, and syphilis. Other sexually transmitted infections are caused by *Mycoplasma genitalium*, human papillomavirus, HIV, and the trichomonas parasite.

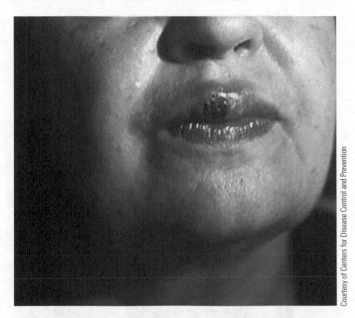

FIGURE 46-7A A sore on the mouth that developed after contact with mucous membranes or genitals with the infection.

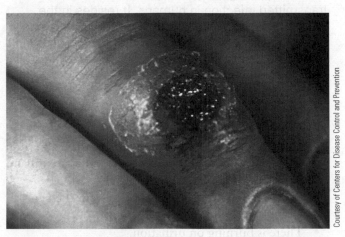

FIGURE 46-7B Although less common, lesions on the hands can develop as a result of contact with the genitalia of an infected person.

Trichomonas Vaginitis

Trichomonas vaginitis is caused by a parasite, *Trichomonas vaginalis*. This condition:

- Is sexually transmitted.
- May affect the male reproductive tract with no signs and symptoms.
- In females, causes a large amount of white, foul-smelling vaginal discharge called **leukorrhea** (Figure 46-8).
- Can be controlled with medication.
- Requires that both sex partners receive treatment.

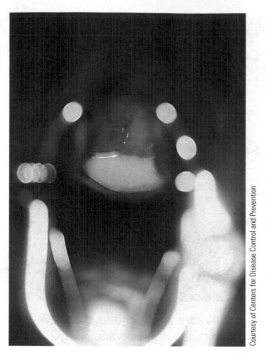

Courtesy of Centers for Disease Control and Prevention

FIGURE 46-8 *Trichomonas vaginalis* is the most common pathogenic protozoan that causes a sexually transmitted infection in humans. It resides in the female lower genital tract and the male urethra and prostate. This is a magnified view of trichomonas vaginitis with copious purulent (puslike) discharge from the cervix of the uterus.

Gonorrhea

Gonorrhea is a serious STI caused by the bacterium *Neisseria gonorrheae*. The disease causes an acute inflammation. In the male:

- Greenish-yellow discharge appears from the penis within two to five days after contact.
- There is burning on urination.
- The disease can spread throughout the reproductive tract, causing **sterility** (inability to reproduce).

In the female:

- Eighty percent may have no signs or symptoms for quite a while. Thus, it is possible to spread the disease before the woman is aware of being infected.
- **Pelvic inflammatory disease (PID)** can lead to formation of abscesses and sterility.

It is important for all sex partners to be treated with antibiotics. When a pregnant woman has gonorrhea, her baby's eyes may be permanently damaged if they are infected by the disease during birth. As a preventive measure, all babies' eyes are routinely treated with silver nitrate drops or antibiotics shortly after birth.

Mycoplasma Genitalium

A 2007 study found that **Mycoplasma genitalium** (MG, Mgen), a little-known sexually transmitted bacteria, was more prevalent than gonorrhea in U.S. adolescents. This pathogen was very difficult to detect until recent technology made identification possible. Most cases of infections caused by *M. genitalium* do not have symptoms. If present, signs and symptoms in females are:

- Vaginal itching
- Burning on urination
- Pain during intercourse

Signs and symptoms in males are:

- Urethral discharge
- Burning on urination
- Joint pain and swelling

This condition is treated with antibiotics. Resistance has become a problem. It is associated with infertility from pelvic inflammatory disease, infection of the uterine lining, and premature births. Additional research is needed for this unusual pathogen.

Syphilis

Syphilis is caused by the microorganism *Treponema pallidum*. Both sexes show the same effects of the disease. If untreated, this disease passes through three stages.

1. *First stage*—a sore (**chancre**) develops within 90 days of exposure. The chancre heals without treatment. Because it is not painful, it may go entirely unnoticed.

2. *Second stage*—may be accompanied by a rash, sore throat, or other mild symptoms suggestive of a viral infection (Figure 46-9A). Again, the signs and symptoms are minor and disappear without treatment. The disease is infectious during the first and second stages and may be transmitted to a sexual partner. By this time, the microorganisms have gained entrance into vital organs such as the heart, liver, brain, and spinal cord.

3. *Third stage*—permanent damage is done to vital organs, though the damage may not appear for many years. Patients in this stage are usually cognitively impaired, but there is no way to differentiate cognitive impairment caused by syphilis from impairment due to other causes. Aside from this, the person usually has no other signs or symptoms, and the diagnosis of tertiary syphilis is usually made after a routine blood test shows an abnormality. Occasionally, the person will develop painless lesions (*gumma*) on various parts of the body (Figure 46-9B). The patient is not infectious in this stage.

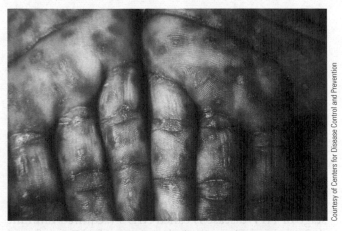

FIGURE 46-9A This rash on the hands is the result of an untreated syphilis infection. The second stage starts when one or more areas of the skin develop a rash that appears as rough, red, or reddish-brown spots. These usually occur on the palms of the hands and the bottoms of the feet. Without treatment, the rash will resolve.

Courtesy of Centers for Disease Control and Prevention

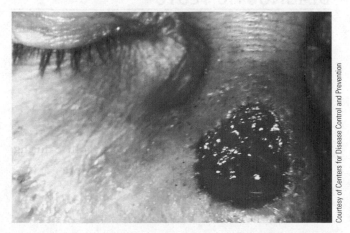

FIGURE 46-9B The signs and symptoms of third-stage syphilis include loss of coordination, dementia, paralysis, numbness, and gradual blindness. This is a picture of a painless, nodular, ulcerative lesion that may develop anywhere on the body. The patient is not contagious in this stage, but the damage is serious enough to cause death.

Courtesy of Centers for Disease Control and Prevention

An additional danger of syphilis during pregnancy is that the microorganism can attack the fetus, causing it to die or be seriously deformed.

Herpes

Herpes simplex II (genital herpes) is an infectious disease caused by the herpes simplex virus. It is transmitted primarily through direct sexual contact. The person who has herpes:

- May develop painful, red, blister-like sores on the reproductive organs.
- Has sores that are associated with a burning sensation.
- Has sores that heal in about two weeks.
- Must remember that the fluid in the blisters is infectious.
- May transmit (shed) organisms even when an outbreak is not present.

One in five American adults has genital herpes and may not know it. People with the herpes infection may have only one episode or may have repeated attacks. In many cases, repeated attacks are milder. Individuals who have weakened immune systems often develop chronic cases. In addition to the local discomfort:

- There seems to be a greater incidence of cancer of the cervix and miscarriages among females with this condition, compared with those who do not have this condition.

🦠 Infection Control **ALERT**

There are several closely related strains of herpes viruses. Oral herpes (Figure 46-10) and genital herpes are caused by different strains. However, they can be cross-infected with each other. Touching a cold sore and then touching the genital area may transmit the herpes virus from the mouth to the genitalia, and vice versa. Because of this, persons with the herpes virus must use very careful handwashing procedures and avoid hand contact with the lesions as much as possible. The virus will occasionally spread when no signs and symptoms are present. The virus usually lies dormant in nerves near the infection site until lesions erupt on the skin during an outbreak. The outbreak may be preceded by tingling, itching, and pain.

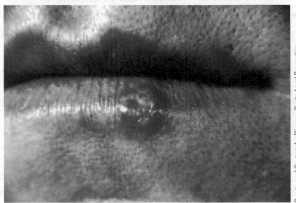

FIGURE 46-10 Oral herpes ulcers are painful. They can be spread to the genital area just as genital herpes can be spread to the mouth.

Courtesy of Centers for Disease Control and Prevention

- Newborn children can be infected when the mother gives birth. This is why the baby of a mother with an active case of herpes simplex II is usually delivered by cesarean section.

Because herpes is caused by a virus, there is no cure. Oral medications are available to stop the replication of the virus, which makes an outbreak subside more quickly. Topical creams are available to relieve discomfort and reduce the danger of spreading the infection.

Venereal Warts

Venereal warts are caused by a virus.

- Lesions develop on the genitals, on both skin and mucous membranes.
- The warts are cauliflower-shaped, raised, and darkened.
- They may be removed by ointments or surgery but often recur.
- They may cause discomfort during intercourse and may cause bleeding when dislodged.
- Warts predispose the person to development of cancerous changes.
- Venereal warts are one of the most rapidly growing forms of STI.

Chlamydia Infection

Chlamydia are small infectious organisms that can invade mucous membranes. These organisms can be:

- Introduced into the eyes, where they infect the conjunctiva. This causes inflammation (*conjunctivitis*) and a more serious condition called *trachoma*. Trachoma can lead to blindness.
- Sexually transmitted; this commonly causes infections of the reproductive tract.
- The cause of serious pelvic inflammatory disease (PID), with scarring and even systemic infections. The scarring can result in sterility.
- Responsible for signs and symptoms similar to those of gonorrhea, except that the discharge is usually yellow to whitish in color.
- Treated with antibiotics.

Patients with pelvic infections are usually checked for gonorrhea. If they are found negative for gonorrhea, they are frequently diagnosed as having nongonorrheal urethritis (NGU) or nonspecified urethritis (NSU), because many different organisms may cause the infection. However, chlamydia organisms are the most common cause.

Human Immunodeficiency Virus (HIV) Disease

HIV is a viral disease that is transmitted primarily through direct contact with the bodily secretions of an infected person. Therefore, it can be transmitted through direct sexual contact when infected blood, semen, or vaginal secretions come in contact with an uninfected person's broken skin or mucous membranes. HIV disease destroys the immune system. There is no cure for this condition, although drugs can slow the damage to the body. If the disease progresses, the immune system is severely weakened. This later stage of HIV disease is called AIDS (acquired immune deficiency syndrome). A discussion of AIDS is found in Chapter 12.

Observation and Reporting

Observations of STIs to make and report are listed in Table 46-1.

DIAGNOSTIC TESTS

Techniques used to diagnose problems of the reproductive system include:

- Cultures for microorganisms.
- Urinalysis for hormone levels.
- **Pap smear**—test using cells from the cervix to detect possible cancer of the cervix. The test:
  - Is painless.
  - Can be performed in the physician's office during the routine pelvic examination.
  - Should be done regularly.

TABLE 46-1 Signs and Symptoms of Sexually Transmitted Diseases to Make and Report

Vaginal or urethral discharge
Vaginal pain or burning
Redness and irritation of genital tissue
Burning on urination
Lower abdominal pain in women
Testicular pain in men
Bleeding between menstrual periods
Painful bowel elimination
Rectal discharge
Sore throat
Skin rash
Fever
Painful joints
Painful lesions on genitalia, throat, or mouth
Burning or itching of external genitalia
Warts on genitalia

- **Dilatation and curettage (D & C)**—a surgical procedure used to help diagnose conditions of the uterus, including tumors. In a D & C, the opening of the cervix is stretched open (dilated), and the uterus is scraped with a surgical instrument known as a *curette*.
- **Biopsy**—examination of a sample of living tissue; used to make a diagnosis. The biopsy sample is obtained through a needle. The procedure may be performed in the physician's office or in the hospital.
- Blood tests for cancer of the prostate.
- MRI and CT scans to help define the presence and extent of tumors.
- Ultrasound, a painless diagnostic tool that uses sound waves to diagnose ovarian cancer and other tumors.
- Cystoscopy—used to evaluate prostate conditions.
- Self-examination.
    - Breast self-examination should be performed by all adult females:
        - Each month on the last day of the menstrual flow.
        - After menopause, on one selected day of the month.
        - Faithfully in a routine manner.
    - Testicular self-examination should be performed by all adult males:
        - At least once each month.
        - During a warm shower so the scrotum will be relaxed.
        - With soapy fingers.
        - By palpating each testis between the fingers and thumb.
- Mammography—X-rays of the breasts. A **mammogram**:
    - Can identify the presence of tumors up to two years before the tumor can be felt during self-examination.
    - Should be performed when the woman is between the ages of 35 and 40 years, to provide a baseline evaluation. Various professional

organizations have different recommendations for when the mammogram should be done.
- According to the American College of Physicians, patient preference is key beginning at age 40. Average risk women who are asymptomatic should discuss it with their physician and have the first mammogram between ages 40 and 50.
- The American Cancer Society recommends an annual mammogram between ages 45 and 55.
- The American Society of Radiology recommends an annual mammogram beginning at age 40.
- Thereafter, a mammogram should be performed every two years for women of average risk from ages 55–74.

Home test kits can be purchased over the counter for:
- Vaginal yeast infection
- HIV
- DNA paternity test
- Pregnancy

Manufacturers recommend using these tests only if the person is under a physician's care.

VAGINAL DOUCHE

A vaginal **douche** is an irrigation of the vagina with fluid or medication. It is done with a physician's order.

A vaginal douche requires the use of standard precautions. The nurse administers medicated douches. Nursing assistants may give nonmedicinal douches if permitted by facility policy. Vaginal douches are given to:
- Remove odor or foul discharge
- Stop bleeding
- Relieve inflammation and pain
- Neutralize vaginal secretions
- Disinfect the vagina
- Cleanse the vagina before surgery or examination
- Administer antiseptic drugs

REVIEW

A. True/False

Mark the following true or false by circling T or F.

1. T F D & C is a surgical procedure that can help establish a diagnosis related to the female reproductive system.
2. T F Following a panhysterectomy, you should check the patient for increased bleeding.
3. T F Salpingectomy is removal of the ovaries.
4. T F Foul-smelling leukorrhea is associated with the condition called trichomonas vaginitis.
5. T F A female with gonorrhea may not know she has been infected with the disease.
6. T F Untreated gonorrhea passes through three stages.
7. T F Syphilis is caused by a bacterium.
8. T F AIDS is a sexually transmitted infection.
9. T F The discharge in gonorrhea is white and very irritating.

B. Matching

Choose the correct term from Column II to match each phrase in Column I.

Column I

10. _____ inability to reproduce

11. _____ inflammation of the vagina

12. _____ painful menstruation

13. _____ removal of a breast

14. _____ whitish discharge

Column II

a. dysmenorrhea

b. mastectomy

c. circumcision

d. leukorrhea

e. sterility

f. vaginitis

C. Multiple Choice

Select the best answer for each of the following.

15. You are to give a nonsterile douche. You will remember to:

a. place the patient in a high Fowler's position.

b. use a solution with a temperature of about 115°F.

c. insert the nozzle about three inches into the vagina.

d. allow the nozzle to touch the vulva.

16. Breast self-examination should be performed:

a. daily.

b. weekly.

c. monthly.

d. yearly.

17. Your patient has just returned from a suprapubic prostatectomy. You know that:

a. there will be no incision.

b. there will be a Foley catheter drain.

c. the patient must be assisted to void every two hours.

d. the patient will be NPO for two to three days.

18. Testicular self-examination should be:

a. done daily.

b. performed while sitting on the commode.

c. performed with soapy fingers.

d. performed only by males over age 50.

D. Completion

Complete the following statements.

19. The type of precautions to be used when caring for patients with STIs is _____. (droplet precautions) (standard precautions) (contact precautions)

20. Human immunodeficiency virus (HIV) disease is transmitted by _____. (indirect contact with a bacterium in body fluids or an environmental surface) (direct or indirect contact with a virus in blood or body fluids) (direct contact with a prion)

21. Testicular self-examination should be done _____. (daily) (monthly) (annually)

22. Breast self-examination should be performed _____. (weekly) (monthly) (yearly)

E. Nursing Assistant Challenge

Mrs. Forstein is 39 and has been admitted for a large pelvic mass. Her doctor suspects that she has a large tumor in her left ovary. She has experienced menorrhagia, dysmenorrhea, and pelvic pain. After tests are complete, she is scheduled for an oophorectomy. Briefly answer the following questions concerning her care.

23. How might you describe her surgical procedure (oophorectomy)?

_____

_____

24. Does the doctor plan to remove the entire uterus, including the cervix?

_____

_____

25. What type of pain would be very significant following surgery?

_____

_____

26. What two areas would you check for drainage?

_____

_____

27. Why is it so important to maintain good circulation postoperatively?

_____

_____

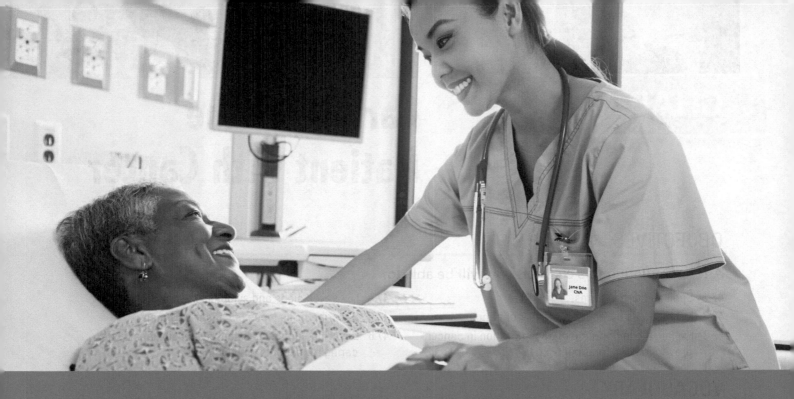

SECTION 12

Expanded Role of the Nursing Assistant

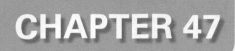

CHAPTER 47

Caring for the Patient with Cancer

OBJECTIVES

After completing this chapter, you will be able to:

47.1 Spell and define terms.

47.2 List methods of reducing the risk of cancer.

47.3 Explain the importance of good nutrition in cancer prevention and treatment.

47.4 List seven signs and symptoms of cancer.

47.5 Describe three types of cancer treatment.

47.6 Describe nursing assistant responsibilities when caring for patients with cancer.

VOCABULARY

Learn the meaning and the correct spelling of the following words and phrases:

alopecia	carcinogen	malignant	radiology precautions sign
anorexia	chemotherapy	metastasis	radiation therapy
benign	dosimeter	palliative care	
cancer	immunotherapy		

INTRODUCTION

Cancer is a disease in which the normal mechanisms of cell growth are disturbed. Cells grow abnormally, invade surrounding tissues, and use oxygen and nutrition intended for normal cells. Cancers that stay in one location and do not spread are **benign**. Benign cancers usually grow slowly. Some types of cancer cells spread to other parts of the body through the blood and lymphatic systems. This is called **metastasis**. When metastasis occurs, a tumor will eventually grow in another area. Cancers that spread to other parts of the body are **malignant**. Many patients die from metastasis instead of the original tumor. Some malignant cancers spread very rapidly.

A **carcinogen** is a substance that causes cancer. Tobacco is one common carcinogen. The incidence of cancer and death rates vary with cause and type of cancer, geographic location, sex, race, and age. Early diagnosis and type of care received also affect the prognosis. Some people do not seek care until the cancer is well advanced. If this is the case, the outcome is usually not good.

Risk Factors

Many factors increase the risk of developing cancer. Some cancers tend to be genetic. This means they run in families. Breast cancer, ovarian cancer, stomach cancer, and pancreatic cancer are examples of cancers that seem to have a hereditary component. Other common risk factors for cancer are:

- Age—this is the most common risk, with most cancers occurring in persons over the age of 55.
- Lifestyle and habits:
  - Smoking and using smokeless or chewing tobacco
  - Alcohol consumption
  - Diet
- Family history and genetics.

- Environmental pollution and other harmful substances in the environment:
  - Asbestos
  - Benzene
  - Chemicals
  - Radiation
  - Secondhand smoke
- Prolonged sun exposure.
- Infections and some viruses.

Nutrition and Cancer

There is a direct relationship between intake of certain foods and the development of certain types of cancers. Table 47-1 lists various types of cancers and their relationship to certain food items. Obesity is associated with cancer of the gallbladder, uterus, colon, and breast. These dietary guidelines will help prevent cancer:

- No more than 30 percent of total calories should come from fat.
- Total cholesterol from the diet should not exceed 300 mg a day.
- At least 55 percent of total calories should come from complex carbohydrates, such as fruits, vegetables, cereals, and grains.
- Salt from all food sources should not exceed 1 teaspoon a day.

TABLE 47-1 Cancer and Food

Type of Cancer	Relationship to Food
Breast	High-fat diet
Prostate	High-fat diet
Colon	High-fat diet, low intake of fruits and vegetables, low fiber, low intake of complex carbohydrates
Esophagus	Low intake of fruits and vegetables, low fiber, low intake of complex carbohydrates; high intake of salt-cured foods; also drinking alcoholic beverages
Bladder	Low intake of fruits and vegetables, low fiber, low intake of complex carbohydrates
Stomach	Low intake of fruits and vegetables, low fiber, low intake of complex carbohydrates; high intake of salt-cured foods
Larynx	Low intake of fruits and vegetables, low fiber, low intake of complex carbohydrates
Lung	Low intake of fruits and vegetables, low fiber, low intake of complex carbohydrates

CANCER PREVENTION AND DETECTION

The American Cancer Society recommends certain lifestyle changes and preventive measures. These include:

- Not smoking
- Limiting the intake of alcoholic beverages
- Eating a healthy diet
- Regular exercise
- Maintaining a healthy weight
- Avoiding sun exposure, particularly between 10:00 a.m. and 3:00 p.m
- Getting genetic testing and counseling if at risk for familial cancers

Some patients take various drugs to reduce the risk of cancer. Natural substances, such as vitamin E and selenium, are being researched for their cancer prevention properties.

Signs and Symptoms of Cancer

Each type of cancer has its own signs and symptoms. General signs and symptoms that may indicate cancer spell the word CAUTION:

C = Change in bowel or bladder habits

A = A sore that does not heal (Figure 47-1)

U = Unusual bleeding or discharge

T = Thickening or lump in the breast, testicles, or any part of the body

I = Indigestion or difficulty swallowing

O = Obvious change in a wart, mole, or skin condition (Figure 47-2)

N = Nagging cough or hoarseness

People with one or more of these warning signs should see a doctor right away.

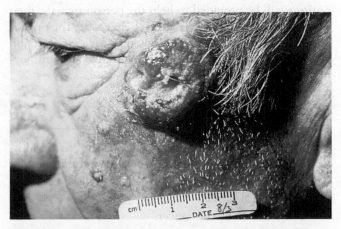

FIGURE 47-1 A sore that does not heal should be examined by a physician.

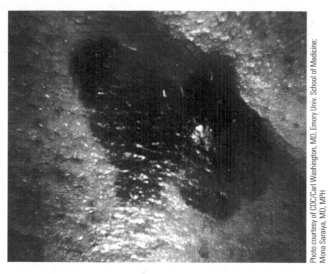

Photo courtesy of CDC/Carl Washington, MD, Emory Univ. School of Medicine; Mona Saraiya, MD, MPH

FIGURE 47-2 A change in a wart or mole requires further medical investigation.

Screening

Regular screening for cancer is a key to survival, because the outcome is better if the disease is detected early. Many different professional organizations have guidelines for cancer screening. These vary slightly from one group to the next. Screening is based on a person's age, gender, risk factors, family history, ethnicity, and history of exposure to carcinogens in the environment. Some personal screening tests are recommended monthly, such as breast self-examination for women and testicular self-examination for men. Other routine screening tests are done by physicians.

Genetic Testing

Mutation of certain genes called BRCA1 and BRCA2 has been linked to hereditary cancer. Blood tests are available to check for the genes. If a harmful BRCA1 or BRCA2 mutation is found, counseling is available, and several options will be provided to help the person manage their cancer risk. Federal and state laws help ensure the privacy of a person's genetic information and provide protection against discrimination in health insurance and employment practices.

TREATMENT

Many different treatments are used for cancer. In addition, some people use alternative and complementary therapies. The type of treatment is determined by:

- The type of cancer.
- The location of the cancer.
- Whether the cancer is malignant.
- The stage (how advanced the cancer is).
- The general condition of the patient.

Surgery

A *biopsy* is a minor surgery that is sometimes done to diagnose a cancer. It involves removing a small piece of tissue from a suspicious area and sending it for laboratory examination. If the biopsy is positive for cancerous cells, a surgical procedure is done with the goal of completely removing the cancer. This may involve removing all or part of an organ, such as a lung, a breast, or the uterus. Lymph nodes in the area may also be removed. The surgeon removes as much cancerous tissue as possible. If it is not possible to remove the entire cancerous area, a portion is left and is usually treated with other methods.

Reconstructive surgery may be done for cosmetic repair of an area. Sometimes this is done early, or even with the initial surgery. Other times reconstruction is done long after the original surgery. An example of reconstructive surgery is breast reconstruction. Preventive surgery may involve a radical procedure when there is a strong genetic link to cancer. For example, the breasts or ovaries may be removed because of a high risk of developing cancer. Preventive surgery is also done to remove areas, such as rectal polyps, that may develop into cancer later.

Hormone Therapy

Hormone therapy is a common cancer treatment. Many different cancers need hormones to grow. During the diagnosis process, testing is done to see if the cancer has certain hormone receptors. If so, hormone therapy may be started immediately, even before other treatments have been selected. Hormones can be used to prevent cancer cells from getting or using the hormones they need to grow and spread. They work with the body's own hormones. The treatment may add, block, or remove hormones from the body to slow or stop the growth of cancer cells. This therapy may be used alone or in combination with other cancer treatments, as well as with supportive care to manage side effects. The type of hormone therapy is determined by many factors. It may be given orally or by injection. It is a systemic therapy, so the hormones circulate throughout the body.

Chemotherapy

Chemotherapy uses medications or drugs to destroy the cancer (Figure 47-3). Unfortunately, healthy cells may also be destroyed. The goals of chemotherapy vary, depending on the type of cancer, stage, and situation. Goals might be to:

- Completely eliminate the cancer.
- Control and slow the growth of cancer to prolong the patient's life.
- Reduce the size of the cancer to eliminate pain and improve quality of life.

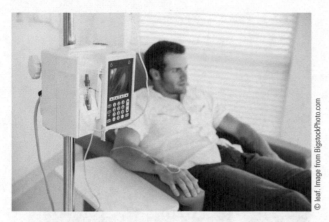

FIGURE 47-3 Intravenous chemotherapy can be provided on an out-patient basis.

Chemotherapy is given by many different routes. Some patients are able to take oral medications. Others must receive the drugs in the muscles, veins, or other organs and body cavities. If the drugs are given intravenously, a central intravenous catheter (Chapter 36) is often inserted to avoid repeated needlesticks and reduce the risk of vein irritation and collapse.

Chemotherapy drugs are very potent and can irritate the skin, eyes, and mucous membranes of caregivers. Because of this, special measures are used to handle the drugs. Never eat, drink, or chew gum in an area where chemotherapy is being prepared. If you accidentally contact a chemotherapy drug with your hands or mucous membranes, flush well with water and seek medical attention. These drugs and the containers they are dispensed in require special handling and disposal.

Side Effects of Chemotherapy

Chemotherapy targets rapidly regenerating cells such as cancer cells. The drugs cannot differentiate cancer cells from normal cells, so other cells that regenerate rapidly may also be affected. Cells that are commonly affected are:

- Blood cells, such as red blood cells, white blood cells, and platelets
- Hair and nail cells
- Gastrointestinal cells

Side effects of cancer drugs can range from mild to life-threatening. Patients receiving these drugs need special monitoring. Sometimes the dose and scheduling must be changed to reduce side effects. Common side effects are:

- **Alopecia** (hair loss)—this usually starts within two weeks after chemotherapy begins. It may take up to five or six months to regrow the hair. To both men and women, this is often the most upsetting of all the side effects associated with chemotherapy.
- Nausea and vomiting, depending on the drugs used—sometimes nausea occurs immediately, but it may be delayed until several days after the drug is given.

- **Anorexia**, or loss of appetite—this sometimes occurs because the drugs cause changes in the taste buds. In other patients, loss of appetite is due to nausea.
- *Anemia*, a deficiency of the red blood cells—this is caused by changes in the body due to the chemotherapy drugs reducing oxygen levels. Sometimes special medications are given to reverse the anemia.
- *Fatigue*—patients often become very tired. This is also related to reduced oxygen to the blood cells. Anemia and the reduced number of red blood cells are the most likely cause.
- Low white blood cell count, which increases the risk of infection—this usually starts within a week of the beginning of therapy, and it may last a long time. Take precautions to prevent exposure to infection.
- A reduction in the number of platelets in the blood, which increases the risk of bleeding. Take precautions to prevent injury.
- Destruction of the mucous membranes of the mouth—this causes burning, pain, redness, and breakdown inside the mouth. An anesthetic mouthwash may be helpful.

Many other side effects are caused by chemotherapy drugs. The nurse will advise you what to watch for in each patient. Having chemotherapy treatments can be physically and emotionally taxing. The patient will need a great deal of emotional support.

Disposal of Body Fluids and Wastes

Patients receiving chemotherapy may excrete the drugs in their waste and body fluids. The care plan will list special instructions for wearing PPE, if any is required, during patient care procedures. Discard gloves and other protective apparel, if worn, in a leakproof container. Follow facility policies for discarding PPE in the biohazardous waste or other contaminated area. Because the drugs are excreted in body waste, linens that have contacted blood, body fluids, or excretions require the use of standard precautions. Place soiled items in specially marked bags before sending them to the laundry.

Special Care of the Patient Undergoing Chemotherapy

Observe patients undergoing chemotherapy for side effects of the drugs and report any possible problems to

Difficult Situations

Monitor the patient undergoing chemotherapy for bruising and abnormal skin lesions. Inform the nurse promptly if fever is present. Encourage fluids of the patient's choice, as tolerated.

the nurse. Provide nursing comfort measures, such as good mouth care and daily bathing. Take precautions to prevent injuries and infection. For example, you may be instructed to remind the patient to cough and deep breathe to keep the lungs clear. You may be asked to take vital signs every four hours. Check with the nurse before taking a rectal temperature, which is contraindicated in some situations. Report a fever over 101°F or chilling to the nurse immediately. Other signs of infection to report are:

- Swelling, redness, or irritation inside the mouth
- Rectal pain or tenderness
- Change in bowel or bladder habits
- Pain or burning on urination
- Redness, swelling, open area, or pain on the skin
- Cough or shortness of breath
- Decreased level of consciousness
- Decreased urine output
- Warm, flushed, dry skin
- Hypotension (below 100/60, or as instructed)

Patients may have to take special precautions, such as blowing the nose gently and using an electric razor to reduce the risk of bleeding. A very soft toothbrush will probably be necessary. Special mouthwash products may be ordered. The care plan and the nurse will provide special directions.

Promoting good nutrition and hydration is very important. You may be asked to serve the patient six small meals a day. High-protein drinks may also be ordered. Encourage fluids, and record intake and output, including emesis. Alternate periods of rest with periods of activity, to reduce fatigue. Plan your care to allow frequent rest periods. Inform the nurse if the patient:

- Has nausea or vomiting.
- Is not eating or drinking.
- Complains of changes in the taste buds, affecting the ability or desire to eat.
- Has constipation or diarrhea.
- Has white patches or unusual areas inside the mouth (Figure 47-4).
- Complains of signs of a vaginal infection.
- Develops bruising or bleeding (which can be massive). Report this promptly.

Observe the patient closely when the patient is receiving chemotherapy drugs. Inform the nurse promptly if there is:

- Any sign of IV infiltration, such as redness, swelling, or pain at the needle insertion site.
- Change in mental status.
- Change in vital signs.

Assisting the Patient with Body Image

Cancer surgery and chemotherapy may change body appearance. This is often very upsetting to the patient.

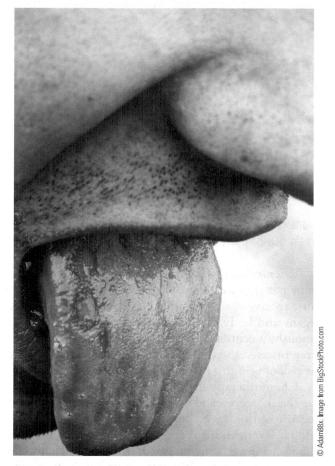

FIGURE 47-4   Monitor for and report white patches in the mouth to the nurse.

Hair loss may be especially traumatic, particularly in females. Be calm and reassuring. The hair will grow back, although the color or texture may be different. Assist the patient to wear a turban, scarf, or wig, if desired.

Radiation Therapy

Radiation therapy involves the use of high-energy, ionizing beams at the site of the cancer (Figure 47-5). The objective is to destroy the cancerous tissue without damaging healthy tissue. Several different types of radiation therapy may be used. Common side effects of radiation that should be reported to the nurse are:

- Fatigue
- Nausea or vomiting
- Loss of appetite
- Diarrhea
- Skin redness, irritation, or peeling
- Change in ability to taste
- Irritation of mucous membranes
- Cough
- Shortness of breath

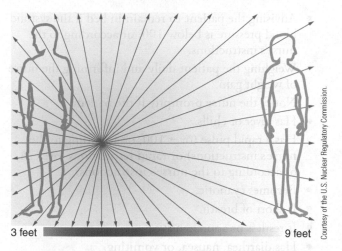

3 feet   9 feet

Courtesy of the U.S. Nuclear Regulatory Commission.

FIGURE 47-5 Radiation therapy is used to treat certain cancers. It may be used alone or in combination with other therapies.

Special Care of the Patient Undergoing Radiation Therapy

The patient may have markings on the skin at the site where radiation is delivered. Do not wash these off. The radiation may be very irritating to the patient's skin. Check the skin daily for problems and report them to the nurse, if found. Special skin care may be listed on the care plan. You may be instructed to:

- Wash the patient with lukewarm water and mild soap, using a soft washcloth; in some situations no soap is used.
- Avoid rubbing or creating friction on the skin.
- Avoid shaving areas near the treatment field.
- Avoid tape on the patient's skin near the treatment field.
- Avoid lotions and cosmetics near the treatment field.
- Avoid tight-fitting garments; dress the patient in loose, comfortable clothing.
- Avoid heat and cold treatments to the irradiated area.

Brachytherapy

Brachytherapy is another form of radiation therapy in which tiny radioactive seeds or pellets are implanted directly inside the patient's body. This treatment is very successful and preferred over traditional radiation therapy for some patients because it has fewer side effects. Brachytherapy is used to treat patients with localized breast, prostate, lung, cervical, and endometrial cancers, and some cancers of the head and neck. The small radioactive seeds are implanted directly into the tumor. The dosage varies with the area being treated and the type of cancer. Treatment may last from several hours to several days. The brachytherapy seeds used to treat prostate cancer may be left in place permanently. Brachytherapy may be used in combination with traditional radiation therapy.

Care of the Patient Receiving Brachytherapy

If a source of radiation is implanted inside the patient's body, you will be instructed in special precautions to follow to reduce your risk of radiation exposure. The patient will be in a private room. Bedrest may be ordered to prevent dislodging the radioactive device(s). Visitors will be restricted with regard to how close they may get to the patient and how long they may stay in the room. Pregnant women and children under the age of 18 are not permitted in the room. A patient who has permanently implanted seeds will be instructed to stay away from pregnant women and children for a designated period of time, such as six months.

You will be assigned a personal monitoring badge, called a **dosimeter** (Figure 47-6), if you will be caring for patients undergoing radiation therapy. This is a small instrument that measures the radiation dose to which

Difficult Situations

A lead-lined container and long-handled forceps will be stored in a corner of the room of a patient with a radiation implant. Radiation safety personnel will mark a "safe line" on the floor with masking tape approximately six feet from the bed. The line is a warning to visitors to minimize their radiation exposure; they should remain behind the line when visiting the patient. The radiation safety department may also place a portable lead shield in the back of the room to use when providing care. If the patient has an implant in the neck or mouth, an emergency tracheotomy tray will be placed in the room. Do not store it in a drawer or cupboard. The tray should be visible at all times.

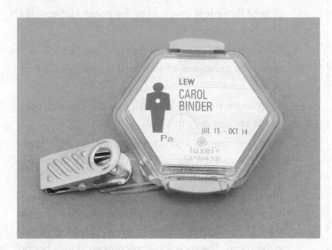

FIGURE 47-6 If caring for a patient receiving brachytherapy, a dosimeter is provided to measure exposure to the radiation.

each individual is exposed. Wear the badge between your waist and collar when you enter the room. Use only the badge that was issued to you. Do not take the badge home. When off duty, store it according to facility policy, away from sources of radiation.

Immunotherapy

Immunotherapy is another treatment that is done to eliminate a cancer. Various biologic agents are given to change the normal immune response. Vital signs must be regularly and closely monitored. Side effects of therapy usually cease within a week after treatment. Care of the patient receiving immunotherapy involves:

- Monitoring vital signs every four hours, or more often if instructed.
- Monitoring capillary refill.

- Advising the patient to remain in bed if the systolic blood pressure is below 100, or according to the nurse's instructions.
- Weighing the patient daily and informing the nurse of weight gain.

Notify the nurse promptly if the patient:

- Has fever or chills.
- Has a rapid pulse (over 100, or according to the nurse's instructions) or rapid respirations (over 24, or according to the nurse's instructions).
- Becomes cyanotic.
- Is short of breath.
- Is restless or apprehensive.
- Has diarrhea, nausea, or vomiting.
- Complains of itching.

GUIDELINES 47-1 Guidelines for Working with Patients Undergoing Radiation Therapy and Brachytherapy

- If you think you may be pregnant, do not enter the room. Inform the nurse.
- Plan and organize your time before entering the patient's room. Provide necessary care, but try to minimize time spent with the patient.
- You may be required to apply gloves and shoe covers when entering the patient's room. Remove them before leaving.
- Wear a mask if the patient has a tracheostomy or signs of a respiratory infection.
- Work behind mobile shields whenever possible.
- Work no closer to the patient than necessary. Stay at least three feet away from the patient unless direct care is being given.
- Think about what you are doing. Conscientiously apply the principles of standard precautions for all patient care.
- A separate sink may be designated for handwashing. If so, use only this sink.
- Follow all special instructions on the patient's care plan. Consult the nurse if you are unsure of something or have questions.
- The care plan, critical pathway, or radiology precautions sign will list where to find special safety precautions, including the maximum length of time to remain in the room. The radiology precautions sign is not an infection control sign. After the radioactive material has

been given to the patient, they will be restricted under "radiology precautions." A sign bearing a radiation symbol (Figure 47-7) will be posted on the door to the room. This sign has a black or magenta triblade on a white or yellow background, with the words "Caution: Radioactive Material." No one should enter the room without consulting medical, nursing, or radiation safety staff. Become familiar with the precautions for each patient, and follow them carefully.

- Monitor the length of time visitors stay in the room. Inform the nurse if they stay beyond the specified time.
- Chairs and other furniture will be located a certain distance away from the patient. Do not move the furniture any closer to the patient. Instruct visitors not to move any furniture closer to the patient.

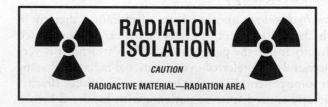

FIGURE 47-7 The radiology precautions sign has a black or magenta triblade on a white or yellow background, with the words "Caution: Radioactive Material." No one should enter the room without first consulting medical, nursing, or radiation safety staff.

(continues)

GUIDELINES 47-1 Guidelines for Working with Patients Undergoing Radiation Therapy and Brachytherapy (continued)

- Explain the purpose of the mobile safety shield and ask visitors to remain behind it.

- Do not allow pregnant women or children under the age of 18 into the radiology precautions room to visit.

- Follow facility policies for cleaning the room, as well as serving and removing meal trays. In many facilities, personnel from the dietary and housekeeping departments are not permitted to enter the room.

- Do not remove items from the room without permission from radiation safety personnel.

- If a radiation source becomes dislodged from the patient, avoid touching it. Ask visitors to leave the room. Try to move the source to a corner by using a tool such as a yardstick. Inform the nurse or radiation safety personnel.

- Find out if special precautions are necessary for handling soiled linens, tissues, or dressings.

- Strain all urine (Chapter 45) of patients with brachytherapy seeds near the bladder. Some seeds may be lost through urination. Follow facility policies for straining urine from a catheter bag. In some facilities, careful visual inspection of the catheter bag is sufficient. If a seed is found, do not attempt to remove it. Inform the nurse or radiation safety personnel.

- Place a small radioactive-labeled container in the patient's bathroom. Do not remove it. The container will be used to dispose of dislodged seeds, if any.

- Follow the nurse's instructions if you are directed to obtain a urine specimen after brachytherapy seeds have been implanted.

- Patients receiving certain types of therapy will require special urine collection. Bottles and special collection shields will be provided. Teach the patient

to be responsible for urine collection, if possible. The urine collection bottles will be removed by radiation safety personnel.

- Notify radiation safety personnel if there is a large spill of urine.

- Contaminated items must be incinerated if possible. A separate container will be used to discard these items, such as tissues, gauze sponges, shoe covers, and gloves.

- Use a separate, designated laundry bag for items that have been contaminated with body fluids, such as vomitus, incontinence, wound drainage, or profuse perspiration.

Discharge

When the patient is discharged:

- Discard disposable utensils, such as bedpans, urinals, and basins, with the radioactive waste.

- You will use the same permanent-equipment items for the patient from admission until discharge. Wash them well with soap and running water. Radiation safety personnel must check the items before they are returned to floor stock.

- Wear utility gloves when washing potentially contaminated equipment. When you have finished, wash the gloves with soap and water, and then dry them *before* removing them. (This is the only exception to the rule that you should never wash your gloved hands. It is a radiology precaution, not an infection control problem.)

- The room will require special cleaning. Follow the radiation safety department's instructions. The room must be cleared by the radiation safety department before it can be used again.

PAIN

Pain is the most common symptom in patients with cancer. It may be caused by the cancer, or be a result of the treatment. The pain may cause difficulty sleeping, loss of appetite, depression, and anxiety. Pain over an extended period of time reduces the patient's quality of life.

Patients with cancer should be evaluated for pain regularly. A pain scale (Chapter 10) is usually used. Narcotic pain-relieving medications may be necessary to control the pain. Some of these patients will use patient-controlled analgesia (Chapter 36). Pain should be treated before it becomes severe and out of control. Remember,

you are only responsible for making and reporting observations. Notify the nurse promptly if a patient complains of pain, tells you that pain medication was ineffective, or has a problem with an IV pump.

MENTAL AND EMOTIONAL NEEDS

Patients with cancer have a life-altering disease. They commonly fear dying. They may be anxious or depressed, and they often go through the grieving process (Chapter 32). Those with a good prognosis may still grieve for loss of function, loss of appearance, loss of their jobs, and so forth.

Communication ALERT

A cancer diagnosis evokes strong feelings and emotions in patients and their families. Patients or families may lash out in anger at you or their loved ones. They are not angry with you. They are angry with their circumstances. Avoid responding with anger. Keep your temper even, and do not take comments personally. Saying, "I see you are upset," or otherwise validating their feelings is the best way to respond. Avoid comments such as "I know" or "I understand." You do not know and understand, and the patient knows it. Providing compassionate care; listening; and giving sincere, solid emotional support will help patients and family members cope with this difficult time.

The point is that they may grieve for something other than death.

Nursing assistant measures to assist with mental and emotional needs include:

- Spending as much time as possible with the patient if they want to talk.
- Allowing the patient to talk about feelings and fears.
- Being proficient at providing physical care and assistance with ADLs.
- Anticipating the patient's needs before they ask.

- Respecting the patient's beliefs and wishes.
- Providing emotional support.
- Respecting the patient's privacy if they want to be alone.
- Making the patient feel respected and valued as a person.

Avoid giving the patient false hope. If you think a patient is losing control, inform the nurse. Just being with the patient and allowing them to talk is very helpful.

PALLIATIVE CARE

Some patients with cancer elect to have **palliative care**. This care is designed to keep the person comfortable without treating the disease. The patient will have an advance directive and do not resuscitate (DNR) order. Hospice (Chapter 32) may be involved in the patient's care. One goal of this type of care is to maintain the patient's quality of life for as long as possible.

You are responsible for keeping the patient clean and comfortable. Use nursing measures, such as positioning and backrubs. Spend time with the patient and allow them to talk, if they want. Respect the patient's wishes and provide emotional support. Inform the nurse if the patient is short of breath, anxious, or complains of pain.

REVIEW

A. True/False

Mark the following true or false by circling T or F.

1. T F Benign tumors spread rapidly to other parts of the body.

2. T F A carcinogen is a cancer-producing substance.

3. T F Most cancers occur in persons over the age of 65.

4. T F In a healthy diet, no more than 30 percent of daily calories should come from fat.

5. T F Lifestyle modification may reduce the risk of cancer.

B. Matching

Choose the correct word from Column II to match each phrase in Column I.

Column I

6. _____ cancer that spreads
7. _____ tissue sample
8. _____ medications or drugs
9. _____ changes immune response
10. _____ comfort care

Column II

a. chemotherapy
b. malignant
c. palliative
d. biopsy
e. immunotherapy

C. Multiple Choice

Select the best answer for each of the following.

11. The most common risk factor for cancer is:
    a. cigarette smoking.
    b. heredity.
    c. poor nutrition.
    d. age.

12. Complex carbohydrates should make up what percentage of the daily caloric intake?
    a. 20 percent
    b. 30 percent
    c. 55 percent
    d. 85 percent

13. Lifestyle changes that can reduce the risk of cancer include:

   a. drinking herbal tea daily.

   b. getting a complete physical exam every five years.

   c. a regular exercise program.

   d. consuming at least 800 mL of water daily.

14. Hereditary cancer:

   a. cannot be identified in advance.

   b. may involve mutation of BRCA genes.

   c. is a low-risk condition for most.

   d. requires very expensive treatment.

15. Reconstructive surgery:

   a. is done for cosmetic repair of an area.

   b. is minor surgery done to diagnose a cancer.

   c. involves removing cancerous tissue.

   d. is a radical preventive procedure.

16. The use of medications to destroy cancer cells is:

   a. brachytherapy.

   b. radiation therapy.

   c. chemotherapy.

   d. complementary therapy.

17. A deficiency of red blood cells that is a common side effect of cancer therapy is:

   a. alopecia.

   b. anemia.

   c. anorexia.

   d. metastasis.

18. Radiation therapy is a cancer treatment that uses:

   a. high-energy ionizing beams.

   b. chemicals.

   c. medication.

   d. a change in the immune response.

19. A patient returns from a radiation treatment with markings on the skin. You should:

   a. wash the markings off with soap and water.

   b. scrub the area vigorously.

   c. apply lotion to the area.

   d. leave the markings alone.

20. The most common symptom of patients with cancer is:

   a. nausea.

   b. vomiting.

   c. pain.

   d. alopecia.

21. Hormone therapy is:

   a. an accepted cancer treatment.

   b. a treatment of last resort.

   c. avoided to prevent tumor spread.

   d. a localized supportive treatment.

22. Which of these is considered a carcinogen?

   a. Water

   b. Broccoli

   c. Cigarette smoke

   d. Grain

23. Tumors that stay in one location and do not spread are:

   a. metastatic.

   b. carcinogens.

   c. malignant.

   d. benign.

24. A dosimeter measures the:

   a. total amount of radiation in the room.

   b. radiation to which the patient is exposed.

   c. level of radiation for effective treatment.

   d. radiation to which the worker is exposed.

25. When immunotherapy treatment is used:

   a. careful monitoring of blood pressure is needed.

   b. keep a lead box and tongs in the room.

   c. apply standard and airborne precautions.

   d. a tracheotomy tray will be placed in the room.

D. Nursing Assistant Challenge

Mr. Weiss is a 37-year-old patient who was recently diagnosed with breast cancer. He had a breast surgically removed and is undergoing chemotherapy. You take his vital signs early in the shift, but he refuses to speak to you. A few hours later, you bring his meal tray to the room and set it on the overbed table. Mr. Weiss sweeps the tray off the table with his arm, and food and dishes fly everywhere. He yells at you, shouting, "You know I am not hungry! Now get out of here and leave me alone!"

26. Why do you think Mr. Weiss is acting this way?

_____

_____

27. Is he mad at you?

_____

_____

28. What action should you take immediately?

_____

29. What will you report to the nurse?

_____

_____

30. Should you leave Mr. Weiss alone for the rest of the shift?

_____

_____

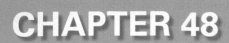

CHAPTER 48

Rehabilitation and Restorative Services

OBJECTIVES

After completing this chapter, you will be able to:

48.1 Spell and define terms.

48.2 Compare and contrast rehabilitation and restorative nursing care.

48.3 Describe the role of the nursing assistant in rehabilitation and restorative care.

48.4 Describe the principles of rehabilitation.

48.5 List the elements of successful rehabilitation/restorative care.

48.6 List six complications resulting from inactivity.

48.7 Identify four perceptual deficits.

48.8 Describe four approaches used for restorative programs.

48.9 List guidelines for providing restorative care.

48.10 Describe monitoring of the resident's response to care.

VOCABULARY

Learn the meaning and the correct spelling of the following words and phrases:

activities of daily living (ADLs)	bowel and bladder retraining (B&B)	mobility skill	restoration
adaptive device	disability	perceptual deficit	restorative
ambulation	geriatric	physiatrist	self-care deficit
		rehabilitation	

INTRODUCTION TO REHABILITATION AND RESTORATIVE CARE

Rehabilitation and **restorative** care are provided to improve and maintain the patient's physical abilities (Figure 48-1). This may include mobility skills and the ability to carry out activities of daily living. **Mobility skills** describe how we move about from one place to another. The most common method is through **ambulation** (walking), but various assistive devices such as a wheelchair may also be used. **Activities of daily living (ADLs)** are the personal hygiene and self-care tasks that we learn as children and do throughout life. These tasks include bathing, oral care, hair and nail care, dressing and undressing, eating, toileting, and mobility. Being independent with daily care promotes self-confidence and positive self-esteem.

    Rehabilitation is a process in which the person is assisted to reach an optimal level of physical, mental, and emotional health. Rehabilitation and restorative care are similar, but there are some differences. These are compared and contrasted in Table 48-1.

    The information in this chapter applies to both rehabilitation and restorative care. These services complement each other. They do not compete. A restorative program is established by the nurse or therapist to complement the rehabilitation program by reinforcing what the therapists are teaching, and the patient masters the skill more quickly. When you follow the program developed by the licensed nurse, you are helping the patient master skills for which nursing is responsible, such as bowel and bladder management. Regardless of whether the service is planned and

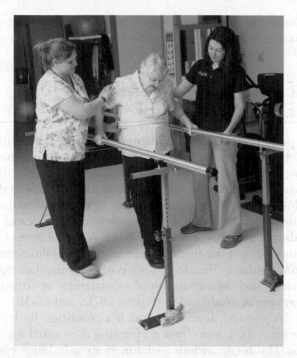

FIGURE 48-1 Rehabilitation is more aggressive and intensive than restorative care.

provided by therapy or nursing, it is a functional service for the patient. For example:

- The speech therapist works with a person who is recovering from a stroke or other condition affecting speech to communicate the need for basic services that are essential to daily life, such as hunger, thirst, pain, and elimination. The therapist would not work with the person to teach words that they are not likely to use on a daily basis, such as *aardvark* or *kumquat*. The speech therapist may also work with a person who has swallowing problems.

- The physical therapist works with a person who, for example, recently had a hip replacement to relearn safe ambulation. In the nursing unit, personnel follows a safe ambulation program to strengthen the patient and complement rehabilitation rather than applying restraints to prevent falls. Generally speaking, the physical therapist works with large muscle groups of the lower extremities, although physical therapy is not strictly limited to problems related to this area.

- The occupational therapist works with a patient to relearn ADL skills, such as toothbrushing. In general, occupational therapy is used for people with

TABLE 48-1 Comparison of Rehabilitation and Restorative Nursing

Rehabilitation	Restorative Nursing
Aggressive and intensive	Slower pace
Requires physician order	Not always scheduled, given 24 hours a day,
Scheduled 1–4 hours a day, 7 days a week	whenever needed
A separate and distinct service	Approaches integrated into regular nursing care
Goal is to improve	Goal is to maintain, improvement is desirable, but not necessary
Person makes rapid, significant progress	Person may or may not make progress, but does not decline
Planned and implemented by therapists	Planned and implemented by nursing
Must have potential for improvement	May participate if no potential for improvement
Provided in any setting, but not required	Required in long-term care; usually provided in home health care, long-term care facilities, subacute care, and long-term acute care hospitals
Licensed personnel provide most services	Both licensed and unlicensed personnel provide services; unlicensed personnel are primary caregivers
Paid by Medicare, Medicaid, private insurance	Inconsistently paid by Medicare and Medicaid in some situations; usually not paid by private insurance

How Rehabilitation and Restorative Nursing Are Alike

- Assists person to attain optimum level of physical, mental, and psychosocial function
- Considers how one weak area can affect the whole person
- Helps person adapt to limitations imposed by illness or injury
- Helps person regain lost skills or learn a new way of doing skills lost due to illness or injury (Figure 48-2)
- Requires initial evaluation and periodic re-evaluation
- Must be verified by measurable documentation
- Safety an important factor
- Patient teaching is part of program; staff and family teaching may also be done
- May use services of others outside the department
- Assists with activities of daily living
- Works toward goals
- Person benefits from service
- Provides a necessary service; not given as an activity or to keep the person occupied
- Prevents complications
- Maintains current abilities
- Improves quality of life

From Acello, B. (2009). *The long-term care restorative nursing desk reference.* Marblehead, MA: HCPro. Used with permission.

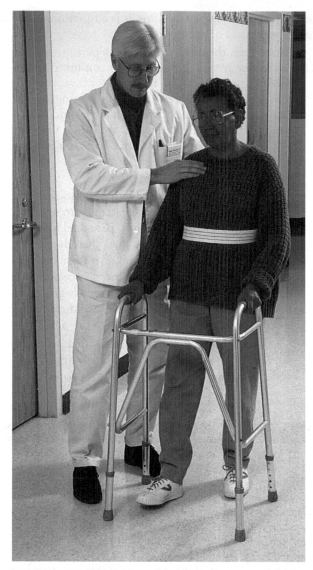

FIGURE 48-2 Rehabilitation and restorative nursing both work on increasing mobility and independence.

problems related to the upper extremities. However, they are not strictly limited to this area. The nursing assistant uses the care plan approaches 24 hours a day, or whenever the skill is needed. In this situation, the patient would brush the teeth during early morning and bedtime care.

- A restorative nursing program may establish a *purposeful* goal, for example, for the person to walk 150 feet with a walker, gait belt, and one assistant. The purpose of the program is to walk to the dining room, which is 150 feet from the patient's room. They would not walk back and forth in the hallway because doing so is not purposeful.

As you can see, both rehabilitation and restorative nursing work with functional skills that the patient needs each day. This process is called **restoration**. The skills are done at the appropriate time of day. For example, most

men shave in the morning. A man who is working on shaving would not be scheduled for this type of restorative care at bedtime.

REASONS FOR REHABILITATION/ RESTORATIVE CARE

A person may need rehabilitation because of a **disability**. A **disability** exists when a person has an impairment that affects the ability to perform one or more activities that a person of that age would normally be able to do. Most adults, for example, are able to dress and undress independently. If a person is unable to do this because of a disease or injury, a disability exists. A disability may be temporary or permanent. Impairments or disabilities result from trauma or disease. Disorders of the musculoskeletal system, such as amputation of an extremity or arthritis, may require rehabilitation (Figures 48-3A and 48-3B).

A physical disability exists if a condition limits or prevents the person from performing their usual role in life. This might include such functions as holding a job, managing a household, and raising a family.

If a disability is permanent, such as tetraplegia (paralysis from the neck down) from a spinal cord injury, it is unrealistic to expect that rehabilitation will enable the person to walk again. In these situations, the goals will be to teach the patient to:

- Adapt to the present circumstances.
- Use adaptive devices to increase independence.
- Learn new ways of doing routine tasks, such as dressing or bathing.
- Become as independent as possible in light of the disability. Patients with severely limiting conditions, such as paraplegia and tetraplegia, are taught to assume responsibility for personal well-being, including verbally directing caregivers to accomplish the results the patient wants. Follow the patient's instructions if they are safe, and do not be insulted if the person's instructions are different from what you are used to.

THE INTERDISCIPLINARY HEALTH CARE TEAM

Physicians who specialize in rehabilitation are called **physiatrists**. Nurses and nursing assistants who work in rehabilitation receive specialized education. Many other disciplines may be involved in the rehabilitation process. For instance, a person who has had a stroke may receive:

- Physical therapy to learn how to walk again.
- Occupational therapy to relearn the activities of daily living.
- Speech therapy to learn new communication or swallowing methods.

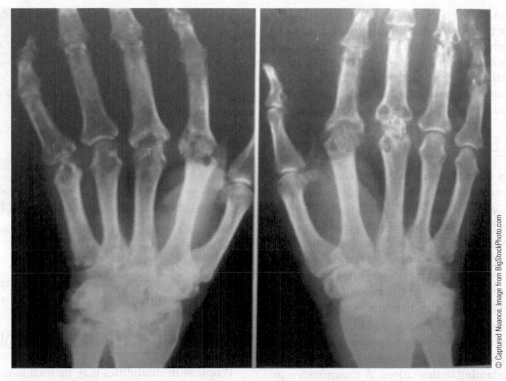

FIGURE 48-3A X-ray of a person with rheumatoid arthritis.

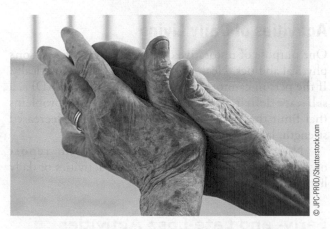

FIGURE 48-3B The hands of an older person with stiff, painful fingers.

- Restorative nursing services for bowel and bladder management, prevention of pressure injuries, and other complications.
- Dietitian services to learn to manage new dietary restrictions for a low-sodium diet (to reduce blood pressure) and to plan and prepare meals.
- Psychological support to adapt to the sudden changes brought about by the stroke.
- Social services to plan for the impending discharge.

All disciplines work together with the patient and family to solve problems and plan care. There are many subspecialties in rehabilitation. Health care professionals may choose to work in **geriatric** (care of the elderly) or pediatric rehabilitation. Others may specialize in the care of patients with strokes, spinal cord injuries, brain injuries, amputations, burns, or arthritis.

THE ROLE OF THE NURSING ASSISTANT

The nursing assistant who works in the rehabilitation and restorative nursing unit will assist with:

- Procedures to prevent complications.
- Procedures to prevent the patient's condition from worsening.
- Mobility skills: transfers and ambulation.
- Bathing and personal care procedures.
- Bowel and bladder management programs.
- Maintaining the patient's nutritional status.
- Programs to increase the patient's independence.
- Modifying circumstances to make it easier for the patient to master a particular skill. For example, a person is working on feeding using their dominant hand. They keep falling over and are wrestling with contractures and deformities in their shoulder, elbow, and hand, making it difficult to scoop their food with a spoon and move the spoon to their mouth. The nursing assistant places a row of pillows and foam cushions at their side, preventing the patient from falling over. They obtain a soup spoon (tablespoon)

and removes the teaspoon from the tray. These changes stabilize the patient, making it possible for them to feed themselves. The assistant gives them verbal cues to guide them through the meal. This enables them to make gradual progress toward their goal. The assistant keeps the nurse informed so the care plan can be updated and others can use the same approaches.

PRINCIPLES OF REHABILITATION

Four principles form the foundation of successful rehabilitation or restorative care.

- *Treatment begins as soon as possible.* This means that services begin as soon as the person's condition is stable. For example, if a patient has had a stroke, passive exercises and positioning techniques are initiated in the critical care unit to prevent contractures, pressure injuries, and other complications that would prohibit or delay rehabilitation.

- *Stress the person's ability, not the disability.* Workers must think in terms of what the person can do, not what they cannot do. The person's strengths are used to help in adapting to limitations. A *strength* refers to anything the person can do. Perhaps a patient whose dominant hand is paralyzed cannot use that hand to feed themselves—but instead of having nursing staff feed them, they can be taught to use the other, stronger hand. Use the restorative philosophy when communicating with patients. Avoid statements such as "You *can't* use your right hand." Instead, say, "You *can* use your left hand." Allow the patient to struggle a little, but avoid letting them progress to the point of frustration before you step in to assist.

- *Activity strengthens and inactivity weakens.* Complications result from physical and mental inactivity. These can cause further disability or even be life-threatening. A rehabilitation or restorative plan of care always includes approaches and goals for physical and mental activity.

- *Treat the whole person.* When we give care to patients, we are concerned with the whole person (Figure 48-4). We must also work with the patients' families. They directly influence patients' emotional and mental health.

Keys to success in rehabilitation and restorative nursing programs are:

- Teamwork—all staff cooperate with each other and other departments involved in the patient's care.
- Using the care plan—all staff are familiar with the patient's problems, goals, and approaches.
- Consistency of care—all staff use the same approaches (as listed on the care plan) when caring for the patient.
- Continuity of care—there is a smooth progression and flow between caregivers and between shifts.

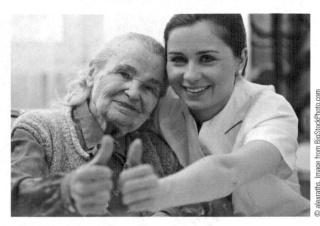

FIGURE 48-4 A patient's mental and emotional status are as important as physical condition.

- Good communication among all caregivers, the patient, and interested family members.

COMPLICATIONS FROM INACTIVITY

People with disabilities may be unable to move about at will. The inactivity or immobility can result in numerous complications affecting body systems, as shown in Table 48-2.

Activities of Daily Living

One purpose of restorative care is to increase the person's physical abilities. Healthy adults do ADLs automatically. If the person cannot complete any or all of the ADLs, a **self-care deficit** exists. Deficits are caused by problems that limit the ability to do self-care, such as decreased strength, lack of endurance, or disorientation.

Nursing assistants should make and report observations of a patient's ability to do activities of daily living, as listed in Table 48-3.

Early- and Late-Loss Activities of Daily Living

Loss of ADL skills due to aging and disease often follows a pattern. Skills that are lost first are *early-loss ADLs*. These are:

- Bathing
- Personal hygiene
- Dressing

Late-loss ADLs are those activities that are likely to be lost last. The person is usually dependent by the time these skills are lost. Late-loss ADLs are:

- Bed mobility
- Transfers
- Feeding/Eating
- Toilet use

TABLE 48-2 Complications of Immobility

System	Complication
Integumentary	Pressure ulcers may develop in a short time from lack of oxygen to the tissues. Pressure ulcers may worsen quickly and be difficult or impossible to reverse.
Muscular	Weakness and atrophy from lack of use. Contractures (Figure 48-5) develop because of the patient's position, freezing the muscle in a permanent state of flexion. Contractures are painful and difficult or impossible to reverse.
Skeletal	Calcium drains from the bones when they are inactive. This contributes to fractures, poor healing, osteoporosis, and other complications.
Respiratory	Fluid and secretions collect in the lungs. The patient has more difficulty expanding the lungs, increasing the risk of pneumonia and other lung infections.
Circulatory	Blood clots caused by pooling of blood and pressure on the legs (Figure 48-6). Edema may be caused by lack of movement. The heart must work harder to pump blood through the body. Changes in the blood vessels may cause dizziness and fainting when the patient is placed in the upright position.
Genitourinary	The extra calcium in the system from bone degradation promotes the development of kidney stones. Retention of urine is common, and is often caused by the patient's position in bed. Overflow of a full bladder leads to incontinence. The patient is at high risk of urinary tract infection.
Gastrointestinal	Indigestion and heartburn may result if the patient is not positioned properly for meals. Loss of appetite may occur from lack of activity, illness, and boredom. Constipation and fecal impaction result from immobility.
Nervous	Weakness and limited mobility. Insomnia may result from sleeping too much during the day, and then being unable to sleep at night.
Mental changes	Irritability, boredom, lethargy, and depression result from the patient's frustration and feelings of helplessness. Lack of social contact and sensory stimulation result in disorientation.

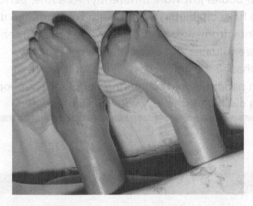

FIGURE 48-5 Contractures are a painful complication of immobility. Foot drop, or a contracture of the feet, can occur.

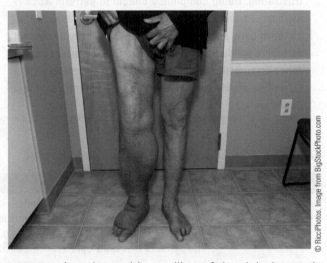

FIGURE 48-6 A patient with swelling of the right leg and foot after a long period of immobility.

Dependence in activities of daily living follows a sequence. People become dependent in early-loss skills first, followed by loss of late-loss ADLs.

Identifying and addressing early- and late-loss ADLs is the best means of prevention. Staff should monitor for ADLs listed on the plan of care and practice preventive approaches.

Perceptual Deficits

Perceptual deficits usually occur because of damage to the brain from disease or injury. Examples of perceptual deficits are:

- Inability to organize a task—ADLs cannot be completed unless the individual is able to prepare for the task, gather the supplies, and then do it.

- Inability to sequence a task—ADLs require doing the steps in the correct order to accomplish the goal. When putting on clothing, for example, underwear must go on before the pants and socks before shoes.
- Lack of judgment—this deficit may be noted if a patient puts on a heavy wool coat in hot weather (when appropriate clothing is available).
- Inability to identify common objects, such as eating utensils and grooming items (*agnosia*)—for example, the patient may try to use a fork to comb their hair.

- Inability to use common items (*apraxia*)—the patient may be able to identify the item but be unable to use it (even though there is no physical reason, such as paralysis).
- Inability to initiate a task.

Patients with self-care deficits are evaluated by therapists and nurses. The results of the evaluations will determine whether the person's functional (physical) abilities can be

Clinical Information ALERT

Patients who are elderly and have one or more chronically illnesses usually lose independence by degrees. Loss of independence as a result of sudden trauma can be devastating for a patient. Imagine being normal one minute, and then having an auto accident that leaves you completely paralyzed. This type of injury immediately changes the lives of the patient and their entire family. Some patients will regain all or part of their independence, but most have to cope with the loss and adjust activities and routines to disability. Because their bodies now work differently, they must learn to do things differently. This is also difficult and frustrating. Being completely unable to perform ADLs is even more frustrating. Despite the best medical and rehabilitative care, some patients will be physically dependent on others for the rest of their lives. One important goal of rehabilitation and restorative nursing is to promote mental and emotional independence, so the person can direct their care.

Difficult Situations

Disabilities can take many forms. Some forms, such as speech, hearing, or language problems, interfere with communication. Other problems, such as physical impairments, missing body parts, or deformities, may make you uncomfortable. You may be unsure of how to avoid offending the patient. Individuals who are newly disabled are more sensitive to their problems than people who have lived with a disability for a long time. People with disabilities are like you are. They have the same wants and needs. Their problems are no different from yours. However, having a disability makes living with these same problems much more difficult and creates additional problems. People with disabilities can do many of the same things you can. However, they may need to adapt the environment to do them. Changing things to meet a patient's needs is called providing *reasonable accommodation*. People with disabilities may perform a task differently than you do. However, the outcome of the task is the same. Their bodies just work differently! As a rule, persons who have disabilities do not want to be treated differently from anyone else. Many are self-sufficient. All are valuable and equal members of society. Emphasize the uniqueness, value, and worth of each patient. Avoid comparing people. Treat people with disabilities the way you like to be treated.

TABLE 48-3 ADL Observations to Make and Report

Activity	Observations
Activities of daily living	• What the person can do independently. • The person's need for assistance, how much assistance, type of assistance needed. • The person's ability to tolerate activity (e.g., Do they become fatigued, short of breath, etc.). • The person's motivation, preferences, abilities.
Bathing	• Does not resist bathing. • Ability for unassisted self-bathing. • Ability for self-bathing with an adaptive device. • Needs partial assistance with bathing. • Needs total assistance with bathing.
Dressing and grooming	• Overall appearance: tidy, untidy, neat, clean. • Ability for unassisted self-dressing. • Ability for self-dressing with an adaptive device. • Needs partial assistance with dressing. • Needs total assistance with dressing. • Requires frequent, but not constant, one-to-one, hands-on assistance for grooming and/or the retrieval and arrangement of clothing. This includes assistance with prostheses. • Requires continuous one-to-one assistance and supervision during the entire activity. If the staff person is not present to guide, teach, motivate, and/or provide hands-on care, person will not complete the activity. • The person does not participate in the dressing/grooming process.

(continues)

TABLE 48-3 *(continued)*

Activity	Observations
Transfers	• Independent; no assistance required, but may use equipment such as railings, trapeze, etc.
	• Requires PRN assistance for transfers.
	• One to transfer; continuously requires one person for physical or verbal assist on 60% or more of transfers. Specify when assistance is required and for what reason.
	• Two to transfer; requires assistance of two or more during the entire activity on 60% or more of transfers. Specify when assistance is required and for what reason.
	• Not transferred; may be transferred to a stretcher or chair once a week or less, excluding transfers to bath or toilet.
Walking	• Difficulty getting up and down.
	• Need for an assistive device, such as a cane or walker.
	• Safety awareness.
	• Gait steady, unsteady, shuffling, rigid, etc.
	• Posture.
	• Sudden onset of falls, difficulty balancing.
	• Walks unassisted. Requires devices such as cane, crutch, or walker.
	• Requires assistance for uneven surfaces or difficult ambulation, such as stairs or ramps.
	• Uses wheelchair and may require physical assistance for difficult maneuvers such as elevators or ramps or longer distances. (May be able to walk, but generally does not.)
Position, movement	• Ability to position/reposition self.
	• Need for staff to reposition.
	• Special positioning aids.
	• Ability to move unassisted.
	• Presence of contractures.
	• Able/unable to move.
	• Movements shaky, jerking, tremors, muscle spasms, etc.
	• Presence or absence of pain upon movement.
	• Deformity, edema.
	• Normal or abnormal range of motion.
	• Ability to sit, stand, move.
	• Independent bed mobility, transfers, ambulation.
	• Paralysis in one or more extremities (hemiplegia, paraplegia, tetraplegia (quadriplegia), diplegia, etc.).
Contractures	• None.
	• One extremity (limb) affected.
	• Two extremities (limbs) affected.
	• Three extremities (limbs) affected.
	• Four extremities (limbs) affected.
	• Fetal position.
	• Note degree and/or stage of contracture.
	• Note measures to prevent additional contractures.
Eating	• Food likes and dislikes, refusals.
	• Feeding ability, need for assistance, how much assistance, type of assistance needed.
	• Requires adaptive device(s) for independent eating.
	• Able to eat finger foods only without assistance; requires assistance with utensils.
	• Percentage of meal consumed.
	• Difficulty chewing or swallowing, coughing, choking.
	• Distracted or wanders at meals, needs to be refocused.
	• Independent or does not receive nutrition (e.g., per advance directive).
	• Intermittent assistance; requires verbal or physical assistance less than 60% of the time.
	• In a restorative feeding program. An assessment of the person's potential should be documented. The restorative program should be provided for at least two meals per day. Verbal cueing must be specific and related to plan of care.
	• Requires assistance to syringe or spoon-feed 60% or more of the time. Specify when assistance is required, the type of assistance provided, and for what reason.
	• Receives non-oral feedings for 60% or more of nutrition, using a tube such as an NG tube, G tube, PEG tube, or administration of TPN via a central line. Document the frequency, amounts, routes, and times the non-oral feedings were administered.

(continues)

TABLE 48-3 *(continued)*

Activity	Observations
Drinking	• Ability to take a drink at will without assistance. • Ability to drink from straw, cup, or need for special device. • Need for assistance, how much assistance, type of assistance needed. • Beverage preferences. • Accepts or refuses water, if offered. • Fluid intake. • Difficulty swallowing liquids, coughing, choking. • Requires I&O monitoring.
Toileting	• Independent, may require special equipment. Performs their own incontinent care, self-catheterization, ostomy care, etc. • Requires assistance but can be left alone for privacy. Assistance may include transferring on and off the commode, cleansing after elimination, adjusting clothing, or washing hands. • Requires physical or verbal assist or supervision during entire toileting process, excluding incontinent care, and cannot be left alone. Document the functional, medical, or behavioral reason the person cannot be left alone. • Incontinent or has an indwelling catheter. Includes staff-administered ostomy care, incontinence care using protective padding, incontinence briefs, changing clothes, or a propped urinal. Document and describe the type of assistance staff provide 60% or more of the time. • Taken to the toilet by the staff every 2 hours during waking hours, or more often if needed, as incontinence management. Stays dry 60% or more of the time as the result of being toileted by staff. Persons who receive in-and-out catheterization by the staff two or more times each day are included in this category. Document and describe the type of assistance staff provide 60% or more of the time.
Urinary elimination	• Frequency of elimination. • Inability to urinate, or voiding frequently in small amounts. • Will the person use the bathroom if given the opportunity? • Color, clarity, odor, amount of urine. • Presence of mucus, sediment, or other abnormalities in urine. • Pain, burning, frequency of urination. • Does the person have a urinary catheter; if so, is it draining properly, leaking, etc.? • Continent. • Incontinent three times a day or less. Includes persons who receive assistance to control dribbling. • Incontinent only at night. • Incontinent 4 or more times in a 24-hour period. Includes persons with external catheters, urostomies, and ileal conduits. • Requires indwelling catheter or intermittent catheterization. • Requires I&O monitoring.
Bowel elimination	• Frequency of elimination. • Will the person use the bathroom if given the opportunity? • Is the person incontinent? • Appearance of stool; presence of blood, mucus, parasites, or foreign matter; liquid or solid stool. • Abnormal color of stool (black, clay color, etc.). • Small or extremely large stool. • Loose, watery stool. • Complaints of pain, constipation, diarrhea, bleeding. • Excessive gas (flatus). • Requires monitoring for tendency toward constipation, fecal impaction. • Continent. • Has an ostomy and is independent with its care. • Is incontinent one to three times per week. • Incontinent four or more times per week. • Requires assistance with an ileostomy or colostomy; includes nursing care or teaching self-care.

increased. In other words, can the interdisciplinary team help this person relearn an activity of daily living? This is discussed with the patient and the family, and a plan of care is then developed.

RESTORATIVE PROGRAMS

A restorative program is planned if the person has the potential to relearn an ADL and is motivated to try. These programs are sometimes called *retraining programs* or *ADL programs*. If the person is in danger of losing the ability to do a task but has no potential to improve, a maintenance restorative program is planned. If the person has a task that is personally very important, this will be the first skill addressed, if possible.

When the patient is unable to do any ADLs independently, it is best to address one at a time. The first step is to find out what the patient wants to work on first, then plan the process with the patient and family to:

- Establish goals. Each ADL consists of several steps, as shown in Table 48-4. The patient will not be able to do all steps right away. Some patients may never be able to do all of the steps. Goals, therefore, are very small. For example, if the patient is in a restorative program for eating, the first goal may be to hold and eat a finger food, such as a piece of bread or a cookie. All goals are functional. Instead of saying the patient will walk 150 feet up and down hallway, the goal will state: "Patient will walk to and from the dining room for breakfast."

- Plan approaches. The approaches include the techniques and procedures carried out by the interdisciplinary team to help the patient relearn the ADL.

Approaches Used in Restorative Programs

The approaches to use will be listed on the care plan. The same approaches must be used in the same order each time. After the patient meets a goal, advance it. When they are able to walk to and from the dining room for breakfast, work on lunch. When they are able to walk to and from the dining room for both breakfast and lunch,

TABLE 48-4 Functional Steps of Activities of Daily Living

Bathing	• Gets to tub/sink/shower • Regulates water flow and temperature • Washes/rinses upper body • Washes/rinses lower body • Dries body
Dressing/ Undressing	• Obtains/selects clothing • Puts on/takes off slipover top • Puts on/takes off cardigan-style top • Manages buttons, snaps, ties, zippers • Puts on/takes off skirt/pants • Buckles belt • Puts on socks/shoes
Eating	• Gets to table • Uses spoon, fork, knife appropriately • Opens/pours • Brings food to mouth • Chews, swallows • Uses napkin
Toileting	• Gets to commode/toilet • Manipulates clothing • Sits on toilet • Eliminates in toilet • Cleans self • Flushes toilet • Gets clothing back in place • Washes hands
Mobility	• Gets self to side of bed • Maintains upright position • Comes to standing position • Places self in position to sit in chair • Locks wheelchair brakes • Turns body to sit • Lowers self into chair • Propels wheelchair • Repositions self in chair • Raises self from chair • Places self in position to sit on edge of bed • Walks alone/with assistance • Uses assistive device

have them walk to and from dinner. Although repetitious, they have met three small, functional goals! For a person with a disability, this is a huge accomplishment.

- *Setup*—patients with self-care deficits are not able to set up or prepare for activities of daily living. Provide the setup, if needed (Figure 48-7).

- *Verbal cues*—use short, simple phrases to prompt the patient. For example, give the patient a prepared toothbrush and then say, "Please brush your teeth" (Figure 48-8). If a complete task, such as brushing the entire mouth, is overwhelming, break it down into a series of smaller tasks until the teeth are clean.

- *Hand-over-hand technique*—example for eating program: Place a spoon filled with food in the patient's hand. Place your hand over the patient's hand. Guide the spoon to the patient's mouth (Figure 48-9).

Clinical Information **ALERT**

We normally think of the grieving process in relation to death and dying. However, the process applies to any major loss. Patients and families experience the grieving process because of disability and loss of independence. The stage of grieving often affects rehabilitation and safety. Some health care workers label patients as being "difficult" or "trying" when in fact they are grieving. Avoid stereotyping and labeling patients. Recognize the stages of the grieving process and use the skills you learned in Chapter 32 to support your patients.

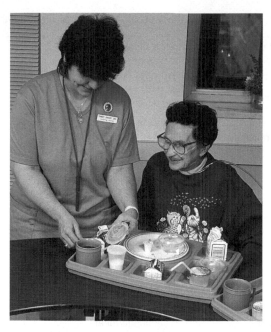

FIGURE 48-7 A patient may be able to self-feed if the tray is set up by the nursing assistant.

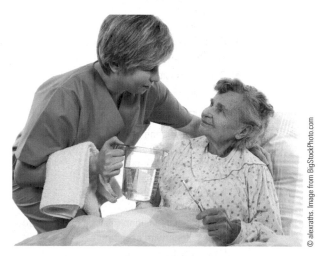

FIGURE 48-8 Verbal cues are used to assist a patient with ADLs.

- *Demonstration*—act out what you want the patient to do; for example, before giving the patient a toothbrush, make the motions of brushing your teeth with the toothbrush.

Adaptive Devices

Adaptive devices are sometimes used to enable a person to do an ADL. These are ordinary items that have been modified for use by persons with various types of problems. A person with a disability may be unable to perform certain ADLs. Adding a device that changes the way the task is done may enable the person to perform it independently. The person is taught to use the device for everyday tasks. Your role as a nursing assistant

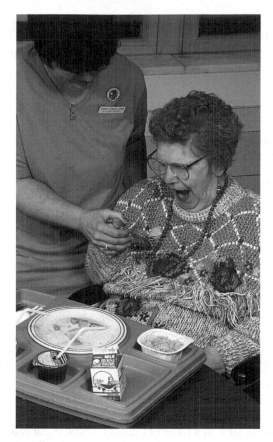

FIGURE 48-9 Hand-over-hand technique is another approach that helps patients relearn essential skills.

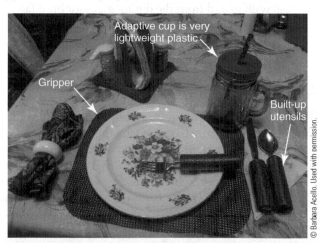

Adaptive cup is very lightweight plastic

Gripper

Built-up utensils

FIGURE 48-10 Adaptive utensils are available to enable patients to self-feed.

is to make sure the device is clean, available, and used by the patient. You may need to work on the skill with the person when they are learning to use the device. The instructions will be listed on the care plan.

Adaptive Devices for Eating

The most common adaptive devices are used to enable patients to feed themselves (Figure 48-10). These include adaptive silverware, plates, plate guards, and cups. Everyday items may also be used. For example, tape the straw to the inside of the glass if you do not have a straw holder. A sliding plate can be a real problem. A wet washcloth on the table under the plate will keep the plate in place and prevent sliding while the person scoops up the food.

Adaptive Devices for Dressing

Dressing aids are also common (Figure 48-11). Using these adaptive devices may seem awkward to you, but for patients, being able to dress themselves is important for self-esteem.

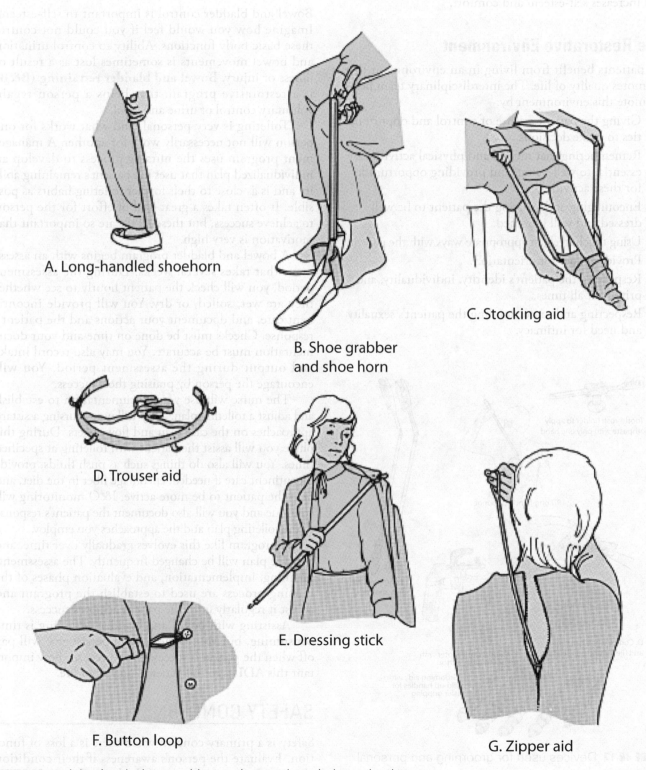

A. Long-handled shoehorn

B. Shoe grabber and shoe horn

C. Stocking aid

D. Trouser aid

E. Dressing stick

F. Button loop

G. Zipper aid

FIGURE 48-11 Adaptive devices enable a patient to dress independently.

Adaptive Devices for Grooming and Hygiene

Grooming and hygiene are very private activities. Bathing and grooming oneself involves important skills. Everyone has a personal hygiene routine. Using adaptive devices (Figure 48-12) enables the person to perform these skills and increases self-esteem and comfort.

The Restorative Environment

All patients benefit from living in an environment that promotes quality of life. The interdisciplinary team helps promote this environment by:

- Giving the patient a sense of control and opportunities to make decisions.
- Remembering that mental and physical activities are essential to well-being, and providing opportunities for these activities.
- Encouraging and assisting the patient to be well dressed and well groomed.
- Using touch freely in appropriate ways with the patient.
- Providing cues for orientation.
- Respecting the patient's identity, individuality, and privacy at all times.
- Respecting and understanding the patient's sexuality and need for intimacy.

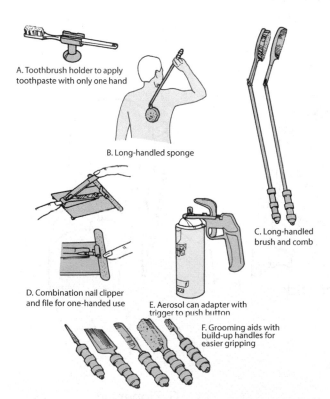

A. Toothbrush holder to apply toothpaste with only one hand

B. Long-handled sponge

C. Long-handled brush and comb

D. Combination nail clipper and file for one-handed use

E. Aerosol can adapter with trigger to push button

F. Grooming aids with build-up handles for easier gripping

FIGURE 48-12 Devices used for grooming and personal hygiene.

- Giving the patient opportunities to help others.
- Encouraging and assisting the patient to remain a part of the community.
- Creating an environment that is safe, serene, and colorful.

BOWEL AND BLADDER RETRAINING

Bowel and bladder control is important to self-esteem. Imagine how you would feel if you could not control these basic body functions. Ability to control urination and bowel movements is sometimes lost as a result of illness or injury. **Bowel and bladder retraining (B&B)** is a restorative program that helps a person regain voluntary control of urine and stool.

Toileting is very personal, and what works for one person will not necessarily work for another. A management program uses the nursing process to develop an individualized plan that uses the patient's remaining ability and is as close to their former toileting habits as possible. It often takes a great deal of effort for the person to achieve success, but these ADLs are so important that motivation is very high.

A bowel and bladder program begins with an assessment that takes several weeks. During the assessment period, you will check the patient hourly to see whether they are wet, soiled, or dry. You will provide incontinent care, and document your actions and the patient's response. Checks must be done on time and your documentation must be accurate. You may also record intake and output during the assessment period. You will encourage the person by praising their success.

The nurse will use your documentation to establish and adjust a toileting plan. They will write nursing assistant approaches on the care plan and flow sheets. During this phase you will assist the patient with toileting at specified times. You will also do things such as push fluids, provide incontinent care if needed, encourage fiber in the diet, and help the patient to be more active. I&O monitoring will continue and you will also document the patient's response to the toileting plan and the approaches you employ.

A program like this evolves gradually over time, and the care plan will be changed frequently. The assessment, planning, implementation, and evaluation phases of the nursing process are used to establish the program and adjust it regularly until the patient achieves success.

Assisting with bowel and bladder retraining is time consuming, but your patience and persistence will pay off when the person is successful and you see how important this ADL is to the patient's quality of life.

SAFETY CONCERNS

Safety is a primary concern when there is a loss of function. Evaluate the person's awareness if their condition changes. Inform the nurse if the level of consciousness and/or mental status have changed. Changes in consciousness and mental status may indicate serious problems. Other important observations that should be reported are:

- Whether the person is aware of the change.
- Whether the person asks for assistance when needed.
- The patient's desire to remain independent despite the increased safety risk.
- Whether the patient denies that there has been a change.
- Any falls that you know of.
- Changes in vision.

- Changes in bowel and bladder control.
- The person's ability to ambulate.
- Problems with standing, balance, or coordination.

The nurse will assess the patient if any of these problems occur. They make other team members aware of the changes. They will reevaluate the care plan and write new approaches, if necessary. The restorative program will be modified as needed, with the changes in mind. Patient safety is the primary goal.

Activity will be increased gradually if the person has been on bedrest for a long time. Inactivity and bedrest cause changes in blood pressure and balance. The nurse will develop a schedule to gradually increase the length of time that the patient will be up.

GUIDELINES 48-1 Guidelines for Restorative Care

- Become familiar with the patient's condition.
- Provide restorative care at the usual time of day for the activity.
- Make sure that the treatment area is ready, equipment is gathered, and the patient's physical needs are met before beginning.
- Follow the instructions on the care plan. Check frequently for changes.
- Provide privacy. The patient will make mistakes and become frustrated. Avoid embarrassing them in front of others.
- Eliminate as many distractions as possible.
- Apply orthotic and prosthetic devices (Figures 48-13A and 48-13B) as ordered. These will be listed on the care plan. *Orthotic devices* improve function and prevent deformities. *Prosthetic devices* are replacements for body parts, such as the eye, breast, hand, leg, or foot.
- Modify the environment to promote independence, if necessary.

- Practice good body mechanics for yourself and the patient.
- Practice safety, and teach the patient safety measures.
- Remember that all ADLs have many steps. If the patient cannot complete one step, they will not be able to complete the activity.
- Treat the patient with dignity.
- Be positive and encouraging. Stress what the patient can do.
- Give the patient as much control as possible by allowing them to make choices and decisions.
- Allow enough time for the activity. Be patient and avoid rushing the patient.
- Work on one step at a time. When the patient masters one step, move to the next.

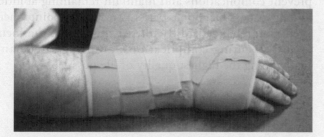

FIGURE 44-13A An orthotic device such as a hand split may be used to maintain alignment and prevent contractures of the hand, wrist, and fingers.

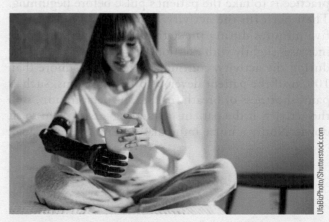

FIGURE 44-13B Advancements have been made in the development of artificial limbs.

(continues)

GUIDELINES 48-1 Guidelines for Restorative Care (continued)

- Remember that the patient's progress may be inconsistent from one day to the next.

- Provide frequent, positive feedback during the procedure.

- Provide simple, clear directions. Demonstrate if the patient does not understand.

- Give verbal cues, whenever necessary, to describe what you want the patient to do.

- If the patient does not respond to verbal cues, use the hand-over-hand technique. Place your hand on top of the patient's hand and guide them to begin the activity. If they do not respond, replace your hand and guide the patient through the activity.

- Encourage and allow the patient to do as much self-care as possible. Show the patient that you are confident in their ability.

- Use adaptive devices, if necessary.

- If the patient cannot complete an ADL, give praise for what they have accomplished. Complete the task without comment or complaint.

- Report your observations to the nurse.

- Notify the nurse if you feel that the patient's condition requires evaluation.

- Document your care immediately after providing it. Avoid documenting in advance.

MONITORING THE PATIENT'S RESPONSE TO CARE

You must observe how the restorative program affects the patient. This is particularly true in the early stages of an illness. The patient may become easily frustrated. Allow them to struggle a little, but intervene before the patient reaches the point of frustration. Remind them that learning takes time. Practice empathy. Tell the patient you understand how frustrated they feel. Be aware of the person's fears. A fear of falling or spilling may prevent the person from participating.

Early in the restorative program, the patient may have an unexpected physical response. You have learned that bedrest, even for a short time, has a negative effect on the body. Any physical activity may cause a change in the physical condition. Monitor for signs of fatigue. Be alert for changes, and report them to the nurse. A good practice is to take the patient's pulse before beginning. Then perform the activity. Monitor the pulse every five minutes during the activity. Normally, the pulse increases slightly with exertion. If the pulse is under 100 during the activity, continue. If the rate is more than 100, or if the patient develops other problems, such as pain, shortness of breath, nausea, or perspiration, stop the activity. If the patient is standing, assist them to sit down. Notify a nurse immediately. Pull the call signal, or send someone else to get help. Do not leave the patient alone.

Upon completion of the activity, check the pulse again. It should return to within 10 beats of the resting pulse rate within five minutes.

Precautions and Special Situations

Patients with certain conditions require special care and handling. Avoid exercising extremities with fractures or dislocations. The bones of patients with osteoporosis or bone cancer break easily. Check with the nurse and the care plan before continuing. Notify a nurse if the patient has a wound, or a red or open area, on the joint you are exercising. Before continuing, inquire if exercise will be harmful. If a patient is combative or resists care, explain why it is important. Try to coax them into participating. Try singing an old song for distraction. Encourage the patient to sing with you. Avoid forcing them. Notify the nurse if the patient continues to refuse.

Not all patients are candidates for restorative programs. For those who are not, the goals are to prevent complications and maintain remaining abilities as long as possible. Some patients reach the point where even maintenance is difficult. At this point, the focus is on preventing complications, ensuring safety, and maintaining the highest quality of life possible.

GUIDELINES 48-2 Guidelines for Implementing Restorative Programs

- Know why the patient has the self-care deficit.
- Do the task at the normal time of day the task should be done.
- Establish small goals and break the task into tiny pieces. Do not expect the patient to master or even remember the steps immediately.
- Make the task part of the regular routine so it is purposeful. Avoid making it look or feel like "busy work."
- Use the restorative care plan approaches each time the task must be done. Some tasks must be done multiple times each day.
- Keep your directions simple but not childish.
- Avoid distractions. Do the ADL in a private area.
- Be consistent. Read the care plan and follow the specific directions each time you work with the

patient. The patient benefits from this consistency. When all staff use the same care plan approaches, the patient masters the task much faster.

- Use adaptive devices consistently and correctly.
- Do not show impatience. Be encouraging and give praise.
- Treat the patient with dignity at all times.
- Realize that the patient's progress may be uneven and inconsistent. Compliment the patient for making progress even if the gains are small.
- It is better for the patient to complete even part of a task than it is for you to do it. Allow the patient to do what they can, and then finish the task. Avoid making the patient feel like a failure because they could not finish the task.

REVIEW

A. True/False

Mark the following true or false by circling T or F.

1. T F Rehabilitation services are provided only in special hospitals.
2. T F OBRA regulations require that restorative services be provided to persons in skilled care facilities.
3. T F Rehabilitation and restorative services both strive to prevent complications.
4. T F Persons with disabilities will never recover their lost skills.
5. T F All persons with disabilities are considered to be handicapped.

B. Multiple Choice

Select the best answer for each of the following.

6. A patient with a permanent disability is:
   a. taught to adapt to the present circumstances.
   b. not a good candidate for rehabilitation.
   c. given much sympathy.
   d. encouraged to be helpless.
7. Disabilities may result from:
   a. too much exercise.
   b. getting inadequate sleep.
   c. spinal cord injury.
   d. not drinking enough water.

8. A patient who is unable to communicate verbally will be treated by a:
   a. physical therapist.
   b. occupational therapist.
   c. nursing assistant.
   d. speech-language pathologist.
9. Physical inactivity is *most likely* to cause:
   a. pressure injuries.
   b. dehydration.
   c. pain.
   d. infection.
10. Agnosia is a perceptual deficit in which the patient cannot:
    a. organize a task.
    b. identify common items.
    c. sequence a task.
    d. initiate a task.
11. Adaptive devices are:
    a. inappropriate for patients receiving rehabilitation.
    b. used by nursing assistants to feed patients.
    c. ordinary items modified for use by patients with self-care deficits.
    d. used only by occupational therapists.

12. Placing your hand over the patient's hand to guide the patient's actions is an approach called:

   a. giving verbal cues.

   b. demonstration.

   c. hand-over-hand technique.

   d. setting up.

13. Early-loss ADLs are:

   a. feeding, toileting, and ambulation.

   b. dressing, bathing, and personal hygiene.

   c. grooming, transfers, and bed mobility.

   d. toileting, bathing, and dressing.

14. Late-loss ADLs are:

   a. bed mobility, transfers, and feeding.

   b. eating, dressing, and grooming.

   c. toileting, bathing, and transfers.

   d. personal hygiene, bathing, and dressing.

15. A person who has had a stroke has a short term goal to be up in a chair for two hours. You are expected to monitor their condition when they are up and complete a written summary of their progress on Thursday. You will monitor them for:

   a. heart rate, nausea, perspiration.

   b. Dilated pupils, cooperation, focus.

   c. applying their gait belt independently.

   d. Willingness to assist with the procedure.

16. Maria Hernandez has a cast on her left arm. She has a nursing order for ROM twice a day. You know this means:

   a. move the cast

   b. resist movement

   c. active range of motion

   d. range of motion

17. A good way to check the patient's response to treatment is to:

   a. check the vital signs

   b. monitor the pulse

   c. monitor the temperature

   d. check the feet for edema

18. You are working with Mr. Mann and he becomes short of breath and dizzy. You will:

   a. Run into the hall to find some help.

   b. Cover his forehead with cool washcloths

   c. Stop the activity and inform the nurse.

   d. Continue the activity because this is normal.

C. Completion

Complete the statements by choosing the correct word from the following list.

   activities of daily living
   atrophy
   contracture
   disability
   geriatric
   handicap
   mobility skills
   physiatrist
   rehabilitation
   self-care deficit
   verbal cueing

19. The process used to help a patient reach an optimal level of ability is _____.

20. Ambulation and transfers are examples of _____.

21. Dressing and undressing are examples of _____.

22. An impairment that affects the ability to perform an activity that a person of that age would normally be able to do is called a(n) _____.

23. When an impairment limits or prevents the person from fulfilling a role that is normal for that person, a(n) _____ exists.

24. A person who chooses to work with rehabilitation of the elderly is specializing in _____ rehabilitation.

25. A physician who specializes in rehabilitation is called a(n) _____.

26. A(n) _____ occurs when a joint is in a permanent state of flexion.

27. _____ occurs when a muscle shrinks and loses strength.

28. A(n) _____ exists when an adult cannot complete one or more activities of daily living.

29. Using short, simple phrases to prompt the patient to complete an activity of daily living is called _____.

D. Nursing Assistant Challenge

You are working as a nursing assistant in the rehabilitation unit of a subacute care section of a skilled nursing facility. Think about what you have learned in this chapter and answer the following questions:

30. What types of patients will you see?

_____

_____

31. What kinds of disabilities will the patients have?

_____

_____

32. What may be the cause of the self-care deficits experienced by your patients?

_____

_____

33. What kinds of problems can limit a patient's ability to do self-care?

_____

_____

34. Explain the significance of early- and late-loss ADLs.

_____

_____

35. What are the differences between rehabilitation and restorative care?

_____

_____

36. What are the responsibilities of the nursing assistant when giving restorative care?

_____

_____

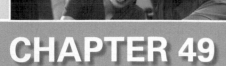

CHAPTER 49

Obstetrical Patients and Neonates

OBJECTIVES

After completing this chapter, you will be able to:

49.1 Spell and define terms.

49.2 Identify the role and responsibilities of the doula as a member of the childbirth team.

49.3 Assist in care of the normal postpartum patient.

49.4 Properly change a perineal pad.

49.5 Recognize reportable observations of patients in the postpartum period.

49.6 Assist in care of the normal newborn.

49.7 Demonstrate three methods of safely holding a baby.

49.8 Describe nursing assistant actions and observations related to the care of the newborn infant.

49.9 List measures to prevent inadvertent switching, misidentification, and abduction of infants.

49.10 Assist in carrying out the discharge procedures for mother and infant.

49.11 Demonstrate the following procedures:

- Procedure 108: Changing a Diaper (Expand Your Skills)
- Procedure 109: Weighing an Infant (Expand Your Skills)
- Procedure 110: Measuring an Infant (Expand Your Skills)
- Procedure 111: Bathing an Infant (Expand Your Skills)
- Procedure 112: Bottle-Feeding an Infant (Expand Your Skills)
- Procedure 113: Assisting with Breastfeeding (Expand Your Skills)
- Procedure 114: Burping an Infant (Expand Your Skills)

VOCABULARY

Learn the meaning and the correct spelling of the following words and phrases:

amniotic fluid	colostrum	isolette	postpartum
amniotic sac	doula	lactation	prenatal
Apgar score	fetus	lochia	status
areola	foreskin	neonate	umbilical cord
circumcision	involution	placenta	

INTRODUCTION TO OBSTETRICS

In this chapter, you will learn to care for a mother and newborn infant. Some facilities will not permit nursing assistants to work in the obstetrics department, but others do. Typical nursing assistant responsibilities in this department are:

- Monitoring and documenting vital signs
- Changing linens
- Assisting mothers with toileting and ADLs
- Cleaning and disinfecting equipment
- Setting up and tearing down rooms for deliveries and procedures such as circumcisions (using standard precautions, medical asepsis, sterile technique, etc.)
- Cleaning and disinfecting instruments
- Cleaning rooms and stocking supplies

- Helping with admissions and discharges
- Transporting patients and supplies
- Passing trays, snacks, fresh drinking water, and the like
- Helping the unit secretary
- Running errands
- Helping in the nursery
- Giving infant baths
- Giving cord care
- Providing circumcision care
- Changing diapers
- Bottle-feeding infants
- Assisting mothers with breast care and breastfeeding
- Weighing mothers and infants
- Measuring infant length and taking other measurements as permitted
- Taking the infants' first pictures
- Taking vital signs of infants and mothers
- Assisting mothers with showers, toileting, and perineal care

Childbirth

When a baby is ready to be born, it is normally upside down in the mother's uterus with its head toward the birth canal (Figure 49-1). Before the baby is born, it is known as a **fetus**. In the uterus, it is surrounded by a membranous bag called an **amniotic sac**. The fetus floats in a liquid called **amniotic fluid**.

The fetus gets nourishment from the mother through the **umbilical cord**. The umbilical cord is attached to the fetus and the **placenta**. The placenta is attached to the wall of the mother's uterus.

After the baby is born and separated from the umbilical cord, the placenta, amniotic sac, and remaining cord are expelled as the *afterbirth*. After a period of time, the mother's uterus, which was greatly stretched during pregnancy, will return to its normal size and shape.

There are three phases of pregnancy:

- **Prenatal** (before birth)
- Labor and delivery
- **Postpartum** (after birth)

Cesarean Birth

Cesarean section is another way of delivering a baby. The baby is delivered through an incision in the abdomen rather than through the birth canal. Between 20 and 30 percent of all births in the United States occur this way. Cesarean deliveries may be performed when there is:

- Fetal distress
- A preterm infant
- Breech (nonheadfirst) presentation
- Prolonged rupture of the membranes
- Prolapsed cord
- Genital herpes
- Premature separation of the placenta
- Placenta previa
- Failure of labor to progress
- A mother who has already had a cesarean section

A spinal or epidural anesthetic is administered before the surgery. This type of procedure introduces drugs into

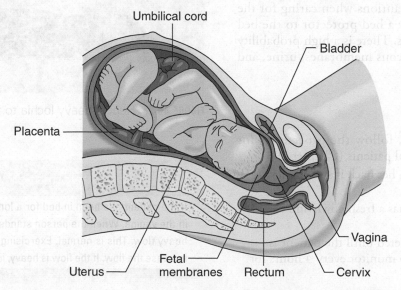

Umbilical cord

Bladder

Placenta

Vagina

Fetal membranes   Rectum   Cervix

Uterus

FIGURE 49-1 The usual position of the fetus at birth. This is known as the *vertex position*.

You may be assigned to monitor patients' vital signs immediately after delivery, and every two to four hours after that. Position the mother in the same position each time. It is not unusual for the blood pressure to drop when the mother changes position from lying to sitting or sitting to standing. Monitor the mother for dizziness.

the cerebrospinal fluid and blocks sensation from the upper abdomen down to the toes. The patient will not be able either to feel or move her legs until the anesthetic wears off.

The Doula

Some patients who come to the hospital in labor may be accompanied by both the spouse and a **doula**. The word *doula* is derived from Greek and means "woman's servant." Doulas are members of the childbirth team. The doula is not a caregiver. Doulas may work for a physician, midwife, or hospital; or they may be self-employed. They are responsible for supporting and comforting the mother and enhancing communication between the mother and hospital staff. Two types of doulas assist families during the childbirth process:

- A *birth doula* provides support and nurtures the mother before, during, and just after childbirth.

- A *postpartum doula* works with a postpartum family to help them care for and enjoy the infant.

POSTPARTUM CARE

You may assist in caring for the mother during the postpartum period. With other team members, you will assist the mother from the stretcher into bed. Apply the principles of standard precautions when caring for the postpartum patient. Apply a bed protector to the bed under the patient's buttocks. There is a high probability of contact with blood, mucous membranes, urine, and breast milk.

Anesthesia

If an anesthetic was used, follow the procedures for postoperative care of surgical patients (Chapter 29).

- Keep the patient flat on her back if spinal anesthesia was used.

- Make sure the patient has a fresh gown and clean bed linens.

- Check vital signs as ordered until the patient is stable, then continue to monitor every 4 hours for 24 hours.

- If the patient complains of being cold, an extra blanket may provide comfort.

- Record the first voiding. Inform the nurse if the patient has not voided by the end of your shift.

Drainage

Carefully check the condition of the perineum and the perineal pad for the amount and color of drainage.

- Always lift the pad away from the body from front to back.

- Red vaginal discharge, called **lochia**, is expected. *Lochia rubra* (Figure 49-2A) is the discharge that occurs during the first three days after delivery. Report the amount of discharge and any clotting.

Initially, the lochia is bright red and moderate in amount. Report heavy lochia to the nurse (Figure 40-2B). Over the next week, the lochia will lessen and become pink to pink-brown in color. A yellowish-white or brown discharge may continue for one to three weeks after delivery and then stop.

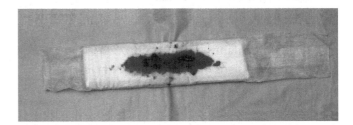

FIGURE 49-2A Moderate lochia is normal during the first few days.

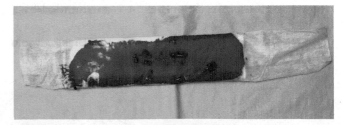

FIGURE 49-2B Report heavy lochia to the nurse promptly.

If the patient has been in bed for a long time, lochia pools in the vagina. When the person stands, she may have very heavy flow. This is normal. Exercising vigorously will also increase the flow. If the flow is heavy, inform the nurse.

Cramping

As the uterus begins to return to its normal size (**involution**), the patient may experience strong cramps. Cramping may also be associated with breastfeeding. This is normal, but be sure to report any complaints of pain to the nurse, who can administer medication for relief.

Voiding

Encourage the new mother to void within the first six to eight hours after the delivery. Check carefully for signs of urine retention.

Toileting and Perineal Care

The mother may be:

- Provided with a squeezable bottle filled with warm tap water.
- Instructed to rinse the genitals and perineum after voiding or defecating.
- Instructed to gently pat, not wipe, the perineal area with tissue or special medicated pads—once only with each piece of tissue or pad, from front to back. Discard the toilet tissue in the toilet. Discard everything else in a plastic trash bag, even if the manufacturer says it can be flushed.
- Taught to wash her hands before applying a fresh perineal pad.
- Taught not to touch the inside of the perineal pad.

If the perineum is very uncomfortable:

- Specially medicated pads may be used for cleansing. The procedure is always the same—front to back and discard.
- Anesthetic sprays may be ordered.
- Ice packs may be used to reduce edema and relieve discomfort.

Instruct patients to apply anesthetic spray after cleansing the perineum to reduce discomfort. If sitting is uncomfortable, instruct the mother to squeeze her buttocks together and hold them in this position until she is seated upright. This reduces tension on the suture line.

BREAST CARE

Teach the mother to wash her breasts daily with soap and water. The mother's first milk is called **colostrum**. The colostrum:

- Is watery.
- Carries protective antibodies to the child.
- Usually begins to flow about 12 hours after delivery. **Lactation**, the flow of milk, does not begin until the second or third postpartum day.

Keeping the breasts clean is especially important when the mother is planning to breastfeed her baby.

- Instruct the mother to wash her hands and nipples just prior to feeding the baby.
- Teach the mother to wash the breasts using a circular motion from the nipples outward.
- Creams are sometimes used between feedings to help the nipples remain supple.
- Breast pads absorb milk leakage. Instruct the mother to change them frequently.
- The breasts should be supported by a well-fitted brassiere even if the mother is not breastfeeding. Medication to suppress milk production may be ordered.

When delivery is uncomplicated, mothers and healthy newborns do not stay in the hospital very long. They are usually able to go home within two days.

GUIDELINES 49-1 Guidelines for Assisting with Breastfeeding

A recent trend holds that "the breast is best," and many mothers elect to breastfeed their newborns. Assist the mother by:

- Instructing her to wash the nipples and **areolae** with a cotton ball moistened with clear water before nursing. She should begin at the nipple, working outward in a circular motion.

- Helping to position the baby. The football hold (Figure 49-3A) or cradle hold (Figure 49-3B) is usually easiest.

- Gently stroking the infant's cheek near the mouth to get the baby to open the mouth and turn toward the breast.

- Instructing the mother to place the nipple and areola into the baby's mouth. The infant should begin to suck and swallow. Advise the mother that she may

feel a tingling sensation in the breasts as milk lets down and is released.

- Checking the position of the breast. Advise the mother to press and hold the breast back, if necessary, so it does not obstruct the baby's nose.

- Allowing the baby to nurse for five to seven minutes, if they have not stopped by then. If the infant has not stopped nursing, avoid pulling it from the breast. Break the infant's suction by placing a finger into the side of the mouth and moving the breast. Instruct the mother to burp the infant.

- Switching to the other breast after the infant has burped. Help the mother reposition the infant and get the baby started nursing on the opposite breast.

- The infant will stop nursing when they are full. Have the mother burp the baby again.

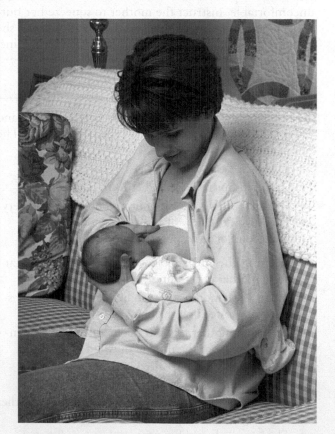

FIGURE 49-3A The football hold is used for breastfeeding and other activities when the baby must be supported well, such as when washing the hair.

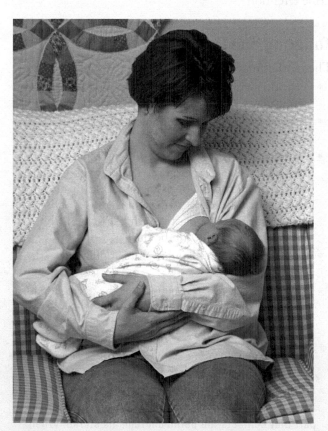

FIGURE 49-3B The cradle hold is also a comfortable position for breastfeeding.

TABLE 49-1 Nursing Assistant Observations of Postpartum Patients

The uterus is unusually high or pushed to one side

Swelling just above the pubis

Complaints of urgency (the need to void), but with voidings of 200 mL or less

Signs of possible urine retention

Inability to void within the first 8 hours postpartum

Voidings of less than 100 mL

Report promptly:

- Temperature of 100.4°F or greater
- Pulse over 100
- Blood pressure of 140/90 or above
- Progressively falling blood pressure
- Signs of inflammation
- Presence of large blood clots
- Foul-smelling lochia
- Saturation of a pad in 15 to 30 minutes
- Bruised appearance of perineum
- Complaints of constipation

Observation and Reporting

Monitor for and report the problems listed in Table 49-1.

NEONATAL CARE

After the newborn is admitted to the nursery, some additional procedures are completed. The physician will examine the baby and evaluate their **status**.

Apgar Scoring

The **Apgar score** is an evaluation of the **neonate**. It is made at 1 minute, 5 minutes, and 10 minutes after birth. The areas evaluated are:

- Heart rate
- Respiratory effort
- Muscle tone
- Reflex, irritability
- Color

A number value is applied to each assessment and recorded on a special form.

Totals indicate the infant's condition. A score of 7 to 10 indicates that the infant is in good condition. A score of 4 to 6 indicates fair condition. A score of 0 to 3 indicates poor (severely depressed) condition. A licensed nurse or physician will make the assessment, but you must understand the score. Refer to Table 49-2.

TABLE 49-2 Apgar Score Chart

SIGN	0	1	2	1 min	5 min
Heart Rate	Absent	Less Than 100	Over 100	2	2
Respiratory Effort	Absent	Slow, Irregular	Good Cry	1	2
Muscle Tone	Limp	Some Flexion	Active Motion	1	2
Reflex Irritability	No Response	Grimace	Cry	1	2
Color	Pale	Body Pink, Extr. Blue	All Pink	1	2
TOTAL SCORE				6	10

Care of the Newborn Infant

The baby's vital signs are determined. The infant is weighed and measured. The infant's temperature is monitored and recorded every 30 to 60 minutes until stable, and then every 4 hours or according to the nurse's instructions. The most desirable and accurate method for taking the infant's temperature is the temporal artery method (on the forehead). When the newborn's status becomes stable:

- The baby is given an admission bath using an antiseptic soap. The umbilical cord is carefully cleaned with a solution prescribed by the facility (Figure 49-4).
- The baby must be kept warm because their temperature has not yet stabilized. The baby is dressed. Cover the head with a stockinette cap because much body heat can be lost through this surface.
- Place the infant in a crib or **isolette** (Figure 49-5).

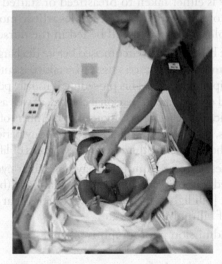

FIGURE 49-4 The cord is carefully cleaned to cause it to dry and to prevent infection.

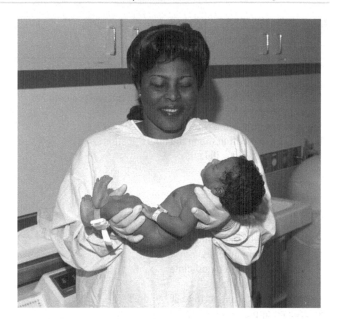

FIGURE 49-6A Always support the infant's bottom and neck.

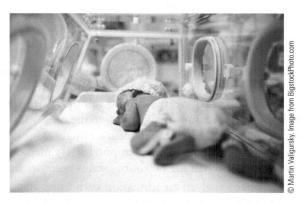

FIGURE 49-5 A stockinette cap is used to prevent heat loss, and the infant stays in the isolette until their temperature is stable.

© Martin Valigursky. Image from BigstockPhoto.com

- Feeding is not usually started for four to six hours after birth. During this time, the baby is monitored and observed carefully. After four to six hours, the baby is either taken to breastfeed or started on feedings of glucose and water. Babies whose mothers are unable to feed them will be fed in the nursery.

- Male babies may be circumcised before discharge. In **circumcision**, the excess tissue (**foreskin**) is cut from the tip of the penis. This procedure is usually performed based on the parents' personal choices, as well as cultural, ethnic, and religious traditions. For members of some faiths, circumcision is a religious ceremony performed at another location within the first few weeks of life.

- Babies who are jaundiced may have their eyes protected and be placed under a special light (bilirubin light [bili light]) in the isolette to help clear the levels of bilirubin in the skin.

- An admission photograph is taken.

Handling the Infant

Take care when lifting, carrying, and positioning an infant. Remember to lift the baby by grasping the legs securely with one hand while slipping the other hand under the baby's back to support the head and neck in

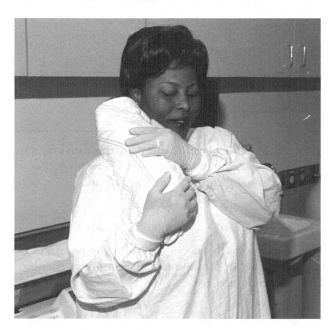

FIGURE 49-6B Shoulder hold.

the shoulder hold (Figures 49-6A and 49-6B). You may also use the cradle hold or football hold. Back through doorways when carrying a baby. Never turn your back when the infant is on an unprotected surface.

Elimination

The passage of urine and stool in a newborn infant are important observations. A normal newborn will urinate 6 to 10 times a day. Elimination is recorded and the color of stool documented. Stools should change from dark, meconium stools (Figure 49-7A) to brown-yellow, pasty transitional stools, and then finally to yellow stools that are slightly loose (Figure 49-7B).

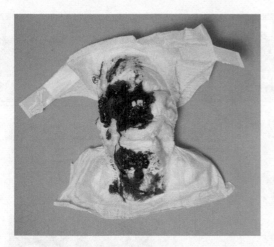

FIGURE 49-7A The first stools are meconium stools.

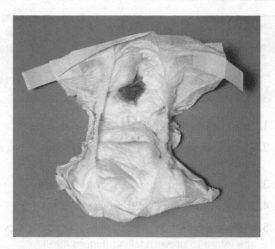

FIGURE 49-7B An infant receiving breast milk will have yellow stool.

Postcircumcision Care

Check the circumcision at each diaper change. Observe the area for bleeding and report anything unusual. You may be instructed to apply petroleum gauze to the area. The crib identification and nursery record will note the circumcision. Document the first voiding after circumcision.

Weighing the Infant

Routine care includes weighing the infant. This procedure should also be done before feeding.

> ### ✎ NOTE
>
> Put clean paper on the scale before using it. Balance the scale with the paper in place. Keep your hand on the infant. Work quickly to prevent heat loss in the infant. Disinfect the scale each time it is used, to prevent cross-contamination.

Measuring Length

Length refers to a measurement taken with the infant in the supine position. Infants move and flex their extremities, so having two people measure is best. Measure the infant twice. The measurements must be within 1/8 inch of each other.

EXPAND YOUR SKILLS

PROCEDURE **108** | **CHANGING A DIAPER** |

1. Carry out initial procedure actions.
2. Assemble equipment:
   - Clean diaper
   - Gloves
   - Plastic bag or container for trash
   - Damp washcloths, wipes, or cotton balls for cleansing
   - Mild soap, if used
   - Supplies for cord care and/or circumcision care, according to facility policy
3. Remove the soiled diaper and observe for color, consistency, and quantity.
4. Roll the soiled diaper so the clean side faces out. Put it in the trash or place it out of reach of the infant.
5. Cleanse the diaper area with wipes or a damp washcloth. Clean from the front toward the back

in a female infant, and from the tip of the penis toward the scrotum for a male infant. Cleanse all folds of the groin and anus. Discard the wipes or washcloth.
6. Lift the buttocks with one hand and slide the new, open diaper underneath.
7. Pull the diaper between the legs. Fold the top edge of the diaper down so it is positioned under the umbilical cord. Fasten the tape snugly on each side.
8. Perform cord care with alcohol or antiseptic according to facility policy.
9. Change other clothing, blanket, or crib linen if soiled or wet.
10. Discard the soiled diaper and your gloves, if not done previously.
11. Carry out ending procedure actions.

ICON KEY:

 = OBRA   = PPE

EXPAND YOUR SKILLS

PROCEDURE 109 WEIGHING AN INFANT ⓞ

1. Wash your hands.
2. Place exam paper or a receiving blanket on the scale and balance the scale.
3. Check the infant's previous weight, if any.
4. Remove the infant's diaper and shirt.
5. Place the infant on the scale, keeping a hand over the infant to prevent falling (Figure 49-8).
6. Move the bar to the correct weight until the scale balances.
7. Return the infant to the crib. Diaper and dress the infant.
8. Record the infant's weight according to hospital policy.
9. Remove the linen from the scale and place it in a laundry hamper.
10. Return the scale to its proper storage place.
11. Wash your hands.

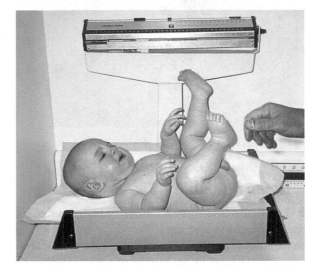

FIGURE 49-8 Keep one hand on the infant except when obtaining the weight.

ICON KEY:
ⓞ = OBRA

EXPAND YOUR SKILLS

PROCEDURE 110 MEASURING AN INFANT ⓞ

1. Wash your hands.
2. Assemble equipment:
   - Paper to cover the surface
   - Calibrated length board, if used
   - Paper tape measure, if used
   - Pen and paper
   - Supplies for disinfecting the measuring surface
3. Check the infant's identification band.

Calibrated length board

Complete steps 1 through 3 above.

4. Position the infant on the back in the center of the length board with the head touching the headrest and the buttocks and shoulders flat against the measuring surface (Figure 49-9A).
5. One person gently holds the infant's head in contact with the headpiece. They gently cup the infant's ears to be sure the infant's chin is not tucked in against the chest or stretched too far back.

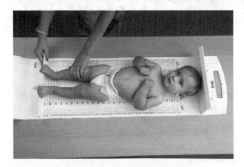

FIGURE 49-9A Align the infant on the board.

6. The other person aligns the infant, extending both legs. Place one hand gently on the knees to keep the legs in extension with the toes pointing upward.
7. Slide the movable footrest up until it rests firmly against the soles of the infant's feet. Read the measurement and write the value on your note pad.
8. Remove the infant and return to their crib.
9. Discard paper cover and sanitize the board.

(continues)

10. Document the value.

11. Carry out ending procedure actions.

Tape measure method #1

Complete steps 1 through 3 above.

4. One person gently holds the infant's head in contact with a solid surface. This person gently cups the ears to be sure the infant's chin is not tucked in against the chest or stretched too far back.

5. The other person aligns the infant, extending both legs. Place one hand gently on the knees to keep the legs in extension with the toes pointing upward.

6. Using a paper tape measure, measure from the top of the head to the soles of the infant's feet. Read the measurement and write the value on your note pad.

7. Remove the infant and return to their crib.

8. Discard the paper and sanitize the surface used.

9. Document the value.

10. Carry out ending procedure actions.

Tape measure method #2

Complete steps 1 through 3 above.

4. Place a piece of exam table paper on a clean surface. Make sure the paper is smooth and wrinkle-free.

5. One person gently holds the infant's head in contact with a solid surface. If not available, this person gently cups the infant's ears while holding the head

to be sure the infant's chin is not tucked in against the chest or stretched too far back.

6. Make a mark on the paper at the center top of the head.

7. Align the infant, extending both legs. Place one hand gently on the knees to keep the legs in extension with the toes pointing upward (Figure 49-9B).

8. Make a mark on the paper at the bottom of the heels. Repeat to verify accuracy.

9. Pick the infant up and return to the crib.

10. Using a paper tape measure, measure the distance between the two marks.

11. Document the value.

12. Discard the paper and sanitize the surface used.

13. Carry out ending procedure actions.

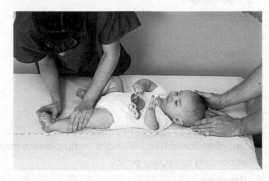

FIGURE 49-9B Make a mark at the head and heels.

ICON KEY:

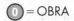 = OBRA

In some facilities, infants are measured by using a calibrated length board with a fixed headrest and movable footrest (similar to the device used for measuring shoe size). This is the most accurate method. In other facilities, the infant is measured using a disposable paper tape measure.

Bathing the Infant

The infant may be bathed after their temperature has stabilized. Bathing is done daily, and as needed. The nurse will teach the parents how to bathe the infant.

 NOTE

Before beginning the bathing procedure, check with the nurse to make sure the infant's temperature is stable enough for bathing. Keep the infant warm throughout the procedure.

Change the crib sheet after bathing the infant. Newborn infants are placed in a plastic bassinette or isolette. Cover the mattress with a pillowcase. Change it after bathing and as needed.

Difficult Situations

Babies are dressed in a long-sleeved T-shirt and a diaper with a stockinette cap on the head, and then covered with a receiving blanket. Despite these measures, some newborns cannot maintain temperature. Try adding a second long-sleeved T-shirt. Place the baby's legs in the armholes and pull the shirt up to create leggings. Keep the head covered at all times, because this is the greatest area of heat loss.

Difficult Situations

You may have trouble rinsing blood from the hair after delivery. Apply a solution of one tablespoon of baby oil to two tablespoons of water to wet hair. Slowly comb the hair with a soft baby comb. Blood is easily removed and the infant will have clean and shiny hair.

EXPAND YOUR SKILLS

PROCEDURE **111** BATHING AN INFANT

1. Carry out initial procedure actions.
2. Assemble equipment:
   - Clean diaper
   - Gloves
   - Washbasin with warm water (98°F to 100°F)
   - Plastic bag or container for trash
   - 2–3 washcloths
   - Towel
   - Cotton balls
   - Liquid infant cleanser/shampoo
   - Supplies for cord care and/or circumcision care, according to facility policy
   - Blankets
   - Sheet
3. Place the infant in a bassinet with sides. Arrange the supplies within reach.
4. Check the infant's skin for dryness, peeling, or signs of infection. If present, notify the nurse and obtain instructions for care.
5. Check the site of the umbilical cord for redness, drainage, drying, and bleeding. If present, notify the nurse and obtain instructions for care.
6. Remove the infant's clothing. Cover the infant with a blanket for warmth.
7. Moisten a cotton ball with plain water. Cleanse the far eye from inside to outside, in one wipe. Repeat with a new cotton ball for the near eye.
8. Wash the outer ears with plain water and a cotton ball or twisted end of the washcloth.
9. Make a mitt with the washcloth. Wash the face and neck with plain water, with attention to areas behind the ears and creases in the neck.
10. Pat the face and neck dry with a towel.

11. Pull the blanket down to expose the upper body.
12. Cleanse the upper body with soap and a washcloth. Rinse soap from the hands quickly, then rinse the rest of the upper body. Pat dry.
13. Cleanse and rinse the area around the umbilicus. Pat dry. Apply alcohol or the drying solution used by the facility.
14. Cover the upper body. Pull the blanket up to expose the lower body.
15. Wash the legs and outer buttocks with soap and water. Rinse well and pat dry.
16. Obtain a fresh washcloth.
17. Cleanse the genitalia with plain water.
    - *Female infant:*
      - Spread the labia gently. Wash from front to back toward the anus. Turn the washcloth so a separate part is used for each wipe.
      - Wash the remaining portions of the labia and the folds in the groin.
      - Rinse and pat dry.
    - *Uncircumcised male infant:*
      - Avoid retracting the foreskin.
      - Wash from the urethra outward, then scrotum and folds in groin.
      - Rinse and pat dry.
    - *Circumcised male infant:*
      - Care for the circumcision according to the nurse's instructions.
      - Check for bleeding.
      - Gently cleanse the area with warm water and cotton balls.
      - Apply petroleum jelly gauze dressing, or according to facility policy.

(continues)

PROCEDURE **111** CONTINUED

18. Cleanse the anal area with soap. Rinse and pat dry.

19. Diaper the infant.

20. Wrap the infant in the blanket.

21. Pick up the infant, using the football hold. Hold the head over the basin.

22. Wet the scalp well with a washcloth and water.

23. Lather and gently wash the scalp with baby shampoo or gentle cleanser.

24. Rinse the scalp by pouring water from a small cup over the scalp and into the washbasin, or rinse well using a washcloth.

25. Pat dry.

26. Comb the infant's hair. Cover the head.

27. Dress the infant.

28. Replace the damp blanket and sheets.

29. Carry out ending procedure actions.

ICON KEY:

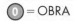 = OBRA 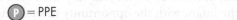 = PPE

Your facility will issue photo identification to all personnel working in the maternity department. Many workers turn the cards around so only the back side shows. This is an unsafe practice that most likely violates hospital policy. Wear the badge on your upper body, with the picture on the front. Some facilities issue a unique identification to staff who are authorized to work with infants, such as a second badge with a pink background or special emblem. The mother will be instructed to check the worker's identification badge if someone tries to remove the infant from the room.

SECURITY

All infants must be identified to prevent inadvertent switching, misidentification, and abduction. The nurse will apply identification bands to the infant's wrist and ankle while in the delivery room. The mother is given a matching wristband. In some facilities, the other parent is also given a wristband. The identification bands must be checked each time the infant is brought to the mother for feeding or rooming-in. Crib cards and other documents are also used for infant identification. Each facility has policies for checking identification. In some, the identification is also checked at the beginning and end of each shift.

Infant Abduction

Unfortunately, a number of infant abductions occur each year. In addition to wearing an identification

badge, reinforce your identity and position to the mother each time you provide care. The mother will be instructed not to hand the infant over to someone she does not know. Hospitals have various security measures in place to prevent abduction. Some apply magnetic-sensor ankle bands in the delivery room. An alarm will sound if the infant is removed from the unit. A few are using Global Positioning Systems (GPS). Some apply a tamper-proof band to the ankle or umbilical cord. If the band is removed or the infant is taken off the unit, doors automatically lock. Infants are transported to other areas of the hospital in a bassinette or crib (Figure 49-10), never carried. A transport identification card may also be used. Nursing staff must remain with the child while they are off the unit.

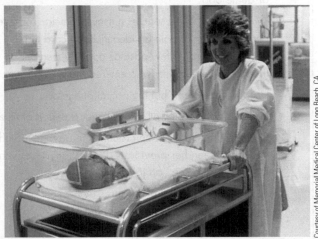

Courtesy of Memorial Medical Center of Long Beach, CA

FIGURE 49-10 Babies are transported in their own bassinet or crib. They are never carried through the hospital.

Code Pink is a frequently used code word signaling that an infant abduction is occurring. Code Purple means a child abduction is taking place. Many hospitals have abduction drills, similar to fire drills. Take these drills seriously. There is no room for error if an abduction is attempted, and the drills help staff react automatically to the emergency, increasing the odds that the infant will be found. Be alert to the people who visit your unit, even if you are busy. Refer to Guidelines 49-2 about the abductor profile and potential abductor behavior.

FEEDING

In addition to providing nutrition, feeding is important to the infant because it satisfies hunger and sucking needs. Sucking provides a pleasant sensation, whether the infant receives food or not. The amount of time an infant needs to suckle will vary with each infant. Provide the infant with the opportunity to suck, even if they cannot eat. Wash your hands well before feeding an infant or assisting a mother with breastfeeding.

🔓 Safety ALERT

Facilities must define the Code Pink and Code Purple classifications. The definitions must be clear to staff. Some facilities define each color by age, such as:

- Code Pink is from birth to 6 months of age.
- Code Purple is from 6 months to 13 years of age.

Some use the codes to specify the location of the abduction, such as:

- Code Pink for newborn nursery.
- Code Purple for the pediatrics unit.

Learn your facility's code designations.

GUIDELINES 49-2 Guidelines for Abductor Profile and Potential Abductor Behavior

- Overweight female between 14 and 48 years of age; average age is 28.

- Usually lives in community, has history of depression and manipulative behavior. Has a record of misdemeanor crimes, such as bad checks; or no criminal record at all.

- Has been telling people she is pregnant over a long period of time. May be abducting the infant in an attempt to save a bad relationship.

- May be carrying a large purse, package, tote bag, or duffle bag.

- Wears scrubs. Impersonates nurse, technician, or other personnel. May create an identification card that is worn backward. A few pose as a family member or friend of other patients who entered the wrong room.

- Usually not violent, but the potential exists.

- Plans the abduction well, usually over a period of time.

- Becomes familiar with unit routines in advance. Staff may have seen her previously. If questioned, says she is there "just to see" an infant.

- Asks questions about procedures and locations during visits, such as "When is feeding time?" "When are babies taken to the mothers?" or "Where are the stairs?"

- During visits, seeks out rooms that are out of view of the nurses' station, and close to means of escape, such as stairs, fire exits, and elevators.

- Usually alone, but may have a partner who will create a disturbance to distract staff.

- Selection of infant is random and opportunistic, but usually targets an infant of the same race.

- Tries to trick mother into letting her think she is taking the infant for a lab test, picture, or other procedure.

- Location of abduction:
  - 57 percent of infants are taken from their mother's room.
  - 15 percent each are taken from the newborn nursery, other pediatric wards, or other parts of the hospital property.

- Studies have shown that most hospital abductions occur Monday through Friday between 8:00 a.m. and 6:00 p.m. More abductions occur in May and December than in other months, but they can occur in any month, at any time of day or night.

When feeding an infant:

- Hold the infant unless there is a medical reason not to. Holding the infant during a feeding allows close, physical contact with the person feeding them.
- Infants breathe through the nose. Nasal congestion will cause feeding problems. Inform the nurse if the newborn experiences nasal congestion or has difficulty during feeding.
- Hold the bottle while the baby eats.
- Never leave an infant in a crib with a bottle propped in the mouth. This is dangerous because the infant could vomit and/or choke.
- Burp the infant during and following feeding.
- If the infant hiccups after feeding, try to get them to swallow a little more formula, or burp the infant to make the hiccups stop.

 NOTE

If an infant cannot be fed, hold and allow them to suck on a pacifier unless a medical reason prevents removal of the infant from the crib.

 Infection Control **ALERT**

The formula and bottle should be sterile for bottle-feeding an infant. Most facilities use prepared, sterile formula in disposable bottles. Avoid touching the nipple or the inside of the cap. Keep the nipple covered until you are ready to begin feeding. Check the expiration date on the bottle to make sure the formula has not expired.

 Safety **ALERT**

Infants can safely drink room-temperature formula. Some facilities warm bottles in commercial bottle warmers. Formula may also be warmed in warm water for about five minutes if providing warm formula is facility policy or infant preference. Avoid heaters such as a microwave. These cause hotspots that may burn the infant. Regardless of the method used, always check the temperature by turning the bottle over and allowing a few drops to drip on your wrist. Do not use it if it is hot. Get another bottle.

Burping

The frequency with which you burp the infant will depend on the infant's age and medical condition. Burping is important because bottle-fed infants swallow a lot of air while sucking. The infant can be burped as frequently as after every half-ounce of formula. Older infants can be burped after one to two ounces during feeding and at the conclusion of feeding. There are three methods of burping an infant.

🔓 Safety **ALERT**

Shake the bottle slightly to ensure that the formula is mixed well. Remove the plastic cap and place it on its side or with the clean inner side up. (The caps for disposable bottles used in hospitals are very lightweight and may fall over if placed upside down.) Invert the bottle and drop a few drops of formula on your wrist to check the temperature of the formula and patency of the nipple. Formula should drip freely, but not come out in a stream. If the formula runs out in a stream, change the nipple. Elevate the infant's head and shoulders slightly during feeding. Keep the nipple filled with formula at all times, to prevent ingestion of air. A steady stream of bubbles should rise in the bottle during feeding. If the infant pushes the nipple out with their tongue, reinsert it. This is a normal reflex and does not mean the infant is full or does not want to eat.

SUMMARY OF NURSING ASSISTANT RESPONSIBILITIES WHEN CARING FOR INFANTS

The overall responsibilities of nursing assistants who care for infants are to:

- Maintain a safe environment.
- Provide information through monitoring of vital signs (temperature, pulse, respiration), weight, length, intake, and output.
- Provide routine care such as bathing, feeding, and changing.
- Assist with treatments, examinations, and procedures.
- Provide warmth, security, and affection.

Observations of newborn infants to make and report are listed in Table 49-3.

TABLE 49-3 Observations of Newborn Infants to Make and Report

Temperature below 97.6°F (36.6°C)	Systolic blood pressure above 80 mm Hg
Temperature above 98.6°F (37.0°C)	Heel stick blood glucose below 40 mg/dL
Apical pulse below 110 when infant is at rest (not crying)	Fewer than 6 wet diapers in 24 hours
Apical pulse above 160 when infant is at rest (not crying)	Flaring of the nostrils
Respiratory rate below 30 when infant is at rest (not crying)	Nasal congestion
Respiratory rate above 60 when infant is at rest (not crying)	Drainage from eyes or ears
Noisy or grunting respirations	Bleeding from circumcision (more than a small amount)
Retractions when breathing (below the sternum, below the ribs, between the ribs, above the sternum, or above the clavicle)	Accepting less than 1 ounce of formula every 3 hours
Systolic blood pressure below 50 mm Hg	

EXPAND YOUR SKILLS

PROCEDURE **112** BOTTLE-FEEDING AN INFANT

1. Wash your hands.
2. Gather the infant's formula and diaper pad, washcloth, or bib.
3. Check the infant's identification band.
4. Pick up the infant and hold them in the crook of your arm, with the head slightly raised.
5. Sit in a chair or rocker.
6. Place a diaper, washcloth, or bib under the infant's chin, covering the chest.
7. You may wish to get a second cloth diaper to protect your own clothing. Place it on your shoulder when you burp the infant or hold it under the infant's chin if you are burping the infant while they are on your lap.
8. Tip the bottle so the nipple is filled with formula.
9. Stroke the side of the infant's cheek closest to you. The infant will automatically turn toward the side stroked and open their mouth. Place the nipple in the mouth.
10. If the nipple is in the mouth but the infant is not sucking, gently lift up under the infant's chin to close their mouth on the nipple.
11. Hold the bottle so the nipple stays filled with formula while the infant feeds (Figure 49-11).

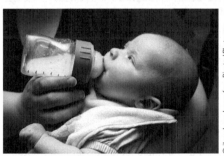
© jlgoodyear. Image from Bigstockphoto.com

FIGURE 49-11 Hold the infant with the head elevated during bottle-feeding. Keep the nipple filled with fluid while the infant sucks to prevent excess air in the stomach.

12. Feed the infant and burp as needed. (See Procedure 114.)
13. If the infant starts to vomit, remove the bottle and turn the infant to the side, with head lowered, to prevent aspiration. Seek help as needed.
14. After feeding, return the child to the crib and place them on their back or side.
15. Pull up the crib side.
16. Carry out ending procedure actions.
17. Record the amount of formula the infant took, according to hospital policy.

ICON KEY:
0 = OBRA

EXPAND YOUR SKILLS

PROCEDURE **113** ASSISTING WITH BREASTFEEDING

1. Wash your hands.
2. Gather supplies:
   - Disposable gloves
   - Sheet (or pillowcase for bassinette)
   - Blanket
   - Shirt
   - Diaper
   - Pad
3. Weigh the infant before the feeding, if this is your facility's policy.
4. Apply the principles of standard precautions as you would with an adult.
5. Instruct the mother to wash the breasts and hands. Provide supplies such as cotton balls moistened with normal saline or a medical-grade wipe, according to facility policy. Ask her to clean by using a circular motion from the nipples outward.
6. Assist the mother into a comfortable position facing the infant.
7. Instruct the mother to support the infant's head and neck.
8. Tell the mother to bring the baby to the breast. Position a pillow under the arm for support, if desired.
9. Help the baby latch on to the nipple. Gently brush the nipple across the cheek closest to the breast. This should cause the infant to turn toward the breast and open the mouth.
10. Wait for the mouth to open and for the tongue to extend.
11. Center the nipple and areola (dark area in the center of the breast) over the mouth.
12. Do not let the child latch on until the tongue is extended. (If the tongue is not extended, the jaw will clamp down on the nipple, which is painful.)
13. When positioned correctly, allow the infant to suck.
14. Instruct the mother to hold the breast back with a finger so the baby can breathe properly.
15. Allow the baby to nurse for 5 to 7 minutes if they have not stopped by then.
16. Place a finger near the infant's mouth and break the suction by placing a finger into the side of the mouth and moving the breast. Instruct the mother to burp the infant.
17. After the infant has burped, switch to the other breast.
18. Help the mother reposition the infant and get the baby started nursing on the opposite breast.
19. Allow the baby to nurse until they stop (usually five to seven minutes).
20. Break the suction, move the infant away from the breast, and burp again.
21. Weigh the infant and document your findings.
22. Change the diaper, shirt, and crib sheet, if needed.
23. Carry out ending procedure actions.

ICON KEY:

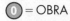 = OBRA

EXPAND YOUR SKILLS

PROCEDURE **114** BURPING AN INFANT

Burping (Method A)

1. Place a diaper or cloth over your shoulder.
2. Lift the infant up to your shoulder, holding the infant close to your chest (Figure 49-12A).
3. Holding the infant with one hand, use the other hand to gently rub or pat the infant's back until the infant burps.

Burping (Method B)

1. Place a diaper, cloth, or bib under the infant's chin.
2. Place the child in a sitting or upright position. Put one hand on the infant's chest and chin, supporting

the infant's weight (Figure 49-12B). With the other hand, gently rub or pat the infant's back until the infant burps.

Burping (Method C)

1. Place a diaper, cloth, or bib under the infant's chin.
2. Place a pillow across your lap.
3. Position the infant in the prone position. Put one hand under the chin and lift the head (Figure 49-12C). With the other hand, gently rub or pat the infant's back until the infant burps.

(continues)

PROCEDURE **114** **CONTINUED**   **0**

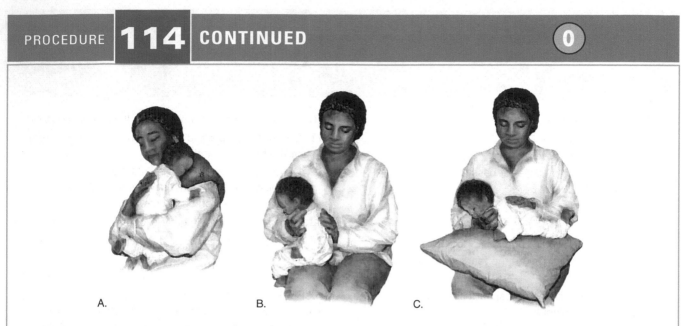

FIGURE 49-12 Burping positions: (A) Supported on the shoulder. (B) Upright on the lap. (C) Face down across the lap.

ICON KEY:

0 = OBRA

DISCHARGE

When delivery is uncomplicated, mothers and healthy newborns are usually able to go home from the hospital within two days. To carry out the discharge procedure:

- Match the baby's identification with the mother's.
- Dress the child in their own clothing.
- Wrap the baby in a blanket, using the technique of "papoosing," as shown in Figures 49-13A through 49-13D.
- Check to be sure that the mother has received and understands any special discharge instructions. If not, inform the nurse.

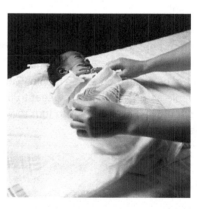

FIGURE 49-13B Fold one side corner over the infant.

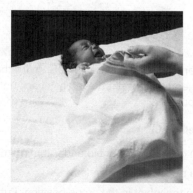

FIGURE 49-13A Position the receiving blanket under the infant so the corners are at the head and feet. Bring the bottom corner up over the infant.

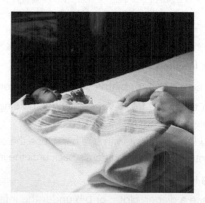

FIGURE 49-13C Bring the corner from the other side over the infant.

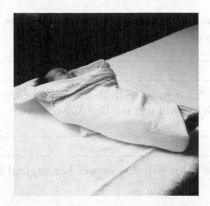

FIGURE 49-13D Tuck the final corner under the infant.

- Check to be sure equipment or needed formula is ready when the parents and newborn are ready to go home.
- Transport the mother, carrying her baby, by wheelchair to the discharge area. Make sure the infant is strapped into a properly secured car seat. Stay with them until they leave. Most facilities will not release an infant unless they are in a car seat that meets state requirements. Know and follow your facility's policies.
- Record the discharge information in the charts of both mother and child. Include the condition of each and the time of release.

REVIEW

A. True/False

Mark the following true or false by circling T or F.

1. T F   You are responsible for noting and reporting the first postpartum voiding.
2. T F   Care of the mother begins in the prenatal period.
3. T F   Immediate postpartum lochia should be yellowish-white.
4. T F   Standard precautions are not necessary when caring for a newborn.
5. T F   The shoulder hold is a safe way to hold and support an infant.
6. T F   The first feeding for the newborn is usually given 12 hours after birth.
7. T F   Assist the mother to wash her hands and nipples before she nurses the baby.

B. Matching

Choose the correct term from Column II to match each phrase in Column I.

Column I

8. _____ maintains an even temperature for the fetus
9. _____ mother's first postpartum breast secretions
10. _____ attachment between baby and placenta
11. _____ vaginal discharge following delivery

Column II

a. lochia
b. umbilical cord
c. fundus

d. lactation
e. colostrum
f. circumcision
g. isolette
h. placenta

C. Multiple Choice

Select the best answer for each of the following.

12. The doula:
    a. is a member of the clinical staff.
    b. actively assists with the birth.
    c. supports and comforts the mother.
    d. provides anesthesia, if needed.

13. The usual vaginal discharge after birth is called:
    a. lochia.
    b. menses.
    c. vernix.
    d. colostrum.

14. Immediately after birth, you would expect the vaginal drainage to be:
    a. brown.
    b. yellow.
    c. yellow-brown.
    d. red.

15. The temperature of a newborn infant is usually:
    a. elevated.
    b. stable.
    c. hypothermic.
    d. unstable.

16. The most desirable and accurate method for taking the infant's temperature is the:

    a. tympanic membrane method.

    b. axillary method.

    c. temporal artery method.

    d. rectal method.

17. The color of the newborn's first stool is expected to be:

    a. brown.

    b. black.

    c. yellow.

    d. red.

18. When caring for a new circumcision, you will wash the area, and then wipe it with:

    a. petroleum jelly.

    b. an alcohol sponge.

    c. disinfectant solution.

    d. povidone iodine.

19. When feeding a newborn infant, the formula and bottle should be:

    a. cold.

    b. clean.

    c. hot.

    d. sterile.

20. After feeding the infant, position her in the crib:

    a. on her abdomen.

    b. with the head elevated.

    c. on her back or side.

    d. with the feet elevated.

21. Burp the newborn infant after every _____ of breast milk or formula they drink drinks:

    a. half-ounce

    b. two ounces

    c. three ounces

    d. four ounces

D. Nursing Assistant Challenge

You are assisting Mrs. Acuff to the bathroom for the first time since she delivered her first child, a nine-pound infant. Answer the following questions.

22. What will you instruct the patient to do before removing the perineal pad?

    _____

    _____

23. You must instruct Mrs. Acuff to remove the perineal pad. What will you tell her?

    _____

    _____

24. Mrs. Acuff starts to flush the toilet before standing up. What will you tell her? Why?

    _____

    _____

25. What color will you expect her vaginal discharge to be?

    _____

    _____

You are working in a busy maternity unit with an average census of 27 per day. You notice the same visitor wandering about on the unit several days in a row. This woman is about 30 years old, short, and very overweight. She wears a ball cap or sunglasses so it is hard to see her face. She never seems to go to a patient's room to visit with any of the mothers. She ends her visit each day by standing at the nursery window for long periods of time watching the babies, and then leaves. Answer the following questions.

26. Is there anything suspicious about her behavior?

    _____

    _____

27. Is there anything about this visitor that fits the profile of a potential abductor?

    _____

    _____

28. Should you do anything about this situation? If so, what action will you take?

    _____

    _____

29. Will you inform the charge nurse about this visitor? If so, what will you report?

    _____

    _____

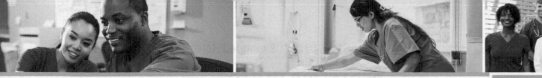

Pediatric Patients

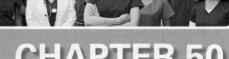

OBJECTIVES

After completing this chapter, you will be able to:

50.1 Spell and define terms.

50.2 Describe how to foster the growth and development of hospitalized pediatric patients.

50.3 Describe how to maintain a safe environment for the pediatric patient.

50.4 Discuss the problem of childhood obesity and identify special problems and complications that occur as a result of this condition.

50.5 Discuss the role of parents and siblings of the hospitalized pediatric patient.

50.6 Describe Munchausen by proxy syndrome (MBPS).

50.7 List signs and symptoms of physical, emotional, and sexual abuse and neglect.

50.8 Demonstrate the following procedures:

- Procedure 115: Admitting a Pediatric Patient (Expand Your Skills)

- Procedure 116: Weighing the Toddler to Adolescent (Expand Your Skills)
- Procedure 117: Changing Crib Linens (Expand Your Skills)
- Procedure 118: Changing Crib Linens (Infant in Crib) (Expand Your Skills)
- Procedure 119: Measuring Temperature (Expand Your Skills)
- Procedure 120: Determining Heart Rate (Pulse) (Expand Your Skills)
- Procedure 121: Counting Respiratory Rate (Expand Your Skills)
- Procedure 122: Measuring Blood Pressure (Expand Your Skills)
- Procedure 123: Collecting a Urine Specimen from an Infant (Expand Your Skills)

VOCABULARY

Learn the meaning and the correct spelling of the following words and phrases:

adolescence	developmental milestones	initiative	Munchausen by proxy
adoptive parent	developmental tasks	legal custody	syndrome (MBPS)
autonomy	family	legal guardian	regress
biological parent	foster parent		stepparent

INTRODUCTION

Children, like adults, get sick and need hospitalization for diagnosis and treatment of their illnesses. But children are different. They are not just small adults. Children differ in age, size, and developmental level. When you work with children, you will also be working with their parents or others who are responsible for their upbringing. When a child is sick and hospitalized, the illness affects the entire family. The family is an important part of the child's life regardless of age.

In today's society, the words *parents* and *family* can have different meanings. A child may live with one or both parents. The words *biological, adoptive, foster,* and *step* refer to the various types of parents that may be part of a child's family. The terms are defined as follows:

- **Biological parent**—birth (genetic) parent
- **Adoptive parent**—person who has legally assumed responsibility for parenting

959

- **Foster parent**—person who carries out parenting duties under the authority of a legal agency
- **Stepparent**—person who assumes the parenting role by marrying a birth or adoptive parent

Families may also include combinations of parents. For example, a child may live with a biological father and an adoptive mother or stepmother. Or a child may live with a single parent, who could be either biological, adoptive, or foster. Other family arrangements may include the child living with a relative while the parent maintains legal custody of the child. **Legal custody** refers to the person who has the right to give consent for hospitalization and for the procedures that may be needed while the child is hospitalized. This person is known as the **legal guardian**. The child may live with someone other than the legal guardian.

The word **family** refers to the household unit in which the child lives. Members of the family may include the parents, siblings (biological, adoptive, foster, or step), and/or other relatives or persons in the household (Figure 50-1).

As a member of the health care team, it is important for you to identify the child's caregivers as well as who has legal custody. Depending on the child's age, some hospitals require at least one family member to remain at the hospital during the child's stay. This person may be required to stay in the room at all times and cannot leave the child alone.

This unit provides guidelines for care of the hospitalized child. Hospitalization may interrupt the child's normal growth and development. This can be a traumatic time for the child. Assist with and encourage the child's development during hospitalization.

Safety is an important part of providing care. This chapter presents guidelines for creating a safe environment for each pediatric age group. Because families are important, suggestions are also made for creating a family-centered approach to pediatric health care.

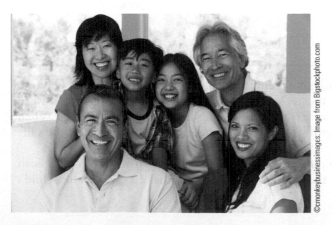

FIGURE 50-1 The family is the child's household unit.

PEDIATRIC UNITS

Pediatric units are typically set up in one of two ways:

- By specific age groups of children
- By types of patient, such as surgical, orthopedic, or cardiac

When a child is admitted to the hospital, you may be involved in the admission procedure. A nurse will obtain a medical and social history from the parents. Once the history is complete, you can continue with the admission procedure.

This chapter gives guidelines for caring for children by age groups:

- Infancy (birth–2 years)
- Toddler (2–3 years)
- Preschooler (3–5 years)
- School-age (5–12 years)
- Adolescent (12–20 years)

DEVELOPMENTAL TASKS

For each age group, it is expected that the child will have reached a certain developmental level. Each level is characterized by physical and psychological tasks that the average child in the group can perform. Review the developmental tasks for the pediatric age groups in Chapter 9. It will be easier to find ways to promote the child's development if you understand the **developmental tasks** for each age group. The approaches suggested here should be personalized for each patient. Some children may appear younger than their stated age due to medical and/or emotional problems. It is also normal for children to **regress** (go backward) when hospitalized.

CARING FOR INFANTS (BIRTH–2 YEARS)

During the first year of life, the normal infant will:

- Double the birth length
- Triple the birth weight
- Show progress in gaining mastery over gross motor behavior, beginning with the head and moving down the trunk toward the feet

The physical development of a normal infant begins by gaining head control (Figure 50-2). The infant then progresses to rolling over, sitting up, crawling, and walking. These motor skills generally occur within specific weeks or months of the infant's life. Achievement of these skills is referred to as reaching the infant's **developmental milestones**.

EXPAND YOUR SKILLS

PROCEDURE **115** **ADMITTING A PEDIATRIC PATIENT**

1. Carry out initial procedure actions.

2. Introduce yourself and escort the child and parents to the child's room and familiarize them with the unit.

3. Explain what you will do.

4. Wash your hands.

5. Place an identification band on the child.

6. Dress the child in their own pajamas or hospital clothing.

7. Obtain the child's height and weight. Record according to facility policy.

8. Measure the child's vital signs.

9. Obtain a urine specimen.

10. Wash your hands.

11. Assist the physician or nurse with examination of the child as necessary.

12. Explain rooming-in and visiting policies to the parents. Comfort the child if parents leave.

13. Carry out ending procedure actions.

ICON KEY:

 = OBRA

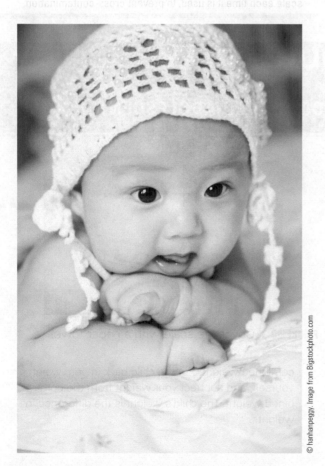

FIGURE 50-2 A picture of an infant who is able to lift the head but does not have the ability to turn over yet.

© hanhanpeggy. Image from Bigstockphoto.com

Communication **ALERT**

An infant's senses of touch and hearing are important. Babies are naturally curious. Talk to babies when you are giving care. Although the infant will not understand the words you are speaking, a tone of calm reassurance in your voice makes the baby feel safe.

Learning to trust is the primary psychosocial developmental task for the infant. All infants depend on others for survival; other people must meet all of the infant's basic needs. How the infant's needs are met lays the foundation for the infant's developing personality.

Typically, the mother is the caregiver and prime source for developing trust. However, when the infant is hospitalized, the hospital staff may assume the role of substitute parent. A caregiver can continue to develop the infant's trust by responding to their cry and needs. Trust is fostered by feeding, holding, touching, and talking to the infant, in addition to keeping them warm and dry.

Communicating with Infants

Working with infants can be challenging because the infant communicates with their cry and body movements. The cry can vary depending on needs. Infants respond to voices, faces, and touch. Talk to the infant whenever you are giving personal care such as bathing, feeding, or holding.

The Waking Hours

When the infant is awake, they need to explore the environment. Provide age-appropriate toys such as colorful mobiles, rattles, and mirrors so that the infant can continue development while in the hospital.

Importance of Families

Siblings of the infant should be allowed to visit while the infant is hospitalized. Toddlers and preschoolers engage in "magical thinking." In other words, they believe that if they wish the infant to be sick, it happens, or if they wish the baby to be gone, they won't be back. Therefore, it is important for both toddlers and preschoolers to see their infant sibling. If a parent is rooming-in with the infant, it is also important for toddlers and preschoolers to see and talk to that parent.

Routine Procedures

When carrying out routine care, hold the infant properly. (Refer to Chapter 49.)

Organize care before feeding so the infant can digest the food and sleep. Moving the infant unnecessarily may cause them to vomit what they have just eaten. Organize the care in this order:

1. Bathe
2. Diaper
3. Dress
4. Change the crib linens
5. Weigh
6. Feed

The routine procedures covered here may apply to all pediatric patients. They include taking vital signs, measuring weight, bottle-feeding, and changing crib linens.

Weighing the Infant

Routine care includes weighing the child. For an infant, this procedure should also be done before feeding. Refer to Chapter 49, Procedure 109.

> **NOTE**
>
> Put clean paper on the scale before using it. Balance the scale with the paper in place. Keep your hand on the infant to prevent accidents. Lift it quickly to measure the weight. Work quickly to prevent heat loss in the infant. Disinfect the scale each time it is used, to prevent cross-contamination.

EXPAND YOUR SKILLS

PROCEDURE 116   WEIGHING THE TODDLER TO ADOLESCENT

1. Use an upright or bathroom scale if the child is able to stand. Place a paper towel on the scale and balance it (Figure 50-3).

2. Wash your hands.

3. Check the child's identification band.

4. Check the child's previous weight.

5. Weigh the child in as few clothes as possible. Remove any diaper and shoes or slippers.

6. Have the child stand on the paper towel. Move the bar until the scale balances.

7. Record the weight according to facility policy.

8. Return the child to bed.

9. Return the scale to its proper storage place.

10. Wash your hands.

Alternate action: If the child is unable to stand on their own, pick them up and step on the scale. Obtain the

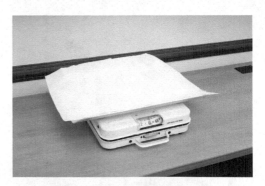

FIGURE 50-3 Cover the scale with a paper towel.

combined weight. Put the child back in bed, weigh yourself, and subtract your weight from the combined weight. The child's weight is the difference in weights.

ICON KEY:

 = OBRA

EXPAND YOUR SKILLS

PROCEDURE **117** **CHANGING CRIB LINENS**

1. Wash your hands.
2. Gather supplies:
   - Disposable gloves
   - Sheet
   - Blanket
   - Shirt
   - Diaper
   - Pad
3. When bathing the infant, apply the principles of standard precautions as you would with an adult.
4. After bathing the infant, diaper and dress them.
5. Place the infant in a stroller, playpen, or other safe place.
6. Strip the linens from the crib. Wear gloves if linens are soiled. Dispose of soiled or used linens according to facility policy.
7. Remove your gloves and discard them according to facility policy.
8. Wash your hands.
9. Place clean linens on the bed and open the sheet, hem side down.
10. Make one side of the crib; miter the corners top and bottom, and tuck in the side (Figure 50-4A).
11. Pull down the crib top (Figure 50-4B). Pull up the crib side (Figure 50-4C).

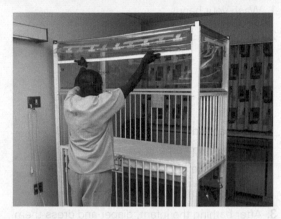

FIGURE 50-4B Pull the crib top down.

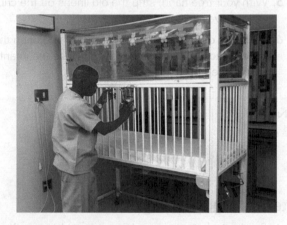

FIGURE 50-4C Pull the side up and check for security.

12. Repeat step 10 on the opposite side of the crib.
13. Place a diaper pad on top of the sheet, according to facility policy.
14. Place a clean blanket at the bottom of the bed.
15. Wash your hands.
16. Return the infant to the crib, cover them with the blanket (if appropriate), and pull up the crib side.

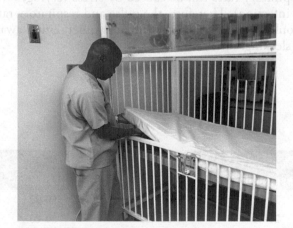

FIGURE 50-4A Make one side of the crib. Miter corners at the top and bottom and tuck under mattress.

ICON KEY:

O = OBRA

EXPAND YOUR SKILLS

PROCEDURE 118   CHANGING CRIB LINENS (INFANT IN CRIB)

1. Wash your hands.

2. Gather linens:
   - Sheet
   - Blanket
   - Shirt
   - Diaper
   - Diaper pad
   - Bathing equipment
   - Disposable gloves

   Do steps 1 and 2 before bathing the infant.

3. After bathing the infant, diaper and dress them.

4. Pick up the infant and hold them in one arm.

5. With your free hand, strip the old linens off the crib. Wear gloves if linens are soiled.

6. Place the clean linens on the mattress and open the sheet, placing the hem side down. Place the infant on the sheet.

7. Place one hand on the infant and keep it on them at all times.

8. Make one side of the crib. Miter the corners, top and bottom, and tuck in the side.

9. Remove your hand from the infant and pull up the crib side.

10. Go around to the other side of the crib.

11. Take down the crib side, place one hand on the infant, and repeat step 8.

12. Place a diaper pad under the infant and cover them with the blanket, if appropriate.

13. Pull up the crib side.

14. Wash your hands.

ICON KEY:

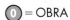 = OBRA

Determining Vital Signs

The infant's vital signs must be measured, as outlined in the care plan. It is normal for an infant's heart to beat faster than an adult's. The normal ranges of heart rates and respiratory rates for each age group are listed in Table 50-1. An increase in the infant's heart and respiratory rates can be caused by stress (crying, fever, or infection). Therefore, the pulse and respiratory rates should be taken when the infant is quiet, either awake or sleeping.

TABLE 50-1 Normal Vital Signs

Age	Temperature	Heart Rate	Respirations	Blood Pressure	
				Systolic	Diastolic
Infants	99.4–99.7	120–160	30–60	74–100	50–70
Toddlers	99–99.7	90–140	24–40	80–112	50–80
Preschoolers	98.6–99	80–110	22–34	82–110	50–78
School-age	98.1–98.6	75–100	18–30	84–119	54–80
Adolescents	97.8–98	60–90	12–24	94–119	62–88

Note: Pulse and respiration are taken for a full minute. The apical pulse is used with infants and young children.

EXPAND YOUR SKILLS

PROCEDURE **119** **MEASURING TEMPERATURE**

Temperatures of children five years of age and younger are usually taken rectally or by the tympanic, temporal artery, or axillary methods. Temperatures are less stable in children and vary slightly with the age of the child. Measure all other vital signs on the pediatric patient before taking the rectal temperature. Select an electronic or digital thermometer.

Rectal Temperature

1. Wash your hands and put on gloves.

2. Check the patient's identification band.

3. Explain to the parents and child what you are going to do.

4. Cover the thermometer with a disposable sheath.

5. Lubricate the thermometer sheath, if it is not prelubricated.

6. Lay the child on their back on bed (Figure 50-5A) or on their stomach across your lap (Figure 50-5B).

7. Insert the thermometer 1/2 inch into the child's rectum and hold. Hold the child securely and gently so the child does not move about.

8. Leave the thermometer in place for the required amount of time (three to eight minutes). Follow your facility's policy for the type of thermometer you are using.

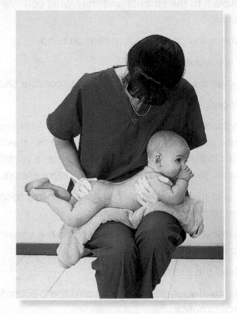

FIGURE 50-5B Infant in prone position.

9. Remove the thermometer when indicated. Discard the sheath according to facility policy.

> 🔓 Safety **ALERT**
>
> Check with the nurse before taking a rectal temperature on a newborn infant. The first rectal temperature must be taken by the nurse, to ensure that the rectum is patent. After that, axillary or tympanic temperature may be the method of choice. Know and follow your facility's policy. When taking a rectal temperature, grasp the child's ankles gently, but firmly, with one hand. Cover the penis of a male infant with a diaper. Insert the lubricated thermometer sheath while holding the ankles. Continue to hold the ankles with one hand and the thermometer with the other throughout the procedure.

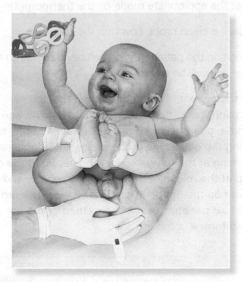

FIGURE 50-5A Infant in supine position.

10. Remove your gloves and wash your hands.

11. Read the thermometer and record the value.

12. Report any deviations from normal according to facility policy.

(continues)

PROCEDURE 119 CONTINUED

Oral Temperature

1. Explain to the parents and child what you will be doing.
2. Check the patient's identification band.
3. Wash your hands.
4. Cover the thermometer with a disposable sheath.
5. Apply gloves.
6. Instruct the child to hold the thermometer under their tongue. If the child cannot hold the thermometer in their mouth, then obtain either a rectal, tympanic, temporal artery, or axillary temperature.
7. Leave the thermometer under the child's tongue for the required amount of time.
8. Remove the thermometer. Discard the sheath according to facility policy.
9. Read the thermometer.
10. Remove your gloves and discard them according to facility policy.
11. Wash your hands.
12. Record the temperature.
13. Report any deviations from normal according to facility policy.

Axillary Temperature

1. Explain to the parents and child what you are going to do.
2. Check the patient's identification band.
3. Wash your hands.
4. Cover the thermometer with a disposable sheath.
5. Place the thermometer in the child's armpit.
6. Hold the child's arm close to their chest for the required amount of time.
7. Remove the thermometer. Discard the sheath according to facility policy.
8. Read the thermometer.
9. Wash your hands and record the temperature value.
10. Report any deviations from normal according to facility policy.

 NOTE

If an electronic thermometer is used, follow the manufacturer's directions supplied with the equipment.

Tympanic Temperature

1. Explain to the parents and child what you are going to do.
2. Check the patient's identification band.
3. Wash your hands.
4. Check the lens on the thermometer to make sure it is clean and intact.

Age-Appropriate Care ALERT

When a tympanic thermometer is used for children under age three, pull the pinna down and back. In children over age three, pull the pinna up and back. This straightens the ear canal, enabling the sensor to detect heat in the eardrum. When the probe is positioned correctly, the probe tip will point at the midpoint between the eyebrow and sideburn on the opposite side of the face.

5. Set the appropriate mode on the thermometer.
6. Place a clean probe cover on the probe.
7. Position the patient so you will have access to the ear you will be using.
8. If the patient is under age three, pull the ear straight back, then down. In children over age three, pull the ear up and back. While gently tugging the ear, fit the probe snugly into the canal, aiming at the tympanic membrane. Point the probe tip at the midpoint between the eyebrow and sideburn on the opposite side of the face. The probe tip should penetrate at least one-third of the ear canal and form a complete seal.

(continues)

NOTE

Tympanic thermometers measure temperature by aiming an infrared light beam on the tympanic membrane. Light does not go around corners. If the ear canal is not fully straightened when the thermometer is inserted, the value will not be accurate. Because of this, step 8 is very important to the accuracy of this procedure.

9. Press the activation button. Leave the thermometer in place until the display blinks or signals that the temperature is final.

10. Remove the thermometer. Discard the probe cover.

11. Wash your hands and record the temperature.

12. Report any deviations from normal according to facility policy.

Temporal Artery Temperature

 NOTE

The guidelines for this procedure vary slightly from state to state, and from one facility to the next. Your instructor will inform you if the sequence in your state or facility differs from the procedure listed here. Know and follow the required sequence for your facility and state.

1. Carry out initial procedure actions.

2. Assemble equipment:
   – Disposable gloves if there may be contact with blood or body fluids, open lesions, or wet linens (gloves are not necessary unless required by facility policy or potential exposure to body fluids)

   – Temporal artery thermometer
   – Probe covers, alcohol sponges, or disinfectant wipes

3. Check the lens to make sure it is clean and intact.

4. Apply a clean probe cover, or wipe the probe with alcohol or a disinfectant wipe.

5. Hold the thermometer as you would a pencil or pen. Gently press the probe (head) of the thermometer against the center of the forehead. Push the switch to the on position with your thumb. Keep this button depressed.

6. Slowly move the probe across the forehead to the hairline on the other side of the head.

7. Push the hair back slightly with the opposite hand, if needed, then lift the probe slightly. Quickly place the probe down just behind the ear lobe on the neck. (Use the area in which perfume is usually applied.) Release the button and remove the thermometer. Note and remember the value on the digital display. The value should remain on the display for about 30 seconds before disappearing.

8. Discard the disposable probe cover, or wipe the probe with an alcohol or disinfectant wipe.

9. Record the temperature on your pad.

10. Carry out ending procedure actions.

ICON KEY:
 = OBRA

EXPAND YOUR SKILLS

PROCEDURE **120** DETERMINING HEART RATE (PULSE)

With infants and children, the easiest way to find the heart rate is to place the stethoscope over the heart (Figure 50-6). This is called the *apical pulse*. It should be done when the child is quiet or at rest because stress and crying can result in a reading that is higher than normal.

1. Wash your hands.

2. Check the patient's identification band.

3. Explain the procedure to the patient and/or their parents. Clean stethoscope earpieces and diaphragm with an antiseptic wipe and allow them to air dry. (Allow a child to play with the stethoscope first, if awake.)

4. Rub the diaphragm of the stethoscope to warm it so that it will not be cold when placed on the child's chest.

5. Place the stethoscope over the child's heart and count the number of beats (1 lub-dub = 1 beat) you hear in a minute.

6. Clean the stethoscope earpieces and diaphragm with an antiseptic wipe and allow them to air dry before using the instrument again.

7. Wash your hands and record the results.

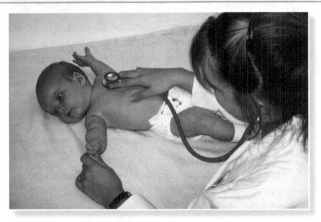

FIGURE 50-6 Measuring the apical pulse.

8. Report rates higher or lower than normal for the appropriate age group, according to facility policy.

 NOTE

The radial pulse can be used for children six years and older. The procedure used is the same as for adults. Refer to Procedure 36 in Chapter 19.

EXPAND YOUR SKILLS

PROCEDURE **121** COUNTING RESPIRATORY RATE

Infants and toddlers use their abdominal muscles for breathing. To count the respiratory rate for this age group, look at the abdomen and chest and count the respirations for a full minute.

To obtain the respiratory rate for preschoolers and older children, follow Procedure 38 in Chapter 19, as for adults, but count the respirations for a full minute.

ICON KEY:

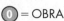 = OBRA

EXPAND YOUR SKILLS

PROCEDURE 122 | MEASURING BLOOD PRESSURE

A blood pressure measurement is not usually required for pediatric patients. If blood pressure is to be recorded, you must have the correct size cuff for the child. The cuff should cover two-thirds of the upper arm.

1. Select the correct cuff size for the patient. The child may have a disposable cuff of the correct size in the room.

2. Assemble all equipment. Clean stethoscope earpieces and diaphragm with an antiseptic wipe and allow them to air dry.

3. Wash your hands.

4. Check the patient's identification band.

5. Explain the procedure to the child, using language such as "This will feel like a tight hug on your arm."

6. Wrap the cuff securely around the upper arm.

7. Feel for the brachial pulse.

8. Place the stethoscope earpieces in your ears and place the diaphragm near the pulse point.

9. Pump up the cuff until you no longer hear the pulse. Release the valve and listen for systolic and diastolic sounds.

10. Wash your hands and record the results according to facility policy.

ICON KEY:

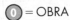 = OBRA

Collecting a Urine Specimen

Urine specimens are needed for various diagnostic tests. Knowing about a urinary tract infection is very important; in infants and small children, the presence of a UTI may indicate an abnormality that was not identified previously. When collecting a specimen from an older child, use the same procedures as those that are used for adults (Chapter 45). To collect a urine specimen from infants and toddlers who are not toilet-trained, use a self-adhesive pediatric urine collection bag (Figure 50-7).

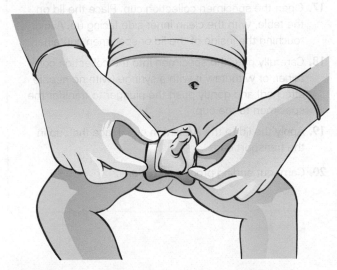

FIGURE 50-7 A pediatric urine collection device has an adhesive backing. The hole in the bag is placed over the external urinary meatus.

👪 Age-Appropriate Care **ALERT**

The pediatric urine collection device is fastened to the perineum with a self-adhesive surface. It should not be used for children with diaper rash or inflamed or broken skin, or for those who are allergic to adhesive tape. If any of these conditions exists, check with the nurse before proceeding. If a clean specimen is needed, another option may be to place several sterile cotton balls directly over the external urinary meatus and then replace the diaper. After the child has voided, collect and use the urine squeezed from the cotton balls into a specimen cup (with your gloved hands). If using the pediatric collection bag or cotton balls is not possible, try applying a disposable diaper inside out. After the child voids, remove the diaper carefully. Pour the urine from the plastic outer surface (which is facing inside) into a specimen collection cup or test tube.

After the child voids, empty the contents of the bag into a specimen collection cup. In some facilities, the specimen is withdrawn into a syringe, then transferred into a urine specimen cup. Some facilities cap the syringe and send it to the lab as is. Follow your facility's policy for specimen handling. Because an infant or toddler cannot urinate on demand, it is a good idea to give the child fluids that they like every 15 to 30 minutes until the specimen is collected.

To keep the urine collection bag in place, make sure the skin is clean, dry, and free of lotions, oils, and powder. Remove the backing from the tape and position the opening over the penis in the male and the labia in the female. Press gently to secure the adhesive. Replace the diaper. Remove the collection bag after the child voids. Carefully pour the contents of the bag into a specimen collection cup. Sometimes the bag becomes dislodged, especially if the infant is active. If you cannot collect a specimen on the first attempt, try again. If you are unsuccessful after two tries, inform the nurse. Ask for the nurse's permission before using other techniques.

EXPAND YOUR SKILLS

PROCEDURE 123 COLLECTING A URINE SPECIMEN FROM AN INFANT

1. Wash your hands.

2. Assemble supplies:
   - At least 2 pairs of disposable gloves
   - Soap and water, or cleanser used by facility
   - Cotton balls or washcloth to cleanse perineum
   - Towel
   - Clean diaper
   - Bed protector
   - Plastic bag
   - Pediatric urine collection bag
   - Syringe to withdraw specimen from collection bag, if this is facility policy
   - Urine specimen cup with label(s)
   - Transport bag

3. Remove the infant's diaper.

4. Wash the perineum with soap and water. Make sure to remove powder or ointment.

5. Rinse the perineum and dry well.

6. Discard the used diaper, cotton balls, and other used supplies in the plastic bag.

7. Apply the urine collection bag by removing the paper backing to expose the adhesive and positioning the center of the hole in the bag over the external urinary meatus in a female, or over the penis in a male.

8. Gently press the bag in place to seal the adhesive.

9. Reapply the diaper, leaving the bag unfolded. In some facilities, the bag is pulled through to the outside of the diaper, or a hole is cut in the diaper so the bag can be pulled through to the outside.

10. Remove your gloves and discard them in the plastic bag.

11. Wash your hands.

12. Prepare the specimen labels and attach them to the specimen cup and transport bag, or according to facility policy. Set aside.

13. Remove the collection device immediately after the child voids.

14. Place the collection device on a bed protector or other clean area. Put the bag down and position the hole in the center carefully to avoid spilling the contents.

15. Cleanse the infant's perineum and apply a clean diaper.

16. Leave the infant in a position of comfort and safety.

17. Open the specimen collection cup. Place the lid on the table, with the clean inner side facing up. Avoid touching the inside of the lid or specimen container.

18. Carefully pour the specimen into the collection container, or withdraw it with a syringe (with no needle attached) and gently push the plunger to transfer the specimen to the cup.

19. Apply the lid to the specimen cup. Place the cup in the transport bag.

20. Carry out ending procedure actions.

ICON KEY:
 = OBRA   ℗ = PPE

Feeding

Feeding satisfies the infant's hunger and sucking needs. Sucking provides the infant with a pleasant sensation, whether they receive food with their sucking or not. The amount of time an infant needs to suckle varies with the child. Provide the opportunity to suck even if the infant cannot eat.

When feeding an infant:

- Hold the infant unless there is a medical reason not to. Holding the infant during a feeding allows close, physical contact with the person feeding them.
- If an infant cannot be held, you should still hold the bottle for them while they eat.
- Never leave an infant in a crib with a bottle propped in the mouth. This practice increases the risk of choking.
- Burp the infant during and after feeding.
- Carefully position the infant on their back or side when they have has finished eating.

> **NOTE**
>
> If an infant cannot be fed, they should still be held and allowed to suck on a pacifier unless a medical reason prevents removal of the infant from the crib.

Summary of Nursing Assistant Tasks and Responsibilities when Caring for Infants

- Maintain a safe environment.
- Provide information to the health care team through monitoring of vital signs (temperature, pulse, respirations), weight, and intake and output.
- Provide routine care such as bathing, feeding, and changing.
- Collect and test specimens.
- Assist with treatments, examinations, and procedures.
- Provide warmth, security, and affection.

CARING FOR TODDLERS (2–3 YEARS)

The second and third years of life can be a difficult time for a child to be hospitalized. This is the age when a child is trying to be independent and in control. The child:

- Increases motor coordination
- Becomes more verbal
- Becomes more curious about the world

At the same time, their parents are trying to toilet-train them. They also are beginning to set limits on the child's behavior. The developmental task for the toddler is **autonomy** (independent action).

Allow the toddler as much independence and choice as possible (within facility policy guidelines). Avoid situations that could create a struggle between the caregiver and the child. Expect delays when the toddler is feeding themselves or bathing. Be sure to allow enough time to do these activities.

The Hospital Environment

When a toddler is hospitalized, it is important to provide an environment that allows as much independence and control as possible while ensuring safety. An example of this is the choice of bed (or crib) for the toddler. If a crib is to be used, it should have a top and sides to prevent the child from climbing out and possibly falling. If the child has been sleeping in a bed at home, then it is more appropriate to provide a child-sized hospital bed with side rails, if available. Facility policies vary, so check your facility's policy with reference to toddlers.

If the child is toilet-trained, it is important to know the words they use for urination and bowel movements. It is also important to know if the child uses a potty chair or the toilet at home. You should try to provide the same arrangement for toileting in the hospital. It is not uncommon for a hospitalized child to regress and return to a previous stage of development. You should not be surprised if a toddler who is toilet-trained starts to have "accidents" while in the hospital. Do not scold the child if this happens.

GUIDELINES 50-1 Guidelines for Ensuring a Safe Environment for Infants

- Always keep crib side rails up.
- Always keep one hand on the infant when a crib side rail is down.
- Use crib bumpers to prevent injury. Some laws prohibit the sale of certain non-mesh crib bumper pads and restricts their use in certain facilities and places of public accommodation, unless a medical professional has

determined a bumper pad is medically necessary for a particular child.

- Never tie balloons or toys to cribs.
- Never use toys with small removable parts or pointed objects.
- Never prop bottles.
- Never tape pacifiers in an infant's mouth.

The Toddler's Need for Autonomy

The toddler is learning to be independent. They may want to feed, dress, and wash themselves while in the hospital. You will be responsible for helping the toddler with these activities. Give toddlers independence. At the same time, you must keep them safe. For example, when bathing a toddler in the bathtub, you must never leave them alone, even for a minute. Check the water temperature before putting the toddler in the bathtub.

Emotional Reaction to Illness

Another important area in the care of toddlers concerns their feelings of responsibility for their own illnesses. Stress that the illness is not the toddler's or anyone else's fault.

To overcome anxiety about routine procedures, allow the toddler to handle equipment whenever possible. A few extra minutes spent familiarizing the toddler with the equipment to be used may make the difference between a frightened child and an interested one (Figure 50-8).

The toddler will have a difficult time if separated from the primary caregiver. One way to prevent this is to permit the parent to room-in. If this cannot happen, either because a parent cannot stay or because facility policy does not permit it, then parents should be encouraged to visit frequently. If a parent is not going to stay, reassure the child that they will not be alone and do all you can to make them feel safe.

Age-Appropriate Care **ALERT**

The child's room and unit playroom should be viewed as "safe places." When painful treatments are necessary, use a special treatment room in the unit or take the child to another area of the hospital for the procedure.

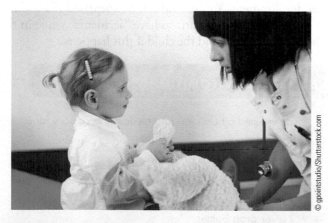

FIGURE 50-8 A hospitalized toddler may be more secure in the environment after having a chance to play with the equipment.

Routine Activities

Routines are important to toddlers. Ask the parents to describe the child's normal day. Try to follow the child's usual schedule as much as possible for eating, naps, toileting, and other activities. Toddlers love to play but, because they have short attention spans, they cannot play with one toy for a long time. Plan a variety of activities to keep the toddler amused.

Educational toys that teach how to dress, button, and zip can also be fun for the toddler. Stethoscopes, masks, and gloves make good hospital toys because they can allow the toddler to work out their fears. Do not leave the child alone with these items, because of the risk of accident or injury.

Toddlers will not play together, but they will play near or next to each other.

Temper tantrums are common with toddlers. If they occur, ignore the tantrum as long as the child cannot hurt themselves, or others. If a toddler is misbehaving, set limits in a firm, consistent manner.

When working with the toddler, remember that they are trying to be independent. Allow the toddler as much choice as possible. For example, at snack time, ask if they want an apple or a cracker. If no choice can be given, be firm and say what will occur (e.g., "It's time to take your nap now"). It is best to be truthful and to give simple explanations to toddlers. If the child is having a blood test, tell them just before it happens. It does not do any good to prepare toddlers in advance because they have very little concept of time. Such advance warning only increases their anxiety.

The toddler has great natural curiosity and loves to explore. It is important to maintain a safe environment in the hospital.

Summary of Nursing Assistant Tasks and Responsibilities when Caring for Toddlers

- Maintain a safe environment.
- Apply standard precautions if contact with blood, body fluids, mucous membranes, or nonintact skin is likely.
- Provide information to the health care team through monitoring of vital signs (temperature, pulse, and respirations), weight, and intake and output.
- Supervise and assist with routine care such as bathing, feeding, and dressing.
- Collect and test specimens.
- Assist with treatments, examinations, and procedures.
- Provide and assist with opportunities for play (Figure 50-9).

GUIDELINES 50-2 Guidelines for Ensuring a Safe Environment for Toddlers

- Keep cleaning products and other poisonous liquids in a locked container or cabinet.
- Store chemicals, disinfectants, and similar products away from food and beverages.
- Make sure that accessible electrical sockets have protective covers.
- Never leave toddlers alone in the bathtub or bathroom.

- Keep crib sides and side rails up when the toddler is in bed.
- Never allow toddlers to play with balloons unless supervised.
- Avoid toys with sharp edges, long strings, or small removable parts.
- Keep doors to utility rooms, housekeeping closets, kitchens, treatment areas, and storage areas closed and locked whenever possible.

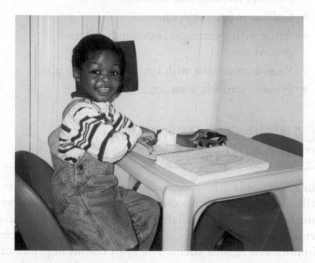

FIGURE 50-9 Toddlers and preschool children often enjoy playing with cars, trucks, and toys with wheels.

- Provide warmth, security, and affection.
- Promote independence by providing opportunities for choices.

CARING FOR PRESCHOOL-AGE CHILDREN (4–6 YEARS)

Between the ages of four and six years, the child's language, fine motor skills, and gross motor skills continue to increase with activity. The preschooler becomes more independent, but the primary developmental task for the age group is **initiative** (doing things themselves). The preschooler needs their independence, but they still need to feel safe and secure. Provide a balance of independence and control.

Emotional Reactions to Illness

Preschoolers normally have many fears. One fear is that their body parts will be injured or changed. For example, a preschooler may fear that body parts will fall out when

a bandage is removed. Use simple, honest explanations when telling the preschooler what to expect.

Fear of the dark and of being alone are other normal fears for a preschooler. You can help reduce this fear by leaving a nightlight on. Another child in the room can also ease fears. Be sure to leave the call signal within reach. Sitting with the child until they fall asleep will also help. Like the toddler, the preschooler can benefit from having their primary caregiver room-in, because they still fear separation.

"Magical thinking" and fantasy are still present in this age group. Stress to the preschooler that it is not their fault that they are sick and that they are not sick because they were bad. The preschooler needs to know that they will return home. They will not be forgotten and left in the hospital. Siblings should be allowed and encouraged to visit (Figure 50-10). In addition to easing separation from the family, this can also be a way of assuring the child that no one is taking their place at home.

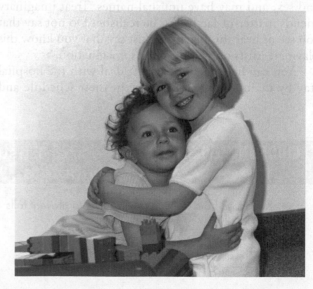

FIGURE 50-10 Having siblings visit the hospitalized child is important.

Explaining Procedures

When telling a preschooler what to expect, simple, honest explanations work best. Choose your words carefully because the preschooler takes things literally (exactly as said).

- If surgery is being planned, show and tell the child what parts of their body will be involved.
- Use time references that are familiar to the child (such as mealtime, nap time, or the time of a favorite TV show). For example, if the child is scheduled for an X-ray in the late morning, tell them that they will have it after breakfast or before lunch.
- Explain what you are going to do. Avoid assuming that the child will remember what you told them before.
- The preschooler needs to maintain some control. Offer choices and allow them to make as many decisions as possible. Encourage independence with care to the extent possible.

Activities

Imagination and fantasy are part of the preschooler's world. Imaginary playmates are normal for the preschooler. These playmates may find their way to the hospital with the child. The playmates can vary in age and sex, and may have unusual names. Treat imaginary friends matter-of-factly, but be realistic. Do not say that you see or hear this playmate. Just say that you know this playmate exists only in the child's imagination.

You can help the preschooler deal with the hospital stay by maintaining consistency in their schedule and setting the limits on their behavior. Use positive reinforcers such as hugs or stickers for appropriate behavior. Behavior that is rewarded is likely to be repeated.

Summary of Nursing Assistant Tasks and Responsibilities when Caring for Preschoolers

- Maintain a safe environment.
- Apply standard precautions if contact with blood, body fluids, mucous membranes, or nonintact skin is likely.
- Supervise and assist with routine care such as bathing, feeding, and dressing.
- Collect and test specimens.
- Assist with treatments, examinations, and procedures.
- Provide and assist with opportunities for play.
- Provide warmth, security, and affection.

CARING FOR SCHOOL-AGE CHILDREN (6–12 YEARS)

In general, the school-age years are a time of exceptionally good health. School-age children are more active, stronger, and steadier than younger children. They have either had most of the childhood illnesses or have been immunized against them. The most common problems of these times involve the gastrointestinal system (e.g., stomach aches) and the respiratory system (e.g., colds and coughs).

Developmental Tasks

In this period, the child is striving to achieve a sense of accomplishment through an increasing number of tasks and completion of projects. They also continue to increase control over their environment and their independence. It is important to remember these tasks when caring for the school-age child.

GUIDELINES 50-3 Guidelines for Ensuring a Safe Environment for Preschoolers

- Keep toys from cluttering walkways, to prevent falls.
- Keep side rails on the bed up at night.
- Keep the bed in low position.
- Keep doors to kitchen and storage areas closed.

- Keep a nightlight on.
- Never leave the child unattended in the tub.
- Never allow children to run with popsicles or lollipops in their mouths.

The school-age child's reaction to hospitalization will be significantly different from that of the younger child. The school-age child is better able to handle the stress of illness and hospitalization. In fact, hospitalization presents the school-age child with an opportunity to:

- Explore a new environment
- Meet new friends
- Learn more about their body

Psychosocial Adjustment

Separation from parents will not be as difficult for the school-age child. However, those just entering this period may regress to a preschool level. These children will need their parents' presence.

The school-age child has left the security of home and entered the school system, where they have has begun to develop relationships with other children. Because of this, they may respond more to the separation from peers than from parents. Help them communicate with schoolmates by writing letters and making phone calls.

Roommate selection is especially important for this age group. A roommate will act as a diversion and enable the child to work on the developmental task of learning to get along with others. The school-age child is seeking more independence and may be reluctant to ask for help even when they need it. Their feelings may show themselves in different ways, such as:

- Irritability
- Hostility toward their siblings
- Other behavior problems

If you observe these behaviors, inform the nurse.

Resistance to bedtime may also become a problem during these years. In the hospital, it is important to be aware of the parents' rules and follow them. Learning rules is another developmental task of the school-age years.

Adjustment to Illness

Fears or stresses associated with an illness and subsequent hospitalization contribute to the school-age child's feelings of loss of control. By involving the child in their own care, you will help them to be a more cooperative patient (Figure 50-11). Procedures that we routinely do without explanation or without providing options, such as using the bedpan, are particularly upsetting to the school-age child. This child is trying hard to act grown up but is not being given the chance. It is also important for this child's self-esteem that you do not scold them when they do lose control. It is best to just overlook the episode.

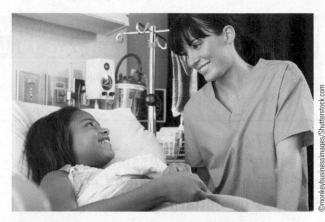

FIGURE 50-11 Explaining the procedure to a school-age child boosts self-esteem, gives the child a sense of independence, and encourages feelings of being a team member.

The school-age child is able to reason. They also understand the impact of their illness and the potential for disability and death. These children take an active interest in health and enjoy acquiring knowledge. You can help them gain information and deal with their fears by explaining all procedures in simple terms. This is also an appropriate age for playing with hospital equipment with supervision.

Pain is passively accepted by the school-age child. They are able to tell you where their pain is located and what it feels like. This child will hold rigidly still, bite their lip, or clench their fists when in pain, in an effort to keep in control and to act brave. This child does well with distraction during painful procedures. Stay with them whenever possible to provide support. This child also tries to postpone all major procedures. For example, when it is time to go to a test, they will need to go to the bathroom. Put limits on the number of postponements allowed.

Activities

Increased physical and social activities are characteristic of this period. School-age children may also miss the activities of school, although they usually deny this. Allow the child time to do schoolwork and visit with friends and other patients.

Age-Appropriate Care ALERT

Children ages 6 to 12 enjoy games. Make up games to teach them how you will perform a procedure, or challenge them to do a task, to reduce fear. Allow them to win, when possible, and praise them for trying and/or doing their best. Take the time to play age-appropriate board games, when possible.

GUIDELINES 50-4 Guidelines for Ensuring a Safe Environment for School-Age Children

- Never leave poisonous materials within reach.
- Keep side rails up when children are in bed.
- Monitor toys to ensure that they are not dangerous.

Summary of Nursing Assistant Tasks and Responsibilities when Caring for School-Age Children

- Maintain a safe environment.
- Apply standard precautions if contact with blood, body fluids, mucous membranes, or nonintact skin is likely.
- Provide information through observation, monitoring of vital signs (temperature, pulse, and respirations), weight, and intake and output.
- Supervise and assist with routine care.
- Collect and test specimens.
- Assist with treatments, examinations, and procedures.
- Provide explanations using proper names of body parts, drawings, books, and medical coloring books and activity sheets.
- Encourage socialization with other children in the same age group.
- Provide time for schoolwork.

USE OF SOCIAL MEDIA BY CHILDREN WHO ARE IN THE HOSPITAL

The use of social media (Facebook, Instagram, Twitter, WhatsApp, Snapchat, etc.) is an important part of most people's lives. Children generally begin exploring social media between the ages of 10 and 12. Teenagers are usually online for more than 70 minutes per day. Teenage girls have the highest use, at about 140 or more minutes per day.

Each health care facility has policies and procedures related to use of social media. Most include setting privacy settings to restrict who can see information, including email address, mailing address and telephone number, photos, identifiable patient information, and financial information.

Employees are not permitted to be social media friends with patients or their families. Do not post your personal information and do not join groups that are open to the public. Avoid taking photos, taking videos, and making audio recordings with patients or their families.

Scammers are tricky and always changing. Take care to avoid scams. You may want to review the information at https://www.consumer.ftc.gov/features/feature-0038-onguardonline to help you avoid online identity theft and scams. You are responsible for protecting the children you care for. If something appears suspicious, notify the nurse and do not be afraid to ask for further help.

CARING FOR THE ADOLESCENT (12–20 YEARS)

Adolescence is the transitional period between childhood and adulthood. The major health problems of this period are usually related to accidents, sports injuries, or chronic and/or permanent disabilities.

Psychosocial Development

Dealing with adolescents is especially challenging for health care providers because:

- The adolescent is developing an identity and becoming increasingly independent.
- Being hospitalized forces the adolescent into a situation where they are dependent on others to meet their needs. Allow the adolescent to make as many of their own decisions as possible.

Adolescents often have a difficult time with authority figures. As a caregiver, you will represent authority to this child. Avoid power struggles with the adolescent. Limit restrictions whenever appropriate.

Adolescents are sometimes uncooperative. Speak with adolescents as you would with adults. Be as flexible as possible. For example, instead of struggling through the morning trying to get the adolescent up and washed, give them a list of things that must be accomplished by a certain time. Then allow the freedom to do things their way and in their order. At the time you decided on, check back with the adolescent to see that the tasks have been completed.

Friends are the most important people to adolescents. A hospital stay makes it more difficult for the adolescent to see friends. It is essential that you:

- Allow the adolescent time for visits
- Permit phone calls
- Introduce them to other patients of their age.

Recognize that adolescents may not want to visit with others if illness has changed their appearance in any way. Body image is important at this age. You can promote a positive image by encouraging the adolescent to continue a normal grooming routine and allowing them to wear their own clothes or pajamas. Teach good hygiene practices if the hospitalized adolescent does not already practice them. Ask a nurse to help if you note that this is a problem for a patient.

Keep in mind that the adolescent is very aware of the changes taking place in their body, whether they can be seen or not. Provide privacy and keep the child covered as much as possible during procedures.

Nutrition and Activity

Adolescents go through a growth spurt. Girls are usually two years ahead of boys. Adequate nutrition and rest continue to be important.

The adolescent often stays up late and likes to sleep late in the morning. Sleep requirements are decreased, but a good night's sleep is essential. It is important to explain the routines of the unit and yet provide flexibility for the adolescent. For example, if the television must be turned off at a certain time, the adolescent should be encouraged to find another quiet activity (such as listening to music with headphones) if they do not want to go to sleep.

Summary of Nursing Assistant Tasks and Responsibilities when Caring for Adolescents

- Maintain a safe environment.
- Apply standard precautions if contact with blood, body fluids, mucous membranes, or nonintact skin is likely.

- Orient the adolescent to the unit and hospital rules.
- Provide information through observations, monitoring of vital signs (temperature, pulse, and respirations), weight, and intake and output.
- Collect and test specimens.
- Assist with treatment, examinations, and procedures.
- Provide simple explanations to the adolescent.
- Assist with body hygiene to help maintain a positive self-image.
- Promote independence; allow adolescents as much control as possible over the schedule of treatments, procedures, and so on.
- Encourage socialization with other adolescents.

CHILDHOOD OBESITY

Some children may be admitted for complications of obesity. According to the WHO, an estimated 38.2 million children under age 5 were obese or overweight worldwide in 2019. The problem is increasing everywhere, including in low- and middle-income countries. An increase in obesity causes an increase in health care costs. Health care professionals are seeing diseases in children that were previously limited to the adult population, such as:

- Type 2 diabetes
- Sleep apnea
- Hypertension
- Skin disorders
- Weight-related orthopedic problems
- Gallstones
- Depression
- Risk factors for atherosclerosis and other cardiac problems

---

GUIDELINES 50-5 Guidelines for Ensuring a Safe Environment for Adolescents

- Carefully check all electrical equipment that the adolescent brings to the hospital—radios, hair dryers, and so on—to ensure that it is appropriate and safe to use. Review with the patient hospital guidelines regarding use of electrical equipment.
- Review smoking policies with all adolescents.
- Reinforce to adolescents that alcohol and other drugs are illegal and are not permitted.

- Provide assistance with showers and bathing if the patient is incapacitated or weakened in any way. The adolescent may not ask for assistance.
- Reinforce the use of shoes or slippers to prevent injuries to the feet.
- Remind adolescents to keep staff informed of their whereabouts.
- Keep beds in low position to prevent falls.

Sleep apnea is a special concern. Researchers have known for years that interrupted sleep inhibits a child's ability to learn. Performance in school, on verbal skills tests, and on IQ tests is not as good as that of children with no sleep problems. It is also suspected that sleep disorders reduce cognitive function. This is important because the damage is being done while the child is growing.

Several studies suggest that children who are obese almost always become obese adults. About half of those studied who were overweight at age 6 became adults who are overweight. About 80 percent of adolescents who are overweight become adults who are overweight. Because of the severity of the problem, childhood obesity is being studied to identify causes and potential solutions to the problem.

Identifying and correcting family eating patterns is often necessary. Educating children and parents about healthy nutrition, exercise, and positive lifestyle choices are some of the methods used to correct overweight. When used in combination with behavior modification, this approach has met with some success in solving the obesity problem. Bariatric surgery (Chapter 31) is a very limited option that is considered only when other methods have failed.

Children who are overweight and obese are often teased and tormented by their peers. Many suffer from low self-esteem. Treat them with compassion and sensitivity when you care for them.

CHILD ABUSE

Child abuse can occur to children of any age. Abuse involves causing harm to a child or failing to do something that protects the child from harm. Abuse can be physical, sexual, or emotional. Neglect is also a form of abuse. Child abuse causes great emotional scars that the abused person carries throughout life. As an adult, the abused child may become an abusive parent. Early identification and treatment are important. In addition to emotional scars, the child is likely to turn to drugs and alcohol or become withdrawn, depressed, suicidal, violent. Other problems include:

- Anxiety
- Anger
- Lack of trust
- Inability to form trusting relationships
- Feelings of being worthless, damaged, stupid, or no good
- Diffculty expressing and regulating emotions

Children need structure, predictability, security, trust, stability, safety, rules, and boundaries. The child who is being abused lives in an unpredictable world. They cannot anticipate how their parents will treat them or how they will act from one day to the next, and they feel insecure, unsafe, and alone. The child does not know when, if, or how the abuse will occur, and feels constant anxiety. Table 50-2 provides an overview of abuse.

Munchausen by Proxy Syndrome (MBPS)

Munchausen by proxy syndrome (MBPS) is a type of child abuse in which a caregiver fabricates illnesses or causes the child to have signs and symptoms of illness. The condition is named after Baron von Munchausen, a public figure in the eighteenth century who made up stories to get attention. "By proxy" means that a parent or other person adult is causing symptoms in a child, not in themselves. Most victims are of preschool age, but there are documented cases in teenagers. The mother is responsible for causing the condition in 85 percent of all cases. Persons with MBPS have a mental illness and need treatment.

The caregiver intentionally deceives health care workers by doing things that cause the child to become ill, such as giving medication or poison, suffocating the child, or withholding food. This person will invent complaints that cannot be verified, falsify tests, inject fecal matter into intravenous lines and feeding tubes, and tamper with medical equipment. They may cause an existing problem to become worse, such as by tampering with a wound so it becomes infected or does not heal.

The child often undergoes painful procedures so the caregiver can appear self-sacrificing and get sympathy and attention. Feelings of jealousy and rage have also triggered MBPS. Occasionally the caregiver will assume a hero role, appearing to rescue or save the child, such as by doing CPR. The syndrome can be life-threatening for the child, and some children have died as a result of this condition.

The offending parent is usually overly attentive and helpful. Hospital staff is busy and appreciates the caregiver's devotion and willingness to give care. Changes in the child's condition always occur in the parent's presence and are seldom witnessed by staff. Typically, the caregiver wants sympathy and attention from doctors, nurses, and other professionals. In addition to getting positive attention, some experts believe that these caregivers derive self-esteem and satisfaction by misleading health care providers, whom they consider to be much more important and powerful than themselves.

As a rule, the caregiver appears to be self-sacrificing, caring, and attentive. It may take several years before health care workers suspect a problem. The condition is very hard to diagnose because these caregivers become skilled in causing symptoms and manipulating health care professionals.

TABLE 50-2 Overview of Child Abuse

Type of Abuse	Examples of Parental Behavior	Signs and Symptoms
Physical	Hitting, kicking, burning, injuring the child with hands or objects. Injuries are often confined to an area of the body that is covered by clothing.	Child may seem fearful. Frequent unexplained injuries, cuts, missing hair. Bruises in various stages of healing; may have a pattern of hand or object on skin; jumps or flinches when touched. Clothing may be inappropriate, such as a long-sleeved sweater in summer heat, to cover injuries.
Emotional	Belittling, humiliating, telling the child they are stupid or no good, making threats, ignoring or rejecting the child, failing to give affection, lack of rules or boundaries, comparing the child unfavorably with others, name-calling, using fear to control behavior, unpredictably lashing out in anger.	Child may be withdrawn, anxious, or fearful. May worry that they are doing something wrong. Lack of attachment to caregiver. May seem inappropriately infantile or inappropriately mature for age. Behavior extremes such as extremely passive or extremely demanding.
Sexual	Abuse usually occurs by an adult the child knows and should be able to trust. Forced sexual contact with parent or other adult. Exposing a child to sexual situations or material, even if there is no touching or physical contact. Child usually instructed to tell no one or harm will come to self or other loved one(s).	Seductive behavior, interest in or knowledge about sex inappropriate for age. New-onset trouble with walking; avoids people for no apparent reason. Injuries to genital or rectal area, pregnancy or STD. Refuses to undress in front of others. Play-acting behavior of a sexual nature.
Neglect	Not meeting child's basic physical, hygienic, mental, or emotional needs; not keeping the child safe.	Poor hygiene (unclean). Clothes fit poorly, or are inappropriate for gender or season. Frequently late to or absent from school. Untreated injuries or illnesses. Left alone without supervision; young child made to babysit for younger siblings. Lives in or left in unsafe environment, unclean living conditions, lack of some or all utilities. Weight loss, malnutrition, dehydration.

Nursing Assistant Responsibilities Regarding Suspected Abuse

Nursing assistants work closely with patients and are in a position to make observations that may be overlooked by others. Make observations of the child's physical condition and interactions with others, and pay careful attention to what the child says. Avoid passing judgment. If you see signs or symptoms suggesting abuse, inform the nurse. Keep your comments objective. Report exactly what you see and hear.

VAPING

An electronic cigarette, also known as e-cigarette and E-cig among other names, is a handheld battery-powered vaporizer that simulates smoking and provides some of the behavioral aspects of smoking, including the hand-to-mouth gratification that is important to smokers.

The E-cig does not burn tobacco. Vaping is popular with adolescents and teens. It is done by inhaling the flavored liquid solution inside an electronic cigarette. It has been implicated in destruction of lung tissue and death. E-cigarettes have also spontaneously caught on fire with no warning in the pockets of users, causing serious burns and other injuries. Much research needs to be done related to vaping devices.

Hospitals do not allow smoking in the facility or on the property. Most are now prohibiting vaping as well. Cigarette smoke has an odor. Some vaping solutions are odor free, but some are scented. The odor does not last as long and does not permeate the clothing or the hair as cigarette smoke does. Inform the nurse if a patient is using a vaping device.

REVIEW

A. True/False

Mark the following true or false by circling T or F.

1. T F   It is normal for a child to regress when hospitalized.

2. T F   The nursing assistant can foster an infant's sense of trust by keeping them warm and dry.

3. T F   The nursing assistant may assume the role of substitute mother.

4. T F   As an adult, an abused child may become an abusive parent.

5. T F   Abused children are unable to form trusting relationships.

6. T F   Weigh the infant daily right after the 10:00 a.m. feeding.

7. T F   Measure pulse and respirations when the child is quiet or asleep.

8. T F   The school-age child has an average heart rate of 90 to 140 beats per minute.

9. T F   The respiratory rate of the toddler averages 30 to 60 respirations per minute.

10. T F   The systolic blood pressure of the child increases with age.

11. T F   Preschoolers normally have many fears.

12. T F   Munchausen by proxy syndrome is a type of child abuse.

13. T F   The most common physical complaints of a school-age child are stomach aches and colds.

14. T F   The offending MBPS caregiver is usually overly attentive and helpful.

15. T F   Vaping is a safe substitute for cigarette smoking.

16. T F   The best way to measure a pulse rate in an infant or child is the apical method.

17. T F   MBPS can be life-threatening for the child.

18. T F   Sucking should be encouraged only when the infant is hungry.

19. T F   It is proper to prop a bottle so an infant can eat in their crib if you are very busy.

20. T F   Carefully position an infant on their back after a feeding.

21. T F   Tie a bright red balloon to the crib to entertain an infant.

22. T F   MBPS is very hard to diagnose because the offending caregiver is good at causing symptoms and manipulating health care personnel.

23. T F   Allow a toddler to play unsupervised in a bathtub for a short time before bathing them, as long as the water is warm.

24. T F   Adolescents have a difficult time dealing with authority figures.

25. T F   Adolescents are particularly sensitive about changes in their body images.

26. T F   Munchausen by proxy syndrome is a hereditary condition that causes mental illness in the child.

27. T F   Neglect is a form of child abuse.

28. T F   Forcing a child to watch a pornographic movie is abusive behavior.

29. T F   Helping a baby learn to trust is an important developmental skill.

30. T F   Overweight is never a problem in children under age 6.

31. T F   Gallstones can be a problem in overweight children.

32. T F   Obese children almost always become obese adults.

33. T F   Magical thinking is a common activity in teenagers.

B. Matching

Choose the correct word from Column II to match each phrase in Column I.

Column I

34. _____ physical and psychological achievements

35. _____ achievement of skills characteristic of a specific age group

36. _____ a person married to a biological parent

37. _____ to move backward developmentally

38. _____ a person who has the right to consent to procedures and the hospitalization of a minor

39. _____ birth parent

40. _____ self-determination

Column II

a. autonomy

b. regress

c. legal guardian

d. developmental tasks

e. biological parent

f. developmental milestone

g. stepparent

C. Nursing Assistant Challenge

You are assigned to take vital signs. The nurse manager just asked the maintenance department to check a problem with the tympanic thermometer, so it is not available. An electronic thermometer is available on the unit, as are oral and rectal glass thermometers. Select the appropriate thermometer and route or method for taking temperatures on the following patients.

41. Joey, a 3-week-old infant who was admitted for surgery

_____

_____

42. Odaysha, a 15-month-old child who was admitted with an upper respiratory infection

_____

_____

43. Saad, a 4-year-old child who was admitted with diarrhea

_____

_____

44. Maria, a 6-year-old with cystic fibrosis who is having difficulty breathing

_____

_____

45. Lisa, an 8-year-old who was admitted with leukemia

_____

_____

46. Robert, a 13-year-old who had his appendix removed earlier today

_____

_____

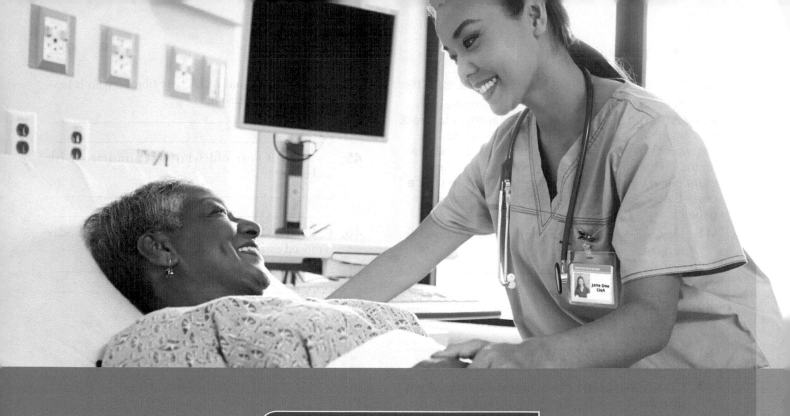

SECTION 13

Recognizing and Responding to Basic Emergencies

CHAPTER 51
Response to Basic Emergencies

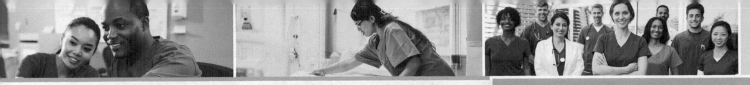

Response to Basic Emergencies

OBJECTIVES

After completing this chapter, you will be able to:

51.1 Spell and define terms.

51.2 Recognize emergency situations that require urgent care.

51.3 Evaluate situations and determine the sequence of appropriate actions to be taken.

51.4 Describe the 11 standardized types of codes.

51.5 Describe how to maintain the patient's airway and breathing during respiratory failure and respiratory arrest.

51.6 Recognize the need for CPR.

51.7 List the benefits of early defibrillation.

51.8 Identify the signs, symptoms, and treatment of common emergency situations such as:

- Brain attack (stroke)
- Seizure
- Vomiting and aspiration
- Thermal injuries
- Poisoning
- Known or suspected head injury

VOCABULARY

Learn the meaning and the correct spelling of the following words and phrases:

adjunctive devices
automatic external
    defibrillator (AED)
cardiac arrest
cardiopulmonary
    resuscitation (CPR)
defibrillation

dislocation
emergency
emergency care
emergency medical
    services (EMS)
first aid
head-tilt, chin-lift maneuver

hemorrhage
jaw-thrust maneuver
pocket mask
recovery position
respiratory arrest
respiratory failure
shock

sprain
strain
vascular
ventilation
victim

DEALING WITH EMERGENCIES

All emergency situations develop rapidly and unpredictably. They can occur at any time to anyone. Examples include:

- Automobile accidents
- Brain attacks (strokes)
- Suddenly feeling weak
- Fainting and falling

An **emergency** is any unexpected situation that requires immediate action and medical attention. In a true emergency, prompt action will prevent complications and may save the life of the **victim** (person needing help). You must know the signs and symptoms of an emergency and be prepared to take immediate action. The following guidelines are basic actions to remember for any emergency.

GUIDELINES 51-1 Guidelines for Responding to an Emergency

- Remember the priorities of any emergency as the ABCs:
  - **A**irway: obstructed or unobstructed?
  - **B**reathing: is the victim able to breathe?
  - **C**irculation: is the heart beating? Is there bleeding?
- Stay calm. Nothing is accomplished and more problems will result if the people at the scene of the emergency become flustered and agitated. If you are calm, you will be a calming influence on the victim and others.
- Know what to do to summon immediate help; you must get the nurse to the scene as soon as possible. Stay with the victim and call out for help. Use a cell phone, if available. If you are out in the community, tell the closest person to call emergency medical services (EMS) (Figure 51-1).
- Do not move the victim unless the person is in danger staying where they are.

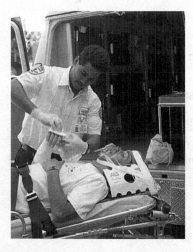

FIGURE 51-1 Know the procedure for activating the EMS system in your community.

- Remain in the room and follow the nurse's instructions. Stay with the victim until the nurse gives you permission to leave.
- Know your limitations and stay within your scope of practice. Be aware of what procedures you are permitted to do.
- Know the procedures to follow for emergencies. Know the code names for various emergencies and how to announce a code. If you are out in the community, know the first aid procedures to apply in emergency situations.
- Know the procedures for activating the **emergency medical services (EMS)** system. In most areas, this is done by dialing 911. You will need to:
  - Give the address.
  - Describe what happened (e.g., the person was burned or has no heartbeat).
  - Give the person's name (if you know this information).
  - Give the telephone number where the call is being made from.
  - Report the number of persons needing help.
- Keep the person warm. Cover with blankets, coats, or other clothing.
- Do not give the person any fluids or food.
- If the person starts to vomit, turn their head to one side to avoid aspiration.
- If the person is conscious, assure them that help is on the way.
- Protect the person's privacy. Keep others away unless they are assisting.
- In all situations, apply standard precautions to prevent exposure to blood, body fluids, mucous membranes, and nonintact skin during the emergency.

BEING PREPARED

Professional medical help is always available when you are working in a health care facility. Professional help is not always available when you are off duty. Whatever course of action you choose, avoid placing yourself or the victim in danger.

FIRST AID

First aid includes:
- Immediate care for victims of injuries or sudden illness
- Care needed if medical help is delayed or is not available

When you give first aid, you deal with the:

- Victim's emotional state
- Victim's physical injuries or problems
- Management of the whole accident situation

Give persons in life-threatening situations immediate attention. Examples of life-threatening situations include those in which a person:

- Has no airway
- Has stopped breathing
- Is in shock
- Has been poisoned
- Is choking
- Is bleeding profusely

Evaluating the Situation

At the scene of an accident:

- Evaluate the situation.
- Find out the extent of injuries.
- Identify the number of victims and their potential injuries.
- Determine whether there are any dangerous factors at the scene.

For example, at the scene of an auto accident, there may be several victims. Some may be trapped in their vehicles; others may be lying on the highway. There may be cars burning and the danger of explosion. In this situation, you must first get yourself and the victims away from further danger.

In the medical facility, unless there is a fire, you usually will be dealing with a single victim. You will be able to focus on the needs of that individual. For example, you might enter a patient's room and find the person lying on the floor, even though the bed side rails are up. Quickly evaluate the situation as you signal for help, giving the patient's name and location and describing the situation.

Emergencies can occur at any time. You can save a life if you know what to do. Basic Cardiac Life Support and First Aid classes are available through the American Red Cross (ARC) and the American Heart Association (AHA). You are responsible for keeping your skills current. This chapter contains only an overview of the skills needed in emergencies. You must successfully complete a certification class offered by the ARC or AHA. These organizations update their guidelines regularly. They are not part of this course. You are responsible for finding the information in your community that is needed for your job. This includes Basic Cardiac Life Support (BCLS) and other certifications required for your job, such as first aid and a food handling course. You can find the most current BCLS information online at ECCguidelines.heart.org. You will find Red Cross BLS and First Aid classes at https://www.redcross.org/ take-a-class/first-aid/first-aid-training/first-aid-online. A Food Handler's Class and others are available at https://www.360training.com. Always look online if something is required specifically for your local community. These classes are all compliant with OSHA requirements.

CODE EMERGENCIES

Most health care facilities call the various types of emergencies *codes*. They have code designations for many situations. The most common of these is a cardiac arrest, which is called a *Code Blue* in many facilities.

In 1999, three employees of a California hospital were killed by an intruder. This tragedy prompted a trade association to survey hospitals regarding how codes were identified and handled. They found that only two codes were standardized, even though most hospitals had code designations, policies, and procedures for many different types of emergencies.

Because codes are high-risk, emergency situations, the California Hospital Association adopted the emergency code words listed in Table 51-1. Many long-term care facilities and hospitals in other states subsequently adopted this list of standardized code words. As a result, these codes are being used in facilities throughout the United States. Make sure to learn the code words and designations used by your facility.

Assisting with a Code

Your duties in a code situation will be determined by the employer, and are set out in your job description. Your responsibilities may also be outlined in the policy and procedure manual. Many facilities have unannounced mock code practices: when personnel respond to the

TABLE 51-1 Example Code Designations

Code Blue Cardiac arrest, medical emergency.
Code Red Fire.
Code Black Bomb threat/evacuation.
Code Green Emergency operations plan activation.
Code White Hospital evacuation.
Code Brown Severe weather.
Code Silver Code Gray may be used interchangeably with Code Silver, a person with a weapon or active shooter situation. May also mean a combative person or geriatric patient who has disappeared from the facility.
Code Orange Hazardous material spill.
Code Purple Child abduction.
Code Pink Infant abduction.
Code Triage Internal for internal disaster.

code page, they find that a manikin is being used. However, the code is conducted as if it were a real patient. This provides all staff with an opportunity to practice their skills, learn their responsibilities, and become comfortable with and proficient in providing life-saving care.

Always follow the directions of the nurse or other licensed health care professional in an emergency. For example, you may be asked to act as a messenger by transporting blood samples to the laboratory, recording the times that procedures begin and end, or recording the times defibrillation was delivered in a CPR situation. A code is a very busy time for everyone. Many tasks must be done in a rapid, orderly manner. However, accuracy is also very important. Become familiar with your facility's policies and your responsibilities so that you are confident in your ability to perform your best in these highly critical situations.

At one time code designations were uniform. However, over time various states and facilities have developed their own list of codes that work best for them. The list here is an example only. Become familiar with the list that is used by your state and facility.

Emergency care is care that must be given right away to prevent loss of life.

- Whether you are out in the community or in the health care facility, ask someone nearby to summon help.
- Do not leave people who need urgent care to get help yourself (exception—CPR).
- As help is on the way, check, in the following order, for the victim's:
  - Degree of responsiveness
  - Airway/breathing ability
  - Presence and rate of heartbeat
  - Signs of bleeding
  - Signs of shock
- Do not move the person if you do not have to.
- Do not allow the person to get up and walk around.
- Check for other injuries.

MAINTAINING THE PATIENT'S BREATHING

The normal respiratory rate is determined by age. Normal respiratory rates for various age groups are listed in Chapter 19.

Respiratory failure occurs when breathing is insufficient to sustain life. **Respiratory arrest** occurs when breathing stops. It is caused by many conditions, including heart attack, brain attack (stroke or CVA), overdose, drowning, electrocution, poisoning, and traumatic injuries. Follow the criteria in Table 51-2 to determine if the patient's breathing is adequate. Abnormal respirations are often a warning of an impending crisis. Stay with the

TABLE 51-2 Monitoring for Breathing Adequacy

- The patient can talk, respirations are between 12 and 20, and there is no apparent distress.
- The rhythm is regular.
- The patient's color is normal, with no cyanosis or gray coloration.
- Look at the patient's chest. It should expand equally with each inspiration.
- Listen for breath sounds, by placing your ear next to the patient's nose and mouth, if necessary. The sounds should be quiet, without gurgling, wheezing, gasping, or other abnormal sounds.
- Feel for breath movement on your cheek and ear.

patient and use the call signal or telephone to request assistance. Report problems to the nurse immediately. (Review Chapter 39 for information on respiratory signs and symptoms to be reported immediately.)

Opening the Airway

If you discover a patient who is in respiratory failure or respiratory arrest, remain in the room and signal or call for immediate help. Open the patient's airway if they cannot do this independently. The most common cause of airway obstruction is the tongue falling back into the throat. Opening the airway lifts the tongue, creating an air passage. Always remove the pillow. Position the patient on the back before beginning.

Because of the nature of the situation, you may not have time to wash your hands or perform other initial procedure actions. Apply gloves and other PPE as soon as you can. Immediately after the patient is safe, wash your hands well. Avoid contact with the patient's secretions if you are not wearing gloves or other personal protective equipment.

The **head-tilt, chin-lift maneuver** is the most common method of opening the airway. Do not perform this procedure if the patient has a neck injury. Instead, use the jaw-thrust maneuver.

The **jaw-thrust maneuver** is used to open the airway of patients with known or suspected neck injuries, and those whose airways cannot be opened using the head-tilt, chin-lift method. In some facilities, this procedure is used for patients with head and facial injuries because they often have neck injuries as well. The purpose of the procedure is to open the airway without moving the head or neck.

Age-Appropriate Care ALERT

Turn the pocket mask upside down to provide a tighter seal on the face if the victim of respiratory arrest is an infant or child.

Mask-to-Mouth Resuscitation

When a patient stops breathing, their respirations must be sustained by artificial means to prevent brain damage and other complications. If you have taken a CPR class, you have learned mouth-to-mouth **ventilation**. This is a technique of breathing for the patient. Avoid using this method on patients because of the risk of disease transmission. Your facility will have various **adjunctive devices** available. An *airway adjunct* is a device used to maintain respirations. This is done by a trained and qualified health care professional.

A **pocket mask** (Figure 51-2) is used for mask-to-mouth ventilation. This is a temporary measure until more advanced airway support becomes available. The mask has a special valve that prevents the patient's exhaled air and secretions from entering the caregiver's mouth. Room air contains approximately 21 percent oxygen. You do not use all the oxygen you take in when you breathe. You exhale extra oxygen, so there is more than enough for the patient to use. Position the person in the supine position with the airway open for effective ventilation. The mask covers both the nose and the mouth. It can be turned upside down for infant resuscitation.

> **🔒 Safety ALERT**
>
> Use the jaw-thrust maneuver for opening the airway when spinal cord injuries are suspected. If the jaw-thrust technique is ineffective, use the head-tilt, chin-lift maneuver.

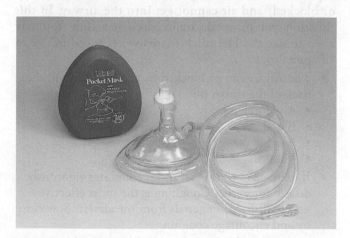

FIGURE 51-2 A pocket mask is a device that provides a one-way barrier if mouth-to-mouth (mask) ventilation is necessary. Supplemental oxygen may be added by connecting the tubing to the male adapter on the mask. However, do not delay resuscitation if oxygen is not available.

Most pocket masks are clear plastic. This enables you to see the position of the patient's mouth. Monitoring the color of the lips will help you see how well the patient is being oxygenated. Sometimes a person will vomit during artificial ventilation. You will see this in the mask. If vomiting occurs, quickly turn the patient on their side, and then clear the mouth and continue ventilation. A licensed professional will suction the patient when suction is available.

CARDIAC ARREST

A respiratory arrest occurs when a person stops breathing but still has a heartbeat. The heart will also stop unless the situation is promptly relieved. **Cardiac arrest** is the term used when the heart has stopped beating and respirations have ceased. Blood and oxygen are not being circulated to the brain and the rest of the body. The person is clinically dead.

Permanent damage to the brain and other organs occurs within four to six minutes. Signs of cardiac arrest are:

- No response from the victim
- Absence of normal breathing
- No pulse

Cardiopulmonary resuscitation (CPR) maintains blood circulation throughout the body until more advanced care is available. *You must never perform CPR unless you have successfully completed an approved course.* The American Heart Association and the American Red Cross both offer such courses in communities across the country. *The information in this book is an overview only and is not intended to take the place of an approved course.* Use these guidelines as a quick reference or refresher.

Some patients will have "do not resuscitate" (DNR) or "no code" orders (see Chapter 32). Full life support measures will be given for cardiac arrest unless the physician has written a DNR order.

THE RECOVERY POSITION

Position a person who is unresponsive, but is breathing and has a pulse, in the **recovery position** to prevent complications. The recovery position is a modified lateral position (Figure 51-3). The patient's position must:

- Be stable.
- Avoid pressure on the chest.
- Avoid pressure on the lower arm.
- Allow the airway to remain open.

Continue to monitor the person frequently to ensure that the pulse and respirations remain adequate. Take vital signs according to the nurse's instructions.

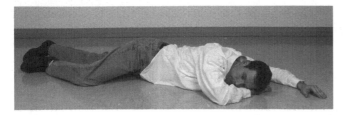

FIGURE 51-3 The recovery position is used for a person who is unconscious but breathing.

EARLY DEFIBRILLATION

Public access to defibrillation has proven to be highly successful. **Defibrillation** is a method of treatment that uses an electric shock to reverse disorganized activity in the heart during cardiac arrest. Early defibrillation has proven to be critical to survival in a victim with cardiac arrest. Defibrillators are placed in various locations in the community and are used in the event of cardiac arrest. Some studies have shown that the chance of survival doubles when early access to defibrillation is available. The speed with which defibrillation is performed is the key to success. Early defibrillation (within five minutes) is a high-priority goal in the community. In health care facilities, the goal is to defibrillate within three minutes.

Automatic external defibrillators (AEDs) are computerized devices that are simple to learn to operate. Several different models are available, and the operating instructions are slightly different for each. The AED is used *only* when a patient is unresponsive, not breathing, and pulseless. When the device is attached to the victim's chest, the unit determines if an electrical shock is necessary to reestablish or regulate the heartbeat. The four basic steps to using the AED are:

1. Turn the power to the unit on.
2. Apply the electrode pads to the patient's chest.
3. Have all rescuers stand back to allow the machine to analyze the heart rhythm.
4. Have all rescuers continue to stand back; the operator of the unit presses the shock button and/or follows the unit's instructions, which are usually audible through a voice-synthesized message (Figure 51-4).

Hospitals normally use manual, portable defibrillators to care for patients who are in cardiac arrest. These defibrillators are operated by qualified, licensed personnel. Although the AED is not routinely used in most hospitals, some facilities with large campuses have purchased AED units for public areas, such as the lobby and cafeteria. Some use semi-automatic AEDs, which can be used either automatically or manually. Many long-term care

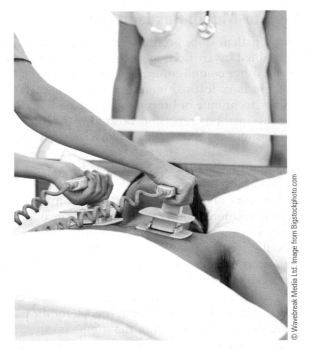

© Wavebreak Media Ltd. Image from Bigstockphoto.com

FIGURE 51-4 Everyone must stand back during defibrillation to prevent accidental shocks.

facilities use AEDs. If your facility uses AEDs, employees will be trained in their use. CPR and use of the AED are included in basic life support classes for health care professionals.

CHOKING

A person chokes when the throat is occluded (closed up or blocked) and air cannot get into the airway. In this situation, you must take quick, decisive action. You may need to use the Heimlich maneuver (Procedure 74 in Chapter 26).

- The airway can be blocked by accumulation in the back of the throat of:
  - Any foreign body
  - Blood
  - Food
  - Vomitus
- If the person can speak and is coughing vigorously, do not intervene. Coughing is the most effective way to dislodge materials from the airway. Stay close by and encourage coughing.
- A person with a complete blockage is unable to speak; they may make high-pitched sounds on inhalation and grasp the throat in the universal distress signal (Figure 51-5).
- Apply standard precautions when assisting a patient who is choking.

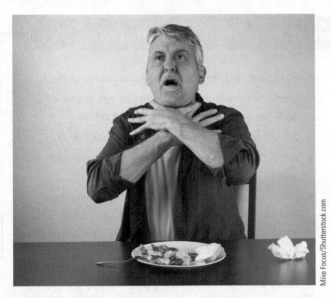

Mike Focus/Shutterstock.com

FIGURE 51-5 The universal sign for choking is placing the hands around the throat.

CPR AND OBSTRUCTED AIRWAY PROCEDURES FOR INFANTS AND CHILDREN

The following procedures for infants and children are only guidelines for emergency treatment of an obstructed airway. An *infant* is a baby from birth to approximately one year of age. A *newly born* infant (newborn) is from the time of birth to approximately one month of age. A *child* is considered to be between one year of age and puberty. Adult guidelines are used at and beyond puberty. You *must* successfully complete an approved CPR course before you perform these procedures.

OTHER EMERGENCIES

For some of the emergencies described here, a patient at home or in a long-term care facility may have to be transported to a hospital emergency department. If the patient is at home, be sure that you know:

- Initial emergency actions to perform
- How and when to notify the EMS system
- How and when to notify the nurse
- How, when, and which family members to notify in the event of emergency

   If the patient is in a long-term care facility, know the initial emergency actions to perform and the procedure to follow for emergencies.

BLEEDING

If the person is conscious, the extent of injuries is likely to be far less severe than if the person is unconscious. Loss of blood is often an imminent threat to life in the unconscious person. Apply gloves and follow standard precautions if you see or suspect that the patient is bleeding. Bleeding is usually easy to see. Sometimes, however, the bleeding is internal. Internal bleeding will only be shown by the signs of shock (described in the next section). Examine the person for evidence of bleeding. Take the following steps to prevent additional loss:

- Identify the area that is bleeding.
- Have the victim apply continuous pressure over the bleeding area, if able.
- If the victim is not able, apply continuous, direct pressure over the bleeding area with a pad and your gloved hand, if necessary.
- Call for help.
- If seepage occurs, increase the padding and pressure.
- If there are no broken bones and there is no pain, raise the wounded area above the level of the heart, but do not release pressure. This will help to reduce bleeding.
- Support the elevated area.

GUIDELINES 51-2 Guidelines for Noncardiac Facility Emergencies

- Anticipate and prevent emergencies whenever possible. Think safety and evaluate the patient and environment for potential safety hazards when you enter the room and again when you leave the room.

- If you discover a patient who is ill or injured, remain in the room and call for help. Your facility will teach you the procedure for getting help. Some facilities instruct employees to call out. Others instruct you to pull the call signal or bathroom emergency signal. Some instruct you to use the telephone in the patient's room.

- Know facility procedures, phone numbers, and names for various code situations for reporting emergencies and completing incident reports.

- Do not move patients who have fallen to the floor unless they are in immediate danger. Movement may worsen an injury. Wait until the nurse checks the patient and gives permission for the move.

- Stay calm and do not panic. Reassure the patient.

- Start emergency measures that you are permitted to do while you are waiting for help to arrive.

- Do not give the patient anything to eat or drink.

- Know the location of emergency equipment and supplies on your unit.

- Many emergencies involve bleeding. Remember that the potential for contact with blood, body fluid, secretions (except sweat), excretions, mucous membranes, and nonintact skin exists. Always remember and apply the principles of standard precautions. Carry extra gloves in your pockets if you are working in an area where they are not immediately available. Know where personal protective equipment is kept.

- Once the nurse arrives, do as they direct.

- Use binding of some kind to hold the padded pressure if there is bleeding from more than one area.
- If you have learned the location of the major blood vessels that control blood flow to an area, and direct pressure seems ineffective, apply pressure over the appropriate pulse point to control **hemorrhage** (heavy bleeding) (Figure 51-6).
- Keep the victim comfortably warm and quiet until help arrives.

🔓 Safety **ALERT**

Do not be distracted by copious bleeding in an unconscious patient. Always check the adequacy of the patient's airway first. If airway, breathing, and circulation (pulse) are adequate, quickly apply gloves and take measures to stop the bleeding.

◇ **NOTE**

Persons who are bleeding are often very frightened. Their anxiety contributes to the development of shock. Continuous reassurance is essential.

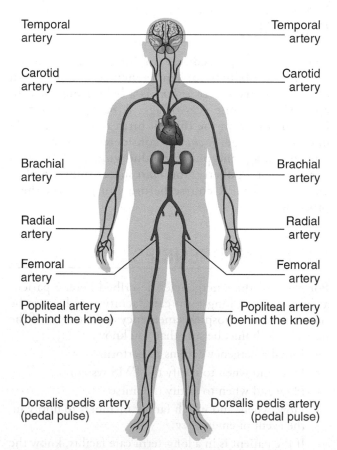

Temporal artery — Temporal artery
Carotid artery — Carotid artery
Brachial artery — Brachial artery
Radial artery — Radial artery
Femoral artery — Femoral artery
Popliteal artery (behind the knee) — Popliteal artery (behind the knee)
Dorsalis pedis artery (pedal pulse) — Dorsalis pedis artery (pedal pulse)

FIGURE 51-6 Pressure on the pulse points is effective for slowing or stopping bleeding.

SHOCK

Shock is defined as a disturbance of the oxygen supply to the tissues and return of blood to the heart. It can follow:

- Any severe injury
- Cardiac arrest
- Acute hemorrhage
- Severe pain
- Excessive loss of body fluids (as in severe burns)
- Serious infection

Signs and Symptoms

Early signs and symptoms of shock include:
- Pale, cold skin that is moist to the touch
- Complaints of weakness
- Weak, rapid pulse
- Rapid and irregular breathing
- Restlessness and anxiety
- Perspiration

Later signs of shock include:
- Mottled skin
- Lack of response
- Sunken eyes with pupils that are dilated, and vacant expression
- Loss of consciousness
- Drop in body temperature
- Low blood pressure

Preventive Measures

Anxiety aggravates the situation, but shock can be prevented if steps are taken early. Prevention of shock includes controlling situations that could trigger it.

- Call for help—activate the emergency medical system.
- Keep the person lying down and quiet.
- Maintain normal body temperature. Provide light warmth if needed.
- Splint fractures before moving or positioning the person, to prevent shock.
- The patient may complain of thirst. Do not give them anything to eat or drink.
- Emergency responders will give intravenous fluids to improve circulatory volume and low oxygen volumes.
- Continue to monitor pulse and respirations.

FAINTING

Fainting (*syncope*) occurs when the blood supply to the brain is reduced for a short time and the person loses consciousness. Fainting is usually a temporary condition that is corrected as soon as blood flow to the brain is restored.

Unfortunately, when consciousness is lost, the person is likely to fall, and injuries can occur. Assist patients who are ambulating for the first time. If fainting occurs, do not try to hold the patient upright. Ease the person to the floor to prevent injury. Assist patients who are *feeling* faint to a safe position. Instruct the sitting patient to lower their head between their knees.

Signs and symptoms indicating that a person might faint are:
- Pallor
- Cold skin
- Perspiration
- Visual changes
- Nausea

To provide assistance to a fainting person:
- Help the person to assume a protected position, sitting or lying down.
- Loosen tight clothing.
- Position the head lower than the heart to increase cerebral blood flow.
- Allow the person to rest for at least 10 minutes.
- Maintain normal body temperature.
- Call for additional help.
- Monitor pulse, respirations, and blood pressure.
- Do not give the patient anything to eat or drink.

HEART ATTACK

Heart attacks can occur in any age group, but the high-risk group includes those who:
- Are overweight.
- Smoke.
- Have atherosclerosis.
- Remain immobile for long periods.
- Are older.
- Have diabetes.
- Have a history of heart disease.

Signs and Symptoms

Signs and symptoms of heart attack include:
- Crushing pain that may radiate up the jaw and down the arm, or heaviness in the chest
- Perspiration; skin cold and clammy
- Nausea and vomiting

- Pale to grayish color of the face
- Difficulty breathing or absence of breathing
- Loss of consciousness
- Irregular pulse or loss of pulse

At other times, the pain of the heart attack may resemble indigestion and the person remains conscious. Do not be fooled into thinking that the degree of pain indicates the severity of the attack. A person with any of these signs or symptoms needs immediate attention.

Action

In the health care facility:

- Immediately signal for help.
- Stay with the patient.
- Have the patient stop any activity and assume a comfortable position.
- Keep the patient calm.
- Elevate the head of the bed to assist breathing.

If the patient is unconscious:

- Check for breathing and heartbeat.
- If necessary, institute CPR (if you have been taught how) until a professional takes charge.

In the community, if the person is conscious, proceed as follows.

1. Evaluate the situation.
2. Activate the EMS.
3. Allow the person to sit up or assume a comfortable position. Loosen clothing around the neck.
4. Keep onlookers away.
5. Provide fresh air but keep the person comfortably warm.
6. Monitor pulse and respirations.
7. Be prepared to initiate CPR.

STROKE

A *brain attack* (cerebral vascular accident or CVA), also called a *stroke*, occurs when there is interference with normal blood circulation to the brain. It usually is caused by a clot that has lodged in a cerebral vessel or by a blood vessel that has ruptured (Figure 51-7).

Signs and Symptoms

The person with a severe stroke usually:

- Experiences seizure activity
- Loses consciousness

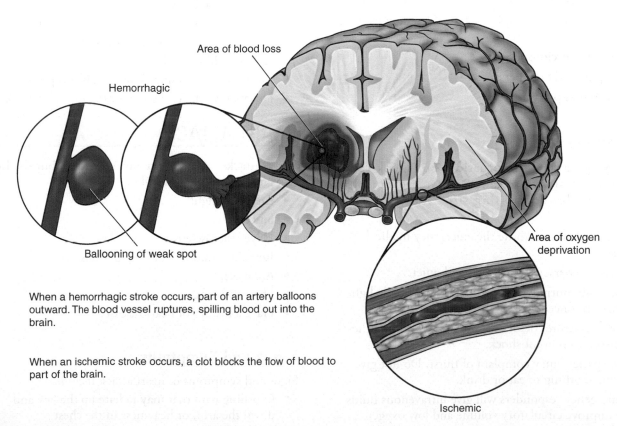

Area of blood loss

Hemorrhagic

Ballooning of weak spot

Area of oxygen deprivation

When a hemorrhagic stroke occurs, part of an artery balloons outward. The blood vessel ruptures, spilling blood out into the brain.

When an ischemic stroke occurs, a clot blocks the flow of blood to part of the brain.

Ischemic

FIGURE 51-7 A stroke occurs when blood flow within the brain is interrupted as a result of a blood clot or rupture of a blood vessel.

- Experiences difficulty breathing
- Develops weakness or paralysis on one side of the body and face
- Has unequal pupil reaction

The patient with a less severe stroke may experience:
- Disorientation
- Dizziness
- Headache
- Slurred speech
- Memory loss
- Loss of consciousness

Action

First aid includes:
- Maintaining an airway
- Providing mask-to-mouth breathing as needed
- Administering CPR, if needed
- Positioning the victim on one side so fluids will drain from the mouth
- Maintaining normal body temperature
- Keeping the person quiet until help arrives or transportation to a medical facility can be arranged

SEIZURES

Seizures or convulsions are sometimes seen when there is:
- Drug overdose.
- Head injury.
- Degenerative brain disease.
- Stroke.
- Infectious disease and fevers.
- Tumors.
- Hypoglycemic reactions.
- Seizure disorder. Seizure disorder is largely controlled with medication, but unusual stress, missed medication doses, and other factors can cause a convulsion.

Signs and Symptoms

Seizures do not always follow the same pattern. Their range may be:
- A momentary loss of contact with the environment (absence seizure, or *petit mal*), in which there are no random or uncontrolled movements but the person seems to stare blankly
- A generalized tonic-clonic seizure (*grand mal*) in which:
  - Consciousness is lost.
  - The person falls and becomes rigid.

- Uncontrolled involuntary movements occur.
- Frothing at the mouth occurs.
- The person becomes cyanotic.
- The person loses control of bladder and/or bowel function.

Gradually the seizure lessens and the person recovers. After a seizure, the person is usually:
- Confused
- Disoriented for a period of time
- Very tired

Action

If you witness someone having a seizure, take the following steps:
- Wear gloves and apply standard precautions, because there is a high probability of contact with blood and body fluids when caring for a patient with a seizure.
- Do not restrain the person's movements.
- Protect the person from injury. For example, move any objects that might break or cause bruising.
- Loosen clothing around the neck.
- Maintain an airway by positioning. Do not try to put anything in the mouth.
- Protect the person's head.
- Observe the seizure.

After seizure activity stops:
- Turn the person to the side so fluid or vomitus can drain freely after the movements subside.
- Give mask-to-mouth resuscitation if breathing is not resumed following the seizure.
- Allow the person to rest undisturbed.
- Stay with the person but summon medical assistance.
- Report and record seizure activity: time, length of seizure, body parts or activity involved.

VOMITING AND ASPIRATION

Food and air are both taken into the body through the mouth. The passageway by which food and air enter is shared. Some diseases and the aging process make swallowing less efficient. Occasionally food, water, vomitus, or other objects accidentally go down the trachea and into the lungs. This is called *aspiration*, and it can occur when a patient is vomiting, bleeding, eating, or drinking. Thick secretions from the mouth may also enter the lungs. Aspiration can cause serious complications.

Signs and Symptoms

Signs and symptoms of aspiration include:

- Coughing
- Choking on food or liquid
- Cyanosis
- Vomiting, especially when lying flat in the supine position
- Inability to swallow
- Inability to spit out vomitus, blood, or secretions from the mouth

Action

If a patient has aspirated anything:

- Stay with the patient and call for help.
- Use standard precautions and select personal protective equipment appropriate to the procedure.
- Do not give the patient any liquids.
- Keep the patient's head elevated if allowed.
- Turn the patient's body to the side if they are vomiting while lying down. If turning the patient's body is not possible, turn the head to the side.
- Provide an emesis basin if the patient is vomiting.
- If the patient begins choking and an airway obstruction occurs, follow the procedure for clearing the obstructed airway.
- After the episode, assist the patient with mouth care.
- Observe any vomitus for color, odor, presence of undigested food, blood, or coffee-ground appearance (coffee-ground appearance suggests blood in the stomach). Save the emesis for the nurse to inspect.
- Measure or estimate the amount of vomitus or blood, and record on the intake and output record.
- Suction, if needed and if possible.

ELECTRIC SHOCK

Electric shock can occur in the:

- Community, when high-tension wires are knocked down in accidents or storms or when electrical appliances are misused or malfunction
- Health facility, because of frayed wires and faulty outlets or fixtures

Severe burns and cardiac and respiratory arrest can result from electric shock (Figure 51-8). You must protect yourself as you try to rescue the victim.

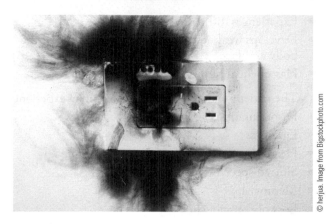

FIGURE 51-8 Electricity can cause serious burns. Use nonconductive material to move the victim away from the source.

Action

- Turn off the electricity at the terminal source, such as at a fuse box, before touching the victim.
- If the source of electricity cannot be controlled, try to move the victim away with some nonconductive material. Dry wood (e.g., a broom handle) is a good nonconductor.
- Once free of the electrical source, check the victim for breathing and pulse.
- Summon medical help.
- Administer CPR, if necessary.
- Once breathing and heart function are restored, check for burns and other injuries. Keep the person lying down and comfortable.
- Give first aid as needed.

⚠️ OSHA **ALERT**

Evaluate the environment carefully. Make sure you are in a safe zone before approaching the patient, away from sources of electricity and water.

 Infection Control **ALERT**

Cool burns with cold water. Avoid ice, which will damage sensitive tissue. Never break blisters on a burn. Cover them loosely with material that will not stick to the tissue.

BURNS

Burns result in loss of skin integrity. They may be caused by heat, chemicals, or radiation. There is a high risk of infection with any burn. Burns are classified as partial thickness or full thickness, depending on the degree of injury. See Chapter 38 for more detail on burns.

Emergency Treatment

all over

1. Call the nurse immediately.
2. If the patient's clothing is on fire, use a coat or blanket to smother the flames.
3. Cool water may be applied to lower skin temperature and to stop further tissue damage. Remove wet clothing (follow the nurse's instructions).
4. Third-degree burns usually require extensive treatment.

ORTHOPEDIC INJURIES

Orthopedic injuries include injuries to bones, joints, muscles, and ligaments.

- A *fracture* is a break in a bone.
- A **sprain** is an injury to a ligament caused by sudden overstretching. A sprained ankle may occur, for example, if a person falls and turns the ankle quickly while falling. Swelling may be noted shortly afterward.
- A **strain** is excessive stretching of a muscle that results in pain and swelling. You may strain the muscles in your back if you use incorrect lifting and moving techniques.
- **Dislocation** occurs in a joint when one bone is displaced from another bone. This can occur in a paralyzed arm that is allowed to hang without support. The weight of the arm pulls the upper arm bone out of position in the shoulder joint. A dislocation can also be caused by improperly lifting a patient under the arms.

Treatment

If you suspect that a patient has suffered a fracture:

- Stay with the patient.
- Immobilize the injured extremity to prevent pain and possible worsening of a fracture and bleeding resulting from tissue damage.
- Do not attempt to move the patient.
- Call the nurse immediately.

The nurse must give permission for moving a patient who is on the floor with a suspected fracture. Have plenty of help available. One staff member should immobilize and move the fractured extremity while others move the rest of the body. Roll the patient onto a sheet, blanket, or backboard and then lift them into bed. This is less traumatic for the patient and reduces the risk of worsening the injury.

Monitor the patient's vital signs as instructed. Report changes to the nurse.

X-rays will be taken if a fracture is suspected. Treatment for a fracture is:

- Casting the extremity
- Using traction
- Surgical repair

If you suspect that a patient has suffered a sprain, strain, or dislocation, notify the nurse at once. You may be instructed to:

- Immobilize the injured extremity to prevent pain and possible worsening of a fracture and bleeding resulting from tissue damage.
- Elevate the injured extremity.
- Apply ice packs to the area.
- After 24 hours, you may be instructed to apply warm packs to the area.

HEAD INJURY

A patient with a known or suspected head injury always requires close observation and monitoring. Bleeding inside the skull commonly occurs when the head strikes a broad, hard object, such as the floor, causing internal bleeding. Serious complications may not be apparent until 72 hours (or more) after a head injury. This is particularly true in elderly persons. The brain shrinks slightly with age. This does not affect the person mentally, but the space between the brain and the skull allows extra room for swelling and bleeding. Therefore, signs and symptoms of an acute bleeding problem may not become apparent for several days until the problem progresses to a point where it increases pressure on the brain. It can take up to six weeks before the patient shows symptoms from a very tiny "bleed." This is usually long after the original injury has been forgotten.

Signs and Symptoms

Signs and symptoms of a possible head injury include:

- Change in the patient's level of alertness or consciousness
- Change in orientation (ability to recognize time, place, person)
- Memory loss

- Unequal pupils
- Visual disturbances
- Blood or clear fluid leaking from ears or nose
- Change in ability to speak or make oneself understood
- Change in ability to follow directions
- No response to verbal stimulation
- Weakness of arms or legs, difficulty maintaining balance
- Headache
- Nausea and/or vomiting

Remember that signs and symptoms of a problem may not appear or become obvious for several days.

Action

If you think a patient has suffered a head injury:
- Stay with the patient and call for help.
- Monitor pulse and respirations while waiting for the nurse to arrive.
- Keep the environment quiet and calm.
- Do not give the patient anything to drink.

- Reassure and orient the patient.
- Elevate the head on a pillow.
- Do not move the patient if they are on the floor.
- Monitor vital signs regularly after the injury, as instructed.

ACCIDENTAL POISONING

Immediate attention is needed if a patient is the victim of accidental poisoning. All potentially harmful substances must be kept in locked cupboards. If you suspect that a poisoning has happened:
- Call the nurse immediately.
- Try to determine what the patient has taken and save the container.
- The nurse may administer a substance that will cause vomiting. (Not all substances can be safely removed from the patient's body by vomiting.)
- Know where to find the telephone number for the regional poison control center.

REVIEW

A. True/False

Mark the following true or false by circling T or F.

1. T F   No special training is needed to give CPR.
2. T F   CPR is needed if breathing and circulation fail.
3. T F   A person in shock should be kept quiet and lying down.
4. T F   A bleeding body part should be elevated.
5. T F   Vomiting should be induced for anyone who has swallowed a poisonous substance.
6. T F   Immediate treatment for burns may include applying cool water to reduce skin temperature.
7. T F   A dislocation occurs when one bone is displaced from another bone.
8. T F   Immediate treatment of orthopedic injuries includes the application of warm packs.
9. T F   Serious complications may not become apparent until 72 hours (or more) after a head injury.

B. Matching

Choose the correct term from Column II to match each phrase in Column I.

Column I

10. _____ person needing first aid
11. _____ excessive bleeding
12. _____ care given when a victim has no breathing or heartbeat
13. _____ signaled by a drop in blood pressure
14. _____ emergency care

Column II

a. arrest
b. first aid
c. victim
d. CPR
e. contraindicated
f. hemorrhage
g. splintered
h. shock

C. Multiple Choice

Select the best answer for each of the following.

15. An organization that offers instruction in CPR is the:

   a. American Diabetes Association.

   b. American Association of Nurses.

   c. Association for Resuscitation.

   d. American Heart Association.

16. First aid is care given:

   a. for nausea and vomiting.

   b. only upon a physician's order.

   c. if immediate help is needed.

   d. for a cough, cold, or sore throat.

17. Which of the following is a life-threatening situation requiring intervention? A person who:

   a. broke a finger.

   b. fell and bruised a knee.

   c. is in shock.

   d. is coughing.

18. The first step you should take when arriving on the scene of an accident is to:

   a. stop a passerby.

   b. evaluate the situation.

   c. move the victims to one side.

   d. help the victims get up and walk.

19. To assist a person who has fainted:

   a. help the person walk to circulate the blood.

   b. cover the person with several blankets.

   c. loosen tight and restrictive clothing.

   d. position the person's head higher than the heart.

20. To assist the person who is experiencing a seizure, you should:

   a. keep the person as active as possible.

   b. restrain the person's movements.

   c. keep the head straight.

   d. maintain an airway and protect the person from injury.

21. You suspect that a patient is in shock because the:

   a. blood pressure is elevated.

   b. face is flushed.

   c. skin is cold and clammy.

   d. pulse is full and bounding.

22. Overstretching of a ligament can result in a:

   a. fracture.

   b. sprain.

   c. strain.

   d. dislocation.

23. The first action to take when an adult is coughing and tells you they are choking is to:

   a. slap the person on the back.

   b. encourage the person to cough.

   c. begin artificial respirations.

   d. begin chest compressions.

24. The first priority in an emergency is:

   a. airway.

   b. bleeding.

   c. circulation.

   d. level of consciousness.

25. When a person suffers cardiac arrest:

   a. the heart has stopped beating.

   b. the respirations are less than 12 per minute.

   c. biological death has occurred.

   d. unconsciousness occurs in about four minutes.

26. In the health care facility, you would initiate CPR for cardiac arrest unless:

   a. the patient has a DNR order.

   b. you think the patient would not want to be revived.

   c. the patient is very old.

   d. the death is unexpected.

27. If you are working in a patient's home and CPR is initiated, you must:

   a. call the EMS system yourself if you are alone.

   b. drive the patient to the closest hospital.

   c. do CPR for 20 minutes, then call EMS.

   d. go next door to have the neighbor call EMS.

28. The procedure to clear an obstructed airway of a conscious infant is to position the infant and:

   a. deliver five abdominal thrusts followed by five back blows.

   b. deliver five back blows followed by five chest thrusts.

   c. perform a blind finger sweep.

   d. perform two ventilations followed by five compressions.

29. Vomiting may be treated as an emergency because of the risk of:

  a. air flow.

  b. aspiration.

  c. hemorrhage.

  d. cardiac arrest.

30. The preferred treatment for external bleeding is to apply:

  a. continuous, direct pressure.

  b. a tourniquet.

  c. pressure to pulse points.

  d. a heat pack.

D. Nursing Assistant Challenge

You and a friend are driving home from work. A car immediately ahead of you goes through a stop sign and is hit on the passenger side by a car going through the intersection. You and your friend park your car to see if your help is needed in this emergency. The people in the car that was ahead of you are conscious, are alert, and deny having any injuries. The passenger in the car that ran the stop sign is unconscious and begins to vomit. You see blood coming from the person's right arm. The driver is conscious but dazed and seems to be disoriented. List, in sequence, the actions you will take.

_____

_____

_____

_____

_____

_____

_____

_____

_____

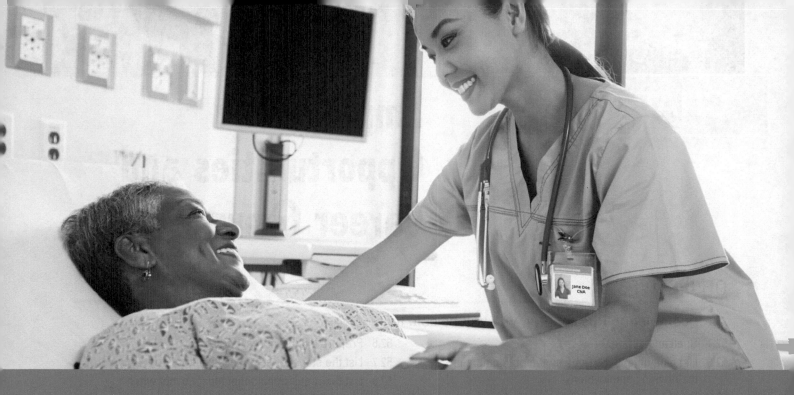

SECTION 14
Moving Forward
CHAPTER 52
Employment Opportunities and Career Growth

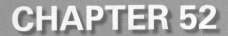

Employment Opportunities and Career Growth

OBJECTIVES

After completing this chapter, you will be able to:

52.1 Spell and define terms.

52.2 List nine objectives to be met in obtaining and maintaining employment.

52.3 Discuss a process for self-appraisal.

52.4 Name sources of employment for nursing assistants.

52.5 Prepare a resume.

52.6 Prepare a letter of resignation.

52.7 List the steps for a successful interview.

52.8 List the requirements that must be met when accepting employment.

52.9 List steps for continuing development in your career.

VOCABULARY

Learn the meaning and the correct spelling of the following words and phrases:

job interview   networking   reference   résumé

INTRODUCTION

Having completed a nursing assistant program, you are now ready to look for employment. You will want to be as successful as an employee as you were as a student. If you meet the objectives presented in this chapter, the task will be made much easier.

Searching for and obtaining a job requires several steps:

- Completing a self-appraisal
- Searching for employment opportunities
- Assembling a résumé
- Validating your references
- Making specific applications for work
- Participating in interviews
- Deciding whether to take the job

OBJECTIVE 1: SELF-APPRAISAL

The first objective is to determine your personal assets and limitations that could influence your choice of employment. To do this, complete the form in Figure 52-1 or:

- Divide a piece of paper into three columns.
- Title one column *assets*, one *limitations*, and one *solutions*.

SELF-EVALUATION WORKSHEET

Respond to the following questions honestly and sincerely. They are meant to assist you in self-assessment.

1. List your three strongest attributes as related to people, data, or things.

    i.e., Interpersonal skills related to people

      Accuracy related to data

      Mechanical ability related to things

    _____ related to _____

    _____ related to _____

    _____ related to _____

2. List your three weakest attributes as related to people, data, or things.

    _____ related to _____

    _____ related to _____

    _____ related to _____

3. How do you express yourself? Excellent, Good, Fair, Poor

    Orally _____ In writing _____

4. Do you work well as a leader of a group or team? Yes _____ No _____

5. Do you prefer to work alone? Yes _____ No _____

6. Can you work under stress/pressure? Yes _____ No _____

7. Do you enjoy new ideas and situations? Yes _____ No _____

8. Are you comfortable with routines/schedules? Yes _____ No _____

9. Which work environment do you prefer?

    Single-provider setting _____   Multiple-provider setting _____

    Small clinic setting _____   Large clinic setting _____

10. Which type of practice do you prefer?

    Pediatrics _____   Obstetrics/Gynecology _____

    Geriatrics _____   General Medicine _____

    Internal Medicine _____   Other _____

11. Which work setting do you prefer?

    Front office (reception) _____   Back office (assisting provider) _____

    Laboratory (phlebotomy) _____   Administrative (coding/billing) _____

FIGURE 52-1 A self-evaluation helps identify strengths, weaknesses, and preferences.

- Review all the positive contributions you can make in an employment situation and list them. For example:
  - Your preference in the care of certain patients
  - Your caring attitude
  - Special skill you have with patients
  - Your personal appearance
- Honestly review all the limitations that might make certain employment less obtainable. For example, consider:

- Home responsibilities
- Specific hours you can work
- Transportation problems
- Physical limitations

- Think of possible solutions so that you reduce the number of limitations. The fewer limitations you have at the beginning of your job search, the more you can expand the possibilities for employment. Make your lists, review them, and add to them over several days.

OBJECTIVE 2: SEARCH FOR ALL EMPLOYMENT OPPORTUNITIES

Having thought through your assets and limitations and found as many solutions to the limitations as possible, you are ready to search for employment. Possible sources for the search process are all the agencies or facilities that employ nursing assistants:

- Physicians' offices
- Blood banks
- Clinics
- Hospices
- Homes for those who are elderly and/or who have disabilities, assisted living, or personal care facilities
- Long-term care facilities
- Hospitals
- Home health care agencies
- Rehabilitation centers

The telephone directory and online search engines will help you select facilities that meet your specific needs for available transportation or specific type of care. You can also use classified ads found in the newspaper, in online search engines, and in social media online.

- Look for facilities in your area.
- Consider the type of work you are willing to do.
- Consider the shifts that have openings.
- Note the person to contact for an interview or additional information.

The facility in which you received your clinical experience can be a valuable resource. Administrators sometimes offer jobs to new nursing assistants who trained

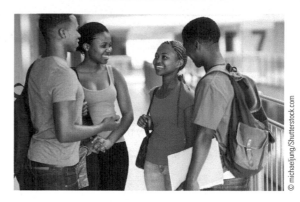

FIGURE 52-2 Friends and classmates are valuable sources of information about potential jobs.

in their facility. Job openings may be posted on the employee bulletin board.

Other resources include friends and colleagues. Friends may know of job openings, and colleagues may be able to put you in touch with others who have potential job connections (Figure 52-2). A term for these activities is **networking**.

Finding employment is a full-time job. You must wake up early and set a time to begin looking for work. It may be helpful to list the steps involved in looking for a job, and preparations you need to make, such as ironing a shirt, finding a babysitter, and preparing a résumé. Apply for jobs early in the day. This makes a good impression and gives you enough time to fill out applications, take tests, or have interviews. Applying at several facilities in the same area will help you organize your time and save time and travel. Follow up on all job leads right away. If you hear of a job opening late in the day, call and schedule an appointment for the next day. It is a good idea to keep a simple contact list (Figure 52-3).

		Company Name/Address	Telephone Number	Contact's Name	Resume Sent	Application/ Cover	Application Form Sent	Follow-up Phone Call	Follow-up Letter	Result	
1	1										
2	2										
3	3										
4	4										
5	5										
6	6										

FIGURE 52-3 A contact list helps with organization of information and prevents confusion.

OBJECTIVE 3: ASSEMBLE A PROPER RÉSUMÉ

A **résumé** is a written summary of work and educational history. You should:

- Prepare several copies.
- Always keep a copy for yourself.
- Type the résumé for a neat appearance, or prepare it on a computer and good printer.
- Carry a copy whenever you seek employment.
- Use the résumé as a ready reference when you fill out forms.
- Update the résumé regularly.

The résumé should be carefully prepared to include:

- Your name, address, telephone number, and email address.
- Your educational background.
  - List your most recent education first.
  - Give dates.
  - Include a brief summary of the content.
- Your work history over the past five years, especially if it gives evidence of successful experiences in the same or related areas as the job for which you are applying.
- Proof of being on the State Nursing Assistant Registry.
- List of any continuing education classes you have attended.
- Other experiences you have had; include jobs that show initiative, reliability, trustworthiness, and worthwhile ways you have spent your time.
- References—a list of three people who know you and can verify your abilities.
- Some personal information that indicates your interests and activities.

It is not necessary to include the following in your résumé:

- Age
- Marital status
- Religion
- Sex
- Height
- Weight

OBJECTIVE 4: VALIDATE REFERENCES

References are people who know you and who would be willing to comment, either in writing or verbally over the telephone, about you and your abilities. Be sure to include accurate titles, names, addresses, and telephone numbers when listing references.

Anyone you use as a reference:

- Should give you permission to use their names and disclose their contact information
- Should know you well enough to make an honest evaluation
- Should not be related to you
- May need to have their memories refreshed about dates of employment or experiences you have stated in your résumé

OBJECTIVE 5: MAKE SPECIFIC APPLICATIONS FOR WORK

Handle this part of the job search process in a business-like way:

- Select three facilities that interest you most.
- Call and ask for the director of nursing or personnel department.
- Tell the person who answers that you are interested in learning if there are any openings for nursing assistants, and if so, what the application procedure is.
- Be prepared to answer questions about your preparation and experience. Have your résumé in your hand.
- Make an appointment for an interview, if possible. A **job interview** is an opportunity for the person applying for a job and the employer's representative to learn about each other. Each person has the opportunity to ask questions to determine if the job seeker has qualifications that match the requirements of the job available.
- Fill out an application form. Use your résumé to be sure you complete the form correctly. Read the directions on the application carefully. Fill out all information. If something on the application does not apply, put "N/A" (not applicable) in the space rather than leaving it blank. List all your previous employers, even if they were not health care providers. If you skip an employer, it looks as if you are hiding something. Complete the application in its entirety. Do not write "see résumé." Although you may attach your résumé to the application, there are legal reasons why you must complete the application. Make sure the information is accurate, spelled correctly, complete, and neat. Use a pen to complete the application. The application represents you on paper. A messy application sends a negative message.
- Learn the names of the persons to whom you speak.
- Thank the person speaking with you by name.
- Repeat the steps until you land the job.

OBJECTIVE 6: PARTICIPATE IN A SUCCESSFUL INTERVIEW

After you have investigated job leads and completed applications, an employer may contact you to schedule an interview. You will be given a date and time to meet. The interview is very important. Most hiring decisions are made during the interview. How you present yourself in the interview is as important as your training, experience, and ability to do the job.

Approach the interview in three steps: preparation, the actual interview, and follow-up after the interview.

Preparation

Plan what you will wear.

- Do not overdress, but be neat and clean.
- Check your clothes for loose or lost buttons or stains.
- Polish your shoes.

Make sure you are well groomed.

- Be sure to take a bath or shower and use deodorant.
- Brush your teeth.
- Make sure your fingernails are short and clean.
- Make sure your hair is neat.
- If you have a beard or a mustache, be sure it is trimmed.

Prepare a list of questions you want to ask. Make sure to have your résumé in hand.

Actual Interview

Be prepared when going to an interview. Go to the interview alone; arrange for babysitters and transportation ahead of time. Use a map, GPS or a smartphone with a map program to get directions to the interview site.

Bring pens and pencils, papers reference information, and your résumé with you. You will also need a photo identification, such as a driver's license, and your Social Security card. If you have completed a nursing assistant program, bring a copy of your certificate and state certification. It is a good idea to arrive a little early so you can complete paperwork, if requested.

- Do not chew gum.
- Offer a firm handshake (Figure 52-4).
- Stand until you are invited to sit.
- Remember that you are "selling" yourself.
- Make sure your body language sends a positive message.
- Make good eye contact with the interviewer. Your eyes should send a message such as "I like you."

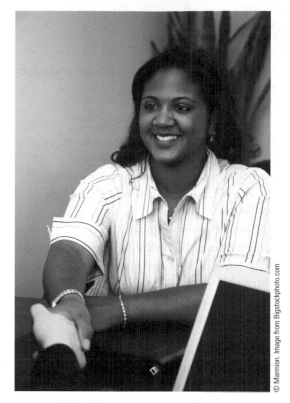

FIGURE 52-4 Dress professionally for the interview and offer a firm handshake.

- Listen carefully to the interview questions and be sure you understand them before you answer. If you do not understand, ask for clarification. Your answers to questions should reflect your positive features.
- Share information willingly with the interviewer.

Use your list of questions to learn information important to you, such as:

- Responsibilities (ask for a job description)
- Hours of work
- Dress code
- Opportunities for future assistance or financial aid to further your education
- Starting salary
- Fringe benefits such as health insurance
- Schedule of raises

Sensitive Issues

Be honest but tactful when discussing former employers. Speak positively of them. Making negative comments about a previous employer is not a good practice. Your answers to questions should reflect your positive features. Avoid discussing negative traits unless you are specifically asked to do so. Be honest with the interviewer. It is easier to defend the truth than it is to be caught in a lie. Avoid discussing your personal life or financial problems. Consider how you will respond to certain questions, such as "Are you available to work every other Sunday?" Avoid responding with excuses such as "My husband will not let me work on Sundays." A better way to respond would be to say, "My husband is a pastor and we are very involved in church activities on Sundays. Working will be a hardship in my personal life, but if it is a job requirement I will do my best to work it out." Remember that health care facilities are open 24 hours a day, 7 days a week. All workers are required to do some weekend, holiday, and shift work. This is one of the requirements of your chosen career.

Discussing Salary and Benefits

Salary and benefits can be sensitive issues. Asking questions about them early in the process gives the employer the impression that you are not really interested in working at the facility but are instead shopping for the highest salary available. This sends a negative message. Save discussions about salary and benefits for late in the interview. Let the employer lead into them. If the interviewer has not discussed salary and benefits by the end of the interview, it is appropriate to ask.

At the end of the interview, shake hands and thank the interviewer, whether you are hired or not.

After the Interview

When you get home:

- Write a short thank-you note to the person who interviewed you, thanking them for their time and the opportunity to be considered for the job.
- Review the interview in your mind. Plan changes you should make to improve future interviews.

OBJECTIVE 7: ACCEPT A JOB

Before accepting a job, think carefully about your employer's expectations of your abilities and job performance. If you accept the job, you must be prepared to follow the policies and procedures of the facility. For example, if the interviewer told you that nursing assistants are scheduled to work every other weekend, do not take the job unless you are willing to do this. There are some additional requirements you will have to complete as you begin your job, as we discuss in this section.

Orientation

Orientation is designed to help you safely perform the duties listed in your job description. It is mandatory and all new employees are required to attend. Keep in mind that even if you were hired to work an evening or night shift, orientation classes may be held during the day. Orientation generally consists of two parts. You will spend at least a day in the classroom learning about the facility's policies and procedures. You will be given printed materials and handbooks that you can refer to in the future. Information presented during the class may include:

- Policies for scheduling and making assignments
- What to do during fire and other emergencies
- How and when performance evaluations are completed
- The organizational chart of the facility
- Safety policies and procedures

⚖ Legal **ALERT**

To work in the United States, you must complete an I-9 form, which proves your legal eligibility to work. To do this, you must provide a copy of your Social Security card and a picture identification. The employer may make a copy of these documents. They will also have to sign the form to confirm that the facility has verified your identity and work eligibility.

A clinical orientation is provided on the nursing unit. An instructor, another nurse, or an experienced nursing assistant will work with you the first few days so that you may learn:

- The routine of the unit
- The location of equipment and supplies
- How to do specific procedures as required by the employer

Health and Safety Requirements

State and federal regulations require new employees to:

- Obtain a physical examination within a specified number of days (some employers will require this before you begin work).
- Receive a two-step Mantoux (tuberculosis) test within a specified number of days (this too may be required before you begin work).
- Indicate whether they wish to receive the hepatitis B vaccine. Health care employers are required by law to offer this vaccination without cost to direct-care

employees. It is the employee's choice whether to take the vaccine. If the employee refuses it at the time of orientation, it can be given at another time if they change their mind.

Health Care Worker Background Check

Most facilities conduct a criminal background check on all potential employees. The procedure should be explained to you during the interview.

Drug Testing

Many employers require that drug testing be performed before you begin work. This procedure too should be explained during the interview.

⚖ Legal **ALERT**

Drug testing is usually done by means of a urine sample. Some prescription drugs, foods, and vitamins may interfere with the urine test results. You will be asked to list prescription and nonprescription medications you are taking. Be honest, and list everything. Collection of the urine specimen is generally monitored to prevent tampering. Some agencies check the temperature of the urine immediately after the specimen is obtained, as a further safeguard. Some facilities will not allow you to take personal items into the bathroom when providing the specimen. Access to water may also be limited, because it is possible to dilute a sample. Some facilities seal the container with tamper-evident tape, which is signed by both the employee and the nurse who assists with specimen collection. Your employer may also have a policy requiring random drug testing if you are involved in a work-related injury or if any use of illicit substances is suspected.

Uniform Requirements

Most health care employers have dress codes that indicate:
- Color and style of uniform to be worn on duty
- Acceptable jewelry that can be worn with the uniform
- Type of shoes and stockings or socks that are safe to wear
- Acceptable hairstyles and makeup (including whether nail polish is permitted)
  Remember that these policies are for the purposes of safety and infection control. Some employers will issue the uniforms to you either at no charge or for a charge that is deducted from your paycheck over a period of time.

OBJECTIVE 8: KEEP THE JOB

You can make your new position secure if you:
- Arrive on time prepared to work. Good attendance is very important. Be at work when you are scheduled and avoid calling off unless you are ill. If you will be unable to work your next scheduled shift, notify your facility as far in advance as possible so they can find a replacement.
- Follow the policies and procedures outlined in your orientation.
- Follow the rules of ethical and legal conduct.
- Recognize your limitations and seek help.
- Have an open and positive attitude.

 Culture **ALERT**

You will work with people from other cultures. Remember, they also have cultural needs, beliefs, and practices. Use cultural competencies and show respect for your co-workers. Do your best to work well with everyone. When staff make the effort to work well together, everyone's job satisfaction increases and patients receive better care.

OBJECTIVE 9: CONTINUE TO GROW THROUGHOUT YOUR CAREER

You will continue to grow if you take advantage of each new experience and opportunity you find.
- Keep your certificate current.
- Seek out knowledgeable staff members and watch and learn by their example.
- Do not be afraid to ask questions at appropriate times.
- Use the nursing literature to learn more about patients' conditions.
- Participate in care conferences with an open mind so that each conference can be a learning experience for you.
- Complete 12 hours of continuing education each year (Figure 52-5), or follow the requirements in your state.
- Investigate the possibilities of advancing your formal education by:
  - Enrolling in general education courses offered at a high school or college in your area.
  - Taking courses in communication, listening, English, and psychology.
  - Participating in in-service education programs at your facility or at nearby hospitals.

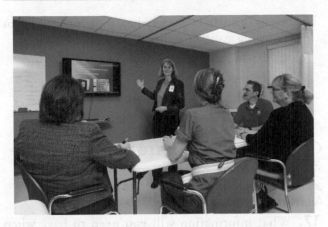

FIGURE 52-5 Attend staff development programs to increase knowledge.

- Enrolling in minicourses offered by hospitals on subjects of general public interest, such as hypertension, weight control, and diabetes.
- Selecting books at the library that pertain to health issues.
- Researching programs that can prepare you for professional advancement into the ranks of LPN/LVN or RN.
- Finding one or more credible sources of information online and staying with them. There is a great deal of medical misinformation online. Staying with major medical centers and other sources you know are credible will help you avoid it. (For example, you can find credible information at the Mayo Clinic, Cleveland Clinic, the CDC, and many other educational and government websites.)

Career Ladders

Many facilities have career ladders available for nursing assistants. The career ladder enables the assistant to progress to a higher position within the organization, such as a restorative assistant. One professional nursing organization has developed the End-of-Life Nursing Education Consortium (ELNEC) Project, which enables direct caregivers, including nursing assistants, to achieve advanced status in providing end-of-life care. Additional education is usually required to move up the career ladder. Completing specialized certificate programs is an excellent way to advance in your career. Explore the possibilities within your facility. Community and junior colleges in your area may also have classes available.

OBJECTIVE 10: RESIGN PROPERLY FROM EMPLOYMENT

When you are ready to leave your present position, you should do so pleasantly and properly. Give as much notice as possible—usually equal to the length of one pay period. Submit a letter of resignation that includes:

- Date
- Salutation (greeting) to the director of nursing
- Brief explanation of your reasons for leaving
- Date your resignation is to be effective
- Thanks for the opportunity to have worked and grown by working in that facility
- Your signature

> **NOTE**
>
> Even if you feel upset by something that happened, make your reasons for leaving positive in nature.

REVIEW

A. True/False

Mark the following true or false by circling T or F.

1. T F The employer may ask your religion during an interview.
2. T F In making a self-appraisal, you only need to list the things you could offer an employer.
3. T F What you wear to an interview is not important.
4. T F The availability of transportation should be considered when you are choosing a job.

5. T F The interviewer should provide you with information about nursing assistant responsibilities in the facility.
6. T F Checking for job possibilities with the facility in which you had your clinical experience is proper.
7. T F If you fail to get the job after the interview, there is nothing left for you to do about the situation.
8. T F At the end of every interview, you should thank the interviewer, even if you were not immediately hired.

9. T F   Participation in care conferences can be a way to continue to grow.

10. T F   Give ample notice if you plan to resign.

B. Multiple Choice

Select the best answer for each of the following.

11. The first step in finding a job is:
    a. making phone calls.
    b. doing a self-assessment.
    c. looking in the paper.
    d. writing letters to friends.

12. A self-appraisal includes:
    a. reading classified ads.
    b. networking with friends.
    c. caring for patients.
    d. listing assets, limitations, and solutions.

13. A compilation of your work history is called a(n):
    a. résumé.
    b. interview.
    c. summary.
    d. application.

14. Which of the following would you include in your résumé?
    a. Marital status
    b. Religion
    c. Weight
    d. Address

15. Before naming a person as a reference:
    a. ask permission.
    b. call the prospective employer.
    c. tell the person you are going to use their name.
    d. get the person's phone number and birth date.

16. Assets that will help you when applying for a job as a nursing assistant include:
    a. having an attractive appearance.
    b. being proficient in skills.
    c. wearing beautiful jewelry.
    d. taking a class the following month.

C. Nursing Assistant Challenge

You have made it! You have completed your course and are eagerly looking forward to employment. Answer these questions.

17. What information will you need to have when completing an application for employment?

    _____

    _____

18. What items do you need to have with you when you go for your interview?

    _____

    _____

19. How will you dress for the interview?

    _____

    _____

20. The interview comes to a close and the interviewer has not given you any information concerning wages and benefits. How would you handle this?

    _____

    _____

2019 novel coronavirus (COVID-19) the 2019 novel coronavirus was initially detected in China in December 2019. The virus has been named SARS-CoV-2, and the disease it causes has been named coronavirus disease 2019, abbreviated as COVID-19. COVID 19 is a highly infectious respiratory illness that spread rapidly, causing a worldwide pandemic. Many people became seriously ill and many died as a result of the virus.

90-90-90 position method of positioning the patient in good posture with the feet at a 90° angle to the lower legs, the lower legs at a 90° angle to the thigh, and the thighs at a 90° angle to the torso.

abbreviation shortened form of a word or phrase.

abdominal distention condition in which the abdomen is bloated and enlarged.

abduction movement away from midline or center.

abduction pillow pillow used to maintain separation between the legs of a patient who has had hip surgery.

ablutions practice of removing sins and diseases and cleansing negative energy from body, mind, and spirit through the use of ritual washing.

abrasion injury that results from scraping the skin.

absence seizure another name for a petit mal seizure.

abuse improper treatment or misuse.

accelerated increased or faster motion, as in pulse or respiration.

acceptance coming to terms with a situation and awaiting the outcome calmly; final stage of dying that some people, but not all, reach.

accreditation voluntary process in which a professional organization recognizes a facility for demonstrating its ability to meet certain quality standards and criteria.

acetone colorless liquid produced during the metabolism of fats because glucose cannot be oxidized in the blood; has a sweet, fruity odor; appears in blood and urine of persons with diabetes.

acquired as applied to developmental disability, indicates that the disability was not present at birth but developed before the age of 22.

acquired immuno deficiency syndrome (AIDS) progressive disease of the immune system caused by the human immunodeficiency virus (HIV). Initially an extremely high mortality rate was the norm for the disease, but now combination drug therapy can slow the disease process and lengthen life expectancy of those infected with HIV.

activities of daily living (ADLs) activities necessary to fulfill basic human needs.

acupuncture insertion of tiny, thin needles in various parts of the body to correct imbalances in energy and treat disease.

acute disease disease that comes on suddenly, requires urgent treatment, and is usually resolved.

acute exacerbation increase in the severity of signs and symptoms of a chronic disease.

acute flaccid myelitis (AFM) serious condition affecting the nervous system and causing the person to become very weak.

acute illness illness that comes on suddenly; requires intensive, immediate treatment.

adaptation adjustment.

adaptive device item altered to make it easier to use by those with functional deficits to perform any activity of daily living.

Addison's disease disease caused by underfunctioning of the adrenal glands.

adduction movement toward midline or center.

adjunctive device secondary device used to maintain the airway and respirations.

admission procedure carried out when a patient first arrives at a facility.

adolescence teenage years.

adoptive parent person who is a parent through a legal adoption procedure.

adrenal glands endocrine glands; one is located on the top of each kidney; secrete hormones, including epinephrine.

advance directive document signed before the diagnosis of a terminal illness, when the individual is still in good health, indicating the person's wishes regarding care during dying.

advocate person who speaks on behalf of the patient.

affective disorders group of mental disorders characterized by a disturbance in mood. They may also be called *mood disorders*, and are usually marked by a profound and persistent sadness.

Affordable Care Act (ACA) law that gives consumers control of their health care.

agitation mental state characterized by irregular and erratic behavior.

aiding and abetting not reporting dishonest acts that are observed.

airborne infection isolation room (AIIR) negative air pressure isolation room in which air enters and leaves the room through a special exhaust system to the outside.

airborne precautions procedures used to prevent the spread of airborne pathogens.

airborne transmission method of spreading disease by breathing tiny pathogens that remain suspended in the air for long periods of time.

akinesia difficulty and slowness in carrying out voluntary muscular activities.

alcoholism dependency on alcohol.

allergen substance that causes sensitivity or allergic reactions.

allergy abnormal and individual hypersensitivity.

alopecia absence of hair where hair normally grows.

alternative choice; option.

alternative medical systems therapeutic or preventive health care practices that are used instead of conventional health care; often involve the use of natural products rather than those derived from chemicals. These systems do not follow generally accepted methods and may not have a scientific explanation for their effectiveness.

alveoli tiny air sacs that make up most of the lungs.

Alzheimer's disease neurological condition in which there is a gradual loss of cerebral functioning.

ambulate to walk.

ambulation process of walking.

a.m. care care given in the early morning when the patient first awakens.

amenorrhea without menstruation.

amino acids basic components of proteins.

amniotic fluid fluid in which the fetus floats in the mother's womb.

amniotic sac sac enclosing the fetus and amniotic fluid.

amputation removal of a limb or other body appendage.

amyotrophic lateral sclerosis (ALS) progressive neuromuscular disease that causes muscle weakness and paralysis.

analgesic pain-relieving medication.

anaphylactic shock extreme, sometimes fatal, sensitivity or allergic reaction to a specific antigen.

anatomic position standing erect, facing observer, feet flat on floor and slightly separated, arms at sides, palms forward.

anatomy study of the structure of the human body.

anemia deficiency of quality or quantity of red blood cells in the blood.

aneroid gauge device for measuring and registering blood pressure.

anesthesia loss of feeling or sensation.

anger feeling of hostility, rage.

angina pectoris acute pain in the chest caused by interference with the supply of oxygen to the heart.

animal-assisted therapy pet therapy; pets visiting in a health care facility for a therapeutic purpose.

anorexia lack or loss of appetite for food.

anorexia nervosa eating disorder in which the patient has a disturbed body image; despite appearing skeletal, he or she views the body as being fat.

antecubital area area on the inner surface of the arm, in front of the elbow.

anterior in anatomy, in front of the coronal or ventral plane.

anteroom small room just inside the entrance to an isolation room; usually has a sink and containers for trash disposal.

anthroposophically extended medicine (AEM) holistic system of natural medicine that treats the whole person, not just the disease or symptoms; treatment is designed to harmonize the relationship of body, mind, and spirit.

antibiotic medication used to treat bacterial infection.

antibiotic stewardship refers to a set of coordinated strategies being used worldwide to prevent antibiotic resistance.

antibodies proteins produced in the body in response to invasion by a foreign agent (antigen); react specifically with the foreign agent.

anticoagulant medication that thins the blood and increases the risk of bleeding.

anti-embolism hose elasticized stockings used to support the leg blood vessels.

antigen marker on cells that identifies a cell as self or nonself; antigens on foreign substances that enter the body, such as pathogens, stimulate the production of antibodies by the body.

anxiety fear, apprehension, or sense of impending danger that is often marked by vague physical symptoms, such as tension, restlessness, and rapid heart rate.

anxiety disorder one of a group of recognized mental illnesses involving anxiety reactions in response to stress.

Apgar score method for determining an infant's condition at birth by scoring heart rate, respiratory effect, muscle tone, reflex irritability, and color.

aphasia language impairment; loss of ability to comprehend or produce language normally.

apical pulse pulse rate taken by placing a stethoscope over the tip of the heart.

apnea period of no respiration.

approach action used by the health care team to help resolve a patient's problems; steps taken to reach a goal.

Aquamatic K-Pad (aquathermia pad) brand name of a unit for applying heat or cold.

areola dark area in the center of the breast.

aromatherapy use of natural scents and smells to promote health and well-being.

art therapy use of art and the various senses to express oneself.

artery vessel through which oxygenated blood moves away from the heart to various parts of the body.

arthritis joint inflammation.

ascites fluid accumulation in the abdomen.

asepsis without infection.

aspirate to withdraw.

aspiration very serious condition in which food, water, gastric contents, or other materials enter the trachea and lungs. It is usually accidental, such as when the patient "swallows down the wrong tube" or accidentally inhales food or fluids. If you suspect that a patient has aspirated, inform the nurse promptly.

assault attempt or threat to do violence to another.

assessment act of evaluating.

assignment specific list of duties; tells you which patients you will care for during your shift and the specific procedures to be performed.

assimilate to absorb.

assisted living facility (ALF) care situation where a person primarily cares for himself or herself but has some help in meeting health care needs or receives health care supervision.

assistive device equipment used to help people be more effective in their physical activity.

asthma chronic respiratory disease characterized by bronchospasms and excessive mucus production.

atelectasis decreased or absent air in all or part of a lung, resulting in loss of lung volume and inability to expand the lung fully.

atheroma degeneration or thickening of artery walls due to formation of fatty plaque and scar tissue.

atherosclerosis degenerative process involving the lining of arteries, in which the lumen eventually narrows and closes; a form of arteriosclerosis.

atrium one of the two upper chambers of the heart.

atrophy shrinking or wasting away of tissues.

attitude external expression of inner feelings about oneself or others.

aura peculiar sensation preceding the appearance of more definite symptoms in a convulsion or seizure.

auscultatory gap sound fadeout for 1–15 mm Hg (millimeters of mercury) pressure, after which sound begins again; sometimes mistaken for the diastolic pressure.

autism developmental disorder that appears during the first three years of life, affecting the person's ability to communicate and interact with others.

autoclave machine that sterilizes articles.

autoimmune presence of antibodies against component(s) of the body.

automatic external defibrillator (AED) computerized device that uses an electric shock to reverse disorganized activity in the heart during cardiac arrest.

autonomic dysreflexia potentially life-threatening complication of spinal cord injury; indicates uncontrolled sympathetic nervous system activity.

autonomy self-determination.

autopsy examination of body after death to determine cause of death.

avulsion fracture fracture caused by a bone fragment pulling off at the point of ligament or tendon attachment.

axilla armpit.

axon extension of neuron that conducts nerve impulses away from the cell body.

Ayurveda natural system of medicine based on the belief that disease is due to an imbalance in the consciousness. Uses lifestyle interventions, natural therapies, and rebalancing among the body, mind, and environment.

bacillus (plural bacilli) rod-shaped bacterium.

bacterium (plural bacteria) form of simple microbes.

bag bath *See* waterless bathing

bag-valve-mask (BVM) device used to support ventilation for patients in respiratory arrest; consists of a face mask and a ventilation bag.

balance bar section of an upright scale that holds the weights used to determine a patient's weight.

bandage fabric, gauze, net, or elasticized material used to cover dressings and keep them securely in place.

bargaining stage of the grieving process in which the individual seeks to make a deal or form a pact that will delay death.

bariatric surgery surgery on the stomach and/or intestines to help the patient with morbid or super obesity and a BMI greater than 40 lose weight. Sometimes used as a treatment for people with a BMI between 35 and 40 who have health problems and potentially serious comorbidities, such as heart disease or type 2 diabetes.

bariatrics relatively new field of medicine that focuses on the treatment and control of obesity and diseases associated with obesity.

baseline measurement of a patient's vital signs or other body functions upon admission; future measurements are compared to these initial measurements to track the patient's progress.

baseline assessment initial observations of the patient and his or her condition.

battery unlawful attack upon or touching of another person.

bedbugs parasites that are difficult to eliminate and have been found throughout the world; they are active mainly at night, seeking a blood meal from a human or animal host.

belief idea based on commonly held opinions, knowledge, and attitudes.

benign nonmalignant (tumor).

benign prostatic hypertrophy noncancerous enlargement of the prostate gland.

bile substance produced by the liver that prepares fats for digestion.

binders fabric or elastic wraps that encircle the abdomen; may be used to hold dressings in place or support a surgical site.

biofeedback method of retraining the mind to consciously control various physical problems and stresses that one would not normally be aware of.

biofilms strong, complex colonies of bacteria and other microbes that attach themselves to environmental surfaces and the human body; they secrete a sticky outer coat that is hard to penetrate.

biohazard waste items or laboratory specimens or materials, and their containers contaminated by body fluids; these have the potential to transmit disease. Discarded items must be labeled. Special precautions are taken to handle and contain this waste.

biological parent natural parent who contributed sperm or an ovum to the development of the fetus.

biological therapy biologically based practices using natural substances and products to promote or regain health.

biopsy removal and examination of a piece of tissue from a living body.

bioterrorism use of biological agents, such as pathogenic organisms or agricultural pests, for terrorist purposes.

bipolar affective disorder mood disorder in which the person has marked mood swings beyond what most people experience (also called *manic depression* or *bipolar depression*).

bisexuality having sexual interest in both genders.

blood pressure pressure of blood exerted against vascular walls.

body alignment position of a human body in which the body can properly function.

body-based therapy practices that are based on direct body contact, including manipulation or movement of one or more parts of the body.

body core center of the body (internal).

body language use of facial expression, body positions, and vocal inflections to convey a message.

body mass index (BMI) mathematical calculation used to determine whether a person is at a healthy, normal weight; is overweight; or is obese. BMI measures body weight relative to a person's height by dividing a person's weight (in kilograms) by his or her height (in meters, squared).

body shell outer surface of the body.

bolus soft mass of food that is ready to be swallowed; also, a dose of medication that is given all at once.

borderline personality disorder (BPD) condition in which the patient feels very unstable. He or she may be manipulative, impulsive, prone to self-injurious behavior, and fear abandonment.

boundaries invisible lines that define healthy relationships and limit the sphere of activity.

bowel and bladder retraining (B&B) restorative program that helps a person regain voluntary control of urine and stool.

Bowman's capsule tubule surrounding the glomerulus of the nephron.

box (square) corner one type of corner used in the making of a hospital bed.

brachial artery main artery of the arm.

brachytherapy form of radiation therapy in which tiny radioactive seeds or pellets are implanted directly inside the prostate gland or tumor site.

bradycardia unusually slow heartbeat.

braille method of communication used by persons with visual impairments, who use fingertips to feel a series of raised dots representing letters and numbers.

brain attack interference with the supply of blood to the brain; also known as *stroke* or *cerebrovascular accident*.

brainstem base of the brain; enlarged extension of the spinal cord, located in the cranium; includes the medulla oblongata, diencephalon, pons, and midbrain.

bridging supporting the body on either side of an affected area to relieve pressure on the area.

bronchi tubal structures connecting the trachea to the lungs.

bronchioles smaller subdivisions or branches at end of the bronchi, located in the lungs.

bronchitis inflammation of the bronchi.

bruxism grinding of the teeth.

bulimia nervosa condition in which patients usually binge-eat in huge amounts, and then vomit (purge) to undo the binge. The binge eating causes feelings of guilt, depression, and self-condemnation.

bullying repeated behavior that makes fun of, embarrasses, scares, threatens, belittles, degrades, offends, or insults another person.

burn traumatic injury to the skin and underlying tissues caused by heat, chemicals, or electricity. Burns are very painful injuries with a high risk of complications. Extensive treatment is often required.

burnout loss of enthusiasm for and interest in an activity.

bursae small sacs of fluid found around joints.

bursitis condition in which the bursae become inflamed and the joint becomes very painful.

cachexia state of malnutrition, emaciation, and debility, usually resulting from a prolonged illness.

cancer disease in which the normal mechanisms of cell growth are disturbed. Cells grow abnormally, invade surrounding tissues, and use nutrition targeted for normal cells.

cannula indwelling tube inserted through a stoma (or into the skin) to maintain patency.

capillary hairlike blood vessel; link between arterioles and venules.

capillary refill quick and painless method of checking a patient's peripheral circulation and oxygenation status; done by pressing on a fingernail and noting the time needed for skin color to return to normal when pressure is released.

carbapenem-resistant *Enterobacteriaceae* (CRE) family of drug-resistant pathogens consisting of more than 70 types of bacteria. This family has the potential to cause life-threatening infections that may be impossible to cure.

carbohydrates energy foods; used by the body to produce heat and energy for work.

carbon dioxide gas that is a waste product of cellular metabolism.

carcinogen cancer-causing substance.

carcinoma malignant tumor made up of connective tissue enclosing epithelial cells.

cardiac arrest sudden and often unexpected stoppage of effective heart action.

cardiac cycle all (mechanical and electrical) events that occur between one heart contraction and the next.

cardiac decompensation another name for congestive heart failure.

cardiac muscle muscle that forms the heart wall.

cardiopulmonary resuscitation (CPR) emergency medical procedure undertaken to restart and sustain heart and respiratory functions.

career ladders programs that provide an opportunity for upward mobility.

care plan nursing plan for care of a resident in a long-term care facility.

care plan conference meeting of members of an interdisciplinary health care team to develop approaches and a plan of care.

caries tooth decay or cavities.

carrier person who hosts infectious organisms without having symptoms of disease. This person can give the disease to others. He or she may not know of the infection.

cartilage type of connective tissue usually found between bones.

case manager registered nurse who coordinates the health care of each home health care client.

cataract opacity of the lens of the eye, resulting in loss of vision.

catastrophic reaction severe and unpredictable violent behavior of a person with dementia.

catheter tube for evacuating or injecting fluids.

causative agent etiology (cause) of a specific disease process.

caustic capable of burning living tissue, including skin, mucous membranes, and internal organs.

cavity enclosed area; space within the body that contains organs.

celibate has no sexual intercourse.

cell basic unit in the organization of living substances.

cellulose basic substance of all plant foods; can supply the body with roughage.

Celsius scale centigrade scale for measuring temperature.

Centers for Disease Control and Prevention (CDC) official public health organization in the United States. Studies disease and makes guidelines and recommendations for preventing and treating infection and keeping the public healthy.

central venous catheter (CVC) tube inserted into a large vein in the area of the clavicle.

cerebellum portion of the brain lying beneath the occipital lobe; coordinates muscular activities and balance.

cerebral palsy (CP) motor control developmental disability caused by an injury or abnormality affecting the immature brain.

cerebrospinal fluid (CSF) watery cushion protecting the brain and spinal cord from shock.

cerebrovascular accident (CVA) more commonly called *brain attack* or *stroke*; disorder of the blood vessels of the brain resulting in impaired cerebral circulation and often causing motor and cognitive deficits.

cerebrum largest part of the brain, consisting of two hemispheres separated by a deep longitudinal fissure; controls all mental activities.

certification inspection process for facilities that accept state or federal funds as payment for health care.

cervical traction use of weights to apply traction in the area of the cervical vertebrae.

chain of infection process of events involved in the transmission and development of an infection.

chancre shallow, craterlike lesion; primary lesion of syphilis.

charting entering information (documentation) in a patient's medical record (chart).

chelation therapy intravenous injection of an amino acid by a licensed professional; commonly used to treat serious circulatory problems, heavy metal poisoning, and reduced blood flow in the legs.

chemical burn injury (burn) caused by exposure to chemicals that damage the skin and mucous membranes.

chemical restraint use of medications to control behavior.

chemotherapy use of medications to treat disease.

chest tubes sterile, clear plastic tubes that are inserted through the skin of the chest, between the ribs, and into the space between the lung and chest wall; used after surgery to drain bloody fluid from the chest and allow air to escape if there is a small leak of air at the suture line after lung surgery.

Cheyne–Stokes respirations periods of apnea alternating with periods of dyspnea.

chiropractic care manual adjustments to keep the vertebrae in good alignment, relieving pressure on nerves, muscles, and joints.

chlamydia type of sexually transmitted infection.

cholecystectomy surgical removal of a diseased gallbladder and stones.

cholecystitis inflammation of the gallbladder.

cholelithiasis formation of stones in the gallbladder.

chorea abnormal, spastic movements that are the primary sign of Huntington disease.

chronic disease, chronic illness incurable illness or disease, but treatable; requires ongoing care.

chronic obstructive lung disease (COLD) any condition, such as emphysema or bronchitis, that interferes with normal respiration over a long period of time.

chronic obstructive pulmonary disease (COPD) *See* chronic obstructive lung disease (COLD)

chronologic in sequential order by date or age.

chyme semiliquid form of food as it leaves the stomach.

circumcision removal of the end of the prepuce by a circular incision.

citation written notice that informs a facility of violations of OSHA rules.

clear liquid diet diet of water and high-carbohydrate fluids given every two to four hours.

client person receiving care in the home; some hospitals also use the designation.

client care record documentation of care provided in the home setting.

Clients' Rights document spelling out rights of persons receiving home health care.

climacteric menopause; the combined phenomena accompanying cessation of the reproductive function in the female or reduction of testicular activity in the male.

clinical thermometer instrument used to measure body temperature.

clitoris small, cylindrical mass of erotic tissue; part of the external female reproductive organs analogous to the penis in the male.

closed bed bed with sheets and spread positioned to the head of the bed; unoccupied.

closed (simple) fracture fracture in which bones remain in proper alignment.

cloud external server for file storage that can be accessed via the Web. Contributing organizations can use all or part of the information.

coccus (plural cocci) round bacterium.

cochlea spiral-shaped organ in the inner ear that receives and interprets sounds.

cochlear implant complex device that helps persons with certain types of hearing loss. An external portion sits behind the ear, while a second part is surgically implanted under the skin. Does not restore hearing, but can help a deaf person understand speech and provides a useful representation of sounds in the environment.

coercion forcing a patient to do something against his or her wishes.

cognitive impairment deficit in intellect, memory, or attention.

coitus sexual intercourse; copulation.

cold pack type of thermal application used to lower the temperature of a portion of the body; often a commercially prepared, disposable item.

colon large intestine.

colony group of organisms derived from a single organism.

color therapy alternative health care practices that use color to affect mood, emotions, relationships, and sense of well-being.

colostomy artificial opening in the abdomen for the purpose of evacuating feces.

colostrum secretion from the lactiferous glands of the mother before the onset of true lactation two or three days after delivery of a baby.

colporrhaphy suturing of the vagina; surgical procedure used to tighten vaginal walls.

combining form word part that can be used with other word parts to form a variety of new words.

comfort state of well-being in which the patient is calm and relaxed, and is not in pain or upset.

comminuted fracture fracture in which the bone is broken or crushed into small pieces.

communicable disease disease caused by pathogenic organisms; can be transmitted from person to person, either directly or indirectly.

communication exchange of messages.

community people who live in a common area and share common health needs.

comorbidities diseases and medical conditions that are either caused by or contributed to by morbid obesity or another medical problem.

compartment syndrome painful condition that occurs when pressure within the muscles builds up, preventing blood and oxygen from reaching muscles and nerves; a very serious complication that may develop following an injury or surgical procedure.

compensate seek a substitute for something unattainable or unacceptable.

complementary/alternative medicine (CAM) group of diverse systems, practices, and products that are not presently considered part of conventional (mainstream) medicine.

complementary medicine treatment regimen in which alternative practices are combined with conventional health care.

complete fracture break across the entire cross-section of the bone.

complication situation that makes the original medical condition more serious.

compound (open) fracture fracture in which part of the broken bone protrudes through the skin.

compression fracture break in a bone with crushing of the bone fragments.

compulsion purposeful, repetitive behavior that is done many times each day and problematic enough to cause distress, be time-consuming, or interfere with the person's normal routine, occupation, social activities, or relationships.

concurrent cleaning daily, routine cleaning of the patient unit.

condom catheter latex sheath that fits over the penis; used for urinary drainage when connected to a urinary collection bag.

confidential keeping what is said or written to oneself; private; not shared.

congenital condition present at birth.

congestive heart failure (CHF) condition resulting from cardiac output inadequate for physiological needs, with shortness of breath, edema, and abnormal retention of sodium and water in body tissues.

conjunctiva mucous membrane that lines the eyelids and covers the eye.

connective tissue tissue that holds other tissues together and provides support for organs and other body structures.

connective tissue cells cells that form connective tissue.

consistent carbohydrate (CHO) diet diabetic meal plan that maintains a consistent carbohydrate content each day without counting calories. The patient receives regular food; about 50 percent of the calories come from carbohydrates, 20 percent from protein, and 30 percent from fat.

constipation difficulty in defecating.

contact precautions practices used to prevent spread of disease by direct or indirect contact.

contact transmission spread of disease by direct or indirect contact with an infected person or a contaminated object.

contagious communicable or easily spread.

contagious disease disease that is communicable; disease that is caused by a pathogenic organism.

contaminated unclean; impure; soiled with microbes.

continuity of care core of practice in which health care is provided on a continuing basis from admission to discharge and beyond.

continuous ambulatory peritoneal dialysis (CAPD) form of dialysis that removes waste products from the patient's blood; performed in subacute care centers and at home.

continuous passive motion (CPM) therapy that prevents stiffness and improves circulation by delivering a form of passive range-of-motion exercise so that the joint is moved without the patient's muscles being used.

continuous positive airway pressure (CPAP) oxygen therapy in which a mask is placed on the patient's face and then connected to a device that creates low levels of pressure to keep the airway open.

continuous sutures special means of closing a wound in which a single thread is used to stitch the wound together.

continuum continuous related series of events or actions.

contracture permanent shortening or contraction of a muscle due to immobility, spasm, or paralysis.

contraindication situation in which a treatment or an action is inappropriate.

contusion mechanical injury (usually caused by a blow) resulting in hemorrhage beneath the unbroken skin.

convulsion seizure or change in electrical brain function.

coping handling or dealing with stress.

core body temperature normal operating temperature of the body center, or *core*. This value reflects the temperature in deep structures of the body such as the liver.

core values deeply held principles and beliefs that guide an organization's or a person's conduct.

cornea transparent portion of the eye through which light passes.

coronary embolism blood clot lodged in a coronary artery.

coronary occlusion closing off of a coronary artery.

coronary thrombosis blood clot within a coronary vessel.

cortex outer portion of a kidney.

countertraction providing opposing balance to traction; used in reduction of fractures.

Cowper's glands pair of small glands that open into the urethra at the base of the penis; part of the male reproductive system.

critical list list that patients are placed on when they are dangerously or terminally ill.

critical (clinical) pathways written documents that detail the expected course of treatment and expected outcomes for a DRG.

critical thinking considering the problem posed by a challenging situation and using what you have learned to solve the problem.

cross-trained educated in several different skills across (health care) disciplines.

crust scab made of dried exudate.

culture views and traditions of a particular group.

culture and sensitivity test to determine what type of microorganisms are causing a disease and the specific antibiotics that can be used to treat the disease.

culture change movement that promotes the transformation of long-term care facilities to treat residents with respect and provide person-directed care.

cumulative collected over a period of time.

cupping use of warmed glass jars to create suction on certain points of the body.

Cushing's syndrome condition that results from an excess level of adrenal cortex hormones.

custodial care providing unskilled services and supplies to assist a person with activities of daily living, such as bathing, eating, and mobility.

cutaneous membrane skin.

cyanosis dusky, bluish discoloration of skin, lips, and nails caused by inadequate oxygen.

cyanotic relating to the condition of cyanosis.

cystitis inflammation of the urinary bladder.

cystocele bladder hernia.

cystoscopy procedure that uses an instrument (cystoscope) for visualization of the urinary bladder and urethra.

dance therapy use of dance to express oneself.

dangling sitting up with legs hanging over the edge of the bed.

debilitating weakening.

debride to remove foreign material and necrotic tissue.

decubitus ulcer older term for a pressure ulcer; open area that develops on the skin over a bony prominence as the result of pressure.

deep vein thrombosis (DVT) blood clot that commonly occurs in the femoral vein, the large blood vessel in the groin.

defamation something harmful to the good name or reputation of another person; slander.

defecation bowel movement that expels feces.

defense mechanism psychological reaction or technique for protection against a stressful environmental situation or anxiety.

defibrillation using an electric shock to reverse disorganized activity in the heart during cardiac arrest.

degenerative joint disease (DJD) deterioration of the tissues of the joints.

dehydration excessive water loss.

delegation transfer of responsibility for the performance of a nursing activity from a nurse to someone who does not already have the authority.

delirium acute, reversible mental confusion due to illness and medical problems.

delirium tremens (DTs) part of a serious withdrawal syndrome seen in persons who suddenly stop drinking alcohol following continuous and heavy consumption; signs and symptoms commonly begin 48 to 96 hours after taking the last drink.

delusion false belief.

dementia progressive mental deterioration due to organic brain disease.

dendrite branch of a neuron that conducts impulses toward the cell body.

denial unconscious defense mechanism in which an occurrence or observation is refused recognition as reality to avoid anxiety or pain.

dentures artificial teeth.

depilatory substance used to remove body hair.

depressant drug that slows down body functions.

depressed fracture fracture in which the bone is depressed and fragments are driven inward; seen only in fractures of the skull and face.

depression morbid sadness or melancholy.

dermal ulcer pressure sore; pressure ulcer.

dermis layer of tissue that lies under the epidermis.

development gradual growth.

developmental disability (DD) permanent condition that occurs before age 22 that changes, delays, or interferes with physical or mental development.

developmental milestones achievement of specific skills at a particular age level.

developmental tasks in psychology, normal steps in personality development.

diabetes mellitus disorder of carbohydrate metabolism.

diagnosis-related groups (DRGs) method used by Medicare to determine the number of hospital days required to treat specific illnesses.

dialect local terminology and usage of a group's common language.

dialysis movement of dissolved materials through a semipermeable membrane, passing from an area of higher concentration to an area of lower concentration; means of cleansing waste or toxic materials from the body.

diaphoresis profuse sweating.

diarrhea condition in which the patient has multiple watery stools.

diastole period during which the heart muscle relaxes and the chamber fills with blood.

diastolic pressure blood pressure during the period of cardiac ventricular relaxation.

diathermy treatment with heat.

digestion process of converting food into a form that can be used by the body.

digital thermometer handheld, battery-operated device that registers temperature and displays the reading as numbers.

dilatation and curettage (D & C) procedure in which the cervical canal is expanded and tissue is scraped from the lining of the uterus.

diplegia paralysis affecting the same region on both sides of the body (such as both arms).

diplo- prefix meaning arranged in pairs, such as diplococci (bacteria that are arranged in groups of two).

dirty anything that has potentially been exposed to pathogens.

disability persistent physical or mental deficit or handicap.

discectomy minimally invasive surgery to repair a back injury.

discharge procedure carried out as a patient leaves the facility; also, an emission of fluid or matter from the body.

disease definite, marked process of illness having characteristic symptoms.

disinfection process of eliminating pathogens from equipment and instruments.

dislocation displacement of the ends of a joint.

disorientation loss of recognition of time, place, or people.

disposable not reusable after one use.

disruption interference with the normal progress of events.

distal farthest away from a central point, such as point of attachment of muscles.

distention state of being stretched out (distended).

diuresis increase in output of fluids by the kidneys.

diverticula small blind pouches that form in the lining and wall of the colon.

diverticulitis inflammation of diverticula.

diverticulosis presence of many diverticula.

DNR do-not-resuscitate order; used when cardiac and respiratory arrest occur.

doctor of osteopathy (DO) physician who receives a complete medical education similar to that of a medical doctor (MD). Additionally, the DO learns how to manipulate the spine for a therapeutic response in the body.

document [noun] legal record; [verb] to record observations and data about a patient's condition.

documentation process of recording the patient's care, response to treatment, and progress in the patient's chart.

dorsal posterior or back.

dorsal lithotomy position position in which the patient is on the back with knees flexed and well separated; feet are usually placed in stirrups.

dorsal recumbent position position in which the patient is flat on the back with knees flexed and slightly separated, with feet flat on the bed.

dorsiflexion toes pointed up.

dosimeter small personal monitoring instrument that measures the radiation dose received by each individual working with patients receiving radiation therapy or brachytherapy.

douche irrigation of the vaginal canal with medicated or normal saline solution.

doula person who accompanies the mother during the childbirth process; responsible for supporting and comforting the mother and enhancing communication between the mother and medical professionals.

Down syndrome congenital condition in which persons are born with 47 chromosomes instead of the usual 46.

drainage systematic withdrawal of fluids and discharge from wounds, sores, or body cavities.

draw sheet sheet folded under the patient, extending from above the shoulder to below the hips.

dressing gauze, film, or other synthetic substance that covers a wound, ulcer, or injury.

droplet precautions procedures used to prevent the spread of disease by droplets in air.

droplet transmission method of spreading infection by inhaling pathogens from the droplets of a patient's respiratory secretions. The droplets do not travel more than three feet from the source patient.

duodenal resection surgical removal of a portion of small intestine (duodenum).

duodenal ulcer ulcer on the mucosa of the duodenum due to the action of gastric juice.

durable power of attorney for health care document stating that a person appointed by the patient can make health care decisions when the patient is unable to do so for himself or herself.

dyscrasia abnormality or disorder of the body.

dysentery infection in the lower bowel.

dysmenorrhea difficult or painful menstruation.

dysphagia difficulty swallowing food and liquids.

dyspnea difficult or labored breathing.

dysuria painful voiding.

eating disorders group of disorders characterized by disturbances in appetite or food intake.

Ebola serious illness caused by the Ebola virus for which there is no cure and 70 percent mortality; 7 out of 10 people with the virus will die.

ecchymosis bruising.

edema excessive accumulation of fluid in the tissues.

ejaculatory duct part of the male reproductive system extending down from the seminal vesicles to the urethra.

elasticity ability to stretch.

electric bed bed operated by electricity.

electrical burn injury (burn) caused by contact with electricity or lightning. Typically deep; the electricity charts an unpredictable path through the body, causing major damage along the path from entrance to exit.

electromagnetic therapy use of various forms of electrical energy to correct imbalances in the body's electrical and magnetic fields; the imbalances are believed to cause illness and disease.

electronic health record (EHR) patient record in digital format; not a complete medical record. The EHR contains data that are part of a larger record collection.

electronic medical record (EMR) digital patient record for a single organization or setting. Information from the nursing assistant contributes to the EHR.

electronic patient record (EPR) term sometimes used to describe an electronic medical record.

electronic thermometer battery-operated clinical thermometer that uses a probe and records the temperature on a viewing screen in a few seconds.

eloping wandering away from a health care facility.

embolus mass of undissolved material carried in the bloodstream; frequently causes obstruction of a vessel.

emergency situation requiring immediate attention or medical treatment.

emergency care medical treatment and nursing care provided to emergency patients (victims).

emergency medical services (EMS) treatment and care provided by specially trained health care personnel during emergencies.

emesis vomiting.

emotional lability unstable emotional status with frequent changes in emotions and mood.

empathy understanding how someone else feels.

emphysema chronic obstructive pulmonary disease in which the alveolar walls are destroyed.

enabler device that empowers patients and assists them to function at their highest possible level.

enabling reacting to a patient in a manner that shields the patient from experiencing the full impact or consequences of his or her actions or behavior.

endocardium lining of the heart.

endocrine gland ductless gland that secretes hormonal substances directly into the bloodstream.

endometrium mucous membrane lining the inner surface of the uterus.

endotracheal intubation inserting a large tube through the trachea and into the lungs to provide complete control over the airway; the procedure is commonly called *intubation*.

endotracheal tube (ET tube) large tube that is passed through the mouth, or less commonly the nose, into the patient's lungs to control the airway; the patient is ventilated and suctioned through the tube.

enema injection of water and/or medications into the rectum and colon; commonly used to help the bowels eliminate feces.

energy therapy alternative and complementary practices that involve working with the energy field that reportedly surrounds and penetrates the body.

enteral feeding giving nutrition through a tube inserted into the digestive tract.

enuresis bedwetting.

environmental safety adaptation of the environment to prevent incidents and injuries.

epidemic rapid spread of infectious disease in a brief period of time.

epidermis top layer of skin.

epididymis elongated, cordlike structure along the posterior border of the testes, in the ducts of which sperm are stored.

epidural catheter tube inserted into the spinal area for delivery of medication.

epilepsy disorder in which temporary abnormal activity occurs in brain cells, causing mild episodic loss of attention, sleepiness, convulsions with loss of consciousness, and various other symptoms.

epithelial cells structures that form protective coverings (epithelial tissue) and sometimes produce body fluids.

epithelial tissue structure formed from epithelial cells; protects, absorbs, produces fluids, excretes wastes.

ergonomics process of adapting the environment and using techniques and equipment to prevent worker injuries.

erythrocyte red blood cell.

eschar slough of tissue produced by burning or by a corrosive application.

Escherichia coli (*E. coli* 0157:H7) strain of bacteria (not found in humans); a pathogen that multiplies rapidly and produces large amounts of toxins that cause serious illness and death.

essential nutrients foods required for normal growth and development and to maintain health.

estrogen hormone produced by the ovaries.

ethical standards guides to moral behavior.

ethnic relating to customs, languages, and traditions of specific groups of people.

ethnicity special groupings within a race.

etiology cause of a disease.

eustachian tube auditory tube; leads from the middle ear to the pharynx.

evaluation assessment, judgment.

eversion turning outward.

evidence-based practice (EBP) approach that guides decision making by identifying evidence for a practice, then rating that practice according to the strength of the evidence.

exacerbation worsening of a chronic medical condition.

exchange list list of measured foods that allows equivalent exchanges between foods within a designated food group.

excoriation superficial injury, such as that produced by scratching the skin.

excrete to eliminate wastes from body.

expectorate to spit (to bring up sputum).

expiration exhalation.

exposure incident occurrence during which there is possible personal contact with infectious material.

expressive aphasia inability to use verbal speech.

extension movement by which the two ends of any jointed part are drawn away from each other.

face shield type of personal protective equipment; protects mucous membranes of eyes, nose, and mouth from pathogens.

facility (health care) agency that provides health care.

Fahrenheit scale system used in the United States to express temperature.

fallopian tube *See* oviduct

false imprisonment unlawfully restraining another person.

family group of persons (usually related by blood or marriage) with common values and traditions.

fasting not eating.

fat nutrient used to store energy.

fecal impaction most serious form of constipation, in which stool is retained in the rectum, where water is absorbed. Over time, the stool becomes hard and dry, and the patient is unable to pass it.

fecal material another term for feces, stool, or solid body waste (bowel movement or BM). Normally brown, but color can be affected by certain foods, medications, and diseases. A BM is normally soft and formed.

feces stool; semisolid waste eliminated from the body.

feedback confirmation that a message was received as intended.

fetus child in the uterus from the third month to birth.

fibromyalgia common pain syndrome for which there is no known cause.

fingerstick blood sugar (FSBS) method of checking blood sugar by collecting a sample of capillary blood with a lancet.

first aid emergency care and treatment of an injured person before complete medical and surgical care can be secured.

fistula abnormal communication between two hollow organs or between a hollow organ and the exterior.

flaccid paralysis loss of muscle tone and absence of tendon reflexes.

flagged marked in a special way to attract attention.

flatulence excessive gas in the stomach and/or intestines.

flatus gas or air in the stomach or intestines; air or gas expelled by way of any body opening.

flexion decreasing the angle between two bones.

flora normal population of organisms found in a given area.

flow sheet clinical record of ongoing patient care and progress.

fluid balance balance between fluid intake and fluid output.

Foley catheter indwelling catheter placed in the urinary bladder to remove urine continuously.

fomite any object contaminated with germs and thus able to transmit disease.

food handler employee who works with unpackaged food, food equipment or utensils, or food contact surfaces.

footboard appliance placed at the foot of the bed so that the feet rest firmly against it and are kept at right angles to the legs.

foot drop neurological problem that causes the foot to point downward.

force fluids notation meaning that the patient must be encouraged to take in as much fluid as possible.

foreskin prepuce; loose tissue covering the penis and clitoris.

foster parent parent figure assigned by an agency.

Fowler's position position in which the patient lies on the back with backrest elevated 45° to 60°.

fracture break in the continuity of bone.

friction rubbing of the skin against another surface, such as bed linens.

full liquid diet diet consisting of all types of fluids.

full weight-bearing (FWB) able to stand on both legs.

fungus (plural fungi) class of organisms to which molds and yeasts belong.

fusion combination into a single unit.

gait manner of walking.

gait belt belt placed around the patient's waist to assist in ambulation.

gait training teaching the patient to walk.

gastrectomy surgical removal of part or all of the stomach.

gastric bypass most common of the six accepted bariatric surgical techniques. In this procedure, the surgeon creates a two-inch-long pouch at the top of the patient's stomach and attaches a portion of small intestine to the stomach pouch.

gastric resection surgical removal of part of the stomach.

gastric ulcer erosion of the lining of the stomach.

gastroesophageal reflux disease (GERD) condition in which stomach contents flow backward into the esophagus.

gastroscopy procedure to examine the inside of the stomach, using a scope for visualization.

gastrostomy feeding nutrition given through a tube inserted into the stomach through the abdominal wall.

gatch bed bed fitted with a jointed backrest and knee rest; patient can be raised to a sitting position and kept in that position by manually adjusting the bed.

general anesthetic medication that induces a state of unconsciousness and reduces or eliminates ability to feel pain.

generalized tonic-clonic seizure another name for grand mal seizure.

generation group of individuals born within the same period of time who have been influenced by the same social markers.

genetic pertaining to or carried by a gene or genes.

genitalia external reproductive organs.

geriatric relating to age or the elderly.

Glasgow Coma Scale system used to monitor neurologic problems after trauma, stroke, and other illnesses and injuries; uses a point score to rank the patient's responses to stimuli.

glaucoma condition in which the pressure is increased within the eye. Untreated, it will lead to blindness.

global aphasia loss of all language ability.

glomerulus blood vessels that branch to form a ball of capillaries in the cortex of the kidney.

glucagon hormone produced by the pancreas that increases blood sugar level.

glucose simple sugar; also called *dextrose*.

glycated hemoglobin (A1C) series of stable minor blood components formed from hemoglobin and glucose. The A1C test is a measurement of glucose levels in the blood over a 90-day period of time.

glycogen polysaccharide that is the chief carbohydrate storage material.

glycosuria sugar in the urine.

goal outcome resulting from implementation of a care plan.

goggles type of personal protective equipment used with standard precautions to protect the eyes.

gonads reproductive organs; ovaries and testes.

gonorrhea sexually transmitted infection that causes an acute inflammation.

gout metabolic disease that results in chronic, painful, inflammatory arthritis and buildup of uric acid deposits in the joints.

graduate container marked in milliliters; used to measure liquids.

graft body tissue used for transplantation.

grand mal seizure major epileptic seizure characterized by loss of consciousness and convulsive movements.

greenstick fracture breaking of a bone on one side only; most often seen in children.

grievance situation in which a consumer feels there are grounds for complaint.

growth physical changes that take place in the body during development.

guided imagery practice in which the patient focuses on and visualizes positive changes, so as to cause the changes to occur.

halitosis bad breath.

handoff communication essential communication that must occur when patient care is transferred from one worker or department to another worker or department.

hand-over-hand technique method in which an instructor or caregiver places his or her hand over the hand of a learner or patient to guide an activity.

hantavirus virus spread by contact with rodents (rats and mice) or their excretions; causes serious illness or death.

harvest to remove donor organs.

head lice parasites that live in the hair and scalp and feed on blood; spread primarily by direct contact with an infected person.

head-tilt, chin-lift maneuver procedure used to open a patient's airway if no neck injury is suspected; pressure is placed on the forehead while the jaw is lifted up.

health state of physical, mental, and social well-being.

health care consumer person requiring health care services.

Health Insurance Portability and Accountability Act (HIPAA) law passed in 1996 that protects privacy, confidentiality, medical records, and other individually identifiable patient information.

health maintenance organization (HMO) group of health care providers and hospitals paid by an insurance company. HMO members must see only certain doctors and go only to designated hospitals, except in emergencies.

heart block condition in which conduction of electrical impulses from atrium to ventricles is impaired and the pumping action of the heart is slowed down (change in rhythm of the heart).

heat exhaustion condition caused by exposure to high temperature that causes the loss and imbalance of body fluids; will progress to heat stroke and death if not treated promptly.

heat stroke serious condition caused by lengthy exposure to high heat that results in the inability to regulate body temperature and progresses to death.

Heimlich maneuver procedure that uses abdominal thrusts to relieve obstruction in the trachea.

hematoma localized mass of blood that is confined to one area.

hematuria blood in the urine.

hemianopsia visual impairment due to stroke; affects one-half of visual field in one or both eyes.

hemiparesis weakness on one side of the body; usually the result of a stroke.

hemiplegia paralysis on one side of the body.

hemodialysis method for circulating blood through semipermeable membranes to remove liquid body wastes.

hemoptysis expectoration of blood.

hemorrhage excessive escape of blood from blood vessels.

hemorrhoids varicose veins in the rectum.

hepatitis inflammation of the liver.

herbal therapy use of herbs to treat pain and illness.

herbs medicines made from plants.

hernia protrusion or projection of a stomach organ through the wall or cavity that normally contains it.

herniorrhaphy surgical operation for hernia.

herpes simplex II virus that causes genital herpes.

heterosexuality sexual attraction between persons of opposite genders.

high-efficiency particulate air (HEPA) filter mask mask used by health care workers that prevents the spread of airborne infection.

high Fowler's position position in which the backrest of the bed is elevated to 90°, with the patient on his or her back.

holistic care practices that consider the whole person, including mind, body, and spirit.

home health assistant nursing assistant who practices under nursing supervision in a client's home.

homemaker aide person hired to perform light housekeeping tasks in a client's home.

homemaker assistant person who provides home management help to a client in the client's home.

homeopathy alternative medicine system that uses a wide range of natural (plant and mineral) substances to stimulate the body's immune system to fight disease.

homosexuality sexual attraction between persons of the same gender.

hormone secretion of an endocrine gland; chemical messenger carried to other parts of the body, where it alters cellular activity.

hospice special facility or arrangement to provide care of persons with a terminally illness.

hospice care health care for persons who are dying.

hospital facility for acute care of the sick or injured.

host animal or plant that harbors another organism.

hot water bottle reusable waterproof canvas or rubber container that can be filled with hot water for a warm application.

human immunodeficiency virus (HIV) virus that causes acquired immune deficiency syndrome (AIDS).

humidifier water bottle that moistens oxygen for comfort and prevents drying of the mucous membranes in the nose, mouth, and lungs; used when oxygen is administered at flow rates of five liters per minute or above.

Huntington disease (HD) also called *Huntington chorea*; a hereditary disease that usually begins when an individual is in his or her 40s or 50s, although some may be younger. The disease is progressive and is marked by involuntary spastic movements called *chorea*; the condition progresses until the person is totally dependent, with cognitive decline or dementia.

hydrochloric (HCl) acid acid produced by the stomach.

hydrocolloid dressing adhesive dressing made from gelatin and pectin that provides a moist environment for wound healing.

hydronephrosis increased pressure of urine on the kidney cells that results in their destruction.

hypercalcemia excess calcium in the bloodstream.

hyperglycemia excessive level of sugar in the blood; high blood sugar.

hyperpyrexia abnormally high body temperature of 104°F (rectal) or above.

hypersecretion excessive secretion.

hypersensitivity state of altered reactivity in which the body reacts to a foreign agent more strongly than normal or in an abnormal way.

hypersomnia disorder characterized by sleeping very late in the morning and napping during the day; causes can be physical or psychological.

hypertension high blood pressure.

hyperthermia hyperpyrexia.

hyperthyroidism excessive functioning of the thyroid gland.

hypertrophy increase in the size of an organ or structure that does not involve tumor formation.

hyperventilation breathing abnormally fast and deep, resulting in excessive amounts of oxygen in the lungs and reduced carbon dioxide levels in the bloodstream.

hypnotherapy practice used to create an altered state of consciousness in which the patient is more open to suggestion.

hypochondriasis abnormal concern about one's health.

hypoglycemia abnormally low level of sugar in the blood.

hyposecretion less than normal production of secretions.

hypotension low blood pressure.

hypothermia lowering of core body temperature to 95°F or below.

hypothermia–hyperthermia blanket (aquathermia blanket) fluid-filled blanket, the temperature of which can be raised or lowered.

hypothyroidism condition due to deficiency of thyroid secretion, resulting in a lower basal metabolism.

hypoxia lack of adequate oxygen supply.

hysterectomy surgical removal of the uterus.

ice bag type of cold treatment.

ideal body weight (IBW) mathematical formula. The concept of ideal body weight developed from life insurance statistics related to life span or longevity and health.

ileostomy incision in the ileum.

immune response response of the body to elements recognized as nonself, with the production of antibodies and rejection of the foreign material.

immunity ability to fight off infectious disease; state of being protected from a disease.

immunization process of making a person more resistant to an infectious agent.

immunosuppression condition in which the immune system is unable to respond to the challenge of infectious disease.

immunotherapy cancer treatment that alters the patient's immune response to eliminate the cancer.

impacted fracture fracture that occurs when the fragment from one bone is wedged into another bone.

implantable cardioverter defibrillator (ICD) implanted device that delivers an impulse similar to a shock when a life-threatening heart rhythm occurs.

implementation putting into effect.

incarcerated (strangulated) hernia abnormal constriction of part of the intestinal tract that has herniated.

incentive spirometer apparatus used to encourage better ventilation.

incident occurrence or event that interrupts normal procedures or causes a crisis.

incident report summary of information about an incident.

incomplete fracture partial break in a bone.

increment amount of increase in measurements.

incubation development of bacteria in a host body between time of exposure and onset of signs and symptoms.

indwelling (retention) catheter Foley catheter that remains in the patient's bladder to drain urine.

infarction death of tissue.

infection invasion and multiplication of any organism and the damage this causes in the body.

infectious capable of transmitting disease.

inferior below another part.

infiltration passage of fluid into the tissues surrounding a vein that occurs when an IV needle or catheter comes out of the vein.

inflammation localized protective reaction of tissue to irritation, injury, or infection; characterized by pain, redness, swelling, and sometimes loss of function.

informed consent permission given after full disclosure of the facts.

initiative action of taking the first step or initial action.

insertion distal point of attachment of skeletal muscle.

insomnia chronic deprivation of quality or quantity of sleep because sleep is ended or interrupted prematurely.

inspiration drawing of air into the lungs; inhalation.

insulin active antidiabetic hormone secreted by the islets of Langerhans in the pancreas; regulates entrance of sugars from the blood into the cells.

insulin-dependent diabetes mellitus (IDDM) form of diabetes mellitus that requires insulin administration as part of the therapy.

intake and output (I&O) recording of the amount of fluid ingested and the amount of fluid expelled by a patient.

integrative (integrated) health care using both mainstream medical treatments and CAM therapies to treat a patient.

integument skin.

intellectual disability (ID) developmental disability that affects about 2 to 3 percent of the U.S. population; persons with this condition have lower-than-average intelligence, limited ability to learn, social immaturity, and a limited ability to adapt to their environment. Formerly called mental retardation (MR).

intention tremor involuntary movement of muscles (particularly hands) that increases when the patient attempts to use the muscles.

interdisciplinary health care team group of professionals from different health care disciplines who each contribute their expertise to the care of a single patient.

intermediate care facility (ICF) place where health care is provided to persons with medically stable conditions.

intermittent care care given periodically, at intervals.

intermittent catheter catheter that is inserted to empty the bladder, then immediately removed.

interpersonal relationships how people interact with each other.

interpreter communication professional who mediates between speakers of different languages.

interrupted sutures special method of closing a wound in which each thread is tied off and knotted separately.

intervention actions that influence the eventual outcome of a situation.

intimacy feelings of closeness and familiarity.

intracranial pressure pressure exerted within the cranium (skull).

intravenous (IV) infusion nourishment given through a sterile tube into a vein.

intravenous pyelogram (IVP) X-ray of the urinary tract following the injection of dye into a vein.

invasion of privacy taking liberties with a person or the personal rights of another.

invasive characterized by invading (penetrating into) or spreading.

inversion turning inward.

involuntary muscle muscle not under conscious control, mainly smooth muscle.

involuntary seclusion separation of a patient from other patients and people, against the patient's will.

involution reduction in the size of the uterus following delivery.

iodine element needed for proper function of the thyroid gland.

iris colored portion of the eye.

ischemia deficient blood supply to body tissues.

ischemic having inadequate blood flow to an area.

islets of Langerhans cells in the pancreas that produce insulin.

isolation place where a patient with an infection disease is separated from others.

isolation technique special procedures carried out to prevent the spread of infectious organisms from an infected person.

isolation unit room used for patients with communicable illness, for protection of other patients, staff, and visitors.

isolette environmentally controlled unit used to house a newborn infant.

jaundice yellow color of the skin and sclera.

jaw-thrust maneuver method of opening the airway of patients with known or suspected neck injuries; involves pushing the jaw forward and upward.

jejunostomy tube (J-tube) long small-bore tube that is threaded through the GI tract until the tip reaches the small intestine. These tubes may be placed through the nose (nasojejunostomy), or surgically through an incision in the abdominal skin. Used for providing enteral nutrition for patients who do not have a stomach and those in whom recurrent formula aspiration is a problem.

job interview discussion between employer and potential employee.

Kaposi's sarcoma type of cancer caused by the herpes virus. It is common in men older than 60 years of age and in those with HIV conditions; can be present even if the person does not have HIV.

Kelly special clamp used to close tubes quickly.

kidney glandular purplish-brown bean-shaped organ situated at back of the abdominal cavity, one on each side of the spinal column; excretes waste matter in the form of urine.

kilogram (kg) metric unit of weight measurement equal to 1,000 grams or 2.2 pounds.

knee-chest position position in which the patient is on the abdomen with knees drawn up toward the abdomen and legs separated; arms are brought up and flexed on either side of the head, which is turned to one side.

labia majora two large hair-covered liplike structures that are part of the vulva.

labia minora two hairless liplike structures found beneath the labia majora.

laceration accidental break in skin; an injury.

lacrimal gland structure that produces tears.

lactation secretion of milk.

laminectomy surgical excision of the rear part of one or more vertebrae, usually done to remove a herniated disk or lesion.

lancet tiny needle.

laryngectomee person who has had a laryngectomy (voice box removal); the patient breathes through an artificial opening in the neck and trachea.

laryngectomy surgical removal of the larynx. The airway is separated from the mouth, nose, and esophagus; there is no longer a connection between the upper and lower airways.

larynx organ located at the upper end of the trachea; part of airway and organ of voice (voice box).

lateral away from the midline.

legal custody condition of having the responsibility for another person (including the right to consent to hospitalization and to give permission for procedures).

legal guardian person who has the legal right to make decisions for another person.

legal standards guides to lawful behavior.

lesions abnormal changes in tissue formation.

leukemia malignant disease of the blood-forming organs; characterized by abnormal proliferation and distortion of the leukocytes in the blood and bone marrow.

leukocyte white blood cell.

leukorrhea white vaginal discharge.

Lhermitte's sign sharp electrical-type sensation felt down the spine when the head is flexed; found in patients with multiple sclerosis.

liable legally responsible.

libel any written defamatory statement.

license state permit allowing a facility to operate.

licensed practical nurse (LPN); licensed vocational nurse (LVN) graduate of a certificate nursing program; must pass a state exam before being permitted to practice nursing.

life-sustaining treatment treatment given to a patient who is injured or who has a critical illness to maintain life and prevent death.

ligament band of fibrous tissue that holds joints together.

light therapy treatment in which patients are exposed to special lights covered with a plastic screen to block ultraviolet rays; used to treat mood and sleep disorders, jet lag, and depression.

Listeriosis illness caused by ingesting the *Listeria monocytogenes* bacterium in contaminated food. The bacterium is found in some raw foods, such as uncooked meats and vegetables, hot dogs, cold cuts, and soft cheeses.

lithotripsy crushing of calculi such as kidney stones.

living will document describing the wishes relating to health care of a person with a terminal illness.

local anesthetic substance that blocks pain receptors or sensation in a specific area.

lochia discharge from the uterus of blood, mucus, and tissue during the puerperal period.

locomotion moving about in a wheelchair.

long-term acute care hospital (LTACH) hospital in which a lengthy stay is anticipated; the accepted patients have medically complex problems but have a good chance of improvement.

long-term care (LTC) health care given to a person in a facility or the person's home for an extended period of time.

long-term care facility facility that cares for persons whose conditions are stable but who need monitoring, nursing care, and treatments.

low bed bed in which the frame is four to six inches from the floor to the top of the frame deck; reduces the risk of injury if the patient falls from the bed.

lumpectomy excision of abnormal tissue, such as a "lump" in the breast.

lymph fluid found in lymphatic vessels.

lymphatic vessel vessel that conveys electrolytes, water, and proteins.

macular degeneration vision impairment due to damage to the macula located at the back of the eye; generally related to aging.

macule flat discolored spot on the skin.

Magnet Program for Excellence in Nursing Services voluntary program that recognizes hospitals for nursing excellence.

maladaptive behavior inappropriate reaction due to mental breakdown.

malignant cancerous.

malodorous having a bad or foul odor.

malpractice improper, negligent, or unethical conduct that results in harm, injury, or loss to a patient.

mammogram X-ray examination of the breasts.

managed care methods used by insurance companies to reduce health care costs.

manual patient handling moving a patient by hand or bodily force, including pushing, pulling, carrying, holding, or supporting the patient or a body part.

massage therapy rubbing various areas of the body to stimulate circulation, promote relaxation, and provide pain relief. Massage increases feelings of well-being and reduces stress and fatigue.

mastectomy excision of the breast.

masturbation sexual self-stimulation.

mechanical lift manually operated hydraulic lift, electrically (or battery-) operated lift, or ceiling-mounted lift. Used to transfer dependent or heavy patients from one surface to another.

mechanical soft diet that includes ground meats; served to patients with no teeth, or those with serious dental problems.

mechanically altered diet in which the consistency and texture of food are modified, making it easier to chew and swallow.

medial close to the midline of the body or structure.

Medicaid federal- and state-funded program that pays medical expenses for those whose income is below a certain level.

medical asepsis procedures followed to keep germs from being spread from one person to another.

medical chart patient record containing all information about that patient.

medical diagnosis name of disease; determination made by a physician.

Medicare federal program that assists persons older than 65 years of age with hospital and medical costs.

meditation calming and quieting the mind by focusing attention.

medulla forms part of the brainstem; also middle area of the kidney.

membranes tissue sheets that line the body cavities.

memo brief written communication to relay information.

meninges three-layered serous membranes covering the brain and spinal cord.

meningitis inflammation of the meninges.

menopause period when ovaries stop functioning and menstruation ceases; female climacteric.

menorrhagia excessive bleeding during menstruation.

menstruation loss of an unneeded part of the endometrium following the release of an ovum and lack of conception.

mental illness behavioral maladaptations.

message information the sender wants to communicate.

metabolism sum total of the physical and chemical processes and reactions taking place in the body.

metabolism rate rate of body function that controls the number of calories needed for the body to function normally.

metastasis spreading of cancer to other body parts or locations.

metastasize to spread (cancer) to other body parts.

methicillin-resistant *Staphylococcus aureus* (MRSA) bacteria resistant to most antibiotics.

metrorrhagia abnormal discharge from the uterus.

microbe *See* microorganism

microorganism tiny organism that can be seen only with a microscope, particularly bacteria.

mind–body therapy practices that use various techniques to enhance the mind's ability to affect bodily function and symptoms.

mineral inorganic chemical compound found in nature; many minerals are important in building body tissues and regulating body fluids.

minimally invasive surgery any surgical procedure that does not require a large incision. It can be done by entering the body through a small cut or incision on the skin, or through a body cavity or other anatomical opening. Miniature scopes and instruments are used to visualize and repair the organs on the inside of the body.

mite microscopic organism that cannot be seen with the naked eye.

mitered corner one type of corner used in making a facility bed.

mobility ability to move or to be moved easily from place to place.

mobility skills ability to move about in bed, out of bed, and walking.

modalities forms of treatment or uses of therapeutic agents or regimens.

mold organism in the fungus family.

monoplegia paralysis affecting one limb only.

Montgomery straps long strips of adhesive attached to the skin on either side of a wound, then tied to hold a dressing in place.

morbid obesity being 100 pounds or more over ideal body weight, or having a BMI of 40 or higher; this condition usually qualifies for surgical treatment.

morbidity incidence or rate at which an illness or abnormality occurs in a given population.

mores customs of ethnic groups.

moribund dying.

mortality being subject to death; the death rate or frequency of deaths in a given population.

movement therapy treatment that combines nonaerobic exercise and breath control to give patients an awareness of how the body moves; alters posture and motion to reduce pain and stress.

moxibustion burning of herbal substances on or near the body.

mucous membrane epithelial tissue that produces fluid called *mucus*; lines body cavities that open to the outside of the body.

mucus secretion of mucous membranes; thick, sticky fluid.

multidrug-resistant organisms (MDROs) bacteria and other microbes that have developed resistance to antibiotics.

multiple sclerosis (MS) disease characterized by hardened patches scattered throughout the brain and spinal cord that interfere with the nerves in those areas.

multisensory stimulation intense stimulation of sight, sound, touch, smell, pressure, pain, and touch to help the patient to awaken and use previously unused portions of the brain.

multiskilled worker worker who is cross-trained to perform additional skills, enabling him or her to do more than one kind of work.

Munchausen by proxy syndrome (MBPS) type of child abuse in which a caregiver (usually the mother) fabricates illnesses or causes the child to have signs and symptoms of illness.

muscle cells cells that form muscle tissue; have ability to shorten or lengthen and to change their shape and the position of parts to which they are attached.

muscle tissue tissue that has the ability to shorten and lengthen.

music therapy therapeutic use of music to address physical, psychological, or cognitive needs and/or social functioning.

Mycoplasma genitalium little-known STDI that is difficult to identify and was found to be more prevalent than gonorrhea in U.S. adolescents.

myocardial infarction (MI) formation of an infarct in the heart muscle due to interruption of the blood supply to the area.

myocardium heart muscle.

N95 respirator mask with small, tightly woven pores that protects the wearer from airborne infection.

narcolepsy condition in which the person has sudden, uncontrollable, unpredictable urges to fall asleep during daytime hours.

narcotic drug that relieves pain and produces sleep.

nasal cannula tubing inserted into nostrils to administer oxygen.

nasogastric feeding (NG feeding) nourishment given through a tube inserted through the nose into the stomach.

nasogastric (NG) tube soft rubber or plastic tube that is inserted through a nostril into the stomach.

nasopharyngeal airway (nasal airway) curved soft rubber device that is inserted through one nostril and extends to the posterior pharynx, keeping the tongue off the back of the throat. May be used in responsive patients, including those with recent oral surgery, loose teeth, or trauma of the mouth, and those who need frequent nasal suctioning.

National Institute of Occupational Safety and Health (NIOSH) federal agency responsible for conducting research and making recommendations for the prevention of work-related disease and injury.

naturopathic medicine medical system that focuses on whole-person wellness, emphasizing prevention and self-care. The doctor looks for the cause of illness, rather than strictly treating symptoms.

nebulizer device used to apply a liquid in the form of a fine spray or mist; may be used to administer medication.

necrosis tissue death.

necrotizing fasciitis serious condition that may be called flesh-eating or man-eating strep. It occurs when bacteria enter the body through minor trauma or a break in the skin, resulting in shock and systemic infection, organ failure, and the need for amputation.

need to know information is disclosed only if workers need it to carry out their duties.

negative air pressure room room with a special ventilation system in which the room air is drawn upward into the ventilation system and is either specially filtered or exhausted directly to the outside of the building.

negative pressure wound therapy (NPWT) provides vacuum-assisted wound closure to remove drainage and potentially infectious materials, relieve edema, improve circulation, and stimulate formation of new tissue.

neglect failing to provide services to patients to prevent physical harm or mental anguish.

negligence failure to exercise the degree of care considered reasonable under the circumstances, resulting in an unintended injury to a patient. Negligence is carelessness that may be caused by hurrying or not focusing on the task at hand.

neonate newborn baby.

neoplasm new growth; tumor.

nephritis inflammation of the kidney.

nephron microscopic kidney unit that produces urine.

nerve bundle of nerve processes (axons and dendrites) that are held together by connective tissue.

nerve cells carry electrical messages to and from different parts of body.

nervous tissue highly specialized tissue capable of conducting nerve impulses.

networking communication between individuals with a common interest or goal.

neuron cell of the nervous system.

neurotransmitter chemical compound that transmits a nervous impulse across cells at a synapse.

nits tiny oval-shaped eggs of head lice; are yellow-white and adhere to the hair. They look like dandruff, but are firmly attached and very difficult to remove.

no-code order order not to resuscitate a patient.

nodule small knotlike protrusion; a small mass of tissue.

non–insulin dependent diabetes mellitus (NIDDM) diabetes controlled by diet and sometimes oral medication, for which insulin is not needed.

noninvasive remaining localized and not spreading; not penetrating.

nonpathogen microorganism that does not produce disease.

nonrapid eye movement (NREM) sleep phase that accounts for 75 percent of the sleep cycle, in which sleep progresses from light to deep.

nonverbal communication communication transmitted without spoken words, such as by facial expression and body language.

nonweight-bearing (NWB) unable to stand or walk on one or both legs.

nosocomial pertaining to or originating in a facility.

nosocomial infection infection acquired in a facility.

nourishments substantial food items given to patients to increase nutrient intake; often planned and ordered by the facility dietitian.

NPO nothing by mouth.

nuclear family consists of parents and their children living in the same household.

Nurse Aide Training and Competency Evaluation Program (NATCEP) test taken by the nursing assistant which, when passed successfully, entitles the nursing assistant to certification.

nurse practice act (NPA) state law that describes the nursing scope of practice and serves as a guide when facilities develop job descriptions.

nurse's notes section of medical record in which nursing staff records procedures, medications, and observations.

nursing assistant person who provides personal care and assists with ADLs under nursing supervision.

nursing diagnosis statement of a patient's problems leading to nursing interventions.

nursing process framework for nursing action.

nursing team members of the nursing staff who provide patient care.

nutrient nourishing substance or food.

nutrition process by which the body uses food for growth and repair, and to maintain health.

nutrition therapy evaluation and modification of the patient's diet and nutrient intake to promote optimal nutrition for health, wellness, and healing.

nystagmus constant involuntary movement of the eyeball.

obese overweight.

obesity being overweight by 20 to 30 percent of the ideal body weight. Being overweight or obese increases the risk for many health conditions, including diabetes, heart disease, and stroke.

objective observation observation made through the senses of the observer.

oblique fracture *See* closed fracture

OBRA *See* Omnibus Budget Reconciliation Act

observation noticing something.

obsession frequent idea, impulse, or thought that usually does not make sense, but cannot be suppressed or eliminated by the person experiencing it.

obsessive-compulsive disorder (OCD) anxiety disorder in which the patient has recurrent obsessions, frequent thoughts, ideas, impulses, or compulsions resulting in repeated ritualistic activity over which the person has no control.

obstetric, obstetrical pertaining to pregnancy, labor, and delivery.

obstruction blockage in a passageway.

occult blood small quantity of blood that can be detected only by microscope or chemical means.

occupational exposure coming into contact with infectious materials during the performance of a person's job.

Occupational Safety and Health Administration (OSHA) federal agency that makes and enforces regulations to protect workers.

occupational therapy therapeutic use of work and activities to help patients regain self-care skills.

oliguria decreased urine production or urination.

ombudsman person who advocates for patients and residents of health care facilities.

Omnibus Budget Reconciliation Act (OBRA) federal law that requires long-term care facilities to provide care that maintains or improves each resident's quality of life, health, and safety. It also requires the education and competency evaluation of nursing assistants in long-term care facilities.

oncology study of cancer.

oophorectomy surgical excision of an ovary.

open bed bed with top bedding fanfolded to the bottom, ready for occupancy.

open (compound) fracture fracture in which part of the broken bone protrudes through the skin.

open reduction/internal fixation (ORIF) surgical procedure to reduce a fractured bone. The skin is opened and the fracture realigned and held in place by screws, plates, and pins.

operative pertaining to an operation.

oral hygiene care of the mouth and teeth.

oral report verbal report.

orchiectomy excision of one or both of the testes.

organ any part of the body that carries out a specific function or functions, such as the heart.

organism any living thing, plant, or animal.

organizational chart guide for communication; spells out lines of authority.

orifice body opening such as the nose or mouth.

origin proximal point of attachment to skeletal muscle.

oropharyngeal airway (oral airway) curved plastic device that is inserted into the mouth to the posterior pharynx to prevent the tongue from falling to the back of the throat and obstructing the airway.

orthopedic concerning the prevention or correction of deformities (orthopedics).

orthopnea need to sit upright to breathe without difficulty.

orthopneic position position in which the patient sits up to breathe comfortably. The patient sits as upright as possible and leans slightly forward, supporting himself or herself with the forearms.

orthostatic hypotension condition that occurs when the blood pressure drops suddenly when changing position from sitting to standing, lying down to sitting, or stretching after standing; causes the person to feel dizzy or light-headed.

orthotic devices (orthoses) devices that restore or improve function and prevent deformity.

ossicles any small bones, such as one of the three bones in the ear.

osteoarthritic joint disease (OJD) degenerative disease of joints.

osteopathic manipulative treatment (OMT) moving the muscles and joints manually by using the hands for stretching, gentle pressure, and resistance. OMT is used in combination with regular medical treatment to relieve pain, promote healing, increase mobility, and enhance blood and oxygen flow throughout the body.

osteoporosis metabolic disorder of the bones in which bone mass is lost, causing the bones to become porous and spongy; affected bones are at very high risk for fracture.

other potentially infectious material (OPIM) includes human body fluids containing visible blood: semen, vaginal secretions, cerebrospinal fluid, synovial fluid, pleural fluid, pericardial fluid, peritoneal fluid, amniotic fluid, saliva in dental procedures, and any other body fluid that is visibly contaminated with blood.

otitis media inflamed condition of the middle part of the ear.

otosclerosis formation of bone in the inner ear that causes the ossicles to become fixed.

Outcome and Assessment Information Set (OASIS) Medicare data collection tool that the case manager must complete and transmit electronically to the government.

ovaries (singular ovary) endocrine glands located in the female pelvis; female gonads.

overweight condition in which a person weighs more than he or she should, according to standards set according to the person's height and bone (frame) size.

oviduct tube in the body between the ovary and the uterus through which an ovum travels; part of the female reproductive system.

ovulation lunar monthly ripening and discharge of an ovum from the cortex of the ovary.

ovum (plural ova) female egg.

oxygen gas that is essential to cellular metabolism and life.

oxygen concentrator device that removes impurities from room air and concentrates oxygen to be delivered to a patient.

oxygen mask device to administer oxygen through the nose and mouth; placed over a patient's face.

oxygenation movement of oxygen from the lungs into the blood; carries the oxygen to body cells.

pacemaker artificial device placed in the body to regulate the heartbeat.

pain state of discomfort; warning signal that something is wrong.

palliative care comfort care; care that treats the symptoms of discomfort, but not the underlying disease.

pallor less color than normal for the skin.

pandemic worldwide spread of a new disease.

panhysterectomy removal of the entire uterus.

panic disorder condition characterized by unexpected chronic panic attacks (bouts of overwhelming fear). The person usually feels that he or she is in danger, but there is no specific cause for the fear. The person may be so fearful that he or she is unable to function.

panniculus fatty apron of abdominal skin seen in most bariatric patients.

Pap smear simple test used to detect cancer of the cervix.

papule solid elevated lesion of the skin.

paralysis loss or impairment of the ability to move parts of the body.

paranoia state in which one has delusions of persecution and/or grandeur.

paraphrasing providing communication feedback by restating one's understanding of what was said.

paraplegia paralysis of the lower portion of the body and of both legs.

parasite organism that lives within, upon, or at the expense of another organism known as the *host*.

parathormone hormone produced by parathyroid glands that regulates calcium and phosphorus levels in the blood.

parathyroid glands two pairs of endocrine glands situated on the posterior of the thyroid gland; produce the hormone parathormone.

paresis weakness of an extremity.

Parkinson disease neurological disorder due to deficiency of dopamine, a neurotransmitter; progressive disease characterized by stiffness of muscles and tremors.

partial weight-bearing (PWB) unable to bear full weight on one or both legs.

partners in practice method of providing care in which a registered nurse works with a nursing assistant as a team.

PASS acronym for fire extinguisher use meaning: Pull the pin; Aim the nozzle; Squeeze the handle; Sweep back and forth.

passive range-of-motion (PROM) exercises exercises performed for the patient by the nursing assistant when independent movement is not possible. Maintains movement and prevents deformities, but does not strengthen muscles.

pathogen microorganism or other agent capable of producing a disease.

pathologic fracture fracture in a diseased bone that occurs as a result of osteoporosis, a tumor, or cancer.

pathology disease.

patient person who needs care; *see also* client; resident.

Patient Care Partnership a booklet given to patients listing their legal rights while they are in the hospital.

patient-controlled analgesia (PCA) administration of pain-relieving medication controlled by the patient, using a special device; amount of medication to be delivered is preset by the nurse.

patient-focused care attention given to mental, physical, and emotional aspects of a person's being.

pediatric patient from birth to 18 years of age.

pediculosis body lice; parasites that feed on humans and animals.

pelvic belt traction form of traction in which a belt that is secured around a patient's hips is attached to weights.

pelvic inflammatory disease (PID) inflammation of the pelvic organs.

pelvis lower portion of the trunk of the body; basin-shaped area bounded by the hip bones, the sacrum, and the coccyx.

penis male organ of copulation and urinary elimination.

pepsin enzyme produced in the stomach that begins protein digestion.

perceptual deficit inability to reason, think systematically, make judgments, or use common items; usually caused by a brain injury.

percutaneous endoscopic gastrostomy (PEG) gastrostomy tube that is surgically placed by a physician by threading the tube through the mouth, then out an incision in the abdominal wall over the stomach.

pericardium membrane that surrounds the heart.

perineal care (peri care) cleansing of genital and rectal areas.

perineum in the male, the area between the anus and the scrotum; in the female, the area between the anus and the vagina.

periodontal disease potentially serious condition that damages the soft tissue and bone that support the teeth.

perioperative occurring in association with an operative procedure.

perioperative hypothermia low body temperature (hypothermia) that develops in the operating room as a result of anesthesia and some other drugs, open body cavities, cold environment, and administration of cold fluids.

peripheral pertaining to the outside or outer part.

peripheral intravenous central catheter (PICC) intravenous line inserted into a vein in the arm and threaded through to a larger vein.

peristalsis progressive wavelike movement that occurs involuntarily in hollow tubes of the body, especially the alimentary canal.

peritoneal dialysis removal of liquid waste by washing chemicals through the abdominal cavity.

peritoneum serous membrane that lines the walls of the abdominal and pelvic cavities.

personal digital assistant (PDA) small handheld computer that operates on battery power. May be used for documentation and storing research information and personal data.

personal health record (PHR) electronic health record that the patient creates and controls.

personal protective equipment (PPE) equipment such as waterproof gowns, masks, gloves, goggles, and other equipment needed to protect a person from infectious material.

personal space physical closeness that a person is comfortable with during interactions with others.

personality sum of the behavior, attitudes, and character traits of an individual.

petit mal seizure type of epileptic attack that is generally short in nature; "absence" attack.

PFR95 respirator mask with very tiny pores that prevents the wearer from breathing in infectious airborne microorganisms.

phagocyte white blood cell that destroys substances such as bacteria, protozoa, and cells.

phantom pain pain experienced in a body part that has been removed from the body, as if the part were still attached.

pharynx muscular membranous tube between mouth and esophagus; throat.

phlebitis inflammation of a vein.

phobia unfounded, recurring fear that causes the person to feel panic.

physiatrist medical doctor specializing in rehabilitation.

physical abuse mistreatment by hitting or other physical contact.

physical restraint device used to prevent a patient from moving about or having access to his or her own body.

physical therapy structured exercise that assists patients to regain mobility skills.

Physician Orders for Life-Sustaining Treatment (POLST) standardized medical order form that specifies the types of life-sustaining treatment a seriously ill patient does or does not want. It is part of the valid medical orders and is transferred with the patient from one health care setting to the next.

physiology science that deals with the functioning of living organisms.

pica condition in which the person eats nonfood items.

piggyback procedure used to administer medication into a vein through an existing intravenous line.

pigmentation coloration of an area by pigment.

pineal body pea-sized endocrine gland located in the brain.

pituitary gland "master" endocrine gland located in the brain at the base of the skull (attached to the hypothalamus); produces hormones that regulate growth and reproduction.

pivot to twist or turn in a swiveling motion.

placenta structure within the womb through which the unborn child is nourished; the afterbirth.

planning establishing possible solutions for a patient's problems (as determined by nursing diagnoses).

plantar flexion extending the foot in a downward movement.

plasma liquid portion of blood.

Platinum Rule "Treat others the way they want to be treated." Guide to behavior that affects feelings and relationships; shifts the focus from treating everyone alike to providing individualized care and treating patients as they want to be treated, in keeping with their plans of care.

pleura membranes that surround the lungs.

pleural effusion fluid that collects around the lungs in patients who have cancer.

p.m. care care given to prepare a patient for sleep.

pneumonia inflammation and infection of the lungs.

pocket mask barrier device used for providing "mouth"-to-mouth resuscitation that prevents the patient's exhaled air and secretions from entering the caregiver's mouth.

point-of-care testing (POCT) testing done at the patient's location that results in action or treatment.

polydipsia excessive thirst.

polyphagia excessive hunger and ingestion of food.

polyuria excessive excretion of urine.

port opening into a catheter where fluid is injected and withdrawn.

portal of entry area of body through which microbes enter and cause disease.

portal of exit area of body through which disease-producing organisms leave the body.

position sense ability to know one's position in space, including how extremities are positioned.

postanesthesia care unit (PACU) room where patients receive immediate care following surgery.

postanesthesia recovery (PAR) area where patients are taken after surgery to recover from anesthesia.

posterior back or dorsal.

postmortem after death.

postmortem care care given to the body after death.

postoperative after surgery.

postpartum after parturition; after birth.

post-polio syndrome (PPS) neurologic disorder marked by increased weakness and/or abnormal muscle fatigue in persons who had paralytic polio many years earlier.

posttraumatic stress disorder (PTSD) development of unusual symptoms, such as nightmares or flashbacks, after a psychologically traumatic event.

postural support device used as an enabler that maintains body position and alignment.

pound (lb) unit of measurement of weight, equivalent to 16 ounces or 453.6 grams.

prayer connection with a person's higher power.

preadolescence years between the ages of 12 and 14.

predisposing factor condition that contributes to the development of disease.

prefix word part that is placed before a word root that changes or modifies the meaning of the word root.

prehypertension condition that means the person is likely to develop high blood pressure in the future; blood pressure range between 120/80 mm Hg and 139/89 mm Hg.

prenatal before birth.

preoperative period before surgery.

pressure injury injuries to the skin associated with open areas from friction, shearing, pressure, and other causes of injury.

private room room in a health care facility that contains only one patient at a time.

probe as used in this text, a long, slender part of an instrument; that portion of an electronic or tympanic thermometer placed into the patient.

procedure practices and processes used when following facility policies in patient care. A procedure prioritizes and orders your responsibilities when doing the task.

proctoscopy inspection of the rectum using a proctoscope.

professional boundaries limits on how a health care worker interacts with patients.

progesterone hormone produced by female ovaries.

prognosis probable outcome of a disease or injury.

projection unconscious defense mechanism by which an individual denies his or her own emotionally unacceptable traits and sees them as belonging to another.

prolapsed uterus also called *pelvic floor hernia;* condition in which the uterus slips downward into the vaginal canal and may protrude from the vaginal opening; usually due to loss of muscle tone and muscle relaxation from normal aging.

pronation placing or lying in a face-downward position; as applied to the hand, indicates the palms facing backward.

prone position in which the patient is on the abdomen, spine straight, legs extended, and arms flexed on either side of the head.

prostate gland gland of the male reproductive system that surrounds the neck of the urinary bladder and the beginning of the urethra.

prostatectomy removal of all or part of the prostate gland.

prosthesis artificial substitute for a missing body part, such as dentures, hand, or leg.

protected health information (PHI) any individually identifiable patient information from facility records.

protein basic material of every body cell; an essential nutrient.

protocol standards of procedure and care developed to prepare a patient for diagnostic tests.

protozoan (plural protozoa) microscopic unicellular organism.

proximal closest to the point of attachment.

pseudomembranous colitis disease caused by overgrowth of *Clostridium difficile*, often after antibiotic therapy has depleted normal bowel flora; results in severe diarrhea and may cause dehydration.

psychiatric relating to mental illness.

psychological abuse mistreatment by threatening, belittling, or otherwise causing mental or emotional harm or upset.

psychosis serious condition that appears in a number of different mental disorders; the person loses contact with reality, hallucinates, and has delusions that seem real.

puberty condition or period of becoming capable of sexual reproduction.

pulmonary embolism blood clot in the lungs.

pulsatile lavage with suction (PLWS) negative pressure therapy in which a wound is irrigated and debrided with normal saline or another solution.

pulse pressure of the blood felt against the wall of an artery as the heart alternately contracts (beats) and relaxes (rests).

pulse deficit difference between contractions of the heart and pulse expansions of the radial artery.

pulse oximetry procedure for measuring level of oxygen in arterial blood.

pulse pressure difference between the systolic and diastolic pressures.

pupil circular opening in the center of the iris; regulates light entering the eye.

pureed diet diet in which foods are blended with gravy or liquid until they are the consistency of pudding.

push fluids to encourage a patient to drink additional fluids.

pustule circumscribed, pus-containing lesion of the skin.

pyloric sphincter muscle at the exit point of the pylorus.

pyuria pus in urine.

qigong physical and mental activities to teach the patient to channel the chi (life force or energy), thereby improving health.

quadrant one of the four imaginary sections of the surface of the abdomen.

quadriplegia *See* tetraplegia

quality assurance (QA) internal review done by facility staff to identify problems and find solutions for improvement.

race classification of people according to shared physical characteristics.

RACE acronym relating to fire emergency procedure, meaning: Remove patient from danger; Activate alarm; Contain fire; Extinguish fire.

radial deviation wrists are turned toward the thumb side.

radial pulse pulse that can be measured by palpating the radial artery.

radiation therapy treatment of cancer with radiation.

radical mastectomy removal of entire breast and adjacent lymph nodes.

radiology precautions sign safety warning sign posted in an area where active radiology is being used for patient care.

rales abnormal respiratory sound heard in auscultation of the chest.

range-of-motion (ROM) exercises series of exercises specifically designed to move each joint through its full range.

rapid eye movement (REM) sleep part of the sleep cycle in which dreams occur.

rate valuation based on comparison with a standard.

reaction formation repressing the reality of an anxiety-producing situation; the individual exhibits behaviors that are opposite to the real feelings.

reality orientation techniques used to help a person remain oriented to environment, time, and self.

receiver person for whom a communication is intended.

receptive aphasia inability to understand written or spoken language.

recovery position modified lateral position used when the patient is recovering from certain emergencies, such as unconsciousness.

recovery room location surgical patients are taken immediately after surgery; they return to their rooms when their condition stabilizes.

rectal prolapse condition that occurs when a large portion of the rectum protrudes from the anus.

rectocele protrusion of part of the rectum into the vagina.

references in a résumé, statements about abilities and characteristics; or persons who give such statements.

reflex activity performed without conscious thought.

reflexology stimulating reflex areas in the hands and feet to reduce stress, stabilize body functions, and correct health problems.

reflux backflow of fluid, such as when stomach juices and food flow back from the stomach into the esophagus and mouth; typically the cause of heartburn.

registered nurse (RN) specially educated person who is licensed to plan and direct the nursing care of patients.

regress to move in a backward fashion.

rehabilitation process of assisting ill or injured person to attain the optimal level of well-being and function.

Reiki using touch on various areas of the body to promote health and well-being, restore energy, and enhance the body's natural healing ability.

relationship danger zone invisible area that threatens a relationship or causes ethical and legal problems.

relaxation techniques and methods of reducing stress.

reminiscing thinking and talking about the past.

remission times in which a chronic disease appears stable.

renal calculi kidney stones.

renal colic spasm in an area near the kidney, accompanied by pain.

renal failure inability of the kidneys to maintain fluid and electrolyte balance, excrete waste products, and regulate essential body functions.

repression involuntary exclusion from awareness of a painful experience or conflict-creating memory, feeling, or impulse.

reservoir storage area; biologically, an animal or source that maintains infectious organisms that periodically can be spread to others.

resident person being cared for in a long-term care facility; *see also* client; patient.

Residents' Rights document that spells out rights of residents receiving care in long-term care facilities.

respiration process of taking oxygen into the body and expelling carbon dioxide.

respiratory arrest cessation of breathing.

respiratory care practitioner (RCP) licensed professional who specializes in the care of patients with disorders of the cardiopulmonary system, respirations, and sleep disorders that affect the patient's breathing.

respiratory failure condition that occurs when breathing is insufficient to sustain life.

respiratory therapy department that provides care for patients with disorders of the cardiopulmonary system, respirations, and sleep disorders.

respite care short-term, time-limited, temporary care that enables an unpaid family caregiver to take a break.

rest state of comfort, calmness, and relaxation.

restoration basic nursing care measures designed to maintain or improve a patient's function and assist the patient to return to self-care.

restorative returning to preexisting level or status.

résumé short account of a job applicant's career and qualifications.

retention inability to excrete urine that has been produced.

retention (indwelling) catheter tube (catheter) that is inserted into the bladder for drainage of urine and is held there by an inflated balloon surrounding the neck of the catheter.

retinal degeneration breakdown and functional loss of the nervous layer of the eye.

retrograde pyelogram backward-moving X-ray picture of a ureter and the renal pelvis.

rheumatoid arthritis (RA) autoimmune response that results in inflammation of the joints.

rhythm repeat interval of measured time or movement.

rigor mortis rigidity of skeletal muscles, developing 6 to 10 hours after death.

risk assessment careful evaluation of problems that have the potential for causing harm to a patient, such as falls or pressure ulcers.

risk factor condition indicating that a problem may develop, causing the patient's health to worsen.

ritual ceremonial acts that reinforce faith.

rotation act of turning about the axis of the center of a body, as in rotation of a joint.

rubeola (measles) highly contagious acute viral illness with fever, runny nose, cough, red eyes, and a spreading rash.

rubra unusual redness or flushing of the skin.

Sacrament of the Sick last rites given by clergy to a person who is terminally ill (dying).

Safety Data Sheet (SDS) information provided by manufacture about a hazardous product; includes health hazards, safe use guidelines, and emergency procedures for chemical exposure.

salpingectomy surgical removal of the fallopian tubes.

sarcoma connective tissue tumor; often highly malignant.

SBAR (situation, background, assessment, recommendation) communication standard structure for concise, factual, effective, and meaningful reporting of patient information. SBAR stands for: Situation; Background; Assessment; Recommendation.

scabies parasitic disease of the skin that causes a rash and severe itching.

schizoaffective disorder condition that is believed to be a combination of schizophrenia and a mood disorder. This chronic, disabling mental illness has symptoms of schizophrenia, alternating with times when the patient also has symptoms of major depression or a manic episode.

scope of practice extent or range of permissible activities.

scrotum saclike pouch that holds the male gonads.

seasonal affective disorder (SAD) depression that recurs each year at the same time, usually starting in fall or winter and ending in spring or early summer. The cause is not known, but it is believed to be related to lack of exposure to sunlight or abnormal melatonin levels.

sebaceous gland gland that produces a lubricating substance for hairs.

seclusion separating a patient from others.

self-care deficit inability to perform an activity of daily living.

self-esteem feeling of confidence about oneself.

self-identity personal knowledge of who one is; personal view of self.

self-quarantine staying at home unless leaving the house to seek a necessary service.

semicircular canal three tubes in the inner ear containing fluid; the function is concerned with balance and detecting motion.

semi-Fowler's position in which the patient is on the back with knees slightly flexed, and the head of the bed is elevated 30° to 45°.

seminal vesicles pair of accessory male sex glands that open into the vas deferens before it joins the urethra; they secrete fluid into seminal fluid.

semiprivate room room in a health care facility that is shared by two patients.

semiprone patient is positioned between the side and the abdomen.

semisupine patient is positioned between the side and the back.

sender person who originates a communication.

senile purpura dark purple bruises on the forearms and back of hands, common in elderly individuals.

sensitivity ability to be aware of and appreciate personal characteristics of others; state of acute or abnormal response to stimuli or allergens.

sepsis presence of pus-forming and other pathogens or their toxins in the blood.

sequential compression therapy postoperative procedure in which pneumatic boots or sleeves are applied to massage the legs using a wavelike milking motion. Prevents blood clots.

seropositive state in which antibodies to HIV exist in the bloodstream.

serous membrane tissue that produces serous fluid, covers organs, and lines closed body cavities.

sexual abuse use of physical means or verbal threats to force a person to perform sexual acts.

sexual harassment unwelcome sexual advances, requests for sexual favors, and other verbal or physical conduct of a sexual nature. The action may be physical, verbal, or nonverbal.

sexuality maleness or femaleness of an individual.

sexually transmitted infection (STI) infection that is passed from one individual to another through sexual contact.

shaman traditional spiritual leader, healer, or medicine man. In some societies, the shaman is expected to heal the sick, escort the souls of the dead into heaven, and meet with gods by taking on the shape or language of an animal or bird.

sharps items that can cut or puncture skin; include needles, knife blades, and the like.

shearing force on skin over bone when the skin remains at the point of contact while the bone moves; causes damage to skin.

shift report information about patients passed from outgoing shift to oncoming shift.

shock condition in which there is a disruption of circulation that results in dangerously low blood pressure and an upset of all bodily functions.

side rails sliding metal bars that may be pulled up on each side of the bed to prevent the patient from falling out of bed.

sigmoidoscopy direct examination of the interior of the sigmoid colon.

sign problem that can be identified by using the senses of seeing, hearing, smelling, and touching.

sign language communication for persons with hearing impairment; uses gestures and forms made with the fingers and hands.

simple (closed) fracture fracture that does not produce an open wound in the skin.

simple goiter thyroid gland hyperplasia unaccompanied by other signs or symptoms.

simple mastectomy removal of the breast tissue without removal of the underlying muscles.

Sims' position position in which the patient is on the left side with left leg extended and right leg flexed; left arm is extended and brought behind the back; right arm is flexed and brought forward.

singultus hiccup.

sitting (lateral) transfer moving patient from one surface to another with patient sitting.

sitz bath method of bathing in which only the pelvic area is immersed; a cleansing or therapeutic bath in a small tub that holds enough water for the patient to sit with the hips covered and the legs and torso above water. Usually done to relieve discomfort following childbirth or perineal or rectal surgery.

skeletal (voluntary) muscle muscle that is attached to bone and allows voluntary movement.

skilled home health nursing care intermittent medically necessary skilled care that is ordered by a physician and given by a nurse, physical therapist, occupational therapist, and/or speech-language pathologist.

skilled nursing facility (SNF) long-term care facility. Skilled nursing facilities provide the most intensive level of care on the residential care continuum. Residents of these facilities have complex medical care and rehabilitation demands. Some are chronically ill and can no longer live independently.

skin tear shallow injury in which the epidermis is ripped or torn.

slander false oral statement that injures the reputation of another person.

sleep period of continuous or intermittent unconsciousness in which physical movements are decreased.

sleep apnea potentially serious condition in which airflow stops for 10 seconds or more while a person is sleeping.

sleep deprivation prolonged sleep loss (inadequate quality or quantity of REM or NREM sleep).

slider device with a slippery, low-friction surface that is used for moving patients.

sliding board plastic or wooden board that is about two feet long with a slippery surface. Used for a sitting, lateral transfer.

slough dead tissue that may be yellow, tan, gray, green, or brown; a wound cannot be staged and the wound will not heal until this dead tissue is removed.

smooth (involuntary, visceral) muscle muscle located in internal organs; responsible for involuntary movement.

social distancing maintaining appropriate physical distance from others so as to stop the transmission of infectious organisms.

social networking sites Internet-based services that enable users to share information.

soft diet intake consisting of low-residue, mildly flavored, easily digested foods.

somnambulism sleepwalking.

source person who has an infection that can be spread to others.

spastic paralysis paralysis in which there is no voluntary movement. The extremities move in an involuntary pattern, similar to muscle spasms. The patient is aware of the movements, but cannot stop or control them.

spasticity sudden, frequent, involuntary muscle contractions that impair function.

spatial-perceptual deficit inability to distinguish between left and right and up and down.

speech therapy treatment to assist a patient to regain communication skills.

sperm male reproductive cell.

sphygmomanometer instrument for determining arterial pressures; blood pressure gauge.

spica cast body cast.

spinal anesthesia technique of providing anesthesia by introducing drugs into the spinal canal.

spiral fracture fracture that twists around the bone.

spirillum (plural spirilla) spiral-shaped bacterium.

spirituality feeling of wholeness resulting from filling the human need to feel connected to the world and to a power greater than oneself.

splint type of orthosis used to maintain position and prevent contractures of the arm and hand.

spores microscopic reproductive bodies that spread infection and are very difficult to eliminate. They can survive in a dormant form until conditions are ideal for reproduction. The spores then multiply and continue to spread infection.

sprain injury to a ligament, resulting in pain and swelling.

sputum matter brought up from the lungs; phlegm.

square corner *See* box corner

stable health condition is steady, predictable, without complications.

staff development process used to educate staff in health care facilities.

standard basis for comparison; a reference point against which performance or a condition can be evaluated.

standard precautions practices used in health care facilities to prevent the spread of infection via blood, body fluids, secretions, excretions, mucous membranes, and nonintact skin.

standing transfer patient is moved from one surface to another while standing.

staphylo- prefix meaning "in clusters."

status condition or state of health.

status epilepticus seizure that lasts for a long time, or repeats without recovery; a very serious medical emergency.

stenosis *See* stricture

stent device that keeps the arteries open.

stepparent person who is married to a child's natural parent.

stereotype rigid belief based on generalizations.

sterile absence of all microorganisms; incapable of reproducing sexually.

sterile field area considered free of all microbes.

sterility inability to produce offspring.

sterilization process that renders an individual incapable of reproduction; process of cleaning equipment to remove all microbes and make equipment sterile.

stertorous snoring-type respirations.

stethoscope instrument used in auscultation to make audible the sounds produced in the body.

stimulant agent that produces stimulation or elicits a response.

stimulus anything that provokes a response in a cell, tissue, or other structure.

stoma artificial, mouthlike opening.

stool another name for feces.

strain injury to a muscle, resulting in pain.

strepto- prefix meaning "in chains."

Streptococcus A bacterium that produces very powerful enzymes that destroy tissue and blood cells. Causes a skin condition that may be called flesh-eating strep or man-eating strep.

stressors situations, feelings, or conditions that cause a person to be anxious about his or her well-being.

stricture narrowing of a passageway in the body, often caused by inflammation or scar tissue.

stroke cerebrovascular accident or brain attack; damage to the blood vessels of the brain.

subacute care comprehensive, goal-oriented care for individuals with acute illness, injury, or worsening of a chronic medical problem.

subcutaneous tissue connective tissue located under the dermis; attaches skin to muscle.

subjective observation observation based on ideas perceived only by the individual involved.

substance abuse disorder characterized by the use of one or more substances (such as alcohol or drugs) that alter mood or behavior, resulting in impairment.

sudoriferous gland gland that secretes perspiration.

suffix word part added to the end of a word root that changes or modifies the meaning of the word root.

suicide self-destruction; killing oneself.

suicide precautions checks and practices a facility follows if a patient indicates that he or she no longer wishes to live and intends to harm himself or herself. May involve modifying the physical environment and securing the assistance of mental health professionals. The facility maintains these procedures until the patient is discharged or believed to be out of danger.

sundowning behavior in which a person becomes more agitated and disoriented during the evening hours.

superior toward the head; upward.

supination act of turning the palm upward.

supine lying with the face upward.

supplement to add.

supplements nutritional substances used to make up a deficiency or strengthen the whole.

supportive care care given to a dying patient that avoids prolonging life; provides comfort measures only.

supportive device used to help maintain a patient's body in a specific position.

suppository medication used to help the bowels eliminate feces.

suppression consciously refusing to acknowledge unacceptable feelings and thoughts.

suprapubic catheter (S/P catheter) urinary catheter that is inserted surgically through the abdominal wall directly into the bladder.

surgical bed bed prepared for a patient returning from surgery.

surgical mask mask worn by health care workers during surgery, sterile procedures, and work in droplet precautions rooms.

survey review and evaluation to ensure that the facility maintains acceptable standards of practice and quality of care.

surveyor representative of a private or governmental agency who reviews facility policies, procedures, and practices for quality of care.

symbols signs, pictures, or other characters used to communicate.

symmetry matching or correspondence in size, form, and arrangement.

symptom any perceptible change in the body or its function that indicates disease or the phases of disease.

synapse space between the axon of one cell and the dendrites of others.

synovial membrane tissue that produces synovial fluid and lines joint cavities.

syphilis chronic infectious venereal disease characterized by lesions that may involve any organ or tissue; usually exhibits cutaneous manifestations; relapses are frequent; may exist asymptomatically for years.

system group of organs organized to perform a specific body function or functions; for example, the respiratory system.

systole contraction or period of contraction of cardiac muscle.

systolic pressure blood pressure exerted by the ventricles during the heart's contraction phase.

tablet PC (TPC) handheld personal computer used for documentation and point of care testing.

tachycardia unusually rapid heartbeat; more than 100 beats per minute.

tachypnea pattern of rapid, shallow respirations.

talisman object used to ward off evil.

tasks accomplishments throughout life that lead to healthy participation in society; work to be done.

tasks of personality development growing stages through which personality is formed, as described by Erickson.

TED hose support hose.

temporal artery thermometer (TAT) battery-operated thermometer that measures temperature of the skin surface over the temporal artery.

tendon fibrous band of connective tissue that attaches skeletal muscle to bone.

tepid lukewarm.

terminal final; life-ending stage.

termination loss of one's job.

testes male gonads; reproductive glands located in the scrotal sac.

testosterone hormone produced by the testes.

tetany nervous condition characterized by intermittent toxic spasms that are usually paroxysmal and involve the extremities.

tetraplegia paralysis of the arms, legs, and trunk below the level of spinal cord injury; also called quadriplegia.

theft taking anything that does not belong to you; stealing.

therapeutic diet treatment through specifically planned nutrition.

therapeutic touch (TT) use of the hands to exchange energy and stimulate healing by restoring the energy field in the body. The practitioner's hands do not touch the patient.

therapy treatment designated to eliminate disease or other bodily disorder.

thermal blanket large fluid-filled blanket used to raise or lower a patient's temperature.

thermal burn injury (burn) caused by heat, fire, or flame.

thready pulse pulse that is challenging to palpate; may feel like a thread or small cord when palpated

thrombocyte blood platelet that is formed in the bone marrow and is important in blood clotting.

thrombophlebitis development of venous thrombi in the presence of inflammatory changes in the vessel wall.

thrombus (plural thrombi) blood clot.

thyrocalcitonin thyroid hormone that lowers calcium in blood.

thyroid gland endocrine gland situated in the base of the neck; has two lobes, one on either side of the trachea; produces the hormones thyrocalcitonin and thyroxine.

thyroxine hormone of the thyroid gland that contains iodine.

TIA *See* transient ischemic attack

time/travel records records kept of the time spent with clients and the distance traveled between client locations.

tissue collection of specialized cells that perform a particular function (e.g., nervous tissue); piece of paper used for cleansing (e.g., toilet tissue, facial tissue).

toddler stage of childhood from one to three years of age.

toe pleat extra space made by folding the top linen over two to three inches at the end of the bed to keep the linen from pulling the feet downward. This is more comfortable for the patient and reduces the risk of contractures, such as foot drop.

total hip arthroplasty (THA) surgical replacement of hip joint with a prosthesis.

total parenteral nutrition (TPN) also called *hyperalimentation*. A complete IV solution containing proteins, carbohydrates, and fats; given to a patient who cannot digest food normally and whose bowel needs complete rest.

toxin microbe that produces poisons that travel to the central nervous system and cause damage.

trachea windpipe.

tracheostomy opening made into the anterior trachea.

traditional Chinese medicine (TCM) complete health care system that treats disease by restoring the balance between the internal body organs and the external elements of earth, fire, water, wood, and metal.

traditions customs and practices followed by a culture and passed from generation to generation.

transcutaneous electrical nerve stimulation (TENS) use of electrical stimulation to relieve pain.

transfer procedure followed when changing a patient's location.

transfer belt gait belt used to assist and support patients during ambulation.

transgender person whose feelings about gender identity do not match the anatomical sex the person was born with. These individuals feel as if they were born with a physical body of the wrong gender.

transient ischemic attack (TIA) temporary reduction of flow of blood to the brain.

transition movement of a patient between various locations in which care is given as the patient's needs change.

transitional care subacute care given after acute care; care that prepares the patient to live in a new setting.

transitional care unit (TCU) nursing care unit that is responsible for setting goals and helping patients move from one level of care to the next. May be a subacute care unit or a block of rooms within a subacute care unit.

transmission transfer from one place or person to another.

transmission-based precautions isolation practices that prevent the spread of infection by interrupting the way in which the disease is spread.

transparent film dressing waterproof adhesive membrane that maintains a moist environment and protects a wound from bacteria.

transverse fracture fracture that breaks completely across the bone.

trapeze horizontal cross bar suspended over the bed to enable the patient to move in bed.

trauma wound or injury.

tremor involuntary trembling.

Trendelenburg position position in which the patient has the head lower than the feet.

trichomonas vaginitis inflammation of vaginal tissues with vaginal discharge caused by a protozoan.

tripod position sitting position that makes the thorax larger on inspiration, enabling the patient to inhale more air.

trochanter roll rolled sheet or bath blanket placed under the patient extending from waist to mid-thigh; positioned against the hip to prevent lateral hip rotation.

tubercle small rounded nodule formed by infection with *Mycobacterium tuberculosis*.

tuberculosis disease condition occurring when tuberculosis bacteria enter the body and damage tissue.

tuberculosis infection condition in which tuberculosis bacteria enter the body but are walled off and contained, and do not cause disease.

tumor neoplasm.

turning (moving) sheet *See* draw sheet

tympanic membrane membrane serving as the lateral wall of the tympanic cavity and separating it from the external acoustic meatus (outer ear).

tympanic thermometer device used to measure temperature at the tympanic membrane in the ear.

ulcer open sore caused by inadequate blood supply and broken skin.

ulcerative colitis inflammation of the colon resulting in the formation of ulcers.

ulnar deviation with hand in supination, lateral movement of the wrist.

ultraviolet germicidal irradiation (UVGI) special lights used to irradiate an isolation room to eliminate pathogens.

umbilical cord attachment connecting the fetus with the placenta. It is severed artificially at the birth of the child.

umbilicus depressed scar marking the site of entry of the umbilical cord in the fetus.

unilateral neglect condition in which the patient ignores one side of body, such as the affected side after a stroke.

upper respiratory infection (URI) infection involving the organs of the upper respiratory tract.

ureter narrow tube that conducts urine from the kidney to the urinary bladder.

urethra mucus-lined tube conveying urine from the urinary bladder to the exterior of the body; in the male, the urethra also conveys the semen.

urgency need to urinate.

urinalysis laboratory analysis of urine.

urinary bladder muscular receptacle for storing urine before it is voided.

urinary incontinence inability to control urination.

urinary meatus external opening to the urethra.

uterus organ of gestation; womb.

vaccine artificial or weakened antigens that help the body develop antibodies to prevent infectious disease.

vagina tube that extends from the vulva to the uterine cervix; female organ of copulation that receives the penis during sexual intercourse.

validation therapy techniques used to help individuals feel good about themselves.

vancomycin-resistant enterococci (VRE) type of bacteria resistant to most antibiotics.

varicose vein enlarged vein in the leg due to an impaired valve in the vein.

vas deferens tube that carries sperm from the epididymis to the junction of the seminal vesicle; ductus deferens.

vascular area of the body that contains many blood vessels and bleeds readily.

vasoconstriction decrease in the inner diameter of the blood vessels.

vasodilation dilation of the blood vessels.

vector carrier, such as an arthropod, that transmits disease.

vein vessel through which deoxygenated blood passes on its way back to the heart.

venereal wart viral condition that can be sexually transmitted.

ventilation process of breathing in oxygen and breathing out carbon dioxide; also, a means of breathing for another person.

ventilator positive-pressure mechanical device that forces air into the patient's lungs; used to facilitate breathing in patients with impaired respiratory or diaphragm function. The ventilator is connected to an endotracheal tube or tracheostomy.

ventral front; anterior.

ventricle small cavity or chamber, as in the brain or heart.

verbal abuse use of speech to humiliate, threaten, or cause fear or anxiety in another person.

verbal communication transmitting messages using words.

vertebrae bones surrounding the spinal cord; the backbone or spine.

vertigo sensation of rotation or movement of or about the person.

vesicle blister-like skin lesion.

victim someone who is injured unexpectedly, as in an accident.

virus tiny living organisms by which some infectious diseases are transmitted.

visceral muscle muscle that operates without conscious control.

visualization form of guided imagery that uses the imagination to form mental pictures to reduce the stress, pain, and symptoms associated with many medical conditions.

vital (living) signs measurements of temperature, pulse, respiration, and blood pressure.

vitamin general term for various unrelated organic substances that are found in many foods in small amounts and are necessary for normal metabolic function of the body.

vocal cords tissue that stretches across the larynx and produces vocal sounds.

void to release urine from the bladder.

volume capacity or size of an object or of an area; measure of the quantity of a substance.

voluntary muscle *See* skeletal muscle

vulva external female genitalia.

vulvovaginitis inflammation of the external female reproductive structures (vulva and vagina).

ward multiple-bed room, usually with three or four beds.

warm soak method of applying moist heat.

waterless bathing system for patient bathing that uses a package of premoistened disposable washcloths; no drying or rinsing is needed.

weight-bearing (WB) having the ability to stand on one or both legs.

wet compress method for applying moist heat or cold.

wheal localized area of edema on the body surface, often associated with severe itching.

wheezing difficult breathing accompanied by a whistling or sighing sound due to narrowing of bronchioles (as in asthma) or an increase of mucus in the bronchi.

word root word form with a basic meaning; used in forming new words by combining it with prefixes or suffixes.

work practice controls procedures used to prevent the spread of disease.

World Health Organization (WHO) global health organization working under the auspices of the United Nations to promote the health of all

Yankauer catheter rigid plastic suction catheter; used only for oral suctioning.

yeast one type of fungus.

yoga system to promote the union between mind and body; involves a combination of breath control, postures, relaxation, and meditation.

zone of helpfulness healthy relationship area in which most patient contact should occur.

Index